Classics in Voice and Laryngology

Classics in Voice and Laryngology

Ryan C. Branski, PhD
Lucian Sulica, MD

With new material from:

Michael S. Benninger, MD, Andrew Blitzer, MD, DDS, Jerrie Cherry, MD, Roger L. Crumley, MD, Herbert H. Dedo, MD, Craig S. Derkay, MD, Charles N. Ford, MD, Bruce R. Gerratt, PhD, Douglas M. Hicks, PhD, James M. Hillenbrand, PhD, Minoru Hirano, MD, PhD, Douglas M. Hicks, PhD, Thomas J. Hixon, PhD, Nobuhiko Isshiki, MD, Uwe Jürgens, PhD, Jamie Koufman, MD, Jody Kreiman, PhD, W. Frederick McGuirt, Sr., MD, Murray Morrison, MD, Lorraine O. Ramig, PhD, Ira Sanders, MD, Stanley M. Shapshay, MD, Gary Y. Shaw, MD, Judith R. Smitheran, MS, Bettie Steinberg, PhD, Marshall Strome, MD, M. Stuart Strong, MD, Susan L. Thibeault, PhD, Robert J. Toohill, MD, Gayle E. Woodson, MD, Steven M. Zeitels, MD

Foreword by Robert T. Sataloff, MD, DMA

PLURAL PUBLISHING INC.
SAN DIEGO
OXFORD
BRISBANE

PLURAL PUBLISHING
INC.

5521 Ruffin Road
San Diego, CA 92123

e-mail: info@pluralpublishing.com
Web site: http://www.pluralpublishing.com

49 Bath Street
Abingdon, Oxfordshire OX14 1EA
United Kingdom

FSC
Mixed Sources
Product group from well-managed forests and other controlled sources

Cert no. SW-COC-002283
www.fsc.org
© 1996 Forest Stewardship Council

Typeset in 10½/13 Palatino book by Flanagan's Publishing Services, Inc.
Printed in the United States of America by McNaughton & Gunn

Library of Congress Cataloging-in-Publication Data

Classics in voice and laryngology / [edited by] Ryan C. Branski and Lucian Sulica.
p. ; cm.
Compilation of papers, 1967-2007, on laryngology and voice science.
Includes bibliographical references.
ISBN-13: 978-1-59756-242-3 (alk. paper)
ISBN-10: 1-59756-242-4 (alk. paper)
1. Voice disorders. 2. Voice—Physiological aspects. 3. Larynx—Diseases. I. Branski, Ryan C. II. Sulica, Lucian.
[DNLM: 1. Voice—Collected Works. 2. Laryngeal Diseases—Collected Works. WV 5 C614 2008]
RF510.C53 2008
616.85′5—dc22

2008038401

Contents

Foreword *ix*
Introduction *xi*
Contributors *xv*
Dedication *xix*

1 Phonatory Anatomy **1**
Introduction 1
Classic Articles 2
Commentary by Minoru Hirano 3
"Morphological structure of the vocal cord as a vibrator and its variations" 5
by M. Hirano
Commentary by Ira Sanders 11
"The innervation of the human larynx" 15
by I. Sanders, B.L. Wu, L. Mu, Y. Li, H.F. Biller
Commentary by Uwe Jürgens 21
"Neural pathways underlying vocal control" 23
by U. Jürgens

2 Perception of Voice **47**
Introduction 47
Classic Articles 47
Commentary by Jody Kreiman and Bruce R. Gerratt 48
"Perceptual evaluation of voice quality: review, tutorial, and a framework for future research" 52
by J. Kreiman, B.R. Gerratt, G.B. Kempster, A. Erman, G.S. Berke
"Test-retest study of the GRBAS scale: influence of experience and professional background on perceptual rating of voice quality" 72
by M.S. DeBodt, F.L. Wuyts, P.H. Van de Heyning, C. Croux

3 Description and Quantification of Voice Production **79**
Introduction 79
Classic Articles 79
Commentary by Thomas J. Hixon and Judith R. Smitheran 81
"A clinical method for estimating laryngeal airway resistance during vowel production" 84
by J.R. Smitheran and T.J. Hixon
Commentary by Douglas M. Hicks 93
"Acoustic correlates of vocal quality" 96
by D.M. Hicks, L. Eskenari, D.G. Childers
"Changes in phonation threshold pressure with induced conditions of hydration" 105
by K. Verdolini-Marston, I.R. Titze, D.G. Druker
Commentary by James M. Hillenbrand 115

"Acoustic correlates of breathy vocal quality" 117
by J.M. Hillenbrand, R.A. Cleveland, R.L. Erickson

4 Clinical Voice Disorders and Voice Therapy **127**
Introduction 127
Classic Articles 127
Commentary by Murray Morrison 129
"Muscle misuse voice disorders: description and classification" 130
by M.D. Morrison and L.A. Rammage
Commentary by Lorraine O. Ramig 137
"Comparison of two forms of intensive speech treatment for Parkinson disease" 144
by L.O. Ramig, S. Countryman, L.L. Thompson, Y. Horii
"Frequency and effects of teachers' voice problems" 164
by E. Smith, S.D. Gray, H. Dove, L. Kirchner, H. Heras

5 Laryngopharyngeal Reflux and Its Sequelae **171**
Introduction 171
Classic Articles 172
Commentary by Jerrie Cherry 174
"Contact ulcer of the larynx" 175
by J. Cherry and S. Margulies
Commentary by Jamie Koufman 179
"The otolaryngologic manifestations of gastroesophageal reflux disease (GERD): a clinical investigation of 225 patients using ambulatory 24-hour pH monitoring and an experimental investigation of the role of acid and pepsin in the development of laryngeal injury" 189
by J.A. Koufman
Commentary by Robert J. Toohill 267
"Role of refluxed acid in pathogenesis of laryngeal disorders" 270
by R.J. Toohill and J.C. Kuhn
"Laryngopharyngeal reflux: position statement of the Committee on Speech, Voice, and Swallowing Disorders of the American Academy of Otolaryngology-Head and Neck Surgery" 277
by J.A. Koufman, J.E. Aviv, R.R. Casiano, G.Y. Shaw

6 Endoscopic Laryngeal Surgery **281**
Introduction 281
Classic Articles 281
Commentary by M. Stuart Strong 282
"Laser surgery in the larynx. Early clinical experience with continuous CO_2 laser" 284
by M.S. Strong and G.J. Jako

7 Benign Laryngeal Lesions **293**
Introduction 293
Classic Articles 293
"Cysts of the larynx—classification" 294
by L.W. DeSanto, K.D. Devine, L.H. Weiland
Commentary by Susan L. Thibeault 326
"Benign pathologic responses of the larynx" 328
by S.D. Gray, E. Hammond, D.F. Hanson

8 Laryngeal Scarring and Stenosis **335**
Introduction 335
Classic Articles 335
Commentary by Michael S. Benninger 336
"Vocal fold scarring: current concepts and management" 338
by M.S. Benninger, D. Alessi, S. Archer, R. Bastian, C. Ford, J. Koufman, R.T. Sataloff, J.R. Spiegel
Commentary by Stanley M. Shapshay 347
"Mitomycin: effects on laryngeal and tracheal stenosis, benefits, and complications" 351
by R. Rahbar, S.M. Shapshay, G.B. Healy

9 Recurrent Respiratory Papillomatosis **357**
Introduction 357
Classic Articles 357
Commentary by Bettie M. Steinberg 359
"Laryngeal papillomavirus infection during clinical remission" 362
by B.M. Steinberg, W.C. Topp, P.S. Schneider, A.L. Abramson
"Intralesional cidofovir for recurrent respiratory papillomatosis in children" 366
by S.M. Pransky, A.E. Magit, D.B. Kearns, D.R. Kang, N.O. Duncan
Commentary by Craig S. Derkay 372
"Recurrent respiratory papillomatosis" 373
by C.S. Derkay

10 Laryngeal Malignancy and Vocal Outcomes **387**
Introduction 387
Classic Articles 387
Commentary by W. Frederick McGuirt, Sr. 389
"Comparative voice results after laser resection or irradiation of T1 vocal cord carcinoma" 392
by W.F. McGuirt, D. Blalock, J.A. Koufman, R.S. Feehs, A.J. Hillard, K. Greven, M. Randall
Commentary by Steven M. Zeitels 397
"Premalignant epithelium and microinvasive cancer of the vocal fold: the evolution of phonomicrosurgical management" 402
by S.M. Zeitels

11 Vocal Fold Paralysis **453**
Introduction 453
Classic Articles 454
"Etiology of bilateral abductor vocal cord paralysis. A review of 389 cases" 455
by L.D. Holinger, P.C. Holinger, P.H. Holinger
Commentary by Gayle E. Woodson 464
"Configuration of the glottis in laryngeal paralysis. I: clinical study" 467
by G.E. Woodson
Commentary by Roger L. Crumley 475
"Evaluation and treatment of the unilateral paralyzed vocal fold" 480
by M.S. Benninger, R.L. Crumley, C.N. Ford, W.J. Gould, D.G. Hanson, R.H. Ossoff, R.T. Sataloff

12 Vocal Fold Augmentation **493**
Introduction 493
Classic Articles 494
Commentary by Charles N. Ford 495

"Role of injectable collagen in the treatment of glottic insufficiency: a study of 119 patients" 498
by C.N. Ford, D.M. Bless, J.M. Loftus
Commentary by Gary Y. Shaw 509
"Autologous fat injection into the vocal folds: technical considerations and long-term follow-up" 511
by G.Y. Shaw, M.A. Szewczyk, J. Searle, J.Woodroof
"Viscosities of implantable biomaterials in vocal fold augmentation surgery" 521
by R.W. Chan and I.R. Titze

13 Laryngeal Framework Surgery **529**
Introduction 529
Classic Articles 530
Commentary by Nobuhiko Isshiki 531
"Thyroplasty as a new phonosurgical technique" 534
by N. Isshiki, H. Morita, H. Okamura, M. Hiramoto
"Arytenoid Adduction for Unilateral Vocal Cord Paralysis" 541
by N. Isshiki, M. Tanabe, M. Sawada
"Silastic medialization and arytenoid adduction: the Vanderbilt experience. A review of 116 phonosurgical procedures" 545
by J.L. Netterville, R.E. Stone, E.S. Luken, F.J. Civantos, R.H. Ossoff

14 Laryngeal Dystonia **557**
Introduction 557
Classic Articles 558
Commentary by Herbert H. Dedo 559
"Recurrent laryngeal nerve section for spastic dysphonia" 562
by H.H. Dedo
Commentary by Andrew Blitzer 571
"Laryngeal dystonia: a series with botulinum toxin therapy" 574
by A. Blitzer and M.F. Brin

15 Laryngeal Transplant **579**
Introduction 579
Classic Articles 579
Commentary by Marshall Strome 580
"Laryngeal transplantation and 40-month follow-up" 582
by M. Strome, J. Stein, R. Esclamado, D. Hicks, R.R. Lorenz, W. Braun, R. Yetman, I. Eliachar, J. Mayes

Foreword

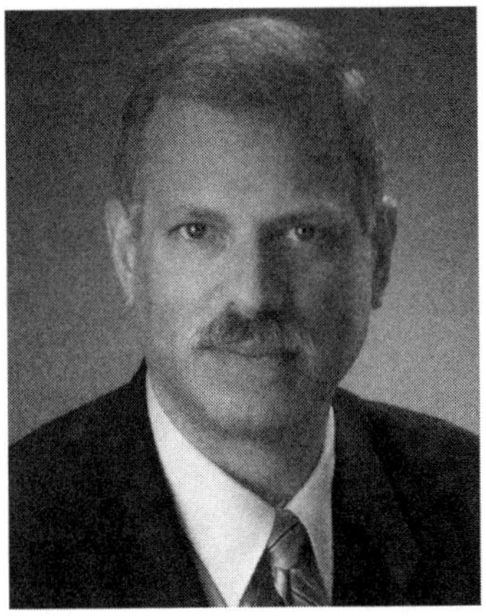

With *Classics in Voice and Laryngology*, Drs. Branski and Sulica have added a unique work to the literature. Their selection of "classics" in laryngology cited 50 times or more would have been valuable even if those articles constituted the entire project. This convenient compilation makes these classic papers easily accessible for laryngologists, fellows, residents, nurses, voice scientists, speech-language pathologists, and other voice professionals who should be familiar with seminal literature, but whose commitments often preclude their gathering such documents even if they have the perspective to know which papers to read. However, in this extraordinary volume, the authors have gone to the trouble of coupling most of the papers with commentary provided by their authors. These informal, personal insights make this volume a true classic, unique in our field. This book belongs in the library of every voice professional.

Robert T. Sataloff, MD, DMA
Professor and Chairman, Department of Otolaryngology-Head and Neck Surgery
Associate Dean for Clinical Academic Specialties
Drexel University College of Medicine
Philadelphia, Pennsylvania

Introduction

Neither the concept for this volume, nor the term "classic" in the context of science is novel. In 1977, Eugene Garfield's essay entitled, "Introducing *Citation Classics:* The human side of scientific papers" was the first to recognize highly-cited manuscripts and their contribution to science (Garfield, 1977). In this essay, published in *Current Contents*, Garfield described his vision for recognizing those investigators who made significant contributions to science in general. In addition, Garfield compiled a list of the 500 most-cited manuscripts published between 1961 and 1975, including Oliver H. Lowry's 1951 paper on protein quantification, the most-cited in the history of science (Lowry et al., 1951). Although the list is interesting, a significant part of the appeal of Garfield's effort was his idea to solicit commentaries from the authors of these landmark papers. Dr. Garfield requested that authors provide insight into "interesting aspects in the development of their techniques, the role played by coauthors or others, and the encouragement received from colleagues." Commentaries included personal anecdotes regarding the scientific process, obstacles encountered, and often, the author's insight into why their paper has been cited so frequently. Garfield's approach in *Citation Classics* was insightful and fundamentally humanistic, bringing out the personalities behind the affectless, impersonal authorial voice typical of scientific papers. In so doing, he explicitly recognized that these seminal contributions to science were made by individuals, encouraged, inspired, constrained, or thwarted by their training, colleagues, mentors, and environment.

With great admiration for Garfield's work and the precedent he set, we present *Classics in Voice and Laryngology*. We recognize that laryngology and voice science represent a small niche within otolaryngology. As such, it is unlikely that seminal works in the advancement of this field will ever be recognized in the context of *science*, in general. However, many publications have significantly altered the way voice production is conceptualized and changed treatment for patients with voice disorders. In fact, in the period covered by this compilation (1967 to 2007), laryngology and voice science have undergone tremendous expansion and change. One recoils from the phrase "paradigm shift," which is used incontinently these days. Yet it obviously and inescapably applies. Laryngology was one of the first medical specialties, brought to life by the development of the laryngeal mirror. Its early practitioners were reviled and not infrequently expelled by the general medical establishment, which found specialization abhorrent. Not only was laryngology an early specialty, but it established the whole concept of specialization in medicine. Then it fell on hard times. The mastery of infectious disease, especially tuberculosis and syphilis, over a very few decades shrank the nonmalignant caseload, and the field atrophied. For a long period, all that was left to it was laryngeal cancer, and it became a minor subdiscipline of head and neck surgery. Its renaissance has been due to the development of surgical endoscopy and microscopic surgical visualization, the resurgence and refinement of framework surgery, stroboscopy, and dramatic and fundamental insights into anatomy and physiology—in fact, by the very authors and papers honored in this volume.

The goals of *Classics in Voice and Laryngology* are three-fold: (1) to recognize great contributions and contributors to the field, (2) to set down in writing aspects of the evolution of voice science and medicine that might fade with time or never be known, and (3) to provide a compilation of landmark manuscripts for both current and future clinician-scientists. As did Garfield, we feel that the author commentaries prepared especially for this volume are as valuable as the papers themselves.

We owe a debt of gratitude to the many leaders in the field that participated in this project. Originally, we hoped to include commentaries from the authors of every manuscript included as a *Classic*. This proved impossible for many reasons. Instead, we attempted to acquire commentaries from a spectrum of investigators, hopefully representing the broad number of research interests encompassed within voice and laryngology. Undoubtedly, we omitted commentaries from many leaders, for which we sincerely apologize and ask for understanding.

What is a Classic?

Although we recognize that pure objectivity is not possible, we tried to develop a rigorous, yet simple formula to determine which articles to include. The number of citations required to be labeled a classic in various fields is highly variable. In botany, for example, 100 citations are required. However, in larger fields such as molecular biology, 500 citations may be required. Recognizing that voice and laryngology represent extremely small fields, the number of relevant citations was set, after consultation with leaders in the field and a review of the results of various thresholds, at 50. On one hand, we sought to identify truly significant papers, but also cover the compass of the field, something not well achieved at higher cutoff points. For instance, had the number of citations required for inclusion increased to 100, virtually the entire volume would have been composed of papers on laryngopharyngeal reflux, which is evidently the most hotly-discussed topic in the voice literature in the past 40 years. Even at 50, some omissions, detailed below, gave us pause. But the number of papers had grown such that we did not dare to expand the field.

A classic, therefore, is defined as a scholarly manuscript in the fields of laryngology, vocology, and/or voice science that has been cited in other work more than fifty times. The program Scopus® was employed to determine manuscript eligibility for the title of *Classic*. Using Scopus®, the following key words were used to generate a list of all articles published between 1967 and 2007: voice, voice disorder, dysphonia, larynx, vocal fold, and vocal cord. Acknowledging that keywords are not included in some scholarly publications, we then undertook a review of the references from the selected articles in addition to an author name search. For example, the most highly-cited manuscript included in this text, Dr. Koufman's paper on the otolaryngologic manifestations of gastroesophageal reflux disease, does not include keywords, and would therefore have been omitted by simply utilizing Scopus® alone.

We debated whether to include review articles, position papers, and the like. The argument against is obvious: these are not original contributions. The argument in favor rests solely on their import. In the end, we decided these merited a place; as a distillation of the standard of care, the state of the art, what have you, at a particular point in time, these are undoubtedly influential and serve as significant and explicit points of reference for practitioners and investigators.

Once the list of *Classics* was compiled, we then attempted to categorize the articles according to topic. This process led us to the development of 15 imperfect and occasionally overlapping areas of voice and laryngology. Although most articles fit nicely into one category, in some cases it seemed as though we were trying to fit a square peg into a round hole.

Originally, we wished to reprint all of the articles that met the criteria of a *Classic*. We quickly altered that plan, as the size of such a book was obviously not feasible, and chose to present selected papers only. Here we used editorial judgment, for which we accept full responsibility, guided by a few principles and external constraints. Where there were multiple related publications for the same investigative group, we chose what seemed to be the broadest and most representative publication. Almost always, our choice was validated by the citation count, higher for our selection than that of other similar papers. Elsewhere, the choice was more challenging. We preserved our preference for overviews of an investigator or investigating group's work where possible. We also gave preference, where possible, to works by authors who agreed to provide commentaries. It is worth mentioning that not everyone that we approached agreed to do so. We do not attempt to present explications of their reasons here. Throughout the entire task of electing articles to include *in toto*, we preserved our respect and consideration for the citation counts as objective markers of significance.

We were subject to the significant limitation that certain journals demanded exorbitant fees for reproduction, amounting to four figure sums for single articles that effectively excluded articles published between their covers from this volume. We do not hesitate to say that we find this to be an injustice to their authors, incompatible with the mission of an academic journal, and also just plain shortsighted.

What's Missing?

We understand that the method cannot be perfect, and may not be entirely just. Some of this is by design. For instance, we excluded a few articles that came up in our search that did not specifically address voice, such as papers on laryngeal cancer that did not concern themselves with voice outcomes. More is by accident. Papers published without abstracts or keywords, like the *New England Journal of Medicine* description of the first laryngeal transplantation, did not register on any of our searches, and were discovered on an incidental crosscheck. We performed such crosschecks for many papers whose omission seemed surprising to us. We hasten to add that neither our surprise nor our estimation were sufficient by themselves to include an article; every one had to meet the citation count. Our ignorance, on the other hand, may have by itself resulted in unfair exclusions. Again, we apologize.

We noted with dismay, but no particular shock, that none of our own papers made the cut. However, we are able to guarantee that these omissions at least are not due to any lack of checking.

By definition, the roster generated for this project is dynamic–the body of classics is constantly shifting by small increments. As time goes on, new publications cite their predecessors, and more papers make the grade. Anyone who wishes to repeat this project in a few years will find either that the resulting volume must be thicker or that the benchmark number of citations will have to change. As a corollary, it takes some maturity and seasoning to be included. Recent developments, such as the angiolytic lasers, at the forefront of discourse now, are invisible in this work. Time will decide whether they are passing fashions or . . . well, classics.

The omission of some topics was puzzling. Microlaryngoscopic surgery—bimanual, magnified endoscopic surgery which takes into account the microanatomic details revealed in recent years—is very poorly represented, for instance. On reflection, though, it becomes clear, no matter how seminal Kleinsasser's book *Microlaryngoscopy and Endolaryngeal Microsurgery*, that these techniques are very poorly represented in the peer-reviewed literature. There are case series justifying its use in various patient groups, papers quibbling over mini-, micro-, and probably nanoflaps, and pieces introducing various pieces of equipment, but none of these are widely cited. Is this because the justification of the technique rests elsewhere, specifically in the paper by Hirano and Sato included in this volume, or because, as we would like to think, the superiority of microlaryngoscopy is so self-evident that it has become the standard of treatment virtually without debate?

Along a similar thread, there are no single reports regarding the efficacy of voice therapy techniques with the exception of Dr. Ramig's LSVT. Given the recent proliferation of high-level behavioral intervention, it is troubling that the literature is essential void of good quality efficacy data. It is also interesting that, in the absence of a single efficacy study, Drs. Ramig and Verdolini provide a comprehensive review of the efficacy data, a true classic manuscript. We hypothesize two potential explanations for this finding. The first is that, until only recently, translational research was unheard of. Communication and collaboration between the ivory tower and the clinic was rare. Looking at the authors on the current list of classics, you can sense the tide of change. Secondly, and perhaps a more persistent issue, is the lack of fundamental metrics by which therapeutic success is determined. The list of classics is relatively sparse on the identification of clinically-viable measures by which to directly or indirectly quantify voice production and the potential for change related to intervention. The reasons are left for another forum; for now, we note the omission.

Obtaining and Assembling Manuscripts

Once the list of articles was compiled and the articles were placed, sometimes awkwardly, into categories, we began the tedious and sometimes disappointing task of obtaining permissions. We wish to acknowledge the many journals and publishers who supported this project and provided permissions for either no charge or for a reasonable rate. A list of these supportive journals and publishing houses is provided below. There are obvious omissions from this list. It is unfortunate that some did not share our vision to recognize those individuals who have shaped our field.

Acta Otolaryngolica
Taylor and Francis Group

Annals of Otology, Rhinology, and Laryngology
Annals Publishing Group

Archives of Otolaryngology-Head and Neck Surgery
American Medical Association

Folia Phoniatricia
Karger Publishing

Journal of Speech, Language and Hearing Research
Journal of Speech and Hearing Research
American Speech, Language, and Hearing Association

Laryngoscope
Lippincott, Williams, & Wilkins

New England Journal of Medicine
Massachusetts Medical Society

Journal of Voice
Otolaryngology-Head and Neck Surgery
American Journal of Medicine
Neuroscience and Biobehavioral Reviews
Elsevier Ltd.

We also wish to thank those individuals who saw merit in the concept of *Classics* for our field and supported it in various ways. Robert T. Sataloff, MD DMA, in his capacity of Editor-in-Chief of *Journal of Voice* and senior statesman in laryngology, intervened with the publisher of several journals to break an impasse in reproduction rights and fees. Tom Murry, PhD provided advice and guidance, and in many respects served as godparent to the project. Last, but in many respects most important, we wish to thank the Singhs and their team at Plural Publishing for their support and encouragement of our vision.

Classics and the Future

As we write, laryngology is gelling into a solid, well-recognized subspecialty in which the clinical and the basic sciences are in communication and in synch to a greater degree than in most other fields of medicine. Various intellectual threads, all represented between these covers, have joined over the past few decades to form an integrated cloth of investigation and patient care. We are excited to be part of it and have found a resonance for our enthusiasm in the many contributors with whom we have interacted in this project. We hope that *Classics in Voice and Laryngology* conveys not only the substance of their contribution, but also some of the intellectual curiosity, process and excitement that has created the momentum that we are benefiting from today. It is certainly a reminder of how far we have come in a very short time, and we hope a touchstone and inspiration for continued advances for the benefit of our patients.

References

1. Garfield E. Introducing citation classics: the human side of scientific reports. *Current Contents.* 1977;3:1–2.
2. Lowry OH, Rosenbrough NJ, Farr AL, Randall RJ. Protein measurement with the Folin phenol reagent. *J Biol Chem.* 1951;193:265–275.

Contributors

Michael S. Benninger, MD
Chairman, Head and Neck Institute, The Cleveland Clinic
Professor of Surgery, The Lerner School of Medicine of Case Western Reserve University
Cleveland, Ohio
Chapter 8

Andrew Blitzer, MD, DDS, FACS
Professor of Clinical Otolaryngology
College of Physicians and Surgeons of Columbia University
Director, New York Center for Voice and Swallowing Disorders
New York, New York
Chapter 14

Ryan C. Branski, PhD
Assistant Attending Scientist
Head and Neck Surgery
Memorial Sloan-Kettering Cancer Center
Assistant Professor of Otorhinolaryngology
Weill Cornell Medical College
New York, New York
Introduction

Jerrie Cherry, MD
Retired
Chapter 5

Roger L. Crumley, MD
Professor and Chairman-Emeritus
Dept of Otolaryngology—Head and Neck Surgery
Director, University Voice and Swallowing Center
University of California, Irvine
Irvine, California
Chapter 11

Herbert H. Dedo, MD
Professor of Otolaryngology
University of California, San Francisco
San Francisco, California
Chapter 14

Craig S. Derkay, MD, FAAP, FACS
Professor and Vice-Chairman, Department of Otoloaryngology and Pediatrics
Eastern Virginia Medical School
Director, Pediatric Otolaryngology, Children's Hospital of the King's Daughters
Norfolk, Virginia
Chapter 9

Charles N. Ford, MD, FACS
Professor, Department of Surgery, Division of Otolaryngology
University of Wisconsin
School of Medicine and Public Health
Madison, Wisconsin
Chapter 12

Bruce Gerratt, PhD
Professor
Division of Head and Neck Surgery
University of California, Los Angeles
Los Angeles, California
Chapter 2

Douglas M. Hicks, PhD, CCC-SLP
Director, The Voice Center
Head, Speech-Language Pathology
Cleveland Clinic
Cleveland, Ohio
Chapter 3

James M. Hillenbrand, PhD
Department of Speech Pathology and Audiology
Western Michigan University
Kalamazoo, Michigan
Chapter 3

Minoru Hirano, MD, PhD, FACS (Hon)
Chancellor Emeritus and Professor Emeritus
Kurume University
Kurume, Japan
Chapter 1

Thomas J. Hixon, PhD, CCC-SLP
Professor Emeritus
Dean Emeritus
University of Arizona
Tucson, Arizona
Chapter 3

Nobuhiko Isshiki, MD, PhD
Head of Isshiki Clinic, KYOTO Voice Surgery Center
Emeritus Professor at Kyoto University
Kyoto, Japan
Chapter 13

Uwe Jürgens, Dr.rer.nat.
Professor Emeritus
University of Göttingen
Göttingen, Germany
Chapter 1

Jamie Koufman, MD
Director, Voice Institute of New York
Professor of Clinical Otolaryngology
New York Medical Center
New York Eye and Ear Infirmary
New York, New York
Chapter 5

Jody Kreiman, PhD
Professor of Surgery
Division of Head and Neck Surgery
University of California, Los Angeles
Los Angeles, California
Chapter 2

W. Frederick McGuirt, MD, FACS
James A. Hanil Professor Emeritus, Wake Forest University and N.C. Baptist Hospital
Department Chair Otolaryngology
Hefner Veterans Administration Hospital, Active Faculty
Wake Forest, North Carolina
Chapter 10

Murray D. Morrison, MD, FCRS (C)
Professor Emeritus of Surgery (Otolaryngology)
University of British Columbia
Director, Pacific Voice Clinic Inc.
Vancouver, British Columbia, Canada
Chapter 4

Lorraine Ramig, PhD, CCC-SLP
University of Colorado—Boulder
National Center for Voice and Speech, Denver
Columbia University, Teachers College, New York City
Boulder, Colorado
Chapter 4

Ira Sanders, MD
Chapter 1

Robert T. Sataloff, MD, DMA, FACS
Professor and Chairman, Dept. of Otolaryngology—Head and Neck Surgery
Associate Dean for Clinical Academic Specialties
Drexel University College of Medicine
Chairman, The Voice Foundation
Philadelphia, Pennsylvania
Foreword

Stanley M. Shapshay, MD
Professor
Division Otolaryngology—Head and Neck Surgery
Albany Medical College
Albany, New York
Chapter 8

Gary Y. Shaw, MD, FACS
Clinical Professor of Surgery, Kansas City University of Medicine and Biomedical Studies
President, Voice and Swallowing Cure Foundation
Kansas City, Kansas
Chapter 12

Judith R. Smitheran, MS, CCC-SLP
Speech/Language Pathologist
St. Vincent Regional Medical Center, Santa Fe, New Mexico
Santa Fe, New Mexico
Chapter 3

Bettie M. Steinberg, PhD
Professor
Chief Scientific Officer, The Feinstein Institute for Medical Research, and
Dean, Elmezzi Graduate School of Molecular Medicine

North Shore—LIJ Health System
Manhasset, New York
Chief, Otolaryngology Research
Long Island Jewish Medical Center
New Hyde Park, New York
Chapter 9

Marshall Strome, MD, MS, FACS
Director, Center for Head and Neck Onocology
Co-Director, Head and Neck Transplantation Program
New York Head and Neck Institute
New York, New York
Chapter 15

M. Stuart Strong, MD
Professor Emeritus, Otolaryngology/Head and Neck Surgery
Boston University
School of Medicine
Boston, Massachusetts
Chapter 6

Lucian Sulica, MD
Director, Voice Disorders/Laryngology
Associate Professor of Otorhinolaryngology
Weill Cornell Medical College
New York, New York
Introduction

Susan L. Thibeault, PhD
Assistant Professor
Division of Otolaryngology—Head and Neck Surgery
Department of Surgery
University of Wisconsin-Madison
Madison, Wisconsin
Chapter 7

Robert J. Toohill, MD, FACS
Professor of Otolaryngology and Communication Sciences
The Medical College of Wisconsin
Milwaukee, Wisconsin
Chapter 5

Gayle E. Woodson, MD
Professor and Chair
Division of Otolaryngology—Head and Neck Surgery
SIU School of Medicine
Springfield, Illinois
Chapter 11

Steven M. Zeitels, MD, FACS
Eugene B. Casey Professor of Laryngeal Surgery
Harvard Medical School
Director: Center for Laryngeal Surgery and Voice Rehabilitation,
Massachusetts General Hospital
Boston, Massachusetts
Chapter 10

We often become engrossed in our academic endeavors without taking the time to appreciate the true genius of a few who created the foundation for our craft. This volume is dedicated to those pioneers who allow me to truly enjoy going to work every day. And to Sarah and TR who make leaving work even sweeter.

—RCB

This volume is dedicated to my teachers, and especially to Roy B. Sessions, MD, who taught me more than any other what it means to take care of patients, and to Andrew Blitzer, MD, DDS, who showed me how little we know and how much more there is left to be done. Without them, clinical practice would have been a profession and not a passion.

—LS

1

Phonatory Anatomy

Introduction

Four cartilages, five muscles, four paired and one unpaired, and two vocal folds—the basics of laryngeal anatomy were established well before the mid-19th century, when it became possible to examine the larynx in vivo. Yet aspects of anatomy that are critical to phonation remained obscure well into the period covered by this compilation. It is a curiosity of our field that Van den Berg's myoelastic-aerodynamic theory of phonation was fully articulated before its microanatomic correlates were described. It is even more interesting that the clinical changes that should have resulted from such a description—the shift to microlaryngoscopic techniques—were underway concurrently, and may even have anticipated it in part.

Nevertheless, the description of the microscopic anatomy of the larynx by Dr. Hirano is a watershed in laryngology that marks the shift of interest from the gross to the cellular level. It is as if the operating microscope has been adjusted to the next higher magnification—the whole field looks different. The consequences are apparent in our notions of pathogenesis of laryngeal disease, in surgical technique, and in the direction of several lines of current laboratory inquiry. It is not an overstatement to say that Dr. Hirano's observations form one of the pillars of modern laryngology. His accompanying commentary recapitulates some of these observations in the context of physiology. It should not be overlooked that two of other classic papers in this section, those of Gray and colleagues, and of Chan and Titze, are direct products of these insights.

Description of laryngeal neuroanatomy has lagged behind vocal fold microanatomy. Perhaps that is not surprising in a field evolved from a surgical tradition. It is well known that laryngeal muscles are small and highly innervated, tasked with finely graded and coordinated motor activity. Yet, important technological limitations prevented an equally sophisticated grasp of the nerve supply. Dr. Sanders describes how these were overcome to enable his team to describe the interesting and highly suggestive arborization of laryngeal nerves, represented here by their 1993 overview paper. In his commentary, his genuine fascination with the work is clear.

Issues of neural control remain only partially explained; the work of Dr. Jürgens is central to what we do know. It points to the direction that work must progress to find a solution to an array of laryngeal diseases of central origin, like spasmodic dysphonia, for which intervention at the end organ is an incomplete treatment. In addition to his review paper, he presents a grand overview of a changing field over 36 years with a particular focus on methodological advances.

Together, these anatomic advances present a picture of a field deeply preoccupied with function. That's not just a reflection of clinical practice, but its fundamental driver. The task of the clinician, whether physician or speech-language pathologist, can be understood entirely as the transformation of these insights and those that have followed since into an ever higher standard of voice rehabilitation.

Classic Articles

● Reprint of article included in this chapter.
♦ Commentary on this article.

●♦Hirano M. Morphological structure of the vocal cord as a vibrator and its variations. *Folia Phoniatr.* 1974;26(2):89–94.

●♦Sanders I, Wu B-L, Mu L, Li Y, Biller HF. The innervation of the human larynx. *Arch Otolaryngol.* 1993; 119(9):934–939.

Chan RW, Titze IR. Viscoelastic shear properties of human vocal fold mucosa: measurement methodology and empirical results. *J Acoust Soc Am.* 1999;106(4 pt 1): 2008–2021.

Gray SD, Titze, IR, Chan R, Hammond TH. Vocal fold proteoglycans and their influence on biomechanics. *Laryngoscope.* 1999;109(6):845–854.

●♦Jürgens U. Neural pathways underlying vocal control. *Neurosci Biobehav Rev.* 2002;26(2):235–258.

Commentary

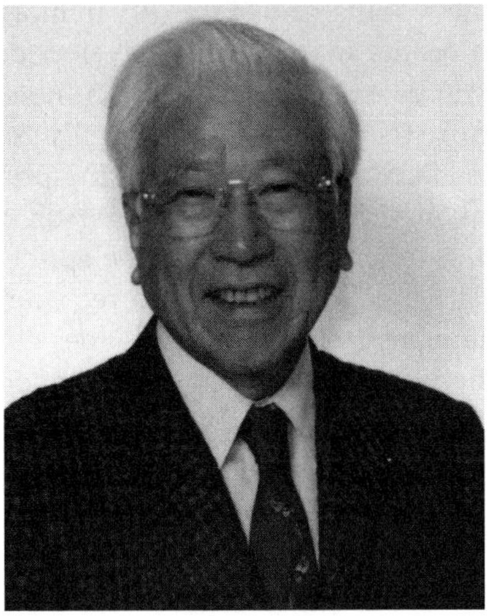

Minoru Hirano, MD, PhD, FACS (Hon)

The original paper[1] was submitted for publication in 1973 and published in 1974. Our studies on the structure and vibration of the vocal fold continued until the end of 1996 when the author retired from his chair as Professor of Otolaryngology. This commentary presents our most recent study results and models.

Morphological Structure of the Human Vocal Fold

The vocal fold comprises the vocalis muscle and mucosa. The mucosa, in turn, is made up of the epithelium and lamina propria. The lamina propria consists of superficial, intermediate and deep layer.

The superficial layer of the lamina propria (Lps), referred to as Reinke's space, is composed chiefly of an amorphous substance and is loose and pliable. The intermediate layer (Lpi) is primarily consists of elastic fibers and the deep layer (Lpd), collagenous fibers. Lps is clearly delineated from Lpi. The border between Lpi and Lpd is not distinct. They together form the vocal ligament. The fibers of Lpd go into the vocalis muscle. Around the edge of the vocal fold, the elastic and collagen fibers in the vocal ligament, as well as the muscle fibers in the vocalis muscle, run roughly parallel to the edge, facilitating vibratory movements.

The findings mentioned above indicate that the vocal fold should be regarded as, at least, a double-layered vibrator consisting of a body made up of the vocalis muscle and the vocal ligament, and the cover consisting of the epithelium and Lps.

Physiological Variations

The mechanical properties of the vocal fold, such as position, shape, mass, tension, and elastic constant, are determined by the intrinsic and extrinsic laryngeal muscles. Among these muscles, the most important in determining the relationship between the body and the cover of the vocal fold are the vocalis and the cricothyroid muscles.

Four typical laryngeal adjustments in terms of the relationship between the body and the cover are proposed in Figure 2 of the reprinted work, which presents schematically frontal sections of the vocal fold during vibration. The vocal fold is deformed to a great extent from the rest state. The first three, Figures 2a, 2b, and 2c, represent condition of heavy or modal register, which is associated with a more or less marked wavelike movement of the mucosa, or mucosal wave, having up-and-down movements. Two ripples in these pictures present the so-called upper and lower lips, respectively.

In Figire 2a, contraction of both the vocalis and cricothyroid muscles is very weak. This occurs in soft phonation at low pitch levels. The elastic constant of both the body and the cover is small because there is little tension in or on the vocal fold. Both the body and the cover are very flexible, and are almost equally involved in the deformation.

In Figure 2b, the vocalis muscle contracts much more powerfully than the cricothyroid. This happens in loud heavy voice at medium pitch levels. The body is stiff and has a high elastic constant. The cover is slackened and associated with a small elastic constant. Deformation during vibration occurs mainly in the cover, especially the wavelike movement involves only the cover.

Figure 2c represents a group of conditions where contraction of the vocalis muscle is a little more dominant than that of the cricothyroid, that is, conditions between Figures 2a and 2b. This is supposedly the case with most phonation in heavy or modal register. Deformation of the vocal fold, especially the wavelike movement, involves both the body and the cover, but more markedly the cover.

Figure 2d represents conditions for light register or falsetto. The vocals muscle is not active or only slightly active, whereas the cricothyroid contracts powerfully. Both the body and the cover are passively stretched and made tense. Both are associated with a high elasticity constant. In this condition, changes in shape during vibration are smaller than in modal register, and the wavelike movement does not appear.

Needless to say, the expiratory force is one of the most important factors which determine the mode of changes in the vocal fold shape during vibration. Figure 2 shows conditions where the expiratory force is at its optimum.

Pathological Variations

Several pathologic conditions are associated with typical changes in mechanical properties of the vocal fold. The changes, in turn, are reflected as variations in the mode of vibration. A slight or moderate degree of edema in Lps results in a decrease in the elastic constant of the cover. This is recognized as a pronounced wavelike movement under a stroboscopic light or in an ultra-high-speed film. The deformation of the vocal fold during vibration seems to involve the cover to a greater extent than the body.

A carcinomatous lesion of the vocal fold, which is first developed in the cover and invades the body later, causes an increase in the elastic constant of the tissue. This usually results in immobility of the affected portion during phonation. A similar state is also caused by papilloma or hyperkeratosis. It is usually developed from the epithelial layer of the cover.

In recurrent laryngeal nerve paralysis, the vocalis muscle does not contract. Because the cricothyroid muscle is not innervated by the recurrent laryngeal nerve but by the superior laryngeal nerve, a condition similar to that in an adjustment for falsetto may result. In typical cases of recurrent laryngeal nerve paralysis, the wavelike movement is not observed, unless there are no other pathologies, such as edema. When the paralysis persists for a long time, the vocals muscle becomes atrophied, the muscular tissue is replaced by fibrous tissue, and the vocal fold becomes thin. The vocal fold presents a movement similar to that of a flag flapping in the wind. When reinnervation of the vocalis muscle begins (at first, usually in only a fraction of the entire motor units of the muscle), gradual recovery of the wavelike movement is observed.

Summary

Histological findings of the human vocal fold indicate that it can be regarded as a double-structured vibrator that consists of a body and a cover. The mechanical properties of the two structures can vary according to different laryngeal adjustments or pathological conditions. This is reflected by changes in the vibratory mode and consequent variations in the acoustical properties of the glottal sound.

References

1. Hirano M. Morphological structure of the vocal cord as a vibrator and its variations. *Folia Phoniatr.* 1974;26: 89–94.
2. Hirano M. Phonosurgical anatomy of the larynx. In: Ford, CN, Bless DM, eds. *Phonosurgery.* Philadelphia, Pa: Raven Press; 1991:26.

Morphological Structure of the Vocal Cord as a Vibrator and its Variations

MINORU HIRANO

Department of Otolaryngology, School of Medicine, Kurume University, Kurume-shi, Kyushu

Various models which simulated vibrating vocal cords have been proposed by several investigators [1, 2, 8, 9, 11]. The degree of similarity of such a model to the real human vocal cord should depend on the purpose of the model. From the physiological or clinical point of view, we need a model which has variable parameters essential to simulate different conditions produced by different laryngeal adjustments or by pathological variations.

In this paper, we will discuss (1) how the morphological structure of the vocal cord should be interpreted, (2) how the mechanical properties of the vocal cord can vary under different laryngeal adjustments, and (3) how the mechanical characteristics of the vocal cord are affected by pathological changes. The discussion is based mainly upon our electromyographic, ultra-high-speed cinematographic and stroboscopic data [3–7] and also upon some previous reports by other investigators [10, 12].

Morphological Structure of the Vocal Cord

Figure 1 presents the histological structure of a human vocal cord in a frontal section. The main part of the vocal cord consists of the vocalis muscle. The vocalis muscle is a stratified, voluntary muscle innervated by the recurrent laryngeal nerve, a branch of the vagus nerve. Its mechanical character varies according to the degree of contraction. The more forceful the degree of contraction becomes, the greater the elasticity constant of the muscle.

Received: February 7, 1973; **accepted:** August 8, 1973.

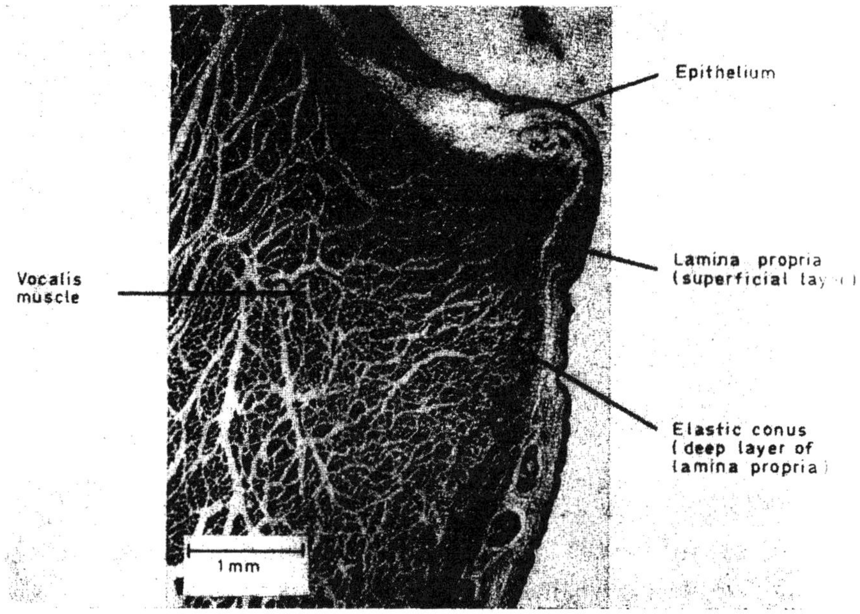

Fig. 1. Histological structure of a human vocal cord. Frontal section. Note that fibers of the elastic conus go into the vocalis muscle, resulting in tight connection of the elastic conus and the vocalis muscle. Note also that the elastic conus and the superficial layer of the lamina propria are connected loosely with each other. The tissue, especially the mucous membrane, should be shrunk by formalin. HE.

The vocalis muscle is covered with the elastic conus. The elastic conus is markedly thick near the edge of the vocal cord. This part is called the vocal ligament. The elastic conus is composed of dense fibrous tissue which in turn consists of collagen and elastic fibers as shown in figure 1. It is important to realize that the fibers of the elastic conus go into the vocalis muscle at many places and merge in the connective tissue between bundles of the muscle fibers. In other words, the elastic conus is tightly connected with the vocalis muscle. Therefore, these two structures appear to move as one unit during vibration.

Superficial to the elastic conus lies the mucous membrane (mucosa) which consists of the very thin epithelial layer and the lamina propria; the latter contains loose connective tissue. The mucous membrane is connected loosely to the elastic conus. Therefore, it can be moved in a different manner from the elastic conus during vibration.

The findings mentioned above indicate that the vocal cord should be regarded as, at least, a double-structured vibrator consisting of a body made up of the vocalis muscle and the elastic conus, and a cover consisting of the mucous membrane.

In many anatomy or laryngology textbooks, the description of vocal cord structure is misleading: the elastic conus is described as a part of the mucous membrane. Although from a histological point of view, the elastic conus might be a part of the mucous membrane, it should be considered as a structure separate from the superficial layer of the mucous membrane when one looks at the vocal cord as a vibrator.

Physiological Variations

The mechanical properties of the vocal cord – such as position, shape, mass, tension, and elastic constant – are determined by the intrinsic and extrinsic laryngeal muscles. Among these muscles, the most important in determining the relationship between the body and the cover of the vocal cord are the vocalis and cricothyroid muscles.

Four typical laryngeal adjustments in terms of the relationship between the body and the cover are proposed in figure 2 which presents schematically frontal sections of the vocal cord during vibration; the vocal cord is deformed to a great extent from the rest state. The first three (fig. 2a, b, c) represent conditions of heavy or modal register which is associated with a more or less

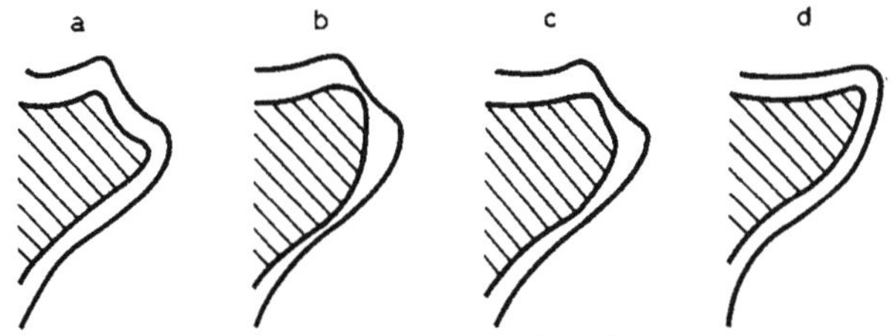

	a	b	c	d
Vocalis	±	⧺+	+ ~ ⧺ ~ ⧺+	− ~ ±
Cricothyroid	±	± ~ +	± ~ + ~ ⧺	⧺ ~ ⧺+
	$K_b = K_c$ (small)	$K_b \gg K_c$	$K_b > K_c$	$K_b = K_c$ (great)

Fig. 2. Four typical laryngeal adjustments in physiological condition which are determined mainly by combinations of different activities of the cricothyroid and the vocalis muscles. K_b = elasticity constant of body; K_c = elasticity constant of cover.

marked wave-like movement of the mucous membrane having an up-and-down movement. Two ripples in these pictures represent the so-called upper and lower lips, respectively.

In figure 2a, contraction of both the vocalis and cricothyroid muscles is very weak. This occurs in soft phonation at low pitch levels. The elastic constant of both the body and the cover is small, since there is little tension in or on the vocal cord. Both the body and the cover are very flexible, and are almost equally involved in the deformation.

In figure 2b, the vocalis muscle contracts much more powerfully than the cricothyroid. This happens in loud heavy voices at medium pitch levels. The body is stiff and has a high elastic constant. The cover is slackened and associated with a small elastic constant. Deformation during vibration occurs mainly in the cover, especially the wave-like movement involves only the cover. This appears to be the condition described by SCHÖNHÄRL [10] based on stroboscopic investigation.

Figure 2c represents a group of conditions where contraction of the vocalis muscle is a little more dominant than that of the cricothyroid – that is, conditions between figure a and b. This is supposedly the case with most phonation in heavy or modal register. Deformation of the vocal cord, especially the wave-like movement, involves both the body and the cover, but more markedly the cover.

The last illustration, figure 2d, represents conditions for light register or falsetto. The vocalis muscle is not active or only slightly active, whereas the cricothyroid muscle contracts powerfully. Both the body and the cover are passively stretched and made tense; both are associated with a high elasticity constant. In this condition, changes in shape during vibration are smaller than in the modal register, and the wave-like movement does not appear.

Needless to say, the expiratory force is one of the most important factors which determine the mode of changes in the vocal cord shape during vibration. Figure 2 shows conditions where the expiratory force is at its optimum.

Pathological Variations

There are several pathological conditions associated with typical changes in mechanical properties of the vocal cord which are, in turn, reflected as variations in the mode of vocal cord vibration.

A slight or moderate degree of edema in the superficial layer of the lamina propria of the mucous membrane results in a decrease in the elastic constant of the vocal cord cover. This is recognized as a pronounced wave-like movement under a stroboscopic light or in an ultra-high-speed film [6, 7, 10]. The deformation of the vocal cord during vibration seems to involve the cover to a greater extent than the body.

A carcinomatous lesion of the vocal cord, which is first developed in the cover and invades the body later, causes an increase in the elastic constant of the tissue. This usually results in immobility of the affected portion during phonation [6, 7, 10]. A similar state is also caused by papilloma or hyperkeratosis. It is usually developed from the epithelial layer of the cover.

In recurrent laryngeal nerve paralysis, the vocalis muscle does not contract. Since the cricothyroid muscle is not innervated by the recurrent laryngeal nerve but by the superior laryngeal nerve, a condition similar to that in an adjustment for falsetto may result. In typical cases of recurrent laryngeal nerve paralysis, the wave-like movement is not observed, unless there are no other pathologies, such as edema [5–7, 10]. When the paralysis persists for a long time, the vocalis muscle becomes atrophied, the muscular tissue is replaced by fibrous tissue, and the vocal cord becomes thin. The vocal cord presents a movement similar to that of a flag flapping in the wind [7]. When reinnervation of the vocalis muscle begins (at first, usually in only a fraction of the entire motor units of the muscle), gradual recovery of the wave-like movement is observed [10, 11].

Summary

Histological findings of the human vocal cord indicate that it should be regarded as a double-structured vibrator which consists of a body and a cover. The mechanical properties of the two structures can vary according to different laryngeal adjustments or pathological conditions. This is reflected by changes in the vibratory mode and consequent variations in the acoustical properties of the glottal sound.

References

1 Flanagan, J. L. and Landgraf, L.: Self-oscillating source for vocal tract synthesizer. 1967 Conf. on Speech Commun. and Processing, pp. 54–62 (1967).

2 Hiki, S.: Personal commun. (1971).

3 Hirano, M.: Regulatory mechanism of voice in singing. 16-mm film (1970).

4 Hirano, M.; Vennard, W., and Ohala, J.: Regulation of register, pitch and intensity of voice. An electromyographic investigation of intrinsic laryngeal muscles. Folia phoniat. *22:* 1–20 (1970).

5 Hirano, M.; Nozoe, I.; Shin, T., and Maeyama, T.: Vibration of the vocal cords in recurrent laryngeal nerve palsy. A stroboscopic investigation. Pract. otol., Kyoto (in press, 1973).
6 Hiroto, I.: The mechanism of phonation; its pathophysiological aspects. Pract. otol. Kyoto *39:* 229–291 (1966).
7 Hiroto, I.: Vibration of vocal cord. 16-mm film (1968).
8 Ishizaka, K. and Matsudaira, M.: Analysis of the vibration of the vocal cords J. acoust. Soc. Jap. *24:* 311–312 (1968).
9 Ishizaka, K. and Matsudaira, M.: What makes the vocal cords vibrate. Proc. 6th Int. Congr. Acoustics, B 9–B 12 (1968).
10 Schönhärl, E.: Die Stroboskopie in der praktischen Laryngologie (Thieme, Stuttgart 1960).
11 Titze, I. R. and Strong, W. J.: Simulated vocal cord motions in speech and singing. Proc. 83rd Meet. Acoust. Soc. Amer., pp. 30–31 (1972).
12 Leden, H. von: The electronic synchron-stroboscope. Its value for the practicing laryngologist. Ann. Otol. Rhinol. Larnyg., St. Louis *70:* 881–893 (1961).

Request reprints from: Minoru Hirano, MD, Department of Otolaryngology, School of Medicine, Kurume University, 67 Asahi-machi, *Kurume-shi* (Japan)

Commentary

Ira Sanders, MD

I was quite surprised to learn that a paper from my laboratory team had been among the most highly cited in laryngeal anatomy, and honored that the editors of *Classics in Voice and Laryngology* asked me to comment on it. This was especially humbling when I learned that one of the other anatomy papers selected, that of Dr. Hirano, I believe to be one of the most influential papers in voice science with implications way beyond laryngeal anatomy.

This commentary is meant to convey the many facets of research; the inspiration for the work, my view of what it meant, and how the field has evolved. Most interesting for me is the request to comment on the human side of research. Most otolaryngologists do not understand how research can be more exciting than clinical practice. Well, it can, and I hope I can convey some of that excitement.

Article Summary

The article describes and demonstrates the nerve supply of the human larynx in detail never seen before. Photographs show the distribution of the superior and recurrent laryngeal nerve from their main trunks to the terminal branching within each muscle. Notable observations included demonstrating new connections between the superior and recurrent nerves, the exact course of nerves within each laryngeal muscle, and the specialized nature of certain terminal nerve branches, particularly the branch to the vocalis part of the thyroarytenoid muscle.

Two technical problems were circumvented. First, this small organ has an extremely complex nerve supply that interweaves extensively. Normal dissection techniques, no matter how careful, cannot trace most of these fine nerves. Second, the most important questions had to be answered by studying human postmortem material. Little help was gained by the many techniques that can be used on animal models. In fact, some of the biggest insights come from the dramatic differences in innervation between human and grossly similar appearing larynges of nonhuman species.

A major contribution was the reintroduction of the Sihler's stain, a powerful technique that makes large anatomical specimens translucent while counterstaining the nerves. The Sihler's stain was adapted by us from an obscure staining technique used during the 19th century to study the peripheral nerves of whole fish. This technique is particularly well suited for human material as it works on postmortem tissue. It has subsequently been used to study the extraocular muscles, tongue, and pharynx.

Notable Observations

Superior Vocalis

One of the most important findings, although not the most obvious finding at the time, was the highly specialized nature of the nerve supply to the vocal fold. More specifically, the nerve distribution to the part of the thyroarytenoid muscle under the vocal ligament is highly complex in humans. This area we refer to as the superior vocalis (SV).

The complex innervation of the SV suggests that this muscle compartment has very small motor units and/or high proprioceptive elements. We subsequently looked at other nonhuman mammals, including monkeys, and found that none of these species has this complex innervation found in the human SV. This suggested that the SV was a specialization found only in human vocal folds, and therefore potentially related to speech.

In other work we examined the SV by many different anatomical techniques. By looking at serial sections of vocal folds we could see that the muscle fiber groups within the SV all originated from the arytenoids cartilage. However, very soon, the more superficial muscle fibers inserted in and around the vocal ligament. In this way, the muscle fibers were capable of controlling the tension and other physical parameters of the vibrating edge of the vocal fold very precisely.

In further work, we carefully looked for muscle spindles and found them to be localized to the human SV at high levels. At least 10 times the level previously reported. Moreover, the muscle fibers of the SV are unique in their size shape, connections, motor endplate number and morphology, and myosin content. Most interesting was the presence of slow tonic muscle fibers, a type of muscle characterized by multiple *en grappe* motor endplates and containing a distinctive slow tonic myosin heavy chain. These fibers had only been described in the eye and middle ear muscles of mammals, two other small but precisely controlled muscle groups. However, the incredible variety and extent of specialization found in the SV compartment is far beyond that seen in these muscles. In fact, we have become convinced that the SV muscle group is an apparently unique type of mammalian muscle.

What is the function of the SV? We can only speculate. Here we overlap into Dr. Hirano's realm. In the classical body cover theory, the layers of the vocal fold are passive structures, their physical properties depend on the overall stretch imparted to the vocal fold. However, the nature of the SV suggests otherwise. It appears to be designed to control the vibration of the edge of the vocal fold very precisely. It appears to us that the human has an active rather then a passive cover.

Nerve Connections

Several remarkable observations were made regarding interconnections between nerves that were normally believed to be separate; the recurrent, internal, and external superior laryngeal nerves.

Around the interarytenoid muscle direct connections could be traced between branches of the internal and recurrent laryngeal nerves. Moreover, nerve connections passed from side to side in this same area. Although relatively small, these nerve connections potentially allow for motor nerves to pass from the superior to recurrent laryngeal nerves. In fact, in later work, we microdissected the motor nerve branch to the human posterior cricoarytenoid muscle and saw that a substantial number of axons were entering from this nerve branch from the superior direction. As most nerve branches to muscles contain both motor and sensory axons, the exact nature of these superior axons innervating the posterior cricoarytenoid muscle is unknown.

Another remarkable observation was the first mention of the communicating nerve, an extension of the external branch of the superior laryngeal nerve that continues within the larynx. In most cases, the communicating nerve could be seen to join with the terminal branches of the recurrent nerve within the thyroarytenoid muscle. However, Dr. Bei-lian Wu followed up with a detailed description in a later manuscript that strongly suggested that the communicating nerve supplied motor innervation to the thyroarytenoid muscle. A further canine study that she never published strongly suggested that the motor innervation that distributed through the communicating nerve supplied double innervation to muscle fibers in a consistent central area of the thyroarytenoid muscle. Moreover, initial nerve tracing experiments using horseradish peroxidase suggested that the motor neurons cell bodies of communicating nerve originated in the retrofacial area. This region is thought to be the site of glossopharyngeal nerve motor neurons innervating the stylopharyngeus muscle. Clearly, the nature and function of the communicating nerve is worthy of further study.

Neuromuscular Compartments

Another notable observation was the "compartmentalized" nature of the nerve supply within laryngeal muscles. As the laryngeal muscles are relatively small, it is surprising that they are composed of even smaller units, called neuromuscular compartments. As these compartments receive their own dedicated terminal nerve branch, they are potentially independently controlled.

Ingredients for Success

The first factor that made this research possible was the environment. The Department of Otolaryngology at the Mount Sinai School of Medicine had a long history of academic contributions in Otolaryngology. A former private attending in the department was Dr Eugene Grabscheid, one of the first otolaryngologists specializing in voice care. When he passed away, he endowed a center for research and treatment of voice disorders.

A second factor was my mentor, Dr. Hugh Biller, the Chairman of the Department of Otolaryngology. Dr. Biller (happily retired in Maine) had a unique style of motivating and inspiring people. A truly exceptional person in both character and surgical skill, he was definitely an inspiration to me. He encouraged research and established an atmosphere that allowed me to pursue a risky and unorthodox strategy.

A third factor was the team. This article was a group effort. The 1990s was a time when many talented individuals were fleeing the oppression of communist China and some of these joined my research team and made invaluable contributions.

Dr. Bei-lian Wu found the original article describing the Sihler's stain and worked to adapt it to human specimens. She became a master of this difficult staining technique. She also made many novel observations on these specimens, particularly involving neural connections. Even more importantly, she continued to work in this area and uncovered a series of surprising and intriguing observations related to laryngeal innervation. Dr. Wu retired before pursuing all these leads.

Dr. Liancai Mu performed the most difficult dissections that are presented in the article. After processing with Sihler's stain anatomical specimens grossly appear to be an amorphous blue blob. Although they can be transilluminated and examined under a microscope, they certainly cannot be photographed. The clarity of the anatomical specimens shown in this article are directly the result of the painstaking work of Dr. Mu. Each specimen reflects weeks, if not months, of meticulous dissection with microsurgical instruments to isolate and show the specific anatomical feature highlighted. Dr. Mu has gone on to have a very successful research career as an independent investigator.

A fourth factor is the nature of Laryngology. Unlike many other medical fields, Laryngology has a long history of clinicians contributing to the basic science of the field. Negus, Harrisson, and Kirschner are just some of the physicians who come to mind.

A fifth factor is myself, the leader of the research group. Most ENT surgeons are not interested in basic research questions. My interest in laryngeal neuroanatomy arose in a roundabout way. I did not set out to study basic science questions. Instead, I spent the first years of my research efforts on trying to develop an implantable stimulator to rehabilitate patients with vocal fold paralysis. As most of the volume of any implant is the battery, there is a strong incentive to make stimulation as efficient as possible. It quickly became apparent that the small posterior cricoarytenoid muscle had multiple parts that abducted the vocal fold in different ways. How these parts were innervated became an important question, as stimulation could then be focused on the most critical nerve branch.

This led me to study the literature regarding laryngeal innervation. Surprisingly, the answers I needed were still controversial. Even more surprising was that I found that this had been a major topic of scientific inquiry early in the 20th and even in the 19th century. Hundreds of articles were written on clinical observations of patients with vocal fold paresis resulting from lesions at all levels of the nervous system and in meticulous postmortem autopsies. Moreover, in that era, meticulous examination of human pathological specimens, so called "experiments of nature" yielded insights that were unavailable today as the diseases that caused them are no longer seen. In many scientific fields, articles 2 years old can be outdated. However, the work of the early anatomists was quite relevant, particularly because aspects of the human upper airway have no animal model. In some cases, there clearly were important observations that had been forgotten.

Studying basic science in a medical school gives the impression that most information is known and well confirmed. This impression is particularly strong in the anatomical sciences, where most important discoveries were made centuries ago. However, after obtaining and reading all of the reprints in the field, I realized that there were real gaps in the knowledge of laryngeal anatomy. At some point, I came to the realization that I had reached the limits of what was known about laryngeal anatomy. I believe that this is a critical realization for all researchers. In a way, it was akin to early explorer who journeyed to the end of the map and realized that no one knows what lies over the edge. It sinks in that here was a chance of contributing to the finite body of human knowledge, even if only a small bit. If you feel this excitement, you may pursue a career in research.

In my case, I found the possibility of adding something truly new to be very motivating. I realized not only that were many areas in Laryngology unknown but the answers could be directly relevant to clinical practice. Laryngology encompassed the main physiological functions of breathing and eating. The failure to separate these functions leads to the pneumonia that has long been the final common pathway humans take to death—"The captain of death" to quote Osler.

Why anatomy? Actually, neurophysiology is more intellectually attractive. However, anatomy is the cornerstone of all other clinically related disciplines. I once heard that "Physiology equals anatomy plus imagination." I have found this to be very true in Laryngology as well as in understanding the tongue, pharynx, and other structures of the human upper airway. Many of these are very complex and anatomical findings point the way toward theories that can be formulated and tested with physiologic techniques.

However, the real surprise was that Laryngology was also of fundamental scientific importance as, along with the tongue, the larynx is one of the main organs of speech. Even now, the evolution and biology of speech is still rank among the top mysteries of science, right alongside the origin of the universe and the nature of consciousness.

Finally, although the tongue has an obvious role in speech articulation, the larynx contributes the more mysterious and beautiful sound of the voice. It provides the character, emotion, and emphasis of speech. It conveys the emotional state directly, a powerful window into the soul. This is why some believe that the pinnacle of art is opera.

In summary, Laryngology, although a small and esoteric field, is the intersection of some of the most critical clinical issues as well as the fundamental questions in science as well as the most revered artist medium. What more could a researcher want?

ORIGINAL ARTICLE

The Innervation of the Human Larynx

Ira Sanders, MD; Bei-Lian Wu, MD; Liancai Mu, MD; Youzhu Li, MD; Hugh F. Biller, MD

Objective: To investigate the gross anatomy of the recurrent and superior laryngeal nerves (RLNs and SLNs) in 10 human larynges.

Methods: Whole larynges were processed to clear all soft tissue while leaving nerves stained. Then the main laryngeal nerves and the muscles they innervate were dissected and analyzed.

Results: It was found that in all larynges the RLNs and SLNs are connected by nerve branches other than Galen's anastomosis. The most consistent connection is in the interarytenoid muscle, where RLNs and internal SLNs combine in a neural plexus. A less consistent connection occurs in the piriform fossa, where a continuation of the external SLN passes from the cricothyroid muscle to the thyroarytenoid muscle.

Conclusion: Based on these findings it is proposed that there are significant neural connections between the RLN and SLN systems. In addition, limited cross-innervation is seen from side to side in the area of the interarytenoid muscle. Other findings concern the innervation patterns within the laryngeal muscles. The posterior cricoarytenoid, cricothyroid, and thyroarytenoid muscles all appear to be composed of separate bellies based on the configuration of their nerve supply. Most notable is the region of the thyroarytenoid muscle at the vocal cord margin that is innervated by a nerve plexus of extreme complexity. The details of the innervation patterns suggest functional differences within and between laryngeal muscles.

(Arch Otolaryngol Head Neck Surg. 1993;119:934-939)

Unanswered questions regarding laryngeal neuroanatomy include possible cross-innervation from side to side in the larynx and between the superior and recurrent laryngeal nerve (SLN and RLN) systems. In addition, the distribution of the nerves within the muscles is almost completely unknown. For example, there is the question of motor unit size in the different muscles. Also, little is known about the distribution of sensory neurons to the joints and muscles. These questions are not only of basic science interest but bear directly on understanding phonation and many clinical issues in neurolaryngology.

Gross dissection has been the traditional method for studying peripheral nerve anatomy. In a complex organ such as the larynx, gross dissection cannot reliably trace the nerve supply into muscles or the small anastomoses between muscles. These nerve slips become so small that they cannot be differentiated from connective tissue or small vessels. This is made even more difficult by the high degree of variation among larynges. Also the multiple nerves in the larynx often cross each other. Therefore, full dissection of one nerve often requires the destruction of its neighbors. As a result, many basic questions regarding laryngeal innervation remain unanswered.

Recently, a nerve staining technique from the previous century, namely, Sihler's, was adapted to investigate the innervation of the larynx in whole canine larynges.[1] Sihler's stain is particularly well suited for this purpose because it renders soft tissue translucent while counterstaining all nerves. Therefore, the innervation of the larynx can

See Materials and Methods on next page

From the Grabscheid Voice Center, Department of Otolaryngology, Mount Sinai Medical Center, New York, NY.

MATERIALS AND METHODS

Ten human larynges were obtained from autopsies. Limited information was available on the specimens; however, most were from the geriatric population and both sexes were represented. Briefly, the six steps of the technique are summarized as follows:

1. *Fixation.* The whole larynx was immersed in 10% unneuralized formaldehyde solution for 1 month or longer.
2. *Maceration.* The fixed specimen was washed with tap water for ½ to 1 hour and then was macerated in 3% potassium hydroxide solution (three drops [approximately 20 μL per drop] of 3% hydrogen peroxide added to each 100 mL of 3% potassium hydroxide) for at least 3 weeks. The potassium hydroxide solution was changed every other day. The specimen was examined daily until the soft tissues looked faded. The duration of maceration varied mainly with the size of the specimen. The maceration was finished when all parts of the specimen were transparent or translucent.
3. *Decalcification.* The macerated specimen was decalcified in Sihler's solution 1 (one part glacial acetic acid, one part glycerin, and six parts 1% aqueous chloral hydrate). Decalcification ended when the calcified cartilage became soft. Duration of decalcification depended on the degree of calcification of the specimen. Generally, this step took 2 weeks to 1 month. The decalcifying solution was changed once weekly during the period of decalcification.
4. *Staining.* The adequately decalcified specimen was put into Sihler's solution 2 (one part stock Ehrlich's hematoxylin, one part glycerin, and six parts 1% aqueous chloral hydrate) for staining until it stained deep purple. This procedure took approximately 3 weeks.
5. *Destaining.* After staining, the specimen was transferred to Sihler's solution 1, with occasional agitation for destaining. The solution was changed when it became purple. The destaining was checked microscopically and was terminated when the soft tissues looked faded and the small nerve branches could still be seen clearly. Ideal destaining would turn muscles light purple and nerve branches dark. The specimen was washed in running tap water for ½ hour and then was immersed in 0.05% lithium carbonate solution for approximately 1 hour.
6. *Clearing.* The destained specimen was washed in running tap water for ½ to 1 hour and then was cleared in increasingly graded glycerin (40%, 60%, 80%, and 100% glycerin) with a few thymol crystals. The specimen was left in each solution for 1 day until the excess of stain was cleared out and then was transferred to 100% glycerin. The nerves and muscles were dissected away from the cartilage and then transilluminated and photographed with a camera (Olympus DM-1, Olympus, Tokyo, Japan) using a 20-mm, 38-mm, or 50-mm lens.

be examined in whole specimens with all of the three-dimensional relationships remaining intact. In a further modification of the technique it was demonstrated that muscles dissected from a whole larynx can be transilluminated to clearly demonstrate the intramuscular branching pattern.[2] In this study the Sihler stain and its modifications were applied to human larynges. The eventual goal of this work is a full description of laryngeal innervation, including the intramuscular distribution of nerves. This article is intended to serve as a preliminary overview of the results.

RESULTS

After processing it was possible to obtain specimens in which the muscles were translucent and the nerves were clearly counterstained. Dissection of the specimens is difficult because all soft tissue, whether fascia, mucosa, or muscle, appears identical. Therefore, most dissections concentrated on removing a single muscle at a time. However, in one case it was possible to obtain both RLNs with their complete intramuscular distributions (**Figure 1**). A second dissection obtained both internal SLNs and their distribution (**Figure 2**). The remainder of the specimens, however, consisted of individual muscles.

In tracing the RLN superiorly, the first branch that arises innervates the posterior cricoarytenoid muscle. In five of 10 specimens the posterior cricoarytenoid was seen to be innervated by two branches that arise separately off the main trunk of the RLN (**Figure 3**). The first branch innervates the lateral aspect of the muscle, while the second branch innervates the medial one. The branch to the posterior cricoarytenoid muscle (PCA) often has some connection to the nerve branch to the interarytenoid muscle (Figures 1 and 3).

The next branch to come off the RLN is the branch to the interarytenoid muscle. This branch passes medially around the cricoarytenoid joint and underneath the PCA to reach the inferior aspect of the interarytenoid muscle. The single midline interarytenoid is innervated by both RLNs, and these nerves anastomose with each other as well as with branches from the SLN (**Figures 4** and **5**). The pattern of the anastomotic plexus is highly variable among specimens.

The terminal branches of the RLN innervate the lateral cricoarytenoid and thyroarytenoid muscles. These two muscles appear almost as a single unit during dissection (Figure 1). The lateral cricoarytenoid is innervated by a single nerve branch. The innervation pattern consists of a dense anastomotic plexus in the center of the muscle (**Figure 6**). The innervation pattern of the lateral cricoarytenoid was found to be similar in all specimens.

The RLN terminates in the thyroarytenoid muscle. Just prior to entering the muscle the nerve branches into multiple fascicles that are distributed throughout the true and false vocal cords (**Figure 7**). The thyroarytenoid innervation is by far the most dense anastomotic network seen in any of the laryngeal muscles. This is especially

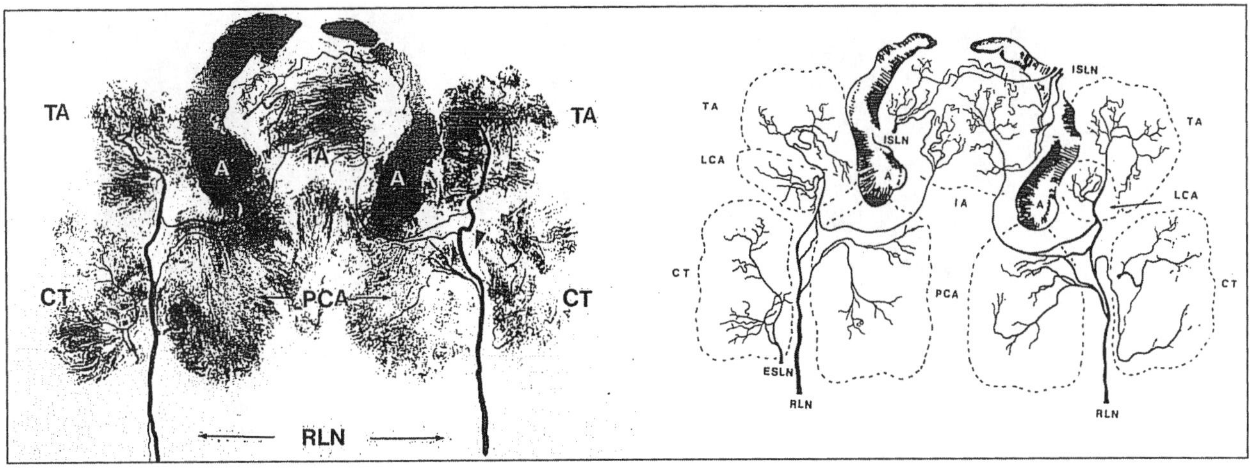

Figure 1. *Recurrent laryngeal nerves (RLNs). Left, In this specimen the entire lengths of both RLNs have been dissected intact. The specimen has been mounted flat, and additional structures, such as the arytenoid cartilages (A), have been retained in an approximation of their normal locations. Note that the distribution of the RLNs is not symmetric from side to side. For example, on the right side the nerve branch to the posterior cricoarytenoid muscle (PCA) also connects with the nerve branches to the interarytenoid muscles (IA). The arrowhead points to a neural communication between the cricothyroid muscle (CT) and the RLN. Right, Line drawing of left side of this figure. TA indicates thyroarytenoid muscle; ISLN, internal superior laryngeal nerve; ESLN, external superior laryngeal nerve; and LCA, lateral cricoarytenoid.*

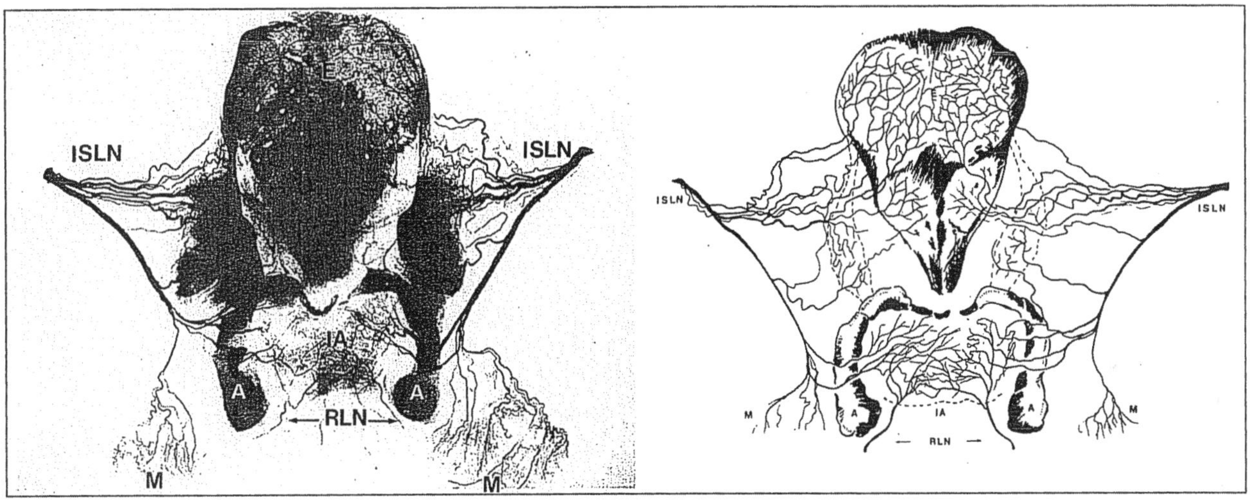

Figure 2. *Internal superior laryngeal nerves (ISLNs). Left, In this specimen both ISLNs and their related structures have been dissected and then arranged in two dimensions. Note that after passing through the thyrohyoid foramen, the ISLN gives off multiple branches that supply the entire supraglottic mucosa. One nerve branch passes behind the arytenoid cartilage (A) to supply the postcricoid mucosa and the interarytenoid muscle (IA). Right, Line drawing of left side of this figure. RLN indicates recurrent laryngeal nerve; E, epiglottis; and M, mucosa.*

true at the medial edge of the thyroarytenoid near the area of the vocal ligament (**Figure 8**).

Communications were often found between the SLNs and the RLNs. The internal branch of the SLN communicates with the RLN within an anastomotic network within the interarytenoid muscle (Figures 4 and 5). This communication is consistent and is found in almost every specimen. The external SLN also communicates with the RLN via a neural connection. The communicating nerve passes out from the posterior surface of the cricothyroid muscle, passes across the piriform sinus, and then enters the thyroarytenoid where it joins with the terminal RLN branches (**Figure 9**). This communicating branch was seen in four of 10 specimens. Neural communications from side to side were not found in the specimens except in the anastomotic plexus of the interarytenoid muscle.

The cricothyroid muscle was dissected intact from all specimens. The cricothyroid muscle is seen to be innervated by two primary nerve branches from the external SLN (**Figure 10**). One branch enters into the oblique belly while the second supplies the rectus. The nerve-branching pattern is characterized by frequent anastomoses. Although the main branches pass through the center of the muscle, secondary extensions travel to the superior and inferior extent of the muscle.

COMMENT

Some of the most important findings in this study involve connections between the RLN and SLN. It is widely accepted that the RLN innervates the intrinsic laryngeal muscles while the external branch of the SLN innervates the cricothyroid

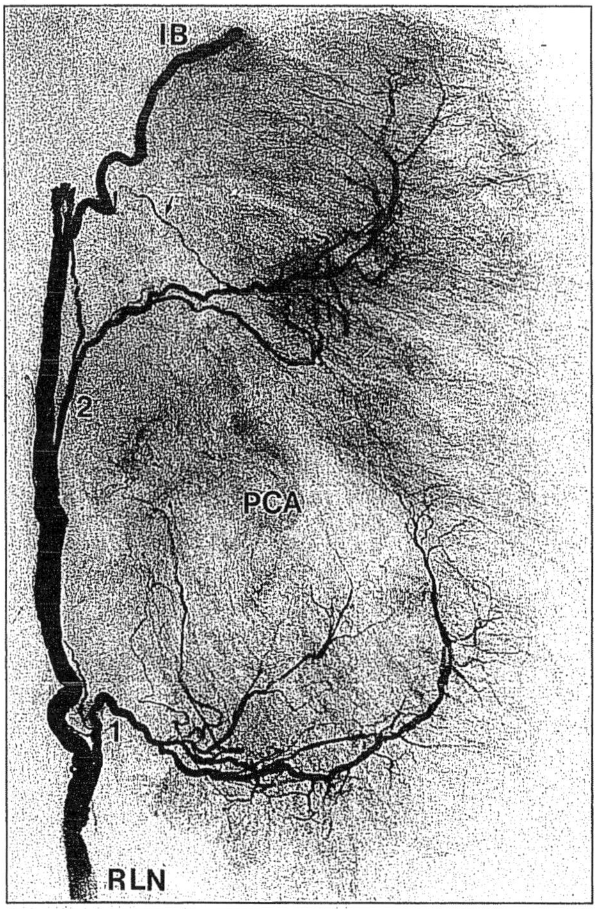

Figure 3. *Posterior cricoarytenoid muscle (PCA). The initial branch of the recurrent laryngeal nerve (RLN) is to this muscle. On entering the larynx, the RLN passes superiorly along the lateral edge of the PCA. In half of the specimens, two branches came off separately from the RLN to innervate two different areas of the muscle. The first branch innervates the lateral half of the muscle (numeral 1), while the second branch innervates the medial half (numeral 2). The arrow points to one of the communicating nerve branches that connect the nerves to the PCA and interarytenoid muscles. IB indicates the nerve branch to the interarytenoid muscle.*

muscle.[3] In this study, we found a variety of exceptions to this view. In the interarytenoid, for example, it was found that RLNs and SLNs converge to form a complex intramuscular plexus. The appearance of the plexus suggests that all four of the main laryngeal nerves are contributing motor innervation to this muscle. That the interarytenoid muscle is innervated by both RLNs has long been accepted; however, although some investigators have claimed that the internal SLN has some motor neurons,[4] this point has never been convincingly demonstrated. Even from our results it is impossible to be sure that the internal SLN neurons are motor in nature. It is conceivable that the neurons from the internal SLN are terminating in proprioceptive elements within the muscle. Also possible is that the internal SLN neurons pass through the intramuscular plexus and exit inferiorly into the RLN nerve branches. Whatever the case, evidence strongly suggests that the area of the interarytenoid muscle is a central meeting area for all the laryngeal nerves. Potentially, it allows crossover of neurons from the SLN to the RLN and to a lesser extent from side to side in the larynx.

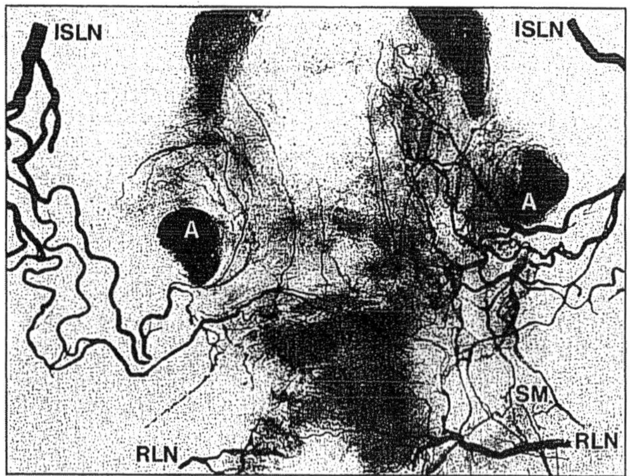

Figure 4. *Interarytenoid muscle (IA). The IA is innervated by nerve branches from both recurrent laryngeal nerves (RLNs) as well as from both superior laryngeal nerves. Note how the nerve branches form a complicated plexus. The IA innervation pattern is one of the most variable of the laryngeal muscles. A indicates arytenoid cartilage; ISLN, internal superior laryngeal nerve; and SM, subglottic mucosa.*

Another area of connection between the RLN and SLN is in the region of the piriform fossa. In four of the specimens an extension of the external SLN is seen to exit from the medial surface of the cricothyroid muscle. The neural branch travels a short distance underneath the piriform mucosa to enter into the lateral surface of the thyroarytenoid muscle. The location of the nerve suggests that it may be the nerve of the fifth cranial arch, a structure that has never been identified by anatomists. Part of this neural connection appears to be sensory, as it terminates in the subglottic mucosa near the vocal process. The other part of the nerve is most likely motor because it terminates within the thyroarytenoid muscle. The function of this nerve is unknown; however, based on the structures it innervates, it may be important for phonation.

The presence of the RLN to SLN connections may have great clinical significance in the understanding of vocal cord paralysis. For example, the position of the vocal cords during unilateral vocal cord paralysis has been controversial since the previous century. On one hand, Semon[5] and Rosenbach[6] believed that the vocal cords go through various stages before reaching complete paralysis. The initial stage always involves loss of the abductor function, then at a later stage the adductor function is lost. On the other hand, Wagner[7] and Grossmann[8] believed that the position of the vocal cords depends on which of the main laryngeal nerves is paralyzed. Isolated RLN paralysis results in a paramedian position of the vocal cords. However, combined RLN and SLN paralysis results in an intermediate position, presumably due to the loss of the unproved adducting action of the cricothyroid muscle. Unfortunately, despite hundreds of reports on the subject, these two theories remain unproven. This controversy may be explainable by the occasional presence of motor neurons from the SLN.

Our other findings concern the distribution pattern of the intramuscular nerves. Each muscle of the larynx has

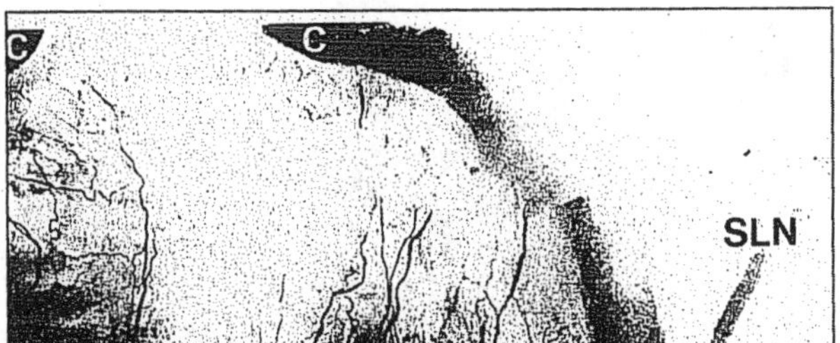

Figure 5. *Interarytenoid muscle (IA). The arrows point to communicating nerve branches between the superior and recurrent laryngeal nerves (SLNs and RLNs). A indicates arytenoid cartilage; IB, recurrent laryngeal nerve branch to the interarytenoid muscle; PCA, posterior cricoarytenoid muscle; and C, corniculate cartilage.*

a distinctive pattern of innervation that reflects the organization of the muscle. Large primary branches to different parts of a muscle suggest that these parts are anatomically separate muscle bellies. This known pattern is seen in the cricothyroid muscle, which is composed of a separate rectus and oblique belly. More surprising, the PCA muscle was also found to have two main nerve branches, and in half of the specimens the branches exited separately from the RLN. Recent work on the canine PCA has demonstrated that the this muscle is separable into different neuromuscular compartments.[9] The lateral half of the muscle is composed of two compartments and appears to be primarily involved with inspiration. These compartments are made up of fast-twitch muscle fibers that travel vertically to insert on the lateral aspect of the arytenoid. The medial half of the PCA appears to be involved with phonation. It has more slow-twitch muscle fibers and is oriented horizontally to insert into the medial aspect of the arytenoid. The canine PCA receives a single nerve branch from the RLN. That the human receives separate nerve branches may indicate that the medial belly in the human has become more specialized to provide fine control during phonation. A final observation regarding the PCA is that its nerve

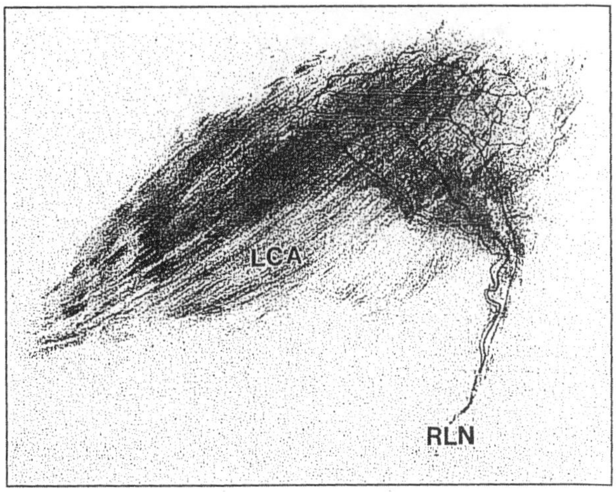

Figure 6. *Lateral cricoarytenoid muscle (LCA). The innervation of the LCA is fairly consistent among specimens. A single branch from the recurrent laryngeal nerve (RLN) enters the muscle near its insertion on the arytenoid cartilage. The intramuscular nerve pattern consists of a plexus that is limited to the superior half of the muscle. Note that the plexus appears to be organized around muscle fascicles.*

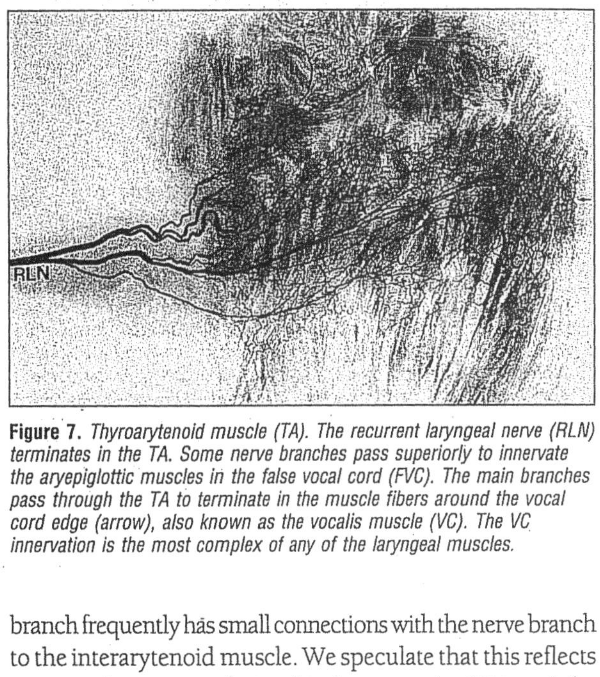

Figure 7. *Thyroarytenoid muscle (TA). The recurrent laryngeal nerve (RLN) terminates in the TA. Some nerve branches pass superiorly to innervate the aryepiglottic muscles in the false vocal cord (FVC). The main branches pass through the TA to terminate in the muscle fibers around the vocal cord edge (arrow), also known as the vocalis muscle (VC). The VC innervation is the most complex of any of the laryngeal muscles.*

branch frequently has small connections with the nerve branch to the interarytenoid muscle. We speculate that this reflects some evolutionary relationship between the PCA and the interarytenoid muscles.

A second level of organization of intramuscular nerve branches involves the terminal branching pattern. The shape of this pattern somehow reflects the architecture of the muscle fibers. A muscle of a given length is not necessarily composed of muscle fibers of the same length. Instead, smaller fibers are connected lengthwise. This may explain why in some muscles the nerve supply courses directly across the middle of a muscle, while in others the nerve branches extend to both ends of the muscle. In the former, the muscle fibers probably span the entire length of the muscle. Since motor end plates are located in the center of muscle fibers, they can easily obtain their axonal connections. In the latter, the muscle fibers are shorter and are distributed through-

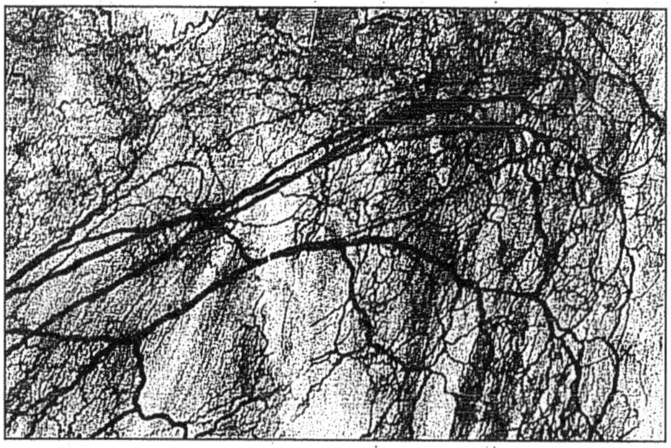

Figure 8. *Vocalis muscle. Magnification of the vocalis muscle shows an extremely dense neural plexus. This density suggests that motor units in this area are extremely small (Sihler).*

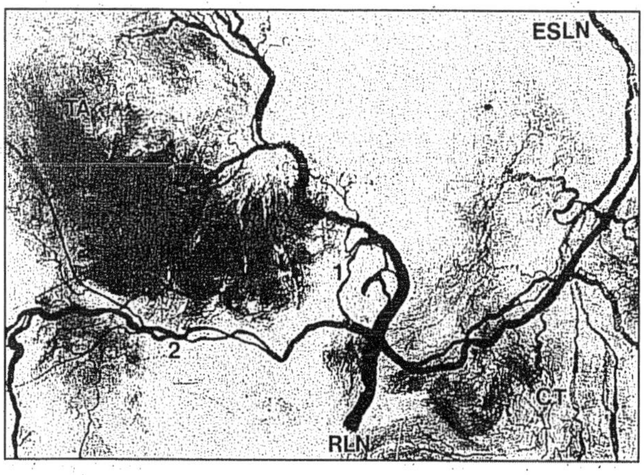

Figure 9. *Communicating nerve branch. A neural communication is often found between the superior laryngeal nerve and the recurrent laryngeal nerve (RLN) in the region of the piriform fossa (arrow). The communication is a continuation of the external superior laryngeal nerve (ESLN) through the cricothyroid muscle (CT). In its most common form, the communicating nerve divides into two parts: one is presumed to be motor and either joins the RLN or terminates in the thyroarytenoid muscle (TA) (numeral 1); the second is sensory and terminates around the vocal process of the arytenoid (numeral 2).*

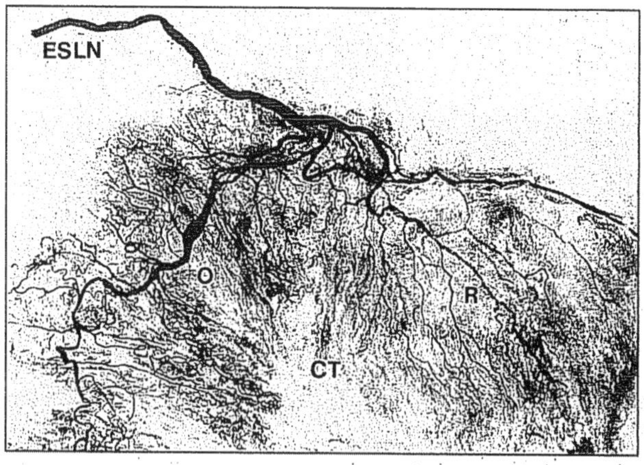

Figure 10. *Cricothyroid muscle (CT). The external superior laryngeal nerve (ESLN) enters the CT near the division between the rectus (R) and oblique (O) bellies. After an initial rearrangement it divides into two main branches that supply the two bellies. Note that in both muscles, but especially in the oblique, the secondary nerve branches appear to extend into the origin and insertions of the muscle fibers.*

out the length of the muscle. This arrangement necessitates extensions of the nerve supply to both ends of the muscle. Short terminal branching is clearly seen in the lateral cricoarytenoid muscle and parts of the PCA. Long terminal branching is seen in the thyroarytenoid and cricothyroid muscles. The interarytenoid muscle is so complex and variable that it is difficult to discern which branches are primary and which are secondary.

A second aspect of the terminal branching pattern is the anastomotic network within the muscle. Muscles such as the lateral cricoarytenoid have neural networks that appear to surround muscle fascicles. In the thyroarytenoid these networks become dense and complicated, especially in the area of the vocalis. This complexity suggests that this area has very small fascicles and a dense innervation. Whether this is due to a large sensory innervation in this area or to very small motor units is impossible to discern in the specimens. However, it does suggest that the vocalis area has an extremely dense innervation that is no doubt related to delicate adjustments during phonation.

In conclusion, a variety of new observations have been presented regarding the innervation of the human larynx. The most interesting findings are of two main types. First is the presence of communicating nerve branches. These are found to connect the RLN and SLN systems in various places. Second is a variety of detail in the intramuscular nerve patterns of all the laryngeal muscles. These may reflect the function of the muscles in ways that have yet to be discovered.

Accepted for publication February 8, 1993.

Reprint requests to Grabscheid Voice Center, Department of Otolaryngology, Box 1189, Mount Sinai Medical Center, New York, NY 10029-6574 (Dr Sanders).

REFERENCES

1. Wu B-L, Sanders I. A technique for demonstrating the nerve supply of whole larynges. *Arch Otolaryngol Head Neck Surg.* 1992;118:822-827.
2. Drake W, Li Y, Rothschild MA, Wu B-L, Biller HF, Sanders I. A new technique for displaying the entire nerve branching pattern of a whole muscle: results in ten canine posterior cricoarytenoid muscles. *Laryngoscope.* 1993;103:141-148.
3. Lemere F. Innervation of the larynx, I: innervation of laryngeal muscles. *Am J Anat.* 1932;51:417-438.
4. Dilworth TFM. The nerves of the human larynx. *J Anat.* 1921;56:48-52.
5. Semon F. Clinical remarks: on the proclivity of the abductor fibers of the recurrent laryngeal nerve to become affected sooner than the adductor fibers or even exclusively, in cases of undoubted central or peripheral injury or disease of the roots or trunks of the pneumogastric, spinal accessory or recurrent nerves. *Arch Laryngol.* 1881;2:197-222.
6. Rosenbach O. Zur Lehre von Doppelseitigen Totalen Laehmung des Nerv Laryngeus Inferior (Recurrens). *Breslauer Aerztliche Z.* 1880;2:14-16, 27-30.
7. Wagner R. Die Medianstellung der Stimmban der bei der Rekurrenslahmung. *Arch Pathol Anat Physiol.* 1890;120:437-459, 124:127.
8. Grossmann M. Experimentelle Beitrage zur Lehre von der 'Posticulslahmung.' *Arch Laryngol Rhinol.* 1897;6:282.
9. Sanders I, Jacobs I, Wu B-L, Biller HF. The three bellies of the canine posterior cricoarytenoid muscle: implications for understanding laryngeal function. *Laryngoscope.* 1993;103:171-177.

Commentary

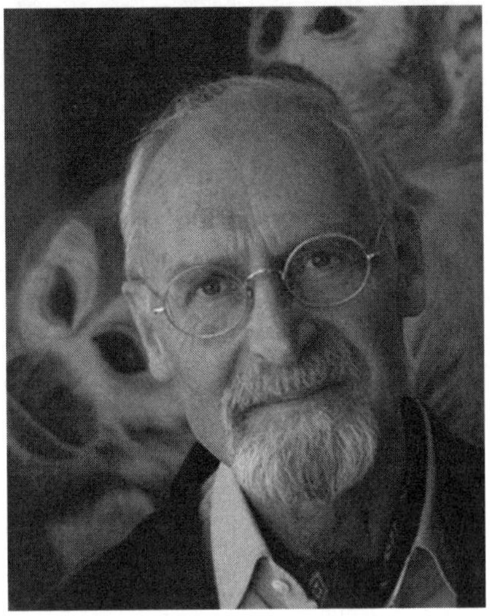

Uwe Jürgens, Dr.rer.nat

The paper included in this collection is a review of 36 years of the author's research in voice physiology, supplemented by the data of various other research groups in the field, with the aim of presenting a coherent picture of central voice control, according to the current state of knowledge. As the author`s education is biological, not medical, the focus of the paper is on animal research. Animals do not have language, nor are they capable of artistic song. This limits the usefulness of animal models to voice phenomena humans and animals have in common; these are the nonverbal emotional vocal utterances and the basic motor coordination processes underlying phonation in general. The strength of animal research, on the other hand, is that a number of methods can be applied which, because of ethical reasons, cannot be applied to humans. Such methods are, for instance, systematic recording of neuronal activity with intracerebral electrodes or mapping of neural pathways using intra-axonally transported tracer substances.

Progress in the life sciences, to a large degree, is determined by the development of new techniques. When I began my first neurophysiological studies on voice control in 1966, a number of techniques regarded as common practice today were simply nonexistent. The functional magnetic resonance imaging technique (fMRI), the positron emission tomography (PET), and the magnetoencephalography (MEG), that is, all those techniques used today to study the relationship between regional brain activity and speech or song production were not yet available. In animal research, the most important technique to correlate local cerebral activities with vocal production is the single-unit recording technique, that is, the recording of the electrical activity of single neurons by the aid of intracerebral microelectrodes. This technique was already available in the 1960s, but it was not applied to vocalization research. The reason for this was that, in order to explore the brain systematically for vocalization-correlated activity, the animal had to produce thousands of vocalizations. However, in the typical single-unit recording situation with the isolated animal sitting in a restraining chair, having the head fixed to prevent relative movements between electrode and neurons, vocalizations are rare and difficult to obtain. Only in the 1990s did we succeed in constructing an implantable single-unit recording device, transmitting the neuronal activity telemetrically. This now allows recording in freely moving animals within their natural social environment, a situation in which gathering of high numbers of vocalizations is no longer a problem.

A classical method to find out which role specific brain structures play in voice control is to study the effects of localized brain lesions on voice production. Here again, methodological developments have markedly promoted our understanding in the last 30 years. In the 1960s, in order to be able to correlate a specific brain lesion with a specific voice deficit, it was necessary to wait until the patient had died and his brain been examined histologically. Today, due to the modern brain imaging techniques, brain lesions can be localized in the conscious patient. Also in animal research, the lesioning approach is characterized by marked methodological advancements. Three decades ago, in order to be able to study the effect of an experimental brain lesion on vocal production, irreversible lesions were produced either electrolytically, thermically, by suction, or direct mechanical intervention. Today, such lesions are replaced by reversible inactivations of small brain regions using intracerebral injections of pharmacologic agents. This saves animals, and in contrast to the irreversible lesions, the pharmacologic approach allows to test many different regions in one and the same animal. In addition, it allows identification of the neurotransmitters underlying specific vocalization-controlling pathways.

Methodological developments of relevance in voice research have also taken place in the field of neuroanatomy. In the 1960s, if one wanted to know to which other brain region a specific region sends its information, the only way was to make a lesion in the region of interest. By the help of silver staining techniques, the degenerating axons then could be followed to their terminations; or by Nissl staining techniques, the site of the degenerating cell bodies, sending their axons to the lesioned region, could be identified. The problem, however, was that the lesions not only damaged nerve cell bodies and axonal terminals, but also axons passing nearby. As a consequence, one never could be sure whether the degenerating axons found in a specific region had their origin really at the lesion site or came from somewhere else and were just passing through the lesion site. The same holds for the retrogradely degenerating nerve cell bodies. Their target structure, to which the information is sent, might be, in fact, not the lesion site, but a region beyond the lesion site, with the latter representing only a through-passage. The problem was solved in the early 1970s when tracer substances became available which were taken up specifically by nerve cell bodies and/or axonal terminals, but not by by-passing axons. This made it possible to follow the course of neural pathways, and even single fibers, from their origin to their target structure, and vice versa.

Finally, one additional methodological development should be mentioned that made an important contribution to voice research; this is the advances in acoustical analysis techniques. When I began my first studies on brain lesion-induced vocal deficits in the late 1960s, vocalizations were recorded on a tape recorder; with the help of a custom-made spectrograph, sonagrams were prepared, and simple acoustic parameters, such as fundamental frequency, frequency range and duration of vocalization were measured with a ruler directly on the sonagram. Today, the whole acoustical analysis process is completely digitalized. Sophisticated computer programs allow us to extract tens of acoustic parameters from the vocal sample, and the preparation of sonagrams is not a matter of minutes, but is made online. Brain lesion- as well as brain stimulation-induced vocal changes thus can be characterized now in a much more fine-grained manner.

Due to these manifold methodological developments, our knowledge about the central voice control has made good progress in the last years, as documented in the accompanying review paper. If progress continues with the same pace, it is conceivable that stuttering, spasmodic dysphonia, and other neurological voice disorders will become accessible to neurosurgical treatment in near future. The question is whether progress will continue in the same way as it did in the past. Pressure of the animal activists is growing. Due to this pressure, the number of laboratories carrying out neurophysiologic voice research in animal models is fading rapidly. Particularly, the research in nonhuman primates virtually has come to an end. If this trend continues, neurosurgical therapies of neurological voice disorders will remain an illusion.

PERGAMON

Neuroscience and Biobehavioral Reviews 26 (2002) 235–258

NEUROSCIENCE AND BIOBEHAVIORAL REVIEWS

www.elsevier.com/locate/neubiorev

Review

Neural pathways underlying vocal control

Uwe Jürgens*

German Primate Centre, Kellnerweg 4, 37077 Göttingen, Germany

Revised 26 November 2001; accepted 26 November 2001

Abstract

Vocalization is a complex behaviour pattern, consisting of essentially three components: laryngeal activity, respiratory movements and supralaryngeal (articulatory) activity. The motoneurones controlling this behaviour are located in various nuclei in the pons (trigeminal motor nucleus), medulla (facial nucleus, nucl. ambiguus, hypoglossal nucleus) and ventral horn of the spinal cord (cervical, thoracic and lumbar region). Coordination of the different motoneurone pools is carried out by an extensive network comprising the ventrolateral parabrachial area, lateral pontine reticular formation, anterolateral and caudal medullary reticular formation, and the nucl. retroambiguus. This network has a direct access to the phonatory motoneurone pools and receives proprioceptive input from laryngeal, pulmonary and oral mechanoreceptors via the solitary tract nucleus and principal as well as spinal trigeminal nuclei. The motor-coordinating network needs a facilitatory input from the periaqueductal grey of the midbrain and laterally bordering tegmentum in order to be able to produce vocalizations. Voluntary control of vocalization, in contrast to completely innate vocal reactions, such as pain shrieking, needs the intactness of the forebrain. Voluntary control over the initiation and suppression of vocal utterances is carried out by the mediofrontal cortex (including anterior cingulate gyrus and supplementary as well as pre-supplementary motor area). Voluntary control over the acoustic structure of vocalizations is carried out by the motor cortex via pyramidal/corticobulbar as well as extrapyramidal pathways. The most important extrapyramidal pathway seems to be the connection motor cortex–putamen–substantia nigra–parvocellular reticular formation–phonatory motoneurones. The motor cortex depends upon a number of inputs for fulfilling its task. It needs a cerebellar input via the ventrolateral thalamus for allowing a smooth transition between consecutive vocal elements. It needs a proprioceptive input from the phonatory organs via nucl. ventralis posterior medialis thalami, somatosensory cortex and inferior parietal cortex. It needs an input from the ventral premotor and prefrontal cortex, including Broca's area, for motor planning of longer purposeful utterances. And it needs an input from the supplementary and pre-supplementary motor area which give rise to the motor commands executed by the motor cortex. © 2002 Published by Elsevier Science Ltd.

Keywords: Vocalization; Speech; Phonatory muscles; Reticular formation; Nucl. ambiguus; Nucl. retroambiguus; Solitary tract nucleus; Periaqueductal grey; Anterior cingulate cortex; Motor cortex; Motor coordination; Pattern generation

Contents

1. Introduction 236
2. Peripheral apparatus 236
   2.1. Larynx 236
   2.2. Respiratory apparatus 238
   2.3. Supralaryngeal tract 238
   2.4. Sensory innervation 239

Abbreviations: Ab, nucl. ambiguus; BC, brachium conjunctivum; BP, brachium pontis; Cb, cerebellum; Cf, nucl. cuneiformis; Cn, nucl. cuneatus; Co, nucl. cochlearis; CoI, colliculus inferior; CoS, colliculus superior; CRf, corpus restiforme; CT, corpus trapezoideum; DG, nucl. dorsalis tegmenti (Gudden); DLM, decussatio lemnisci medialis; DPy, decussatio pyramidum; DR, nucl. dorsalis raphae; DV, nucl. dorsalis n. vagi; FLM, fasciculus longitudinalis medialis; FRM, formatio reticularis myelencephali; FRPc, formatio reticularis pontis caudalis; FRPo, formatio reticularis pontis oralis; GC, griseum centrale (periaqueductal grey); LC, locus coeruleus; LLd, nucl. dorsalis lemnisci lateralis; LLv, nucl. ventralis lemnisci lateralis; LM, lemniscus medialis; MV, nucl. motorius n. trigemini; NCS, nucl. centralis superior; NSV, nucl. spinalis n. trigemini; NTS, nucl.tractus solitarii; OI, oliva inferior; OS, oliva superior; PbL, nucl. parabrachialis lateralis; PbM, nucl. parabrachialis medialis; Pp, nucl. praepositus; PV, nucl. principalis n. trigemini; Py, tractus pyramidalis; Rab, nucl. retroambiguus; RL, nucl. reticularis tegmenti pontis; TSc, tractus spinocerebellares; Ves, nucl. vestibularis; VR, nucl. ventralis raphae; IV, nucl. trochlearis; V, n. trigeminus; VI, nucl. abducens; VII, nucl. and n. facialis; VIII, n. acustico-vestibularis; XII, nucl. hypoglossus

Reproduced with permission from *Neurosci Biobehav Rev.* 2002;26:235–258. Copyright 2002 Elsevier Science Ltd. All rights reserved.

3. Brainstem mechanisms 240
3.1. Premotor neurones 240
3.2. Periaqueductal grey 242
3.3. Lateral midbrain–pons transition 245
4. Cortical pathways 246
4.1. Mediofrontal cortex 246
4.2. Motor cortex 247
4.3. Pyramidal and extrapyramidal pathways 248
4.4. Cerebello-thalamo-cortical pathway 249
4.5. Ascending somatosensory pathway 249
4.6. Further speech-related cortical areas 250
5. Conclusion 251
References 252

1. Introduction

Vocal behaviour can take place on different levels of complexity. The lowest level is represented by a completely genetically determined vocal reaction. An example is the infant's pain shrieking. A heavy blow against the body, for instance, elicits shrieking from birth on. An infant does not need prior experience with this stimulus in the form of a pairing with another, unconditioned stimulus. It also does not need to hear shrieking from other humans in order to be able to produce it. The infant's shrieking reaction to a painful stimulus thus may be considered as a reflex behaviour, comparable to coughing induced by an irritating stimulus in the glottis or swallowing elicited by a food bolus entering the pharynx.

When the child has grown up, pain does not automatically elicit shrieking. In adolescents and adults, shrieking can be suppressed, even if pain is severe; and, on the other hand, shrieking can be produced in the complete absence of pain—for instance, on the stage by an actor mimicking pain. As we will see in the following, this higher level of vocal behaviour depends on brain structures dispensable for the production of reflex-like vocal reactions.

Another type of higher-level vocal behaviour is vocal imitation. An example are the songs of humpback whales [1]. In this case, there is not only voluntary control over the initiation process of an (innate) vocal pattern, but also a voluntary control over the acoustic structure of the pattern, that is, vocal plasticity. This level of vocal behaviour, although common in birds, is only rarely found in mammals. The behaviour is dependent on a number of brain areas in addition to those involved in voluntary control of innate vocal patterns.

Finally, the most complex level of vocal behaviour is represented by human speech. In this case, there is not only voluntary control on initiation and acoustic structure of the vocal utterances, but also attribution of specific meanings to these utterances. The utterances, furthermore, are organised in the form of long sequences structured according to syntactical and grammatical rules.

The present review is an attempt to identify brain areas involved in the control of vocal behaviour at each of the aforementioned complexity levels.

2. Peripheral apparatus

Vocal behaviour, irrespective of its innate or learned character, represents a complex motor pattern made up of essentially three components: vocal fold adduction, respiratory activity (usually expiration) and supralaryngeal movements (articulation).

2.1. Larynx

Control of vocal fold movements is carried out mainly by five intrinsic and three extrinsic laryngeal muscles (Fig. 1). The thyroarytenoid muscle makes up the body of the vocal folds. Its isometric contraction gives the vocal folds stiffness, thus ameliorating regular vibration. The interarytenoid and lateral cricoarytenoid muscles are the classical adductor muscles. By tilting and rotating the arytenoid cartilages toward the midline, respectively, these muscles control the degree of glottis closure. The posterior cricoarytenoid muscle is the only abductor muscle of the larynx. It has been reported to be active, together with the thyroarytenoid muscle, during hissing in cats [2] and also during articulation of consonants in human speech [3]. The function of the cricothyroid muscle is to pull the cricoid cartilage toward the thyroid cartilage, thus stretching the vocal folds by increasing the distance between the anterior (thyroid) and posterior (arytenoid) fixation points of the vocal folds [4]. Its activity is directly correlated with the pitch of a vocalization. Its deactivation causes a loss of high-pitched sounds.

The cricothyroid muscle is innervated by the external branch of the superior laryngeal nerve which leaves the brain via the n. vagus roots. The corresponding motoneurones are located in the rostral part of the nucl. ambiguus [5]. The remaining intrinsic laryngeal muscles are innervated by the recurrent nerve. Its fibres leave the brain via the n. accessorius roots, but join the vagal nerve from the foramen jugulare on. The corresponding motoneurones are located in the caudal part of the nucl. ambiguus. The

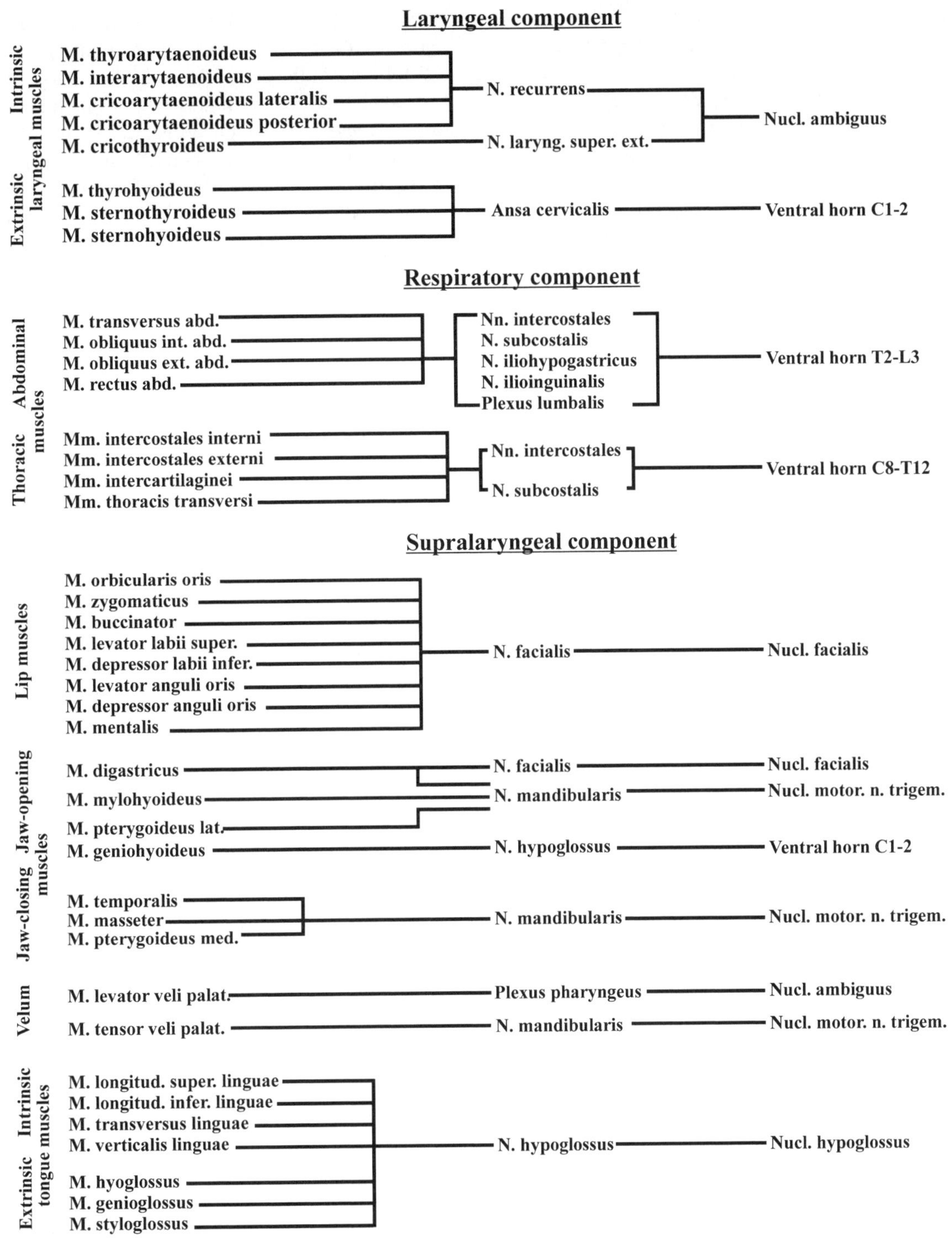

Fig. 1. Scheme of phonatory muscle innervation. On the left, the muscles are listed for which there is evidence that they are involved in one or the other type of vocalization. In the middle, the peripheral nerves innervating those muscles are listed. On the right, the sites of the corresponding motoneurones are given.

innervation of the laryngeal muscles by the nucl. ambiguus is strictly ipsilateral. Some of the motoneurones, however, innervate more than one muscle [6].

Apart from the intrinsic laryngeal muscles, connecting the different laryngeal cartilages with each other, there are five extrinsic laryngeal muscles, connecting the larynx directly and indirectly with surrounding structures (hyoid bone, sternum, pharynx). Only three of them play a major role in phonation. These are the thyrohyoid muscle, connecting thyroid cartilage and hyoid bone; sternothyroid muscle, connecting thyroid cartilage with sternum; and sternohyoid muscle, connecting sternum with hyoid. The main function of these muscles is to stabilize the thyroid cartilage within the neck, so that it can act as an abutment against which the intrinsic laryngeal muscles can exert their forces. In humans, it has been shown that during singing, the external laryngeal muscles increase their activity with increasing fundamental frequency in the high-frequency range and increase their activity with decreasing fundamental frequency in the low-frequency range. In other words, the more the fundamental frequency deviates from the value of a normal, relaxed voice, the stronger is the activation [7]. The sternohyoid muscle, in addition, is correlated in its activity with sound intensity [8]. Its activity is also influenced by articulation: lowering the jaw or pulling back the tongue during phonation increases its activity [9]. Deactivation of the external laryngeal muscles has only minor effects on normal speech, but severely reduces the frequency range during singing [9].

The thyrohyoid and sternohyoid muscles are innervated via the ansa cervicalis by fibres leaving the central nervous system with the n. hypoglossus and first cervical spinal nerve [10]. The motoneurones of the thyrohyoid muscle are located ventrolateral to the caudal hypoglossal nucleus. The motoneurones of the sternohyoid muscle form a cell column running from just ventral of the caudal pole of the nucl. hypoglossus down into the ventral horn of the first cervical segment [10,11]. The sternothyroid muscle is innervated via the first cervical spinal nerve and ansa cervicalis. The corresponding motoneurones are located in a cell column partially overlapping with that of the sternohyoid muscle. The column begins caudoventral to the hypoglossal nucleus and ends in the ventral horn of the second cervical segment [10,11].

2.2. *Respiratory apparatus*

Only if there is an airflow passing the glottis, phonation occurs. This airflow, normally, is an expiratory one. Systematic electromyographic studies have revealed that both abdominal and intercostal muscles are involved in the respiratory component of phonation [12–15]. Among the abdominal muscles, the internal and external oblique muscles are activated before the mm. transversus and rectus abdomini. While the oblique muscles and the m. transversus are well correlated in their activity with the amplitude envelope of phonation, there is only a loose relationship between m. rectus activity and amplitude envelope. The exact time these muscles become active in relation to phonation onset, depends upon the type of phonation, intensity and volume of inhaled air [12,13].

The motoneurones innervating the abdominal muscles lie in the ventral horn of the thoracic and upper lumbar spinal cord. The distribution of these motoneurones differs somewhat between muscles and species. In an anatomical dissection study, Sakamoto et al. [16] report that in humans the internal oblique muscle is innervated by spinal nerves T10–L1, the external oblique muscle by nerves T5–12, the transversus muscle by nerves T6–L1 and the rectus muscle by nerves T7–L1. In a retrograde tracing study in the squirrel monkey, we found obliquus internus motoneurones in the spinal segments T8–L3, obliquus externus motoneurones in the segments T4–L3, transversus motoneurones in the segments T7–L2 and rectus motoneurones in the segments T2–L4 [17]. In the cat, obliquus internus motoneurones are located in T13 to L3, obliquus externus motoneurones in T6 to L3, transversus motoneurones in T9 to L3 and rectus motoneurones in T4 to L3 [18,19]. In the cat as well as in the squirrel monkey, the density of motoneurones innervating a specific muscle is not constant along the spinal cord. Some segments contain a much higher number of motoneurones than others [17,18].

With respect to the intercostal muscles, electromyographic recordings in humans and monkeys have shown that internal as well as external intercostals are activated during phonation [12,20]. The external intercostals traditionally are considered as inspiratory muscles. A more recent study, however, has argued that due to the mechanics of the thorax, inspiratory effects can be exerted only by the most rostral external intercostals [21]. Contraction of caudal external intercostals (VI to VIII), in contrast, would produce expiratory effects. This is in harmony with electromyographic observations made in the squirrel monkey, according to which rostral external intercostals were found to be active immediately before vocalization, while caudal external intercostals were active during vocalization [12]. Similar holds for the intercartilagineus muscles which also have been considered traditionally as inspiratory. They, as well, show a pre-phonatory activity in the rostral intercostal spaces and a phonation-correlated activity in the caudal intercostal spaces. Expiratory effort during phonation is supplemented by a fourth thoracic muscle, the m. thoracis transversi (also called m. triangularis sterni) [15,22].

The different thoracic muscles are innervated by the nervi intercostales and the nervus subcostalis, the perikaya of which are located in the ventral horn of C8–T12 (Fig. 1).

2.3. *Supralaryngeal tract*

The primary sound generated at the glottis is modulated in its spectral properties by the resonance characteristics of the supralaryngeal tract. The resonance characteristics are determined by the length and shape of the supralaryngeal tract. In many mammals, one or both can be changed. Vocal tract lengthening, for instance, can be obtained by protruding the lips or lowering the larynx. Protruding the lips is brought about by an activation of the m. orbicularis together with the m. mentalis [23]. Lowering the larynx is brought about by the mm. sternothyroideus and sternohyoideus [24]. Vocal tract shortening can be obtained by drawing back the mouth corners or lifting the larynx. Drawing back the mouth corners is brought about by the conjoint action of the mm. buccinator, zygomaticus major and depressor anguli oris [23]. Lifting of the larynx is brought about by the mm. thyrohyoideus and mylohyoideus [24]. Innervation of the muscles controlling vocal tract length is made by the facial and mandibular nerves and the ansa cervicalis. The corresponding motoneurones are located in the facial nucleus, trigeminal motor nucleus and the ventral horn of the first and second cervical segments (Fig. 1). Within the facial nucleus, the lip muscles are represented ventrolaterally and laterally [25]. The mylohyoid motoneurones, which indirectly control the larynx height (by controlling the hyoid position), are located in the ventromedial part of the trigeminal motor nucleus [11]. The position of the other larynx height-controlling motoneurones (innervating mm. thyrohyoideus, sternothyroideus, sternohyoideus) has been described already earlier.

A second factor influencing the resonance characteristics of the supralaryngeal tract is the degree of mouth-opening. Jaw-opener muscles are the mm. digastricus, mylohyoideus, pterygoideus lateralis and geniohyoideus; jaw-closer muscles are the mm. temporalis, masseter and pterygoideus medialis. During normal speaking, only the lateral and medial pterygoid muscles and the anterior belly of the m. digastricus are activated [26]. The latter three are innervated by the trigeminal motor nucleus via the mandibular nerve. The remaining jaw-opener/closer muscles are innervated partly by the trigeminal motor nucleus (mm. temporalis, masseter, mylohyoideus), partly by the facial nucleus (m. digastricus posterior) and partly by the ventral horn of C1-2 (m. geniohyoideus) (Fig. 1). Within the trigeminal motor nucleus, the motoneurones innervating the anterior belly of the m. digastricus are located in the dorsomedial part, the pterygoideus lateralis motoneurones are located in the ventromedial part, the pterygoideus medialis motoneurones in the ventral part, the masseter motoneurones in the ventrolateral part and the temporalis motoneurones in the dorsal part [27]. The posterior belly of the digastric muscle is innervated from the most dorsal part of the facial nucleus [28].

Another factor influencing the resonance characteristics of the supralaryngeal tract is the position of the velum. If the velum is lowered, the nasal cavity is coupled to the oropharyngeal cavity and gives the sound a nasalized character. If the mouth is closed—as it is in many animal vocalizations—coupling of the nasal to the oropharyngeal passage is the only way to allow phonation. The position of the velum is determined by the mm. levator and tensor veli palatini, with the first playing the dominant role, at least in human speech [29]. The m. levator veli palatini is innervated from the rostral nucl. ambiguus via glossopharyngeal nerve and pharyngeal plexus; the m. tensor veli palatini receives its innervation from the ventral trigeminal motor nucleus via n. mandibularis [30,31].

A fourth way to change resonance frequencies in the supralaryngeal tract is by tongue movements. In human speech, the tongue is in fact the most important articulatory organ. Tongue movements are controlled by a number of intrinsic and extrinsic muscles (Fig. 1). While the first determine the shape of the tongue, the latter, in addition, determine the position of the tongue within the mouth. The vowel 'i', for instance, is produced by pulling the tongue forward and upward; a movement induced mainly by activation of the m. genioglossus. The vowel 'u', in contrast, is formed by pulling the tongue backward and upward, and the vowel 'a' by pulling it downward, involving in the first case the m. styloglossus, and in the second the m. hyoglossus [32]. Both intrinsic and extrinsic muscles are controlled by the hypoglossal nucleus via the hypoglossal nerve. Within the hypoglossal nucleus, the genioglossus motoneurones are located in the dorsomedial part, the hyoglossus and styloglossus motoneurones in the dorsolateral part; the intrinsic tongue muscles are represented throughout the hypoglossal nucleus [33].

2.4. Sensory innervation

All three subsystems of the phonatory apparatus, that is, laryngeal, respiratory and articulatory, also have sensory innervation in addition to their motor innervation. The larynx contains in its mucosal part numerous corpuscular mechanoreceptors as well as plexiform and free unmyelinated nerve endings [34]. Some of these receptors react to vibratory stimuli in a 1:1 manner up to frequencies of 600 Hz [35]. There are, furthermore, muscle spindles and spiral nerve endings in the laryngeal muscles measuring muscle length, and there are mechanosensitive nerve endings in the cricoarytenoid and cricothyroid joints registering relative movements of the laryngeal cartilages against each other [36]. The sensory innervation of the larynx is made in the subglottic part by the recurrent nerve and in the supraglottic part by the internal and external branch of the superior laryngeal nerve [5]. Recording of the electrical activity of single fibres of these nerves reveals that only the sensory fibres in the internal branch of the superior laryngeal nerve change their activity with phonation [37]. If the internal branch of the superior laryngeal nerve is cut in the squirrel monkey or cat, both of which do not carry motor fibres in this branch, dysphonia in the form of hoarseness and a drop of fundamental frequency emerges [38,39]. The sensory fibres of the larynx project into the interstitial and medial subnuclei of the solitary tract nucleus and, to a smaller degree, into the spinal trigeminal nucleus and the parvocellular reticular formation between the latter two nuclei [40–43]. The corresponding perikarya are located in the ganglia nodosum, jugulare and glossopharyngeus inferior [41].

With respect to the respiratory system, Nakazawa et al. [44] have shown that the somatosensory feedback from the lungs is essential for phonation. If left and right vagal nerves are cut distal to the superior laryngeal nerve separation, vocalization cannot be elicited anymore by electrical stimulation of the periaqueductal grey of the midbrain. Obviously, the central vocalization-controlling structures are not able to generate vocal motor patterns without information about the current air volume in the lungs. This information is gained via pulmonary stretch receptors and reaches the brain via fibres which have their cell body in the nodose ganglion and terminate in the subnuclei ventrolateralis, ventralis, intermedius and interstitialis of the solitary tract nucleus [45,46].

Somatosensory feedback also plays a role in the supralaryngeal control of vocalization. Elimination of part of this feedback by trigeminal nerve-block anaesthesia distorts articulation in humans [47–49]. Apart from the trigeminal nerve, also the glossopharyngeal and vagal nerves are involved in the sensory innervation of the articulatory organs. The oral proprioceptive and tactile information is sent to the principal and spinal trigeminal nuclei, the solitary tract nucleus and, to a minor degree, into the parvocellular reticular formation, nucleus cuneatus and dorsal horn of the first few cervical segments [42,43,50–53]. All intraoral articulatory structures project to both, the solitary tract nucleus as well as the spinal trigeminal nucleus [42,43].

3. Brainstem mechanisms

3.1. Premotor neurones

The production of a specific vocal pattern requires that the widely dispersed phonatory motoneurone groups are coordinated in their activity. Principally, this could be done in two ways: either by reciprocal interconnections between all the motoneurone groups involved in phonation, or by superordinate structures controlling the motoneurones differentially. Neuroanatomical studies show that direct interconnections between the different phonatory motoneurone pools are almost completely absent [54–56]. There are, however, premotor areas which are connected with all phonatory motoneurone pools conjointly. These areas are shown in Fig. 2. They comprise the ventrolateral parabrachial region (including the Kölliker–Fuse nucleus) (AP O), the lateral pontine reticular formation just above the superior olive (AP O), the parvocellular and gigantocellular nuclei of the rostral medulla (AP-1.5 and -3) and the dorsal and ventral reticular nuclei of the caudal medulla (AP-4.5 and -6). All these structures have been shown to contain retrogradely labeled neurones after tracer injections into the nucl. ambiguus, ventral horn of thoracic and lumbar spinal cord, trigeminal motor nucleus, facial and hypoglossal nuclei [54,55,57–62]. The projections to the phonatory motor nuclei are bilateral [63]. Double-labeling experiments have shown that there are single reticular cells projecting to the trigeminal motor nucleus as well as the facial nucleus, to the facial as well as the hypoglossal nucleus and to the hypoglossal as well as the trigeminal motor nucleus [64]. The ventrolateral parabrachial region and parts of the reticular formation are not only connected with the phonatory motor nuclei, but also receive an input from the most important somatosensory nuclei involved in phonation, that is, the solitary tract nucleus and the spinal trigeminal nucleus [65–68]. In an electrophysiological study, Ezure et al. [69], furthermore, showed that there are neurones in the reticular formation dorsomedial to the nucl. ambiguus which are activated by electrical stimulation of the superior laryngeal nerve with short latency (7.7 ms) and which project to the nucl. ambiguus and hypoglossal nucleus at the same time.

The strategic neuroanatomical position of the reticular formation and ventrolateral parabrachial region suggests that these areas play a crucial role in vocal motor coordination. This suggestion is supported by a number of observations. If, for instance, in the squirrel monkey, the lower brainstem is stimulated with focal glutamate injections, sites are found yielding vocalizations [70]. All positive sites are located within that part of the reticular formation maintaining direct connections with the phonatory motor nuclei (Fig. 2). In another squirrel monkey study, a systematic exploration of the brainstem was carried out, looking for sites affecting ongoing phonation when electrically stimulated [71]. Sites distorting the acoustic structure of ongoing phonation were found throughout the phonatory premotor areas, reaching from the ventrolateral parabrachial region through the lateral pons into the caudal medullary reticular formation (Fig. 3). Lesioning studies in the squirrel monkey showed that lesions in the parvocellular reticular formation cause dysphonia [72] (Fig. 4). Single-cell recording studies in the squirrel monkey, finally, revealed vocalization-correlated neuronal activity in the ventrolateral parabrachial region, lateral pons and large parts of the medullary reticular formation [73,74]. In the parvocellular part of the medullary reticular formation as well as in the dorsal reticular nucleus, a greater number of neurones were found the discharge rate of which correlated with the rate of frequency modulation of the fundamental frequency (Fig. 5). These neurones started firing before vocalization onset and did not react to acoustic stimuli. This suggests that these neurones are involved in a very direct way in vocal pattern control.

A group of premotor neurones playing a special role in the respiratory component of phonation is found in the nucl. retroambiguus. The nucl. retroambiguus is a slender cell column, bordering rostrally at the nucl. ambiguus and extending caudally to the end of the brain. It contains the highest number of expiratory bulbospinal neurones in the brain [75]. Some of these neurones contact directly the intercostal and abdominal motoneurones [76,77]. The majority, however, is connected with the motoneurones indirectly via spinal interneurones in layers V–VIII [78–80]. If the activity of single retroambiguus cells is recorded during vocalization, an increase in spike rate is found in some of them that is correlated with m. obliquus externus activation [81]. Bilateral destruction of the nucl. retroambiguus abolishes vocalizations electrically elicited from the periaqueductal grey [82]. From the fact that destruction of the nucl. retroambiguus does not only eliminate the respiratory component of electrically elicited vocalization, but also the laryngeal one, and the fact that nucl. retroambiguus and nucl. ambiguus are reciprocally connected with each other, some authors concluded that the nucl. retroambiguus is responsible for expiratory muscle as well as vocal fold

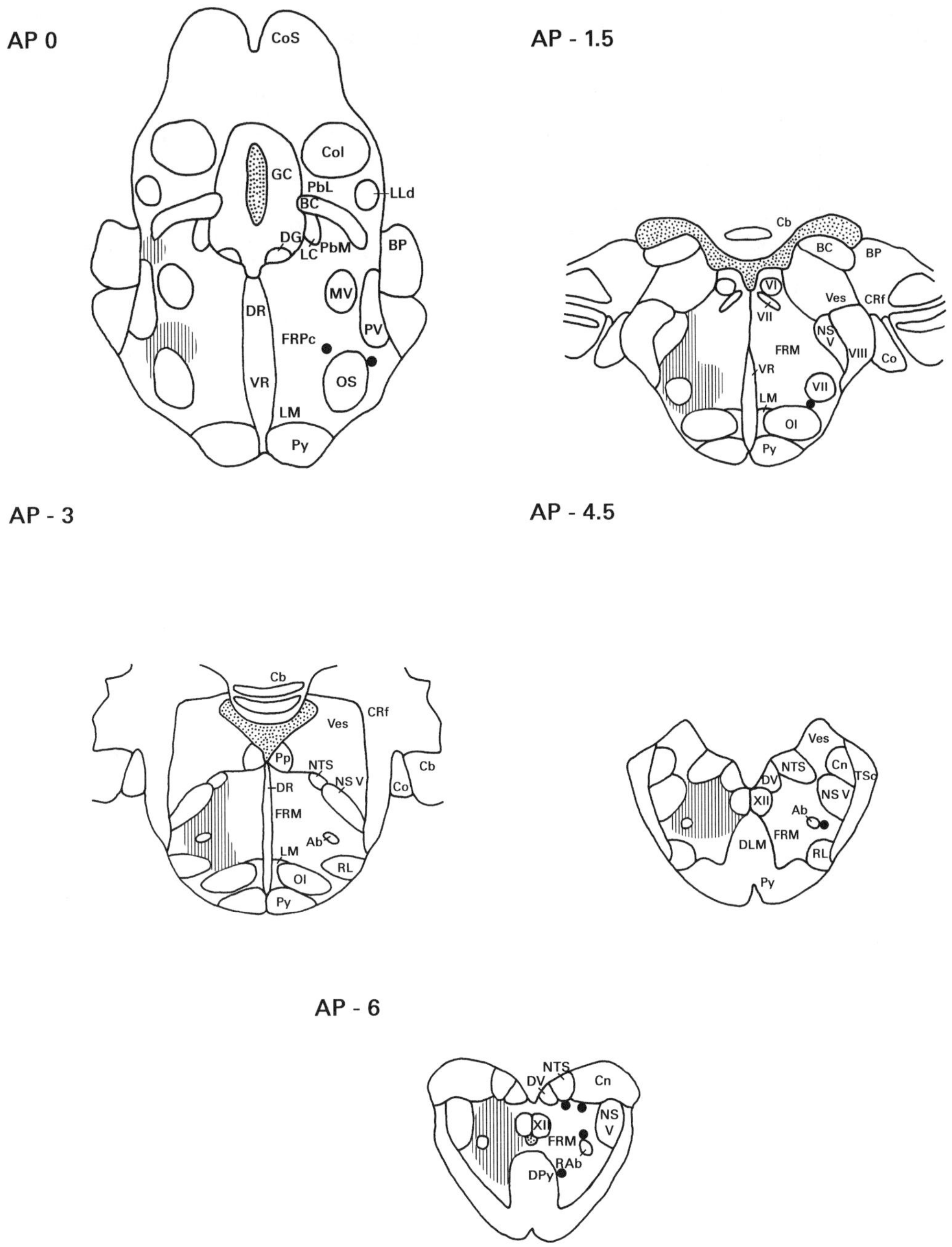

Fig. 2. Frontal sections of the squirrel monkey's brainstem. Hatched areas on the left side indicate brain areas with direct projections to the phonatory motor nuclei. Black circles on the right side indicate sites the glutamatergic stimulation of which produces vocalization. The coordinates in the upper corner indicate the Horsley–Clarke stereotactic anterior–posterior planes in mm.

control during phonation [82–84]. This conclusion can be accepted only with reservation. The lesions of Shiba et al. [82] were not limited to the nucl. retroambiguus, but invaded the surrounding reticular formation. The effects on laryngeal muscles thus might be due to destruction of the peri-retroambigual reticular formation and not the nucl. retroambiguus itself. Single-unit recordings of the author revealed that there are only very few cells in the nucl. retroambiguus the activity of which reflects pitch changes [73]. Such cells, however, are common in the nearby reticular formation. The latter, furthermore, contains cells that, like those in the nucl. retroambiguus, receive an input from the periaqueductal grey and project into the nucl. ambiguus, but unlike those in the nucl. retroambiguus, are non-respiratory [82]. This is not to exclude the possibility that the nucl. retroambiguus interacts directly with the nucl. ambiguus during phonation. Such an interaction, however, might rather serve to adapt vocal fold adduction and tension to the expiratory force than to convey pattern-specific motor comands to the laryngeal motoneurones.

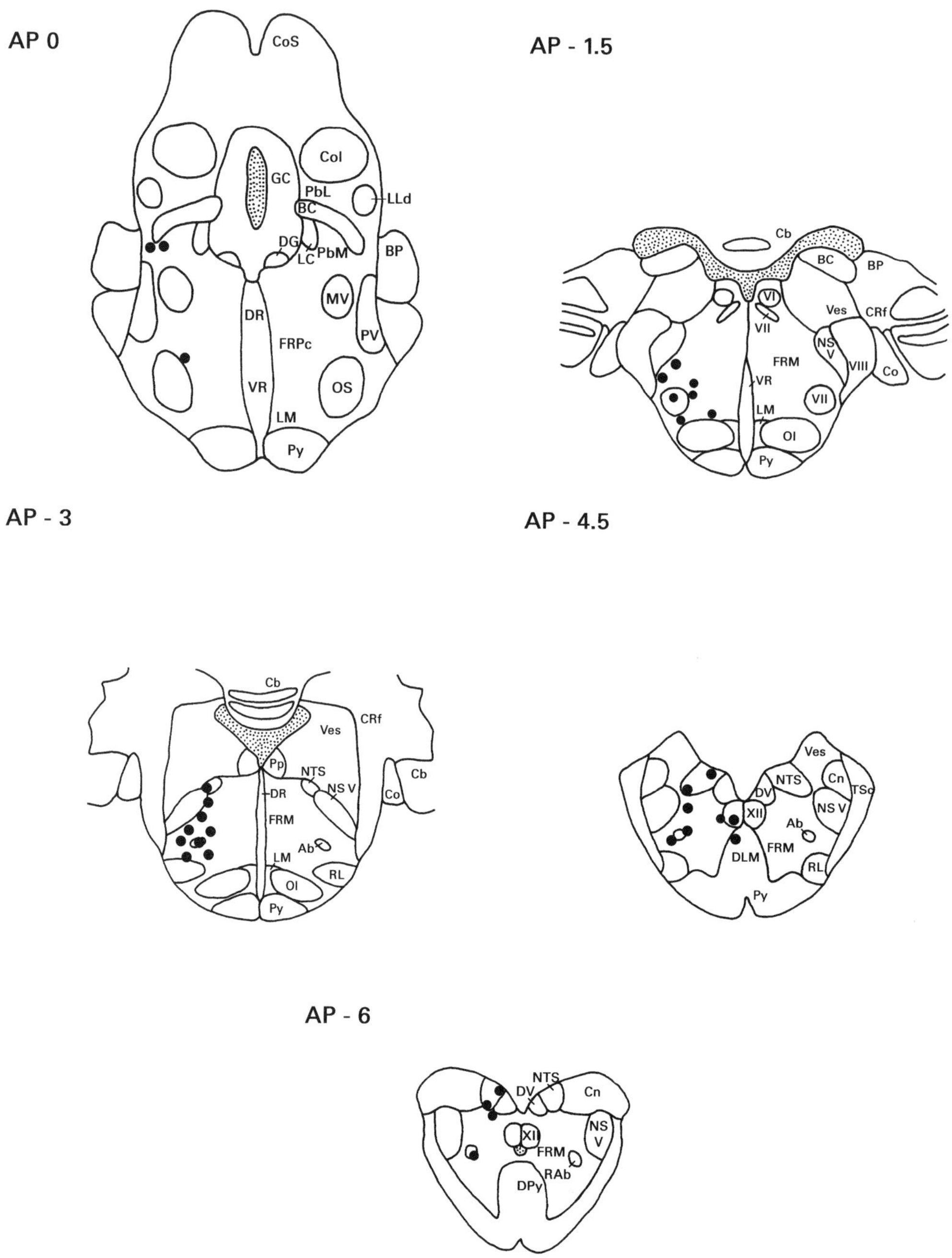

Fig. 3. Black circles indicate sites which, when electrically stimulated during ongoing vocalization, cause a change in acoustic structure in the squirrel monkey.

3.2. Periaqueductal grey

Electrical stimulation of the periaqueductal grey of the midbrain has been reported to produce vocalizations in the rat [85,86], guinea pig [87–89], bat [90,91], cat [92], squirrel monkey [93], rhesus monkey [94], gibbon [95], chimpanzee [96] and man [97]. The elicited vocalizations generally resemble natural, species-specific calls. The majority of them are of agonistic kind, e.g. hissing, growling, screaming and howling in the cat or shrieking, yelling, yapping and cackling in the squirrel monkey. Non-agonistic calls, however, also are obtained, such as meowing in the cat [94], trilling in the squirrel monkey [93], echolocation sounds in the bat [90] and laughing in humans [97]. Sometimes agonistic as well as non-agonistic calls are obtained from one and the same site. The fact that vocalizations cannot only be produced by electrical stimulation, but also injections of glutamate agonists and GABA antagonists (Fig. 6), makes clear that the elicited vocalizations are not due to activation of by-passing fibres, but of inherent periaqueductal neurones [98,99].

Self-stimulation experiments in the squirrel monkey have

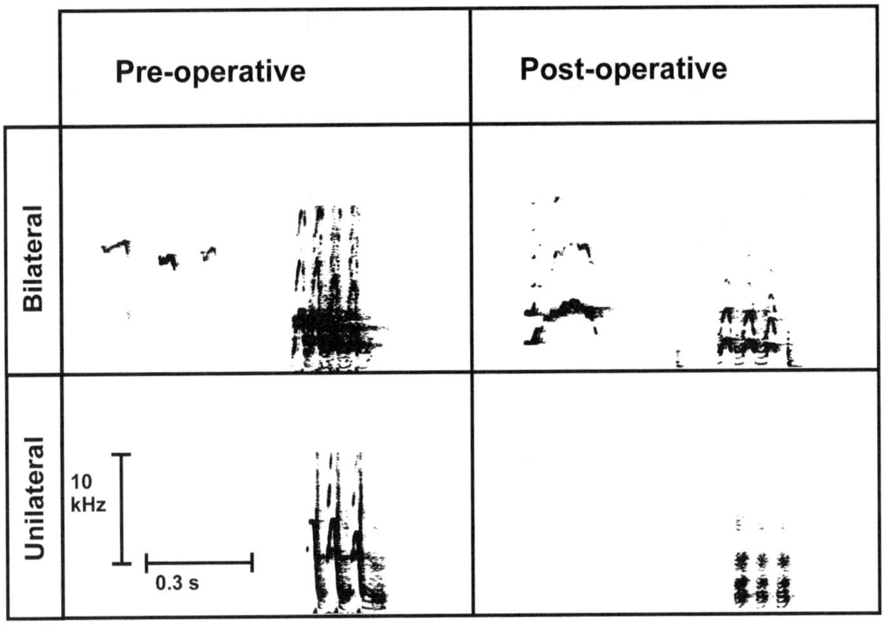

Fig. 4. Sonagraphic representation of squirrel monkey calls before (Pre-operative) and after (Post-operative) experimental lesions in the medullary parvocellular reticular formation. It can be seen that bilateral as well as unilateral lesions severely affect the acoustic structure of the calls.

shown that the periaqueductally elicited vocalizations do not represent secondary reactions to stimulation-induced motivational changes, but are elicited rather directly. If the animal is given the opportunity to switch on or off the vocalization-eliciting brain stimulation itself, no correlation is found between call type and self-stimulation behaviour; that is, one and the same call type elicited in the periaqueductal grey can be associated with aversive emotional states (switch-off behaviour) as well as hedonistic emotional states (positive self-stimulation behaviour), depending upon the exact site of stimulation [100]. This lack of correlation between vocalization and motivation excludes a motivation-based explanation. Further arguments for a rather direct control of vocalization by the periaqueductal grey are (a) the short latency with which vocalization is obtained. In the macaque, electromyographic activity in the laryngeal muscles has been detected as early as 12 ms after stimulation onset [101]. (b) The periaqueductally elicited vocal

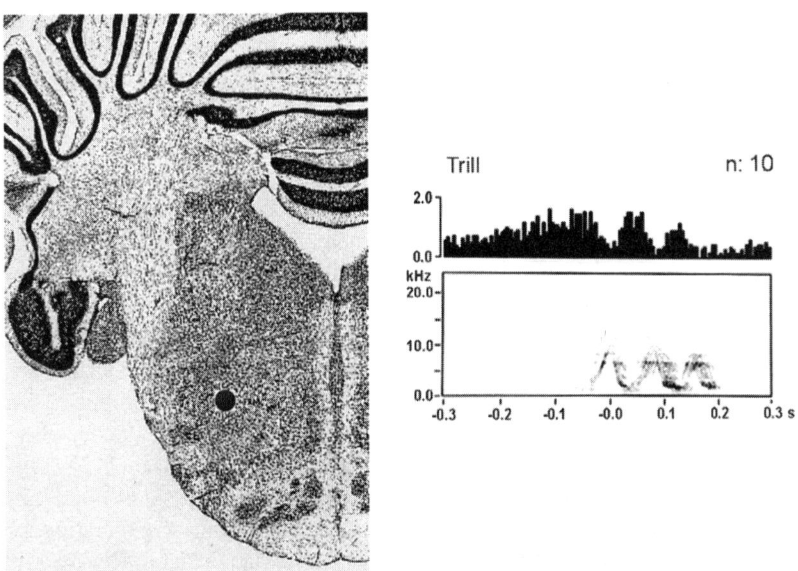

Fig. 5. Vocalization-related neuronal activity in the parvocellular reticular formation just above the nucl. ambiguus. Left: Frontal section of the squirrel monkey's brain indicating the recording site (black circle). The section corresponds to the Horsley–Clarke stereotactic plane AP-3. Right: Averaged neuronal activity at the site indicated on the left during the production of 10 trill calls. Upper part shows a peri-event time histogram (PETH) with 10 ms bin width; trigger point is the first maximum of fundamental frequency. Lower part represents the superimposed sonagrams of the 10 trills underlying the PETH shown above.

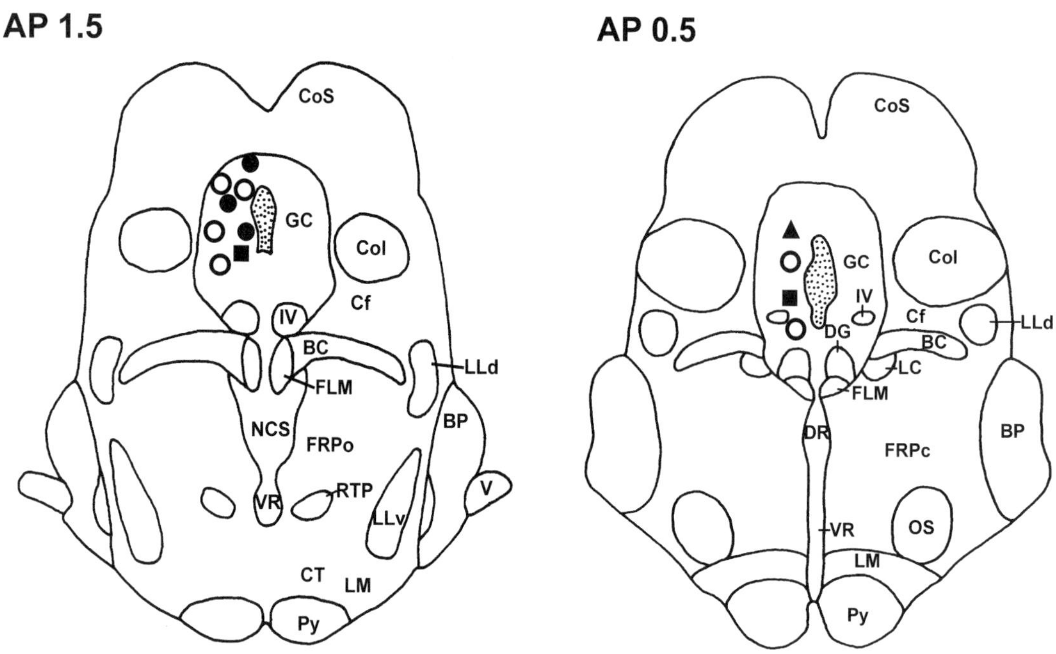

Fig. 6. Vocalization-eliciting sites in the periaqueductal grey of the squirrel monkey. Black circles: sites producing vocalization when injected with glutamate agonists and GABA antagonists. Black squares: sites producing vocalization with glutamate agonists only. Black triangle: site producing vocalization with GABA antagonists only. White circles: sites producing vocalization only when electrically, but not when pharmacologically stimulated.

reaction shows a low habituation; that is, by extending the stimulation, very long sequences of vocalizations can be obtained [93]. (c) Destruction of the periaqueductal grey, together with the laterally bordering tegmentum, causes mutism. Such lesion-induced mutism has been reported for the rat [102], cat [103–106], squirrel monkey [107] and man [108,109].

Partial destruction of the periaqueductal grey does not change the acoustic structure of the calls—as it does in the lower brainstem—but leads to a complete loss of some vocal reactions, leaving others intact. In the squirrel monkey, for instance, a lesion limited to the dorsomedial periaqueductal grey abolishes a vocal alarm reaction (yapping) to a visual stimulus (dummy leopard), but leaves intact a vocal protest reaction (shrieking) to a tactile stimulus (gripping the animal) [107]. The animal still reacts to the visual stimulus with a non-vocal reaction, namely flight. Kelly et al. [103] report that destruction of the dorsal periaqueductal grey and adjacent superior colliculus changed the vocal response of a cat encountering a dog in such a way that, instead of the preoperative hissing, howling was uttered. Another example is given by Skultety [104]: a periaqueductally lesioned cat did not react to painful stimuli with vocalization anymore, but meowed spontaneously. The loss of the vocal pain reaction, in this case, was not due to a general analgesia as the animal still reacted to the pain stimulus with flight.

Single-unit recording studies in the periaqueductal grey revealed vocalization-correlated activity changes in the cat [110], bat [111], squirrel monkey [112] and macaque (*Macaca fascicularis*, *M. nemestrina*) [113]. The responsive cells lie in the dorsal and lateral part of the caudal two thirds of this structure. The cells can be classified into 4 reaction types: (a) cells showing an increased activity immediately before, but not during vocalization; (b) cells showing an increased activity immediately before and during vocalization; (c) cells increasing their activity at or shortly after vocalization onset; (d) cells decreasing their activity during vocalization [114]. If a cross-correlation analysis of neuronal activity with laryngeal and respiratory electromyographic activity is carried out, cells are found the activity of which correlates with the activity of specific laryngeal adductor and/or abdominal expiratory muscles [114]. This points to a quite direct involvement of the periaqueductal grey in vocal motor control. On the other hand, a systematic search for cells reflecting in their activity changes in fundamental frequency has been unsuccessful [112]. Most of the cells found, do not even differentiate different call types (Fig. 7). In the squirrel monkey, furthermore, cells have been reported which are specifically active in the interval between a perceived vocalization (produced by a group mate) and the self-produced vocal response. In other words, there are periaqueductal neurones behaving like an audio–vocal interface [112] (Fig. 8). These observations suggest that the periaqueductal grey has a gating function rather than a pattern-generating function.

The periaqueductal grey receives input from a number of motivation-controlling limbic structures, such as the anterior cingulate cortex, septum, amygdala, nucleus of the stria terminalis, preoptic region, hypothalamus and midline thalamus [107,115–118]. It also receives direct input from various sensory structures, such as the superior

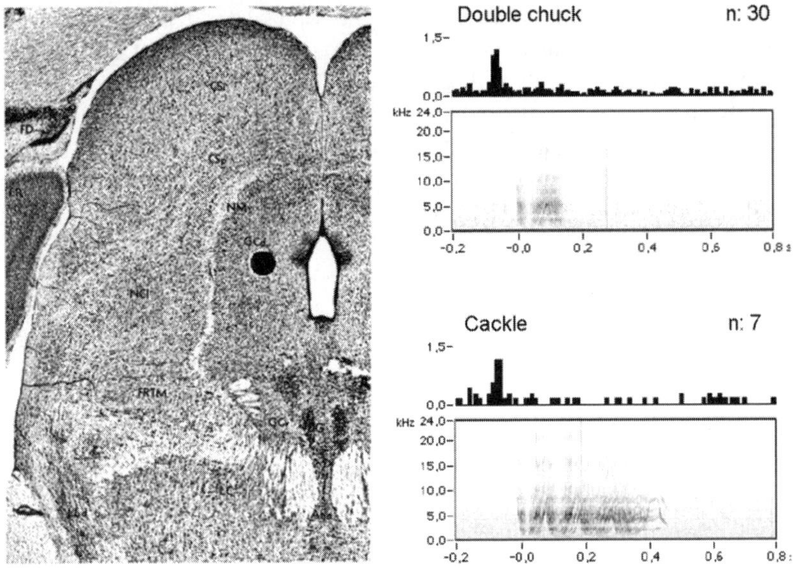

Fig. 7. Vocalization-related neuronal activity in the periaqueductal grey of the midbrain. Left: frontal section of the squirrel monkey's midbrain indicating the recording site (black circle). The section corresponds to the Horsley–Clarke plane AP1. Right: averaged neuronal activity (PETH) at the site indicated on the left during the production of two different call types ('double chuck', 'cackle'). Further explanation, see Fig. 5.

and inferior colliculi, spinal trigeminal and solitary tract nuclei, and dorsal horn of spinal cord [119–124]. This combined input could provide the periaqueductal grey with the necessary information to fulfill its gating function.

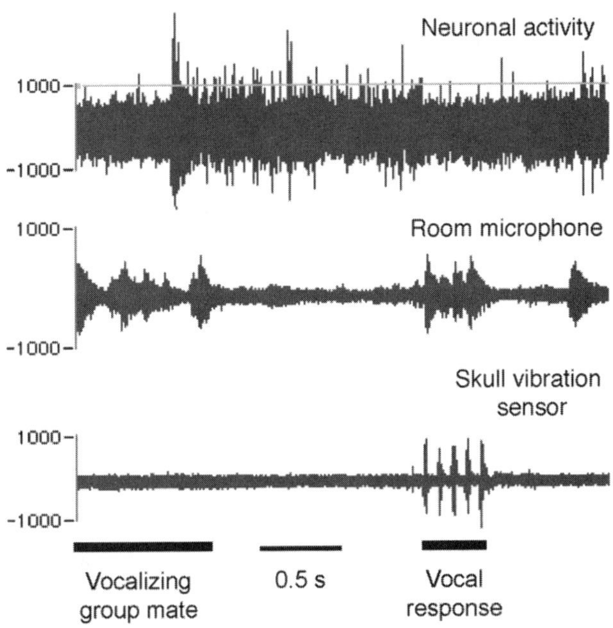

Fig. 8. Neuronal activity in the periaqueductal grey during audio–vocal interactions in the squirrel monkey. First trace shows the telemetrically recorded multi-unit activity. Second trace shows the output of the room microphone, displaying the vocal activity within the monkey group, including the experimental animal. Third trace shows the signal from the piezoceramic vibration sensor implanted on the skull of the experimental animal. This trace displays the vocal activity exclusively of the experimental animal. It can be seen that there is an increased neuronal activity in the interval between the vocalization uttered by a group mate and the vocal response of the experimental animal.

The output of the periaqueductal grey does not reach the phonatory motoneurone pools directly. Only in the case of the nucl. ambiguus, a weak projection has been found [55,121,125–129]. There are, however, numerous projections to structures which themselves project to the phonatory motor nuclei. Such structures are the lateral parabrachial area, parvocellular, gigantocellular and paragigantocellular reticular formation, nucl. reticularis dorsalis and ventralis, nucl. retroambiguus and solitary tract nucleus [127–131]. In a combined stimulation/lesioning study, the pathway via which the periaqueductal grey exerts its vocalization control was traced [107]. In this study, vocalization-eliciting electrodes were implanted into the periaqueductal grey, and lesions were placed in various parts of the lower brainstem. Lesions capable of blocking periaqueductally elicited vocalization could be followed from the caudolateral periaqueductal grey into the lateral tegmentum underneath the inferior colliculus. From here, the lesions descended along the medial edge of the lateral lemniscus into the ventrolateral pons and, from there, into the periambigual reticular formation.

3.3. *Lateral midbrain–pons transition*

Electrical stimulation along the vocal output pathway of the periaqueductal grey has been reported to produce vocalization in several species (see Ref. [90] for the bat, Ref. [132] for the cat, Ref. [70] for the squirrel monkey and Ref. [94] for the rhesus monkey). More specifically, species-specific calls cannot only be obtained by stimulation of the periaqueductal grey itself, but also of the dorsolateral midbrain tegmentum bordering the periaqueductal grey and the paralemniscal area between inferior colliculus and superior olive. Several observations suggest that the periaqueductal vocalization pathway does not only pass through these areas, but also synapses there. There are, for instance, sites along this pathway which produce vocalization not only when electrically stimulated, but also when injected with glutamate [70]. At the ventral end of the paralemniscal area, a site has been found in the squirrel monkey which when injected with a glutamate antagonist (kynurenic acid) blocks periaqueductally elicited vocalization [133]. Not all call types elicitable from the periaqueductal grey can be blocked, however; only calls showing a characteristic frequency modulation are affected. The effective blocking site is located in an area comprising the nucleus of the central acoustic tract in bats. Electrical as well as chemical stimulation of this nucleus with a glutamatergic agonist (kainic acid) produces vocalization [134]. Destruction of the nucleus abolishes the bat's capacity to adjust the pitch of the echolocation sounds in a way that the returning echo frequencies fall within the optimal hearing range (Doppler shift compensation) [134]. Furthermore, single-unit recordings in the bat have shown that there are numerous cells in the paralemniscal area just above the nucleus of the central acoustic tract, which are activated during and immediately before vocalization [135]. Electrical stimulation of this area produces echolocation sounds with lower threshold and shorter latency than stimulation in the periaqueductal grey [90]. It therefore, has been proposed that in the bat the paralemniscal area plays a similar role in vocalization control as does the periaqueductal grey in non-echolocating mammals [136].

Immediately caudal to the paralemniscal area, there is another area participating in vocal control: the ventrolateral parabrachial region (corresponding to the Kölliker–Fuse nucleus of rats,cats and dogs). Single-unit recording studies in the cat [137] and squirrel monkey [74] have revealed vocalization-correlated activity in this region. In the cat, 30% of the recorded cells increased their firing rate after vocalization onset, 15% showed an increased activity shortly before and during vocalization, 3% decreased their activity during vocalization [137]. Most of the vocalization-correlated cells also changed their activity in relation to quiet respiration. The majority increased its activity during expiration or in the late inspiratory phase. Glutamate injections into the ventrolateral parabrachial region have been reported to change the respiratory rhythm, causing either hyperpnea or deceleration of the respiratory cycle—depending upon the exact injection site [138]. Electrical stimulation with short pulse trains induces phase-switching from inspiration to expiration and from expiration to inspiration [139]. Prolonged stimulation elicits abdominal straining movements [140]. Destruction is followed by apneustic breathing [141]. Anatomically, the ventrolateral parabrachial region receives a heavy input from the solitary tract nucleus [65,142] and projects massively into the nucl. retroambiguus [143–145]. These findings suggest that the ventrolateral parabrachial region participates in the respiratory component of vocalization control. More specifically, it seems to be involved in the gating of vocal onset on the basis of the momentary respiratory status.

4. Cortical pathways

4.1. Mediofrontal cortex

The cortex within the interhemispheric fissure contains two areas that have been related to vocal behaviour: one is the anterior cingulate gyrus, the other the supplementary motor area (SMA). Both areas have been reported to produce vocalization when electrically stimulated. The SMA, however, has been found to produce vocalization only in humans, not in other mammals. The anterior cingulate gyrus, in contrast, produces vocalization in non-human mammals, such as the rhesus monkey, squirrel monkey, cat and bat, but not in humans [93,146–154]. As the vocalizations of monkeys, cats and bats are almost completely genetically determined in their acoustic structure, while the vast majority of human vocal utterances are more or less completely learned, the difference in cortical representation might reflect the different role motor learning plays in vocal behaviour of these species.

Bilateral destruction of the anterior cingulate gyrus in macaques abolishes the capacity to master a vocal operant conditioning task [155,156]. This means that the animals are no more able to increase vocalization rate for obtaining a food reward or postponing an electroshock in a Sidman avoidance task. The animals, however, still react vocally to unconditioned stimuli, such as grasping them. In the squirrel monkey, a bilateral destruction of the anterior cingulate and bordering subcallosal cortex has been reported to abolish spontaneously uttered long-distance contact calls in socially isolated animals. These animals, however, still produced long-distance contact calls in response to contact calls uttered by other conspecifics [157]. Lesions in the SMA do not affect spontaneous vocal behaviour in the squirrel monkey [158]. Lesions invading the pre-SMA, an area bordering the SMA rostrally, however, decrease the number of spontaneous vocalizations. This holds for the squirrel monkey as well as the rhesus monkey [158,159]. Vocal operant conditioning tasks are still mastered after pre-SMA lesions, but the vocalizations show a marked increase in the latency with which they are produced. In humans, bilateral lesions limited to the anterior cingulate gyrus or SMA, to the author's knowledge, have not been reported in the literature. Lesions invading anterior cingulate gyrus as well as SMA and/or pre-SMA usually are characterized in the beginning by an akinetic mutism which, after some time, changes into transcortical motor aphasia [160,161]. In this state, the patient has recovered the ability to produce well-articulated, grammatically correct sentences. There is a severe reduction in the number of speech utterances, however. Most of the utterances represent responses to questions of the partner; there are only very few spontaneous utterances. If the patient is asked to produce short sentences with different emotional intonations, the sentences are all spoken in the same monotonous manner [161].

Single-unit recording experiments in macaques have shown that about 7% of the neurones in the anterior cingulate gyrus change their activity during vocalization in a vocal operant conditioning task [162]. The activity preceded vocalization onset up to 1200 ms (average 303 ms). Vocalization-correlated activity in the anterior cingulate cortex was also found in a study in which field potentials were recorded in macaques [163]. In this study, it was found that only those vocalizations were associated with cingular activity that were produced as an operant response to obtain food reward. Vocalizations produced as a protest reaction to the withdrawal of food reward in the extinction phase were not associated with cingular activity [163]. Activity measurements in humans, using the positron emission tomography (PET) or functional magnetic resonance imaging (fMRI) techniques, show that the SMA is regularly activated during speech and singing [164–172]. This is not the case for the anterior cingulate gyrus which is activated only in few speech-related tasks [164,168]. The anterior cingulate gyrus, however, is regularly activated in non-vocal emotion-related tasks, such as the volitional imagination of emotional states [173–175]. These findings suggest that the anterior cingulate gyrus is involved in the volitional control of emotional states and that of innate motor patterns, while the SMA is involved in the volitional control of learned motor patterns. Both areas have in common that they control the initiation rather than the pattern generation of vocal utterances.

The periaqueductal grey is an obligatory relay station of the cingular vocalization-controlling pathway. If a glutamate antagonist (kynurenic acid) is injected into the periaqueductal grey, no vocalizations can be elicited anymore from the anterior cingulate gyrus [176]. If, in contrast, the anterior cingulate gyrus is inactivated, vocalizations can still be elicited from the periaqueductal grey. The course of the cingular vocalization-controlling pathway has been determined with a combined stimulation/lesioning technique [177]. The pathway enters the internal capsule at the level of the genu of the corpus callosum and follows this structure down to the caudal diencephalon. Here, the pathway leaves the cerebral peduncle dorsally and crosses the substantia nigra and rostral midbrain tegmentum to finally reach the periaqueductal grey. After having synapsed in this structure, the pathway continues into the lower brainstem along the route described earlier for the periaqueductal vocalization pathway. The periaqueductal grey does not seem to play a major role in the SMA's control of vocal behaviour as there is a complete lack of direct connections between these structures [178].

4.2. Motor cortex

One of the first structures that has been related to phonation control was the face area of the motor cortex. In primates, this area is located in the lateralmost part of the precentral gyrus, bordering the Sylvian fissure. Its electrical stimulation produces movements of the lips, jaw, tongue and vocal folds, with the lip representation farthest away from the Sylvian fissure and the tongue and vocal fold representation directly bordering it. The vocal folds are represented rostral to the tongue [179–184]. While movements of the lips, tongue and jaw have been obtained in all species tested, isolated movements of the vocal folds could be produced only in primates, including man [179–186].

Bilateral destruction of the facial motor cortex in humans causes pseudobulbar palsy, a syndrome characterized by a complete loss of voluntary control over the speech apparatus [187–190]. As a consequence, the patients are no more able to speak and sing. If the facial motor cortex is destroyed bilaterally in non-human primates, no significant effects are found in the production of species-specific calls [155,156,191,192]. This discrepancy in the effects of motorcortical lesions on the vocal communication of humans on the one hand and monkeys on the other is probably due to differences in the degree of innateness/learnedness of the two communication systems. Kaspar–Hauser studies in squirrel monkeys [193] as well as hybridisation studies in gibbons [194,195] and cross-fostering experiments in macaques [196] have made clear that monkeys do not need to learn their species-specific calls from conspecifics. In other words, the acoustic structure characterizing the different call types is genetically preprogrammed. Human speech and song, in contrast, represent learned motor patterns. Not all human utterances are learned, however. The crying of a newborn or the laughing of a congenitally deaf infant also have to rely on genetically preprogrammed motor commands [197]. It fits with the innateness/learnedness hypothesis that crying and laughing can still be produced by patients with pseudobulbar palsy [189,190]. On the other hand, if monkeys are trained a learned oral motor task, namely to press the protruded tongue with a definite pressure against a plate for 0.5 s, bilateral deactivation of the facial motor cortex causes a severe deterioration of performance [198]. These observations suggest (a) that monkey calls can be used as models for non-verbal emotional vocal utterances of humans, but not for speech and song; (b) that the motor cortex plays a crucial role in the control of learned vocal patterns, but is dispensable for the production of innate vocal patterns.

PET and fMRI studies have reported a bilateral activation in the motor cortex during speaking and singing [165,168,170–172,199–201]. Two activation foci have been found: one in the face area, representing the laryngeal and articulatory components of phonation; the other in the trunk area, representing the respiratory component. The fMRI technique, with its higher spatial resolution, even allows to discriminate the activation foci of different phonemes [201]. Magnetoencephalographic studies show that the activation in the facial motor cortex occurs 150 ms before vocalization onset and 60 ms before perioral electromyographic activity [202,203]. If immediately before vocalization onset (production of the vowel 'a'), a short transcranial magnetic stimulation pulse is delivered to the facial motor cortex, vocalization onset is delayed [204]. This effect is stronger on the left side, if the stimulus is delivered 50–100 ms before vocalization onset, and is stronger on the right side, if the stimulus is delivered 0–50 ms before vocalization onset. Simultaneous bilateral stimulation has a stronger effect than unilateral stimulation only if delivered 0–50 ms before vocalization onset. These findings suggest that the initial phase of vocal preparation is dominated by the left hemisphere, while the following phase is characterized by a more bilateral involvement. Apart from the preparatory phase, also the executive phase shows a hemispheric asymmetry. fMRI data indicate that the left facial motor cortex shows a stronger activation during speech, while the right is more activated during song [205,206]. This functional differentiation is supported by lesion data. While left-sided lesions in the region of the facial motor cortex affect speech to a much higher degree than song, the contrary holds for right-sided lesions [207–210]. Right-sided lesions, furthermore, have a more severe effect on the prosodial than the linguistic component of speech [209,211,212].

Hemispheric asymmetries do not only exist in humans. If the squirrel monkey's vocal fold area in the motor cortex is stimulated during ongoing vocalization, a more or less pronounced change in the acoustic structure occurs. The magnitude of change depends upon the side of stimulation. In 40% of the animals, the left side produces the larger effect; in another 40%, the right side is more effective; the remaining 20% do not show an asymmetry [213]. As it is still unclear whether the squirrel monkey's vocal fold area is involved in vocal behaviour at all or rather serves non-vocal functions, such as abdominal straining or stabilization of the thorax during forceful pulling or jumping, the question remains open of whether the asymmetry is a truly vocal one or not.

4.3. Pyramidal and extrapyramidal pathways

Direct connections between the motor cortex and the phonatory motor nuclei have been found only in primates, not in other mammals [214–221]. Direct connections with the nucl. ambiguus seem to exist only in humans [222–224]. The cortico-motoneuronal projections are bilateral, with a contralateral dominance. The projection fibres run through the corona radiata, enter the internal capsule at a level somewhat rostral to the anterior commissure and descend within the ipsilateral internal capsule and cerebral peduncle down to the pontine and medullary level. Here, the fibres leave the pyramidal tract dorsally. The major part crosses to the contralateral side. Ipsilateral and contralateral fibres traverse the ventromedial pontine and medullary reticular formation to finally reach the trigeminal motor, facial and hypoglossal nuclei, and, in the case of humans, also the nucl. ambiguus. In humans, furthermore, direct projections into the anterior horn of the thoracic and upper lumbar cord have been found [223]. In non-primate mammals, the motor cortex is connected with the phonatory motor nuclei via interneurones in the reticular formation [215,219,225]. Such interneurones are found in the supra- and inter-trigeminal nuclei, the parvocellular reticular formation and the dorsal reticular nucleus. These areas receive a direct input from the facial motor cortex via the corticobulbar tract. The indirect projection is not only found in non-primate mammals, but in primates as well. Obviously, this indirect connection is the phylogenetically older pathway. The course of the indirect pathway through forebrain and brainstem is identical with the direct cortico-motoneuronal pathway, except for the fact that the fibres do not end in the motor nuclei, but in the reticular formation close by. A combined interruption of the direct and indirect cortico-motoneuronal pathways has a similar effect as motor-cortex lesions [226–228].

The facial motor cortex and the phonatory motor nuclei are not only interconnected via the corticobulbar and corticospinal tracts, respectively, but also a number of extra-pyramidal tracts. Neuroanatomical studies show that there is a massive projection of the facial motor cortex into the ventral putamen at about the level of the anterior commissure [222,229], The ventral putamen projects into the dorsolateral substantia nigra pars reticulata which, in turn, projects to the parvocellular reticular formation, an area directly connected with the phonatory motoneurones [230]. Lesions in the putamen have been reported in the neurological literature to cause dysarthria and dysphonia [231–233]. PET and fMRI studies have revealed a speech-related activity in the putamen [166,167,170,234]. With respect to the substantia nigra, neurones have been identified in its dorsolateral part which are specifically active during oral movements [235,236]. Furthermore, Parkinson patients with their characteristic loss of substantia nigra cells and resulting decrease of dopaminergic input into, among others, the putamen, also show speech affection. The deficit is characterized by a reduction in volume and articulatory distinctness [237,238]. The parvocellular reticular formation, finally, has been shown (Section 3.1) to be a crucial structure for vocal production. These observations suggest that the pathway running from the facial motor cortex via putamen and substantia nigra to the parvocellular reticular formation is involved in speech control.

Anatomically, three additional extrapyramidal pathways have been described from the facial motor cortex. One connects the facial motor cortex directly with the dorsolateral substantia nigra, pars reticulata and then continues into the parvocellular reticular formation [219]. A second runs from the facial motor cortex to the deep layers of the

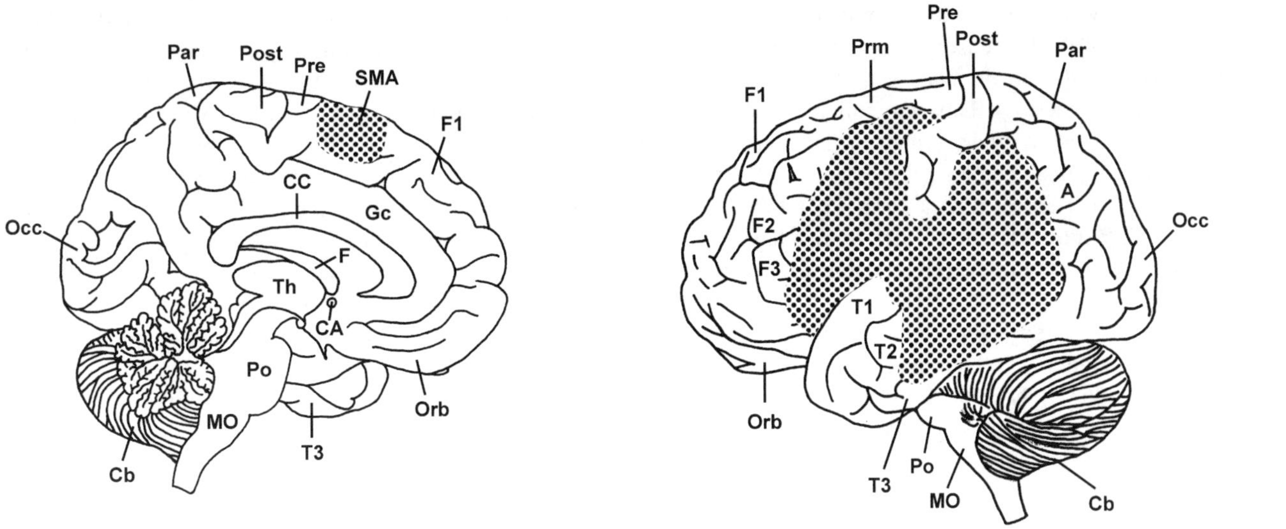

Fig. 9. Regions of the human cortex which, when electrically stimulated, interfere with normal speech production (drawing based on data from Ref. [257]). Left: medial view; right: lateral view. Abbreviations: A, gyrus angularis; Cb, cerebellum; F1, gyrus frontalis superior; F2, gyrus frontalis medius; F3, gyrus frontalis inferior; MO, medulla oblongata; Occ, occipital cortex; Orb, orbital cortex; Par, parietal cortex; Po, pons; Post, gyrus postcentralis; Pre, gyrus praecentralis; Prm, premotor cortex; SMA, supplementary motor area; T1, gyrus temporalis superior; T2, gyrus temporalis medius; T3, gyrus temporalis inferior.

lateralmost superior colliculus and from there to the parvocellular reticular formation [219,239,240]. A third can be followed from the facial motor cortex via the dorsal nucl. ruber to the parvocellular reticular formation [241–243]. Finally, there are connections between these pathways, in the form of direct projections from the dorsolateral substantia nigra into the dorsal nucl. ruber and the lateral superior colliculus [239,241]. Whether one or more of these pathways take part in speech production is still unclear.

4.4. Cerebello-thalamo-cortical pathway

One of the main input structures of the motor cortex is the ventrolateral thalamus; and one of the main input structures of the ventrolateral thalamus is the cerebellum. Lesions in the ventrolateral thalamus and cerebellum severely affect speech production. In the case of ventrolateral thalamus, the voice becomes breathy and monotonous; in articulation, the distinction between voiced and unvoiced phonemes is lost; the fundamental frequency is raised and shows an increased jitter [244–247]. Cerebellar lesions are characterized by irregular changes in fundamental frequency and intensity, explosive voice onset, scanning speech rhythm and slowed speech tempo [248–250]. The severest effects are found after lesions in the paramedian portions of the posterior lobe and in the middle part of the vermis. PET and fMRI studies have reported speech- and song-related activity in the ventrolateral thalamus as well as the cerebellum [165–167,169–172]. The activity is bilateral in both structures. In the cerebellum, two foci have been reported: one in the vermis and one in the lobulus VIa of the lateral hemisphere. Lobulus VI–VII has been reported in another fMRI study to contain the tongue representation [251]. The cerebellar cortex projects to the ventrolateral thalamus via the nuclei dentatus and interpositus [252]. In the ventrolateral thalamus, the facial muscles are represented medial to the upper extremities, trunk and lower extremities [253]. Accordingly, many neurones are found in the medial part of the ventrolateral thalamus which increase their activity during vocalization [254]. The number of neurones reacting to somatosensory stimuli in the mouth region decreases from caudal to rostral parts of the ventrolateral thalamus, while the number of cells being activated exclusively during active movements increases from caudal to rostral [253]. It fits with this distribution that in the rostral part of the ventrolateral thalamus, there is a larger number of cells becoming active already before vocalization onset [254]. The ventrolateral thalamus does not only project to the primary motor cortex, but also to the Broca area and supplementary motor area [255,256]. All four areas have been found to produce vocalization when electrically stimulated in man [151,247,257].

In the macaque, cerebellar lesions have only mild effects on vocalization [163,258]. The characteristic acoustic structure of the species-specific calls remains intact [259]. Cerebellar lesions, however, have been reported to abolish the vocalization-correlated field potentials in the motor cortex of macaques [163].

4.5. Ascending somatosensory pathway

Proprioceptive and tactile information from the larynx and articulatory organs, after having been relayed in the solitary tract nucleus, spinal and principal trigeminal nuclei, is transmitted via the parabrachial area to the nucl. ventralis posterior medialis of the thalamus, and from there to the primary and secondary somatosensory cortices [65,130,260–264]. The sensory trigeminal nuclei are also directly connected with the nucl. ventralis posterior medialis. Direct connections between solitary tract nucleus and thalamus exist only in primates. There is evidence from the neurological literature that lesions in the primary somatosensory cortex cause dysarthria, i.e. articulatory disturbances [265,266]. PET and fMRI studies have reported speech-related activity in the primary somatosensory cortex [165,168,172,201].

Vocalization-related activity also has been found in the form of field potentials in the primary somatosensory cortex of macaques [267]. These field potentials preceded vocalization onset by ca. 700 ms. In contrast to the field potentials recorded from the primary motor cortex, the field potentials from the primary somatosensory cortex could not be abolished by cerebellar lesions [163]. Bilateral destruction of the primary somatosensory cortex in the squirrel monkey does not affect the acoustic structure of species-specific calls significantly [268]. The same holds for the nucl. ventralis posterior medialis [268]. Electrical stimulation of the latter during ongoing vocalization, however, causes small, but distinct, changes in acoustic structure [71]. Single-unit recordings in the nucl. ventralis posterior medialis of humans revealed speech-related activity [269]. The same cells that were activated by speech, also were activated by touching the tongue or lips. The nucl. ventralis posterior medialis receives input from both sides of the face. Input from the ipsilateral side is relayed in the ventral part of the nucleus, input from the contralateral side in the dorsal part [260].

4.6. Further speech-related cortical areas

PET and fMRI studies have made clear that the sensorimotor cortex together with the supplementary motor area and anterior cingulate gyrus are not the only cortical areas being active during speech and song. Depending upon the specific vocal task, the number and type of additionally activated areas vary. If the task is simply to pronounce sequences of meaningless phonemes, there is, apart from the sensorimotor cortex and supplementary motor area, an activation of the insula and auditory cortex [172]. The auditory cortex is activated by the auditory feedback of the produced sounds. It is also activated during passive listening to an external sound [171]. Bilateral destruction of the auditory cortex causes the syndrome of cortical deafness in humans, a marked increase in auditory threshold in non-human primates and a negligible increase in auditory threshold in other mammals [270–277]. The role of the insula in vocal behaviour is less clear. The insula is activated during loud speaking as well as singing, but remains inactive during silent speaking and singing [165,206]. In contrast to the auditory cortex, it is not activated by listening to speech or tone sequences [278]. Lesions in the insula cause speech apraxia [279]. This syndrome is characterized by articulatory disturbances which cannot be explained by a paralysis of the articulatory muscles (as is the case after motor cortex lesions) nor by word-finding problems (as they occur in aphasic disorders). Habib et al. [280] have proposed that the insula plays a mediating role between auditory input, speech output and communicative motivation. Their conclusion is based on the anatomical fact that the insula is directly connected with the facial sensorimotor cortex, Broca area, primary and secondary auditory cortex as well as several limbic structures, such as the anterior cingulate gyrus, orbital cortex and amygdala.

If the task is not to repeat meaningless phonemes but words, there is, in addition, an activation of the posterior part of the superior and middle temporal gyri [165,168, 172,200]. This region which represents auditory association cortex is also activated by passive listening to words or speech [168,200,278,281]. The difference between the fMRI activation during listening to speech and that during listening to meaningless sounds is also greatest in this region [278]. This suggests that the posterior upper temporal cortex is involved in attributing significance to sounds. This fits with lesion studies. Bilateral destruction of the auditory association cortex in humans produces auditory agnosia, that is, an inability to identify sounds with only minor deficits in auditory threshold [271,282, 283]. Left-sided lesions, depending on the exact lesion site, cause sensory (Wernicke) aphasia or word deafness, that is, an inability to understand speech with retained ability to read; right-sided lesions cause sensory amusia or aprosodia, that is, an impairment to recognize melodies, emotional intonations and complex non-verbal acoustic stimuli [284–288].

If the task is not to name an acoustical stimulus or to repeat a word presented by ear, but to name a visually presented object or to read a word, additional activation is found in the visual cortex (areas 17, 18 and 19) and the visual association cortex (areas 20, 21, 37 and 39) [166,200].

Whenever a spoken utterance does not only consist of a short simple word, but of a longer sequence of syllables or words, there is in addition to the activation of the sensorimotor cortex, supplementary motor area, insula and temporal cortex, an activation of the inferior parietal cortex (including the parietal operculum) and the posterior part of the inferior frontal gyrus [168–170,202]. The latter has been associated with speech control since the early lesion studies of Paul Broca (1861). More recent studies have made clear that lesions restricted to the posterior part of the inferior frontal gyrus (areas 44 and 45 = Broca area) do not cause Broca's aphasia for more than a few days [289–295]. Persistent Broca aphasia is only obtained, if the lesions invade, in addition, bordering structures, such as the facial motor cortex, fronto-opercular cortex, insula, white matter underneath the cortex (capsula extrema and externa) or putamen. There is general agreement, however,

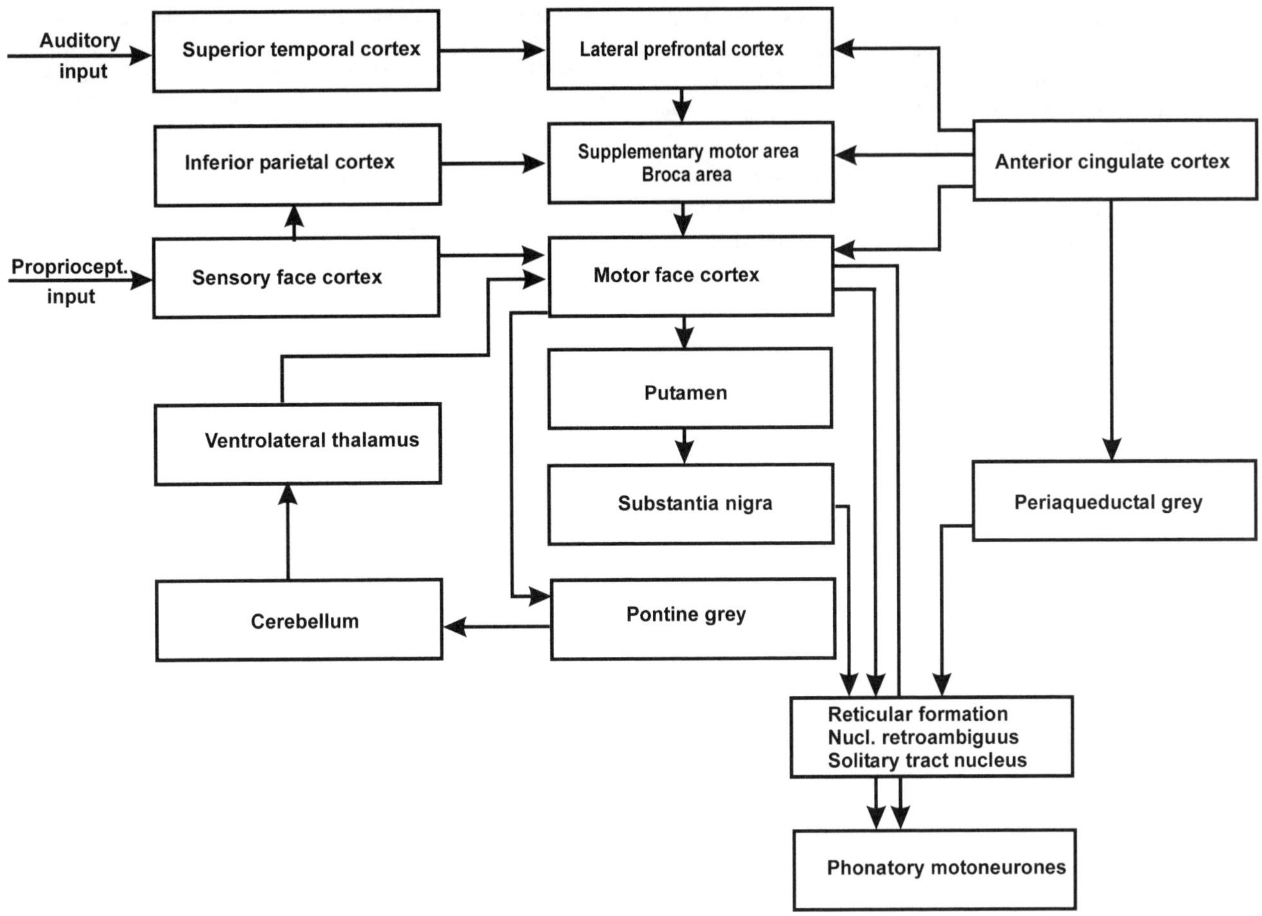

Fig. 10. Circuit diagram summarizing the most important structures for which there is evidence from lesion, stimulation, single-unit recording and brain imaging studies that they are involved in speech production. The arrows indicate anatomically verified direct connections. If there is more than one structure in a box, the arrows relate to at least one, but not necessarily all structures. The structures within a box are directly connected with each other.

that lesions in Broca's area cause a persistent reduction in verbal fluency. This points to a motor planning function of this area. PET studies have demonstrated that Broca's area is not only active during production of speech, but also during listening to speech [167,281]. It is in harmony with this finding that lesions in Broca's area often are associated with more or less pronounced deficits in speech comprehension [290].

Lesions in the inferior parietal cortex also have been reported to affect speech. The typical errors occurring after such lesions are phonemic substitutions (paraphasia) and neologisms (production of new words by combining parts of two or more non-congruent words) [296]. Electrical stimulation of the inferior parietal cortex during ongoing speech interrupts speech or causes phonemic errors [257] (Fig. 9). These observations suggest that the inferior parietal cortex is involved in the word formation process. Its task seems to be to transform the word representations stored in the Wernicke area by aid of proprioceptive feedback information from the articulatory organs into a form that can be used by the motor cortex to generate the verbal motor patterns.

Finally, if the task is not only to repeat a word or name an object, but to use language in a more complex way, such as generating as many words as possible beginning with a given letter or associating an appropriate verb to a given noun, additional activations are found in the prefrontal cortex, especially in its ventrolateral part [164,297–301].

5. Conclusion

The central control of vocal behaviour is hierarchically organized (Fig. 10). The lowest level is represented by a neural network consisting of essentially the parvocellular and dorsal medullary reticular formation, nucl. retroambiguus and solitary tract nucleus. This network serves to integrate laryngeal, respiratory and articulatory activity. In the case of innate vocal patterns, it also seems to be involved in pattern generation. The network has direct access to the phonatory motoneurones. Its input is of two different kinds: one input serves motor coordination of learned vocal patterns. This input comes from the motor cortex and basal ganglia via the pyramidal and extrapyramidal pathways. The other input controls the release of vocal patterns, that is, it has a gating function. This input comes from the periaqueductal grey and anterior cingulate cortex, with both structures representing different levels of gating control. The anterior cingulate cortex is involved in voluntary initiation and suppression of vocal utterances, while the periaqueductal grey exerts a more basic gating function, relating to voluntary as well as unconditioned vocal reactions. Future studies will have to clarify on the one hand, in which way pattern generation of innate as well as learned vocal utterances takes place in detail. On the other hand, more knowledge is needed on the processes underlying vocal gating, that is, the way in which vocalization/speech-eliciting external and internal (motivational) stimuli are coupled to the motor-coordinating mechanism.

References

[1] Payne K, Payne R. Large scale changes over 19 years in songs of humpback whales in Bermuda. Z Tierpsychol 1985;68:89–114.

[2] Zhang SP, Davis PJ, Bandler R, Carrive P. Brain stem integration of vocalization: role of the midbrain periaqueductal gray. J Neurophysiol 1994;72:1337–56.

[3] Hiroto I, Hirano M, Toyozumi Y, Shin T. Electromyographic investigation of the intrinsic laryngeal muscles related to speech sounds. Ann Otol Rhinol Laryngol 1967;76:861–72.

[4] Stone RE, Nuttall AL. Relative movements of the thyroid and cricoid cartilages assessed by neural stimulation in dogs. Acta Otolaryng 1974;78:135–40.

[5] Yoshida Y, Tanaka Y, Saito T, Shimazaki T, Hirano M. Peripheral nervous system in the larynx. An anatomical study on the motor, sensory and autonomic nerve fibers. Folia Phoniatr 1992;44:194–219.

[6] Gauthier P, Barillot JC, Dussardier M. Mise en évidence électrophysiologique de bifurcations d'axone dans le nerf recurrent laryngé. J Physiol 1980;76:39–48.

[7] Roubeau B, Chevrie-Muller C, Saint Guily JL. Electromyographic activity of strap and cricothyroid muscles in pitch change. Acta Oto-Laryngol 1997;117:459–64.

[8] Hirano M, Koike Y, von Leden H. The sternohyoid muscle during phonation. Acta Oto-Laryngol 1967;64:500–7.

[9] Ohala J, Hirose H. The function of the sternohyoid muscle in speech. Res Inst Logoped Phoniatr, Ann Bull 1970;4:41–4.

[10] Ueyama T, Satoda T, Tashiro T, Mizuno N. The distribution of infrahyoid motoneurons in the cat: a retrograde horseradish peroxidase study. Anat Embryol 1988;177:445–50.

[11] Kirzinger A, Jürgens U. Motoneuronal location of external laryngeal and hyoid muscles involved in primate phonation. J Brain Res 1994;35:559–65.

[12] Jürgens U, Schriever S. Respiratory muscle activity during vocalization in the squirrel monkey. Folia Primatol 1991;56:121–32.

[13] Draper MH, Ladefoged P, Whitteridge D. Respiratory muscles in speech. J Speech Hear Res 1959;2:16–27.

[14] Newsom Davis J, Sears TA. The proprioceptive reflex control of the intercostal muscles during their voluntary activation. J Physiol 1970;209:711–38.

[15] Estenne M, Zocchi L, Warl M, Macklem PT. Chest wall motion and expiratory muscle use during phonation in normal humans. J Appl Physiol 1990;68:2075–82.

[16] Sakamoto H, Akita K, Sato T. An anatomical analysis of the relationships between the intercostal nerves and the thoracic and abdominal muscles in man. Acta Anat 1996;156:132–50.

[17] Schriever S, Jürgens U. Location of respiratory motoneurons involved in phonation. An HRP study in the squirrel monkey. J Hirnforsch 1989;30:521–7.

[18] Miller AD. Localization of motoneurons innervating individual abdominal muscles of the cat. J Comp Neurol 1987;256:600–6.

[19] Holstege G, van Neerven J, Evertse F. Spinal cord location of the motoneurons innervating the abdominal, cutaneous maximus, latissimus dorsi and longissimus dorsi muscles in the cat. Exp Brain Res 1987;67:179–94.

[20] Hoshiko M. Electromyographic investigation of the intercostal muscles during speech. Arch Phys Med Rehabil 1962;43:115–9.

[21] Wilson TA, Legrand A, Gevenois PA, De Troyer A. Respiratory effects of the external and internal intercostal muscles in humans. J Physiol 2001;530:319–30.

[22] De Troyer A, Ninane V, Gilmartin JJ, Lemerre C, Estenne M. Triangularis sterni muscle use in supine humans. J Appl Physiol 1987; 62:919–25.

[23] Leanderson R, Persson A, Öhman S. Electromyographic studies of facial muscle activity in speech. Acta Otolaryng 1971;72:361–9.

[24] Shipp T. Vertical laryngeal position during continuous and discrete vocal frequency change. J Speech Hear Res 1975;18:707–18.

[25] Welt C, Abbs JH. Musculotopic organization of the facial motor nucleus in *Macaca fascicularis*: a morphometric and retrograde tracing study with cholera toxin B-HRP. J Comp Neurol 1990; 291:621–36.

[26] Tuller B, Harris KS, Gross B. Electromyographic study of the jaw muscles during speech. Haskins Lab Status Report Speech Res 1979;56:83–102.

[27] Mizuno N, Matsuda K, Iwahori N, Uemura-Sumi M, Kume M, Matsushima R. Representation of the masticatory muscles in the motor trigeminal nucleus of the macaque monkey. Neurosci Lett 1981;21:19–22.

[28] Matsuda K, Uemura M, Takeuchi Y, Kume M, Matsushima R, Mizuno N. Localization of motoneurons innervating the posterior belly of the digastric muscle: a comparative anatomical study by the HRP method. Neurosci Lett 1979;12:47–52.

[29] Lubker JF. Normal velopharyngeal function in speech. Clin Plast Surg 1975;2:249–59.

[30] Strutz J, Hammerich T, Amedee R. The motor innervation of the soft palate. An anatomical study in guinea pigs and monkeys. Arch Otorhinolaryngol 1988;245:180–4.

[31] Furusawa K, Yamaoka M, Kogo M, Matsuya T. The innervation of the levator veli palatini muscle by the glossopharyngeal nerve. Brain Res Bull 1991;26:599–604.

[32] Duchin LE. The evolution of articulate speech: comparative anatomy of the oral cavity in Pan and Homo. J Human Evol 1990; 19:687–97.

[33] Uemura-Sumi M, Mizuno N, Nomura S, Iwahori N, Takeuchi Y, Matsushima R. Topographical representation of the hypoglossal nerve branches and tongue muscles in the hypoglossal nucleus of macaque monkeys. Neurosci Lett 1981;22:31–5.

[34] Adzaku FK, Wyke B. Innervation of the subglottic mucosa of the larynx, and its significance. Folia Phoniatr 1979;31:271–83.

[35] Davis PJ, Nail BS. Quantitative analysis of laryngeal mechanosensitivity in the cat and rabbit. J Physiol 1987;388:467–85.

[36] Wyke B. Deus ex machina vocis. An analysis of the laryngeal reflex mechanisms of speech. Br J Dis Communic 1969;4:3–25.

[37] Clark KF, Farber JP. Recording from afferents in the intact recurrent laryngeal nerve during respiration and vocalization. Ann Otol Rhinol Laryngol 1998;107:753–60.

[38] Shiba K, Yoshida K, Miura T. Functional roles of the superior laryngeal nerve afferents in electrically induced vocalization in anesthetized cats. Neurosci Res 1995;22:23–30.

[39] Thoms G, Jürgens U. Role of the internal laryngeal nerve in phonation: an experimental study in the squirrel monkey. Exp Neurol 1981;74:187–203.

[40] Altschuler SM, Bao X, Bieger D, Hopkins DA, Miselis RR. Viscerotopic representation of the upper alimentary tract in the rat: sensory

ganglia and nuclei of the solitary and spinal trigeminal tracts. J Comp Neurol 1989;283:248–68.

[41] Patrickson JW, Smith TE, Zhou S-S. Afferent projections of the superior and recurrent laryngeal nerves. Brain Res 1991;539:169–74.

[42] Hayakawa T, Takanaga A, Maeda S, Seki M, Yajima Y. Subnuclear distribution of afferents from the oral, pharyngeal and laryngeal regions in the nucleus tractus solitarii of the rat: a study using transganglionic transport of cholera toxin. Neurosci Res 2001; 39:221–32.

[43] Travers SP, Norgren R. Organization of orosensory responses in the nucleus of the solitary tract of the rat. J Neurophysiol 1995;73: 2144–62.

[44] Nakazawa K, Shiba K, Satoh I, Yoshida K, Nakajima Y, Konno A. Role of pulmonary afferent inputs in vocal on-switch in the cat. Neurosci Res 1997;29:49–54.

[45] Kalia M, Richter D. Morphology of physiologically identified slowly adapting lung stretch receptor afferents stained with intra-axonal horseradish peroxidase in the nucleus of the tractus solitarius of the cat. I. A light microscopic analysis. J Comp Neurol 1985;241: 503–20.

[46] Kalia M, Mesulam M-M. Brainstem projections of sensory and motor components of the vagus complex in the cat. J Comp Neurol 1980;193:435–508.

[47] Scott CM, Ringel RL. Articulation without oral sensory control. J Speech Hear Res 1971;14:804–18.

[48] Putnam AHB, Ringel RL. Some observations of articulation during labial sensory deprivation. J Speech Hear Res 1972;15:529–42.

[49] Prosek RA, House AS. Intraoral air pressure as a feedback cue in consonant production. J Speech Hear Res 1975;18:133–47.

[50] Segade LAG, Quintanilla JS, Cobos AR. Contralateral projections of trigeminal mandibular primary afferents in the guinea pig as seen by transganglionic transport of horseradish peroxidase. Brain Res 1990;506:267–80.

[51] Takeuchi Y, Hayakawa T, Ozaki HS, Kito J, Satoda T, Matsushima R. Afferent fibers in the hypoglossal nerve: a horseradish peroxidase study in the cat. Brain Res Bull 1990;24:81–7.

[52] Shigenaga Y, Chen IC, Suemune S, Nishimori T, Nasution ID, Yoshida A, Sato H, Okamoto T, Sera M, Hosoi M. Oral and facial representation within the medullary and upper cervical dorsal horns in the cat. J Comp Neurol 1986;243:388–408.

[53] Marfurt CF, Rajchert DM. Trigeminal primary afferent projections to non-trigeminal areas of the rat central nervous system. J Comp Neurol 1991;303:489–511.

[54] Cunningham ET, Sawchenko PE. Dorsal medullary pathways subserving oromotor reflexes in the rat: implications for the central neural control of swallowing. J Comp Neurol 2000;417:448–66.

[55] Thoms G, Jürgens U. Common input of the cranial motor nuclei involved in phonation in squirrel monkey. Exp Neurol 1987;95: 85–99.

[56] Manaker S, Tischler LJ, Bigler TL, Morrison AR. Neurons of the motor trigeminal nucleus project to the hypoglossal nucleus in the rat. Exp Brain Res 1992;90:262–70.

[57] Miller AD, Tan LK, Lakos SF. Brainstem projections to cats' upper lumbar spinal cord: implications for abdominal muscle control. Brain Res 1989;493:348–56.

[58] Kolta A, Westberg K-G, Lund JP. Identification of brainstem interneurons projecting to the trigeminal motor nucleus and adjacent structures in the rabbit. J Chem Neuroanat 2000;19:175–95.

[59] Li YQ, Takada M, Kaneko T, Mizuno N. GABAergic and glycinergic neurons projecting to the trigeminal motor nucleus: a double labeling study in the rat. J Comp Neurol 1996;373:498–510.

[60] Li YQ, Takada M, Kaneko T, Mizuno N. Distribution of GABAergic and glycinergic premotor neurons projecting to the facial and hypoglossal nuclei in the rat. J Comp Neurol 1997;378:283–94.

[61] Sahara Y, Hashimoto N, Nakamura Y. Hypoglossal premotor neurons in the rostral medullary parvocellular reticular formation participate in cortically-induced rhythmical tongue movements. Neurosci Res 1996;26:119–31.

[62] Takada M, Itoh K, Yasui Y, Mitani A, Nomura S, Mizuno N. Distribution of premotor neurons for the hypoglossal nucleus in the cat. Neurosci Lett 1984;52:141–6.

[63] Li YQ, Takada M, Mizuno N. Identification of premotor interneurons which project bilaterally to the trigeminal motor, facial or hypoglossal nuclei. A fluorescent retrograde double-labeling study in the rat. Brain Res 1993;611:160–4.

[64] Li YQ, Takada M, Mizuno N. Premotor neurons projecting simultaneously to orofacial motor nuclei by sending their branched axons. A study with a fluorescent retrograde double-labeling technique in the rat. Neurosci Lett 1993;152:29–32.

[65] Ezure K, Tanaka I, Miyazaki M. Pontine projections of pulmonary slowly adapting receptor relay neurons in the cat. Neuroreport 1998;9:411–4.

[66] Beckstead RM, Morse JR, Norgren R. The nucleus of solitary tract in the monkey: projections to the thalamus and brain stem nuclei. J Comp Neurol 1980;190:259–82.

[67] Fort P, Luppi PH, Jouvet M. Afferents to the nucleus reticularis parvicellularis of the cat medulla oblongata: a tract-tracing study with cholera toxin B unit. J Comp Neurol 1994;342:603–18.

[68] Slugg RM, Light AR. Spinal cord and trigeminal projections to the pontine parabrachial region in the rat as demonstrated with Phaseolus-vulgaris leucoagglutinin. J Comp Neurol 1994;339:49–61.

[69] Ezure K, Oku Y, Tanaka I. Location and axonal projection of one type of swallowing interneurons in cat medulla. Brain Res 1993;632: 216–24.

[70] Jürgens U, Richter K. Glutamate-induced vocalization in the squirrel monkey. Brain Res 1986;373:349–58.

[71] Dressnandt J, Jürgens U. Brain stimulation-induced changes of phonation in the squirrel monkey. Exp Brain Res 1992;89:549–59.

[72] Kirzinger A, Jürgens U. The effects of brain stem lesions on vocalization in the squirrel monkey. Brain Res 1985;358:150–62.

[73] Lüthe L, Häusler U, Jürgens U. Neuronal activity in the medulla oblongata during vocalization. A single-unit recording study in the squirrel monkey. Behav Brain Res 2000;116:197–210.

[74] Kirzinger A, Jürgens U. Vocalization-correlated single-unit activity in the brain stem of the squirrel monkey. Exp Brain Res 1991; 84:545–60.

[75] Ellenberger HH, Feldman JL. Brainstem connections of the rostral ventral respiratory group of the rat. Brain Res 1990;513:35–42.

[76] Hardy SGP, Horecky JG, Presley KG. Projections of the caudal medulla to the thoracic spinal cord in the rat. Anat Rec 1998;250: 95–102.

[77] Billig I, Foris JM, Card JP, Yates BJ. Transneuronal tracing of neuronal pathways controlling an abdominal muscle, rectus abdominis, in the ferret. Brain Res 1999;820:31–44.

[78] Puskar Z, Antal M. Localization of last-order premotor interneurons in the lumbar spinal cord of rats. J Comp Neurol 1997;389:377–89.

[79] Miller AD, Ezure K, Suzuki I. Control of abdominal muscles of brain stem respiratory neurons in the cat. J Neurophysiol 1985;54: 155–67.

[80] Lipski J, Merrill EG. Inputs to intercostal motoneurones from ventrolateral medullary respiratory neurones in Nembutal-anaesthetized cats. J Physiol 1983:25P–6P.

[81] Katada A, Sugimoto T, Utsumi K, Nonaka S, Sakamoto T. Functional role of ventral respiratory group expiratory neurons during vocalization. Neurosci Res 1996;26:225–33.

[82] Shiba K, Umezaki T, Zheng Y, Miller AD. The nucleus retroambigualis controls laryngeal muscle activity during vocalization in the cat. Exp Brain Res 1997;115:513–9.

[83] Zhang SP, Bandler R, Davis PJ. Brain stem integration of vocalization: role of the nucleus retroambigualis. J Neurophysiol 1995;74: 2500–12.

[84] Holstege G. Anatomical study of the final common pathway for vocalization in the cat. J Comp Neurol 1989;284:242–52.

[85] Waldbillig RJ. Attack, eating, drinking, and gnawing elicited by electrical stimulation of rat mesencephalon and pons. J Comp Physiol Psychol 1975;89:200–12.
[86] Yajima Y, Hayashi Y, Yoshii N. The midbrain central gray substance as a highly sensitive neural structure for the production of ultrasonic vocalization in the rat. Brain Res 1980;198:446–52.
[87] Martin JR. Motivated behaviors elicited from hypothalamus, midbrain, and pons of the guinea pig (*Cavia porcellus*). J Comp Physiol Psychol 1976;90:1011–34.
[88] Panksepp J, Normansell L, Herman B, Bishop P, Crepean L. Neural and neurochemical control of the separation distress call. In: Newman JD, editor. The physiological control of mammalian vocalization, New York: Plenum Press, 1988. p. 263–99.
[89] Kyuhou S-I, Gemba H. Two vocalization-related subregions in the midbrain periaqueductal gray of the guinea pig. Neuroreport 1998; 9:1607–10.
[90] Schuller G, Radtke-Schuller S. Neural control of vocalization in bats: mapping of brainstem areas with electrical microstimulation eliciting species-specific echolocation calls in the rufous horseshoe bat. Exp Brain Res 1990;79:192–206.
[91] Suga N, Schlegel P, Shimozawa T, Simmons J. Orientation sounds evoked from echolocating bats by electrical stimulation of the brain. J Acoust Soc Am 1973;54:793–7.
[92] Hunsperger RW. Affektreaktionen auf elektrische Reizung im Hirnstamm der Katze. Helv Physiol Pharmacol Acta 1956;14:70–92.
[93] Jürgens U, Ploog D. Cerebral representation of vocalization in the squirrel monkey. Exp Brain Res 1970;10:532–54.
[94] Magoun HW, Atlas D, Ingersoll EH, Ranson SW. Associated facial, vocal and respiratory components of emotional expression: an experimental study. J Neurol Psychopath 1937;17:241–55.
[95] Apfelbach R. Electrically elicited vocalizations in the gibbon *Hylobates lar* (Hylobatidae), and their behavioral significance. Z Tierpsychol 1972;30:420–30.
[96] Brown TG. Note on physiology of basal ganglia and midbrain of anthropoid ape especially in reference to act of laughter. J Physiol 1915;49:195–207.
[97] Sem-Jacobsen C, Torkildsen A. Depth recording and electrical stimulation in the human brain. In: Ramey ER, O'Doherty DS, editors. Electrical studies on the unanesthetized brain, New York: Paul B. Hoeber, 1960. p. 275–87.
[98] Bandler R, Carrive P. Integrated defence reaction elicited by excitatory amino acid microinjection in the midbrain periaqueductal grey region of the unrestrained cat. Brain Res 1988;439:95–106.
[99] Lu C-L, Jürgens U. Effects of chemical stimulation in the periaqueductal gray on vocalization in the squirrel monkey. Brain Res Bull 1993;32:143–51.
[100] Jürgens U. Reinforcing concomitants of electrically-elicited vocalizations. Exp Brain Res 1976;26:203–14.
[101] Ortega JD, DeRosier E, Park S, Larson CR. Brainstem mechanisms of laryngeal control as revealed by microstimulation studies. In: Fujimura O, editor. Vocal physiology: voice production, mechanisms and functions, New York: Raven Press, 1988. p. 19–28.
[102] Chaurand JP, Vergnes M, Karli P. Substance grise centrale du mésencéphale et comportement d'aggression interspécifique du rat. Physiol Behav 1972;9:475–81.
[103] Kelly AH, Beaton LE, Magoun HW. A midbrain mechanism for faciovocal activity. J Neurophysiol 1946;9:181–9.
[104] Skultety FM. Clinical and experimental aspects of akinetic mutism. Arch Neurol 1968;19:1–14.
[105] Adametz J, O'Leary JL. Experimental mutism resulting from periaqueductal lesions in cats. Neurology 1959;9:636–42.
[106] Randall WL. The behavior of cats (*Felis* catus) with lesions in the caudal midbrain region. Behaviour 1964;23:107–39.
[107] Jürgens U, Pratt R. Role of the periaqueductal grey in vocal expression of emotion. Brain Res 1979;167:367–78.
[108] Botez MI, Carp N. Nouvelles données sur le problème du mécanisme de déclenchement de la parole. Rev Roum Neurol 1968;5: 153–8.
[109] Esposito A, Demeurisse G, Alberti B, Fabbro F. Complete mutism after midbrain periaqueductal gray lesion. Neuroreport 1999;10: 681–5.
[110] Adams DB. Cells related to fighting behavior recorded from midbrain central gray neuropil of cat. Science 1968;159:894–6.
[111] Suga N, Yajima Y. Auditory-vocal integration in the midbrain of the mustached bat: periaqueductal gray and reticular formation. In: Newman JD, editor. The physiological control of mammalian vocalization, New York: Plenum Press, 1988. p. 87–107.
[112] Düsterhöft F, Häusler U, Jürgens U. On the search for the vocal pattern generator. A single-unit recording study. Neuroreport 2000;11:2031–4.
[113] Larson CR, Kistler MK. Periaqueductal gray neuronal activity associated with laryngeal EMG and vocalization in the awake monkey. Neurosci Lett 1984;46:261–6.
[114] Larson CR. On the relation of PAG neurons to laryngeal and respiratory muscles during vocalization in the monkey. Brain Res 1991; 552:77–86.
[115] Marchand JE, Hagino N. Afferents to the periaqueductal gray in the rat. A horseradish peroxidase study. Neuroscience 1983;9:95–106.
[116] Meller ST, Dennis BJ. Afferent projections to the periaqueductal gray in the rabbit. Neuroscience 1986;19:927–64.
[117] Mantyh PW. Forebrain projections to the periaqueductal gray in the monkey, with observations in the cat and rat. J Comp Neurol 1982;206:146–58.
[118] Beitz AJ. The organization of afferent projections to the midbrain periaqueductal gray of the rat. Neuroscience 1982;7:133–59.
[119] Mantyh PW. The ascending input of the midbrain periaqueductal gray of the primate. J Comp Neurol 1982;211:50–64.
[120] Bianchi R, Tredici G, Gioia M. The spinal terminals into the midbrain periaqueductal gray of the rat. A light and electron microscope study of the projections ascending via the ventro-lateral funiculus. J Hirnforsch 1990;31:349–58.
[121] Carrive P. The periaqueductal gray and defensive behavior. Functional representation and neuronal organization. Behav Brain Res 1993;58:27–48.
[122] Keay KA, Feil K, Gordon BD, Herbert H, Bandler R. Spinal afferents to functionally distinct periaqueductal gray columns in the rat: an anterograde and retrograde tracing study. J Comp Neurol 1997; 385:207–29.
[123] Bandler R, Tork I. Midbrain periaqueductal grey region in the cat has afferent and efferent connections with solitary tract nuclei. Neurosci Lett 1987;74:1–6.
[124] Li J-L, Ding Y-Q, Xiong K-H, Li J-S, Shigemoto R, Mizuno N. Substance P receptor (NK1)-immunoreactive neurons projecting to the periaqueductal gray: distribution in the spinal trigeminal nucleus and the spinal cord of the rat. Neurosci Res 1998;30:219–25.
[125] Ennis M, Xu SJ, Rizvi TA. Discrete subregions of the rat midbrain periaqueductal gray project to nucleus ambiguus and the periambigual region. Neuroscience 1997;80:829–45.
[126] Gaytan SP, Pasaro R. Connections of the rostral ventral respiratory neuronal cell group: an anterograde and retrograde tracing study in the rat. Brain Res Bull 1998;47:625–42.
[127] Van der Horst VGJM, Terasawa E, Ralston HJ, Holstege G. Monosynaptic projections from the lateral periaqueductal gray to the nucleus retroambiguus in the rhesus monkey: Implications for vocalization and reproductive behavior. J Comp Neurol 2000;424:251–68.
[128] Cameron AA, Khan IA, Westlund KN, Cliffer KD, Willis WD. The efferent projections of the periaqueductal gray in the rat: a Phaseolus vulgaris leucoagglutinin study. J Comp Neurol 1995;351:568–601.
[129] Meller ST, Dennis BJ. Efferent projections of the periaqueductal gray in the rabbit. Neuroscience 1991;40:191–216.
[130] Fay RA, Norgren R. Identification of rat brainstem multisynaptic

connections to the oral motor nuclei in the rat using pseudorabies virus. Brain Res Rev 1997;25:255–311.
[131] Mantyh PW. Connections of midbrain periaqueductal gray in the monkey. J Neurophysiol 1983;49:567–94.
[132] Kanai T, Wang SC. Localization of the central vocalization mechanism in the brainstem of the cat. Exp Neurol 1962;6:426–34.
[133] Jürgens U. Localization of a pontine vocalization-controlling area. J Acoust Soc Am 2000;108:1393–6.
[134] Behrend O, Schuller G. The central acoustic tract and audiovocal coupling in the horseshoe bat, *Rhinolophus rouxi*. Eur J Neurosci 2000;12:4268–80.
[135] Metzner W. An audio-vocal interface in echolocating horseshoe bats. J Neurosci 1993;13:1899–915.
[136] Pillat J, Schuller G. Audiovocal behavior of Doppler-shift compensation in the horseshoe bat survives bilateral lesion of the paralemniscal tegmental area. Exp Brain Res 1998;119:17–26.
[137] Farley GR, Barlow SM, Netsell R. Factors influencing neural activity in parabrachial regions during cat vocalizations. Exp Brain Res 1992;89:341–51.
[138] Chamberlin LN, Saper CB. Topographic organization of respiratory responses to glutamate microstimulation of the parabrachial nucleus in the rat. J Neurosci 1994;14:6500–10.
[139] Cohen MJ. Switching the respiratory phases and evoked phrenic responses produced by rostral pontine electrical stimulation. J Physiol 1971;217:133–58.
[140] Fukuda H, Fukai K. Location of the reflex center for straining elicited by activation of pelvic afferent fibres of decerebrate dog. Brain Res 1986;380:287–96.
[141] Von Euler C, Marttila J, Remmers JE, Trippenbach T. Effects of lesions in the parabrachial nucleus on the mechanisms for central and reflex termination of inspiration in the cat. Acta Physiol Scand 1976;96:324–37.
[142] Herbert H, Moga MM, Saper CB. Connections of the parabrachial nucleus with the nucleus of the solitary tract and the medullary reticular formation in the rat. J Comp Neurol 1990;293:540–80.
[143] Smith JC, Morrison DE, Ellenberger HH, Otto MR, Feldman JL. Brainstem projections to the major respiratory neuron populations in the medulla of the cat. J Comp Neurol 1989;281:69–96.
[144] Chen S, Aston-Jones G. Extensive projections from the midbrain periaqueductal gray to the caudal ventrolateral medulla: a retrograde and anterograde tracing study in the rat. Neuroscience 1996;71:443–59.
[145] Gerrits PO, Holstege G. Pontine and medullary projections to the nucleus retroambiguus: a wheat germ agglutinin horseradish peroxidase and autoradiographic tracing study in the cat. J Comp Neurol 1996;373:173–85.
[146] Kaada BR. Somato-motor, autonomic and electrocorticographic responses to electrical stimulation of rhinencephalic and other structures in primates, cat and dog. Acta Physiol Scand, Suppl 1951; 83:1–285.
[147] Hunsperger RW, Bucher VM. Affective behaviour produced by electrical stimulation in the forebrain and brain stem of the cat. In: Adey WR, Tokizane T, editors. Structure and function of the limbic system, Amsterdam: Elsevier, 1967. p. 103–27.
[148] Fried I, Katz A, McCarthy G, Sass KJ, Williamson P, Spencer SS, Spencer DD. Functional organization of human supplementary motor cortex studied by electrical stimulation. J Neurosci 1991; 11:3656–66.
[149] Robinson BW. Vocalization evoked from forebrain in *Macaca mulatta*. Physiol Behav 1967;2:345–54.
[150] Brickner RM. A human cortical area producing repetitive phenomena when stimulated. J Neurophysiol 1940;3:128–30.
[151] Penfield W, Welch K. The supplementary motor area of the cerebral cortex. Arch Neurol Psychiatry 1951;66:289–317.
[152] Gooler DM, O'Neill WE. Topographic representation of vocal frequency demonstrated by microstimulation of anterior cingulate cortex in the echolocating bat, *Pteronotus parnelli parnelli*. J Comp Physiol A 1987;161:283–94.
[153] Talairach J, Bancaud J, Geier S, Bordas-Ferrer M, Bonis A, Szikla G, Rusu M. The cingulate gyrus and human behavior. Electroencephalogr Clin Neurophysiol 1973;34:45–52.
[154] Erickson TC, Woolsey CN. Observations on the supplementary motor area of man. Trans Am Neurol Assoc 1951;76:50–6.
[155] Sutton D, Larson C, Lindeman RC. Neocortical and limbic lesion effects on primate phonation. Brain Res 1974;71:61–75.
[156] Aitken PG. Cortical control of conditioned and spontaneous vocal behavior in rhesus monkeys. Brain Lang 1981;13:171–84.
[157] MacLean PD, Newman JD. Role of midline frontolimbic cortex in production of the isolation call in squirrel monkeys. Brain Res 1988;450:111–23.
[158] Kirzinger A, Jürgens U. Cortical lesion effects and vocalization in the squirrel monkey. Brain Res 1982;233:299–315.
[159] Sutton D, Trachy RE, Lindeman RC. Discriminative phonation in macaques: effects of anterior mesial cortex damage. Exp Brain Res 1985;59:410–3.
[160] Rubens AB. Aphasia with infarction in the territory of the anterior cerebral artery. Cortex 1975;11:239–50.
[161] Jürgens U, von Cramon D. On the role of the anterior cingulate cortex in phonation: a case report. Brain Lang 1982;15:234–48.
[162] West RA, Larson CR. Neurons of the anterior mesial cortex related to faciovocal activity in the awake monkey. J Neurophysiol 1995; 74:1856–69.
[163] Gemba H, Miki N, Sasaki K. Cortical field potentials preceding vocalization and influences of cerebellar hemispherectomy upon them in monkeys. Brain Res 1995;697:143–51.
[164] Paus T, Petrides M, Evans AC, Meyer E. Role of the human anterior cingulate cortex in the control of oculomotor, manual, and speech responses. A positron emission tomography study. J Neurophysiol 1993;70:453–69.
[165] Herholz K, Pietrzyk U, Karbe H, Wurker M, Wienhard K, Heiss WD. Individual metabolic anatomy of repeating words demonstrated by MRI-guided positron emission tomography. Neurosci Lett 1994; 182:47–50.
[166] Bookheimer SY, Zeffiro TA, Blaxton T, Gaillard W, Theodore W. Regional cerebral blood flow during object naming and word reading. Hum Brain Mapp 1995;3:96–106.
[167] Price CJ, Wise RJS, Warburton EA, Moore CJ, Howard D, Patterson K, Frackowiak RSJ. Hearing and saying. The functional neuroanatomy of auditory word processing. Brain 1996;119:919–32.
[168] Petersen SE, Fox PT, Posner MI, Mintun MA, Raichle ME. Positron emission tomographic studies of the cortical anatomy of single-word processing. Nature 1988;331:585–9.
[169] Hirano S, Kojima H, Naito Y, Honjo I, Kamoto Y, Okazawa H, Ishizu K, Yonekura Y, Nagahama Y, Fukuyama H, Konishi J. Cortical speech processing mechanisms while vocalizing visually presented languages. Neuroreport 1996;8:363–7.
[170] Paus T, Perry DW, Zatorre RJ, Worsley KJ, Evans AC. Modulation of cerebral blood flow in the human auditory cortex during speech: role of motor-to-sensory discharges. Eur J Neurosci 1996;8:2236–46.
[171] Perry DW, Zatorre RJ, Petrides M, Alivisatos B, Meyer E, Evans AC. Localization of cerebral activity during simple singing. Neuroreport 1999;10:3979–84.
[172] Bookheimer SY, Zeffiro TA, Blaxton TA, Gaillard W, Theodore WH. Activation of language cortex with automatic speech tasks. Neurology 2000;55:1151–7.
[173] Partiot A, Grafman J, Sadato N, Wachs J, Hallett M. Brain activation during the generation of non-emotional and emotional plans. Neuroreport 1995;6:1397–400.
[174] Damasio AR, Grabowski TJ, Bechara A, Damasio H, Ponto LLB, Parvizi J, Hichwa RD. Subcortical and cortical brain activity during the feeling of self-generated emotions. Nat Neurosci 2000;3:1049–56.

[175] Bartels A, Zeki S. The neural basis of romantic love. Neuroreport 2000;11:3829–34.
[176] Jürgens U, Zwirner P. The role of the periaqueductal grey in limbic and neocortical vocal fold control. Neuroreport 1996;7:2921–3.
[177] Jürgens U, Pratt R. The cingular vocalization pathway in the squirrel monkey. Exp Brain Res 1979;34:499–510.
[178] Jürgens U. The efferent and afferent connections of the supplementary motor area. Brain Res 1984;300:63–81.
[179] Foerster O. In: Bumke O, Foerster O, editors. Motorische Felder und Bahnen, Handbuch der Neurologie, vol. 4. Berlin: Springer, 1936. p. 1–448.
[180] Welker WJ, Benjamin RM, Miles RC, Woolsey CN. Motor effects of stimulation of cerebral cortex of squirrel monkey. J Neurophysiol 1957;20:347–64.
[181] Hines M. Movements elicited from precentral gyrus of adult chimpanzees by stimulation with sine wave currents. J Neurophysiol 1940;3:442–66.
[182] Hast MH, Fischer JM, Wetzel AB, Thompson VE. Cortical motor representation of the laryngeal muscles in *Macaca mulatta*. Brain Res 1974;73:229–40.
[183] Leyton ASF, Sherrington CS. Observations on the excitable cortex of the chimpanzee, orang-utan, and gorilla. Quart J Exp Physiol 1917;11:135–222.
[184] Penfield W. Mechanisms of voluntary movement. Brain 1954;77:1–17.
[185] Jürgens U. On the elicitability of vocalization from the cortical larynx area. Brain Res 1974;81:564–6.
[186] Penfield W, Rasmussen T. The cerebral cortex of man. New York: Macmillan, 1952.
[187] Foix C, Chavany JA, Marie J. Diplégie facio-linguo-masticatrice d'origine cortico-souscorticale sans paralysie de membres. Rev Neurol 1926;1:214–9.
[188] Alajouanine T, Thurel R. La diplégie faciale cérébrale forme corticale de la paralysie pseudobulbaire. Rev Neurol 1933;60:441–58.
[189] Groswasser Z, Korn C, Groswasser-Reider I, Solzi P. Mutism associated with buccofacial apraxia and bihemispheric lesions. Brain Lang 1988;34:157–68.
[190] Mao C-C, Coull BM, Golper LAC, Rau MT. Anterior operculum syndrome. Neurology 1989;39:1169–72.
[191] Jürgens U, Kirzinger A, von Cramon D. The effects of deep-reaching lesions in the cortical face area on phonation. A combined case report and experimental monkey study. Cortex 1982;18:125–40.
[192] Myers RE. Comparative neurology of vocalization and speech: proof of a dichotomy. Ann NY Acad Sci 1976;280:745–57.
[193] Winter P, Handley P, Ploog D, Schott D. Ontogeny of squirrel monkey calls under normal conditions and under acoustic isolation. Behaviour 1973;47:230–9.
[194] Brockelman WY, Schilling D. Inheritance of stereotyped gibbon calls. Nature 1984;312:634–6.
[195] Geissmann T. Inheritance of song parameters in the gibbon song analysed in 2 hybrid gibbons (Hylobates pileatus × Hylobates lar). Folia Primatol 1984;42:216–35.
[196] Owren MJ, Dieter JA, Seyfarth RM, Cheney DL. Food calls produced by adult female rhesus (*Macaca mulatta*) and Japanese (*M. fuscata*) macaques, their normally-raised offspring, and offspring cross-fostered between species. Behaviour 1992;120:218–31.
[197] Eibl-Eibesfeldt I. The expressive behaviour of the deaf-and-blind-born. In: Von Cranach M, Vine I, editors. Social communication and movement, London: Academic Press, 1973. p. 163–94.
[198] Murray GM, Lin LD, Moustafa EM, Sessle BJ. Effects of reversible inactivation by cooling of the primate face motor cortex on the performance of a trained tongue-protrusion task and a trained biting task. J Neurophysiol 1991;65:511–30.
[199] Ramsay SC, Adams L, Murphy K, Corfield DR, Grootoonk S, Bailey DL, Frackowiak RSJ, Guz A. Regional cerebral blood flow during volitional expiration in man. A comparison with volitional inspiration. J Physiol 1993;461:85–101.
[200] Price CJ. The anatomy of language: contributions from functional neuroimaging. J Anat 2000;197:335–59.
[201] Lotze M, Seggewies G, Erb M, Grodd W, Birbaumer N. The representation of articulation in the primary sensorimotor cortex. Neuroreport 2000;11:2985–9.
[202] Sasaki K, Kyuhou S, Nambu A, Matsuzaki R, Tsujimoto T, Gemba H. Motor speech centre in the frontal cortex. Neurosci Res 1995;22:245–8.
[203] Gunji A, Kakigi R, Hoshiyama M. Spatiotemporal source analysis of vocalization-associated magnetic fields. Cognit Brain Res 2000;9:157–63.
[204] Terao Y, Ugawa Y, Enomoto H, Furubayashi T, Shiio Y, Machii K, Hanajima R, Nishikawa M, Iwata NK, Saito Y, Kanazawa I. Hemispheric lateralization in the cortical motor preparation for human vocalization. J Neurosci 2001;21:1600–9.
[205] Wildgruber D, Ackermann H, Klose U, Kardatzki B, Grodd W. Functional lateralization of speech production at primary motor cortex: a fMRI study. Neuroreport 1996;7:2791–5.
[206] Riecker A, Ackermann H, Wildgruber D, Dogil G, Grodd W. Opposite hemispheric lateralization effects during speaking and singing at motor cortex, insula and cerebellum. Neuroreport 2000;11:1997–2000.
[207] Alcock KJ, Wade D, Anslow P, Passingham RE. Pitch and timing abilities in adult left-hemisphere-dysphasic and right-hemisphere-damaged subjects. Brain Lang 2000;75:47–65.
[208] Yamadori A, Osumi Y, Masuhara S, Okubo M. Preservation of singing in Broca's aphasia. J Neurol Neurosurg Psychiatry 1977;40:221–4.
[209] Botez MI, Wertheim N. Expressive aphasia and amusia following right frontal lesion in a right-handed man. Brain 1959;82:186–202.
[210] Gordon HW, Bogen JE. Hemispheric lateralization of singing after intracarotid sodium amylobarbitone. J Neurol Neurosurg Psychiatry 1974;37:727–38.
[211] Ross ED. Language-related functions of the right cerebral hemisphere. In: Rose FC, Whurr R, Wyke MA, editors. Aphasia, London: Whurr Publ, 1988. p. 188–209.
[212] Ross ED, Mesulam M-M. Dominant language functions of the right hemisphere? Prosody and emotional gesturing. Arch Neurol 1979;36:144–8.
[213] Jürgens U, Zwirner P. Individual hemispheric asymmetry in vocal fold control of the squirrel monkey. Behav Brain Res 2000;109:213–7.
[214] Kuypers HGJM. Some projections from the peri-central cortex to the pons and lower brain stem in monkey and chimpanzee. J Comp Neurol 1958;110:221–55.
[215] Alipour M, Chen Y, Jürgens U. Anterograde projections of the cortical tongue area of the tree shrew (Tupaia belangeri). J Brain Res 1997;38:405–23.
[216] Enomoto S, Kohase H, Nakamura Y. Dual brain stem projection from the cortical masticatory area in guinea pig. Neuroreport 1995;6:1573–7.
[217] Shriver JE, Noback CR. Cortical projections to the lower brain stem and spinal cord in the tree shrew (Tupaia glis). J Comp Neurol 1967;130:25–54.
[218] Yasui Y, Itoh K, Mitani A, Takada M, Mizuno N. Cerebral cortical projections to the reticular regions around the trigeminal motor nucleus in the cat. J Comp Neurol 1985;241:348–56.
[219] Zhang G, Sasamoto K. Projections of two separate areas for rhythmical jaw movements in the rat. Brain Res Bull 1990;24:221–30.
[220] Sirisko MA, Sessle BJ. Corticobulbar projections and orofacial and muscle afferent inputs of neurons in primate sensorimotor cerebral cortex. Exp Neurol 1983;82:716–20.
[221] Travers JB, Norgren R. Afferent projections to the oral motor nuclei in the rat. J Comp Neurol 1983;220:280–98.
[222] Jürgens U. Projections from the cortical larynx area in the squirrel monkey. Exp Brain Res 1976;25:401–11.
[223] Iwatsubo T, Kuzuhara S, Kanemitsu A, Shimada H, Toyokura Y.

Corticofugal projections to the motor nuclei of the brainstem and spinal cord in humans. Neurology 1990;40:309–12.
[224] Kuypers HGJM. Corticobulbar connections to the pons and lower brain-stem in man. Brain 1958;81:364–88.
[225] Newman DB, Hilleary SK, Ginsberg CY. Nuclear terminations of corticoreticular fiber systems in rats. Brain Behav Evol 1989;34: 223–64.
[226] Bauer G, Gerstenbrand F, Heugl W. Involuntary motor phenomena in the locked-in-syndrome. J Neurol 1980;223:191–8.
[227] Urban PP, Hopf HC, Connemann B, Hundemer HP, Koehler J. The course of cortico-hypoglossal projections in the human brainstem. Functional testing using transcranial magnetic stimulation. Brain 1996;119:1031–8.
[228] Furstenberg AC. Anatomical and clinical study of central lesions producing paralysis of the larynx. Ann Otol Rhinol Laryngol 1937;46:39–54.
[229] Künzle H. Bilateral projections from precentral motor cortex to the putamen and other parts of the basal ganglia. An autoradiographic study in *Macaca fascicularis*. Brain Res 1975;88:195–209.
[230] Iwata K, Yagi J, Tsuboi Y, Koshikawa N, Sumino R, Cools AR. Anatomical connections of the ventral, but not the dorsal part of the striatum with the parvicellular reticular formation. Implication for the anatomical substrate of oral movements. Neurosci Res Commun 1996;18:71–8.
[231] Lee MS, Lee SB, Kim WC. Spasmodic dysphonia associated with a left ventrolateral putaminal lesion. Neurology 1996;47:827–8.
[232] Pickett ER, Kuniholm E, Protopapas A, Friedman J, Lieberman P. Selective speech motor, syntax and cognitive deficits associated with bilateral damage to the putamen and the head of the caudate nucleus: a case study. Neuropsychologia 1998;36:173–88.
[233] Metter EJ, Jackson C, Kempler D, Riege WH, Hanson WR, Mazziotta JC, Phelps ME. Left hemisphere intracerebral hemorrhages studied by (F-18)-fluorodeoxyglucose PET. Neurology 1986;36:1155–62.
[234] Klein D, Zatorre RJ, Milner B, Meyer E, Evans AC. Left putaminal activation when speaking a second language: evidence from PET. Neuroreport 1994;5:2295–7.
[235] DeLong MR, Crutcher MD, Georgopoulos AP. Relations between movement and single cell discharge in the substantia nigra of the behaving monkey. J Neurosci 1983;3:1599–606.
[236] Mora F, Mogenson GJ, Rolls ET. Activity of neurons in the region of the substantia nigra during feeding in the monkey. Brain Res 1977;133:267–76.
[237] Ackermann H, Ziegler W. Articulatory deficits in Parkinsonian dysarthria: an acoustic analysis. J Neurol Neurosurg Psychiatry 1991;54:1093–8.
[238] Aronson AE. Clinical voice disorders. An interdisciplinary approach. Stuttgart: Thieme, 1980.
[239] Tsumori T, Ono K, Kishi T, Yasui Y. Demonstration of the corticobulbar pathway from the orofacial motor cortex to the parvicellular reticular formation in the rat. Brain Res 1997;755:151–5.
[240] Tokuno H, Takada M, Nambu A, Inase M. Direct projections from the orofacial region of the primary motor cortex to the superior colliculus in the macaque monkey. Brain Res 1995;703:217–22.
[241] Yasui Y, Tsumori T, Ando A, Domoto T. A nigro-rubro-bulbar pathway to the parvicellular reticular formation in the rat. Neuroreport 1996;7:1157–60.
[242] Hartmann-von Monakow K, Akert K, Künzle H. Projections of precentral and premotor cortex to the red nucleus and other midbrain areas in *Macaca fascicularis*. Exp Brain Res 1979;34:91–105.
[243] Humphrey DR, Gold R, Reed DJ. Sizes, laminar and topographic origins of cortical projections to the major divisions of the red nucleus in the monkey. J Comp Neurol 1984;225:75–94.
[244] Ackermann H, Ziegler W, Petersen D. Dysarthria in bilateral thalamic infarction. A case study. J Neurol 1993;240:357–62.
[245] Samra K, Riklan M, Levita E, Zimmerman J, Waltz JM, Bergmann L, Cooper IS. Language and speech correlates of anatomically verified lesions in thalamic surgery for parkinsonism. J Speech Hear Res 1969;12:510–40.
[246] Mazaux JM, Orgogozo JM. Etude analytique des trouble de langage par lésion du thalamus gauche: l'aphasie thalamique. Cortex 1982; 18:403–16.
[247] Schaltenbrand G. The effects on speech and language of stereotactical stimulation in thalamus and corpus callosum. Brain Lang 1975;2:70–7.
[248] Brown JR, Darley FL, Aronson AE. Ataxic dysarthria. Int J Neurol 1970;7:302–18.
[249] Ackermann H, Ziegler W. Cerebellar voice tremor: an acoustic analysis. J Neurol Neurosurg Psychiatry 1991;54:74–6.
[250] Lechtenberg R, Gilman S. Speech disorders in cerebellar disease. Ann Neurol 1978;3:285–90.
[251] Nitschke MF, Kleinschmidt A, Wessel K, Frahm J. Somatotopic motor representation in the human anterior cerebellum. A high-resolution functional MRI study. Brain 1996;119:1023–30.
[252] Kyuhou S, Matsuzaki R, Gemba H. Cerebello-cerebral projections onto the ventral part of the frontal cortex of the macaque monkey. Neurosci Lett 1997;230:101–4.
[253] Vitek JL, Ashe J, DeLong MR, Alexander GE. Physiologic properties and somatotopic organization of the primate motor thalamus. J Neurophysiol 1994;71:1498–513.
[254] Farley GR. Neural firing in ventrolateral thalamic nucleus during conditioned vocal behavior in cats. Exp Brain Res 1997;115:493–506.
[255] Nakano K, Tokushige A, Kohno M, Hasegawa Y, Kayahara T, Sasaki K. An autoradiographic study of cortical projections from motor thalamic nuclei in the macaque monkey. Neurosci Res 1992;13:119–37.
[256] Rouiller EM, Liang F, Babalian A, Moret V, Wiesendanger M. Cerebellothalamocortical and pallidothalamocortical projections to the primary and supplementary motor cortical areas: A multiple tracing study in macaque monkeys. J Comp Neurol 1994;345: 185–213.
[257] Penfield W, Roberts L. Speech and brain mechanisms. Princeton: Princeton University Press, 1959.
[258] Larson CR, Sutton D, Lindeman RC. Cerebellar regulation of phonation in rhesus monkey (*Macaca mulatta*). Exp Brain Res 1978;33:1–18.
[259] Kirzinger A. Cerebellar lesion effects on vocalization of the squirrel monkey. Behav Brain Res 1985;16:177–81.
[260] Rausell E, Jones EG. Histochemical and immunocytochemical compartments of the thalamic VPM nucleus in monkeys and their relationship to the representational map. J Neurosci 1991;11:210–25.
[261] Pritchard TC, Hamilton RB, Morse JR, Norgren R. Projections of thalamic gustatory and lingual areas in the monkey. J Comp Neurol 1986;244:213–28.
[262] Pritchard TC, Hamilton RB, Norgren R. Projections of the parabrachial nucleus in the Old World monkey. Exp Neurol 2000; 165:101–17.
[263] Norgren R, Leonard CM. Taste pathways in rat brainstem. Science 1971;173:1136–9.
[264] Nishikawa Y, Koyama N, Yokota T. Ipsilateral somatosensory tongue representation within the lateral subdivision of the nucleus ventralis posteromedialis parvocellularis of the cat thalamus. Brain Res 1988;458:394–6.
[265] Luria AR. Aspects of aphasia. J Neurol Sci 1965;2:278–87.
[266] Luria AR. Language and cognition. Washington: Winston, 1981.
[267] Gemba H, Kyuhou S, Matsuzaki R, Amino Y. Cortical field potentials associated with audio-initiated vocalization in monkeys. Neurosci Lett 1999;272:49–52.
[268] Jürgens U, Kirzinger A. The laryngeal sensory pathway and its role in phonation. A brain lesioning study in the squirrel monkey. Exp Brain Res 1985;59:118–24.
[269] McClean MD, Dostrovsky JO, Lee L, Tasker RR. Somatosensory

neurons in human thalamus respond to speech-induced orofacial movements. Brain Res 1990;513:343–7.

[270] Bahls FH, Chatrian GE, Mesher RA, Sumi SM, Ruff RL. A case of persistent cortical deafness: clinical, neurophysiologic and neuropathologic observations. Neurology 1988;38:1490–3.

[271] Ho KJ, Kileny P, Paccioretti D, McLean DR. Neurologic, audiologic, and electrophysiologic sequelae of bilateral temporal lobe lesions. Arch Neurol 1987;44:982–7.

[272] Adams AE, Rosenberger K, Winter H, Zoellner C. A case of cortical deafness. Arch Psychiatry Nervenkr 1978;224:213–20.

[273] Leicester J. Central deafness and subcortical motor aphasia. Brain Lang 1980;10:224–42.

[274] Heffner HE, Heffner RS. Hearing loss in Japanese macaques following bilateral auditory cortex lesions. J Neurophysiol 1986;55:256–71.

[275] Massopust LC, Wolin LR, Frost V. Increases in auditory middle frequency discrimination thresholds after cortical ablations. Exp Neurol 1970;28:299–307.

[276] Goldberg JM, Neff WD. Frequency discrimination after bilateral ablation of auditory areas. J Neurophysiol 1961;24:119–28.

[277] Cranford JL, Igarashi M, Stramler JH. Effect of auditory neocortex ablations on pitch perception in the cat. J Neurophysiol 1976;39: 143–52.

[278] Binder JR, Frost JA, Hammeke TA, Bellgowan PSF, Springer JA, Kaufman JN, Possing ET. Human temporal lobe activation by speech and nonspeech sounds. Cereb Cortex 2000;10:512–28.

[279] Dronkers NF. A new brain region for coordinating speech articulation. Nature 1996;384:159–61.

[280] Habib M, Daquin G, Milandre L, Royere ML, Rey M, Lanteri A, Salamon G, Khalil R. Mutism and auditory agnosia due to bilateral insular damage. Role of the insula in human communication. Neuropsychologia 1995;33:327–39.

[281] Schlosser MJ, Aoyagi N, Fulbright RK, Gore JC, McCarthy G. Functional MRI studies of auditory comprehension. Hum Brain Mapp 1998;6:1–13.

[282] Lhermitte F, Chain F, Escourolle R, Ducame B, Pillon B, Chedru F. Etude des troubles perceptifs auditifs dans les lésions temporales bilatérales. Rev Neurol 1971;124:329–51.

[283] Guard O, Couailler JF, Dumas R, Romanet P, Richard D, Mauguière F. Agnosie auditive. Lyon Méd 1980;243:311–7.

[284] Ross ED. The aprosodias. Arch Neurol 1981;38:561–9.

[285] Metz-Lutz M-N, Dahl E. Analysis of word comprehension in a case of pure word deafness. Brain Lang 1984;23:13–25.

[286] Fujii T, Fukatsu R, Watanabe S, Ohnuma A, Teramura K, Kimura I, Saso S, Kogure K. Auditory sound agnosia without aphasia following a right temporal lobe lesion. Cortex 1990;26:263–8.

[287] Peper M, Irle E. Categorical and dimensional decoding of emotional intonations in patients with focal brain lesions. Brain Lang 1997;58:233–64.

[288] Ligeois-Chauvel C, Peretz I, Babai M, Laguitton V, Chauvel P. Contribution of different cortical areas in the temporal lobes to music processing. Brain 1998;121:1853–67.

[289] Marcie P, Hécaen H, Constans JP, Chodkiewicz JP. Etude spectrographique de la parole chez deuz malades après ablation de méningiome de la region du pied de la troisième circonvolution frontal gauche. Rev Neurol 1969;120:350–2.

[290] Hécaen H, Consoli S. Analyse des troubles du langage au cours de lésions de l'aire de Broca. Neuropsychologia 1973;11:377–88.

[291] Henschen SE. Klinische und anatomische Beiträge zur Pathologie des Gehirns. Stockholm: Nordiska Bokhandeln, 1920.

[292] Mohr JP, Pessin MS, Finkelstein S, Funkenstein HH, Duncan GW, Davis KR. Broca aphasia: pathologic and clinical. Neurology 1978; 28:311–24.

[293] Levine DN, Sweet E. The neuropathologic basis of Broca's aphasia and its implications for the cerebral control of speech. In: Arbib MA, Caplan D, Marshall JC, editors. Neural models of language processes, New York: Academic Press, 1982. p. 299–326.

[294] Masdeu JC, O'Hara RJ. Motor aphasia unaccompanied by faciobrachial weakness. Neurology 1983;33:519–21.

[295] Knopman DS, Selnes OH, Niccum N, Rubens AB, Yock D, Larson D. A longitudinal study of speech fluency in aphasia: CT correlates of recovery and persistent nonfluency. Neurology 1983;33:1170–8.

[296] Cappa S, Cavalotti G, Vignolo LA. Phonemic and lexical errors in fluent aphasia: correlation with lesion site. Neuropsychologia 1981; 19:171–7.

[297] Buckner RL, Raichle ME, Petersen SE. Dissociation of human prefrontal cortical areas across different speech production tasks and gender groups. J Neurophysiol 1995;74:2163–73.

[298] Herholz K, Thiel A, Wienhard K, Pietrzyk U, von Stockhausen HM, Karbe H, Kessler J, Bruckbauer T, Halber M, Heiss WD. Individual functional anatomy of verb generation. Neuroimage 1996;3:185–94.

[299] Yetkin FZ, Hammeke TA, Swanson SJ, Morris GL, Mueller WM, McAuliffe TL, Haughton VM. A comparison of functional MR activation patterns during silent and audible language tasks. Am J Neuroradiol 1995;16:1087–92.

[300] Binder JR, Frost JA, Hammeke TA, Cox RW, Rao SM, Prieto T. Human brain language areas identified by functional magnetic resonance imaging. J Neurosci 1997;17:353–62.

[301] Chee MWL, Ocraven KM, Bergida R, Rosen BR, Savoy RL. Auditory and visual word processing studied with fMRI. Hum Brain Mapp 1999;7:15–28.

2

Perception of Voice

Introduction

Regardless of the technological advances in the field of laryngology, the simple act of perceiving and rating voice quality continues to be elusive. No doubt, the classic articles presented below shed some light on this intriguing topic, but as eloquently described by Drs. Kreiman and Gerratt, fundamentally, humans perceive the human voice differently. In addition, it is clear that clinicians have likely employed perceptual voice analyses as a component of the management schema for patients with dysphonia for centuries. However, as elucidated in the list of articles below, the first classic article in this area of investigation was published in 1990, likely an acknowledgment to the inherent complexity associated with the task of perceiving the human voice. Furthermore, perceptual evaluation of voice has been historically labeled more "subjective" than acoustic measures, although we now recognize this is not the case.

Drs. Kreiman and Gerratt provide thorough and interesting insight into their multidisciplinary collaboration and progression from the simple observation that the variability of perceptual ratings of voice vastly exceeded expectations to a formal algorhythm for the standardization of perceptual voice evaluation. Their dynamic interactions as well as significant contributions to the field are captured in the following commentary.

Classic Articles

●Reprint of article included in this chapter.
♦Commentary on this article.

Kreiman J, Gerratt BR, Precoda K. Listener experience and perception of voice quality. *J Speech Hear Res.* 1990; 33(1):103–115.

Klatt DH, Klatt LC. Analysis, synthesis, and perception of voice quality variations among female and male talkers. *J Acoust Soc Am.* 1990;87(2):820–857.

Childers DG, Lee CK. Vocal quality factors: analysis, synthesis, and perception. *J Acoust Soc Am.* 1991;90(5):2394–2410.

Kreiman J, Gerratt BR, Precoda K, Berke GS. Individual differences in voice quality perception. *J Speech Hear Res.* 1992;35(3):512–520.

●♦Kreiman J, Gerratt BR, Kempster GB, Erman A, Berke GS. Perceptual evaluation of voice quality: review, tutorial, and a framework for future research. *J Speech Hear Res.* 1993;36(1):21–40.

Gerratt BR, Kreiman J, Antonanzas-Barroso N, Berke GS. Comparing internal and external standards in voice quality judgments. *J Speech Hear Res.* 1993;36(1):14–20.

Dejonckere PH, Obbens C, de Moor GM, Wieneke GH. Perceptual evaluation of dysphonia: reliability and relevance. *Folia Phoniatr.* 1993;45(2):76–83.

Dejonckere PH, Remacle M, Fresnel-Elbaz E, Woisard V, Crevier-Buchman L, Millet B. Differentiated perceptual evaluation of pathological voice quality: reliability and correlations with acoustic measurements [Evaluation perceptuelle differentielle de la qualite de la voix pathologique: La fiabilite et les correlations avec dex mesures acoustiques]. *Revue de Laryngol Oto Rhinol.* 1996;117(3):219–224.

●De Bodt MS, Wuyts FL, Van De Heyning PH, Croux C. Test-retest study of the GRBAS scale: influence of experience and professional background on perceptual rating of voice quality. *J Voice.* 1997;11(1):74–80.

Commentary

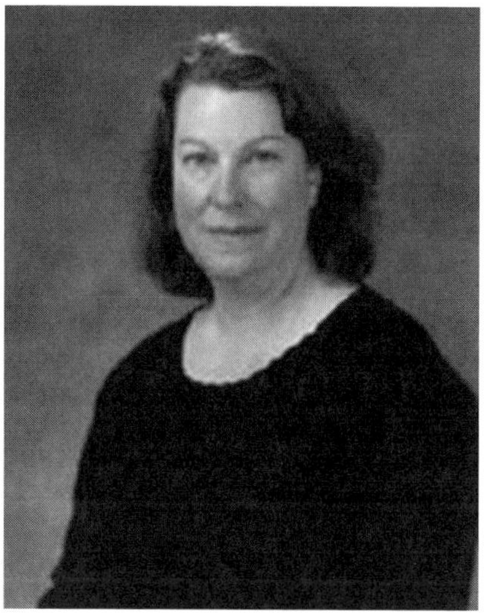

Jody Kreiman, PhD

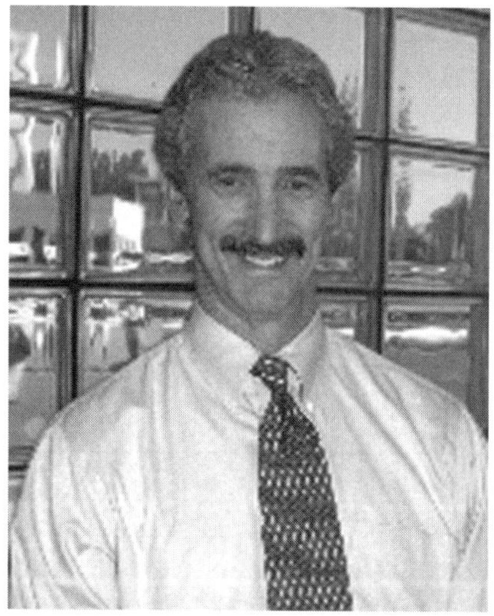

Bruce R. Gerratt, PhD

The papers included in this volume are part of a long series of investigations that all began with the question, "Why?" Although we have different training (Bruce in speech-language pathology and Jody in phonetics), at the beginning of our collaboration we were brought together by our shared interest in voice quality. Bruce mentioned to new postdoctoral student Jody that he (and others) had observed very large differences among raters in their use of traditional rating scales for qualities like breathiness, roughness, and strain. Some of the research we had been reading reported high levels of agreement among listeners, whereas many other studies reported much lower levels, and still others recommended using acoustic measures that were "more objective" to avoid these "inherently subjective" perceptual rating scale measures altogether. Jody (who at the time knew something about speaker recognition, but almost nothing about voice quality per se) asked, "Why such variability? Where is it all coming from?" Almost 20 years later, we think we have finally answered this question. This essay describes the long path and the answers we found.

Our attack on this question involved three lines of inquiry that ran more or less simultaneously. In the first, we attempted to determine how much raters really do vary in their voice quality ratings. We noticed that most studies reported the overall variability in ratings across raters and voices, but not how ratings vary for a single voice, which seemed to us to be of more relevance. When we calculated the likelihood that any two raters would agree in their ratings of a single voice, we found a pattern of results we called "smileygrams:" Listeners agreed relatively well about the quality of voices that were near-normal or severely disordered, but they never agreed consistently for voices with average ratings in the midrange of a scale (so that plots of the likelihood of agreement against the mean rating were U shaped, with agreement in the midrange averaging about 0.21 when chance equals 0.14.[1] In fact, in all our data over all these years, we have never found a single instance in which raters as a group agreed that a voice was a "4" on a 7-point scale for any quality, although these data sets meet conventional standards for interrater reliability (ie, high intraclass correlations or Cronbach's alpha values). These findings suggested that average ratings in the middle of a scale do not mean that the voice is moderately disordered. Instead, such scores merely indicate that listeners disagreed about the extent of disorder (so that the average is in the middle of the scale). When we used analysis of variance to determine how much of the difference in ratings was due to actual differences among voices in the quality being rated, and how much was error, we found that only about 32% of rating variability was related to differences among voices—the remaining 78% was error.[1] Because it appeared that using traditional rating scale protocols produced more error than data, we concluded that it was unlikely that protocols using scales like "breathy" and "rough" were generating valid measures of voice quality. These findings also show that the magnitude of the attribute being rated has a consistent effect on listener agreement levels, and must be included in a model of the voice rating process.

Given these results, our second line of inquiry was an attempt to determine what dimensions or features listeners actually pay attention to when they judge voice quality. Like everyone else at the time, we did not question the assumption that linguistic-style features like "breathy" and "rough" were a good way to describe voice quality, and we reasoned that listeners would be more accurate and reliable in their ratings if we asked them to make judgments about dimensions that were "psychologically real." Because evidence for the validity or psychological reality of different traditional scales for voice was generally lacking, we needed data about how listeners actually perceive voice quality, so we used multidimensional scaling (MDS), a technique that does not require a priori assumptions about what aspects of voice quality are perceptually important, and that allows investigation of individual differences in perceptual strategy. Listeners judge the similarities between pairs of voices, and the algorithm determines the dimensions of the best-fitting perceptual space that underlies the observed similarities (so that similar voices are close together in the space).

The results of these studies caused something of a crisis of faith in the lab. Contrary to our expectation, all of our MDS studies pointed to large differences between listeners in the features they paid attention to when judging voice quality. We found systematic differences between groups of listeners in their average perceptual strategies: Naive listeners all attended primarily to F0 (and thus were alike in their quality judgments), whereas experts differed from one another in the vocal attributes they used when judging quality.[2] We also found that, within a given listener, perceptual strategies shifted according to the characteristics of the stimuli under study: The likelihood that listeners will pay attention to some dimension is partly related to how much the stimulus set varies on that dimension.[3] On reflection, this is not especially surprising, but it demonstrated that the perceptual importance of a given dimension in a voice pattern varies with listening context. We also found that the ratings a voice receives on a specific scale depends on listening context as well.[4] Listeners' ratings can drift significantly across a single rating session, such that voices sound much rougher over time in the context of very many mildly rough voices. Worst of all, we found that linguistic-style "dimensions" for quality only emerged when we studied small sets of voices. When large sets (n = 80) were used, the voices did not disperse in a perceptual space along continuous scale-like dimensions, but instead clustered together in groups that lacked subjective unifying percepts.[5] Clusters did not correspond to traditional qualities like breathiness or roughness. Instead, the spaces seemed structured by "family resemblances," so that each voice in a cluster resembled others with respect to some property, but no one property linked all the voices within a cluster. Furthermore, different clusters of voices emerged from each listener's data, so that two voices were never consistently treated as similar in the perceptual spaces. The only consistent distinction across listeners was the difference between extremely severe pathology and moderate to mild pathology. We were forced to conclude that, in rating scale tasks, variability in perceptual strategies is a major source of listener unreliability, and that dimensional or rating scale approaches might not be appropriate for these complex auditory stimuli.

We found ourselves in a depressing situation: listeners from different populations used different perceptual strategies, experts differed so much that it did not appear possible to define a single set of perceptual features that would apply to all voices, and the validity of traditional scales like "breathy" and "rough" appeared limited to the most extreme cases of pathology. How, under such circumstances, could we hope to standardize voice quality assessments? The answer, we thought, was in our original question: We could only devise a reliable and valid voice rating protocol if we understood the sources of variability in voice quality ratings. Once those sources were identified and their relative importance quantified, we would be able to design a quality assessment tool that would control for each source of variability, and thus would be both reliable and valid. This effort constitutes our final line of inquiry, and it was a relief to have positive results to report after a long line of papers whose primary messages were "listeners don't agree" and "the traditional methods don't work." Our original theoretical framework[6] was a first pass at specifying the sources of interrater disagreements, based on a review of the literature and some original data. We originally proposed that rating vocal quality is a kind of matching task, in which listeners compare the externally presented stimulus to their own internal standard for both the quality of interest and the different levels of that quality. In this view, variability can arise because of differences between listeners in experience (through which standards develop), sensitivity (or lack thereof) to the quality being rated, problems related to the psychological reality of the scale, scale resolution issues, listening context, vagaries of attention to individual dimensions of a complex pattern,[7] "error" factors like fatigue.

This theoretical framework suggested that an ideal protocol for voice quality assessment would (1) provide listeners with external references, eliminating dependence on internal standards; (2) provide good scale resolution; and (3) help listeners focus their attention on one dimension of quality at a time. The first protocol we evaluated that met these criteria was an anchored rating task, in which listeners compared the voices to be rated to exemplars for the different levels of a scale. This task eliminated reliance on internal standards for the particular quality or for the different levels of the quality, because these are presented explicitly; it focused attention on a specific dimension; and the problem of scale resolution could be resolved empirically for each scale. Our preliminary test of this approach was very encouraging.[4] Use of the anchored protocol resulted in a significant increase in reliability compared to responses from a matched unanchored paradigm. We also found that ratings from the anchored task did not drift across the test session, but did drift significantly in the unanchored protocol. Using anchor stimuli thus appeared to control for several kinds of error.

The problem, of course, given the results reviewed above, was that we were unable to find any evidence about what qualities we should develop anchored scales *for*. This problem seemed insurmountable, and we came to view our attempts to develop an anchored protocol for specific qualities like breathiness and roughness as futile. However, a second protocol—a method of adjustment task—shared the desirable characteristics of the anchored protocol while avoiding its fatal limitations.[8] In this task, listeners vary parameters in a speech synthesizer to create an acceptable auditory match to a natural voice stimulus—in essence, creating custom anchor stimuli to match the target voice sample from an infinitely variable, multidimensional acoustic palette. This approach does not require the use of individual scales for qualities like hoarseness or strain; it incorporates an explicit matching task, thus eliminating reliance on unstable internal standards; it provides scale resolution to the limits of auditory resolution; and it helps listeners focus attention on individual aspects of voice quality, because adjusting each parameter brings that aspect to the perceptual foreground (in the same way that a camouflaged object becomes visible when it moves). In theory, then, this task should improve agreement among listeners because it controls all the major sources of variance in quality judgments. At the time that Bruce first proposed this task to Jody, she was not enthusiastic, in part because the technical hurdles to implementing it were enormous. We would have to develop both analysis and synthesis tools to model pathological voice quality in great detail, and we did not have any idea about what a starter set of control parameters might be. However, Bruce was right and Jody was wrong. The hurdles were worked through one by one, thanks to many years' effort and the help of our talented colleagues. Our reward was that the task seems to do what it is designed to do. In studies to date, listeners consistently agree when using the method of adjustment task, which they find very easy to perform, even when manipulating several parameters at once.[8–10]

The success of this method is consistent with the model we proposed about the sources of variability in voice quality ratings, but it did not test that model directly. To do this, we completed one additional study[10] in which listeners performed anchored and unanchored rating tasks using continuous or 7-point scales, and anchors that did or did not match the test stimuli. We then examined the likelihood that listeners would agree exactly, to determine how much each of four theoretical factors (instability of internal standards; difficulty isolating individual attributes in complex vocal patterns; scale resolution; and the magnitude of the attribute being measured) contributed to interlistener agreement. These factors accounted for 84.2% of the variance in agreement levels, so we conclude that as a set they are a very good model of the sources of interrater disagreements. When these sources of error are all controlled (as they are in the method of adjustment task), listeners agreed exactly 96% of the time, consistent with this view. This also shows that there is very little random error in voice quality ratings—almost all of it is related to factors that can be controlled experimentally. The most important of these factors is the relative ease of isolating the quality under consideration in the different tasks, corresponding experimentally to provision of anchor stimuli that match or do not match the target voice. When comparison stimuli matched the test voices, the likelihood that listeners would agree exactly in their assessment of voice quality more than doubled compared to an unmatched context.

A tool like the voice synthesizer makes it possible to ask all sorts of other questions about voice, because the approach provides a direct, causal link between the acoustic signal and perceived voice quality (unlike older rate-and-correlate approaches, which cannot demonstrate causality). For example, using this approach we can test the perceptual importance of individual acoustic parameters in natural, multidimensional contexts, so that we can determine how importance varies depending on other vocal attributes. In one study like this,[9] we found that listeners are very sensitive to changes in the signal-to-noise ratio, but not at all sensitive to changes in levels of jitter and shimmer, suggesting that these latter parameters do not contribute to voice quality to any significant extent. In this way, we may eventually derive a perceptually validated set of acoustic measures that truly reflect voice quality, fulfilling the old dream of "objective" measures of a subjective attribute. One additional possibility deserves mention. The synthesizer allows us to demonstrate experimentally how changes in the acoustic signal result in changes in perceived voice quality (although there are many, many details of this mapping still to investigate). As additional studies reveal more about how changes in patterns of vocal fold vibration produce changes in the acoustic signal, it may become possible to determine how physiological changes result in changes in vocal quality. This greater dream—the "big theory of everything vocal"—remains as a challenge for the future.

Acknowledgments

The research described in this essay was supported by grant DC01797 from the National Institutes of Health. Synthesizer software is available for download as open source shareware at http://www.surgery.medsch.ucla.edu/glottalaffairs/, or by request to the authors. Additional documented software for voice analysis and inverse filtering is available at the same URL.

References

1. Kreiman J, Gerratt BR. Validity of rating scale measures of voice quality. *J Acoust Soc Am.* 1998;104:1598–1608.
2. Kreiman J, Gerratt BR, Precoda K. Listener experience and perception of voice quality. *J Speech Hear Res,* 1990;33:103–115.
3. Kreiman J, Gerratt BR, Precoda K, Berke GS. Individual differences in voice quality perception. *J Speech Hear Res,* 1992;35:512–520.
4. Gerratt BR, Kreiman J, Antoñanzas-Barroso N, Berke GS. (1993). Comparing internal and external standards in voice quality judgments. *J Speech Hear Res,* 1993;36:14–20.
5. Kreiman J, Gerratt BR. (1996). The perceptual structure of pathologic voice quality. *Acoust Soc Am.* 1996;100:1787–1795.
6. Kreiman J, Gerratt BR, Kempster GB, Erman A, Berke GS. Perceptual evaluation of voice quality: review, tutorial, and a framework for future research. *J Speech Hear Res.* 1993;36:21–40.
7. Kreiman J, Gerratt BR. Sources of listener disagreement in voice quality assessment. *J Acoust Soc Am.* 2000;108:1867–1879.
8. Gerratt BR, Kreiman, J. Measuring vocal quality with speech synthesis. *J Acoust Soc Am,* 2001;110:2560–2566.
9. Kreiman J, Gerratt BR. Perception of aperiodicity in pathological voice. *J Acoust Soc Am.* 2005;117:2201–2211.
10. Kreiman J, Gerratt BR, Ito M. When and why listeners disagree in voice quality assessment tasks. *J Acoust Soc Am.* 2007;122:2354–2364.

Perceptual Evaluation of Voice Quality: Review, Tutorial, and a Framework for Future Research

Jody Kreiman
Bruce R. Gerratt
VA Medical Center, West Los Angeles and UCLA School of Medicine Los Angeles, CA

Gail B. Kempster
Governors State University University Park, IL

Andrew Erman
Gerald S. Berke
VA Medical Center, West Los Angeles and UCLA School of Medicine Los Angeles, CA

The reliability of listeners' ratings of voice quality is a central issue in voice research because of the clinical primacy of such ratings and because they are the standard against which other measures are evaluated. However, an extensive literature review indicates that both intrarater and interrater reliability fluctuate greatly from study to study. Further, our own data indicate that ratings of vocal roughness vary widely across individual clinicians, with a single voice often receiving nearly the full range of possible ratings. No model or theoretical framework currently exists to explain these variations, although such a model might guide development of efficient, valid, and standardized clinical protocols for voice evaluation. We propose a theoretical framework that attributes variability in ratings to several sources (including listeners' backgrounds and biases, the task used to gather ratings, interactions between listeners and tasks, and random error). This framework may guide development of new clinical voice and speech evaluation protocols, ultimately leading to more reliable perceptual ratings and a better understanding of the perceptual qualities of pathological voices.

KEY WORDS: voice quality, perception (voice), agreement, reliability

Voices can be objectively measured in many ways (see, e.g., Baken, 1987; Hirano, 1981). However, voice *quality* is fundamentally perceptual in nature. Patients seek treatment for voice disorders because they do not sound normal, and they often decide on whether treatment has been successful based on whether they sound better or not. For this and other reasons, speech clinicians use and value perceptual measures of voice and speech far more than instrumental measures (Gerratt, Till, Rosenbek, Wertz, & Boysen, 1991). Further, listeners' judgments are usually the standard against which other measures of voice (acoustic, aerodynamic, and so on) are evaluated (e.g., Coleman, 1969, 1971; Deal & Emanuel, 1978; Emanuel & Sansone, 1969; Fukazawa & El-Assuooty, 1988; Hillenbrand, 1988; Klatt & Klatt, 1990; Kojima, Gould, Lambiase, & Isshiki, 1980; Ladefoged, Maddieson, & Jackson, 1988; Sansone & Emanuel, 1970; Takahashi & Koike, 1975; Wendahl, 1966b; Wendler, Doherty & Hollien, 1980). For perceptual ratings to be meaningful, listeners must use scales consistently: A given rater must rate a voice sample the same way every time he or she hears it. Additionally, for ratings to be clinically useful, interrater agreement must be high: Each rater who hears a voice sample must rate it similarly. Thus, the reliability of such judgments is a central issue in the study of voice quality and voice disorders.

Unfortunately, it is unclear which of the many scales, procedures, and statistics that have appeared in the literature are best suited to measuring voice quality and evaluating the reliability of such measurements. Research in this area has proceeded without benefit of a consistent theoretical approach to the voice perception process. Consequently, authors have had no particular basis for selecting one or another of the many possible protocols and analyses when designing studies. Both methodology and estimates of listener reliability have varied widely from study to study. However, because research questions have not been motivated by a model or unified approach to the problems at hand, basic questions such as "How reliably *can* listeners judge voices in clinical settings?" and "What is the *best* method for gathering voice ratings and measuring rater agreement?" remain unanswered. A better understanding of the factors that affect intrarater and interrater agreement and reliability would lead to improved protocols for voice quality assessment, a cornerstone of the diagnosis and treatment of voice disorders.

This paper examines the issues of how voice quality can most appropriately be assessed, what reasonable standards for intra- and interrater reliability of perceptual judgments might be, and how reliability of ratings and levels of agreement within and among listeners might be maximized. A review of the literature on voice quality judgments describes the range of reported levels of agreement and variability, examines how methodological variables might affect listener agreement and reliability, and attempts to determine what de facto model of voice ratings underlies previous research. We describe the various statistics and scales that have appeared in the literature and discuss how appropriate these different measures of reliability might be for generalizing results to clinical settings. Experiments designed to evaluate the adequacy of the models implied by previous research are reported, and the suitability of the various methods for gathering voice quality ratings is evaluated. Finally, we propose an alternate theoretical framework that accounts for the present findings and for others in the literature.

Methodological Preliminaries

Because we are concerned with the most effective measurement of perceived vocal quality, we begin by reviewing a number of statistical concepts that are important for deciding how to gather and evaluate listeners' ratings.

Types of Rating Scales

Perceived voice quality has been measured using a variety of tasks. *Categorical ratings* involve assigning speech or voice samples to discrete, unordered categories (e.g., breathy, rough). *Equal-appearing interval* (EAI) scales require listeners to assign a number between 1 and n to a voice sample, where n in the number of points on the scale. Points on EAI scales are *assumed* to be equidistant, so measurements are generally treated as interval level and parametric statistics applied. *Visual analog* (VA) scales are undifferentiated lines, often 100 mm long. Listeners rate voices on these scales by making a mark on the line to indicate the extent to which a voice possesses a given characteristic. In *direct magnitude estimation* (DME), listeners assign a number to a voice sample to indicate the extent to which it possesses the quality being rated. The range of possible numbers generally is not restricted. In anchored DME, listeners are provided with a reference voice sample assigned a specific magnitude (usually 100) of the quality being rated. In unanchored paradigms, listeners make their judgments with reference to their own criteria. Finally, in *paired comparison* tasks listeners compare two stimuli. They may judge the extent of difference on some dimension, similarity/difference, relative roughness, and so on.

Other tasks may be used to measure perceived vocal quality (see, e.g., Dunn-Rankin, 1983, for discussion of many psychometric procedures). For example, Kempster, Kistler, and Hillenbrand (1991) recently used triadic comparisons to evaluate the similarity of dysphonic female voices. However, these other methods are not common in voice quality research and did not appear in any of the 57 papers reviewed below.

Agreement and Reliability of Judgments

The terms *reliability* and *agreement* are frequently treated as synonymous in common usage and in the literature, and are often referred to jointly as "reliability." However, in statistical usage they are technical terms with different meanings (e.g., Berk, 1979). Listeners are in *agreement* to the extent that they make exactly the same judgments about the voices rated. Ratings are *reliable* when the relationship of one rated voice to another is constant (i.e., when voice ratings are parallel or correlated), although the absolute rating may differ from listener to listener. The number of ratings that agree exactly or within ± one scale value is a common measure of agreement; the intraclass correlation is one measure of rating reliability (Ebel, 1951; Tinsley & Weiss, 1975).

The distinction between these two concepts is clinically as well as statistically important. *Agreement* implies that two listeners assign identical meanings to each scale point: their idea of what constitutes extreme roughness or breathiness (for example), their definitions of normal (nonrough or nonbreathy), and the distance between intervening points on the scale are all the same. *Reliability* implies only that listeners rate the voices in a parallel fashion, without implying that scale values have the same meaning. Thus, knowing that a set of ratings is reliable does not necessarily allow prediction of one listener's ratings from another's, unless their relative levels of rating are also known (e.g., A always rates voices one point lower than B).

There is no necessary relationship between levels of agreement and reliability. A rater whose standards drift within a listening session may have high test-retest reliability but low test-retest agreement. Similarly, two raters who use a scale in parallel ways but whose ratings consistently differ by some number of scale values will not be in agreement, but will be reliable relative to one another. Further, good agreement does not necessarily imply good reliability. If the range of ratings is restricted (for example, because listeners consistently avoid the endpoints of an EAI scale, or if stimuli vary very little with respect to the quality rated), reliability coefficients may be low, even if raters agree well with one another (Tinsley & Weiss, 1975).

In general, speech and voice researchers have required high levels of intrarater agreement from their listeners. Reliability, rather than agreement, has often been the standard for between-rater evaluations. In this case, agreement has been viewed by some as too strict a requirement (e.g., Sheard, Adams, & Davis, 1991). However, in clinical situations where voices are evaluated one at a time, information about a clinician's general level of rating is not usually available. Because the absolute level of the ratings must be meaningful to another rater for rating information to be clinically useful, reporting reliability without including a measure of agreement may be inappropriate for studies with clinical applications.

Focus of the Evaluation

Depending on the experimenter's purpose, measures of reliability and agreement may compare ratings for pairs of raters or may reflect the overall coherence of an entire group of listeners.[1] For example, Pearson's *r* is frequently calculated across all possible pairs of raters and then reported as a single, average value (e.g., Moran & Gilbert, 1984; Nieboer, De Graaf, & Schutte, 1988; Samar & Metz, 1988). Calculation of agreement/reliability across all possible pairs of raters can reveal the number of raters who disagree with the majority and the extent of their disagreement, both of which may be masked by use of a single estimator of interrater agreement/reliability. Use of pairwise measures can also help identify which raters differ substantially from the group. However, averaging many pairwise measures to produce a single measure of reliability tends to amplify the error inherent in the individual statistics. These measures are also subject to inflation or deflation due to several factors, including the probability of chance agreement and levels of occurrence of the quality being rated, as discussed in the following section (see also Berk, 1979).

In contrast, the intraclass correlation (ICC) always reflects the overall coherence of an entire group of listeners. Two formulas are commonly used (although several others exist; see Shrout & Fleiss, 1979). ICC(2,1) reflects the average agreement between one observer and another (also called the reliability of a single listener).[2] ICC(2,k) reflects the reliability of the average of k observations (or the average agreement between the single random sample of observers used in a study and a theoretical set of other random samples drawn from the same universe of raters). This second measure is sometimes referred to as the reliability of the average rating. The value of ICC(2,k) will always be larger than that of ICC(2,1), provided ICC(2,1) is positive (Shrout & Fleiss, 1979). In addition, increasing the number of raters will increase the value of ICC(2,k), because the larger sample size improves the estimate of the mean rating. Because of this, it is misleading to report ICC(2,k) without identifying it as a measure of the reliability of the mean and without justifying the use of mean ratings as the unit of reliability.

Because individual raters, rather than average ratings, are usually of interest in clinical voice evaluations, as a rule ICC(2,k) is not appropriate for measuring reliability in this area. In research applications, however, experimenters may sometimes wish to generate a single average rating of a voice (for example, to study the correlation between average voice ratings and objective measures of voice). If use of mean ratings is appropriate, ICC(2,k) should also be used to assess the reliability of the estimate of those means. Because considerable interrater variability can underlie a stable mean, especially if *n* is large, we feel this statistic is not a substitute for ICC(2,1), even in research applications.

Chance Levels of Agreement and Reliability

Statistically significant coefficients do not necessarily demonstrate a strong relationship between two sets of measurements, just as large correlations or percent agreement values are not necessarily statistically significant. When evaluating a measure of agreement or reliability, it is important to consider the chance level associated with the statistic and the precision of the estimate of that measure (usually with reference to the 95% confidence interval). Particularly when samples are small, reliability coefficients are only guesses (e.g., Ebel, 1951). Confidence intervals and chance values permit assessment of the goodness of the guess.

Unfortunately, most measures of listener agreement do not correct for chance agreement and are subject to inflation or deflation if the set of voices includes very many or very few voices at the extremes of the scale (Berk, 1979). It has been shown (Hopkins & Hermann, 1977; Kearns & Simmons, 1988) that measures of agreement and reliability may also be inflated or deflated due to the rate of occurrence of the quality being rated. That is, listeners frequently agree about what constitutes normal phonation or severe pathology, but disagree more about the extent of mild-to-moderate behaviors. If the stimulus set includes a large number of normal voices, agreement levels may be misleadingly high.

Because listeners seldom agree perfectly, agreement on equal-appearing interval (EAI) scales is often measured as the percentage of ratings that agree within plus or minus one scale value. Assuming all scale values are equally probable (used equally often by each listener), the chance probability of listeners responding within ± one scale value equals $[n + 2(n - 1)]/n^2$, where n = the number of points in the scale (N. Antonanzas-Barroso, personal communication, November 1990). Thus for a 7-point EAI scale, 38.8% of ratings would be expected to fall within ± one scale value by chance alone. For a 5-point scale, chance equals 52%. Thus, "70% agreement within ± one scale value" is at most 18% above chance for a 5-point EAI scale. In practice, many listeners avoid scale extremes; chance levels of agreement are even higher in these cases. When the 95% confidence intervals about "70% agreement" are calculated, it is possible that agreement levels will not differ significantly from chance (see Cullinan, Prather, & Williams, 1963).

---

[1]Measures may also reflect the reliability with which an individual voice is rated, averaged across raters, rather than the usual focus on the reliability of a rater, averaged across voices. This is not commonly done (but see Kearns & Simmons, 1988).

[2]In this notation, the first number refers to the ANOVA model used to calculate the ICC. A value of 2 indicates that judges are included as a factor in a 2-way ANOVA (vs. model 1, which uses a 1-way ANOVA) and that judges are treated as a random effect (vs. model 3, which treats judges as fixed). The second value represents the unit of reliability: a single judge (1), or the mean of k judges (k). See Shrout & Fleiss (1979) for discussion of other models.

Methods for calculating chance probability levels and confidence intervals are not available for every statistic used to evaluate reliability and agreement (Tinsley & Weiss, 1975). Because the intraclass correlation is based on analysis of variance, confidence intervals can be calculated for this statistic (Ebel, 1951; Shrout & Fleiss, 1979). Additionally, the confidence intervals around the mean rating for a single voice can be calculated, and can indicate the extent to which average ratings reflect the underlying data (e.g., Cullinan et al., 1963).

Fixed Versus Random Samples of Judges and Voices

Whether measures of reliability and agreement can be generalized beyond a given study depends in part on whether the voices and raters are treated statistically as fixed or random factors (Ebel, 1951; Shrout & Fleiss, 1979). When samples of raters or voices are treated as fixed, we assume that we have sampled the entire population of interest, that is, every voice or every rater. Thus no conclusions can be drawn about other groups of raters or voices. When samples are treated as random, we attempt to draw conclusions about differences between raters in general (for example) based on a limited sample selected at random. (See, e.g., Hays, 1973, or Winer, 1971, for more discussion of these issues.)

Most statistics used to assess reliability and agreement do not distinguish between fixed and random effect models (Berk, 1979). However, the intraclass correlation can be calculated to reflect fully fixed, fully random, or mixed effects models, as appropriate (Ebel, 1951), and thus is often the preferred measure of reliability (Berk, 1979). Many authors recommend treating judges as a random effect and stimuli (e.g., voices) as a fixed effect (e.g., Shrout & Fleiss, 1979; Tinsley & Weiss, 1975). However, application of experimental results to clinical settings may in fact require a fully random ANOVA model, so that results will be generalizable to other raters *and* other voices. In any case, authors should specify and justify the ANOVA model used. Unfortunately, this information often is not supplied (see below).

Review of the Literature

This review included 57 papers randomly selected from those published between 1951 and 1990. All papers were concerned with assessment of speech and voice quality, although the studies had many different purposes and utilized a wide variety of qualities, speakers, listeners, and rating tasks. Speech, phonetics, and otolaryngology journals were included in the survey, which was meant to be thorough but not exhaustive. Details of the studies reviewed are given in the Appendix. The discussion below summarizes research practices during this period.

Study Designs

Listeners. The number of raters included in the studies reviewed ranged from 1 to 461, with a median of 11, a mean of 30, and a standard deviation of 63. The distribution of group sizes was roughly trimodal, with modes at 5, 8, and 11 raters. Judges have included experts (experienced clinicians, teachers, and scientists: 28 papers), graduate students in speech pathology (19 papers), undergraduate students (14 papers), naive adults (3 papers), and children (1 paper).[3] One paper did not identify the listeners used.

Rating instruments. "Categorical" ratings,[4] equal-appearing interval scales (with 4, 5, 6, 7, 8, or 9 points), visual analog scales, direct magnitude estimations (with and without anchor stimuli), and paired comparison tasks were all used in the studies reviewed here to gather perceptual judgments of speech and voice quality. EAI scales were by far the most prevalent, appearing in 82.5% of the studies (47/57). Seven-point scales were most common (18 studies), followed by 5-point scales (16 studies). Four studies varied the number of scale points with the quality being rated. Anchored DME was used in 7 studies; one of these also included an unanchored DME task. Six studies used paired comparison tasks; two used "categorical" ratings, and one used a visual analog scale.

Listener training. Task-specific listener training varied from none to years of formal practice and discussion. To simplify our analyses, training was divided into three levels: none, orientation, and extensive training. Orientation was defined as providing listeners with definitions of scale terms, sample or anchor stimuli, and/or a limited number of practice trials (fewer than 20, or less than 25% of experimental trials). Extensive training was any training in excess of orientation. Six studies (10.5%) provided listeners with no training, 29 (50.9%) provided orientation, and 8 (14.0%) included extensive training. Training procedures were not reported in nearly 30% of the papers sampled (15 studies).

Intrarater Agreement and Reliability

The number of repeated trials underlying the different estimates of intrarater agreement/reliability ranged from 3 to 224 (3.3 to 100% of trials). The mean across studies was 49.4% of trials repeated, with a standard deviation of 38.5%. Two studies did not specify the number of repeated trials, and 17 (29.8%) did not report test-retest reliability.

Seven different statistics were used to evaluate intrarater agreement and reliability. The most common was Pearson's *r*, the correlation between the first and second ratings (19 papers). Other statistics included the number of trials whose ratings agreed exactly or within ± one scale value (14 studies), Pearson's *r* for the means or medians of the two sets of ratings (7 studies), an "ANOVA technique" or "test-retest procedure" (4 studies), a t-test or one-way ANOVA for a (directional) difference between the means of the two sets of ratings (3 studies), Kendall's rank-order coefficient (1

[3]Throughout this discussion, totals may exceed 57 because some papers included more than one listener group or protocol.

[4]Although the authors of these studies (Anders, Hollien, Hurme, Sonninen, & Wendler, 1988; Sapir, Aronson, & Thomas, 1986) describe their rating instrument as categorical, both use parametric statistics to evaluate listener reliability. This suggests they actually used equal-appearing interval scales. However, we have maintained the original terminology here.

study), and the Phi correlation, a nonparametric measure of association related to Chi-squared analysis (e.g., Hays, 1973; 1 study). Seven studies reported both Pearson's *r* and the percentage of ratings within ± one scale value. The statistic(s) used varied within as well as across scales. All seven statistics were used with EAI scales, and four of the seven were used with other rating instruments.

Intrarater reliability was not obviously related to the scale type or statistic used, although comparisons must be made with caution because many scales and statistics appeared infrequently. For EAI scales, Pearson's *r* ranged from .66 to .74 for a 4-point scale (one study), from .37 to .98 across seven studies using 5-point scales, and from .73 to .97 for 7-point scales (5 studies). The percentage of ratings within ± one scale value ranged from 55 to 100% for 5-point EAI scales (7 studies), and from 80 to 95% for 7-point scales (2 studies). A single study reported 85% agreement within ± one scale value for a 9-point scale. Pearson's *r* for the means or medians of the first and second ratings ranged from .93 to .98 across 5 studies using 5-point EAI scales. The possible increase in reliability with the number of points in an EAI scale is probably artifactual. Values for Pearson's *r* for the 4-point scale may be depressed by the limited range of the scale; and results for the 5-point scale include one study using very young children as subjects (Deal & Belcher, 1990).

No obvious effect of listener training on intrarater reliability is apparent from the literature, although conclusions are again limited by the small number of observations in some cells. In particular, studies in which listeners were extensively trained did not report higher levels of intrarater reliability than did studies that employed only orientation to the task and/or stimuli. Across scales, Pearson's *r* varied from .86 to .98 for extensively trained listeners (3 studies), from .66 to .98 for listeners who received orientation (9 studies, not including one using small children as subjects (Deal & Belcher, 1990)). Similarly, 86 to 100% of ratings agreed within ± one scale value for extensively trained subjects (2 studies), and 80 to 96% agreed within ± one scale value for subjects who received orientation training (4 studies). A single study reported 85% agreement within ± one scale value for subjects who received no training.

Finally, no clear relationship emerged between intrarater reliability and a rater's experience. Correlations between the first and second rating (Pearson's *r*) ranged from .66 to .98 for expert listeners (10 papers), and from .59 to .95 for graduate students (5 papers). A single paper reported a correlation of .97 for undergraduate students. Similarly, 80 to 95% of ratings were within ± one scale value for experts (3 papers), and 55 to 100% for graduate students (6 papers). A single paper reported 85% agreement within ± one scale value for undergraduates.

Interrater Reliability

Nine different statistics were used to measure interrater reliability and agreement in the papers reviewed. The most common were intraclass correlations (12 papers), the percentage of ratings within ± one scale value (10 papers), and Pearson's *r* for pairs of listeners (7 papers). Other statistics included Cronbach's alpha and coefficient Q (2 papers each), Spearman's rho, Kendall's Coefficient of Concordance, Friedman 2-way ANOVAs, and the Phi correlation (one paper each). All nine statistics were used with EAI scales. Only intraclass correlations were used with VA and DME scales. Interrater reliability was not reported in 40% of papers reviewed (23/57).

The relationship between scale type and interrater reliability is difficult to determine, due to the variety of methods used and the limited number of observations in each cell. For EAI scales, values of Pearson's *r* for pairs of raters varied widely both within and across studies. For 5-point scales, values ranged from .56 to .98 across three studies. A single study using a 7-point scale reported values ranging from .18 to .66, and two studies using 8-point scales reported values from .17 to .87. Across six studies using 5-point scales, listener agreement ranged from 72 to 100% of ratings within ± one scale value. For 7-point scales, values ranged from 58 to 84% (3 studies); a single study using a 9-point scale reported 75% interrater agreement. Values of ICC(2,1) varied from .57 to .83 across five studies that distinguished between ICC models. Listener reliability for direct magnitude estimation tasks was comparable to that for EAI scales: ICC(2,1) values ranged from .58 to .65 (2 studies).

Task-specific training does not obviously improve agreement among raters. Values of Pearson's *r* ranged from .62 to .89 for extensively trained listeners, from .18 to .98 for listeners who received orientation training, and from .17 to .78 for listeners who received no training. Values were derived from at most two studies in each of these cases, and differences probably represent sampling error. Interrater agreement levels (± one scale value) support this suggestion. For extensively trained listeners, values ranged from 58 to 82% (2 studies), and from 75 to 100% for listeners receiving orientation (6 studies). A single study reported 75% agreement within ± one scale value for listeners who received no training.

Finally, no consistent relationship between listeners' background and levels of interrater reliability is apparent from the studies reviewed. For experts, a single study reported ICC(2,1) = .79. Values for graduate students ranged from .58 to .83 across 3 studies, and a single study using undergraduate students reported ICC values from .57 to .74. Values for other statistics followed similar patterns (see Appendix for details).

Discussion

An answer to the question, "Can listeners make reliable judgments about voice quality?," is not readily forthcoming from the literature. Across scales and statistics, reliability and agreement levels ranged from very low (a correlation of .18 indicates less than 4% of variance common to the raters) to extremely high (100% of ratings within ± one scale value). However, methods also varied widely across studies, and neither intrarater nor interrater reliability varied consistently with any of the methodological factors examined here. Unfortunately, it is not possible to conclude that any one factor does or does not contribute to rating reliability.

Thus the literature does not further our understanding of the sources of variability in ratings of voice quality in any substantial way. Several factors contribute to the present situation. First, methodological problems are not uncommon in this research area. For example, many studies failed to report reliability at all; others used the authors as the only raters. Second, inadequate or inappropriate statistical techniques for estimation of rater reliability and agreement limit the conclusions that may be drawn from the literature. In particular, the lack of confidence interval data and/or consideration of chance probability levels seriously limits the conclusions that may be drawn from previous studies.

Finally, the literature as a whole lacks a clear theoretical approach to perceptual and rating processes. Although in some cases design features are motivated by study concerns (e.g., Bassich & Ludlow, 1986), in the majority of cases the choice between scale types, rater population, sample size, and statistical approaches is not based on clearly stated goals or theoretical considerations. Further, with the exception of studies using ICC(2,1), previous research has treated all intra- and interrater variability as unpartitioned error. Because possible sources of consistent variation in reliability and/or agreement are not considered, authors have no basis for deciding what procedures are likely to result in maximally stable and reliable ratings. A better understanding of this variability is a necessary step in the development of methods that yield judgments that are reliable and valid across clinicians, voices, and occasions.

In order to begin systematically examining the sources and extent of rater variability, we gathered ratings of vocal roughness from experienced listeners. This study examines the effects of differences among voices, listeners, and tasks on rating reliability. By applying a variety of statistical approaches to the data, we hoped to determine (a) which sources of intra- and interrater variability may be consistent and thus potentially controllable, and (b) which statistical approaches best reflect both the central trend and the extent of variation in listeners' judgments. Finally, these data will serve as an empirical basis for a more adequate approach to voice quality perception.

EXPERIMENT 1

Method

Listeners

Twenty clinicians participated in the listening tests. Four were otolaryngologists, and 16 were speech pathologists. Each listener had a minimum of 2 years' postgraduate experience evaluating and treating voice quality disorders, with a mean of 9.0 years (*SD* = 6.4 years; range = 2–20 years).

Stimuli

The voices of 22 males with voice disorders were selected at random from a library of recordings. Speakers ranged in age from 24 to 77 years (mean age = 54.6 years; *SD* = 14.4 years). In the judgment of the authors, these voices sampled the entire range of vocal roughness: Five were mildly rough, 6 were severely rough, and 11 were moderately rough. (This impression was later confirmed by examination of listeners' mean roughness ratings, which spanned the entire scale and were approximately normally distributed.) An additional 8 voices were selected at random from a similar library of normal voices, except that the normal speakers were roughly matched in age to the pathological speakers (range 30–70 years; mean age = 56.6 years; *SD* = 14.2 years). All speakers were recorded using the same procedures and equipment. They were asked (among other tasks) to sustain the vowel /ɑ/ at comfortable levels of pitch and loudness for as long as possible.

Voice samples were low-pass filtered at 8 kHz and then sampled at 20 kHz using a 12-bit A/D converter. A 3-sec segment was extracted from the middle of each speaker's vowel. These digitized segments were normalized for peak voltage. The onsets and offsets were multiplied by a 50 msec ramp to reduce click artifacts. Stimuli were then output at 20 kHz through a 12-bit D/A converter, again using an 8 kHz low-pass filter.

Tapes

Two stimulus tapes were constructed. Each included two repetitions of each stimulus voice (so test-retest reliability could be evaluated) for a total of 60 trials per tape. For each tape, the 30 stimulus voices were randomized, played out, rerandomized, and played out again. Trials were separated by 6 sec. Listeners were not informed that any voices were repeated.

Tasks

Each listener participated in two listening sessions. At the first, he or she judged the roughness of the voices using a 7-point equal-appearing interval (EAI) scale. This scale was selected because it is commonly used in voice perception research. At the second listening session, listeners judged the voices using a 10 cm visual analog (VA) scale. This scale was selected because pilot studies (e.g., Kempster, 1987) suggested it is more reliable than EAI scales.

Procedure

Because knowing how (and how much) listeners differ in their voice ratings is a first step toward understanding why they differ, our primary interest in this study was to compare the voice ratings of individual listeners. Given this perspective, it was important that differences among listeners within a task not be confounded with possible learning effects associated with different task presentation orders. For this reason, tape and task presentation orders were not counterbalanced across listeners in this first experiment. Instead, all listeners made judgments using the EAI scale first, followed by VA scale judgments; and all listeners heard tape 1 before tape 2. Thus the effects of task order and tape order, if any, were constant across listeners, and all listeners within a condition could be compared without any confounding effects. (These effects are examined separately in Experiment 2 below.) Test sessions were separated by at least 1 week to minimize learning effects across tasks.

Listeners received no formal training or instruction in the use of either scale. For the EAI scale task, they were asked to circle a single number to indicate the degree of roughness for each voice sample. They were asked not to circle between numbers and to try to use the whole scale. For the VA scale they were asked to make a single clear, unambiguous mark on an undifferentiated 10 cm line to indicate the roughness of each sample. The left and right endpoints of both the EAI and VA scales were labeled "not rough at all" and "extremely rough," respectively. However, listeners were offered no definition of roughness, but were asked to apply whatever standards or criteria they normally used in their practices when making their judgments.

For both tasks, separate answer sheets were provided for every voice, to minimize interactions among ratings. Listeners were asked not to refer to any previous ratings when judging the voices, and they were not permitted to change answers after hearing subsequent voices.

Listeners were tested individually in a sound-treated booth. Tapes were played at a comfortable listening level (approximately 75 dB SPL) in free field over two speakers equidistant from the listener. Each experimental session lasted approximately 15 minutes.

Results

Intrarater Reliability

Table 1 lists values of the most common measures of test-retest agreement and reliability, calculated from our data. On the average, ratings of these voices did not vary much from first to second rating. Squared values of Pearson's *r* (which measure the amount of variance common to two sets of ratings) suggest that overall about 74% of variance is consistent across rating occasions. Most statistics give approximately the same estimates of intrarater agreement and reliability, with the exception of Pearson's *r* for the medians of the first and second ratings. This statistic inflated reliability levels relative to the others examined here, because calculating median values prior to correlations removes most of the variance from the data before measuring reliability. Thus this statistic is not a good measure of intrarater reliability.

Although average statistics indicate reasonable intrarater agreement and reliability, individual listeners did vary in their performance. For both scales, squared correlations between the first and second ratings were below .75 for 8 of the 20 raters. Squared correlations were above .9 for only one rater. For the worst rater, r^2 was .55 for the EAI scale and only .41 for the VA scale.

TABLE 1. Measures of intrarater (test-retest) reliability.

Statistic	EAI ratings	VA ratings
Exact agreement	47.5%	
SD	11.1%	
Range	20–63.3%	
Mean ratings ± one scale value	84.7%	
SD	8.39%	
Range	68–93%	
Mean Pearson's *r*	.86	.86
SD	.06	.07
Range	.74–.95	.64–.97
Pearson's *r* for medians of 1st and 2nd rating	.95	.98
Mean Spearman's rho	.86	.86
SD	.06	.06
Range	.74–.96	.69–.96
Mean gamma coefficient	.86	.71
SD	.07	.08
Range	.72–.95	.50–.88
Significant *t*-test: 1st vs. 2nd rating	9/20	0/20

T-tests reveal a consistent trend in the EAI ratings for many listeners: Voices were rated as rougher when presented the second time during that listening session than they were the first time they were rated. Differences were significant when all listeners were combined in a single analysis (paired samples *t*-test, $t(359) = -6.65, p < .01$) and for 9 out of 20 individual listeners. Eight of these 9 clinicians had less than 3 years' experience evaluating voice quality. Ratings for the other 11 listeners showed the same trend, but the differences did not reach statistical significance. VA scale ratings showed no such effects, either for the group (paired samples t (359) $= -0.57$, $p > .01$) or for any individual listeners.

No other significant relationship was found between measured intrarater agreement and reliability and the amount of experience listeners had evaluating voice quality, for either scale. For the EAI ratings, the correlation between agreement (± one scale value) and years experience was .38 ($p > .01$). For exact agreement, the correlation was .31 ($p > .01$). For reliability measured with Pearson's *r*, the correlation was .38 ($p > .01$). For the VA scale, the correlation between Pearson's *r* values and years of experience was .29 ($p > .01$). Scatterplots confirmed that listeners varied in intrarater reliability at every level of experience. It was not the case that listeners with relatively little experience varied in reliability and more experienced listeners were consistently reliable.

Interrater Agreement and Reliability

Measures of interrater agreement and reliability are given in Table 2. The intraclass correlation was calculated using the formula for ICC(2,1) and a fully random effects ANOVA

TABLE 2. Measures of interrater reliability.

Statistic	EAI ratings	VA ratings
Mean exact agreement	33.7%	
SD	8.3%	
Range	6.7–56.7%	
Mean ratings ± one scale value	74.5%	
SD	8.52%	
Range	50–91.7%	
Mean Pearson's *r*	.78	.78
SD	.07	.07
Range	.55–.92	.56–.92
Mean Spearman's rho	.78	.78
SD	.07	.06
Range	.55–.92	.57–.90
Intraclass correlation		
Reliability of single rating	.79	.78
95% confidence interval	$.70 < \rho < .87$	$.69 < \rho < .87$
Reliability of mean rating	.99	.99
Kendall's Coefficient of Concordance	0.76	0.79

model. Squaring values of ICC(2,1) and average Pearson's *r* indicates that roughly 60% of variance in roughness ratings is explainable in terms of shared variance. Note that the 95% confidence intervals for the intraclass correlation suggest that our estimate of this parameter is not particularly precise: The true ICC value for the EAI ratings is probably between .7 and .87, and for the VA ratings it is probably between .69 and .87. Levels of exact agreement between pairs of listeners are consistently lower than are correlation values, indicating that listeners agreed about the relative roughness of the voices, but differed in the precise meaning assigned to each scale value. The value of ICC(2,20), which measures the reliability of the mean ratings of the voices, is nearly unity for both scales, suggesting that stable average ratings may be obtained with fewer than 20 listeners. Note that these values are considerably higher than those of other measures of the reliability of individual raters, as discussed above.

Despite the levels of average agreement, the range of values for these statistics indicates that many pairs of listeners are not in good agreement with one another in their judgments of vocal roughness. Only 12 out of 190 (6.3%) pairs of raters agreed with r^2 greater than .75 for the EAI scale. For the VA scale, only 20 of 190 pairs of raters (10.5%) agreed at r^2 levels greater than .75. In contrast, for the EAI scale 29 of 190 pairs of raters (15.3%) agreed at r^2 levels below .5 (less than half the variance in ratings shared by the two raters); 26 of 190 (13.7%) pairs of raters shared less than half the variance in ratings for the VA scale. Measures that represent an average of many pairwise comparisons (e.g., average Pearson's *r* or the average number of ratings within ± one scale value) mask the low probability of two individuals agreeing closely and the substantial probability of poor agreement between individuals.

TABLE 3. Intrarater agreement for EAI ratings of pathological and normal voices.*

	Pathological voices	Normal voices
% Exact Agreement	42.7	60.6
SD	11.1	20.8
Range	18.2–63.6	25.0–100
% ± One Scale Value	81.6	93.1
SD	9.1	11.1
Range	63.6–95.5	62.5–100

*Based on 20 individual raters. For the pathological voices, $n = 22$; for the normal voices, $n = 8$.

Pathological Versus Normal Voices

Table 3 shows intrarater agreement levels for EAI ratings of pathological and normal voices. Levels of exact test-retest agreement are given first, followed by agreement within ± one scale value. Due to the highly restricted range of ratings for the normal voices, other measures of agreement/reliability, such as Pearson's *r*, could not be meaningfully calculated. These analyses therefore include only ratings on the EAI scale. Although ranges of agreement levels overlap considerably, test-retest agreement was significantly greater for normal than for pathological voices, for both measures of agreement (exact agreement: paired samples $t = -3.90$, $df = 19$, $p < .01$; agreement within ± one scale value: paired samples $t = -4.71$, $df = 19$, $p < .01$).

Table 4 shows levels of interrater agreement for EAI ratings of pathological and normal voices. As above, agreement levels were significantly greater for normal than for pathological voices (exact agreement: paired samples $t = -12.46$, $df = 189$, $p < .01$; agreement within ± one scale value: paired samples $t = -27.18$, $df = 189$, $p < .01$).

Agreement Levels for Individual Voices

When examined voice by voice, listeners' ratings appear extremely variable. Ratings for 4 of the 22 pathological voices spanned the entire 7-point scale. Six additional voices received nearly the full possible range of ratings; ratings ranged from 2 to 7 for one voice, and from 1 to 6 for

TABLE 4. Interrater agreement for pathological and normal voices.*

	Pathological voices	Normal voices
% Exact Agreement	29.3	46.1
SD	9.7	16.3
Range	6.8–52.3	6.3–81.3
% ± One Scale Value	68.0	90.5
SD	10.1	8.5
Range	40.9–88.6	62.5–100

*Based on 190 pairs of raters. For the pathological voices, $n = 44$ (22 voices, each rated twice); for the normal voices, $n = 16$ (8 voices, each rated twice).

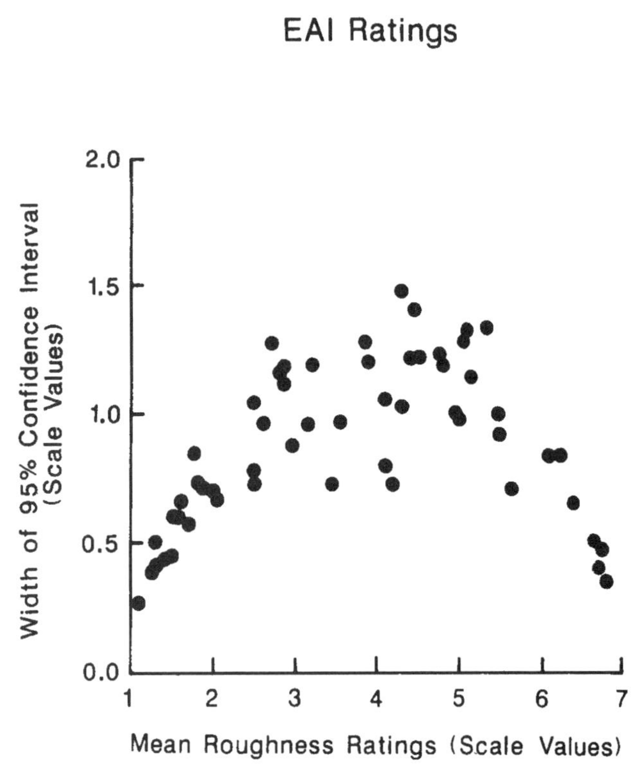

FIGURE 1. The width of the 95% confidence interval for a voice's mean rating vs. the mean rating for that voice on the EAI scale. Wider confidence intervals indicate more variance in ratings across listeners. Listeners agreed best (i.e., ratings were least variable) for voices rated normal or extremely rough; ratings varied most (confidence intervals were widest) for voices whose average rating was near the middle of the scale.

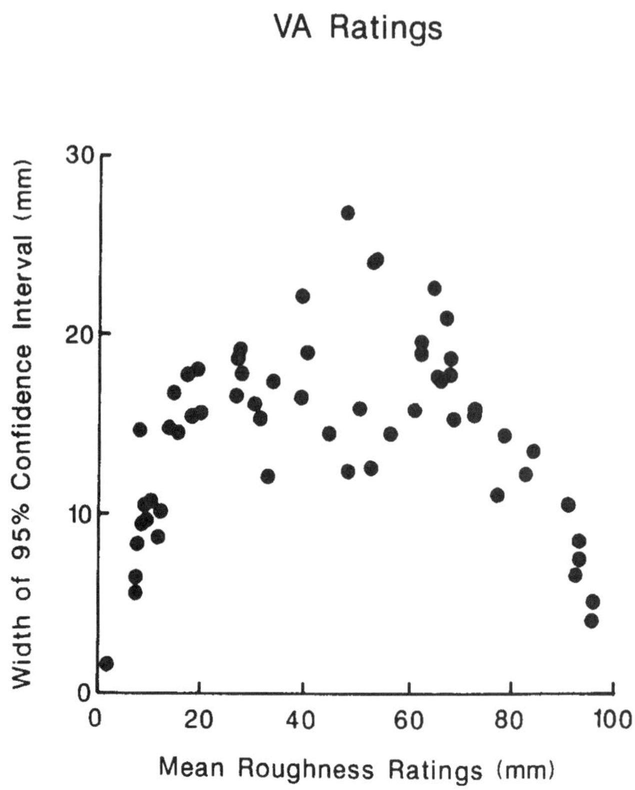

FIGURE 2. The width of the 95% confidence interval for a voice's mean rating vs. the mean rating for that voice on the VA scale. As for the EAI scale, ratings are most variable in the middle range of average roughness and least variable for voices that are near-normal or extremely rough.

five others. Across listeners, the range of ratings was three scale values or less for only three pathological voices (one whose ratings ranged from 1 to 3, one from 5 to 7, and one from 6 to 7). Agreement was not appreciably better for the normal voices. Ratings spanned three scale values or less for only 4 of the 8 speakers (from 1 to 2 or from 1 to 3).

The average range for the VA ratings of pathological voices was 69.5 mm (out of a possible 100). Ratings for three voices spanned more than 90 mm. The maximum range was 95.5 mm, and the minimum range was 32.5 mm. Ratings for the normal voices were not less variable than those for the pathological voices (an average range of 59.6 mm; $F(1, 28) = 2.05$, $p > .01$). The minimum range for the normal voices was 34 mm; the maximum was 75 mm.

Confidence intervals were calculated as a measure of the variability in ratings for each individual voice, using the large-sample formula: 95% confidence interval = mean rating ± (1.96* standard error of the mean) (e.g., Hays, 1973). For EAI ratings, confidence intervals ranged in width from .27 scale values to 1.48 scale values. For the VA scale, they ranged from 1.71 mm to 26.77 mm. The average confidence interval widths (.85 scale values for the EAI ratings and 14.4 mm for the VA ratings) again reflect the overall variability in ratings of individual voices across raters.

Figures 1 and 2 show the 95% confidence interval plotted against the mean rating for each voice for the EAI and VA scales, respectively. These figures show that ratings are much more variable in the midrange of vocal roughness (cf. Arends, Povel, van Os, & Speth, 1990; Kearns & Simmons, 1988). Confidence intervals for near-normal and extremely rough voices are markedly narrower than are those for mildly to moderately rough voices.

Discussion

As suggested by the literature review above, listeners varied widely in their levels of reliability and agreement, and some individual voices were much more likely to receive consistent ratings across listeners than others. Because all listeners in this experiment performed the tasks in the same order, reliability and agreement scores within a task condition are not confounded with presentation orders. Thus, comparisons among subjects and voices in reliability/agreement levels within a task reflect the range of expert skills on that scale under identical conditions. Had task order been randomized across subjects, within-task variability in reliability would include effects of different task orders, making it difficult to draw conclusions about the range of listener performance within a task.

Listener performance appeared quite similar overall on the EAI and VA tasks. However, between-task comparisons in this study are confounded with the fixed presentation order. For example, reliability for VA ratings may be inflated by learning effects, making findings of similar reliability levels for

TABLE 5. Measures of intrarater (test-retest) reliability: Experiment 2.

Statistic	EAI ratings	VA ratings
% Exact agreement	39.7	
SD	13.57	
Range	26.7–66.7	
Mean % ratings ± one scale value	81.0	
SD	13.70	
Range	56.7–100	
Mean Pearson's *r*	.80	.81
SD	.09	.05
Range	.66–.90	.73–.88
Pearson's *r* for medians of 1st and 2nd rating	.95	.96
Mean Spearman's rho	.80	.79
SD	.10	.06
Range	.59–.91	.68–.88
Mean gamma coefficient	.80	.62
SD	.12	.07
Range	.56–.96	.5–.67
Significant *t*-test: 1st vs. 2nd rating	4/10	1/10

the two scales incorrect. Further, drift may have occurred in the EAI task because it was presented first, whereas learning effects prevented such drift in the VA task. Thus it is not possible to determine from the present results if drift is a characteristic of EAI scales or an artifact of our design. Experiment 2 was undertaken to examine directly the role of task order in our results.

EXPERIMENT 2

Method

Ten additional subjects participated in this experiment. Eight were otolaryngologists and two were speech-language pathologists/voice researchers. None had participated in Experiment 1. They averaged 6 years' postgraduate experience evaluating and treating voice disorders (*SD* = 5.37 years; range = 3 to 20 years).

These listeners heard the same experimental tapes as in Experiment 1, but performed the tasks in the reverse order (i.e., VA task first, followed by the EAI task). Test sessions were again separated by at least 1 week. All other methods were as described in Experiment 1 above.

Results and Discussion

Intrarater reliability and agreement levels for Experiment 2 are reported in Table 5. Ranges of scores are comparable to those observed in Experiment 1. One-way ANOVAs showed no significant effect of task presentation order on levels of within-subject agreement on the EAI task (exact agreement: $F(1, 28) = 0.83$, $p > .01$; agreement within ± one scale value: $F(1, 28) = 2.87$, $p > .01$). A two-way ANOVA (experimental order × task) compared average values of Pearson's *r* for intrarater reliability on the VA and EAI tasks for the two presentation orders. The subjects in Experiment 2 were significantly less reliable overall on this measure than those in Experiment 1 [$F(1, 56) = 13.39$, $p < .01$]. However, the two tasks did not differ in intrarater reliability [$F(1, 56 = 0.06$, $p > .01$], and no experiment-by-task interaction was observed. Note that 95% confidence intervals for ICC(2,1) in Table 6 blanket those in Table 2, indicating that on this measure the two subject groups did not differ significantly in overall interrater reliability for either task.

Table 6 shows interrater agreement and reliability for Experiment 2. Again, ranges of scores are comparable to those in Experiment 1. For the EAI scale, listeners in this second experiment agreed less well on the average than those in Experiment 1, for both exact agreement [$F(1, 233) = 14.63$, $p < .01$] and agreement within ± one scale value [$F(1, 233) = 13.06$, $p < .01$]. A two-way ANOVA (experiment × task) showed that subjects in Experiment 2 were less reliable overall than those in Experiment 1 [$F(1, 466) = 80.45$, $p < .01$]. The two tasks did not differ significantly [$F(1, 466) = 0.24$, $p > .01$], and there was no task × experiment interaction [$F(1, 466) = 0.90$, $p > .01$]. In contrast, 95% confidence intervals for the ICC show no significant differences between tasks in levels of interrater reliability.

Finally, ratings showed the same patterns of "drift" when tasks were presented in the reverse order. Across the entire set of raters, voices were rated rougher the second time they were heard than the first for the EAI task (matched pairs *t* =

TABLE 6. Measures of interrater reliability: Experiment 2.

Statistic	EAI ratings	VA ratings
Mean % exact agreement	28.4	
SD	8.05	
Range	10.0–46.7	
Mean % ratings ± one scale value	68.8	
SD	13.01	
Range	33.3–93.3	
Mean Pearson's *r*	.71	.69
SD	.11	.08
Range	.39–.89	.44–.83
Mean Spearman's rho	.71	.70
SD	.12	.09
Range	.36–.90	.45–.84
Intraclass correlation		
Reliability of single rating	.71	.64
95% confidence interval	$.57 < \rho < .83$	$.48 < \rho < .79$
Reliability of mean rating	.96	.95
Kendall's Coefficient of Concordance	.71	.73

-4.23, $df = 179$, $p < .01$), but not for the VA task (matched pairs $t = -0.75$, $df = 179$, $p > .01$). Results were significant for 4 of the 10 individual raters for the EAI task (compared to 9 of 20 in Experiment 1), and for only 1 rater in the VA task (versus 0 in Experiment 1).

These results confirm our finding that experienced listeners vary widely in their ratings of the same voices. No evidence of a significant effect of presentation order was observed. We therefore conclude that differences between the two tasks in patterns of drift were due to differences between the rating scales themselves and were not artifacts of a fixed presentation order.

GENERAL DISCUSSION

Our findings may be summarized as follows. Previous studies using listener ratings to evaluate speech and voice quality have varied widely in the methods applied. Many studies suffer from methodological weaknesses, including failure to evaluate listener reliability, inadequate samples of raters, too few repeated trials for intrarater reliability estimates, failure to report confidence intervals, and use of inappropriate statistics. Across studies, no clear relationship between methods and reliability/agreement has emerged, and no model of voice perception or the rating process has been developed.

Although the present research examined ratings of a single perceptual quality (roughness), many of our findings are consistent with the literature on voice and speech ratings. Thus, we feel our findings may be generalized to ratings of other voice and speech qualities. Our results suggest that average levels of intra- and interrater reliability are relatively high, but that considerable variability underlies average values (see, e.g., Cullinan et al., 1963; Kempster, 1984). EAI ratings—but not VA ratings—drifted significantly during a single listening session, with voices sounding rougher the second time they were evaluated. Ratings for individual voices varied widely across raters. Ratings varied more for pathological than for normal voices and more for mild-to-moderately rough voices than for voices at scale extremes. Order of task presentation had no significant effect on listener performance.

To account for these findings, we propose the following descriptive theoretical framework for perceptual evaluations of voice quality. It includes factors drawn from the literature and from the studies described above. Although this framework is clearly preliminary and includes elements that are speculative, we feel it provides a useful format for conceptualizing the voice perception process and may allow a coherent experimental approach to be developed.

A Conceptual Framework for Voice Quality Perception

When listeners rate a voice on some dimension (e.g., breathiness or roughness), they compare the stimulus presented to an internal standard or scale. We suggest that listeners develop individual internal standards for vocal qualities through their experience with voices (Kreiman, Gerratt, Precoda, & Berke, 1992). These standards represent "average" or "typical" exemplars for some level of the quality being rated, based on that listener's experience.

Listeners may differ in where along the severity continuum they place their internal standards. Individuals may also differ in the amount of detail present in their internal representation of vocal qualities. Accordingly, the precise number of severity levels represented in memory probably differs from listener to listener. Scant evidence regarding the nature of internal representations for voices has been published. To date, arguments have been based on patterns of confusions in short-term memory (Kreiman & Papcun, 1991) and long-term memory (Papcun, Kreiman, & Davis, 1989) and spatial representations from multidimensional scaling (Kreiman, Gerratt, & Precoda, 1990; Kreiman et al., 1992). Clearly many more such studies are needed.

Existing evidence from multidimensional scaling provides support for the existence of individual internal standards for voice quality. Kreiman et al. (1992) have argued that all listeners have similar, relatively stable internal standards for "normal" voice quality, because all listeners have extensive and approximately equal experience with normal voices (through their everyday contact with normal speakers). Therefore, similarity ratings (and ratings of specific qualities in the present study) consistently show relatively little variation within and across listeners for normal and near-normal voices.

Expert listeners (particularly less-experienced ones) differ in their experience with pathological voices, so internal standards for pathological qualities differ from listener to listener (Kreiman et al., 1992). Naive listeners, on the other hand, have no formal exposure to pathological voices and thus appear to lack specific internal standards for judging pathological qualities. Naive listeners apparently judge pathological speakers according to standards better suited to normal voices. Their perceptual strategies are therefore quite similar. In contrast, expert listeners vary widely in their perceptions of pathological voices (Kreiman et al., 1990; Kreiman et al., 1992).

The results presented in this paper further suggest that internal standards for vocal qualities are inherently unstable and that a listener's notion of the extent of roughness or breathiness may be influenced by factors other than the acoustic characteristics of the voice being judged. As reported above, EAI ratings drifted significantly in a consistent direction within a listening session. The stimulus set used here contained a number of normal (8/30) and near-normal (5/30) voices. We suggest that this unbalanced context systematically influenced listeners' internal standards for roughness. That is, over time the rougher voices began to sound worse by comparison to the large number of normal and near-normal samples. Although all listeners in this study had at least 2 years' experience rating voices, eight of the nine clinicians whose ratings drifted significantly in Experiment 1 (and two of the four in Experiment 2) were relatively inexperienced. This suggests listeners need many years to develop a stable set of criteria for this kind of rating. This is consistent with the failure of extensive training to improve the reliability of voice quality ratings in the literature reviewed above.

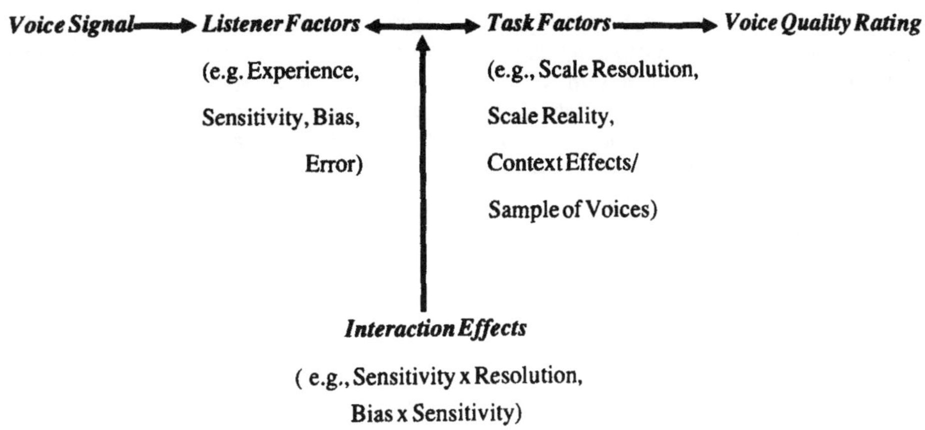

FIGURE 3. Factors involved in mapping an acoustic signal onto a voice quality rating.

Similar drift in ratings was not observed for the VA scale. This asymmetry, which has also been reported in studies evaluating the quality of synthetic speech (Rossi, Pavlovic, & Espesser, 1990), may be related to the relative coarseness/fineness of the two scale types. The EAI scale required listeners to distinguish seven levels of roughness; however, the VA scale (an undifferentiated line) in principle assumes listeners can distinguish a very large number of levels of roughness. When a scale is fine relative to a listener's ability to make judgments, measurements will include some random error related to the mismatch between scale resolution and the listener's perceptual acuity. For example, if a listener can reliably distinguish only five levels of breathiness, but breathiness is measured on a 100-point scale, the difference between ratings of 40, 45, and 52 may not be meaningful, and these numbers may be assigned to the same stimulus. This sort of error may have made drift difficult to detect on a VA scale.

The number of levels of roughness listeners can reliably distinguish and identify is not known. The 7-point EAI scale is probably slightly coarse relative to listeners' acuity, and the continuous 100 mm VA scale (with responses measured to the nearest 0.5 mm) is probably too fine. Further research may clarify these issues.

Sources of Variability in Voice Quality Ratings

The above discussion suggests that several factors are involved in mapping an acoustic signal onto a voice quality rating (Figure 3). The first is the acoustic voice signal being rated. Most studies of voice quality in the literature apparently assume that mapping between physical signals and psychological qualities is a constant, linear process and thus treat any variation in ratings as random error by raters. However, our findings indicate that several consistent—and thus potentially controllable—factors also contribute to observed voice ratings.

The rated quality a listener derives from a signal may be systematically affected by several factors related to the listeners. These factors include listeners' experience with voices (which will shape their particular internal standard[s] for the quality being judged), their individual perceptual habits and biases (Kreiman et al., 1990; Kreiman et al., 1992), and presumably overall sensitivity to the quality being judged. These factors change relatively slowly over time and thus hypothetically affect interrater reliability more than intrarater reliability. Additional factors related to listeners include fatigue, attention lapses, and mistakes. These "error" terms should affect both intra- and interrater reliability.

Factors related to the task of rating also systematically affect measurements of voice quality. If the quality to be rated is poorly defined or lacks perceptual reality, listeners will not be able to rate it consistently. Our results suggest perceptual context may cause systematic drift in ratings, presumably because of its effect of altering a listener's internal standards. We test this hypothesis directly in a companion paper (Kreiman, Gerratt, & Berke, 1993). These (and possibly other) factors can affect ratings within a given session and thus affect both intra- and interrater reliability.

Several systematic interactions among listener and task factors may also occur. Listener sensitivity may interact with scale resolution, and mismatches may add noise to the data or result in information loss. Also, listener biases may interact with "scale specificity." If the quality being rated is multidimensional in nature but is rated on a unidimensional scale, listeners may selectively focus on one dimension or another, reducing apparent agreement levels. For example, recent findings (Kreiman, Gerratt, & Berke, 1992) suggest that breathiness and roughness are related, multidimensional constructs. These investigators demonstrated that listeners' differential attention to various aspects of each quality is a significant source of interrater unreliability in voice quality ratings.

Conclusions and Implications for Research Design

Our findings paint a rather bleak picture of the current state of voice quality ratings. A review of the literature suggests that existing protocols do not consistently result in reliable ratings. Although intrarater and interrater reliability varied considerably across studies, they did not vary consistently with any of the methodological factors reviewed, including levels of task-specific training or the actual rating task used.

The present experimental results suggest that even highly experienced listeners frequently disagree completely about what they hear. Finally, the presence of an error term in our theoretical framework suggests that perfect reliability and agreement are not achievable, even in theory. It appears that nearly 30 years of research have returned us to the point articulated by Jensen in 1965: "... the assumption that the perceptual characteristics of a person's voice provide sufficient information for a reliable description of vocal deviation and its severity appears to be hazardous" (p. 82).

Nevertheless, the theoretical framework presented above does offer a potential remedy for this situation. It suggests that variability in voice quality ratings might be reduced by replacing listeners' idiosyncratic, unstable, internal standards with fixed external standards or "reference voices" for different vocal qualities. A voice rating protocol using fixed reference voices would reduce listener-related rating variability by providing all raters with a constant set of perceptual referents. Similar protocols using explicitly presented standards have improved listener performance in other kinds of auditory judgment tasks (for example, ratings of the intensity of tones: Berliner, Durlach, & Braida, 1978). Such a protocol for rating voice quality would also control context-related variability, because external standards remain constant from trial to trial.[5] (See the companion paper, Gerratt et al., 1993, for further discussion of anchored protocols for voice quality ratings.)

Pending development of new protocols, several other improvements may be made to existing research techniques. First, both intra- and interrater reliability must be reported in all studies using voice quality ratings. Our findings and the discussion above suggest that there is no one best measure of "listener concordance." Rather, statistics should be chosen on the basis of the characteristics of the application and of the data. In cases where the exact value of the ratings is not important, reliability should be assessed with the intraclass correlation (using the appropriate ANOVA model). However, if it is important that the meaning of each scale value be constant across raters (for example, in studies with strong clinical implications), agreement should also be assessed. If the stimulus voices vary little on a given quality (for example, if patients with a single diagnosis are studied), then statistics like Pearson's r that are sensitive to the range of values should be avoided. In all cases, authors should report ranges and confidence intervals for any measures used and should explicitly justify their selection of reliability and/or agreement measures.

Our results suggest that traditional voice rating methods may never generate ratings that consistently meet strict standards for reliability. However, new rating protocols may be developed to control some of the sources of variability in listeners' perceptions of vocal quality. In particular, main and interaction effects involving task factors can be eliminated by designing scales and protocols (possibly using fixed reference voices) that eliminate context effects and unnecessary rating noise from measures of voice quality. Such protocols might also benefit research aimed at developing instrumental measures of voice. For example, more valid and reliable perceptual measures of voice quality may facilitate the search for acoustic correlates of perceived vocal qualities. As our methods of voice assessment improve with further research, voice ratings will approach maximum reliability and validity.

[5]Random error may also be reduced by careful attention to listening conditions, by motivating subjects adequately to pay attention, and by limiting the number of judgments made at any one session.

Acknowledgments

We thank our expert listeners Mary J. Bacon, Steven Bielamowicz, Robert Block, Nancy Brough, Hong-Shik Choi, S. Trey Fyte, Patricia Gomeztrejo, Susanne Hildebrand, Leona Hubatch, Ann E. Kalec, Daniel Kempler, Ming Ye, Julianne Morlock, Lee Nguyen, Janet Novak, Clare Anne Paskiet, Douglas Ross, Shimon Sapir, Joel Sercarz, Steven Sloan, Julie Trautmann, Diana Van Lancker, and Mary Walsh, for volunteering their time. This work was supported in part by grant # DC 00855-01 from the NIDCD and Merit Review funds from the DVA.

References

Anders, L., Hollien, H., Hurme, P., Sonninen, A., & Wendler, J. (1988). Perception of hoarseness by several classes of listeners. *Folia Phoniatrica, 40,* 91–100.

Arends, N., Povel, D-J., Os, E. van, & Speth, L. (1990). Predicting voice quality of deaf speakers on the basis of certain glottal characteristics. *Journal of Speech and Hearing Research, 33,* 116–122.

Arnold, K. S., & Emanuel, F. (1979). Spectral noise levels and roughness severity ratings for vowels produced by male children. *Journal of Speech and Hearing Research, 22,* 613–626.

Askenfelt, A. G., & Hammarberg, B. (1986). Speech waveform perturbation analysis: A perceptual-acoustical comparison of seven measures. *Journal of Speech and Hearing Research, 29,* 50–64.

Baken, R. J. (1987). *Clinical measurement of speech and voice.* Boston: College Hill.

Bassich, C., & Ludlow, C. (1986). The use of perceptual methods by new clinicians for assessing voice quality. *Journal of Speech and Hearing Disorders, 51,* 125–133.

Berk, R. (1979). Generalizability of behavioral observations: A clarification of interobserver agreement and interobserver reliability. *American Journal of Mental Deficiency, 83,* 460–472.

Berliner, J.E., Durlach, N. I., & Braida, L. D. (1978). Intensity perception IX: Effect of fixed standard on resolution in identification. *Journal of the Acoustical Society of America, 64,* 687–689.

Brancewicz, T. M., & Reich, A. R. (1989). Speech rate reduction and "nasality" in normal speakers. *Journal of Speech and Hearing Research, 32,* 837–848.

Coleman, R. F. (1969). Effect of median frequency levels upon the roughness of jittered stimuli. *Journal of Speech and Hearing Research, 12,* 330–336.

Coleman, R. F. (1971). Effect of waveform changes upon roughness perception. *Folia Phoniatrica, 23,* 314–322.

Coleman, F., & Wendahl, R. (1967). Vocal roughness and stimulus duration. *Speech Monographs, 34,* 85–92.

Cullinan, W. L., Prather, E. M., & Williams, D. E. (1963). Comparison of procedures for scaling severity of stuttering. *Journal of Speech and Hearing Research, 6,* 187–194.

Darley, F., Aronson, A., & Brown, J. (1969). Differential diagnostic patterns of dysarthria. *Journal of Speech and Hearing Research, 12,* 246–269.

Deal, R. E., & Belcher, R. A. (1990). Reliability of children's ratings of vocal roughness. *Language, Speech, and Hearing Services in Schools, 21,* 68–71.

Deal, R., & Emanuel, F. (1978). Some waveform and spectral features of vowel roughness. *Journal of Speech and Hearing Research, 21,* 250–264.

Dunn-Rankin, P. (1983). *Scaling methods.* Hillsdale, NJ: Lawrence Erlbaum Associates.

Ebel, R. (1951). Estimation of the reliability of ratings. *Psychometrica,16,* 407–424.

Emanuel, F., Lively, M. A., & McCoy, J. (1973). Spectral noise levels and roughness ratings for vowels produced by males and females. *Folia Phoniatrica, 25,* 110–120.

Emanuel, F., & Sansone, F. (1969). Some spectral features of "normal" and simulated "rough" vowels. *Folia Phoniatrica, 21,* 401–415.

Emanuel, F., & Scarinzi, A. (1979). Vocal register effects on vowel spectral noise and roughness: Findings for adult females. *Journal of Communication Disorders, 12,* 263–272.

Emanuel, F., & Smith, W. (1974). Pitch effects on vowel roughness and spectral noise. *Journal of Phonetics, 2,* 247–253.

Fritzell, B., Hammarberg, B., Gauffin, J., Karlsson, I., & Sundberg, J. (1986). Breathiness and insufficient vocal fold closure. *Journal of Phonetics, 14,* 549–553.

Fukazawa, T., & El-Assuooty, A. (1988). A new index for evaluation of the turbulent noise in pathological voice. *Journal of the Acoustical Society of America, 83,* 1189–1193.

Gelfer, Marylou P. (1988). Perceptual attributes of voice: Development and use of rating scales. *Journal of Voice, 2,* 320–326.

Gerratt, B. R., Kreiman, J., Antonanzas-Barroso, N., & Berke, G. (1993). Comparing internal and external standards in voice quality judgments. *Journal of Speech and Hearing Research, 36,* 14–20.

Gerratt, B. R., Till, J. A., Rosenbek, J. C., Wertz, R. T., & Boysen, A. E. (1991). Use and perceived value of perceptual and instrumental measures in dysarthria management. In C. A. Moore, K. M. Yorkston, & D. R. Beukelman (Eds.), *Dysarthria and apraxia of speech* (pp. 77–93). Baltimore, MD: Brookes.

Hammarberg, B., Fritzell, B., Gauffin, J., & Sundberg, J. (1986). Acoustic and perceptual analysis of vocal dysfunction. *Journal of Phonetics, 14,* 533–547.

Hammarberg, B., Fritzell, B., Gauffin, J., Sundberg, J., & Wedin, L. (1980). Perceptual and acoustic correlates of abnormal voice qualities. *Acta Otolaryngologica, 90,* 441–451.

Hammarberg, B., Fritzell, B., & Schiratzki, H. (1984). Teflon injection in 16 patients with paralytic dysphonia: Perceptual and acoustic evaluations. *Journal of Speech and Hearing Disorders, 49,* 72–82.

Hays, W. L. (1973). *Statistics for the social sciences* (2nd ed.). New York: Holt, Rinehart and Winston.

Heiberger, V. L., & Horii, Y. (1982). Jitter and shimmer in sustained phonation. In N. J. Lass (Ed.), *Speech and language: Advances in basic research and practice* (Vol. 7, pp. 299–332). New York: Academic Press.

Hillenbrand, J. (1988). Perception of aperiodicities in synthetically generated voices. *Journal of the Acoustical Society of America, 83,* 2361–2371.

Hirano, M. (1981). *Clinical examination of voice.* Vienna: Springer.

Hopkins, B. L., & Hermann, R. J. (1977). Evaluating interobserver reliability of interval data. *Journal of Applied Behavior Analysis, 10,* 2141–2150.

Isshiki, N., Okamura, H., Tanabe, M., & Morimoto, M. (1969). Differential diagnosis of hoarseness. *Folia Phoniatrica, 21,* 9–19.

Isshiki, N., & Takeuchi, Y. (1970). Factor analysis of hoarseness. *Studia Phonologica, 5,* 37–44.

Jensen, P. J. (1965, December). Adequacy of terminology for clinical judgment of voice quality deviation. *The Eye, Ear, Nose and Throat Monthly, 44,* 77–82.

Kane, M., & Wellen, C. J. (1985). Acoustical measurements and clinical judgments of vocal quality in children with vocal nodules. *Folia Phoniatrica, 37,* 53–57.

Kearns, K., & Simmons, N. (1988). Interobserver reliability and perceptual ratings: More than meets the ear. *Journal of Speech and Hearing Research, 31,* 131–136.

Kempster, G. (1984). *A multidimensional analysis of vocal quality in two dysphonic groups.* Unpublished doctoral dissertation, Northwestern University, Chicago.

Kempster, G. (1987, November). *A comparison of two scales for measuring vocal quality.* Paper presented at the Annual Meeting of the American Speech-Language-Hearing Association, New Orleans, Louisiana.

Kempster, G. B., Kistler, D. J., & Hillenbrand, J. (1991). Multidimensional scaling analysis of dysphonia in two speakers groups. *Journal of Speech and Hearing Research, 34,* 534–543.

Klatt, D. H., & Klatt, L. C. (1990). Analysis, synthesis, and perception of voice quality variations among female and male talkers. *Journal of the Acoustical Society of America, 87,* 820–857.

Klich, R. J. (1982). Relationships of vowel characteristics to listener ratings of breathiness. *Journal of Speech and Hearing Research, 25,* 574–580.

Kojima, H., Gould, W., Lambiase, A., & Isshiki, N. (1980). Computer analysis of hoarseness. *Acta Oto-Laryngologica, 89,* 547–554.

Kreiman, J., Gerratt, B. R., & Berke, G. S. (1992). The multidimensional nature of pathologic vocal quality. Unpublished manuscript.

Kreiman, J., Gerratt, B. R., & Precoda, K. (1990). Listener experience and perception of voice quality. *Journal of Speech and Hearing Research, 33,* 103–115.

Kreiman, J., Gerratt, B. R., Precoda, K., & Berke, G. S. (1992). Individual differences in voice quality perception. *Journal of Speech and Hearing Research, 35,* 512–520.

Kreiman, J., & Papcun, G. (1991). Comparing discrimination and recognition of unfamiliar voices. *Speech Communication, 10,* 265–275.

Kreul, E. J., & Hecker, M. H. L. (1971). Description of the speech of patients with cancer of the vocal fold. Part II: Judgments of age and voice quality. *Journal of the Acoustical Society of America, 49,* 1283–1287.

Ladefoged, P., Maddieson, I., & Jackson, M. (1988). Investigating phonation types in different languages. In O. Fujimura (Ed.), *Vocal fold physiology: Voice production, mechanisms and functions* (pp. 297–317). New York: Raven Press.

Lively, M., & Emanuel, F. (1970). Spectral noise levels and roughness severity ratings for normal and simulated rough vowels produced by adult females. *Journal of Speech and Hearing Research, 13,* 503–517.

Martin, R. R., Haroldson, S. K., & Triden, K. A. (1984). Stuttering and speech naturalness. *Journal of Speech and Hearing Research, 49,* 53–58.

Monsen, R. B. (1979). Acoustic qualities of phonation in young hearing-impaired children. *Journal of Speech and Hearing Research, 22,* 270–288.

Montague, J. C., & Hollien, H. (1973). Perceived voice quality disorders in Down's Syndrome children. *Journal of Communication Disorders, 6,* 76–87.

Moody, D. K., Montague, J., & Bradley, B. (1979). Preliminary validity and reliability data on the Wilson Voice Profile System. *Language, Speech, and Hearing Services in Schools, 10,* 231–240.

Moran, M. J., & Gilbert, H. R. (1984). Relation between voice profile ratings and aerodynamic and acoustic parameters. *Journal of Communication Disorders, 17,* 245–260.

Nieboer, G. L., De Graaf, T., & Schutte, H. K. (1988). Esophageal voice quality judgments by means of the semantic differential. *Journal of Phonetics, 16,* 417–436.

Papcun, G., Kreiman, J., & Davis, A. (1989). Long-term memory for unfamiliar voices. *Journal of the Acoustical Society of America, 85,* 913–925.

Prosek, R. A., Montgomery, A. A., Walden, B. E., & Hawkins, D. B. (1987). An evaluation of residue features as correlates of voice disorders. *Journal of Communication Disorders, 20,* 105–117.

Ptacek, P. H., & Sander, E. K. (1963). Breathiness and phonation length. *Journal of Speech and Hearing Disorders, 28,* 267–272.

Rees, M. (1958). Some variables affecting perceived harshness. *Journal of Speech and Hearing Research, 1,* 155–168.

Reich, A., & Lerman, J. (1978). Teflon laryngoplasty: An acoustical and perceptual study. *Journal of Speech and Hearing Disorders, 43,* 496–505.

Rossi, M., Pavlovic, C., & Espesser, R. (1990, November). *Reduc-*

ing context effects in the subjective evaluation of speech quality. Paper presented at the 120th Meeting of the Acoustical Society of America, San Diego, California.

Samar, V., & Metz, D. (1988). Criterion validity of speech intelligibility rating-scale procedures for the hearing-impaired population. *Journal of Speech and Hearing Research, 31,* 307–316.

Sansone, F., Jr., & Emanuel, F. (1970). Spectral noise levels and roughness severity ratings for normal and simulated rough vowels produced by adult males. *Journal of Speech and Hearing Research, 13,* 489–502.

Sapir, S., & Aronson, A. E. (1985). Clinician reliability in rating voice improvement after laryngeal nerve section for spastic dysphonia. *Laryngoscope, 95,* 200–202.

Sapir, S., Aronson, A. E., & Thomas, J. E. (1986). Judgment of voice improvement after recurrent laryngeal nerve section for spastic dysphonia: Clinicians versus patients. *Annals of Otology, Rhinology, and Laryngology, 95,* 137–141.

Schiavetti, N., Metz, D. E., & Sitler, R. W. (1981). Construct validity of direct magnitude estimation and interval scaling of speech intelligibility: Evidence from a study of the hearing impaired. *Journal of Speech and Hearing Research, 24,* 441–445.

Schiavetti, N., Sacco, P. R., Metz, D. E., & Sitler, R. W. (1983). Direct magnitude estimation and interval scaling of stuttering severity. *Journal of Speech and Hearing Research, 26,* 568–573.

Sheard, C., Adams, R. D., & Davis, P. J. (1991). Reliability and agreement of ratings of ataxic dysarthric speech samples with varying intelligibility. *Journal of Speech and Hearing Research, 34,* 285–293.

Sherman, D., & Linke, E. (1952). The influence of certain vowel types on degree of harsh voice quality. *Journal of Speech and Hearing Disorders, 17,* 401–408.

Shipp, T., & Huntington, D. (1965). Some acoustic and perceptual factors in acute-laryngitic hoarseness. *Journal of Speech and Hearing Disorders, 30,* 350–359.

Shrout, P., & Fleiss, J. (1979). Intraclass correlations: Uses in assessing rater reliability. *Psychological Bulletin, 86,* 420–428.

Smith, B., Weinberg, B., Feth, L., & Horii, Y. (1978). Vocal roughness and jitter characteristics of vowels produced by esophageal speakers. *Journal of Speech and Hearing Research, 21,* 240–249.

Stoicheff, M. L., Ciampi, A., Passi, J. E., & Fredrickson, J. M. (1983). The irradiated larynx and voice: A perceptual study. *Journal of Speech and Hearing Research, 26,* 482–485.

Stone, R. E., & Sharf, D. J. (1973). Vocal change associated with the use of atypical pitch and intensity levels. *Folia Phoniatrica, 25,* 91–103.

Takahashi, H., & Koike, Y. (1975). Some perceptual dimensions and acoustic correlates of pathological voices. *Acta Otolaryngologica* (Suppl. 338), 2–24.

Tinsley, H., & Weiss, D. (1975). Interrater reliability and agreement of subjective judgments. *Journal of Counseling Psychology, 22,* 358–376.

Toner, M. A., & Emanuel, F. W. (1989). Direct magnitude estimation and equal appearing interval scaling of vowel roughness. *Journal of Speech and Hearing Research, 32,* 78–82.

Wendahl, R. W. (1966a). Some parameters of auditory roughness. *Folia Phoniatrica, 18,* 26–32.

Wendahl, R. W. (1966b). Laryngeal analog synthesis of jitter and shimmer auditory parameters of harshness. *Folia Phoniatrica, 18,* 98–108.

Wendler, J., Doherty, E. T., & Hollien, H. (1980). Voice classification by means of long-term speech spectra. *Folia Phoniatrica, 32,* 51–60.

Whitehead, R. L., & Emanuel, F. W. (1974). Some spectrographic and perceptual features of vocal fry, abnormally rough, and modal register vowel phonations. *Journal of Communication Disorders, 7,* 305–319.

Winer, B. J. (1971). *Statistical principles in experimental design* (2nd ed.). New York: McGraw-Hill.

Wolfe, V., & Ratusnik, D. (1988). Acoustic and perceptual measurements of roughness influencing judgments of pitch. *Journal of Speech and Hearing Disorders, 53,* 15–22.

Yumoto, E., Sasaski, Y., & Okamura, H. (1984). Harmonics-to-noise ratio and psychophysical measurement of the degree of hoarseness. *Journal of Speech and Hearing Research, 27,* 2–6.

Received May 12, 1992
Accepted July 10, 1992

Contact author: Jody Kreiman, PhD, VAMC, West Los Angeles, Audiology and Speech Pathology (126), Wilshire and Sawtelle Boulevards, Los Angeles, CA 90073.

Appendix

LITERATURE REVIEWED

Key to abbreviations: (Training) E = Extensive; O = Orientation (see text for definitions). (Scale) EAI = equal-appearing interval scale; DME = direct magnitude estimation; paired comp = paired comparison task. (Interrater reliability) ICC = Intraclass correlation.
[a]Not significant.

Study	Raters	Training	Scale	Intrarater reliability	Interrater reliability
Anders et al. (1988)	34 naive, 79 expert	not reported	4 categories hoarseness	40/40 rerated. t = 0.02–0.57[a]	not reported
Arends et al. (1990)	10 expert	"a few sessions" (E)	5 pt. EAI 4 scales	not reported	Pearson's r = .62–.89
Arnold & Emanuel (1979)	11 grad students	not reported	5 pt. EAI roughness	20/200 rerated. 55–100% ± 1 scale value	72–95% ± 1 scale value
Askenfelt & Hammarberg (1986)	6 expert	4 years min. (E)	5 pt. EAI 12 scales	8/41 rerated. Pearson's r = .86–.98; 86% ± 1 scale value	not reported
Bassich & Ludlow (1986)	4 grad students	8 hours (E)	n pt. EAI (varied with scale) 13 scales	4/21 rerated. 100% ± 1 scale value 75% exact agreement	Mean ICC = .8 across all scales for normal voices; = .71 for pathological voices
Brancewicz & Reich (1989)	10 expert	9 practice trials (O)	100 mm visual analog scale nasality	26/120 rerated. Pearson's r = .84–.90	ICC(3,10) = .66–.75
Coleman (1969)	32 psychology students	none	paired comp; 7 pt. EAI roughness	not reported	not reported
Coleman (1971)	15 undergrads	none	anchored DME roughness	not reported	not reported
Coleman & Wendahl (1967)	18 undergrads	not reported	paired comp roughness	not reported	not reported
Cullinan et al. (1963)	15–20 undergrads in each of 7 groups	samples of extremes provided (O)	5, 7, 9 pt. EAI; anchored DME severity of stuttering	27/27 rerated. "ANOVA technique"; reliability of 1 judge making 1 rating = .74–.80 across tasks	"ANOVA technique"; reliability of 1 judge making 1 rating = .48–.75 across tasks
Darley et al. (1969)	3 authors	discussed ratings during study (O)	7 pt. EAI 38 scales	30/212 rerated. 80–95% ± 1 scale value	84% ± 1 scale value
Deal & Belcher (1990)	30 children 1, 3, 5 grade	4 anchor stimuli; discussed 1st 5 ratings (O)	5 pt. EAI roughness	15/40 rerated. Pearson's r = .37–.95; 60–100% ± 1 scale value	Pearson's r = .56–.98; 75–100% ± 1 scale value
Emanuel et al. (1973)	11 grad students	20 item training tape heard 2× (O)	5 pt. EAI roughness	100/400 rerated. Pearson's r for medians of 1st & 2nd ratings = .98; > = 95% ± 1 scale value	> = 92% ± 1 scale value
Emanuel & Scarinzi (1979)	15 grad students	not reported	5 pt. EAI roughness	20/90 rerated. Pearson's r = .59–.95; 94% ± 1 scale value; 59% exact agreement	ICC adjusted for between-rater variance = .83 reliability of average rating = .98

LITERATURE REVIEWED

Key to abbreviations: (Training) E = Extensive; O = Orientation (see text for definitions). (Scale) EAI = equal-appearing interval scale; DME = direct magnitude estimation; paired comp = paired comparison task. (Interrater reliability) ICC = Intraclass correlation.
[a]Not significant.

Study	Raters	Training	Scale	Intrarater reliability	Interrater reliability
Emanuel & Smith (1974)	8 grad students	20 practice trials (O)	anchored DME roughness	20/80 rerated. Pearson's *r* for mean of 1st/2nd ratings = .80	not reported
Fritzell et al. (1986)	21 expert	not reported	5 pt. EAI breathiness	not reported	not reported
Gelfer (1988)	19 expert, 18 naive	none	9 pt. EAI 22 scales	not reported	Kendall's coefficient of concordance = .17–.69 for experts; = .14–.57 for naive
Hammarberg et al. (1986)	11 expert	terms discussed/ defined (O)	5 pt. EAI 25 scales	3/22 rerated. Pearson's *r* = .76–.98; 86% ± 1 scale value	not reported
Hammarberg et al. (1980)	14 expert	not reported	5 pt. EAI 28 scales	3/17 rerated. Pearson's *r* for means of 2 ratings on 28 scales = .93–.97	not reported
Hammarberg et al. (1984)	10 expert	not reported	5 pt. EAI 11 scales	6/16 rerated. Pearson's *r* = .68–.97	not reported
Heiberger & Horii (1982)	A: 25	not reported	anchored DME roughness	unspec. number rerated. Pearson's *r* for medians = .78–.96;	not reported
	B: 52 students (grad & undergrad)	2 demonstration trials; 20 practice trials (O)	paired comp roughness	20/138 rerated. Pearson's *r* = .96; exact agreement = 68–93%	not reported
Isshiki et al. (1969)	5 expert	not reported	4 pt. EAI 4 scales	not reported	not reported
Isshiki & Takeuchi (1970)	34 students, 6 expert	3 example stimuli repeated 2× (O)	7 pt. EAI 17 scales	not reported	not reported
Kane & Wellen (1985)	1 expert	not reported	7 pt. EAI severity	not reported	N/A (single rater)
Kearns & Simmons (1988)	5 expert	3 1-hour sessions (E)	7 pt. EAI 40 scales	not reported	82% ± 1 scale value overall; 68% ± 1 scale value for voices not rated as normal
Klatt & Klatt (1990)	5 expert	14 practice trials (O)	6 pt. EAI change in breathiness	12/12 repeated 5×. "rarely" exceeded ± 1 scale value	not reported
Klich (1982)	27 undergrads	10 minutes (O)	7 pt. EAI breathiness	40/40 rerated. ANOVA: no sig. presentation effect	ICC > .92 for all voice samples
Kojima et al. (1980)	5 expert	not reported	4 pt. EAI hoarseness	not reported	not reported

LITERATURE REVIEWED

Key to abbreviations: (Training) E = Extensive; O = Orientation (see text for definitions). (Scale) EAI = equal-appearing interval scale; DME = direct magnitude estimation; paired comp = paired comparison task. (Interrater reliability) ICC = Intraclass correlation.
[a]Not significant.

Study	Raters	Training	Scale	Intrarater reliability	Interrater reliability
Kreul & Hecker (1971)	22 under-grads	none	9 pt. EAI 5 scales	10/50 rerated. Kendall rank-order coefficients = .4–.95 for path voices; = .4–1.0 for normal voices	Friedman 2-way ANOVA: all F ratios significant
Lively & Emanuel (1970)	11 grad students	samples of scale extremes played 2× before each block of trials (O)	5 pt. EAI roughness	50/200 repeated. Pearson's r for medians of 1st/2nd ratings = .98; 96% ± 1 scale value	92% ± 1 scale value
Martin et al. (1984)	30 under-grads	none	9 pt. EAI naturalness	30/30 rerated. 85% ± 1 scale value	ICC: reliability of average rating = .98; reliability of single rater = .57–.74; 75% ± 1 scale value
Monsen (1979)	10 expert	short practice tape (O)	4 pt. EAI adequacy of voice quality	100% rerated. Pearson's r = .66–.74	not reported
Montague & Hollien (1973)	31 naive, 17 expert	definitions; example stimuli; 25 practice items (E)	7 pt. EAI 3 scales	40/40 rerated. "ANOVA technique" correlation = .70–.94	"ANOVA technique" correlation = .35–.96
Moody et al. (1979)	11 grad students	workshop plus 1 training session (E)	Wilson voice profile (7 scales)	5/11 judges; 20/40 rerated. Phi correlation = −.11–.96	Phi correlation = −.18–.97
Moran & Gilbert (1984)	4 expert, 3 grad students	not reported	Wilson voice profile (4 scales)	5/25 rerated. Pearson's r = .85–.95	"ANOVA technique" coefficient = .77–.93
Nieboer et al. (1988)	34 undergrad, 51 grad students	15 example stimuli; 2 practice trials (O)	7 pt. EAI 13 scales	not reported	Mean Pearson's r = .18–.66; ICC: reliability of average rating = .94–.99
Prosek et al. (1987)	9 expert	90 practice trials (E)	7 pt. EAI severity	90/90 rerated. Pearson's r = .86–.93	Cronbach's coefficient of generalizability = .82
Ptacek & Sander (1963)	8 expert	anchor stimuli, 16 practice trials (O)	7 pt. EAI breathiness	20/240 rerated. Pearson's r = .73	not reported
Rees (1958)	32 grad students	definitions; sample of each scale value repeated 3×; 30 practice (O)	7 pt. EAI harshness	100/1080 rerated. Pearson's r = .90 Difference between 2 means sig. by t-test	Q = .79
Reich & Lerman (1978)	20 grad students	trained to use EAI scale (O)	5 pt. EAI hoarseness 7 pt. EAI rough, pleasant	unspec. number rerated. Pearson's r = .73–.83	not reported
Samar & Metz (1988)	4 panels of 3 experts	not reported	5 pt. EAI intelligibility	84/84 rerated. Pearson's r = .975	Pearson's r = .95

LITERATURE REVIEWED

Key to abbreviations: (Training) E = Extensive; O = Orientation (see text for definitions). (Scale) EAI = equal-appearing interval scale; DME = direct magnitude estimation; paired comp = paired comparison task. (Interrater reliability) ICC = Intraclass correlation.
[a]Not significant.

Study	Raters	Training	Scale	Intrarater reliability	Interrater reliability
Sansone & Emanuel (1970)	11 grad students	4 scale extremes played several times (O)	5 pt. EAI roughness	50/200 rerated. Pearson's *r* for medians of 1st/2nd ratings = .96	>95% ± 1 scale value for 46 pairs of raters; lowest value = 80%
Sapir & Aronson (1985)	3 expert (inc. 2 authors)	not reported	8 pt. EAI severity of dysphonia	224/224 rerated. Pearson's *r* = .94–.96	Pearson's *r* = .83–.87
Sapir et al. (1986)	3 authors	not reported	7 pt. categorical scale	25/25 rerated. Pearson's *r* = .87–.95	Pearson's *r* = .80–.88
Schiavetti et al. (1981)	40 grad students	5 example stimuli (O)	7 pt EAI; anchored DME intelligibility	not reported	not reported
Schiavetti et al. (1983)	45 grad students	3 example stimuli (O)	7 pt EAI; anchored & unanchored DME severity of stuttering	not reported	ICC: reliability of mean ratings = .98 (EAI ratings); = .96 (anchored DME); = .97 (unanchored DME). Reliability of single rating = .75 (EAI scale); = .61 (anchored DME); = .65 (unanchored DME)
Sherman & Linke (1952)	35 students	examples of scale extremes played several times (O)	7 pt EAI harshness	30/90 rerated. Pearson's *r* = .97	mean Q = .77
Shipp & Huntington (1965)	4 expert	none	8 pt. EAI hoarseness, breathiness	not reported	Pearson's *r* = .17–.78
Smith et al. (1978)	9 grad students; 8 expert	stim. tape played 1× (O)	paired comp roughness	36/36 rerated. % agreement = .69–.89	not reported
Stoicheff et al. (1983)	8 expert	examples of scale extremes played several times (O)	7 pt. EAI dysphonia	50/150 rerated. "test-retest reliability" = .91	ICC(2,1) = .79
Stone & Sharf (1973)	5 grad students	60 actual stimuli (E)	7 pt. EAI "extent of change"	15/450 rerated. Pearson's *r* = .75	58% ± 1 scale value; 86% ± 2 scale values
Toner & Emanuel (1989)	20 grad students	10 practice trials (O)	5 pt. EAI; anchored DME roughness	60/60 rerated. mean Pearson's *r* = .76 (EAI); = .775 (DME)	ICC: reliability of mean rating = .975 (EAI); = .965 (DME). Reliability of single rating = .685 (EAI); = .575 (DME)
Wendahl (1966a)	461 undergrads	10 practice pairs (O)	paired comp roughness	3/15 rerated. .93 "by test-retest procedures"	not reported

LITERATURE REVIEWED

Key to abbreviations: (Training) E = Extensive; O = Orientation (see text for definitions). (Scale) EAI = equal-appearing interval scale; DME = direct magnitude estimation; paired comp = paired comparison task. (Interrater reliability) ICC = Intraclass correlation.
[a]Not significant.

Study	Raters	Training	Scale	Intrarater reliability	Interrater reliability
Wendahl (1966b)	97 undergrads	20 practice pairs (O)	paired comp roughness	not reported	not reported
Whitehead & Emanuel (1974)	11 grad students	15 practice trials (O)	5 pt. EAI roughness	50/300 rerated. Pearson's *r* for medians of 1st/2nd ratings = .98	> = 90% ± 1 scale value
Wolfe & Ratusnik (1988)	8 grad students	15 sample stimuli presented (O)	7 pt. EAI roughness	40/102 rerated. 89% ± 1 scale value	Cronbach's alpha = .95
Yumoto et al. (1984)	8 expert	Standard training tape (O)	4 pt. EAI hoarseness	2 judges rerated 87/87. Results not reported	Spearman's rho = .51–.79

Test-Retest Study of the GRBAS Scale: Influence of Experience and Professional Background on Perceptual Rating of Voice Quality

*†Marc S. De Bodt, *Floris L. Wuyts, *Paul H. Van de Heyning, and ††Christophe Croux

*Department of Otolaryngology, Head and Neck Surgery, and Communication Disorders, University Hospital; ‡Department of Mathematics, University of Antwerp, UIA, Belgium; and †Belgian National Science Foundation (NFWO)

Summary: Perceptual evaluation was performed by means of the GRBAS scale for a series of nine pathological voice samples that were presented twice to a group of 23 judges, consisting of experienced and inexperienced otolaryngologists (ENTs) and speech-language pathologists (S/LPs). The time interval between ratings was 14 days. Test-retest reliability was moderate. The best agreement between the observers was obtained for the G (grade) parameter and the worst for the S (strained) parameter. Considering the medians of the GRBAS ratings, no significant influence was measured for level of experience or professional background. Yet, based on means, the results show that professional background has a greater impact on perceptual rating than experience. **Key Words:** Perceptual evaluation—Voice quality—Test-retest—GRBAS scale.

Perceptual evaluation is fundamental to assessment of vocal quality, overall severity of defects, and their impact on communication skills. Nevertheless, it is one of the most controversial subjects in voice evaluation, because of poor correlation among raters. Review of the literature reveals a wide variety of rating scales and reliability data that fluctuate from study to study (1–3). Multiple factors contribute to this phenomenon.

First, there is inadequate internationally accepted terminology in describing voice quality (4). Some researchers have tried to make order from chaos. Several of the better known perceptual judgment protocols are those of Hammarberg (5), Wilson (6), Laver (7,8), Gelfer (9), and the Japan Society of Logopaedics and Phoniatrics (10). At the present, there is no universally accepted system for the perceptual assessment of voice quality. The GRBAS scale of the Japan Society of Logopaedics and Phoniatrics received its international introduction and reputation through the publication of Hirano's *Clinical examination of voice* in 1981 (10). It seems to have become the most widely used scaling method (11).

The GRBAS system for describing vocal quality contains five well-defined parameters (10,12): G (overall grade of hoarseness); R (roughness); B (breathiness); A (asthenic), and S (strained quality) of the voice. A four-point scale, from 0 to 3, is used for each parameter. "0" equals nonhoarse or normal, "1" slight, "2" moderate, and "3" severe. Results are denoted as $G_1R_1B_1A_0S_0$. The GRBAS scale is probably the most compact of all perceptual rating systems and was conceived for daily use by all members of the voice team. The Japan Society has made a standardized tape with typical voice samples represented by the GRBAS scale.

Accepted July 2, 1996.
Address correspondence and reprint requests to Dr. M. S. De Bodt at University Hospital Antwerp, Department of Otolaryngology and Communication Disorders, Wilrijkstraat 10, B 265 EDEGEM, Belgium.

A second issue is the difference in perceptual strategies between judges as discussed by Kreiman et al. (13). Most perceptual tasks involve comparing voices to internal standards. These internal standards are fluctuating and unstable and cause variability in rating. Kreiman et al. (13) suggest the use of explicit comparisons between stimuli (anchored protocols) to improve reliability. It is not clear how these modifications are to be operationalized in clinical practice.

Finally, interrater agreement is influenced by methodological aspects such as types of scale, speech sample, and rater.

To date, research concerning factors influencing perceptual ratings of voice quality has focused on training scales, listening experience, cultural background, and speech fragments. Several authors emphasize the importance of training and experience (3,4,12). Anders et al. (14) studied the effects of training (i.e., classes of auditors) and of culture (language) on the perception of hoarseness. They found small but not significant differences between classes of listeners in favor of trained listeners. They conclude that training and professional and cultural background do not have major influence on perceptual rating. Experienced listeners (speech-language pathologists) in Gelfer's study judged somewhat more consistently than untrained raters (9). In contrast, Kreiman et al. (15) showed that naive and expert listeners use different perceptual strategies. They found that expert listeners show less agreement than naive listeners about the relative importance of various aspects of voice quality. They suggest that care must be taken when using data averaged across all clinicians (15). Bassich and Ludlow (3) reported that 8 h of training were required for previously inexperienced listeners to attain 80% interjudge reliability using a 13-dimension perceptual rating system.

With regard to the GRBAS scale, Abe et al. (16) found that reproducibility differs according to listeners and scales. High reproducibility is possible when listeners are selected prudently. Recent work of Dejonckere et al. (17) showed that in a perceptual score list of 15 items, the GRBAS scale parameters appear to be the most interesting, because they show favorable combinations of low intra- and interjudge variance and high intervoice variance. In the comparison of judgments of two different judges, the best correlation was found for G ($p = 0.7$). Impressions about A and S were less consistent.

The GRBAS scale was introduced in our voice clinic to standardize perceptual evaluation of voice quality and to improve the descriptive communication between speech-language pathologists (S/LPs) and otolaryngologists (ENTs) with differing levels of experience. The current literature is not clear about the extent to which perceptual rating by means of the GRBAS scale can be influenced by experience and profession. The primary purpose of this study was to determine the test-retest reliability of S/LPs and ENTs' judgments of voice using the GRBAS scale. A second purpose was to investigate the influence of experience and professional background.

MATERIALS AND METHODS

Voice Samples

Recordings were made of 12 patients from the voice clinic. We used three recordings as trials and the remaining nine for the study. All patients (3 men, 6 women) complained of dysphonia. Age ranged between 22 and 65 years. The voice sample consisted of sustained vowels /a/ and /i/ and the reading of a phonetically balanced text (115 words). We instructed patients to read at a comfortable pitch- and loudness level. High-quality recording was made in a silent room with an ambient noise level <45 dB. The recording equipment consisted of a Sony TCD-D3 digital audiotape recorder and a dynamic microphone (Prologue Series 14 dynamic microphone, model 14HLC). Mouth-to-microphone distance was standardized to 30 cm. We performed acoustic analysis of the sustained vowel /a/ using the Computerized Speech Lab (Kay Elemetrics, Model 4300) and did calculations of F_o (Hz), jitter (%), shimmer (dB), and H/N ratio (dB) for each recorded sample. The voice sample characteristics are described in Table 1.

Judges

Twenty-three judges participated in this study; they all reported normal hearing. Thirteen were ENTs; five of them were experienced. The 10 remaining judges were certified S/LPs with ≥2 years of experience. All S/LPs had intensive voice training. This is not characteristic of the training given to the ENTs in this study. Although all judges assessed voice disorders on a regular basis, most of them were not familiar with the GRBAS system. For the statistical analysis, we denoted two groups: "experienced" and "inexperienced" containing 12

TABLE 1. *Voice sample characteristics*

Sample	Gender	Age	Fo Hz	Jitter (%)	Shimmer (dB)	H/N ratio (dB)	G[a]	R[a]	B[a]	A[a]	S[a]
1	M	57	129	4.538	1.252	−11.682	3	2	3	3	1
2	M	55	140	6.650	1.645	−13.187	1	1	1	0	1
3	F	22	187	0.592	0.621	6.778	2	2	1	1	2
4	M	53	143	0.637	0.442	5.996	3	2	2	1	3
5	F	70	251	0.882	0.683	−1.318	1	1	2	1	1
6	F	58	258	0.486	0.307	11.451	3	2	3	3	2
7	F	65	188	3.107	1.037	−7.097	1	0	1	0	0
8	F	51	200	0.580	0.284	8.547	2	2	2	1	2
9	F	64	253	1.460	0.822	7.398	2	2	1	1	2

Rating scale: G, grade; R, rough; B, breathiness; A, asthenic; S, strained.
[a] Medians calculated for the "experienced" group. Four-point grading: 0, normal; 1, slight; 2, moderate; 3, severe.

and 11 judges, respectively. Judges were considered experienced when they had been confronted with voice pathology over at least one third of their professional life and during ≥3 years. Otherwise, we considered them inexperienced. Both groups contained ENTs as well as S/LPs.

Listening Task

Before the first rating session, all judges received theoretical and clinical instructions about the GRBAS system and the scoring procedure from an experienced instructor. A training tape composed by the same instructor, using Dutch spoken speech samples, was used to ensure that judges were listening to the same percept. The rating of the nine different samples selected for this study was preceded by three trial judgments of samples that were not included in the study. Judges were allowed to ask questions during the trials. We presented all nine patient voices successively to the entire group at one time. The voice samples were presented only once to the listeners and interrupted by a short break allowing the judges to score the sample. We did not allow contact or discussion between judges during the listening task.

All judges used the same preprinted rating sheet that included a brief specification of the GRBAS parameters as described by Hirano (10). A second rating, occurring 14 days after the first rating and using an identical procedure, took place. None of the judges were informed about their first rating.

RESULTS

The GRBAS ratings were evaluated by means of nonparametric statistics because they are on an ordinal scale. Comparison of related groups was performed using the Wilcoxon Matched-Pairs Signed-Ranks Test and comparison of independent groups by the Wilcoxon Mann-Whitney statistic. Test-retest reliability was measured by the kappa statistic (18,19); this method gives the most appropriate measure of reliability for ordinal data (20).

The data for statistical analysis consisted of 2,070 ratings: 5 GRBAS parameter scores for 9 voices by 23 judges at two different times. We divided the judges into four subsets according to their level of experience in voice rating: experienced (E) (n = 12) or inexperienced (I) (n = 11); and according to their professional background: ENT (n = 13) or S/LP (n = 10). The data are equally distributed between both professional groups (χ^2: p = 0.28).

The first goal of this study was the assessment of test-retest reliability between the first and second ratings. This reliability was evaluated by the kappa statistic. The calculations were based on frequency tables as in Table 2, where the scores are shown for the G parameter, rated by all judges. The Table illustrates on the diagonal how many times the first and second scores were equal. Of the 207 G ratings made on the nine voices by the 23 judges, G3 was assigned 48 times both on the first rating and the second rating done 2 weeks later. The kappa statis-

TABLE 2. *Frequency table for the first and second rating of G, assessed by all judges*

	Second rating			
First rating	0	1	2	3
0	3	3	0	0
1	4	50	15	0
2	0	9	50	15
3	0	0	10	48

G, grade.

TABLE 3. *Test-retest reliability value (κ) between the first and second score, assessed by experienced (E) and inexperienced (I) judges, otolaryngologists (ENTs) and speech-language pathologists (S/LPs), and all examiners together*

κ	I	E	ENT	S/LP	All
G	0.50	0.70	0.62	0.58	0.60
R	0.29	0.40	0.27	0.43	0.35
B	0.29	0.45	0.30	0.46	0.38
A	0.51	0.28	0.42	0.36	0.39
S	0.30	0.36	0.32	0.35	0.34
GRBAS	0.40	0.45	0.41	0.44	0.43

Rating scale: G, grade; R, rough; B, breathiness; A, asthenic; S, strained.

tic was used to evaluate the test-retest reliability of the GRBAS scale between the first and second ratings. Each individual GRBAS parameter, as well as the entire scale, was evaluated, and the judges were divided into four groups according to experience and professional background. We also considered them all together in one pool. These results are in Table 3. In this table, the κ values indicate the agreement between the scores from both trials. In the case of the experienced listeners, κ equals 0.7 for G, which reflects that 70% of the difference between perfect agreement (κ = 1) and the real agreement expected purely by chance (κ = 0) is accounted for by the agreement between the scores for trial 1 and trial 2. Altman (21) provides a good discussion of interpretation of κ, as expressed in Table 4.

The agreement between the 23 observers was equally calculated by means of the kappa statistic (18). Again we performed the calculations for four observer categories: experienced versus inexperienced listeners, ENT versus SP. Successively, we pooled all groups together. As an example, the ratings of the 12 experienced listeners are listed in Table 5, indicating that for the second voice sample, one observer assessed this voice as normal (G_0), nine judges assigned a G_1, and two judges assigned a G_2.

Based on this method, agreement was calculated

TABLE 4. *κ interpretation table*

Value of κ	Strength of agreement
<.20	Poor
0.21–0.40	Fair
0.41–0.60	Moderate
0.61–0.80	Good
0.81–1.00	Very good

TABLE 5. *Example of scoring by the 12 experienced observers for the G parameter for all nine voices*

Voice score	0	1	2	3
1	0	0	0	12
2	1	9	2	0
3	0	4	8	0
4	0	0	4	8
5	0	7	5	0
6	0	0	1	11
7	1	11	0	0
8	0	1	10	1
9	0	1	8	3

G, grade.

for each individual GRBAS parameter as reported in Table 6. In all cases, $p < 0.001$.

The values for kappa should be interpreted using Table 4. The best agreement among the judges was elicited for G; for the other parameters, only poor to fair agreement was reached. Except for G, experience does not much improve the agreement among the observers. S/LPs in this study had better inter-rater agreement than ENTs.

The next hypothesis of the study concerned the experience of the listeners assessing voice quality. To investigate the different possible rating behaviors, due to the amount of experience, we calculated per GRBAS parameter and per voice the median score of the 12 experienced listeners and the median score of the 11 inexperienced listeners. For each GRBAS parameter, we then compared these 9 median scores for the experienced with those of the inexperienced judges. We used the Wilcoxon Matched-Pairs Signed Rank Test for this analysis. This offered the following significance levels (p) for the GRBAS parameters: G, $p = 0.18$; R, $p = 0.7$; B, $p = 0.32$; A, $p = 0.32$; and S, $p = 0.6$. We observed no significant difference between the medians. A similar statistical analysis for the medians by ENTs and S/LPs revealed the following signifi-

TABLE 6. *Agreement between the observers, divided into subgroups, according to their experience or profession*

κ	I	E	ENTs	S/LPs	All
G	0.39	0.49	0.45	0.46	0.44
R	0.16	0.20	0.14	0.25	0.17
B	0.21	0.20	0.19	0.31	0.21
A	0.33	0.27	0.26	0.28	0.27
S	0.11	0.17	0.12	0.12	0.10

κ, test-retest reliability value; I, inexperienced judges; E, experienced judges; ENT, otolaryngologists; S/LP, speech-language pathologists; (rating scale) G, grade; R, rough; B, breathiness; A, asthenic; S, strained.

cance levels: G, p = 0.36; R, p = 0.11; B, p = 0.18; A, p = 0.32; and S, p = 0.11, indicating no influence of professional background on the medians for the GRBAS scale.

We also calculated the mean score of four new judge groups: experienced and inexperienced ENTs as well as experienced and inexperienced S/LPs. For these groups, we calculated an average based on all GRBAS scores attributed to all patients. Although these averages have no physiological meaning because all voices were averaged, it was expected that the averages of the four groups would be distributed closely around the grand average. This was not the case. Figure 1 shows the grand average (±95% confidence interval) of all scores for all GRBAS parameters and voice samples by the entire collection of judges, as well as the subgroup averages and their standard errors.

Figure 2 shows, for example, the average G score of the nine voices, ordered by their G rating for the four subgroups of judges.

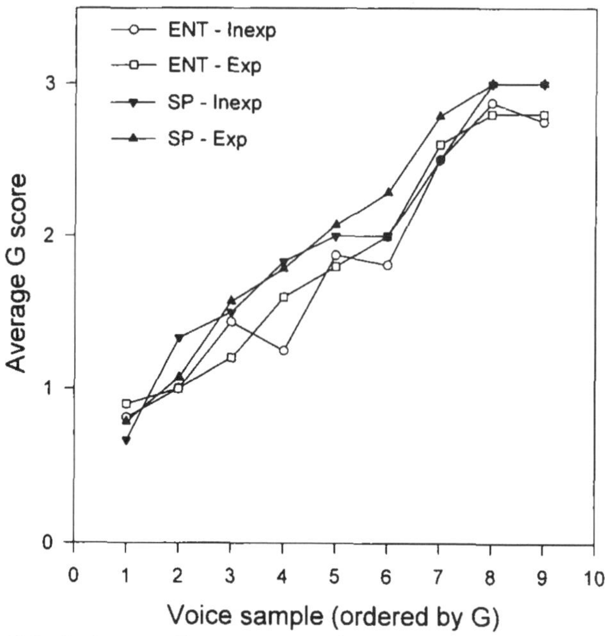

FIG. 2. Average G (grade) score for the nine voice samples, divided per subgroup of judges. The results are ordered with increasing degree of G score. ENT, otolaryngologist; SP, speech-language pathologist.

DISCUSSION

A wide variety of perceptual rating scales has been described in literature. In comparison with other systems, the GRBAS scale has the advantage of practical use in a daily clinical environment. This is mainly because of the simplicity of the scale, with only five parameters (GRBAS) and four categories: normal, slight, moderate, and severe. This advantage is offset by the lack of accuracy and precision of the scale. In this study, we raised the following issues concerning the GRBAS scale: test-retest reliability between successive ratings over time, the degree of agreement between observers, and the influence on the scale of professional background and experience of the raters.

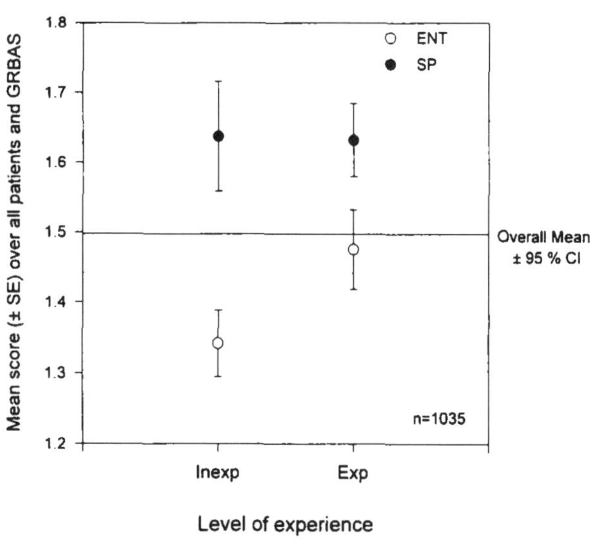

FIG. 1. Mean scores of the four subgroups of judges, compared to the overall mean of the GRBAS score for all voices. G, grade; R, rough; B, breathiness; A, asthenic; S, strained; ENT, otolaryngologists; SP, speech-language pathologists.

It must be emphasized that all of the voice samples were dysphonic, two severely. No normal voices were included in this study. Kreiman et al. (13) found that listeners differed more from one another in their judgments of pathological voices than they did for normal voices. Yet, the kappa statistic for extremes (normal or very pathologic) is much more favorable than for intermediate cases, which means that the results for κ are the lower limits of actual clinical practice.

The reliability of the scale was tested by assessing the test-retest reliability between two successive ratings with a time lapse of ⩾2 weeks, and by the test-retest reliability among 23 judges. The influence on the variability of the GRBAS scale by professional background as well as experience level was also investigated.

The overall test-retest reliability of the GRBAS scale when assessing scores at two distinct times was moderate (κ = 0.43). Professional background or experience level did not influence this reliability.

Considered apart, the reliability between time 1 and time 2 was good for the assessment of the overall grade of voice disorder (G). Moreover, both professional groups showed similar test-retest reliability. Yet, the influence of experience level is more prominent on the test-retest reliability, ranging from moderate (0.5) to good (0.7). For roughness (R) and breathiness (B), S/LPs seemed to be more reliable in their judgment than ENTs. Reliability for these parameters increased with the level of experience. The test-retest reliability decreased for the asthenic property of the voice with increasing experience. Clearly, this indicates that the A parameter is susceptible to interpretation error. Loss of reliability with experience was also described by Kreiman et al. (15). In their study, clinical training and experience caused listeners to differ more. The strained property (S) of the voices also showed rather low test-retest reliability.

The best test-retest reliability can be expected in a group of experienced listeners (4,14,22), which was confirmed in our study (Table 3). The parameters G, R, B, and S were reliable, whereas A showed much more variability over time. Dejonckere et al. (17) have described similar findings. This result indicated that the interpretation of G, B, R, and S was less ambiguous among the judges than the interpretation of A.

Another quality of the GRBAS scale was investigated by measuring the agreement among the different judges. Table 6 indicates that the G parameter was most unambiguously interpreted among the listeners. Furthermore, the agreement among the judges was not influenced by level of experience or professional background. These findings are in accord with those of Dejonckere (17) and Anders et al. (14).

In clinical application, it is of interest to know whether two judges would similarly rate a certain patient's voice. Therefore, we calculated the medians (discrete variable), because the scores are whole integers and not a figure in between, as is the case in visual analog scales. The statistical results showed that there was no difference between these medians in the different groups of judges, irrespective of their profession or experience. Thus, most observers gave the same categorical value of 0 to 3 to the same patients for each of the GRBAS parameters.

Although no statistically significant differences were found, we demonstrated different tendencies among the four classes of listeners when the averages, based on a large data pool, were calculated. Figure 1 illustrates the deviation from the grand average of GRBAS scores for experienced and inexperienced ENTs and S/LPs. Overall, the experienced listeners scored higher than the inexperienced listeners, suggesting that the later "underestimated" and the former "overestimated" the severity of the voice disorder. Also, using this criterion, ENTs "underestimated" and S/LPs "overestimated" the dysphonia. Moreover, the difference between experienced and inexperienced listeners was smaller than that between ENTs and S/LPs. It should be emphasized that the absolute deviations around the grand average are only 3% of the full scale (0–3). Figure 1 illustrates that the experience factor is more influential in the ENT than in the SLP group. In their rating, experienced ENTs clearly best approached the overall mean.

The results of this study show that test-retest reliability of the GRBAS scale is moderate. The G parameter seems to be the most reliable. Based on the statistical results of the medians, we concluded that no statistically significant differences were evident between different judges, irrespective of their experience or profession. Based on analysis of the means, small differences appeared among judges depending on level of experience and professional background. These differences are small enough (Fig. 2) to permit useful evaluation and reporting of voice quality by clinicians with different levels of experience or professional background using the GRBAS scale.

REFERENCES

1. Kreiman J, Geratt BR, Kempster GB, Erman A, Berke GS. Perceptual evaluation of voice quality: review, tutorial, and a framework for future research. *J Speech Hear Res* 1993; 36:21–40.
2. Blaustein S, Asher B. Reliability of perceptual voice assessment. *J Commun Disord* 1983;16:157–61.
3. Bassich CJ, Ludlow CL. The use of perceptual methods by new clinicians for assessing voice quality. *J Speech Hear Disord* 1986;51:125–33.
4. Fex S. Perceptual evaluation. *J Voice* 1992;6:155–8.
5. Hammarberg B. Pathological voice qualities. Perceptual and acoustic characteristics of a set of Swedish "reference" voices. *Bull Audiophonology* 1992;8:39–52
6. Wilson DK. *Voice problems of children*. Baltimore: Williams & Wilkins, 1987.
7. Laver J. *The phonetic description of voice quality*. Cambridge University Press, 1980.
8. Wirz S, Mackenzie Beck J. Assessment of voice quality: the Vocal Profiles Analysis Scheme. In: Wirz S, ed. *Perceptual approach to communication disorders*. London: Whurr Publishers, 1995:39–55.

9. Gelfer MP. Perceptual attributes of voice: development and use of rating scales. *J Voice* 1988;2:320–326.
10. Hirano M. *Clinical examination of voice*. New York: Springer Verlag, 1981:81–4.
11. Dejonckere PH, Wieneke GH. GRBAS-scaling of pathological voices: reliability, clinical relevance and differentiated correlation with acoustic measurements, especially with cepstral measurements. *Proceedings of the 22nd IALP Congress*. Hannover, Germany: 1992.
12. Hirano M. Clinical applications of voice tests, assessment of speech and voice production: research and clinical applications. NIDCD monograph. *Proceedings of a conference of the National Institute of Health*. Bethesda: 1990:196–203.
13. Kreiman J, Geratt BR, Precoda K, Berke GS. Individual differences in voice quality perception. *J Speech Hear Res* 1992;35:512–20.
14. Anders LC, Hollien H, Hurme P, Soninnen A. Wendler J. Perception of hoarseness by several classes of listeners. *Folia Phoniatrica* 1988;40:91–100.
15. Kreiman J, Geratt BR, Precoda K. Listener experience and perception of voice quality. *J Speech Hear Res* 1990;33: 103–15.
16. Abe H, Yonekawa H, Ohtq F, Imaizumi S. Reproducibility of hoarse voice psychoacoustic evaluation. *Jpn J Logop Phoniatr* 1986;27:168–77.
17. Dejonckere PH, Obbens C, De Moor GM, Wieneke GH. Perceptual evaluation of dysphonia: reliability and relevance. *Folia Phoniatr* 1993;45:76–83
18. Cohen J. A coefficient of agreement for nominal scales. *Educ Psych Measurement* 1960;20:37–46.
19. Siegel S, Castellan JN. *Nonparametric statistics for the behavioral sciences*. New York, McGraw-Hill, 1988.
20. Fleis JL. *The design and analysis of clinical experiments*. New York: Wiley, 1986:1–32.
21. Altman DG. *Practical statistics for medical research*. London: Chapman & Hall, 1991.
22. Rabinov CR, Kreiman J, Geratt BR, Bielamowics S. Comparing reliability of perceptual ratings of roughness and acoustic measures of jitter. *J Speech Hear Res* 1995;38: 26–32.

3

Description and Quantification of Voice Production

Introduction

The largest and most diverse chapter in this compilation, this section likely requires its own volume to do it justice. Reviewing the authors of the articles below is like a who's who of the voice and speech sciences. We must first apologize. Readers will likely notice that the *Journal of the Acoustical Society of America* (JASA) is well represented among the *classic* articles. There is no question that the inherent productivity in this area of investigation was mediated through the collaborative spirit promoted by JASA. Unfortunately, the publishers of JASA categorically rejected all attempts to obtain reprint permissions (the only publisher to do so). In spite of this unfortunate omission, these 29 manuscripts provide an interesting historical perspective on the evolution of the speech and voice sciences throughout the past 4 decades.

The commentaries provided by Drs. Hicks, Hillenbrand, and Hixon and Mrs. Smitheran provide an interesting framework for the contemporary developments in the speech and voice sciences. In addition, these commentaries provide insight into the fundamental concepts in acoustic and aerodynamic analyses largely overlooked in both the clinic and laboratory today. Furthermore, in spite of these advances, objectively defining voice and voice quality remains elusive.

Classic Articles

●Reprint of article included in this chapter.
♦Commentary on this article.

Rothenberg M. A new inverse filtering technique for deriving the glottal air flow waveform during voicing. *J Acoust Soc Am.* 1973;53(6):1632–1645.

Klatt DH. Voice onset time, frication, and aspiration in word initial consonant clusters. *J Speech Hear Res.* 1975;18(4):686–706.

Hammarberg B, Fritzell B, Gauffin J. Perceptual and acoustic correlates of abnormal voice qualities. *Acta Otolaryngol.* 1980;90(5–6):441–451.

●♦Smitheran JR, Hixon TJ. A clinical method for estimating laryngeal airway resistance during vowel production. *J Speech Hear Res.* 1981;46(2):138–146.

Yumoto E, Gould WJ, Baer T. Harmonics-to-noise ratio as an index of the degree of hoarseness. *J Acoust Soc Am.* 1982;71(6):1544–1549.

Ramig LA, Ringel RL. Effects of physiological aging on selected acoustic characteristics of voice. *J Speech Hear Res.* 1983;26(1):22–30.

Hanson DG, Gerratt BR, Ward PH. Cinegraphic observations of laryngeal function in Parkinson's disease. *Laryngoscope.* 1984;94(3):348–353.

Milenkovic P. Least mean square measures of voice perturbation. *J Speech Hear Res.* 1987;30(4):529–538.

Titze IR. The physics of small-amplitude oscillation of the vocal folds. *J Acoust Soc Am.* 1988;83(4):1536–1552.

Titze IR. On the relation between subglottal pressure and fundamental frequency in phonation. *J Acoust Soc Am.* 1989;85(2):901–906.

Hirano M. Objective evaluation of the human voice: clinical aspects. *Folia Phoniatr.* 1989;41(2–3):89–144.

Gauffin J, Sundberg J. Spectral correlates of glottal voice source waveform characteristics. *J Speech Hear Res.* 1989;32(3):556–565.

Titze IR. Physiologic and acoustic differences between male and female voices. *J Acoust Soc Am.* 1989;85(4): 1699–1707.

●♦Eskenazi L, Childers DG, Hicks DM. Acoustic correlates of vocal quality. *J Speech Hear Res.* 1990;33(2):298–306.

●Verdolini-Marston K, Titze IR, Druker DG. Changes in phonation threshold pressure with induced conditions of hydration. *J Voice.* 1990;4(2):142–151.

Baer T, Gore JC, Gracco LC, Nye PW. Analysis of vocal tract shape and dimensions using magnetic resonance imaging: vowels. *J Acoust Soc Am.* 1991;90(2 pt 1):799–828.

Titze IR. Phonation threshold pressure: a missing link in glottal aerodynamics. *J Acoust Soc Am.* 1992;91(5): 2926–2935.

Titze IR, Liang H. Comparison of F(o) extraction methods for high-precision voice perturbation measurements. *J Speech Hear Res.* 1993;36(6):1120–1133.

●♦Hillenbrand J, Cleveland RA, Erickson RL. Acoustic correlates of breathy vocal quality. *J Speech Hear Res.* 1994;37(4):769–778.

Herzel H, Berry D, Titze IR, Saleh M. Analysis of vocal disorders with methods from nonlinear dynamics. *J Speech Hear Res.* 1994;37(5):1008–1019.

Berry DA, Herzel H, Titze IR, Krischer K. Interpretation of biomechanical simulations of normal and chaotic vocal fold oscillations with empirical eigenfunctions. *J Acoust Soc Am.* 1994;95(6):3595–3604.

Story BH, Titze IR. Voice simulation with a body-cover model of the vocal folds. *J Acoust Soc Am.* 1995;97(2): 1249–1260.

Steinecke I, Herzel H. Bifurcations in an asymmetric vocal-fold model. *J Acoust Soc Am.* 1995;97(3):1874–1884.

De Krom G. Some spectral correlates of pathological breathy and rough voice quality for different types of vowel fragments. *J Speech Hear Res.* 1995;38(4): 794–811.

Story BH, Titze IR, Hoffman EA. Vocal tract area functions form magnetic resonance imaging. *J Acoust Soc Am.* 1996;100(1):537–554.

Svec JG, Schutte HK. Videokymography: high-speed line scanning of vocal fold vibration. *J Voice.* 1996; 10(2):201–205.

Holmberg EB, Hillman RE, Perkell JS. Glottal airflow and transglottal air pressure measurements for male and female speakers in soft, normal, and loud voice. *J Acoust Soc Am.* 1998;84(2):511–529.

Fitch WT, Giedd J. Morphology and development of the human vocal tract: a study using magnetic resonance imaging. *J Acoust Soc Am.* 1999;106(3 pt 1): 1511–1522.

Dejonckere PH, Bradley P, Clemente P, et al. A basic protocol for functional assessment of voice pathology, especially for investigating the efficacy of (phonosurgical) treatments and evaluating new assessment techniques: guideline elaborated by the Committee on Phoniatrics of the European Laryngological Society (ELS). *Eur Arch Otorhinolaryngol.* 2001;258(2): 77–82.

Commentary

Thomas J. Hixon, PhD and Judith R. Smitheran, MS

Our article had its conceptual beginnings in classroom teaching in a graduate course titled Experimental Phonetics taught by one of us (TJH) at the University of Wisconsin between 1965 and 1976. The idea for the method grew out of a clinical need and an interest in applying speech science principles to clinical endeavors. The principles were vetted through videotaped demonstrations to students that included Diane Bless, Gary Weismer, Jim Abbs, Steve Barlow, and others, who had biomechanical interests in speech and voice production. The conceptual seed was carried to the University of Arizona where the other of us (JRS) learned about the idea in a similar course and became intrigued with more fully developing it as a method and then testing it for possible application. What started out as a classroom interest, turned into a master's thesis, and then found routine clinical application in the voice and neuromotor clinics at the University of Arizona and many other places throughout the world.

As much, or more, work went into piloting the project than went into gathering the data published in the article. We tried a wide variety of instrumentation arrays, speech samples, measurement approaches, and subject monitoring techniques before arriving at the final clinical protocol. Response to the published version of the method was instantly positive. The article was selected for the 1981 Editor's Award of the *Journal of Speech and Hearing Disorders*. It took off quickly and spawned a large number of applications in various studies of normal function and in clinical studies of voice disorders. We took this as evidence of the general thirst for practical means for quantifying voice production mechanism. Subsequent incorporation of the method into commercial applications also proved to be encouraging. One of us recalls how a salesperson at a corporate booth at a national convention eagerly explained how the method worked and what information it provided, not knowing to whom he was talking. It all sounded really quite clever and plausible.

When we prepared the manuscript for publication, we did the usual trimming of things here and there to fit the format and length requirements of the journal. We debated about whether or not to include a formal definition that emphasized that resistance is a property of the airway and not of the structures that bound the airway. We ultimately decided to leave out such a definition, because, in the thinking of one of us, it was something that "any schoolboy would know." Well, as it turned out, this was not the case. We greatly regret not making it explicit in the manuscript that resistance is a property of the airway, because it would have avoided some of the confusion we have seen about what the method actually quantifies. Fortunately, we meticulously used the phrase "laryngeal airway resistance" throughout the article, but many who have followed us have applied terms to the method that do not embrace what we intended or what they thought they were calculating. For example, some authors have suggested that the method enables the calculation of "glottal resistance" "vocal fold resistance," "laryngeal resistance," or this or that "other-named resistance." These labels are misleading. Laryngeal airway resistance is not a measure of the mechanical status of the vocal folds, nor is it a measure of the size of the opening designated as the glottis.

Laryngeal airway resistance can certainly change, and does change, with changes in the positioning of structures within the larynx. But laryngeal airway resistance also can change with no change in the glottis, vocal folds, or interior of the larynx. The reason is that airway resistance is airflow dependent and may change with a change in airflow without any changes brought on by the larynx. A more concrete understanding of this concept (pun intended) can be gained by thinking of a plaster cast of the interior of the larynx. Nothing in such a cast is adjustable. Everything is rigid and immovable. Nevertheless, resistance to the flow of air through the cast is airflow dependent. Force air through the cast (in either direction) and it may be found (especially at higher airflows) that laryngeal airway resistance goes up and down as airflow goes up and down. The specific relation approximates that of a general second-order resistor. The dependence of laryngeal airway resistance on airflow for a fixed laryngeal airway is portrayed graphically in Figure 3–1 for expiratory airflow—that of more importance to speech and voice utterances.[1] Laryngeal airway resistance is not something you can look at and measure. It is something you must calculate. And, it is something that reflects the opposition to the

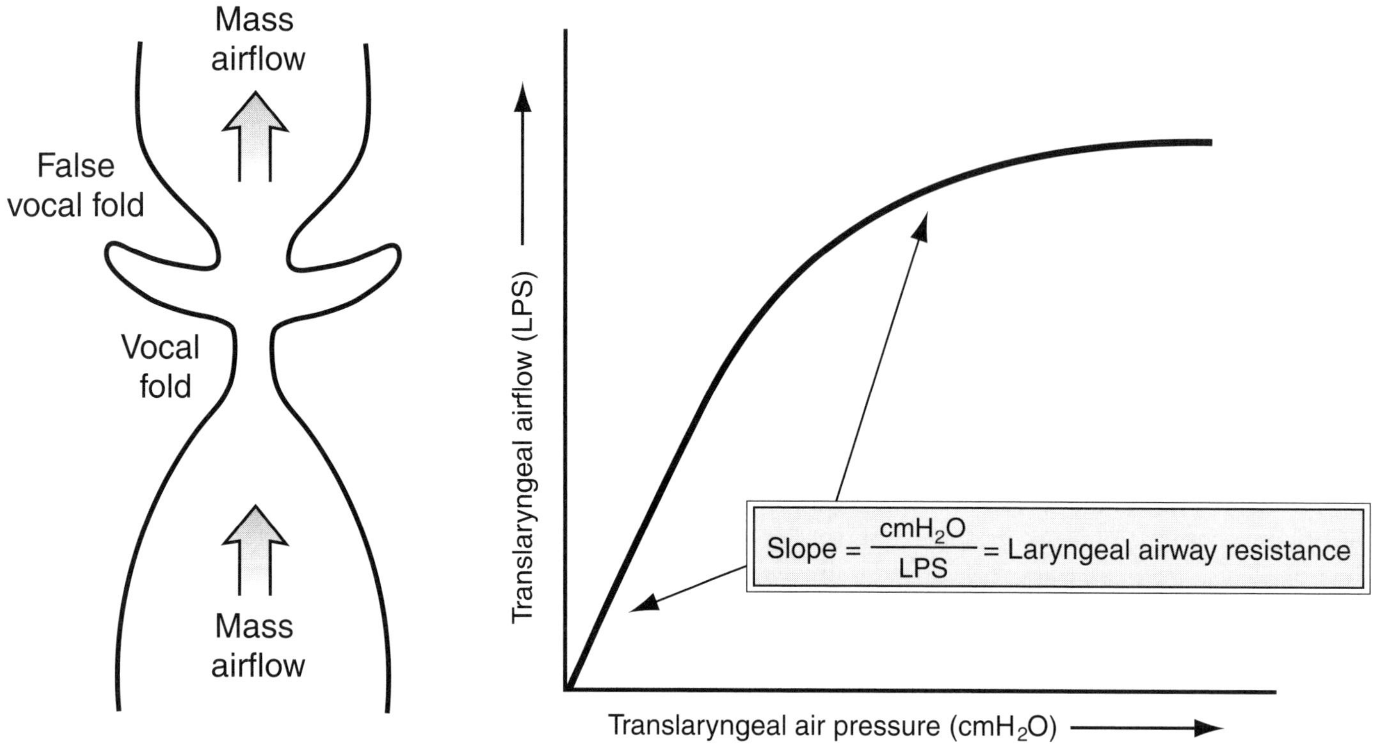

Fig 3–1. Graphic depiction of the dependence of laryngeal airway resistance on airflow. (Reproduced with permission from *Preclinical Speech Science: Anatomy, Physiology, Acoustics, Perception.* By T. Hixon, G. Weismer, & J. Hoit, 2008, San Diego, Calif: Plural Publishing, Inc. Copyright 2008 by Plural Publishing, Inc.

movement of air across the entire length of the laryngeal airway, not just the glottis or the vocal folds.

When we developed the method we were careful to ascribe the driving pressure in the formula to translaryngeal air pressure and defined it as the pressure differential between the trachea and pharynx. Many who have used the method subsequently have used the term subglottal air pressure in place of our use of the term tracheal air pressure. We don't like this term and encourage others to eschew it for a number of reasons in favor of the term tracheal pressure. The following excerpt, from a piece titled "Throttle Subglottal," considers several of those reasons:

> Most readers will be familiar with the term "subglottal pressure." Although popular, it has problems. The "sub" part of the term is not site-specific. For example, bronchial and alveolar pressures are also "sub" glottal. The "glottal" part of the term is also problematic. The term glottis means hole. There are times during voicing when the vocal folds are approximated. How can anything then be "sub" glottal? There is no way to be below a hole when there is no hole. Respiratory physiologists would use the term tracheal pressure for the pressure of interest. Such a term specifies the site of the pressure. And the term is accurate regardless of the state of the laryngeal airway (whether it is open or closed). Finally, it removes the ambiguity involved in the use of "sub" as a location.[2(p92)]

We notice that on occasion the term "lung pressure" is also used in place of our choice of tracheal pressure. We equally dislike this term because of its ambiguity. Respiratory physiologists usually consider the pressure developed by the lung as only one component of the pressure developed by the respiratory apparatus, usually as the static recoil pressure of the pulmonary apparatus alone. Thus, so-called "lung pressure" is never delivered to the larynx alone, but always in combination with the recoil pressure and/or the muscular pressure of the chest wall. Thus, we come again to our liking of the term "tracheal pressure."

Finally, while we are concerned with terms, one other usage has caught our attention over the years from discussions of the use of our method. That is that writers often talk about opening and closing the vocal folds. This can only be done with a scalpel and sutures, respectively. It is the laryngeal airway that is opened and closed by way of laryngeal adjustments. Language can sometimes be maddening, but ask yourself whether or not you have ever opened and closed a door. Maybe you have with an axe and plastic wood filler, respectively. But most readers have ever only opened and closed a "doorway."

We are pleased that our article has been chosen for inclusion in this volume and that it is considered to have had a significant impact since its publication. This research was fun for us and we are glad to see that the results of our work have a continuing life.

As Hoffmann[3] has expressed so well, facts are mute, human beings do science, and science and stories are not only compatible but also inseparable. The theme of this volume seems to reinforce this perspective.

References

1. Hixon T, Weismer G, Hoit J. *Preclinical Speech Science: Anatomy, Physiology, Acoustics, Perception.* San Diego, Calif: Plural Publishing, Inc; 2008.
2. Hixon T. *Respiratory Function in Singing: A Primer for Singers and Singing Teachers.* Tucson, Ariz: Redington Brown; 2006.
3. Hoffmann R. Storied theory. *Am Scientist.* 2005;93: 308–310.

A CLINICAL METHOD FOR ESTIMATING LARYNGEAL AIRWAY RESISTANCE DURING VOWEL PRODUCTION

JUDITH R. SMITHERAN THOMAS J. HIXON
University of Arizona, Tucson, Arizona

A noninvasive clinical method for estimating laryngeal airway resistance during vowel production is described. Resistance is calculated from the ratio of translaryngeal pressure to translaryngeal flow, the first determined from measurement of oral pressure and the second determined from measurement of airway-opening flow made during the production of a specially designed utterance. Application of the method to the study of vowels resulted in a calculated mean laryngeal airway resistance of 35.7 cm H_2O/LPS for 15 normal adult males. This resistance value is remarkably similar to mean values obtained in previous research using complex invasive experimental methods. Clinical use of the method is illustrated in case studies that highlight both evaluation and management potentials. It is concluded that the method proposed is clinically practical, that the data it provides are both valid and reliable, and that the method shows great promise of becoming a routine clinical tool for estimating laryngeal airway resistance during vowel production.

The larynx is a mechanical valve situated between the lower and upper airways. Much can be inferred about the function of this valve during vowel production from knowledge of the magnitude of coupling the larynx permits between the trachea and pharynx. Such knowledge can be obtained in different but related forms, one of the most pertinent being the extent to which the larynx offers opposition to the flow of air through it. In technical parlance, this opposition is termed laryngeal airway resistance (R_{law}). Laryngeal airway resistance cannot be measured but must be calculated from the ratio of translaryngeal pressure (P_{tl}) (the difference between tracheal and pharyngeal pressures) to translaryngeal flow ($\dot{V}_{tl}$) (the flow through the larynx). Restated, $R_{law} = P_{tl}/\dot{V}_{tl}$.

The relevance of information on laryngeal airway resistance during vowel production is apparent for three clinical endeavors: (1) the understanding of disordered function; (2) the evaluation of disordered function; and (3) the management of disordered function. Unfortunately, current clinical technology does not enable the easy acquisition of data on laryngeal airway resistance. Clearly, the greatest difficulty in this regard has to do with the fact that to obtain the translaryngeal pressure data needed to calculate resistance, the pressure in the trachea must be known. Continuous direct recording or continuous indirect estimation of this pressure requires one of the following: (1) that a sensing probe (catheter, miniature transducer, or hypodermic needle) be positioned within the trachea; (2) that a sensing probe (catheter-balloon or miniature transducer) be positioned within the esophagus; or (3) that the subject be encased in a whole-body chamber. Tracheal and esophageal probes are invasive, cause discomfort, have physical risks, and require the assistance of a physician. Whole-body encasement requires plethysmographic systems that are rare, cumbersome, call for technical sophistication, and demand complex calibration maneuvers by the subject.

In this article, the development and testing of a new, simple, noninvasive clinical method for estimating laryngeal airway resistance during vowel production is presented. The need to base resistance determinations on data that include continuous direct recording or continuous indirect estimation of tracheal pressure is circumvented in this method. In the sections to follow, consideration is given to the conceptual development of the method, the salient features of the method, data obtained from use of the method on a group of normal-speaking subjects, and implications pertaining to the general clinical application of the method.

Judith R. Smitheran, M.S., and Thomas J. Hixon, Ph.D., are affiliated with the University of Arizona, Tucson.

CONCEPTUAL DEVELOPMENT

The conceptual development of the present method has its roots in general fluid dynamics theory. Such theory predicts that in many fluid-filled systems, certain combinations of valving adjustments enable estimates of upstream pressure-flow events from measurements of pressure-flow events made at sites that are substantially downstream of the measurement sites of interest. Upon application of this same theory to the air-filled respiratory passages, it becomes apparent that certain combinations of valving adjustments of the larynx, velopharynx, and oral segment enable estimates of tracheal pressure, pharyngeal pressure, and translaryngeal flow from measurements of pressure-flow events made downstream of the trachea, pharynx, and larynx. Furthermore, upon viewing speech production from this perspective, it becomes apparent that these same combinations of valving adjustments occur naturally in the aeromechanical scheme associated with the production of certain speech-sound subsets of the English language.

Given these aeromechanical and phonetic realizations, it was reasoned that these two areas of knowledge could be combined in a manner that would enable the noninvasive determination of laryngeal airway resistance during vowel production. The key to this combination is the construction of an utterance which, when elicited from a subject, will call up and serially order various combinations of valving adjustments, such that it is possible to make discontinuous estimates of tracheal pressure, pharyngeal pressure, and translaryngeal flow associated with the vowel elements in the utterance from the simultaneous and continuous recording of relevant downstream pressure-flow events.

The simplest utterance in this regard is that which repeatedly alternates voiceless stop-plosives and voiced vowels. These two types of segments involve different combinations of valving adjustments. For voiceless stop-plosives, two sets of adjustments occur: one constituting a "closed" phase and one constituting a "release" phase. The closed phase finds the laryngeal valve open and the velopharyngeal and oral valves closed. The release phase, by contrast, maintains the open laryngeal valve and the closed velopharyngeal valve, but involves an abrupt opening of the oral valve. For vowels, a single set of adjustments occurs in which the laryngeal valve is relatively highly constricted on the average (through repeated opening and closing of the glottis), the velopharyngeal valve is closed, and the oral valve is open such that the oral airway is relatively unconstricted.

When this type of utterance is produced, two downstream variables—oral pressure and airway-opening flow—can be used as measurement substitutes for upstream tracheal pressure, pharyngeal pressure, and translaryngeal flow. Oral pressure can be used to obtain discontinuous estimates of tracheal pressure and pharyngeal pressure at different moments during such an utterance, and airway-opening flow can be used to obtain a discontinuous estimate of translaryngeal flow.

An estimate of tracheal pressure can be obtained from the measurement of oral pressure by taking into account the following: for one instant during the production of voiceless stop-plosives, oral pressure and tracheal pressure are identical. This correspondence occurs during the closed phase of voiceless stop-plosives, when the upper airway is sealed airtight, except for its laryngeal entry. During the latter part of the closed phase, the pressure within the oral cavity behind the site of airway occlusion equilibrates with the pressure within the lower airways, the trachea included. More specifically, this moment of oral-tracheal pressure equilibration is coincident with the occurrence of the peak oral pressure associated with voiceless stop-plosives (Netsell, 1969; Shipp, 1973). Thus, the peak oral pressure during the production of a voiceless stop-plosive can be taken as an estimate of the tracheal pressure existing at the corresponding moment. Based on evidence for the type of utterance referenced above, one that repeatedly alternates between voiceless stop-plosives and voiced vowels, it is possible to use the data from successive oral pressure peaks to infer the presumed tracheal pressure contour for the utterance. This can be done by linearly interpolating the pressure between adjacent oral pressure maxima and then constructing an underlying contour from the successive linear interpolations. Thereafter, it is possible to estimate the tracheal pressure associated with voiced vowel segments that occur between adjacent pairs of voiceless stop-plosives.

Turning to oral pressure as an estimate of pharyngeal pressure, attention focuses on a different moment during the production of the type of utterance discussed. Specifically, an estimate of the pharyngeal pressure associated with each vowel production can be obtained from the measurement of oral pressure made during each vowel. The direct substitution of oral pressure for pharyngeal pressure is possible because the pressure drop between the pharynx and the oral cavity is essentially nil during voiced vowels, the oral airway being relatively unconstricted and the flow through it being relatively low. In fact, under most circumstances of normal voiced vowel productions, where flows through the upper airway are relatively low, little precision would be lost in the calculation of laryngeal airway resistance were pharyngeal pressure and oral pressure both assumed to be zero.

The use of airway-opening flow as a discontinuous estimate of translaryngeal flow during voiced vowel production is made possible because of the continuity of mass flow through the upper airway when the mouth is open. Structural displacements of the upper airway (that is, articulatory motions) generate small flows during vowel production, but these are trivial, and can be neglected, in comparison to the flow related to the displacement of air through the larynx. In any event, the contribution of such "airway" flows is zero if airway-opening flow measurements are made during moments when the airway is in a quasi-static state, such as prevails during the middle portion of vowels produced in the type of utterance considered here.

METHOD

This method evolved from an extensive pilot investigation that considered different utterances, equipment arrays, testing procedures, and data analyses. Seven normal-speaking adult males served as pilot subjects in one or more of the areas considered. In the following subsections, a fully-developed clinical protocol is offered. Where appropriate, this protocol is justified on pilot experiences. Subjects described in the next subsection are those for whom data are presented in the *Results* section, and on whom the protocol was tested.

Subjects

Fifteen adult males served as test subjects. These individuals ranged in age from 21 years, 10 months, to 40 years, six months. Ages were distributed relatively evenly within this range. Subjects met the following criteria: normal speech and voice, hearing reported to be normal, no known structural or neurological disorders, and no known respiratory infections or allergies at the time of testing. All subjects were monolingual, white, and English-speaking. Choice of the subject group was prompted by the desire to infer the validity of the present method via comparisons of data from the present subjects with similar subjects studied previously by others with experimental methods.

Utterance Design

Utterance design was guided by the desire to provide a task that met the following: (1) fulfilled the constraints imposed by the underlying theory; (2) was simple for the subjects to perform and would have widespread application to other subjects, including children, difficult-to-test individuals, and persons with structural or neuromuscular disorders of the speech apparatus; (3) was of a character akin to conversational speech but controlled for variables that might influence resistance; (4) would yield data that could be analyzed easily and quickly in a clinical setting; (5) minimized potential measurement artifacts; and (6) minimized the complexity of subject-equipment interfacing.

The utterance employed was the syllable /pi/ repeated in three separate trains of seven productions each. For each train, subjects were instructed to take a breath of twice normal depth and to produce the seven productions on a single, continuous expiration at normal loudness, pitch, and quality, with equal stress on each syllable, with each of the seven vowels in the train prolonged slightly, and at an utterance rate of 1.5 syllables/sec. (as paced externally). The rationale for the selection of these particular utterance features is considered below.

At the segmental level, the voiceless stop-plosive /p/ and the voiced vowel /i/ were chosen for inclusion. The consonant /p/ offered the following merits for selection from among the three voiceless stop-plosive candidates in the English language (/p, t, k/): (1) it has been shown empirically that oral pressure and tracheal pressure equilibrate at the moment of occurrence of peak oral pressure during /p/ production (Shipp, 1973), so that /p/ meets one of the important constraints of the method's theoretical basis; (2) it has been shown empirically that /p/ is the first of the voiceless stop-plosives to emerge in the sequence of speech-sound development (Prather, Hedrick, and Kern, 1975), so that it may have the widest potential applicability in subject testing; (3) the place of production of /p/ is the most anterior of the three voiceless stop-plosives in the English language, so that the measurement of oral pressure can be accomplished with the least degree of insertion of a sensing probe, with the least complex insertion pathway for a probe, with the least likelihood of recording artifact from blockage of a probe by saliva, and with the least likelihood of recording artifact from articulatory interference with a probe; (4) the compression compliance between the airway-occluding structures (that is, the two lips) at the place of production for /p/ is greater than that for the other voiceless stop-plosives in the English language, so that on peroral insertion of a sensing probe there is the greatest likelihood of an airtight seal being formed around the sensing probe during consonant closed-phases, and there is the least likelihood of encumbrance to the normal articulatory process; and (5) the adequacy of closure of the oral segment, a necessity in application of the method, is more easily determined at the lips on /p/ production than on other voiceless stop-plosives in persons with structural or neuromuscular disorders.

The /i/, a high, front, unrounded vowel, offered the following merits for selection from among the many vowel candidates: (1) it has been shown empirically that velopharyngeal closure is airtight during /i/ and other high vowels produced in non-nasal phonetic contexts (Thompson & Hixon, 1979), so that /i/ meets one of the important constraints of the method's theoretical basis; (2) the front place of production of /i/, in combination with /p/, puts the focus of articulatory activity for utterance in a single region (anterior) of the upper airway, so that the performance task is simplified for normal-speaking subjects and for those persons who are neuromuscularly impaired and may have difficulty performing a more demanding set of gestures; (3) the production of /i/ does not involve lip-rounding, or extensive excursions of either the tongue or the mandible, so that flow artifacts (even though miniscule) related to articulatory motions are minimized; and (4) the production of /i/ does not involve extensive articulatory motions in the facial region, so that there is little likelihood of an air leak around the border of the oronasal mask (see *Equipment*) due to subject-mask interfacing problems.

Finally, considerations of a supra-segmental nature were also taken into account in utterance design. An attempt was made through instruction to the subject to influence the form of the breath group used. That is, by telling the subject to take a breath of twice normal depth before utterance and to produce utterance on a single, continuous expiration, it was reasoned that breath group conditions would be similar to those of conversational speech. During such speech, subjects make pre-utterance inspirations to about 60% of the vital capacity and then produce utterances on uninterrupted expirations that extend through the mid-range of the vital capacity (Hixon, Goldman, & Mead, 1973). Having the subjects perform utterances at normal loudness, pitch, and quality was intended to establish conditions that were routinely natural to the subjects and closely approximated their "normal" manner of using the larynx during vowel production. The choice of the syllable as the fundamental utterance unit was prompted by its simplicity from the viewpoint of subject performance and the ease with which it could be monitored for linguistic stress and utterance rate. With regard to the former, it was desired that stress be the same on each syllable to maximize the consistency of the drive provided to the larynx and upper airway by the respiratory apparatus (that is, to maintain a relatively flat tracheal pressure contour) and to maximize the consistency of the laryngeal adjustment associated with successive vowels in the syllable train. With regard to the latter, it was deemed important to control utterance rate to maximize the consistency of the laryngeal adjustment associated with successive vowels and to provide vowel productions of sufficient duration to have the larynx assume quasi-static resistances during their midpoints. Selection of the repetition rate of 1.5 syllables/sec. was influenced by a compromise between the issues just mentioned and the need to insure that airtight velopharyngeal closure would be maintained during the utterance sample. It has been demonstrated empirically that utterance rates below 1.5 syllables/sec. are often accompanied by intermittent velopharyngeal openings (Thompson & Hixon, 1979), which would be unacceptable were it desired to make measurements with the present method.

Equipment

Two aspects were recorded: oral air pressure (hereinafter called pressure) and airway-opening flow (hereinafter called flow).

Pressure was tapped and transmitted via a polyethelene catheter (1.5 mm bore, 20.0 cm length) with the proximal end positioned in the oral cavity (see *Procedure*) and with the distal end coupled to a differential air-pressure transducer. The output signal of the transducer was led to a carrier amplifier where it was amplified and low-pass filtered such that components above 30 Hz were attenuated markedly. The resulting pressure-analog was displayed on one channel of a two-channel storage oscilloscope for monitoring, and on one channel of a two-channel thermal recorder for permanent recording.[1] The latter was operated at a paper speed of 20 mm/sec. System calibration was performed against a U-tube water manometer arranged in parallel with the polyethelene catheter.

Flow was channeled through a large, hard-rubber, anesthesia mask positioned over the mouth and nose. Flow from the mask was sensed by a double-coned, one-square inch, Silverman-type pneumotachometer coupled to a second differential air-pressure transducer matched to the one used to sense oral pressure.[2] The output signal of this transducer was conditioned (amplified and filtered) through a second carrier amplifier in the same manner as for pressure. The resulting flow-analog was monitored and recorded permanently on the remaining channels of the storage oscilloscope and the thermal recorder, respectively. System calibration was performed with a continuously variable, vane air pump whose output was directed through an air rotameter arranged in series with the pneumotachometer.

An electronic metronome was used to aid subjects in the pacing of their utterances. This metronome was operated at a rate of 1.5 beats/sec. and provided a synchronous light-flash and audible click to guide the subjects.

Procedure

Each subject was seated upright and positioned so that the monitoring and recording systems were out of his visual field. Next, the anesthesia mask was placed over the subject's mouth and nose so as to form a comfortable and airtight seal between it and the subject's face. The pressure-sensing catheter then was threaded through a small opening in the side of the mask, and its proximal end was positioned in the midline of the oral cavity approximately 1.0 cm behind the central incisors. Following this, the subject was informed of the nature of the task to be performed and was instructed to model his performances after those generated by an investigator. Utterances made by each subject had to meet the criteria discussed previously. Subject utterances judged inappropriate copies of the model provided by the investigator were not accepted, and additional samples were elicited until appropriate copies were obtained. Repeated requests for utterances were made of the subject until three acceptable syllable-trains were obtained. Those subject performances that met the utterance criteria were culled from the permanent thermal recordings for analysis.

Record Analysis

Figure 1 is an example of the pressure-flow records obtained. Oral pressure and airway-opening flow are shown in the upper and lower parts of the figure, respectively.

The seven maxima in the upper part of the figure correspond to the peak oral pressures obtained during the seven /p/-segments of the utterance. These peaks are relatively consistent and hover in the neighborhood of 7.0 cm H_20 on the average. Increase in pressure to each maximum is rapid and has its beginning closely time-locked to closure of the oral airway at the lips. Decrease in pressure from each maximum is also rapid and has its beginning time-locked to release of oral airway closure. The seven pressure minima following the /p/-segments in Figure 1 correspond to the pressures associated with the seven /i/-segments of the utterance. These minima are in the form of pressure plateaus that are highly consistent and of a magnitude of less than 0.1 cm H_20.

[1]During pilot study, a three-channel thermal recorder was used so that speech audio could be recorded simultaneously with pressure and flow. Recording was accomplished with a three-component equipment set-up: (1) a contact throat-microphone; (2) a DC amplifier; and (3) one channel of the thermal recorder. It was intended that speech audio be used as an aid to the temporal segmentation of phonetic events. Use of this recording was abandoned because points of measurement interest in the pressure and flow recordings proved validly and reliably identifiable from the pressure and flow data alone.

[2]Resistance offered by the flow-channeling and sensing equipment was measured as less than .5 cm H_20/LPS over the range of flows observed in the present study. This value is negligible in comparison to the resistances measured for subject utterances, and so equipment resistance has been neglected in all considerations.

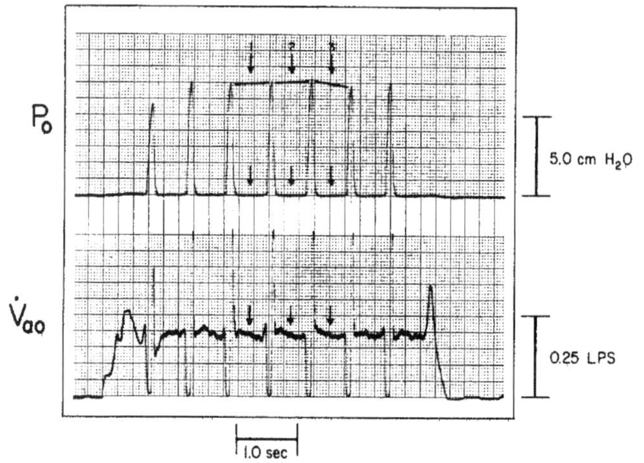

FIGURE 1. Example of the pressure-flow records obtained. P_o = oral pressure and $\dot{V}_{ao}$ = airway-opening flow.

The seven plateau-like portions of the record in the lower part of Figure 1 correspond to the flows obtained during the same seven /i/-segments just mentioned. These flows are relatively consistent and of an approximate magnitude of 0.19 LPS on the average. Flow minima between the vowel segments represented in Figure 1 are at zero and coincide with closures of the oral airway. The extremely rapid increases in flow following these moments of zero flow are associated with the opening of the oral airway upon plosive release. The flow maxima associated with these releases are greater than those shown in those cases in which the tracing reaches recording-pen limitation beyond full-scale deflection.

Records were analyzed as follows: First, to preclude performance end-effects, the first two and last two vowel segments in each syllable train were discarded and only the middle three vowels in the train were considered. Next, an estimate of tracheal pressure at the approximate mid-point of each vowel was determined as follows. The peak oral pressures on the third, fourth, fifth, and sixth productions of /p/ were identified on the records and interconnected with those for their adjacent mates by straight lines. The contour formed as a result of this linear interpolation between the four oral pressure peaks was taken to represent the prevailing tracheal pressure associated with the middle portion of the syllable train. Next, the time points midway between the designated pressure peaks on the records were identified and the corresponding interpolated pressures were noted. Thus, a separate estimate of tracheal pressure was provided for each of the three vowels analyzed. In Figure 1, points of measurement for these three vowels are indicated by the numbered arrows. Pressures were expressed in cm H_2O.

An estimate of pharyngeal pressure at the approximate midpoint of each vowel was determined by noting the magnitude of the oral pressure coincident with the moments of tracheal pressure estimation. Thus, a separate estimate of pharyngeal pressure was provided for each of the three vowels of interest. Pressures were expressed in cm H_2O.

An estimate of translaryngeal flow at the approximate midpoint of each vowel was determined by noting the magnitude of airway-opening flow coincident with the moments of tracheal-pressure and pharyngeal-pressure estimation. Thus, a separate estimate of translaryngeal flow was provided for each of the three vowels studied. Flows were expressed in LPS.

Laryngeal airway resistance was calculated for each vowel studied as follows: translaryngeal pressure was determined as the difference between estimated tracheal and pharyngeal pressures; this difference was then divided by the measured translaryngeal flow. Calculation yielded a separate resistance value, expressed in cm H_2O/LPS, for the three vowels studied in the three syllable trains analyzed for each subject. (In Figure 1, the three resistance values are 37.4, 37.9, and 36.8 cm H_2O/LPS for vowels 1, 2, and 3, respectively.) The mean resistance was determined for each syllable train (for the three vowels in Figure 1, this value is 37.4 cm H_2O/LPS), and the grand mean, the mean of the three means, was then determined as the criterion score for each subject on the utterance.

RESULTS

Reliability of Criterion Scores

The reliability of the criterion scores for the utterances was determined through intraclass correlation technique. The obtained reliability coefficient associated with data derived from the mean of three performances of the utterance by the subjects was .96. A coefficient of this magnitude indicates that the mean of three determinations is a highly reliable estimate of the true value for the resistances of interest.

Criterion Scores

Table 1 presents the criterion scores obtained for the 15 subjects studied. Subjects are listed down the table in order of increasing chronological age. The resistance values for the subject group yield a mean of 35.7 cm H_2O/LPS, with a range of 30.0 cm H_2O/LPS to 43.1 cm H_2O/LPS, and a standard deviation of 3.3 cm H_2O/LPS. Inspection of the data in Table 1 suggests that no relationship exists between chronological age and the magnitude of laryngeal airway resistance during vowel production. This impression is corroborated statistically through the computation of a Spearman rank-order coefficient of .16 between the two data sets.

DISCUSSION

Adequacy of the Method

The present data strongly support the reliability and validity of the proposed clinical method for estimating laryngeal airway resistance during vowel production. An

TABLE 1. Subject identifications, ages, and criterion scores.

Subject (Initials)	*Age (Years-Months)*	*Resistance (cm H_2O/LPS)*
DM	21-10	30.0
JB	23-8	35.5
KG	24-2	41.7
DB	24-8	35.8
JT	24-11	36.1
DS	27-0	43.1
JL	28-8	34.6
JK	31-8	32.3
JM	32-4	34.4
RC	32-5	36.0
RW	34-4	32.1
TG	38-5	33.0
KW	38-8	37.3
TH	40-0	36.8
DW	40-6	37.4
	Mean	35.7
	Range	30.0-43.1
	SD	3.3

estimate of reliability, as statistically evaluated through intraclass correlation technique, resulted in a highly satisfactory coefficient based on the mean of three sets of measurements on three repetitions of the utterance. Validity is inferred from the magnitude of the airway resistances calculated, the low intersubject variability on the resistance values, the extent to which the data agree with the theoretical basis for the method itself, and the very close agreement between data obtained on the subjects studied here and subjects studied in earlier reports where invasive experimental procedures were used.

The average laryngeal airway resistance calculated for the 15 adult males of the present study was 35.7 cm H_2O/LPS. Several investigations include mean data that allow for a reasonable comparison to the present data in terms of subject and utterance-sample comparability. The three most extensive of such investigations include the works of Kunze (1962), Sant & Logemann (1970), and Shipp & McGlone (1971). Each of these investigations used puncture of the trachea with a hypodermic needle to obtain records of tracheal pressure. Each also used an oronasal anesthesia mask to trap airway-opening flow. In Kunze's study, flow was derived from the recordings of a respirometer coupled to the mask, while in the Sant and Logemann and the Shipp and McGlone studies flow was determined through use of a pneumotachometer coupled to the mask. Each of the three investigations was based on the study of a sizeable group of adult male subjects producing sustained vowels. For comparison with the present findings, the following data have been considered: from Kunze (1962)—the data for 10 subjects producing the vowels /æ, ɑ, o, u, i/ at 50% of their vocal intensity ranges and at 30% of their vocal fundamental frequency ranges; from Sant and Logemann (1970)—the data for 18 subjects producing the vowel /ɔ/ at the "medium" point of their vocal sound pressure level ranges and at 25% of their vocal fundamental frequency ranges; and, from Shipp and McGlone (1971)—the data for 14 subjects producing the vowel /ɑ/ at a presumed average 50% of their vocal sound pressure level ranges (data collapsed across the 25% and 75% levels) and at 30% of their vocal fundamental frequency ranges.

Data from the present study and from the three investigations mentioned are in Figure 2. The data shown are mean laryngeal airway resistances (expressed in cm H_2O/LPS) calculated from the data provided in the various reports. The mean resistance obtained with the present clinical method is remarkably similar to the mean resistances obtained in the earlier invasive investigations. In fact, when the mean data from the present study are compared to the weighted mean data from the earlier three investigations indicated in Figure 2, the two sets of data (the present for 15 subjects and the earlier for 42 subjects) differ by only 1.5 cm H_2O/LPS. The closeness in value of the present data to those provided by invasive procedures bears forcefully on the face validity of the present method and suggests strongly that it is fully adequate as a means for estimating laryngeal airway resistance during vowel production.

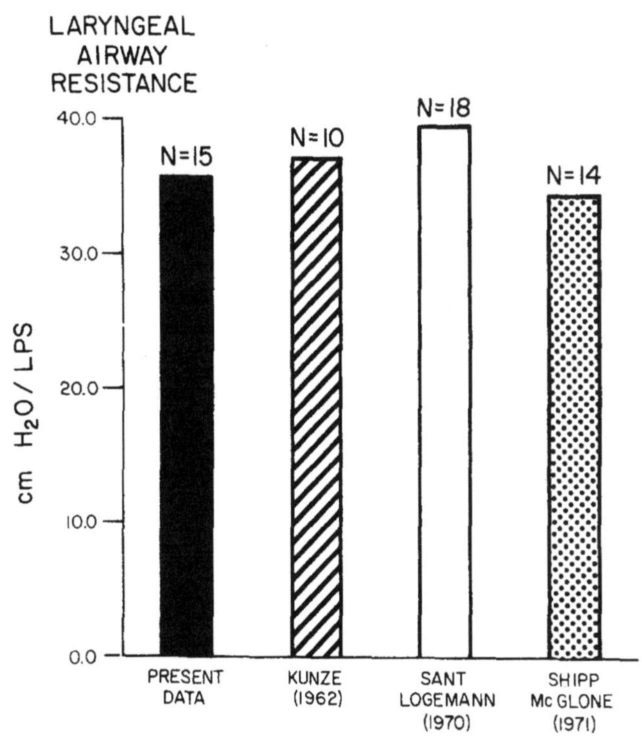

FIGURE 2. Graphic representation of the mean laryngeal airway resistances obtained in the present and earlier investigations.

The Method as a Routine Clinical Tool

The results of the present study are very encouraging with regard to the potential usefulness of the present method as a routine clinical tool. An important aspect of the resistance data reported is the low intersubject variability (that is, the small standard deviation). Pending further needed research on large groups of normal-speaking subjects and on subjects with demonstrated laryngeal airway resistance control problems during voicing, this low intersubject variability suggests that it should be possible to use the present method to obtain data that will discriminate between individuals with normal laryngeal function and those with disordered laryngeal function.

A second important aspect of the resistance data reported here is that a highly stable criterion score (that is, a high intrasubject reliability) results from analyses made on only three performances of the utterance specified in the protocol. This means that the present method is clinically practical with regard to the time required to collect the needed pressure-flow data, to analyze the records, and to calculate the airway resistance offered by the larynx. More specifically, once the examiner is intimately familiar with the method, the time required to obtain a criterion score is typically only five minutes. Beyond the present study, it would seem a relatively simple task to computerize the method such that the required pressure-flow values could be machine-read and the resistance calculations done automatically. This modification of the method would reduce its running-time to essentially that taken to collect the data for three acceptable utterances.

There are other practical aspects of the method. The utterance required of the subject is simple and easy to perform, involving only the repetition of a single syllable over and over in the same fashion. Although the present study was restricted to adult male subjects, it seems reasonable to assume that even young children and many difficult-to-test individuals would be capable of performing the utterance called for in the method. The present method causes no discomfort to the subject during data collection and it must be considered essentially noninvasive. Furthermore, encumbrance to the normal speech-production process from use of the method appears minimal, and at no time is the subject placed at physical risk.

Important practical aspects from the examiner's point of view include that a physician is not required for protective supervision during data collection. In addition, there are no special ethical considerations to be dealt with beyond those routinely associated with the practice of speech-language pathology. Examiners with very limited experience in the use of clinical equipment can be trained easily and quickly in use of the present method. Fortunately, the method, as it has been described, capitalizes on measurement technology that is currently available in many speech-language pathology clinics, particularly those found in hospital environments. With regard to the specific equipment used, that required by the method is of only moderate expense and when appropriately configured is reasonably portable. A wide variety of laryngeally-based clinical disorders can be studied with the present method (see next section) and the same basic equipment required by the method can be used to both evaluate and manage disorders manifested in the resistance parameter. Not only does the method provide precise data on laryngeal airway resistance, it also provides permanent records of the aeromechanical behavior of the larynx that can be used to track the status of the resistance parameter. Such data can be used to document and chart changes in function, to make numerical comparisons between subject performances and baseline norms, to compare values among disordered populations, to compare values from clinic to clinic, and to quantify the success of various mechanical management programs (for example, teflon injection of a paralyzed vocal fold). Data provided by the present method also complement data obtained by other methods of observation with which most clinicians are already familiar. In summary, as a clinical tool, the present method would appear to be extremely powerful, useful, and welcomed.

It is relevant to close this section of the discussion by considering examples of the use to which the method has been put subsequent to its standardization. At the time of this writing, the method has been used clinically with six individuals exhibiting voice dysfunction. Two of these individuals, one presenting resistance values above and one presenting resistance values below the presumed normal laryngeal airway resistance continuum, have been chosen for consideration.

BT, a healthy 21-year-old female university student, was referred for functional dysphonia. She exhibited a low-pitched, harsh, breathy voice, the quality of which had become unacceptable to her. Indirect laryngoscopic examination revealed bilateral vocal fold nodules. Information in her case history suggested vocal abuse as the probable cause of her nodules, and in turn, her presenting dysphonia. An inordinately heavy vocal schedule as a drama student, an active social life in noisy environments, and continuing nightly performances as a singer in stage musicals, were judged the principle aggravating factors associated with her dysphonia. As a part of the evaluation of BT's laryngeal function during voice production, the present method was used to determine her laryngeal airway resistance on vowels. Resistance was calculated to be 22.9 cm H_2O/LPS. This value is 35.9% lower than the average value obtained for the subject group studied here and 23.7% lower than the value obtained for the subject with the lowest resistance in the same group.[3] It seemed reasonable to assume that BT's low laryngeal airway resistance was related to the presence of her bilateral vocal fold nodules and the likelihood that they were precluding her from attaining a firm approximation of the vocal folds along their entire length. An intensive voice-therapy program was used with BT. This program was conventional with regard to the identification and elimination of her abusive laryngeal behaviors and with regard to the use of symptomatic voice modification procedures to raise her vocal pitch and reduce her harshness and breathiness. Coupled with these standard procedures, BT was given training in the use of the present method as a biofeed-

[3]It should be noted that the subject group used for this comparison included only adult males. In lieu of needed normative data on adult female subjects, it has been assumed that this comparison is appropriate for two reasons: first, BT demonstrated typical adult-male resistance values once her voice had returned to a quality adequate for release from therapy, and second, preliminary findings on a small number of adult females show them to fall within the range of values determined for the adult males studied here.

back means of obtaining information concerning her laryngeal airway resistance during vowel production. This information was provided on the thermal recorder display. (The two-channel storage oscilloscope is also convenient for this purpose.) Approximately three months following the initial airway resistance evaluation, with its result of 22.9 cm H_20/LPS, BT was dismissed from therapy and placed on a self-monitoring vocal-hygiene program. At that time, indirect laryngoscopic examination revealed that the bilateral vocal fold nodules were no longer present. Determination of laryngeal airway resistance immediately before dismissal revealed a value of 34.3 cm H_20/LPS, a resistance of approximately the average magnitude for the subject group studied here and an increase for BT of 33.2% in the magnitude of her airway resistance from the time of her initial evaluation.

BT's case is significant for at least two reasons. She is the first individual on whom laryngeal airway resistance changes have been documented in response to a management program and the first individual to use laryngeal airway resistance in a biofeedback mode as a part of a program of rehabilitation. From even this one case, it is clear that the present method can play an important role in the evaluation and management of dysphonias that have functional bases.

LD, a 57-year-old male who had had multiple, bilateral, cerebral-vascular accidents two years before, was referred for evaluation of his speech production capabilities. Study revealed that LD had a mixed dysarthria with perceptual correlates that included hypernasality, articulatory imprecision, short phrases, and a marked strained-strangled voice quality. The latter was judged the most prominent deviant characteristic of his speech behavior. Included within a battery of physiological examinations for motor-speech integrity, was the present method for estimating laryngeal airway resistance. Application of the method revealed a laryngeal airway resistance of 66.0 cm H_20/LPS for vowel utterances. This value is 84.9% higher than the average resistance determined for adult males studied here and 53.1% higher than that obtained for the subject with the highest calculated resistance. The high resistance determined for LD was consistent with his prominent strained-strangled voice quality and was assumed related to a probable spastic component of his laryngeal control problem. Noticeable improvement in LD's voice quality was achieved when he raised his fundamental frequency level, rotated his head backward, or initiated his utterance from a high lung volume. Determination of laryngeal airway resistance under these three conditions revealed values that were lower than usual for LD, the most marked improvement being a decrease in resistance to 52.0 cm H_20/LPS when utterance was initiated from a high lung volume. It was assumed that this improvement was related to passive abduction of the vocal folds brought about by the tracheal tug associated with a lower diaphragm position at a high lung volume. In LD's case, it was recommended that he be started on a voice modification program that was behavioral, and that the present method be used as a means of revealing those conditions that optimally reduce his laryngeal airway resistance during voicing.

LD's case illustrates the value of the present method in the detailed evaluation of individuals with laryngeally based dysarthrias and the extent to which the specification of laryngeal airway resistance can be used as an aid to determining fruitful avenues of management.

Future Considerations

The present study was methodological and exploratory. Study of laryngeal airway resistance for the 15 adult males used as subjects was intended to determine the face validity of the present method and to present a small initial pool of data for the benefit of further research considerations. Additional laryngeal airway resistance data are needed to establish further the efficacy of the present method as a routine clinical tool for the quantification of laryngeal function.

Specifically, the need remains to determine the range and central tendencies of laryngeal airway resistance values exhibited by the full variety of normal-speaking subjects. Such study necessitates the collection of normative information on large groups of males and females encompassing all age ranges. With the collection of such data, it should be possible to differentiate between those individuals with normal and disordered laryngeal function as it pertains to resistance control. To this end, various types of voice disorders warrant systematic study with the present method for the purpose of discovering how the resistance parameter is influenced by disordered production of voice and of evaluating changes with management. Some of the more obvious areas of study in this regard include so-called hyperfunctional and hypofunctional voice disorders without organic bases, neurologically-based voice disorders, and voice control problems associated with such disorders as profound hearing impairment. The ultimate hope is the establishment of approximate cut-off points for the normal range of laryngeal airway resistance values during vowel production, below and above which dysfunction in control of laryngeal airway resistance could be assumed. In this regard, it may even be possible eventually to designate more efficiently those individuals with borderline resistance control skills.

Another group of studies that could be done using the present method involves observations of changes in laryngeal airway resistance under a wide variety of conditions of voicing. For example, the present method provides a useful and simple tool for the study of factors believed to influence laryngeal airway resistance, such as vocal sound pressure level, vocal fundamental frequency, voice quality, and whispering. Thus, studies of normal control mechanisms are seemingly more readily achieveable for the researcher than has been the case with invasive procedures.

Those wishing to use the present method routinely in a clinical setting might well consider several factors that expand the method's universality. First, the oronasal anesthesia mask used in the present study provides an adequate fit for the subjects chosen for study here but not for all subjects. Those wishing to use the method with women, children, or individuals with various orofacial disorders are well advised to obtain masks similar to the one used in the present study, but of different sizes.

A second consideration to extend the general applicability of the method pertains to rendering the technique useful on those persons with valving incompetence at either the velopharynx or the lips. Recall that airtight seals need to be made at these two sites coincident with laryngeal opening to enable a moment of pressure equilibration for accurate tracheal pressure estimation. Failure to meet this requirement leads to a tracheal pressure estimate that is lower than the actual tracheal pressure, so that the resistance value calculated will be lower than the actual resistance. In the case of either the velopharynx or the lips, valving incompetence is manifested in the recording obtained with the present method by flow not returning to zero during the closed phase of voiceless stop-plosive production. This problem is easily solved in the case of the velopharynx by placing a nose clip on the subject before placing the mask over the mouth and nose. This modification creates an infinite resistance along the nasal pathway so that flow escape through the incompetent velopharyngeal valve is precluded. In the case of LD, data were obtained in this fashion to counteract a velopharyngeal leak that was a contributing factor to his speech disorder. In the case of valving incompetence of the lips around the pressure-sensing tube, one should consider the option of selecting a voiceless stop-plosive with a more posterior placement in the oral airway and the positioning of the pressure-sensing tube via other routes. Placement at the midline of the oropharyngeal cavity by way of pernasal insertion or by way of insertion along the buccogingival sulcus are two alternatives. While these two placements are far more invasive and difficult than simply positioning the pressure-sensing tube behind the lips for /p/, they nonetheless provide the data that are required to make useful laryngeal airway resistance calculations.

A third area of consideration for extending the applicability of the method clinically involves a compromise to the actual method proposed here, but one that seems acceptable considering that a reasonably close approximation of the true resistance is better than none. Clinical experience with use of the method has shown that in a small number of subjects the simultaneous measurement of oral pressure and airway-opening flow is difficult to achieve. This is occasionally the case with a very young subject or with a subject who shows a substantial degree of neuromuscular involvement in the orofacial region. As an alternative to abandoning data acquisition, it has been found useful to record oral pressure and airway-opening flow during separate repetitions of the utterance task. Recordings of the two variables are then measured from the separate records and are combined to determine an approximate value for laryngeal airway resistance. Under these circumstances, it seems advisable to average a greater number of resistance calculations on a greater number of syllable repetitions in an attempt to estimate more accurately the subject's mean laryngeal airway resistance.

ACKNOWLEDGMENT

Requests for reprints should be directed to Thomas J. Hixon, Ph.D., Department of Speech and Hearing Sciences, Building 25, University of Arizona, Tucson, Arizona 85721.

REFERENCES

HIXON, T., GOLDMAN, M., & MEAD, J. Kinematics of the chest wall during speech production: Volume displacements of the rib cage, abdomen, and lung. *Journal of Speech and Hearing Research*, 1973, *16*, 78-115.

KUNZE, L. An investigation of the changes in subglottal air pressure and rate of air flow accompanying changes in fundamental frequency, intensity, vowels, and voice registers in adult male speakers. Unpublished doctoral dissertation, University of Iowa, 1962.

NETSELL, R. Subglottal and intraoral air pressures during the intervocalic contrast of /t/ and /d/. *Phonetica*, 1969, *20*, 68-73.

PRATHER, E., HEDRICK, D., & KERN, C. Articulation development in children aged two to four years. *Journal of Speech and Hearing Disorders*, 1975, *40*, 179-191.

SANT, L., & LOGEMANN, J. An investigation of the variations in air flow and subglottal pressure with changes in pitch and intensity of phonation. Paper presented to the Annual Convention of the American Speech-Language-Hearing Association, New York, 1970.

SHIPP, T. Intraoral air pressure and lip occlusion in midvocalic stop consonant production. *Journal of Phonetics*, 1973, *1*, 167-170.

SHIPP, T., & MCGLONE, R. Laryngeal dynamics associated with voice frequency change. *Journal of Speech and Hearing Research*, 1971, *14*, 761-768.

THOMPSON, A., & HIXON, T. Nasal air flow during normal speech production. *Cleft Palate Journal*, 1979, *16*, 412-420.

Received June 23, 1980.
Accepted August 4, 1980.

Commentary

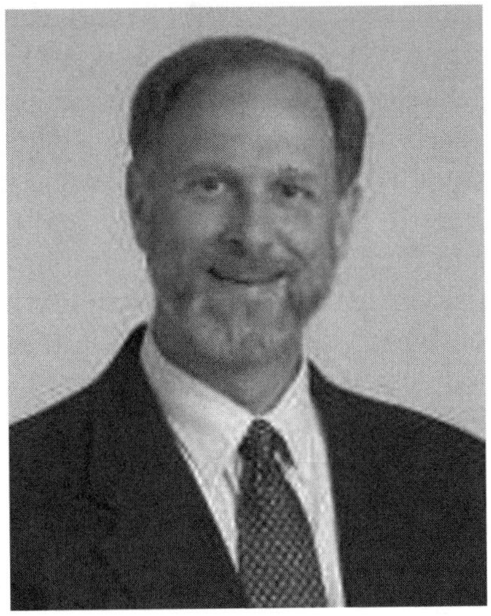

Douglas M. Hicks, PhD

Rarely does one have or take the time to reflect on past work in terms of its lasting significance or its place in one's overall career. The opportunity to do that reflection is an unexpected and enjoyable journey. The following commentary is testimony to that process. Critical review of our published study must be placed in the context of the knowledge base at that point in time. During the 1970s and 1980s, there was an explosion of interest in laryngeal anatomy and vocal physiology, coinciding with the development of assessment technology—both dedicated units and software programs. The clamor for acoustic, aerodynamic, and movement measurements that would define voice led to the emergence of many contenders—many of them ultimately rendered pretenders. It was a time when clinicians were confronted with too many choices regarding measures, protocols and equipment to feel comfortable with their decision-making process. Many investigators, both individuals and teams, attempted to identify key measures that would operationally define voice performance—our University of Florida (UF) research team was part of that process.

For this particular study, our stated goal was "to find the acoustic correlates of voices spanning a wide range on the vocal quality continuum." That continuum included normal voices to severely dysphonic ones. Like other researchers, we were seeking quantitative measures of vocal performance that would correlate perceptual (subjective) attributes like "quality" with objective parameters. At the time, our motivation was twofold: (1) advance the quest for developing effective speech processing systems, and (2) identify objective tools for the clinical assessment of voice disorders. This research project represented one of more than a dozen publications between the mid-1980s and early 1990s emerging from our UF group effort to address phonatory function. Many of those studies were supported by two major grants: (1) NIH; Laryngeal Function: Objective-Perceptual Classification (1985–1988); and (2) NSF; Two Channel (EGG and Speech) Analysis-Synthesis for Voice Recognition (1985–1988).

There are several unusual aspects of this article worth noting. First, we utilized a study design theme in which both disordered patients and normal subjects (providing both a control and reference point) were included in data collection. The investigation of "normal," as well as the inclusion of normal performance when investigating patient performance, remains a strategy in much of my research. As an illustration, our recent Cleveland Clinic Foundation (CCF) work on laryngopharyngeal reflux (LPR) benefited from studying the normal population before tackling the population of ultimate interest—voice patients. Second, we employed a unique twist with our disorder population by including both real patient and mimicked pathologic voices. The latter subgroup was determined to be authentic and consistent with voices of real patients. Our motivation to pursue this subplot related to our voice recognition modeling efforts, and ultimately allowed some improved control of dysphonic severity. Third, our prior work with operationally defining laryngeal quality led to confidence in the quality categories of breathy, rough, and hoarse. Although those terms were not unique to us, our combined high-speed and EGG investigations established a real physiologic basis for these perceptual categories. Breathy was defined by incomplete medial compression of the true vocal folds (membranous portion) with associated excessive escaping of air, whereas rough required a disruption in the periodicity of vocal fold vibration. Hoarseness was a combination of the other two quality defects, including a combination of their disrupted physiology. Subsequently, I have found this perceptual classification system (breathy, rough, and hoarse) to be an effective clinical tool—being finite enough to be manageable but robust enough to represent the majority of disordered vocal quality.

A lasting contribution from our work is the conclusion that time-domain measures are among the most useful acoustic measures for differentiating disordered voices. This suggests that timing characteristics of the glottal waveform can be helpful in assessing vocal quality. Although both pitch amplitude (PA) and harmonics-to-noise ratio (HNR) were specifically identified as useful parameters, they have not emerged as "the" key measures. In fact, looking 17 years forward, many of the same research questions and physiology dilemmas from the past still exist. Despite many excellent research efforts, both before and after our publication, the challenge to succinctly define voice performance by a single (or small group of) measures is still beyond our grasp. The multidimensional nature of voice performance and the unknown factors of perceptual assessment likely account for our continued lack of answers into the early 21st century. I suspect that the criteria utilized by listeners in evaluating voice include different parameters than are represented by the current set of acoustic options, both past and present. Therefore, future research endeavors will need to both expand the relevant acoustic signal attributes, and address the complicated correlation between sound and the cognitive process of perception.

The final commentary relates to a broader professional and career focus. A lifetime theme of my research journey has been effective multidisciplinary collaboration. The UF team joining me for the various voice and laryngeal physiology projects was Don Childers (Electrical Engineering), Nick Cassissi (ENT), Paul Moore (SLP), and various graduate students (both master's and doctoral from both SLP and engineering). The first author on this article was one of Dr. Childers' doctoral students. I had the privilege of sitting on the thesis or dissertation committee for several of his outstanding students. As many were internationals, exposure to different cultures and disciplines (math, physics, engineering) provided a stimulating environment in which to plan/execute research. That collaboration stretched me professionally as I was occasionally involved in research outside of my mainstream expertise. Conversely, my unique clinical/scientific perspective was invaluable in brokering the application of basic science to practical applications (military, industry, and clinical care). The essence of effective collaboration is the unique mix of ideas in a nonthreatening, collegial atmosphere from which emerges robust ideas and creative research designs. Those professional relationships foster professional challenge, intellectual reward, and scientific value. During my UF years (1980–1989), I had the distinct privilege of being involved with various research collaborations in my capacity as member or Fellow of The Center for Gerontological Studies, The Mind-Machine Interaction Research Center, and the Institute for Advanced Study of Communication Processes. The collaborative model is signature for me and continues to the present with my recent reflux (LPR) investigations. My CCF team involved colleagues from ENT, SLP, GI, and Surgery working on various projects spanning eight years. Almost 20 publications and dozens of presentations emerged from that joint venture.

Another lifetime career theme has been interest in and investigation of laryngeal physiology. Its importance is reflected in the operational definition of all voice disorders being compromised of three components: symptoms, physiology, and etiology. Physiology is the key component that reconciles the other two—explaining why a particular patient sounds a particular way given the etiology or pathology. That triad definition was championed by Dr. G. Paul Moore and is unavoidably linked to his pioneering work with high-speed photography. The critical "bridge" role of physiology justifies its attention for research efforts—particularly with the voids of understanding that still exist in our knowledge base. That void was one of the driving forces behind our study of the focus for this article, vocal quality. Laryngeal or vocal quality represents one of the more complicated of the performance parameters of all voices. (The other parameters being pitch, loudness, and nasal resonance.) Within the voice disorder population, laryngeal quality is the parameter most often compromised. Given the complexity of physiology responsible for quality (both respiratory, laryngeal, and vocal tract dynamics), research focus on vocal quality is logical. Ironically, almost 2 decades after publishing this article, our insight into the "acoustic correlates of vocal quality" is not much advanced. This dilemma says less about our research commitment and more about the complexity of human voice. It defies being defined simply; it is worthy of our continued research effort.

Final comment relates to our ability to conduct that future research. Will there be enough new scientists to receive the proverbial baton from an older cohort? The current manpower shortage, reflected in ASHA's focused initiative for recruitment of scientists, suggests a potential "brain drain" crisis. In the 1960s and 1970s, our own trained speech pathology/science colleagues provided the majority of knowledge. By the 1980s, the trend toward abdicating that responsibility to other disciplines was beginning. My own UF experience confirms that, as much of our physiology work (including this article) was bound to nontraditional scientists—in this case, electrical engineers. That trend has accelerated to the point that few speech science students are being trained in our own communicative disorder and science graduate programs. There is a decline of senior faculty, as well, that disrupts the time-honored mentoring process that creates the next generation of scientific investigators. There should be legitimate concern about our ability to continue to study this important area of speech science.

In summary, the featured article "Acoustic Correlates of Vocal Quality" allows reflection on several levels. It represents one of many investigations attempting to better understand voice performance and its underlying physiology. The relative lack of improved insight with this topic, almost 2 decades after publication, highlights the complexity of the problem to be addressed. The critical involvement of vocal quality in the differential diagnosis and treatment of voice disorders justifies it to be the continued focus of future research investigation. A multidisciplinary approach holds the best prospect for answers. The measure of research success is not strictly the number of scientific questions answered. Equally important is an investigation process reflecting patience, tenacity, scientific rigor, intellectual integrity, creativity, and collegial communication. In my research journey, I have been privileged to experience that process in great measure by collaboration with outstanding professional colleagues. This featured article represents just one such project in my 3 decades of research endeavor.

ACOUSTIC CORRELATES OF VOCAL QUALITY

L. ESKENAZI
Department of Electrical Engineering, University of Florida

D. G. CHILDERS
Thomson CSF, Malakoff, France

D. M. HICKS
Communicative Disorders, The Cleveland Clinical Foundation

We have investigated the relationship between various voice qualities and several acoustic measures made from the vowel /i/ phonated by subjects with normal voices and patients with vocal disorders. Among the patients (pathological voices), five qualities were investigated: overall severity, hoarseness, breathiness, roughness, and vocal fry. Six acoustic measures were examined. With one exception, all measures were extracted from the residue signal obtained by inverse filtering the speech signal using the linear predictive coding (LPC) technique. A formal listening test was implemented to rate each pathological voice for each vocal quality. A formal listening test also rated overall excellence of the normal voices. A scale of 1–7 was used. Multiple linear regression analysis between the results of the listening test and the various acoustic measures was used with the prediction sums of squares (PRESS) as the selection criteria. Useful prediction equations of order two or less were obtained relating certain acoustic measures and the ratings of pathological voices for each of the five qualities. The two most useful parameters for predicting vocal quality were the Pitch Amplitude (PA) and the Harmonics-to-Noise Ratio (HNR). No acoustic measure could rank the normal voices.

KEY WORDS: vocal quality, vocal disorders, acoustic measures, residue signal

Analytic methods and commercial devices exist for measuring certain vocal characteristics, for example, the common measures of fundamental frequency of voicing (F_0), intensity, flow rate and flow volume, and the less common measures of F_0 jitter perturbations (Davis, 1976; Hillenbrand, 1987; Hollien, Michel, & Doherty, 1973; Horii, 1979; Klinholz & Martin, 1985; Koike & Markel, 1975; Koike, Takahashi, & Calcaterra, 1977; Lieberman, 1961, 1963; Milenkovic, 1987; Smith, Weinberg, Feth, & Horii, 1978; Sorensen & Horii, 1984; Wendahl, 1966), shimmer perturbations (Horii, 1980; Kasuya, Ogawa, Kikushi, & Ebihara, 1986; Klinholz & Martin, 1985; Ludlow, Bassich, Connor, Coulter, & Lee, 1987; Sorensen & Horii, 1984), spectral noise levels and harmonics-to-noise ratio (Kasuya, Masubuchi, Ebihara, & Yoshida, 1986; Kitajima, 1981; Yumoto, Gould, & Baer, 1982; Yumoto, Sasaki, & Okamura, 1984), breathiness (Fukazawa, El-Assuoofy, & Honjo, 1988), long term spectral average (Hammarberg, Fritzell, Gauffin, Sundberg, & Wedin, 1980), and others. From these measures normative ranges for F_0 and several other measures have been established. However, acoustic profiles of vocal quality are lacking, despite the fact that speech quality has been the focus of considerable research (Childers & Wu, 1990; Colton & Estill, 1981; Eskenazi, 1988; Klatt, 1987; Laver, 1980; Murry & Singh, 1980; Pinto, Childers, & Lalwani, 1989; Quackenbush, Barnwell, & Clements, 1988; Singh & Murry, 1978). Researchers have also attempted to determine those vocal qualities most common and significant. To achieve this goal various quality scales have been used, such as GRBAS in Japan (Imaizumi, 1986) and diagnostic acceptability measure (Voiers, 1977). Numerous studies have examined the possibility of obtaining quantitative information concerning vocal fold function and voice quality; however, the performance of the various measures considered has been found to depend on the type of pathology, the speaker's gender, and the condition of analysis (Kasuya, Kobayashi, & Kobayashi, 1983; Kasuya, Masubuchi, Ebihara, & Yoshida, 1986; Kasuya, Ogawa, Kikushi, & Ebihara, 1986; Muta, Muraoka, Wagatsuma, Fukuda, Takayama, Fujioka, & Kanou, 1987). Although a single measure of assessing vocal quality may be ineffective, a combination of measures may prove satisfactory (Prosek, Montgomery, & Hawkins, 1987; Sansone & Emanuel, 1970; Yumoto, Gould, & Baer, 1982).

One indirect procedure often used for studying vocal fold vibratory characteristics and their relationship to vocal quality is inverse filtering to obtain an estimate of the volume-velocity waveform (Hillman & Weinberg, 1981; Javkin, Antonanzas-Barroso, & Maddieson, 1987; Koike & Markel, 1975; Markel & Gray, 1976; Rothenberg, 1973; Rothenberg & Zahorian, 1977). Several disadvantages of using this approach are: (a) it is difficult to determine the parameters for the inverse filter model from the speech signal, (b) the volume-velocity waveform obtained by inverse filtering contains only low-frequency information, and (c) the vocal tract is assumed to be a linear model, which may not always be valid for large glottal openings (Koike & Markel, 1975; Rothenberg & Zahorian, 1977). For these reasons researchers have considered alternative procedures, for example the error or residue signal at the output of the inverse filter (Davis, 1976; Prosek et al., 1987). The residue signal has a broad frequency spectrum and for speakers with normal voices the residue signal typically contains clear spikes at glottal closure (Markel & Gray, 1976). Speakers with pathological voices often have incomplete glottal closure contrib-

Reproduced with permission from *J Speech Hear Res.* 1990;33:298–306.

uting to a less distinct pattern of periodic spikes (Koike & Markel, 1975; Prosek et al., 1987). Figures 1 and 2 show illustrative examples of the speech and residue signals for a normal and pathological speaker respectively. We decided to use the residue signal in our studies because it required less interactive judgment on the part of the investigator, contained more high-frequency spectral information than the glottal volume-velocity waveform, provided information about the timing of vocal fold vibratory events, and removed the effects of the vocal tract. Most of the previous studies have attempted to identify acoustic features that could distinguish a normal voice from a voice with a vocal disorder. As in the study by Prosek et al. (1987) we wanted to examine the possibility of using features of the residue signal to predict vocal quality, including vocal disorders. A listening test was conducted to confirm the usefulness of one or more of these acoustic measures for predicting and objectifying the assessment of vocal quality. The listening test was not conducted to justify the machine classification of vocal quality, rather, it was to serve as a method for validating the possible clinical utility of any of the acoustic measures we assessed. Thus, in brief, the purpose of our study was to relate the parameters of the residue signal obtained by analyzing the speech signal to the perceived vocal qualities judged by trained listeners. The acoustic parameters were evaluated as possible predictors of vocal quality using multiple linear regression analysis.

PROCEDURES

Acoustic Measures

Following the completion of a pilot study by Eskenazi (1988), six measures were implemented.

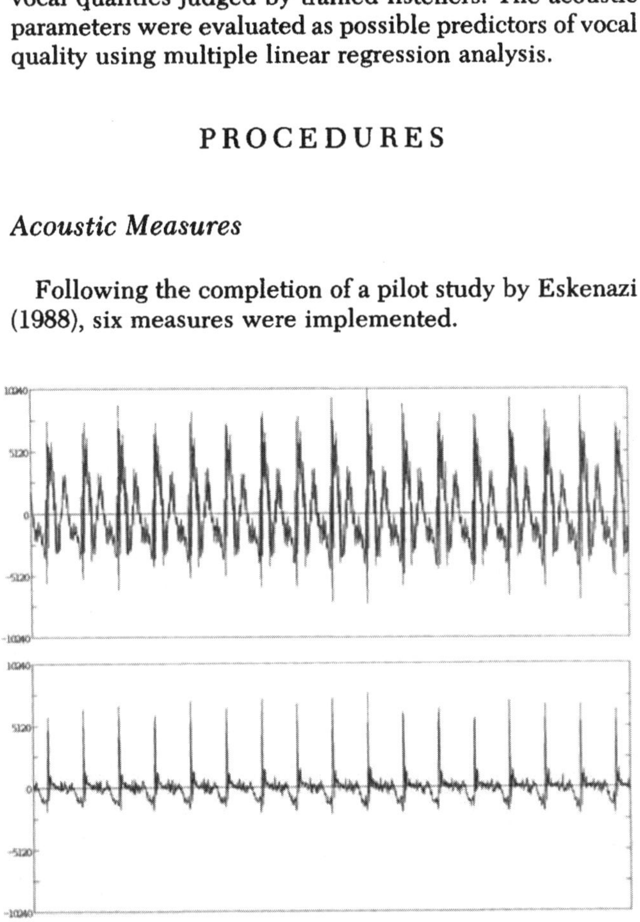

FIGURE 1. Speech (top panel) and residue signals (bottom panel) for a normal male speaker (M1). The time scale is from 0 to 128 ms.

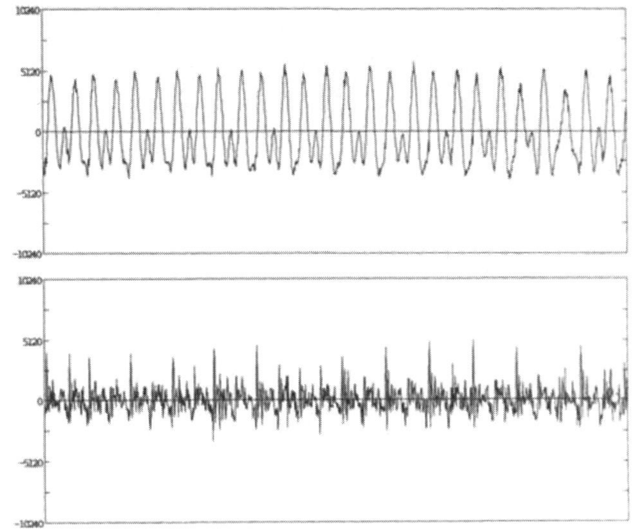

FIGURE 2. Speech (top panel) and residue signals (bottom panel) for a pathological speaker (P13). The time scale is from 0 to 128 ms.

Spectral Flatness of the Residue Signal (SFR). As defined by Markel & Gray (1976), the flatness of the magnitude spectrum (in decibels) is the logarithm of the ratio of the geometric mean of the spectrum to the arithmetic mean of the spectrum. The SFR is a negative quantity, and a large negative number corresponds to a "good voice," whereas a small negative number corresponds to a "bad voice." Davis (1976) and Prosek et al. (1987) suggested that the SFR measures the masking of fundamental frequency harmonics by noise.

Pitch Amplitude (PA). The PA is the maximum amplitude of the normalized autocorrelation function of the residue signal that does not appear at the origin (Rabiner & Schafer, 1978). This maximum peak usually corresponds to the second peak in the normalized autocorrelation function. The first peak is unity amplitude and occurs at the origin. Figure 3 presents examples of PAs for normal and pathological voices. Since the PA represents the degree of voicing, it is expected to be lower for abnormal (e.g., breathy) voices than for normal voices. It will also be low for normal voices phonating unvoiced sounds and voiced fricatives. Prosek et al. (1987) employed the PA in their measurement battery as well.

Harmonics-to-Noise Ratio. A spectrogram of a normal voice typically shows well-developed harmonics, whereas a hoarse voice will fail to show strong harmonics (Yanagihara, 1967). Based on this observation, Yumoto, Gould, & Baer (1982) derived a new measure, the Harmonics-to-Noise Ratio (HNR), which is the ratio of the acoustic energy of the stable harmonic to that of the noise. The Harmonics-to-Noise Ratio is believed to be well correlated with the index of hoarseness (Yumoto, Gould, & Baer, 1982). By its nature, this measure takes into account the jitter and shimmer present in the signal, which is one of its advantages, because jitter affects the spectrum of a sustained vowel by reducing the amplitudes of the harmonics and introducing noise between

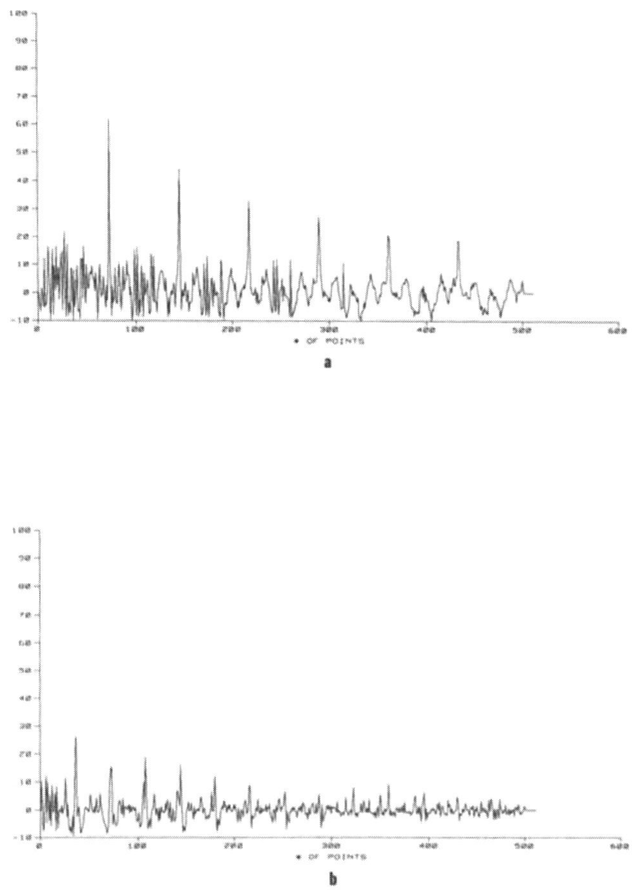

FIGURE 3. Autocorrelation of residue signal a: normal male speaker (M4), b: pathological speaker (P22).

them. The HNR is the only measure in this study to be extracted directly from the speech signal.

Perturbation Measures. Koike et al. (1977) indicated that steady vowel sounds normally exhibit slow and relatively smooth changes in the period and suggested that perturbations be measured from a smoothed trend line when investigating rapid variations in periodicity. This leads to the concept of Perturbation Quotients. The Pitch Perturbation Quotient, or PPQ, is the ratio of a moving average of fundamental period differences to the average fundamental period, where the length of the moving average is equal to five periods. The Amplitude Perturbation Quotient (APQ) is defined as the variation in signal amplitude measured at the fundamental period divided by the mean amplitude. A moving average of five amplitude values is used for this calculation. These perturbation quotients are computed using first the positive peaks of the residue signal, then the negative peaks, with the smallest result being kept (Davis, 1976). The PPQ and APQ represent the amount of deviation from the mean period and the mean amplitude, respectively. Both quantities are expressed in percent. Prosek et al. (1987) also included PPQ and APQ in their study.

Percent Jitter. This term is derived by dividing the mean jitter in ms by the mean period in ms times one hundred, where the mean jitter is

$$\textit{Mean Jitter} = 1/(N-1) * \sum_{i=1}^{N-1} \left| P_i - P_{i+1} \right|$$

where P_i is the period of the *i*th cycle and N is the number of consecutive cycles analyzed. This measure was introduced by Horii (1979, 1980).

Most of the above measures require a precise evaluation of the pitch period, which we measured using the location of the highest peak of the autocorrelation of the residue signal (not counting the peak at the origin). The results of this latter algorithm were compared to another algorithm that measured the pitch period as the difference between the negative peaks of the differentiated electroglottogram (DEGG). The two algorithms gave comparable results (Eskenazi, 1988).

Voice Data Base

The data base of speakers with no vocal disorders (normal) consisted of 25 normal male speakers with an average age of 34 years, ranging from 21–51, and 25 normal female speakers, with an average age of 28 years, ranging from 20–53. None of the speakers had a history of laryngeal disease.

One finds it difficult to define a "normal voice." Moore (1971) has pointed out that there are many normal voices based on such characteristics as gender and age. The location of the threshold that separates the normal from the abnormal voice is judged by each listener on the basis of his or her cultural standards, education, environment, vocal training, and similar factors, but wherever the separation between adequate and inadequate is placed, it is obvious that each individual has acquired concepts of normalcy and defectiveness (Moore, 1971). Our definition of normal voice was given by one of the authors (Hicks) as a voice with no apparent pathology (either functional or organic) and no unusual voice characteristics or habits.

Each subject performed a number of vocal tasks, including counting from 1 to 10, singing the musical scale, reading three sentences, and phonating vowels and fricatives. For this study, we examined the data for the vowel /i/, which each subject phonated for approximately 2 s at a comfortable loudness and pitch. The speech and electroglottographic signals were recorded with an Electrovoice, type *RE-10* dynamic cardoid microphone and a Synchrovoice electroglottograph. The microphone was located 6 in. from the mouth. The signals were directly digitized via a Digital Sound Corporation (DSC) 200 A/D system and stored on a disk for further processing on a VAX 11/750 computer. The speech signal was sharply low-pass filtered at 4800 Hz and sampled at 10 kHz with each sample being represented by 16 bits. Sampling began before the initiation of the vowel and continued for about 1 s after vowel cessation. All recordings were made in an IAC sound-treated booth. For this study we examined only the speech data.

The pathologic voice data base consisted of 16 patients with vocal disorders. Two patients were remeasured twice and 3 patients were remeasured once after treatment. A description of the vocal disorders can be found in Table 1. The range of voices varied from mildly deviant to very deviant as determined by one of the authors (Hicks). The patients were asked to phonate the vowel /i/ for about 2 s. The vowel /i/ was chosen for this study because we have found this vowel particularly useful for ultra high-speed laryngeal photography (Childers & Krishnamurthy, 1985; Childers, Naik, Larar, Krishnamurthy, & Moore, 1983). Consequently, we had extensive data for this vowel.

Listening Test

The panel of listeners consisted of seven judges (four males and three females). All judges were faculty in the University of Florida Speech Department familiar with the various voice qualities evaluated in this study. For this listening test, the vowel /i/ was used. A training signal representative of the average quality of the vowel /i/ to be judged was presented before each listening task. Each task signal (token) was 2 s in duration and was presented two times with an interval of 2 s between the two tokens. Prior to the presentation of each pair of test tokens a sinusoidal tone of 2 s was presented to cue the listener that a test token was about to be presented. The tokens were generated by computer via a digital-to-analog converter and were presented via headphones in a professional IAC sound room. In all, six tasks were implemented. There were five tasks for the ratings of the pathological voices: 1) overall severity, 2) hoarseness, 3) breathiness, 4) roughness, and 5) vocal fry; and 6) an additional task to judge the overall excellence of the 50 normal voices. The definitions we used for these six listening tasks were:

Overall severity. Defined as a comprehensive evaluation of the voice taking into account such factors as hoarseness, breathiness, roughness, and vocal fry.
Hoarseness. Defined as breathy plus rough; it is, therefore, a result of a combination of excessive air escapage and an aperiodicity of vocal fold vibration.
Breathiness. Defined as audible escapage of air through the glottis due to insufficient glottal closure; the degree of breathiness severity is inversely proportional to the length of the closed glottal phase.
Roughness. Defined as low-pitched noise, presumably due to irregular vocal fold vibrations.
Vocal fry. Defined perceptually to be a low-pitched, rough-sounding phonation.
Excellence of normal voice. An excellent normal voice was defined as one that appeared to have professional speech training, for example, a voice with good glottal closure, thus providing a good excitation of the vocal tract. The normal voice was defined above.

The scale used for pathological voices was from 1 to 7 with 1 denoting the absence of the quality to be judged (e.g., no breathiness) and 7 denoting an extreme example of the quality to be judged (e.g., extreme breathiness). For normal voices, a value of 1 denoted a poor quality voice whereas a 7 denoted an excellent quality voice. Most previous studies used either a 4-point scale (Moran & Gilbert, 1984), a 5-point scale (Kuwabara & Ohgushi, 1984; Sapozhkov, 1972), a 7-point scale (Prosek et al., 1987), a 9-point scale (Hecker & Kreul, 1971; Kreul & Hecker, 1971), a 10-point scale (Rothauser, Urbauer, & Pachl, 1971). In our case, due to the relatively wide range of vocal qualities present in the data base, a 7-point scale was appropriate. In order to test the reliability of each judge, a selected number of tokens, unknown to the judges, were repeated for each task. We then graded each judge on ability to make consistent judgments on the repeated tokens.

TABLE 1. Characteristics of pathological speakers.

Patient code	*Gender*	*Symptoms*
P1	F	Mild Hoarseness
*P2	F	Hyper Functional
*P3	F	Vocal Fry
P4	F	P3 1 month post injection
P5	F	P3 3 months post injection
*P6	F	Enlarged muscle
P7	M	Breathy; Hoarse
P8	M	P7 1 month post injection
P9	M	Hoarse
P10	M	P9 5 months post injection
*P11	F	Posterior cyst
P12	M	True Vocal Cords (TVC) contact ulcer
*P13	M	Hoarse unilateral TVC carcinoma
P14	M	Vocal Fry
P15	F	Nodules
*P16	F	Right TVC unilateral paralysis
*P17	F	Unilateral paralysis
P18	F	P17 1 month post injection
*P19	F	P17 4 months post injection
P20	F	Breathy, Weak
P21	F	P20 1 month post injection
*P22	M	Bilateral paralysis of TVC
P23	F	Bilateral nodule

*Very deviant voices.

Conditions of Analysis

Based on the studies by Davis (1976) and Prosek et al. (1987), we adopted the following conditions of analysis:

Sampling frequency: 10 kHz
Filter order: 14
No preemphasis
Starting point: 384 ms after start of utterance
Length of interval of analysis: 128 ms with no overlap between successive frames.

The vocal intensity was not controlled. Each subject phonated at a comfortable pitch and intensity level. Intensity was not considered a factor because all signals analyzed were approximately the same magnitude after digitization. No recording or post recording amplification adjustments of gain were made.

The short interval of analysis resulted in a relatively small number of pitch periods being analyzed. This

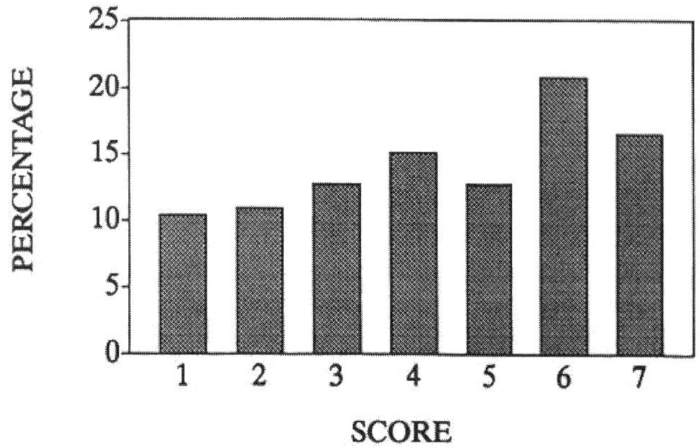

FIGURE 4. Histogram of the distribution for the 7 scores for overall severity. The coefficient of concordance is .63.

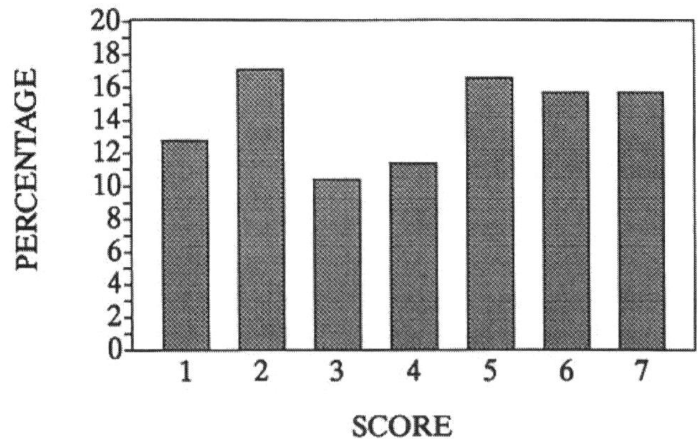

FIGURE 5. Histogram of the distribution for the 7 scores for hoarseness. The coefficient of concordance is .65.

required further investigation. We examined the influence of the number of periods analyzed on the perturbation measures and the HNR and found that there were variations depending on the number of pitch periods in the data record analyzed (Eskenazi, 1988). We concluded that an interval of 50 periods was the best compromise, which was in agreement with the findings of Yumoto, Gould, & Baer (1982). Hence, for the multiple linear regression analyses between the listening test ratings and the acoustic measures, we analyzed data intervals containing at least 50 pitch periods and updated the inverse filter coefficients every 25.6 ms. For those measures that required a peak picking algorithm, we used parabolic interpolation (Markel & Gray, 1976). This counterbalanced the effect of using a relatively low sampling frequency of 10 kHz (Titze, Horii, & Scherer, 1987). To further confirm our use of the 10 kHz sampling frequency we investigated the effect on our data analysis of using a 100 kHz sampling frequency for three representative patients. The results of our analysis were not affected by the sampling frequency.

RESULTS

Analysis of the Listening Test

Recall that the seven judges rated the 50 normal voices on a 1-to-7 scale of overall excellence, and the 23 pathological voices using the same 1-to-7 scale for five voice quality conditions: overall severity, hoarseness, breathiness, roughness, and vocal fry. We evaluated the listeners' agreement by computing a histogram of the distribution of the seven scores for the six listening tasks. In addition, we calculated the coefficient of concordance for each task (Winer, 1971). These data are presented in Figures 4–9. As the coefficients of concordance indicate, the listeners tended to agree for the pathological listening tasks and disagreed on the evaluation of "normal" voices. The histograms tended to be uniformly distributed across the scoring scale for the pathological tasks, whereas the distribution for the normal task tended to be bell shaped with a slight skewing toward the excellence end of the scale.

In addition to the above listener evaluation we graded each judge's consistency for scoring repeated tokens in each listening task. If a particular judge did not achieve at least a 60% consistency score for a given task, then his or her ratings for that task were not included in the calculations of the means. This happened only four times for three different tasks. We believe this indicated a good intrajudge consistency, given the difficulty of the listening tasks.

Pathological voices. Since we expected that each vocal quality was in fact correlated to more than just one acoustic parameter, the following procedure was adopted for each task: a multiple linear regression analysis was performed, and the acoustic parameters obtained by this regression were recorded. The selection criterion we used was the prediction sum of squares (PRESS) (Allen & Cady, 1982). The acoustic parameters were used as predictors with the quality scale as a criterion. The best PRESS model (i.e., the model with the lowest PRESS value) was adopted. The acoustic correlates of each vocal quality are summarized in Table 2 along with the square of the multiple linear correlations (R^2). The correspond-

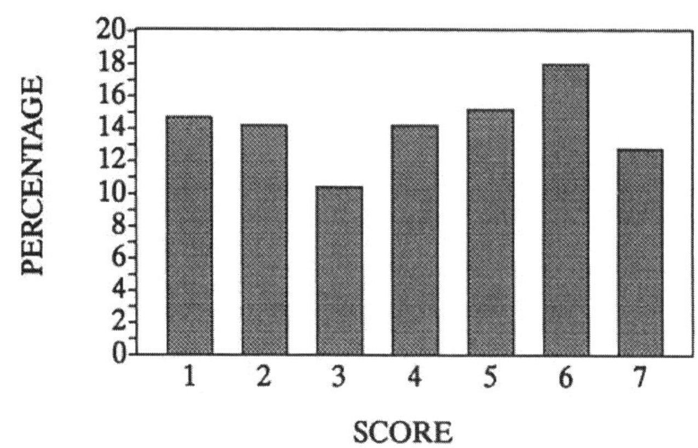

FIGURE 6. Histogram of the distribution for the 7 scores for breathiness. The coefficient of concordance is .54.

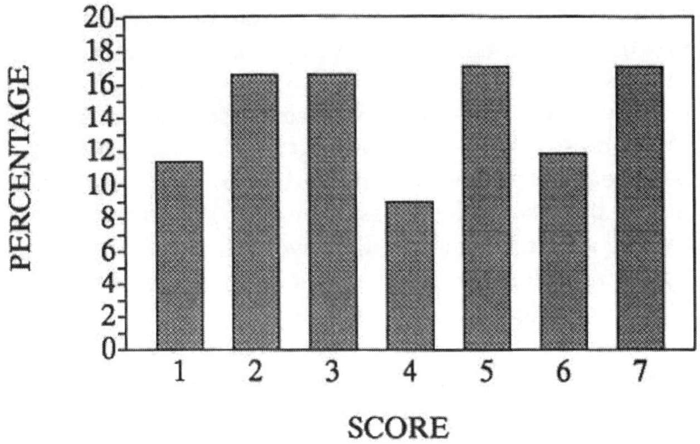

FIGURE 7. Histogram of the distribution for the 7 scores for roughness. The coefficient of concordance is .71.

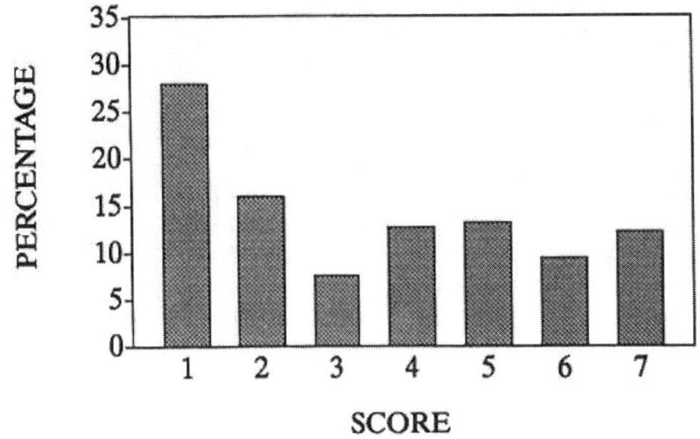

FIGURE 9. Histogram of the distribution for the 7 scores for the normal speakers. The coefficient of concordance is .26.

ing multiple linear regression models are presented in Table 3.

Normal voices. A mentioned earlier, the interjudge reliability was low for normal voices, preventing us from considering the means of the ratings across all judges for the single rating of overall excellence of the voice. We conducted multiple linear regressions for each vocal quality as evaluated by each judge using the acoustic parameters as predictors. The results indicated that the important parameters varied from judge to judge, and no definite trend could be derived from these results. These results suggest that each judge relied on different parameters, and apparently the parameters studied here represent only a small subset of the set of parameters used by the judges. Consequently, the only conclusions we considered were for the pathological voices

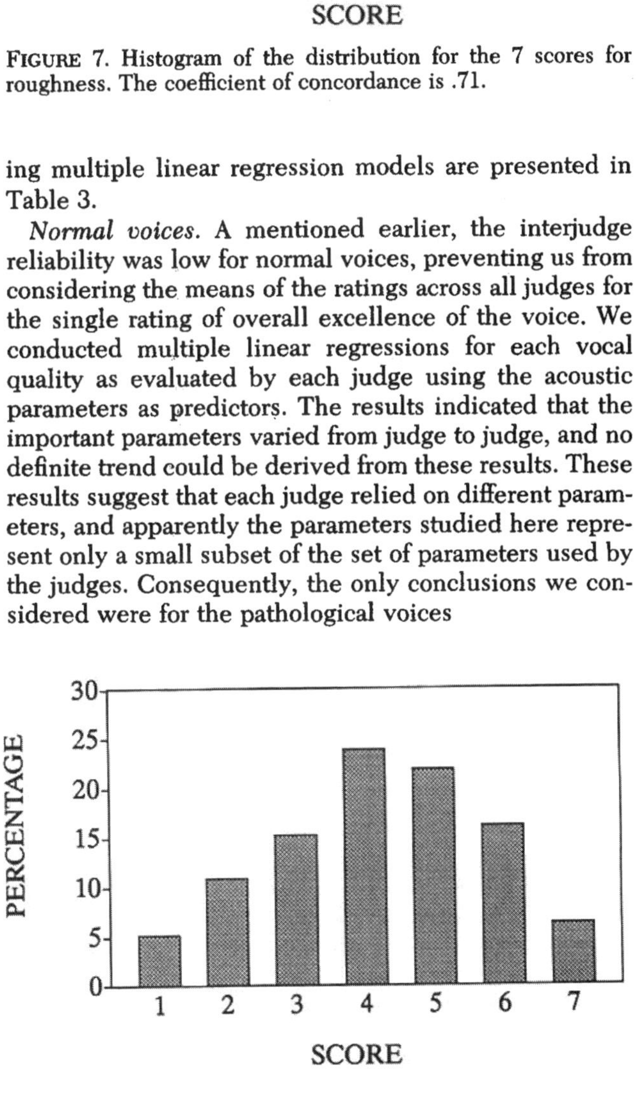

FIGURE 8. Histogram of the distribution for the 7 scores for vocal fry. The coefficient of concordance is .51.

DISCUSSION

The selection of the model order in regression analysis is known to involve a "trade-off between including variables that will reduce the residual sum of squares from the use of an insufficient model, and including variables that have little effect on the residual sum of squares but will increase the variance of a predicted value" (Allen & Cady, 1982, p. 254). The prediction sum of squares (PRESS) is recommended as a more realistic criterion than the residual sum of squares (Allen & Cady, 1982). For a particular set of variables PRESS is obtained by predicting each observation using all the *other* observations. The resulting residuals (PRESS residuals) are squared and summed to form PRESS (Allen & Cady, 1982). The PRESS criterion is to find the lowest value of the PRESS residuals. When we applied the PRESS criterion to our data we found that each vocal quality (severity, hoarseness, breathiness, roughness, and vocal fry) could be modeled by a first or second order model as listed in Table 3. Lower and higher order models had larger prediction sum of squares residuals. We also calculated the R^2 as shown in Table 2 for the PRESS condition. When we used the R^2 as the model selection criterion (instead of PRESS) we calculated the model orders up to and including six and listed the residual sum of squares for comparison purposes. Although the R^2 always increased in this case the increase was not very great over that for the second order model (or first order model in the case of breathiness) selected by the PRESS criterion.

The results of the regression analyses performed for the various vocal qualities brought out several points. Among the six acoustic parameters considered, the most impor-

TABLE 2. Main factors for the prediction of the quality of pathological voices (using means of listening test) with PRESS as the selection criterion.

	Overall severity	*Hoarseness*	*Breathiness*	*Roughness*	*Vocal fry*
Main Factors	PA, HNR $R^2 = 0.57$	PA, %JIT $R^2 = 0.56$	%JIT $R^2 = 0.30$	SFR, HNR $R^2 = 0.59$	PA, HNR $R^2 = 0.54$

TABLE 3. Models derived from regression analyses for various quality scales with PRESS as the selection criterion.

Quality (Y)	*Equation of the model*
Overall severity	Y = 6.37 − 4.18 * PA − 0.06 * HNR
Hoarseness	Y = 4.8 − 4.26 * PA + 0.1 * %JIT
Breathiness	Y = 2.27 + 0.19 * %JIT
Roughness	Y = 6.49 + 0.20 * SFR − 0.13 * HNR
Vocal fry	Y = 5.06 − 2.55 * PA − 0.09 * HNR

tant was the PA, which was a predominant factor for three of the pathological vocal qualities. The second most important factor was the HNR, which was also a factor for three of the vocal qualities. However, HNR was always a second factor. The parameter %JIT was a predictor for both hoarseness and breathiness. The PPQ and the APQ did not play a role in the judges' evaluation of vocal quality of pathological speakers.

The results obtained contradict previous studies concerning the HNR. It is interesting to note that in our study the HNR did not play a role in the prediction of hoarseness, contrary to other studies (Yumoto et al., 1982; Yumoto et al., 1984). As a result of their research, Yumoto et al. (1982) concluded that pathological voices had an HNR smaller than 7.4 dB. Our results do not support this conclusion; 70% of the pathological voices analyzed had an HNR larger than 7.4 dB, and 19% of the normal voices had an HNR smaller than 7.4 dB. This finding is similar to that given by Moss & Hicks (1985). Also, contrary to the findings of Yumoto et al. (1982), female voices had a larger HNR than male voices, and this difference was statistically significant (Eskenazi, 1988).

The model obtained for the prediction of breathiness was the poorest because the R^2 was lower than any of the other voice qualities. The R^2 never exceeded 0.5 even when all six acoustic parameters were included. Furthermore, the PRESS criterion did not vary greatly as other acoustic parameters were added to increase the model order. In other words, %JIT was the best predictor for breathiness according to the PRESS criterion. It appears that breathiness has not been studied as extensively as hoarseness. Klich (1982) noted that the number of discernible harmonics decreased as breathiness increased. This is not in contradiction with our findings because, unlike Klich (1982), we used speakers with vocal disorders for the study of breathiness, and the effects and relationship of spectral parameters may differ from normal speakers to pathologic ones. Furthermore, HNR was a factor for breathiness in our study if we considered a higher order prediction model. In their research, Wolfe and Steinfatt (1987) found that the fundamental frequency and a jitter-related measure were the only significant predictors of breathiness, with the logarithm of the period standard deviation being the most important one. It has been observed (Hammarberg et al., 1980; Issihiki, Yanagihara, & Morimoto, 1966) that the loss of high frequency components in the overall spectrum was an acoustic correlate of breathiness, which was attributed to an increase in the open phase of the laryngeal vibratory cycle. This explains why the spectrographic classification system (Yanagihara, 1967), based on noise components increasing in intensity in the higher portion of the frequency range, was not very effective for the detection of breathiness. Wolfe and Steinfatt (1987) conjectured that laryngeal irregularities contributing to turbulent airflow in breathiness might be less complex than in the production of a hoarse quality. This would mean that breathy voices are closer to normal voices than are other voice types, and might explain why the prediction of breathiness is almost as difficult as the prediction of the quality of normal voices.

In a study of roughness, Imaizumi (1986) concluded that the acoustic correlates of roughness include the multiplicative variations that occur over several pitch periods, as well as those that are synchronous with the vocal pitch period; he also noted that an irregularity in the speech waveform was not essential for perceptual roughness. Our results suggest that pitch perturbation measures as reflected in the HNR and SRF are indeed an important correlate of roughness.

The primary goal of this study was to find the acoustic correlates of voices spanning a wide range on the vocal quality continuum. The perceptual evaluation of pathologic voices on five different scales yielded some results that were readily interpretable. On the other hand, the perceptual evaluation of normal voices was inconclusive because each judge apparently used his or her own criteria, possibly using perceptual factors not covered by the set of acoustic measures studied here. Our finding with respect to normal voices agrees with that of Prosek et al. (1987).

It is likely that a vocal disorder could affect more than one dimension of the voice simultaneously. This makes the task of estimating specific attributes of the voice using acoustic parameters difficult. To be more conclusive, more information concerning the effects of specific pathologies on vocal fold vibration is needed and a more comprehensive study of larger speech samples is needed. Furthermore, a larger set of subjects should be used so that the statistics would be more meaningful.

Despite these weaknesses, the results obtained in this study for pathological voices were sufficient to derive models to predict the various vocal qualities with a reasonable level of reliability. One of the weaknesses of our study and that of others resides in the fact that the acoustic measures used as predictors of quality appear to represent only a fraction of the set of all measures used by a human listener. However, our results suggest that the set of acoustic measures chosen for this study was adequate. The values of R^2 obtained for the various regressions were slightly inferior to those obtained by Prosek et al. (1987) in a similar study, but this was due to the fact that by using multiple linear regression with PRESS as the selection criterion we used fewer acoustic parameters as predictors.

Our conclusions for the patient data are similar to those of Prosek et al. (1987, p. 115) who suggested that "it may be possible to develop a vocal index of degree of impairment based on these (their) measurements." These authors also suggested (p. 115) that their results "indicate how difficult it will be to develop an acoustically based vocal index that includes a quantification of specific voice qualities." Our results for the normative data also agree with this latter observation.

The main conclusion of our study was that the two best predictors for vocal quality were Pitch Amplitude (PA) and Harmonics-to-Noise Ratio. This result is consistent with the findings of Prosek et al. (1987). The results concerning pathological voices were:

1. overall quality was characterized by a low PA and a low HNR,
2. a hoarse voice exhibited a low PA and a high %JIT,
3. a breathy voice was characterized by high %JIT,
4. a rough voice was characterized by a low SFR and a low HNR,
5. vocal fry was characterized by a low PA and a low HNR.

This study showed that various patient vocal qualities can be predicted with some acoustic measures, and that the degree of reliability of this prediction may be improved by adding other efficient and independent acoustic measures to the list of predictors.

ACKNOWLEDGMENTS

This research was primarily supported by NIH grants NIDCD R01 DC00577 and NINCDS R01 NS17078 with additional support from the University of Florida Center of Excellence Program in Information Transfer and Processing, and the Mind-Machine Interaction Research Center.

REFERENCES

ALLEN, D. M., & CADY, F. B. (1982). *Analyzing experimental data by regression.* Belmont, CA: Wadsworth.

CHILDERS, D. G., & KRISHNAMURTHY, A. K. (1985). A critical review of electroglottography. *CRC Critical Reviews in Biomedical Engineering, 12,* 131–161.

CHILDERS, D. G., NAIK, J. M., LARAR, J. N., KRISHNAMURTHY, A. K., & MOORE, G. P. (1983). Electroglottography, speech and ultra-high speed cinematography. In I. R. Titze & R. Scherer (Eds.), *Vocal fold physiology and biophysics of voice* (pp. 202–220). Denver, CO: Denver Center for the Performing Arts.

CHILDERS, D. G. & WU, K. (1990). Quality of speech produced by analysis-synthesis. *Speech Communication, 9*(1).

COLTON, R. H., & ESTILL, J. A. (1981). Elements of voice quality: Perceptual, acoustic, and physiologic aspects. *Speech and Language, 5,* 311–403.

DAVIS, B. S. (1976). *Computer evaluation of laryngeal pathology based on inverse filtering of speech.* Speech Communication Research Laboratory, Monograph Number 13, Santa Barbara, CA.

ESKENAZI, L. (1988). *Acoustic correlates of voice quality and distortion measure for speech processing.* Unpublished doctoral dissertation, University of Florida, Gainseville.

FUKAZAWA, T., EL-ASSUOOFY, A., & HONJO, J. (1988). A new index for evaluation of the turbulent noise in pathological voice. *Journal of the Acoustical Society of America, 83*(3), 1189–1193.

HAMMARBERG, B., FRITZELL, B., GAUFFIN, J., SUNDBERG, J., & WEDIN, L. (1980). Perceptual and acoustic correlates of abnormal voice qualities. *Acta Otolaryngology, 90,* 441–451.

HECKER, M. H., & KREUL, E. J. (1971). Descriptions of speech of patients with cancer of the vocal folds. Part I: Measures of fundamental frequency. *Journal of Acoustical Society of America, 49,* 1275–1282.

HILLENBRAND, J. (1987). A methodological study of perturbation and additive noise in synthetically generated voice signals. *Journal of Speech and Hearing Research, 30,* 448–61.

HILLMAN, R. E., & WEINBERG, B. (1981). Estimation of volume velocity waveform properties. A review and study of some methodological assumptions. In N. Lass (Ed.), *Speech and language: Advances in basic research and practice* (pp. 411–473). New York: Academic Press.

HOLLIEN, H., MICHEL, J., & DOHERTY, E. T. (1973). A method for analyzing vocal jitter in sustained phonation. *Journal of Phonetics, 1,* 85–91.

HORII, Y. (1979). Fundamental frequency perturbation observed in sustained phonation. *Journal of Speech and Hearing Research, 22,* 5–19.

HORII, Y. (1980). Vocal shimmer in sustained phonation. *Journal of Speech and Hearing Research, 23,* 202–209.

IMAIZUMI, S. (1986). Acoustic measures of roughness in pathological voice. *Journal of Phonetics, 14,* 457–462.

ISSHIKI, N., YANAGIHARA, N., & MORIMOTO, M. (1966). Approach to the objective diagnosis of hoarseness. *Folia Phoniatrica, 18*(6), 393–400.

JAVKIN, H. R., ANTONANZAS-BARROSO, N., & MADDIESON, I. (1987). Digital inverse filtering for linguistic research. *Journal of Speech and Hearing Research, 30,* 122–129.

KASUYA, H., KOBAYASHI, Y., & KOBAYASHI, T. (1983). Characteristics of pitch period and amplitude perturbations in pathological voice. *Proceedings of the International IEEE Conference on Acoustics, Speech, and Signal Processing.* New York, NY: Institute of Electrical and Electronic Engineers, 1372–1375.

KASUYA, H., MASUBUCHI, K., EBIHARA, S., & YOSHIDA, H. (1986). Preliminary experiments on voice screening. *Journal of Phonetics, 14,* 463–468.

KASUYA, H., OGAWA, S., KIKUSHI, Y., & EBIHARA, S. (1986). An acoustic analysis of pathological voice and its application to the evaluation of laryngeal pathology. *Speech Communications, 5,* 171–181.

KITAJIMA, K. (1981). Quantitative evaluation of the noise level in the pathological voice. *Folia Phoniatrica, 33,* 115–124.

KLATT, D. H. (1987). Review of text-to-speech conversion for English. *Journal of the Acoustical Society of America, 82,* 737–793.

KLICH, R. J. (1982). Relationships of vowel characteristics to listener ratings of breathiness. *Journal of Speech and Hearing Research, 25,* 574–580.

KLINHOLZ, F., & MARTIN, F. (1985). Quantitative spectral evaluation of shimmer and jitter. *Journal of Speech and Hearing Research, 28,* 169–174.

KOIKE, Y., & MARKEL, J. (1975). Application of inverse filtering for detecting laryngeal pathology. *Annals of Otology, Rhinology and Laryngology, 84*(1), 117–124.

KOIKE, Y., TAKAHASHI, H., & CALCATERRA, T. C. (1977). Acoustic measures for detecting laryngeal pathology. *Acta Otolaryngologica, 84,* 105–117.

KREUL, E. J., & HECKER, M. H. L. (1971). Description of the speech of patients with cancer of the vocal folds. Part II: Judgements of age and voice quality. *Journal of the Acoustical Society of America, 49,* 1283–1287.

KUWABARA, H., & OHGUSHI, K. (1984). Experiments of voice quality of vowels in males and females and correlation with acoustic features. *Language and Speech, 27,* 135–145.

LAVER, J. (1980). *The phonetic description of voice quality.* Cambridge: Cambridge University Press.

LIEBERMAN, P. (1961). Perturbation in vocal pitch. *Journal of the Acoustical Society of America, 33,* 597–603.

LIEBERMAN, P. (1963). Some acoustic measures of the fundamental periodicity of normal and pathological larynges. *Journal of the Acoustical Society of America, 35,* 344–353.

LUDLOW, C. L., BASSICH, C. J., CONNOR, N. P., COULTER, D. C., & LEE, Y. J. (1987). The validity of using phonatory jitter and shimmer to detect laryngeal pathology. In T. Baer, C. Sasaki, & K. Harris (Eds.), *Laryngeal function in phonation and respiration* (pp. 492–508). Boston, MA: College-Hill Press.

MARKEL, J. D., & GRAY, A. H. (1976). *Linear prediction of speech.* New York: Springer-Verlag.

MILENKOVIC, P. (1987). Least mean square measures of voice perturbation. *Journal of Speech and Hearing Research, 30,* 529–538.

MORAN, M. J., & GILBERT, H. R. (1984). Relation between voice profile ratings and aerodynamic and acoustic parameters. *Journal of Communication Disorders, 17,* 245–260.

MOORE, G. P. (1971). *Organic voice disorders.* Englewood Cliffs, NJ: Prentice-Hall.

MOSS, S. E., & HICKS, D. M. (November 1985). *Acoustical analysis of three phonatory behaviors in adducted spastic dysphonia.* Papers presented at the American Speech-Language-Hearing Association Convention, Washington, DC.

MURRY, T., & SINGH, S. (1980). Multidimensional analysis of male and female voices. *Journal of the Acoustical Society of America, 68*(5), 1294–1300.

MUTA, H., MURAOKA, T., WAGATSUMA, K., FUKUDA, H., TAKAYAMA, E., FUJIOKA, T., & KANOU, S. (1987). Analysis of hoarse voices using the LPC Method. In T. Baer, C. Sasaki, & K. Harris (Eds.), *Laryngeal function in phonation and respiration* (pp. 463–474). Boston, MA: College-Hill Press.

PINTO, N. B., CHILDERS, D. G., & LALWANI, A. (1989). Formant speech synthesis: Improving production quality. *IEEE Transcripts on Acoustics, Speech, and Signal Processing, 37,* No. 12, 1870–1887.

PROSEK, A. R., MONTGOMERY, B. E., & HAWKINS, D. B. (1987). An evaluation of residue features as correlates of voice disorders. *Journal of Communication Disorders, 20,* 105–117.

QUACKENBUSH, S. R., BARNWELL, T. P., & CLEMENTS, M. A. (1988). *Objective measures of speech quality.* Englewood Cliffs, NJ: Prentice-Hall.

RABINER, L. R., & SCHAFER, R. W. (1978). *Digital processing of speech signals.* Englewood Cliffs, NJ: Prentice-Hall, Inc.

ROTHAUSER, E. H., URBAUER, G. E., & PACHL, W. P. (1971). A comparison of preference measurement methods. *Journal of the Acoustical Society of America, 49,* 1291–1308.

ROTHENBERG, M. R. (1973). A new inverse-filtering technique for deriving the glottal air flow waveform during voicing. *Journal of the Acoustical Society of America, 53,* 1632–1645.

ROTHENBERG, M. R., & ZAHORIAN, S. (1977). Nonlinear inverse filtering technique for estimating the glottal-area waveform. *Journal of the Acoustical Society of America, 61*(4), 1063–1071.

SANSONE, F. E., JR., & EMANUEL, F. W. (1970). Spectral noise levels and roughness severity ratings for normal and simulated rough vowels produced by adult males. *Journal of Speech and Hearing Research, 13,* 489–502.

SAPOZHKOV, M. A. (1972). Method of investigative and rating speed-transmission equipment. *Society of Physics-Acoustics, 18,* 80–83.

SINGH, S., & MURRY, T. (1978). Multidimensional classification of normal voice qualities. *Journal of the Acoustical Society of America, 64*(1), 81–87.

SMITH, B. E., WEINBERG, B., FETH, L. F., & HORII, Y. (1978). Vocal roughness and jitter characteristics of vowels produced by esophageal speakers. *Journal of Speech and Hearing Research, 21,* 240–249.

SORENSEN, B. E., & HORII, Y. (1984). Directional perturbation factors for jitter and shimmer. *Journal of Communication Disorders, 17,* 143–151.

TITZE, I. R., HORII, Y., & SCHERER, R. C. (1987). Some technical considerations in voice perturbation measurements. *Journal of Speech and Hearing Research, 30,* 252–260.

VOIERS, W. D. (1977). Diagnostic acceptability measure for speech communications systems. *Proceedings of the 1977 International IEEE Conference on Acoustics, Speech, and Signal Processing.* New York: Institute of Electrical and Electronic Engineers, 204–207.

WENDAHL, R. W. (1966). Laryngeal analog synthesis of jitter and shimmer—Auditory parameters of harshness. *Folia Phoniatrica, 18,* 98–108.

WINER, B. J. (1971). *Statistical principles in experimental design.* New York: McGraw-Hill.

WOLFE, V. I., & STEINFATT, T. M. (1987). Prediction of vocal severity within and across voice types. *Journal of Speech and Hearing Research, 30,* 230–240.

YANAGIHARA, N. (1967). Significance of harmonic changes and noise components in hoarseness. *Journal of Speech and Hearing Research, 10,* 531–541.

YUMOTO, E., GOULD, W. J., & BAER, T. (1982). Harmonics-to-noise ratio as an index of the degree of hoarseness. *Journal of the Acoustical Society of America, 71,* 1544–1550.

YUMOTO, E., SASAKI, Y., OKAMURA, H. (1984). Harmonics-to-noise ratio and psychophysical measurement of the degree of hoarseness. *Journal of Speech and Hearing Research, 27,* 2–6.

Received December 13, 1988
Accepted December 11, 1989

Requests for reprints should be sent to D. G. Childers, University of Florida, Mind-Machine Interaction Research Center, Department of Electrical Engineering, Gainesville, FL 32611.

Changes in Phonation Threshold Pressure with Induced Conditions of Hydration

Katherine Verdolini-Marston, *†Ingo R. Titze, and *David G. Druker

*Department of Psychology, Washington University, St. Louis, Missouri; *Voice Acoustics and Biomechanics Laboratory, Department of Speech Pathology and Audiology, The University of Iowa, Iowa City, Iowa; and †The Recording and Research Center, Denver Center for the Performing Arts, Denver, Colorado, U.S.A.*

Summary: The purpose of this pilot study was to investigate the relationship between phonation threshold pressure and level of hydration in human subjects. Six adult subjects produced consonant-vowel-consonant strings as quietly as possible at low, medium, and high pitches in no-treatment, hydrated, and slightly dehydrated conditions. Average oral pressures for these trials were used to estimate minimal subglottal pressures required for phonation (phonation threshold pressure). Main effects for hydration and for pitch were significant, as was the interaction of hydration times pitch. Overall, the lowest pressures were seen for the hydrated (or "wet") condition, and reduction in baseline pressures was greatest for high pitches in this condition. The highest pressures were found for the dry condition, and the greatest increase in pressure relative to the baseline was found at low pitches for this condition. Threshold pressures for intermediate (speaking) pitches were not affected by hydration condition. The findings are consistent with previously reported theoretical predictions regarding the relationship between oscillation threshold pressures and tissue viscosity. They are also consistent with previous empirical reports on the effect of direct hydration of vocal fold tissue in nonhuman subjects. **Key Words:** Vocal folds—Oscillation—Larynx—Phonation—Hydration

There has been some speculation about the importance of hydration in vocal fold tissue for normal voice production. Clinicians emphasize the presence of a mucosal wave on the superior surface of the folds as a sign of healthy tissue. When this mucosal wave disappears in certain dysphonias, vocal fold vibration is either impeded or requires considerably greater pulmonary effort. A general hypothesis is that the ease with which vocal fold vibration can be initiated and maintained depends on the mobility and deformability of the vocal fold mucosa, which in turn depend on how well this tissue is irrigated with body fluids. In a previous article, Titze (1) proposed a theory of vocal fold oscillation based on mucosal wave propagation. The results of this theory apply to small-amplitude oscillations that build up around slightly abducted vocal folds, such as those occurring in phonation threshold events. Within the framework of this theory, it was possible to predict how *phonation threshold pressure* (PTP), i.e., the lung pressure required to initiate vibration of the vocal folds, would vary with viscous energy losses. For the special case of a rectangular glottis, the lung pressure P_L had to be greater than a certain threshold value:

$$P_L \geqslant (2k/T)\,(Bc)\,(w/2) \tag{1}$$

where k is a transglottal pressure coefficient that has a dimensionless value of about 1.1, T is the thickness of the vocal folds, B is the damping coef-

Address correspondence and reprint requests to Dr. Verdolini-Marston, Department of Psychology, Washington University, St. Louis, MO, 63130, U.S.A.

ficient of the tissue, c is the velocity of the mucosal wave during vocal fold oscillation, and w is the prephonatory glottal width. The equality in Eq. (1) defines the PTP.

According to this formula, PTP is inversely proportional to vocal fold thickness but directly proportional to the amount of damping, the velocity of the mucosal wave, and the prephonatory glottal width. The damping coefficient B is a lumped-element representation of the tissue viscosity, which we assume to be dependent on hydration. Some preliminary test of this dependence was made on excised canine larynges by Finkelhor et al. (2). It was shown that PTP decreased with hydration induced by osmotic gradients across the mucus membrane.

The principal focus of this study is again the relationship between PTP and damping, but more specifically, the empirical relationship between PTP and the degree to which the vocal folds are kept moist by internal and external means. A major difference between this and the previous Finkelhor et al. study is the use of human subjects. Thus, the manner in which hydration was induced is quite different. It was again predicted that increased hydration would lower the PTP.

A second focus was to empirically investigate another factor that might affect PTP, fundamental frequency (F_0). Although F_0 does not appear explicitly in the formula given earlier, it may affect PTP indirectly in a variety of ways. First, as the vocal folds are lengthened for increased frequencies of vibration, they are stiffened, and this increases the mechanical impedance of the tissue, requiring greater driving pressures for oscillation. Second, when the vocal folds become stiffened for the production of higher F_0, there is a reduction in thickness, which is theoretically inversely proportional to PTP. Third, the increase in the tension of the mucosal cover may result in an increase in the velocity of propagation of the mucosal wave during oscillation, which is theoretically directly proportional to PTP. In all of these instances, an increase in fundamental frequency of vibration should result in an increase in PTP. This prediction was borne out rather clearly in the previous Finkelhor et al. study, where a uniform increase in PTP was measured with increased vocal fold length on excised larynges. In this study, empirical confirmation of the relationship between PTP and fundamental frequency was also sought on human subjects. Vocalizations were produced at different pitch levels as PTP was measured.

METHODS

Subjects

Six adult subjects, three men and three women, were recruited from the faculty, staff, and graduate program of the Department of Speech Pathology and Audiology of the University of Iowa. All denied a history of voice or hearing disorders, as well as the presence of risk factors associated with the experimental medications (high blood pressure, high blood pressure medications, various psychotropic medications, or pregnancy, all of which are risk factors related to decongestant agents).

Subjects' ages ranged from 25 to 46 years, and the average age was 36.7 years. All subjects were healthy at the time of data collection, and only one was taking medications (birth control pills) beyond the ones administered for the experiment.

Two of the men, IT and SA, were classically trained singers, both tenors, with 8 and 13 years of formal voice training, respectively. Another man, DD, and one woman, AP, had initiated classical voice training about 1–2 months prior to the time of testing. They classified themselves as tenor and soprano. One woman, SP, had received minimal voice training in a high school choir several years ago and considered herself a mezzo soprano. The remaining woman, NR, had never received vocal training of any sort and did not know what her voice classification was.

Only NR and SP were completely naive to the experimental hypotheses for this preliminary study.

Manipulation of vocal fold hydration

It was assumed that hydration to vocal fold tissue could be affected by manipulating three different factors: relative humidity of the air, ingestion of decongestant mucolitics, and amount of liquid intake. Specifically, for the "dry" (or "decreased hydration") condition, commercial dehumidifiers were used to decrease relative environmental humidity to 30–35%, and all subjects were exposed to this environment for a period of 4 h. (Using commercial dehumidifiers, it was not possible to obtain lower levels of environmental humidity in our geographical location.) For the dry condition, subjects also ingested three teaspoons of Dimetapp, a nonprescription decongestant, approximately 1 h prior to leaving the dry environment for testing. (Peak effect for this drug occurs 1–1½ h following ingestion, according to pharmaceutical specifications.) For this condition, subjects were asked not to drink any liquids unless they felt a strong need to do so. All subjects reported that they did not, in fact, drink any liquids during this period. On a different day, commercial vaporizers were used to increase relative environmental humidity to 85–100%, and subjects were exposed to this environment for 4 h. For this treatment, they ingested 2 teaspoons of Robitussin syrup, a nonprescription mucolitic expectorant, at the beginning of the 4-h exposure period and again approximately 30 min prior to leaving the wet environment for testing. (Peak effect for this drug reportedly occurs 30–60 min following administration.) During the 4-h exposure to increased environmental humidity, pitchers of water were provided, and subjects were asked to drink as much as they could comfortably tolerate. The range of water consumed by subjects during this period ranged from 16 to 64 oz. This was called the "wet" or "increased hydration" condition. For both the wet and the dry conditions, relative humidity was measured and monitored with an Abbeon Cal Cras Certified Hygrometer and Temperature Indicator, Model HTAB-176. For the "normal" (or "no-treatment") condition, there was no manipulation of environmental humidity, no medications were taken, and the amount of liquid intake was not controlled. On the no-treatment days, the hygrometer indicated that environmental humidity in our laboratory ranged from approximately 40 to 55%.

There were no restrictions on talking or other activities while subjects were exposed to the experimental conditions.

The "wet" and "dry" manipulations were assumed to affect the viscosity of vocal fold tissue. As a point of reference, the viscosity of pure water is 0.01 poise (P). The average viscosity of vocal fold tissue is estimated at 0–10 P, and the viscosity for human surface tissues (skin, fat, muscle) is on the order of 100 P (3). The assumption is that if water is added to tissue, there is a decrease in the net tissue viscosity, although homogeneous mixing may not occur. There is some indirect support for this assumption. In Reinke's space, a considerable amount of edema can accumulate. This can be removed by suctioning through a small incision in the mucous membrane. Thus, liquid can presumably be added and subtracted in Reinke's space. Further, while the viscosity of mucus and sputum normally ranges from approximately 0.1 to 1.0 P (4), mucolitics are believed to decrease these values and decongestants are believed to increase them. In this study, however, it is not known by what mechanisms the experimental manipulations might have affected the viscosity of laryngeal tissue itself, and there are no independent measures of tissue viscosity that have been made on live subjects. Therefore, for the purposes of this experiment, it was necessary to assume that the experimental manipulations did affect the viscosity of vocal fold tissue in the directions indicated.

Manipulation of pitch

For all conditions, subjects produced consonant-vowel-consonant (CVC) strings at "low," "intermediate," and "high" pitches. The specific pitches were determined individually for each subject prior to his or her initial threshold pressure measurements: the total pitch range for singing was determined using a portable electric keyboard, and the number of semitones was counted. The "low" pitch for each subject was the lowest note produced plus 10% of the total range in semitones, and the "high" pitch was the lowest note plus 80% of the total pitch range in semitones. The "intermediate" pitch was the average pitch produced by the subject during rote speech (counting), as estimated using the portable keyboard. Once these pitches had been determined for each subject, they were used as "low," "intermediate," and "high" pitches for all subsequent measurements for that individual subject.

Estimation of PTP, equipment, and experimental design

Several authors have reported that it is possible to noninvasively estimate subglottal pressures from oral pressures generated during voiceless stop consonants (5–7). This is because lung and oral pressures become temporarily equalized during these productions. For oral pressures to reflect subglottal pressures during longer speech strings, it is necessary for subglottal pressure to be grossly constant for the duration of the string. This occurs when constant pitch and loudness levels are maintained.

In our study, oral pressures occurring during phonation were obtained using a translabial catheter housed within a circumferentially vented face mask

→

FIG. 1. Individual average phonation threshold pressures for each pitch times hydration condition, in centimeters of H_2O. Dash lines, dry condition; solid lines, no-treatment condition; dot-dash lines, wet condition. L, low; M, medium; and H, high.

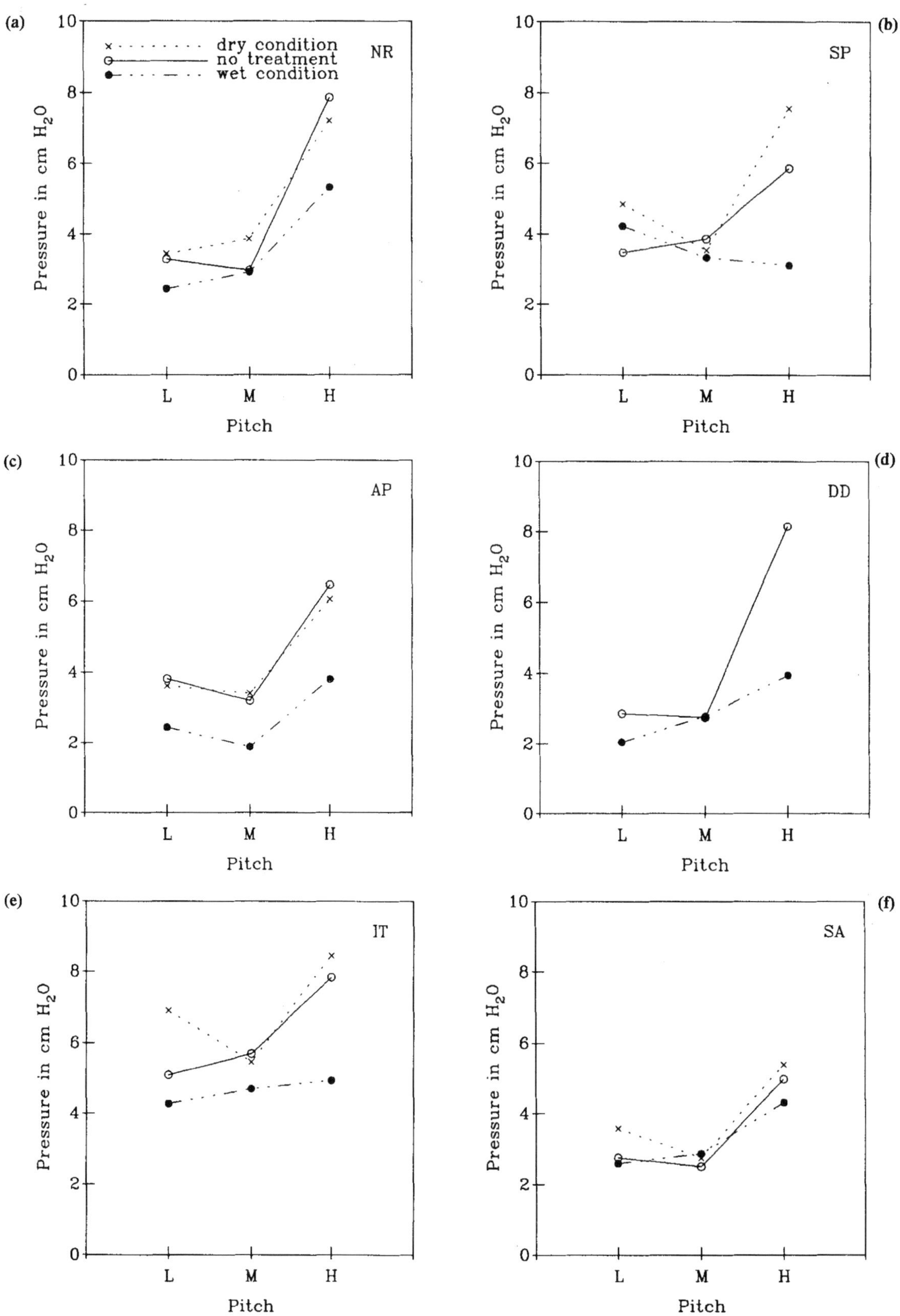
(a)
dry condition
no treatment
wet condition
NR
(b)
SP
(c)
AP
(d)
DD
(e)
IT
(f)
SA
Pressure in cm H_2O
0
2
4
6
8
10
L
M
H
Pitch

and attached to a pressure transducer. The mask, air-flow, and pressure transducers and attached amplifier were a Glottal Enterprises MS100 system. The system determines AC and DC flow by measuring the pressure drop across the mesh screens in the mask with a very sensitive pressure transducer; the pressure signal is the output of another transducer attached to the translabial catheter. The pressure signal is low-pass filtered, and both signals are amplified. As an aid in analyzing data, a small condenser microphone was attached to the outside of the mask to record audio signals. Subjects were also videotaped.

The subjects stood in a sound-isolated booth during experimental vocalizations. A window and intercom allowed experimenter and subject to see and speak with each other during the experiment. Before each production, the experimenter struck the key of the electronic keyboard at the appropriate pitch as an audible cue to the subject.

Flow and pressure signals were digitized and stored on a Data 6000 Universal Waveform Analyzer during the experiment. The experimenter also monitored the signals on the Data 6000. Subsequently, the data were recalled to the screen and analyzed as described later.

Using a similar experimental setup to obtain various oral measurements, Holmberg et al. (8) reported that the mode of CVC production as well as the rate could significantly affect the validity and reliability of transglottal pressures estimated from oral pressure values. They noted that if oral pressure traces were "choppy," i.e., if steady state values were not obtained, there might not be equalization in pressure along the vocal tract, and the implication is that oral pressures might underestimate subglottal pressures in this instance. Table 1 in their article shows that choppy pressure contours resulted in a lower average oral pressure value than smooth contours, and that the standard deviation was larger for peaked productions for one subject. They further found that if their subjects produced CVC strings at a rate of about 1.4/s, not only oral pressure traces but also oral flow contours tended to achieve steady state values, and both of these were necessary for the validity and reliability of various measurements in which they were interested. They reported that traces of this type were most easily obtained by restricting the number of syllables per trial to five.

In our estimates of subglottal pressure, we attempted to take these restrictions into account. Following approximately 5–10 min of training, measurements were initiated. For each hydration times pitch condition, subjects first repeated the syllable /pæ/ five times at a loudness level they felt was just above the phonation threshold, at a rate of 1.5/s. This rate was indicated by a metronome set at 92 beats/min. Subjects then repeated /pæ/ five times at a level just below threshold, at the same rate, and finally, five /pæ/s were produced at a level between these, which subjects believed to be the threshold of phonation. These, too, were produced at a rate of 1.5/s. The cycle of suprathreshold, subthreshold, and threshold trials was repeated a total of five times for each hydration times pitch condition. The experimenter repeated the instruction to "phonate as softly as possible" before almost every threshold trial and monitored all practice and experimental trials on a digital oscilloscope (Data Precision Data 6000 Universal Waveform Analyzer). Smooth contours were verbally reinforced (e.g., "good"), and subjects were asked to repeat trials that had resulted in very choppy contours. These traces were excluded from later analysis (approximately 5%). For each pitch condition, the target pitch was provided by an electric keyboard prior to initiation of each trial.

It was found that for threshold tasks, most of our subjects were not able to consistently produce pressure traces as smooth as those reported by Holmberg et al. (8) for suprathreshold trials. When our subjects repeated the tasks to obtain smoother traces, it was often noted that loudness increased to levels that were clearly above phonation threshold. These trials were not included in subsequent analyses and were repeated to reduce loudness to threshold levels while obtaining acceptably smooth pressure traces.

In virtually all instances, minimal oscillations were noted in oral flow traces for threshold trials, while they were not present in subthreshold trials. These oscillations were generally noticeably smaller than those for trials where the target was to phonate "just above threshold." These observations confirmed that subjects were in fact fairly successful at approaching phonation threshold with this approach.

Subjects removed the face mask between all trials to allow for zeroing of pressure and flow readings, and they were reminded to reapply the mask firmly to the face before initiating subsequent trials.

A 3 × 3 factorial design of hydration condition (no-treatment, dry, and wet) times pitch (low, intermediate, and high) was utilized. For each hydration condition, suprathreshold, subthreshold, and threshold trials were performed at low, intermediate, and high pitches. All subjects except one were exposed to each hydration times pitch condition; this subject declined participation in the dry condition. The equipment was calibrated before each hydration times pitch condition and was also recalibrated during the condition, if necessary (this was rarely the case). The order of pitch as well as humidity conditions was varied to control for order effects.

It was noted that the men tended to produce high pitches in falsetto register. This is not surprising, given that threshold phonation is at very low intensity. The tendency was also seen in the women.

Data extraction and analysis

Only oral pressures were evaluated; flow data were stored for later analysis, should this become relevant. For each threshold trial of five repetitions of /pæ/, pressure peaks 2–5 were used to estimate subglottal pressure for the three middle syllables. All five peaks were visualized on the Data 6000 screen, then the display was magnified so that only the second peak appeared on the screen. The maximum value in volts was then extracted for the screen, and the procedure was repeated for the third peak. The average voltage was calculated from the two peaks, and this was recorded as the voltage for the second syllable. The same procedure was repeated to obtain average voltages for syllables 3 and 4 of a single threshold trial. As there were five threshold trials for each pitch condition and three syllables were analyzed for each trial, a total of 15 syllables were analyzed for each pitch condition. The voltage values were averaged and converted to pressure in centimeters of H_2O, and these pressure averages were used for statistical analysis.

Two types of standard deviations were calculated for each subject, for each pitch times hydration condition. The first, $\overline{SD_w}$, is the average within-trial standard deviation for the condition for that subject. It reflects average peak-to-peak instability in measured oral pressures. The second, SD_b, is the overall between-trial standard deviation for the same subject in the same condition, derived from the average PTPs for each of the five trials in the condition. It is a measure of between-trial instability of oral pressures for a given pitch times hydration condition.

For the subject who declined exposure to the dry treatment (DD), average group pressures for low, intermediate, and high pitches in the dry condition were utilized in data analysis as substitutes for his missing values.

RESULTS

Data for individual subjects shown in Fig. 1 indicate that estimated PTPs tended to be higher for the dry condition (dash lines) and lowest for the wet condition (dot–dash lines). This trend was quite consistent across subjects, with minor exceptions. Differences in pressures as a function of hydration tended to be greatest at high pitches, less accentuated at low pitches, and minimal at intermediate pitches for most subjects. Group averages are shown in Fig. 2. Note that group PTPs differed on the order of approximately 1–3 cm of H_2O between the wet and dry conditions.

Average PTPs and standard deviations for individual subjects and for the group as a whole are given in Table 1; group standard deviations are also shown graphically in Fig. 3A and B. As is evident in these figures, average within-trial standard deviations did not vary as a function of hydration but were slightly higher for low and high pitches than for intermediate pitches. However, average be-

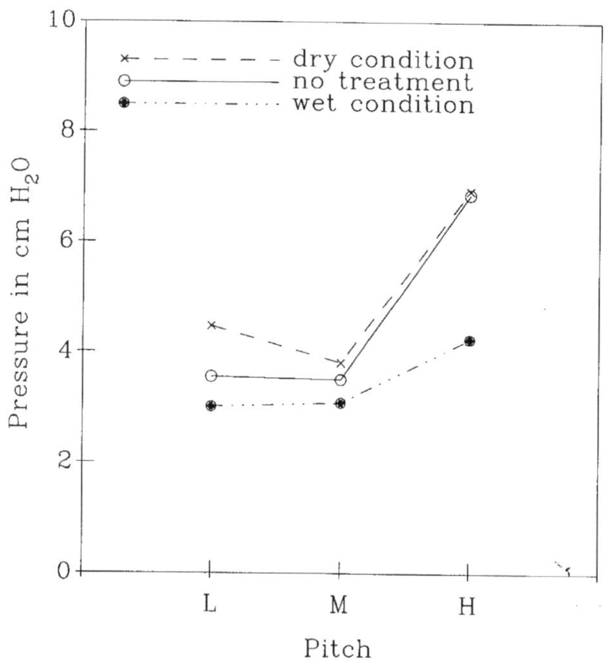

FIG. 2. Group average phonation threshold pressures for each pitch times hydration condition, in centimeters of H_2O. Dash lines, dry condition; solid lines, no-treatment condition; dot-dash lines, wet condition. L, low; M, medium; and H, high.

TABLE 1. *Individual and group data. For individuals, the average phonation threshold pressure for each pitch times hydration condition is given ($\overline{X}$), as well as average within-trial standard deviation ($\overline{SD}_w$) and standard deviation for the five separate trials in the condition ("between-trial" standard deviation, SD_b). Group values for these statistics are also given ($\overline{\overline{X}}$, $\overline{\overline{SD}}_w$, and $\overline{SD}_b$).*

Subject	Dry, pitch			No treatment, pitch			Wet, pitch		
	Low	Intermediate	High	Low	Intermediate	High	Low	Intermediate	High
NR									
$\overline{X}$	3.43	3.86	7.20	3.28	2.96	7.86	2.44	2.91	5.32
$\overline{SD}_w$	0.13	0.14	0.21	0.07	0.11	0.61	0.24	0.13	0.27
SD_b	0.31	0.24	0.97	0.40	0.43	1.29	0.43	0.54	0.19
SP									
$\overline{X}$	4.85	3.54	7.55	3.47	3.86	5.87	4.22	3.33	3.11
$\overline{SD}_w$	0.24	0.20	0.56	0.32	0.32	0.63	0.19	0.31	0.43
SD_b	0.64	0.28	1.79	0.58	0.43	0.53	0.42	0.26	1.11
AP									
$\overline{X}$	3.61	3.40	6.05	3.81	3.19	6.46	2.44	1.89	3.80
$\overline{SD}_w$	0.18	0.28	0.29	0.28	0.22	0.46	0.23	0.18	0.30
SD_b	0.36	0.18	1.34	0.32	0.46	0.90	0.16	0.34	0.27
DD									
$\overline{X}$	4.47[a]	3.81[a]	6.93[a]	2.86	2.75	8.15	2.05	2.78	3.94
$\overline{SD}_w$	0.25[a]	0.21[a]	0.37[a]	0.20	0.11	0.33	0.10	0.13	0.40
SD_b	0.46[a]	0.30[a]	0.93[a]	0.24	0.19	0.39	0.34	0.27	0.64
IT									
$\overline{X}$	6.90	5.47	8.46	5.09	5.70	7.84	4.28	4.70	4.94
$\overline{SD}_w$	0.51	0.28	0.45	0.34	0.39	0.32	0.66	0.43	0.35
SD_b	0.44	0.56	0.36	0.37	0.43	0.32	0.27	0.18	0.39
SA									
$\overline{X}$	3.58	2.76	5.39	2.76	2.51	4.98	2.60	2.87	4.31
$\overline{SD}_w$	0.18	0.14	0.36	0.09	0.20	0.31	0.21	0.11	0.34
SD_b	0.53	0.22	0.20	0.24	0.25	0.50	0.15	0.09	0.27
$\overline{\overline{X}}$	4.47	3.81	6.93	3.55	3.50	6.86	3.01	3.08	4.24
$\overline{\overline{SD}}_w$	0.25	0.21	0.37	0.22	0.23	0.44	0.27	0.22	0.35
$\overline{SD}_b$	0.46	0.30	0.93	0.36	0.37	0.66	0.30	0.28	0.48

[a] Group averages used.

tween-trial standard deviations did vary with hydration as well as with pitch: overall, PTPs were the most stable from trial to trial for the wet condition and were least stable for the dry condition. Differences in between-trial standard deviations for the three hydration conditions were greatest at high pitches.

Table 2 shows average PTP values as a function of pooled pitch and pooled hydration conditions. As indicated in this Table, low and intermediate pitches were produced with similar average pressures across the different humidity conditions, whereas high pitches were produced with higher average pressures. Likewise, PTPs were similar for dry and no-treatment conditions across all pitches and were lowest for the wet condition.

Repeated measures analysis of variance, using subjects' estimated PTP values for each threshold utterance, revealed that both main effects, hydration and pitch, were significant (F = 26.13, $p < 0.001$ and F = 49.87, $p < 0.001$, respectively.) The hydration times pitch interaction was also significant (F = 7.16, $p < 0.001$). Inspection of group averages (Fig. 2) shows that the interaction was of the uncrossed type.

DISCUSSION

Phonation threshold pressures were lowest for the subjects as a group in the hydrated or "wet" condition and increased somewhat relative to baseline for the dry condition. This trend was seen across all subjects, trained and untrained voice us-

TABLE 2. *Pooled average phonation threshold pressures as a function of hydration and pitch*

	Average pressure, cm of H_2O
Hydration condition	
dry	4.95
no treatment	4.64
wet	3.44
Pitch	
low	3.64
intermediate	3.44
high	5.96

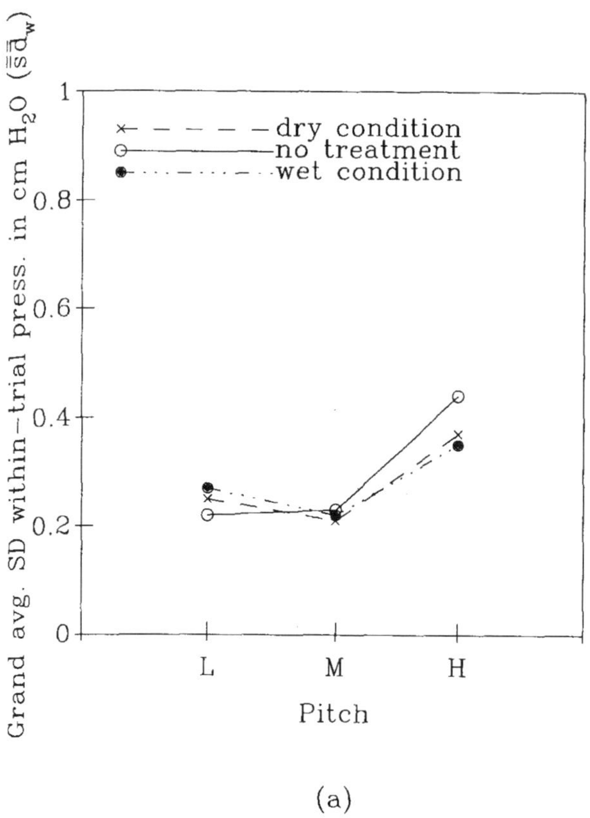

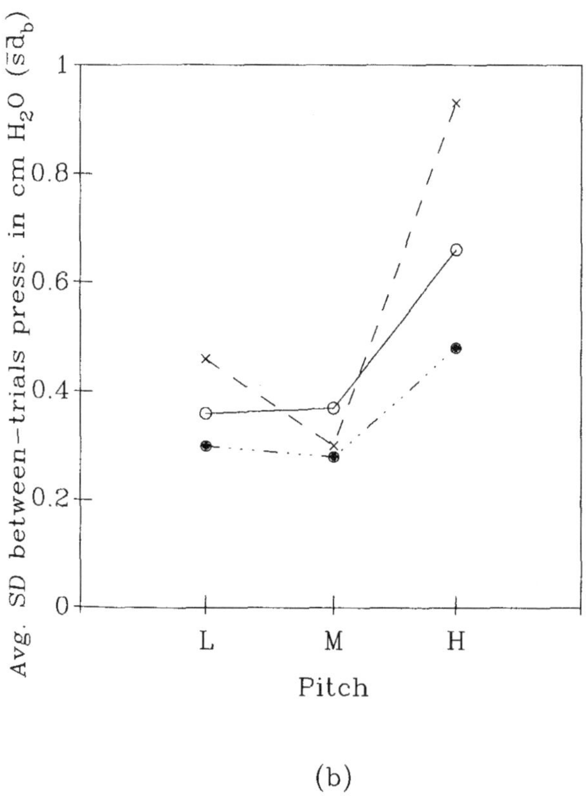

ers, naive and informed, for most conditions. The change in PTP relative to no-treatment measures was greatest for the wet condition, at high pitches. This can be taken as preliminary support for the theoretical prediction that PTP is affected by tissue viscosity. It also lends credence to the likelihood that fluid content in the vocal folds can be changed by the combined experimental manipulations.

The distinction between PTPs was less clear for the dry versus the no-treatment condition than for the wet versus the no-treatment condition. This may be a reflection of the fact that, for the dry condition, environmental humidity was not as effectively decreased as it was increased for the wet condition. In fact, for the dry condition, environmental humidity was only decreased by 5–25% (from 40–55% to 30–35%), while for the wet condition, there was a change of 30–60% (from 40–55% to 85–100%). An environmental humidity of 30–35% is clearly not extremely dry for certain geographical locations. However, the focus of this study was not to quantify changes in PTP across a full range of hydration levels. Rather, the intention was to examine relative changes in PTP as a function of relative changes in hydration. Changes in PTP were in fact observed as hydration was increased and decreased, and these changes were in the predicted direction. The issue of whether greater effects might be obtained following exposure to extremely dry environments is an empirical one that we later propose to evaluate experimentally.

The finding that PTPs tend to be lowest for the wet condition is consistent with previous reports that water-infused excised canine laryngeal tissue oscillated with lower pressures than noninfused tissue (Finkelhor et al., (2). It is also consistent with observations made by Baer (9) and Durham et al. (10) that excised tissue will not oscillate if the humidity of forced air systems is too low. Finally, it agrees with common clinical wisdom about body hydration.

The PTPs were also higher, on average, for high pitches than for other pitches. This trend was seen for all subjects. This finding agrees with the theoretical formulation that an increase in stiffness and mucosal wave velocity and a decrease in the thick-

FIG. 3. Group standard deviations for each pitch times hydration condition, in centimeters of **A:** grand average within-trial standard deviations ($\overline{\overline{SD}}_w$); **B:** average between-trial standard deviations ($\overline{SD}_b$). Dash lines, dry, condition; solid lines, no-treatment condition; dot-dash lines, wet condition. L, low; M, medium; and H, high.

ness of the vocal folds associated with higher pitches leads to greater PTPs. It is also a replication of various other empirical reports that subglottal or driving pressures tend to be highest for high pitches in humans as well as for excised larynges (e.g., Finkelhor et al., 2, van den Berg, (11); and Isshiki, (12). In particular, our data for the no-treatment condition closely replicate those reported by Gramming (13) for a similar task. It was noted that both our men and women tended to produce high pitches in falsetto. Therefore, the pitch effect may actually be underestimated because it takes less pressure to phonate in falsetto register than chest register (e.g., Kunze, (14).

It should be underlined that there was a significant interaction between the degree of humidification and pitch; most notably, whereas there was a reduction in average PTP relative to the no-treatment condition for all pitches in the wet condition, the effect was greatest for high pitches. Similarly, whereas average PTPs were greater than no-treatment values for the dry condition, this effect appeared to be greatest for low pitches. There were minimal differences between dry, no-treatment, and wet PTPs at the intermediate, or speaking, pitch.

The effects of humidification and pitch were seen not only in actual PTP values but also in average between-trial standard deviations ($\overline{sd}_b$s). As shown in Fig. 3B, $\overline{SD}_b$s were the smallest, overall, for the wet condition, and greatest for the dry condition. Therefore, between-trial stability in PTP was greatest for the wet conditions, $\overline{SD}_b$s were greatest at the high pitch, showing the greatest instability in PTP for high pitches. As was found for average PTP values, there appeared to be an uncrossed humidification times pitch interaction: differences in $\overline{SD}_b$s relative to the no-treatment condition were greatest at the high pitch.

The between-trial standard deviations were greater than the average within-trial standard deviations. For low and intermediate pitches, the mean average within-trial standard deviations ($\overline{SD}_w$s) given in Table 1 and shown in Fig. 3A are equivalent to those reported by other authors for suprathreshold trials at spontaneous pitches. Holmberg et al. (8) reported a within-trial standard of 0.22 cm of H_2O for one subject performing a suprathreshold task at a comfortable pitch and loudness level in a way they argued produced reliable and valid results. Our $\overline{SD}_w$s ranged from 0.21 to 0.27 cm of H_2O for low- and intermediate-pitched threshold tasks performed with the same methodology. Individual $\overline{SD}_w$s exceeded 0.5 cm of H_2O in only two of a possible 34 instances for low and intermediate pitches in our study. Our $\overline{SD}_w$s were somewhat greater for the high pitch, ranging from 0.35 to 0.44 cm of H_2O. Therefore, it may be that PTPs are less stable in general for high as compared to low and intermediate pitches.

It is tentatively concluded that our results may have theoretical as well as practical significance. They provide an initial validation of the theoretically proposed relationship between phonation threshold pressure and viscosity of vocal fold tissue in human subjects, as well as between PTP and pitch. It may also be that the degree of "ease" experienced by singers and speakers producing higher and lower pitches is related to the viscoelastic status of the vocal folds. Our conclusions are tentative at this point, due to the small number of subjects and the inclusion of several nonnaive subjects. However, the fact that similar trends were seen in naive and informed subjects allows us to be optimistic about their potential generality.

Further investigation is needed to verify and generalize results. A greater number of subjects is needed, with greater numbers of both trained and untrained voice users, all of whom should be naive to the experimental hypotheses. Better manipulation of environmental humidity should be obtained for the dry condition to assess effects across the full range of humidities. Further, high-pitch trials could be performed in both chest and falsetto (or "head") registers, to determine relative threshold pressure requirements for high pitches in the two registers. If the relationships found in this preliminary study were verified, it would be appropriate to determine what proportion of the variance in PTP is due to changes in environmental humidity and what proportion is due to the ingestion of the pharmaceutical agents and liquid intake.

Acknowledgment: We are grateful to Linnie Southard for her help with the typing of this manuscript and to our subjects for their willingness to participate.

This research was partially supported by NIH grant #NS16320-08.

REFERENCES

1. Titze IR. The physics of small-amplitude oscillation of the vocal folds. *J Acoust Soc Am* 1988;83:1536–52.
2. Finkelhor BK, Titze IR, Durham PL. The effect of viscosity changes in the vocal folds on the range of oscillation. *J Voice* 1988;1:320–5.
3. Titze IR, Talkin DT. A theoretical study of the effects of

various laryngeal configurations on the acoustics of phonation. *J Acoust Soc Am* 1979;66:60–74.

4. Fung YC. *Biomechanics: mechanical properties of living tissues.* New York: Springer-Verlag, 1981.
5. Rothenberg MR. Measurement of air flow in speech. *J Speech Hearing Res* 1977;13:155–76.
6. Smitheran JR, Hixon TJ. A clinical method for estimating laryngeal airway resistance during vowel production. *J Speech Hearing Dis* 1981;46:138–46.
7. Löfqvist A, Carlborg B, Kitzing P. Initial validation of an indirect measure of subglottal pressure during vowels. *J Acoust Soc Am* 1982;72:633–4.
8. Holmberg E, Perkell J, Hillman R. *Methods for using a non-invasive technique for estimating glottal functions from oral measurements.* Cambridge, Massachusetts: Speech Communication Group, Research Laboratory of Electronics, Massachusetts Institute of Technology, 1987:47–58.
9. Baer T. *Investigation of phonation using excised larynges* [Dissertation]. Cambridge, Massachusetts: Massachusetts Institute of Technology, 1975.
10. Durham PL, Scherer RC, Druker DG, Titze IR. *Development of excised larynx procedures for studying mechanisms of phonation.* Iowa City, Iowa: Voice Acoustics and Biomechanics Laboratory, University of Iowa, 1987. (Technical Report No. VABL-1.)
11. Van den Berg J. Direct and indirect determination of the mean subglottic pressure. *Folia Phoniatr* 1957;9:65–71.
12. Isshiki N. Regulatory mechanism of vocal intensity variation. *J Speech Hearing Res* 1964;7:17–29.
13. Gramming P. *The phonetogram: an experimental and clinical study.* Malmö, Sweden: Dept. of Otolaryngology, University of Lund, Malmö General Hospital, 1988:133–41.
14. Kunze LH. *An investigation of the changes in subglottic air pressure and rate of airflow accompanying changes in fundamental frequency, intensity, vowels, and voice register in adult male speakers* [Dissertation]. Iowa City, Iowa: University of Iowa, (1962).

Commentary

James M. Hillenbrand, PhD

As a beginning graduate student, one of the first bits of advice I can recall receiving from my mentor is that good research is programmatic. Begin with a problem that is both interesting and difficult, she told me, break it into a manageable set of subproblems, and have at it. Tough problems typically do not respond well to the short attention spans characterized by what my advisor called hit-and-run research. This was good advice, of course, and although I have tried to follow it over the years this particular study on breathy voice is not at all a good example. My primary interest when we began work on this project was, and still is, speech perception, with a primary focus on trying to understand the auditory mechanisms and mental computations that are involved in phonetic recognition. Along with colleagues Bob Houde and Rob Gayvert, we had for some time been working on two closely related source-filter speech synthesizers that were needed for a series of experiments that were designed to learn something about the acoustic correlates of phonetic features. Along with many other measures, both synthesizers required estimates of the glottal source function from naturally spoken utterances, which in turn depended on measures of fundamental frequency and degree of periodicity. Finding a faithful representation of the degree of periodicity—needed for determining whether the speech signal being reconstructed was voiced, unvoiced, or somewhere in between—proved to be by far the most difficult problem in developing the synthesizers. Although we eventually found several measures that worked reasonably well, degree of periodicity remains to this day the weakest link in the resynthesis algorithm.

The possibility of applying the periodicity measures we had developed for the synthesis project to the quantification of voice quality, especially breathy voice, had occurred to me early on. The primary application that I had in mind for these periodicity measures was the characterization of dysphonic vocal quality. The fact that this thought occurred to me at all can be attributed not to any training I received as a graduate student, as I had had very little exposure to clinical problems such as these, but rather to the simple fact that in my first academic job at Northwestern University I was surrounded by doctoral students who were interested in finding better methods to characterize this great zoo of sound qualities produced by speakers suffering from both functional and organic laryngeal disorders. I am especially grateful to Bruce Gerratt, who served as my unpaid tutor in this area while completing work on his doctoral thesis. (He would later be joined in this uncompensated duty by his UCLA colleague, Jody Kreiman.)

For the next year or so the idea of applying our periodicity measures (along with several others that we knew little about until we hit the books) remained just that—we were working full tilt collecting data to support a grant application in phonetic perception and had no time to pursue it. Then along came Ron Cleveland, a bright and energetic graduate student who was shopping around for a master's thesis topic. Although Ron was pursuing a degree in audiology, he came to our department with an undergraduate degree in music, with a specialty in vocal performance, and therefore had a strong interest in voice. The last and, in many respects, most important remaining piece to fall into place involved persuading Bob Erickson to join the project. Bob, who passed away quite recently, was a skilled and extraordinarily experienced voice clinician with a great ear and was the only member of the project with any real experience in vocal pathology.

Although we are obviously pleased that our paper received some attention, we ended up viewing our project as essentially an extension and formalization of a study by Klatt and Klatt,[1] which, unknown to us at the time, was nearly complete when we began data collection for our study. This beautiful paper—Dennis Klatt's last publication, as it turned out was a revelation to us. This was the first paper to attempt to understand breathy voice in a comprehensive way by stringing together all of the key components: the underlying laryngeal vibratory patterns, the aerodynamic and acoustic consequences of those movement patterns, measurement of their acoustic correlates, perceptual judgments of naturally spoken utterances showing normal (and, most impressively to us, rather slight) variations in breathiness, the correlation of those perceptual findings with the acoustic measurements and, as if all that were not enough, ending with a synthesis experiment validating the major hypotheses that were generated by all of the above. Our paper added some useful methods, particularly periodicity algorithms that correlated strongly with the perception of breathiness, and in a later paper we were able to show that the methods worked well even with ragged, marginally periodic utterances spoken by dysphonic speakers.[2] But much of the heavy lifting, it turned out, had been done at MIT by Dennis Klatt and his daughter Laura.

There are, of course, many aspects of dysphonic voice quality that remain quite poorly understood. Toward the top of our list are questions about the specificity of measures of periodicity of the kind we used. Although it is clear both from our evidence and from other literature that features other than periodicity play a role in the perception of breathy voice (eg, first harmonic amplitude and measures of spectral balance), reductions in signal periodicity appear to be especially important. Our study focused on breathy voice, but what we do not know is whether periodicity measures—alone or in combination with other measures—can separate the breathiness percept from the many other irregular sounding percepts that are associated with laryngeal dysfunction. Although we have not pursued this question, we are doubtful that this can be done in the absence of a much better understanding than we currently have of the psychoacoustics of vocal quality.

References

1. Klatt DH, Klatt LC. Analysis, synthesis, and perception of voice quality variations among female and male talkers. *J Acoust Soc Am.* 1990;87:820–857.
2. Hillenbrand JM, Houde RA. Acoustic characteristics of breathy vocal quality: dysphonic voices and continuous speech. *J Speech Hear Res.* 1996;39:311–321.

Acoustic Correlates of Breathy Vocal Quality

James Hillenbrand
Ronald A. Cleveland
Robert L. Erickson
Department of Speech Pathology and Audiology
Western Michigan University, Kalamazoo

The purpose of this study was to evaluate the effectiveness of several acoustic measures in predicting breathiness ratings. Recordings were made of eight normal men and seven normal women producing normally phonated, moderately breathy, and very breathy sustained vowels. Twenty listeners rated the degree of breathiness using a direct magnitude estimation procedure. Acoustic measures were made of: (a) signal periodicity, (b) first harmonic amplitude, and (c) spectral tilt. Periodicity measures provided the most accurate predictions of perceived breathiness, accounting for approximately 80% of the variance in breathiness ratings. The relative amplitude of the first harmonic correlated moderately with breathiness ratings, and two measures of spectral tilt correlated weakly with perceived breathiness.

KEY WORDS: acoustic analysis, breathy voice, voice quality, cepstrum, autocorrelation

This study was designed to improve our understanding of the acoustic correlates of breathy vocal quality. Breathy voice plays an important role in both normal and disordered speech production. Breathiness is a prominent feature of numerous pathological conditions affecting the laryngeal mechanism, including neoplasms, abductor spasmodic dysphonia, vocal cord paralysis, and laryngeal trauma (Aronson, 1971, 1990; Colton & Casper, 1990). Breathiness can also be associated with vocal misuse and other functional conditions (Aronson, 1990; Boone & McFarlane, 1988), and there is evidence that the physiological effects of aging may include breathy voice (Hollien, 1987; Ryan & Burk, 1974). Breathy (murmured) voice quality also plays an important role in the phonological systems of many of the world's languages (Fischer-Jorgensen, 1967; Huffman, 1987; Ladefoged, 1975, 1983). Finally, there is some evidence that breathy quality may be a social marker of female gender among English speakers (Klatt & Klatt, 1990; McKay, 1987). Despite the widespread occurrence of breathy voice, a good deal remains to be learned about the acoustic features underlying the perception of breathiness.

Acoustic Correlates of Breathy Voice

First harmonic amplitude. Breathiness is thought to be due to incomplete glottal closure during the "closed" phase of the phonatory cycle (Fairbanks, 1940; Hillenbrand et al., 1990; Zemlin, 1968). Breathy glottal source signals obtained through inverse filtering typically show more symmetrical opening and closing phases with little or no complete closed phase (Bickley, 1982; Fischer-Jorgensen, 1967; Huffman, 1987). The rounded, more nearly sinusoidal shape of breathy glottal waveforms is responsible for increases in the relative amplitude of the first harmonic.

Enhanced H1 amplitude in the spectra of breathy speech signals has been observed by a number of investigators (Bickley, 1982; Fischer-Jorgensen, 1967; Huffman, 1987; Klatt & Klatt, 1990; Ladefoged, 1983). Huffman (1987) used inverse filtering to derive glottal waveforms from samples of four phonation types used in

Hmong. Breathy (murmured) samples showed stronger first harmonics than nonbreathy samples.

Fischer-Jorgensen (1967) used a variety of techniques to study the acoustic characteristics of Gujarati murmured vowels. She considered the high intensity of H1 to be the most salient spectral feature of murmured vowels and conducted a listening experiment to measure the effects of filtering on the perception of breathy vocal quality. Highpass filtering at 230 Hz was used to reduce H1 amplitude by about 25 dB. Contrary to the expected outcome, correct identification of murmured vowels was not significantly decreased. Despite her belief that the relative amplitude of H1 was "the most obvious and constant feature" (p. 133–134), Fischer-Jorgensen concluded that no single acoustic feature was sufficient to produce the sensation of breathiness.

A perceptual study by Bickley (1982) used synthetic Gujarati breathy and clear word pairs varying in aspiration noise and H1 amplitude. Identification of the stimuli as breathy or clear by native Gujarats was affected by H1 amplitude only, with no effect for aspiration noise. However, as was noted by Klatt & Klatt (1990), the H1 enhancement that was needed to effect a decisive shift from clear to breathy greatly exceeded measured H1 amplitude differences between naturally produced breathy and clear word pairs.

Ladefoged (1983) reported enhanced H1 amplitudes for breathy vowels in !Xóõ. A follow-up study by Ladefoged & Antonanzas-Barroso (1985) found that the breathiness judgments of American listeners were more strongly correlated with H1 amplitude than aspiration noise, as measured by a waveform variability index.

Klatt & Klatt (1990) used a variety of acoustic and perceptual techniques to investigate male-female differences in voice quality. In general, women were judged to be breathier than men. H1 amplitude measures were also generally greater for women than men. A variety of acoustic measures were evaluated by measuring correlations with breathiness ratings. Only two were found to be significantly correlated with breathiness ratings: H1 amplitude and the degree of aspiration noise present in band-limited signals. In a second listening experiment using synthetic speech, a number of synthesis parameters were manipulated in order to measure their effect on the perception of vocal quality. Increases in H1 alone were heard as breathy by some listeners and nasal by many others. Signals were never judged to be nasal when H1 amplitude increases were accompanied by aspiration noise. Contrary to previous investigators, Klatt & Klatt concluded that the sensation of breathiness is controlled primarily by aspiration noise in the middle and upper portion of the spectrum.

Additive noise. When a portion of the breathstream passes through a persistent and relatively narrow glottal chink it results in the generation of noise. The higher frequency harmonics are reduced in amplitude and the upper portion of the spectrum becomes dominated by dense aspiration noise (Klatt & Klatt, 1990).

Based on spectrographic observations, Fischer-Jorgensen (1967) believed differences in spectral noise between murmured and clear vowels were small and inconsistent. Similarly, Bickley (1982) found no correlation between breathiness ratings and increases in additive noise in synthetic vowels. In contrast, a synthesis study by Hillenbrand (1988a) found a strong relationship between breathiness ratings and additive noise.

Klatt & Klatt (1990) used a bandpass filter centered at F3 to isolate the third formant of [ha] samples. Unfiltered signals, which tend to be dominated by low-frequency periodic components, were judged to be unsuitable for noise estimation. (A similar observation was made by Kasuya, et al., 1986, who noted that even pathological voices sometimes exhibit well defined harmonic structure in the lower frequencies.) The degree of periodicity in the band-limited signals was judged by visual inspection of time-domain waveforms using a five-point rating scale. The noise ratings accounted for approximately 60% of the variance in listener ratings of breathiness. A follow-up synthesis study found that increases in spectral noise were the single most important cue to perceived breathiness.

Spectral tilt. Several investigators have noted that breathy signals tend to have more high-frequency energy than normally phonated signals. For example, Klich (1982) reported strong correlations between perceived breathiness and several measures of spectral tilt calculated as energy ratios of low-, mid-, and high-frequency bands. A similar energy ratio method was described by Frokjaer-Jensen & Prytz (1976), who showed a reduction in high-frequency energy in the long-term average spectra of voice patients following treatment.

A closely related spectral tilt measure described by Fukazawa, El-Assuooty, and Honjo (1988) was defined as the ratio of the energy in the second derivative of a signal to the energy in a nonderived signal. The index is conceptually similar to the ratios described by Klich (1982) and Frokjaer-Jensen & Prytz (1976), except that the Fukazawa et al. technique produces a global measure of spectral tilt that does not require arbitrary cutoffs for low-, mid-, or high-frequency bands. Fukazawa et al. reported that the spectral tilt measure accounted for approximately half of the variance in breathiness ratings obtained from the sustained vowels of speakers with various laryngeal pathologies.

In contrast to these findings, Klatt & Klatt (1990) reported no significant correlations between breathiness ratings and two measures of spectral tilt. Further, a synthesis study by Hillenbrand (1988a) found that breathiness ratings were affected only by the level of aspiration noise, with no effect for spectral tilt.

In summary, previous work on breathy voice suggests that the perception of breathiness is affected by first harmonic amplitude and the presence of aspiration noise. There are conflicting findings on the relative importance of these two cues. Some investigators (e.g., Bickley, 1982; Fischer-Jorgenson, 1967; Ladefoged & Antonanzas-Barroso, 1985) have concluded that H1 amplitude is the primary cue to breathiness, with aspiration noise playing little or no role. More recently, Klatt & Klatt (1990) have suggested that the presence of aspiration noise is the primary cue to breathiness, with H1 amplitude playing a secondary role. There are also conflicting findings on the relationship between spectral tilt and breathiness, with some studies (e.g., Frokjaer-Jensen & Prytz, 1976; Fukazawa et al., 1988; Klich, 1982) suggesting that breathiness is associated with greater amounts of high frequency energy, and other studies (e.g., Hillenbrand, 1988a; Klatt & Klatt, 1990) suggesting that spectral tilt plays little or no role in the perception of breathy voice.

The primary purpose of the present study was to measure the relationship between breathiness ratings and a relatively large set of acoustic measurements. The measurements fell into three categories: (a) measures of signal periodicity, (b) measures of first harmonic amplitude, and (c) measures of spectral tilt. A second purpose was to introduce two fully automatic measures of signal periodicity. These automated periodicity measures were intended to supplement or replace the subjective, visual rating method used by Klatt & Klatt (1990).

Methods

Recording of Voice Samples

Subjects and training. Voice samples were provided by eight men and seven women between the ages of 22 and 37 with no reported history of voice, speech, or hearing problems. Nine additional subjects were recorded who proved to be unable to perform the speaking task.

A sample recording of a naturally produced normal, moderately breathy, and very breathy [u] was used to familiarize talkers with the speaking task. Each talker was trained to produce three voicing variations (normal, moderately breathy, and very breathy) at estimated average fundamental frequency. Average fundamental frequency was estimated by asking each subject to read a portion of the Rainbow Passage (Fairbanks, 1940). Average fundamental frequency was calculated from this reading with a Kay Elemetrics Visi-Pitch/IBM PC Interface (Horii, 1983).

Recordings. Recordings were made in a sound-treated chamber using a unidirectional microphone (Audio-Technica 250XL) at a distance of 7–10 cm in front of the lips and 3 cm above the breath stream. The signals were recorded with a Sony PCM-F1 digital audio processor. A portable electronic keyboard was used to provide talkers with the target pitch determined previously through the Rainbow Passage analysis. The Visi-Pitch was used again to provide talkers with visual feedback regarding fundamental frequency and duration during the recording of vowel tokens. Speech materials included the four vowels [a], [i], [æ] and [o]. A randomized list of these vowels was provided for each talker. Talkers were asked to sustain each vowel for approximately 3 seconds. Each utterance was recorded at least twice during a 45–60 minute recording session. A total of 12 vowel samples (4 vowels × 3 voicing variations) was selected from each talker's recordings, yielding 180 vowel stimuli.

The signals were low-pass filtered at 7.2 kHz and digitized at 20 kHz using a 12-bit A/D board (Data Translation DT3382). The 3 sec sustained vowels were then digitally edited to the most stable 1 sec segment. A preliminary estimate of the maximally stable 1 sec interval was derived by computing a non-pitch-synchronous amplitude variability measure over consecutive 1 sec segments of the signal at intervals of 100 msec (e.g., 0–1000 msec, 100–1100 msec, etc.). The amplitude variability measure was essentially a shimmer calculation (Horii, 1980), except that it was computed non-pitch-synchronously using adjacent 10 msec intervals. The 1 sec segment of the signal showing the lowest amplitude variability was taken as a preliminary estimate of the maximally stable segment. The signal was then edited at the zero-crossings so that it included an integer number of pitch periods. In a few cases, the 1 sec segment extracted in this way did not appear by ear to be the most steady in terms of pitch. In these cases, a more appropriate interval was chosen by listening to different 1 sec segments of the signal. After editing, the signals were ramped on and off with a 20 msec inverted and lifted cosine function to eliminate onset and offset transients.

Breathiness Ratings

Twenty listeners (19 women, 1 man) were recruited from among graduate students and faculty in the Speech-Language Pathology Department at Western Michigan University. Listeners were audiometrically screened at 20 dB HL at five frequencies (0.5, 1, 2, 4, 6 kHz). Listening experiments were conducted in a sound-treated room. The stimuli consisted of 180 vowels (15 talkers × 3 breathiness levels × 4 vowels). Signals were low-pass filtered at 7.2 kHz, amplified and presented free field at approximately 80 dBA over a single loudspeaker (Boston Acoustics A60).

Listeners were asked to rate each signal according to the amount of perceived breathiness. Subjects were allowed to repeat each signal as often as they wished before entering their responses on a computer terminal. The direct magnitude estimation procedure required the listeners to determine their own numerical rating scales. Subjects were simply told to "enter a large number if the signal is very breathy and a small number if the signal shows little or no breathiness." Ratings were later linearly rescaled so that each listener's ratings for the 180-stimulus set ranged from 0.0 to 1.0.

Listeners participated in two 30–45 minute listening sessions at least 24 hours apart. In each listening session signals were presented in random order within three blocks including all 180 signals. A practice session of 60 trials began all listening sessions to familiarize subjects with the task and the range of breathiness percepts. The practice trials were identical to the listening session except that ratings from these trials were disregarded.

Acoustic analysis

The six acoustic measures that were used are described below. The measures were based on three assumptions about breathy voice: (a) the more rounded glottal waveforms for breathy signals should produce stronger first harmonics, (b) breathy signals should be less periodic, especially in the mid and high frequencies where aspiration noise is most prominent, and (c) breathy signals should show more high frequency energy than normally phonated signals. With the exception of first harmonic amplitude, the measures were fully automatic. Explanations of some of the signal processing techniques can be found in Parsons (1986) and Witten (1982).

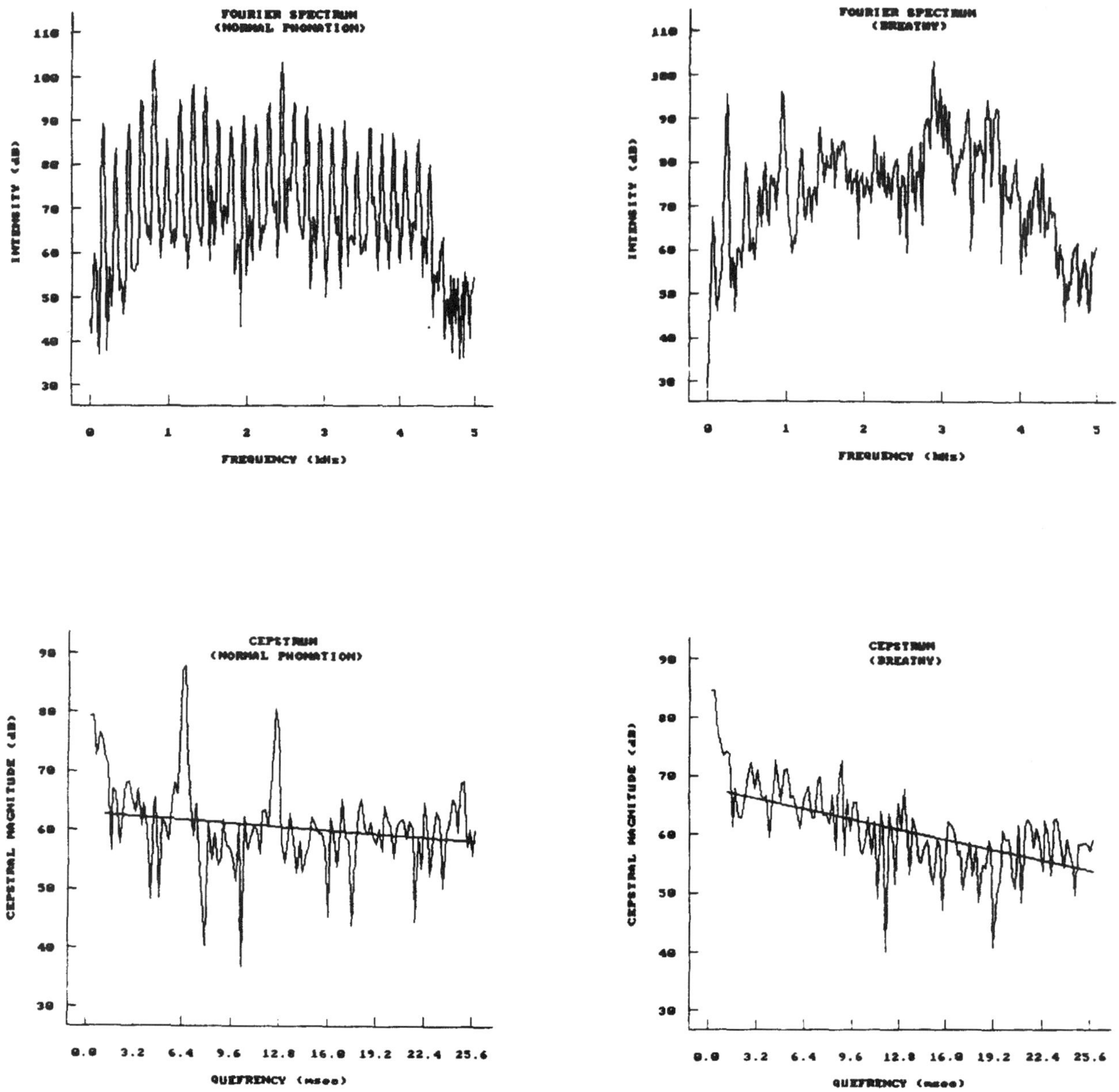

FIGURE 1. Fourier power spectra and cepstral representations for normally phonated and breathy signals. The linear regression line relating quefrency to cepstral magnitude is used in the CPP measure to normalize the cepstral peak for overall amplitude (see text).

CPP (Cepstral Peak Prominence): This is a measure of cepstral peak amplitude normalized for overall amplitude. Figure 1 shows examples of Fourier spectra and cepstral analyses from normally phonated and breathy signals. The cepstral peak in both cases corresponds to the fundamental period. The idea behind the CPP measure is that a highly periodic signal should show a well defined harmonic structure and, consequently, a more prominent cepstral peak than a less periodic signal. What is needed is a measure of the *prominence* of the peak rather than its absolute amplitude. This is because the amplitude of the cepstral peak is affected not only by the degree of periodicity but also by overall energy and the window size of the cepstrum analysis. Any number of methods might be used to normalize for overall amplitude. The method that we adopted involved fitting a linear regression line relating quefrency to cepstral magnitude. The line is computed between 1 msec and the maximum quefrency. (Quefrencies below 1 msec are ignored since these components are primarily sensitive to the envelope of the spectrum shape rather than signal periodicity.) The CPP measure is the difference in amplitude between the cepstral peak and the corresponding value on the regression line that is directly below the peak (i.e., the predicted cepstral magnitude for the quefrency at the cepstral peak). In other words, the CPP measure represents how far the cepstral peak emerges from the cepstral "background noise." Since breathy signals often retain a good deal of periodicity in the low frequencies, the CPP measure was computed not only from unfiltered signals but also from signals that were: (a) bandpass filtered between 2.5 and 3.5 kHz, and (b) highpass filtered at 2.5 kHz. The measure was made every 10 msec using a 25.6 msec analysis window. The CPP measure for a signal was averaged over all analysis frames.

It is important to note that this method is fully automatic, and no attempt was made to verify that the peak in the cepstrum actually corresponded to the fundamental period. Comparison of the fundamental period extracted using this method with hand measurements of the same signals showed that the technique frequently produced pitch tracking errors, especially for the breathy signals. As will be noted below, this method provided accurate predictions of breathiness ratings in spite of these errors.

RPK (Pearson r at Autocorrelation Peak): This measure is based on a standard autocorrelation pitch tracker (Hillenbrand, 1988b). The tracker computes the correlation between the signal and a delayed version of itself at delays between the minimum expected fundamental period and the maximum expected fundamental period (period limits of 3.3 and 16.7 msec were used in the present study). For periodic signals, a peak occurs in the autocorrelation function at a delay corresponding to the fundamental period.

The idea behind the RPK measure is that highly periodic signals should show more prominent autocorrelation peaks than breathy signals. Since the correlation at each delay is calculated as the sum of the cross-product between the signal and the delayed copy, the peak amplitude will be strongly affected by overall signal amplitude and autocorrelation window length. Consequently, as with the cepstral measure, a method is needed to normalize for overall amplitude. A variety of amplitude normalization schemes were tested, including the regression-line method used in CPP. The method that was the most successful in predicting breathiness ratings involved computing a Pearson product-moment correlation coefficient between the signal and a delayed copy at a delay corresponding to the peak in the autocorrelation function. For an accurately tracked signal, this is simply a normalized measure of the degree of correlation between adjacent pitch pulses. The expectation was that adjacent periods would be less highly correlated for breathy signals. The RPK measure was calculated every 10 msec using a 30 msec analysis window. The RPK measure for a signal was averaged over all analysis frames. RPK was calculated from bandpass, highpass, and unfiltered signals. As with CPP, no attempt was made to correct tracking errors, which were quite common for breathy signals.

P/A (Peak-to-Average ratio): This very simple measure is based on a suggestion made by Klatt & Klatt (1990; see also Koike & Markel, 1975, and Davis, 1981, for related measures). P/A is the ratio of peak amplitude to average amplitude from full-wave rectified time-domain signals (see Figure 2). The expectation was that highly periodic signals would show relatively large peak-to-average ratios. P/A measures were averaged over successive nonoverlapping 10 msec segments of bandpass, highpass, and unfiltered signals.

BRI (Breathiness Index): This is a slightly modified version of the spectral tilt measure described by Fukazawa et al. (1988). The measure was calculated every 10 msec using a 25.6 msec analysis window. The BRI measure for a signal was averaged over all analysis frames. (The Fukazawa et al. implementation made a single spectral tilt measure at approximately the center of the signal.) The expectation was that breathy signals would show more high frequency energy and, consequently, larger BRI values. The measure was calculated from unfiltered signals only.

H/L (ratio of High- to Mid/Low-Frequency energy): This a measure of the average spectral energy at or above 4 kHz to the average energy below 4 kHz. The energies were calculated from 128-point (6.4 msec) Fourier spectra computed every 3.2 msec. The H/L measure for a signal was averaged over all analysis frames, using unfiltered signals.

H1A (First Harmonic Amplitude): This measure is simply the dB amplitude of the first harmonic relative to the second harmonic. The measure was made by visual inspection of 512-point (25.6 msec) Fourier spectra taken at approximately the center of the signal (see Figure 3).

Conspicuously absent from the list above are the extensively studied measures of jitter (Lieberman, 1963), shimmer (e.g., Horii, 1980), and harmonics-to-noise ratio (Yumoto, Gould, & Baer, 1982). There were several reasons for this decision. First, as was pointed out by Klatt and Klatt (1990), measures such as these are primarily influenced by low-frequency signal components that tend to dominate waveform characteristics because of their relatively high energy. Aspiration noise, on the other hand, is most prominent in the mid and high frequencies. There is also evidence from synthesis studies that variations in jitter produce a sensation of roughness rather than breathiness (Hillenbrand, 1988; Wendahl, 1966a, 1966b). Finally, the problem of reliably and automatically identifying the oscillographic landmarks used by these measures in noisy voice signals is not trivial, and it is known that these measures can be quite sensitive to relatively small errors in detecting these landmarks (Hillenbrand, 1987).

Listener Reliability

Intra-judge reliability was assessed by measuring the correlation between ratings in the first listening session and ratings for the same signals in the second listening session. As can be seen in Table 1, correlations between the two sessions were relatively high, with an average session-to-session correlation of 0.91.

Between-subject reliability was computed using Cronbach's Coefficient Alpha (Cronbach, 1951). This method involves measuring the correlation between each individual listener's mean rating for each stimulus with the group mean of all the other listeners. Table 2 summarizes the results. The correlations ranged from 0.88 to 0.98 with a mean of 0.95.

Effects of Phonation Type, Vowel, and Gender

An analysis of variance was performed in order to investigate the effects of talker gender, phonation type, and vowel ([a], [æ], [i], or [o]) on breathiness ratings. There was a highly significant effect for phonation type [$F(2,156) = 330.94$, $p = 0.0001$], no effect for vowel [$F(3,156) = 1.31$, p NS], a significant effect for gender [$F(2, 156) = 4.83$, p 0.05], and

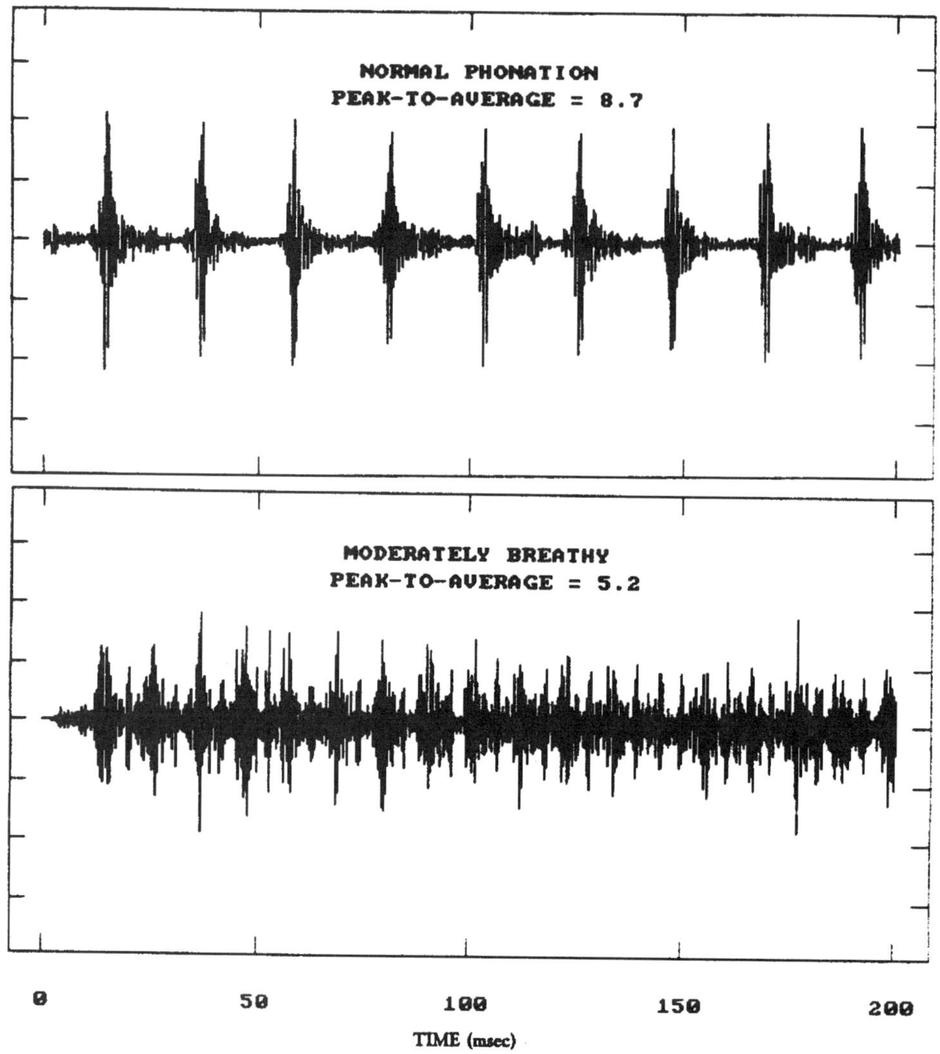

FIGURE 2. Bandpass filtered signals (2.5–3.5 kHz) from normally phonated and breathy vowels.

no significant interactions. The gender effect was due to higher breathiness ratings for men than women. However, additional analyses found no differences between men and women in breathiness ratings for normally phonated or moderately breathy signals (cf. Klatt & Klatt, 1990). Consequently, the gender effect simply indicates that men tended to produce higher levels of simulated breathiness than women for the very breathy condition. It might also be the case that listeners allowed for greater breathiness in female talkers, whereas the breathy male voice was perceived as being more abnormal.

Prediction of Breathiness Ratings

Table 3 shows the correlation of each measure with breathiness ratings and with all other acoustic measures. *Squared* correlations between the acoustic measures and the breathiness ratings are displayed in Figure 4. All correlations with breathiness ratings were significant at the 0.05 level or better. It can be seen that the cepstrum- and autocorrelation-based measures of signal periodicity accounted for a large proportion of the variance in breathiness ratings. The autocorrelation measure worked well only with filtered signals, while the CPP measure produced accurate predictions of breathiness ratings for unfiltered signals as well. For both of these measures it appears not to matter whether a bandpass or highpass filter is used. Breathiness predictions with CPP and RPK were somewhat more accurate than the predictions reported by Klatt & Klatt (1990) for a subjective visual method of rating the degree of periodicity in bandpass filtered signals.

The very simple peak-to-average measurement suggested by Klatt & Klatt (1990) correlated weakly with breathiness ratings. Examination of the scatter plot showed some indication of a nonlinear relationship between P/A and breathiness ratings. A log transform of the P/A measures resulted in slight improvements in prediction accuracy for all three types of signals, but prediction accuracy remained considerably lower than that for CPP and RPK.

Contrary to the findings of Fukazawa et al. (1988), spectral tilt correlated weakly with breathiness ratings. This was true both for BRI and H/L. This finding is in agreement with Klatt

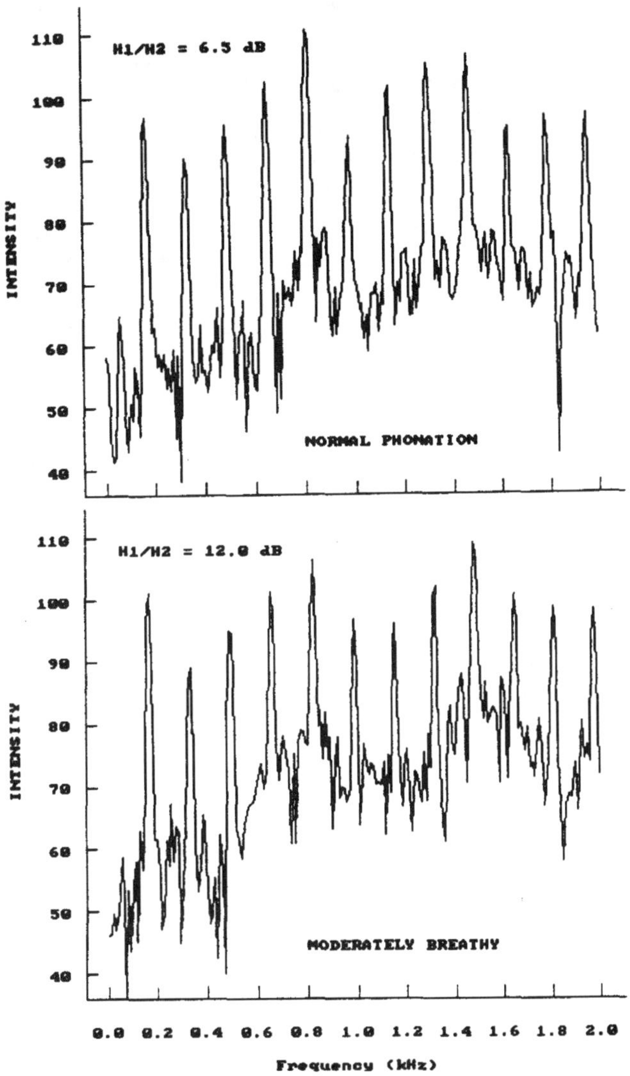

FIGURE 3. Sample spectra showing H1/H2 ratios for normal and moderately breathy phonation.

& Klatt (1990) who reported weak correlations between breathiness ratings and two measures of spectral tilt. We experimented with several variations of both BRI and H/L with limited success. For example, using a highpass filter to remove the fundamental frequency resulted in a slight improvement in prediction accuracy for BRI. We also experimented with a variety of frequency bands for the H/L calculation (including several bands that excluded the low frequency components of the spectrum) but did not find anything that worked better than the bands described previously. For the set of signals used in this study we consider it unlikely that additional tinkering with the measures would result in significant improvements in prediction accuracy. Examination of long-term average spectra for these signals simply did not show consistent breathiness-related differences in spectral tilt.

TABLE 1. Within-subject reliability measured as the correlation of average breathiness ratings between two listening sessions.

Subject	Pearson r	Subject	Pearson r
1	0.91	11	0.91
2	0.94	12	0.95
3	0.85	13	0.92
4	0.87	14	0.93
5	0.88	15	0.91
6	0.95	16	0.86
7	0.94	17	0.87
8	0.89	18	0.97
9	0.94	19	0.81
10	0.91	20	0.87

TABLE 2. Between-subject reliability measured with Cronbach coefficient alpha.

Subject	Correlation with set of all others	Subject	Correlation with set of all others
1	0.95	11	0.92
2	0.96	12	0.96
3	0.94	13	0.96
4	0.96	14	0.96
5	0.94	15	0.95
6	0.93	16	0.92
7	0.96	17	0.95
8	0.95	18	0.98
9	0.97	19	0.88
10	0.96	20	0.95

The measure of first harmonic amplitude correlated moderately with breathiness ratings. The 0.66 correlation is somewhat lower than the 0.83 correlation reported by Klatt & Klatt (1990). This might be related to the fact that Klatt & Klatt's talker group contained more women (n = 10) than men (n = 6). Further analysis of our measurements showed that H1A produced somewhat better predictions of breathiness ratings for women than men. We experimented with several methods for representing H1 amplitude (e.g., H1 amplitude relative to F1 amplitude and H1 amplitude relative to overall amplitude) but did not find anything that worked better than H1 relative to H2.

A stepwise multiple regression (SPSS-X, Version 4.00) was performed to determine if some linear combination of acoustic variables would improve prediction accuracy. Results are shown in Table 4. It can be seen that combining the acoustic measures results in relatively modest improvements in prediction accuracy. This is not surprising given the large proportion of the variance accounted for by CPP and RPK and the strong correlations between these two measures.

Discussion

Listening Experiment

Our results are in close agreement with those of Klatt & Klatt (1990), who reported that the best predictors of breathiness ratings were measures of: (a) periodicity in band-limited signals, and (b) first harmonic amplitude. The CPP and RPK measures are essentially automated versions of the subjective visual rating method used by Klatt & Klatt to represent periodicity. The CPP measure is similar in principle to a cepstrum-based signal-to-noise ratio calculation described

TABLE 3. Intercorrelation matrix for acoustic measures.* All correlations with breathiness ratings are significant at 0.05 or better.

	BR	CPP	CPPb	CPPh	RPK	RPKb	RPKh	P/A	P/Ab	P/Ah	BRI	H/L	H1A
BR	—	−0.92	−0.90	−0.89	−0.54	−0.91	−0.89	−0.30	−0.54	−0.58	0.41	0.51	0.66
CPP		—	0.98	0.98	0.42	0.92	0.91	0.32	0.51	0.56	−0.23	−0.37	−0.58
CPPb			—	0.98	0.38	0.93	0.91	0.30	0.46	0.52	−0.24	−0.40	−0.52
CPPh				—	0.36	0.93	0.92	0.37	0.53	0.59	−0.22	−0.39	−0.53
RPK					—	0.39	0.36	−0.21	0.22	0.23	−0.28	−0.24	−0.31
RPKb						—	0.97	0.36	0.55	0.59	−0.25	−0.42	−0.57
RPKh							—	0.40	0.57	0.60	−0.28	−0.48	−0.58
P/A								—	0.48	0.48	−0.04	−0.19	−0.33
P/Ab									—	0.95	−0.19	−0.32	−0.43
P/Ah										—	−0.14	−0.27	−0.42
BRI											—	0.81	0.20
H/L												—	0.25
H1A													—

*BR = breathiness rating, CPP = cepstral peak prominence, RPK = Pearson r at autocorrelation peak, P/A = peak-to-average ratio, BRI = breathiness index, H/L = ratio of high- to mid/low-frequency energy, H1A = first harmonic amplitude; b = bandpass filtered between 2.5 and 3.5 kHz; h = highpass filtered at 2.5 kHz.

recently by de Krom (1993), but is considerably simpler. It is somewhat surprising that CPP and RPK performed as well as they did since, as noted earlier, the very simple pitch trackers upon which they are based are not particularly accurate in identifying the fundamental period for breathy signals that are band-limited well above the fundamental frequency. In pilot work not reported here we attempted to improve the accuracy of the tracker in locating the fundamental period by constraining the search for the cepstral or autocorrelation peaks to relatively narrow limits around the average fundamental period determined from hand measurements. For reasons that are not clear, CPP and RPK measures obtained in this way were somewhat more weakly correlated with breathiness ratings than were measures obtained by the unconstrained method. Although we do not have an explanation for this finding, it is encouraging that these techniques do not depend on accurate tracking of the fundamental period. This is quite important since reliable measurement of fundamental frequency for marginally periodic signals is an extremely difficult and quite possibly unresolvable problem.

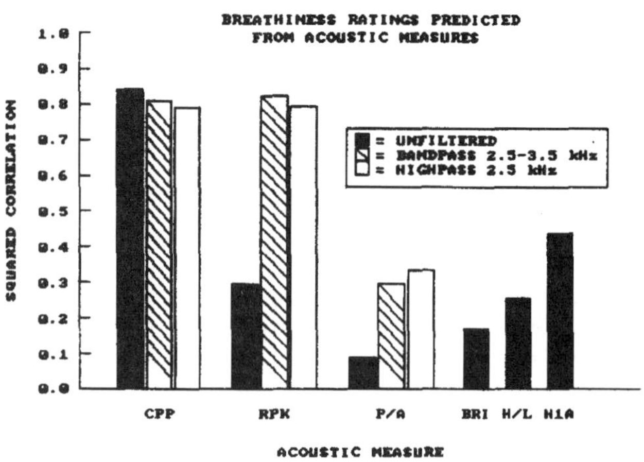

FIGURE 4. Squared correlation coefficients between acoustic measures and breathiness ratings.

It should be noted that the present results are purely descriptive and do not provide any direct evidence about the cues used by listeners in making breathiness judgments. However, our findings are quite consistent with the synthesis study of Klatt & Klatt (1990), which demonstrated that listener judgments of breathiness were more strongly influenced by aspiration noise than first harmonic amplitude. This conclusion is at odds with that reached by Bickley (1982) and Fischer-Jorgensen (1967). A detailed discussion of these conflicting findings can be found in Klatt & Klatt (1990).

Potential clinical applications of these techniques include the use of such acoustic measures as: (a) visual feedback in the treatment of vocal pathologies involving breathy voice, (b) a method of tracking progress throughout the course of a treatment program, and (c) indices to evaluate the relative effectiveness of alternative treatment approaches. Viewed in relation to these kinds of applications the CPP and RPK measures appear to be the most promising, in part because they provide accurate predictions of perceived breathiness, but also because they operate automatically and appear to be insensitive to pitch tracking errors. Although H1A correlated moderately with breathiness ratings, this measure appears to be much less promising as a clinical tool because of the difficulty of producing a reliable automatic algorithm that is capable of handling signals that are marginally periodic. We recently developed a semiautomatic algorithm that produces accurate measurements of H1A when given an estimate of fundamental frequency. However, the measure-

TABLE 4. Stepwise multiple regression analysis showing the prediction of breathiness ratings from various combinations of acoustic measures.

Step	Acoustic measure	Variance explained
1	CPP	0.84
2	BRI	0.88
3	H1A	0.90
4	RPK	0.92
5	RPK-BP	0.94

ments become unreliable if the estimated fundamental frequency is off by more than about 5%.

Development of an acoustically based feedback device would obviously require that the signal processing algorithms operate in real time. While the software used in this study operates in many times real time, none of the techniques are particularly computationally intensive. Real-time implementations of these algorithms are well within the capabilities of current digital signal processing hardware.

An important limitation of the present findings concerns the fact that the signals were produced by normal talkers who were simulating various levels of breathiness. The advantage of this method is that it ensured that the signals varied primarily in a single voice quality dimension. It was almost certainly the nearly univariate nature of the stimulus variations, in addition to the broad range of breathiness percepts, that accounted for the high degree of reliability in the listener ratings of breathiness. However, it remains to be determined whether the acoustic methods that were used in this study will provide accurate predictions of perceived breathiness in naturally occurring rather than simulated breathiness. Naturally occurring breathy voices will almost certainly present a more complicated picture, particularly in the voices of dysphonic speakers, which are seldom simply breathy and often show rather complex laryngeal vibratory patterns (e.g., von Leden, Moore, & Timcke, 1960).

A second limitation, common to many studies in this area, is the exclusive reliance on monotone, sustained vowels. The use of these simple signals greatly simplifies the measurement of phenomena such as aspiration noise since it is not necessary to separate waveform and spectral changes that are due to aspiration from those that might be due to intonation or supraglottal articulatory dynamics. However, since breathiness is quite easy to detect auditorily in continuous speech, it is clear that perceptual mechanisms exist to extract this quality from more complex speech signals. A challenge for future research will be to extend acoustic methods developed for sustained vowels to continuous speech.

Acknowledgments

We are grateful to William Dawson for his technical help with the instrumentation used to record the voice samples. This work was supported by a research grant from the National Institutes of Health (1-R01-DC01661).

References

Aronson, A. E. (1971). Early motor unit disease masquerading as psychogenic breathy dysphonia: A clinical case presentation. *Journal of Speech and Hearing Disorders, 36,* 115–124.

Aronson, A. E. (1990). *Clinical voice disorders* (3rd ed.). New York: Thieme.

Bickley, C. (1982). *Acoustic analysis and perception of breathy vowels.* (Speech Communication Group Working Papers I). Cambridge, MA.: Research Laboratory of Electronics.

Boone, D. R., & McFarlane, S. C. (1988). *The voice and voice therapy.* 4th ed. Englewood Cliffs, NJ: Prentice Hall.

Colton, R. A., & Casper, J. K. (1990). *Understanding voice problems: A physiological perspective for diagnosis and treatment.* Baltimore: Williams and Wilkins.

Cronbach, L. J. (1951). Coefficient alpha and the internal structure of tests. *Psychometrica, 16,* 297–334.

Davis, S. B. (1981). Acoustic characteristics of normal and pathological voices. *ASHA Reports, 11,* 97–115.

de Krom, G. (1993). A cepstrum-based technique for determining a harmonic-to-noise ratio in speech signals. *Journal of Speech and Hearing Research, 36,* 254–266.

Fairbanks, G. (1940). *Voice and articulation drillbook.* New York: Harper and Brothers.

Fischer-Jorgensen, E. (1967). Phonetic analysis of breathy (murmured) vowels in Gujarati. *Indian Linguistics, 28,* 71–139.

Frokjaer-Jensen, B., & Prytz, S. (1976). Registration of voice quality. *Bruel and Kjaer Technical Review, 3,* 3–17.

Fukazawa, T., El-Assuooty, A., & Honjo, I. (1988). A new index for evaluation of the turbulent noise in pathological voice. *Journal of the Acoustical Society of America, 83,* 1189–1192.

Hillenbrand, J. (1987). A methodological study of perturbation and additive noise in synthetically generated voice signals. *Journal of Speech and Hearing Research, 30,* 448–461.

Hillenbrand, J. (1988a). Perception of aperiodicities in synthetically generated voices. *Journal of the Acoustical Society of America, 83,* 2361–2371.

Hillenbrand, J. (1988b). *MPITCH: An autocorrelation fundamental-frequency tracker.* [Computer Program]. Kalamazoo, MI.: Western Michigan University.

Hillenbrand, J., Metz, D. E., Colton, R. A., & Whitehead, R. L. (1990). *A high-speed film and acoustic study of breathy voice.* Paper presented at the meeting of the American Speech-Language-Hearing Association, Seattle, WA.

Hollien, H. (1987). "Old voices": What do we really know about them? *Journal of Voice, 1,* 2–17.

Horii, Y. (1980). Vocal shimmer in sustained phonation. *Journal of Speech and Hearing Research, 23,* 202–209.

Horii, Y. (1983). Automatic analysis of voice fundamental frequency and intensity using a Visi-Pitch. *Journal of Speech and Hearing Research, 26,* 467–471.

Huffman, M. K. (1987). Measures of phonation type in Hmong. *Journal of the Acoustical Society of America, 81,* 495–504.

Kasuya, H., Ogawa, S., Kazuhiko, M., & Satoshi, E. (1986). Normalized noise energy as an acoustic measure to evaluate pathologic voice. *Journal of the Acoustical Society of America, 80,* 1329–1334.

Klatt, D. H., & Klatt, L. C. (1990). Analysis, synthesis, and perception of voice quality variations among female and male talkers. *Journal of the Acoustical Society of America, 87,* 820–857.

Klich, R. J. (1982). Relationships of vowel characteristics to listener ratings of breathiness. *Journal of Speech and Hearing Research, 25,* 574–580.

Koike, Y., & Markel, J. D. (1975). Application of inverse filtering for detecting laryngeal pathology. *Annals of Otology, Rhinology and Laryngology, 84,* 117–124.

Ladefoged, P. (1975). *A course in phonetics.* New York: Harcourt Brace Jovanovich.

Ladefoged, P. (1983). The linguistic use of different phonation types. In D. M. Bless & J. H. Abbs (Eds.), *Vocal fold physiology: Contemporary research and clinical issues* (pp. 351–360). San Diego: College Hill.

Ladefoged, P., & Antonanzas-Barroso, N. (1985). *Computer measures of breathy phonation.* (Working Papers in Phonetics, 61). University of California, Los Angeles, 79–86.

Lieberman, P. (1963). Some acoustic measures of the fundamental periodicity of normal and pathologic larynges. *Journal of the Acoustical Society of America, 35,* 344–353.

McKay, I. R. A. (1987). *Phonetics: The science of speech production* (2nd ed.). Boston: College Hill.

Parsons, T. W. (1987). *Voice and speech processing.* New York: McGraw-Hill.

Ryan, W. J., & Burk, K. W. (1974). Perceptual and acoustic correlates of aging in the speech of males. *Journal of Communication Disorders, 7,* 181–192.

von Leden, H., Moore, P., & Timcke, R. (1960). Laryngeal vibra-

tions: Measurements of the glottic wave. *AMA Archives of Otolaryngology, 71*, 26–45.
Wendahl, R. (1966a). Some parameters of auditory roughness. *Folia Phoniatrica, 18*, 26–32.
Wendahl, R. (1966b). Laryngeal analog synthesis of jitter and shimmer: Auditory parameters of harshness. *Folia Phoniatrica, 18*, 98–108.
Witten, I. H. (1982). *Principles of Computer Speech.* London: Academic Press.
Yumoto, E., Gould, W. J., & Baer, T. (1982). Harmonics-to-noise ratio as an index of the degree of hoarseness. *Journal of the Acoustical Society of America, 71*, 1544–1550.
Zemlin, W. (1968). *Speech and hearing science: Anatomy and physiology.* Englewood Cliffs, NJ: Prentice-Hall.

Received September 27, 1993
Accepted February 28, 1994

Contact author: James Hillenbrand, Speech Pathology and Audiology, Western Michigan University, Kalamazoo, MI 49008.

4

Clinical Voice Disorders and Voice Therapy

Introduction

Laryngology and voice pathology as subspecialties among both otolaryngologists and speech pathologists continue to increase in popularity with new voice centers popping up at academic institutions across the globe. Given the boom in expertise and clinical service, the fact that only 17 manuscripts met the criteria for the designation of classic was, frankly, shocking. Seventeen articles provide the foundation for the clinical management of patients with voice disorders and the provision of voice therapy. Also interesting is the fact that less than 20% of the classic manuscripts were published prior to 1990, further confirming the emergence of this field over the past 2 decades.

This section is diverse and likely warrants additional stratification. Among others, this section includes epidemiological studies, meta-analyses of voice therapy, and interestingly, one paper on the quantification of the impact of voice disorders on quality of life. Drs. Morrison and Rammage, in their classic paper, were the first to provide a framework for what is contemporarily referred to as muscle tension dysphonia. As described in his commentary, Dr. Morrison began to notice that patients with "functional" voice disorders appear to misuse voluntary muscles, and established a collaboration to describe and classify these postures. This topic remains relatively controversial to this day.

From reviewing the list of classic articles, one will appreciate the the significant contributions made by Dr. Lorraine Ramig. A debt of gratitude is owed to Dr. Ramig for her landmark work in patients with Parkinson disease. Her work represents the bulk of voice therapy efficacy studies, and has led to Lee Silverman Voice Treatment (LVST) becoming a household term among voice professionals. Although many of us know of LSVT and are impressed with its impact, few understand the story behind the technique and the evolution of LSVT to its current state. Dr. Ramig provides her insight into the evolution of LSVT into the international phenomena it is today.

Classic Articles

● Reprint of article included in this chapter.
♦ Commentary on this article.

Logemann JA, Fisher HB, Boshes B, Blonsky ER. Frequency and cooccurrence of vocal tract dysfunctions in the speech of a large sample of Parkinson patients. *J Speech Hear Dis.* 1978;43(1):47–57.

Honjo I, Isshiki N. Laryngoscopic and voice characteristics of aged persons. *Arch Otolaryngol.* 1980;106(3): 149–150.

Williams AJ, Baghat MS, Stableforth DE, Cayton RM, Shenoi PM, Skinner C. Dysphonia caused by inhaled steroids: recognition of a characteristic laryngeal abnormality. *Thorax.* 1983;38(11):813–821.

Fuhrman GM, Stieg III FH, Buerk, CA. Blunt laryngeal trauma: classification and management protocol. *J Trauma.* 1990;30(1):87–92.

Sataloff RT, Spiegel JR, Hawkshaw MJ. Strobovideolaryngoscopy: results and clinical value. *Ann Otol Rhinol Laryngol.* 1991;100(9 pt 1):725–727.

Sapir S, Keidar A, Mathers-Schmidt B. Vocal attrition in teaches: survey findings. *Eur J Disord Comm.* 1993; 28(2):177–185.

Gotaas C, Starr CD. Vocal fatigue among teachers. *Folia Phoniatr.* 1993;45(3):120–129.

●♦Morrison MD, Rammage LA. Muscle misuse voice disorders: description and classification. *Acta Otolarygol.* 1993;113(3):428–434.

Sataloff RT, Bough Jr ID, Spiegel JR. Arytenoid dislocation: diagnosis and treatment. *Laryngoscope.* 1994;104 (11 pt 1):1353–1361.

Dromey C, Ramig LO, Johnson AB. Phonatory and articulatory changes associated with increased vocal intensity in Parkinson disease: a case study. *J Speech Hear Res.* 1995;38(4):751–764.

Smith ME, Ramig LO, Dromey C, Perez KS, Samandari R. Intensive voice treatment in Parkinson disease: laryngostroboscopic findings. *J Voice.* 1995;9(4):453–459.

●♦Ramig LO, Countryman S, Thompson LL, Horii Y. Comparison of two forms of intensive speech treatment for Parkinson disease. *J Speech Hear Res.* 1995;38(6):1232–1251.

Ramig LO, Countryman S, O'Brien C, Hoehn M, Thompson L. Intensive speech treatment for patients with Parkinson's disease: short- and long-term comparison of tow techniques. *Neurology.* 1996;47(6): 1496–1504.

●Smith E, Gray SD, Dove H, Kirchner L, Heras H. Frequency and effects of teachers' voice problems. *J Voice.* 1997;1(1):81–87.

Ramig LO, Verdolini K. Treatment efficacy: voice disorders. *J Speech Lang Hear Res.* 1998;41(1):S101–S116.

Benninger MS, Ahuja AS, Gardner G, Grywalski C. Assessing outcomes for dysphonic patients. *J Voice.* 1998;12(4):540–550.

Russell A, Oates J, Greenwood KM. Prevalence of voice problems in teachers. *J Voice.* 1998;12(4):467–479.

Hogikyan ND, Sethuraman G. Validation of an instrument to measure voice-related quality of life (V-RQOL). *J Voice.* 1999;13(4):557–569.

Commentary

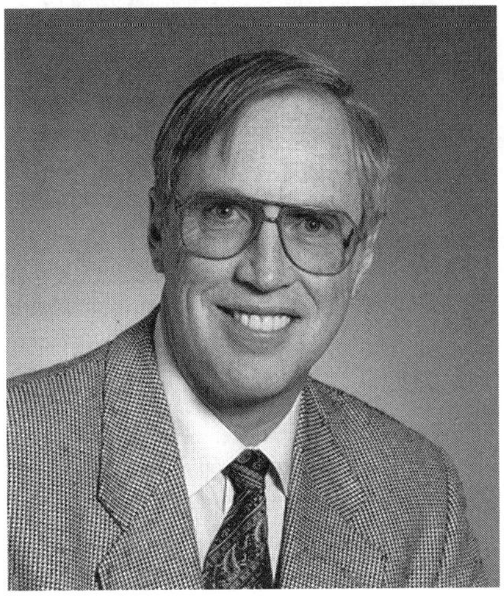

Murray Morrison, MD

Timing is important. In the late 1970s, innovation in rigid and flexible laryngoscopy, coupled with a stroboscope and the ability to record the images on videotape, brought laryngeal and voice evaluation to a new level. It was just at that time, in the fall of 1980, that I, having acquired these tools, started our voice clinic. Speech-language pathologist Linda Rammage and I began regular joint patient evaluations and like others using the new tools began to see things unknown at that time, like sulcus vocalis and loss of mucosal wave after vocal cord surgery. We were also intrigued by the many ways the larynx posture changed in the so-called "functional" voice disorders. Recognizing that many of these patients were suffering from psychological distress, we became aware that we needed help in that aspect of evaluation and care. My being called to the emergency room to treat a psychiatric patient with a self-inflicted wound of the larynx led to a meeting with his psychiatrist, Hamish Nichol. Dr. Nichol was interested in emotionally based misuse of muscle systems and he agreed to be the voice clinic's psychiatric consultant. Recognizing that people with "functional" voice disorders produce dysphonia by misusing voluntary muscles, we collaborated on our early attempts to describe and classify the sorts of misuse postures that we were seeing. The first paper on "muscular tension dysphonia" (MTD) was published in 1983, and the more often cited "muscle misuse voice disorders: description and classification" in 1992.

Linda Rammage, Hamish Nichol, and I have continued our very rewarding collaboration to the present. Our textbook *The Management of the Voice and Its Disorders* is in its second edition. We are currently extending the concept of central nervous system hypersensitivity and how laryngeal disorders including MTD and vocal cord dysfunction relate to illness such as fibromyalgia and irritable bowel. This is described in our paper "The Irritable Larynx Syndrome" published in 1999 in the *Journal of Voice*.

Muscle Misuse Voice Disorders: Description and Classification*

MURRAY D. MORRISON and LINDA A. RAMMAGE

From the Division of Otolaryngology, University of British Columbia, Vancouver General Hospital, Vancouver, British Columbia, Canada

Morrison MD, Rammage LA. *Muscle misuse voice disorders: description and classification.* Acta Otolaryngol (Stockh) 1993; 113: 428–434.

It is apparent that voice disorders frequently labelled "functional" are associated with laryngeal muscle misuse. This use of the word "functional" is, however, intrinsically ambiguous, and so we propose an alternative term based on descriptive features of dysfunction: "muscle misuse voice disorders". Persistent phonation with an abnormal laryngeal posture can lead to organic changes such as nodules or polyps, particularly in females with posterior glottic chink. We hypothesized that the chink was related to an overall increase in laryngeal muscle tension, and more directly due to inadequate relaxation of the posterior crico-arytenoid muscle during phonation. We employed the term "muscular tension dysphonia" (MTD) to note this condition, but it may be that the term "laryngeal isometric" is superior since there are other misuses of the larynx that obviously are manifestations of abnormalities of muscular tension. With this in mind we have evolved a new classification based on the laryngeal isometric, glottic and supraglottic lateral contraction states, antero-posterior contraction states, conversion aphonia, phychogenic bowing, and adolescent transitional dysphonia. *Key words: functional dysphonia, psychogenic voice disorders, muscular tension dysphonia, glottic posture.*

INTRODUCTION

Patients with so-called "functional dysphonia" who have structurally normal larynges and demonstrate muscle misuse in the larynx, and those with several interacting causes including habituated muscle tension, are probably better defined as having a "muscle misuse voice disorder".

Commonly occuring organic triggers of muscle misuse voice disorders are upper respiratory tract infections and gastro-esophageal reflux. The task of the voice team is a difficult one: to define and "sort out" pathological processes that are predisposing, precipitating and perpetuating an individual's dysphonia, and to apply terminology that best describes the relevant ongoing pathophysiological processes for each patient.

The clinician's diagnostic task may be further complicated by signs of organic change secondary to misuse. Vocal nodules are mucosal changes thought to be secondary to vocal abuse and misuse. Nodules often can be identified with a laryngeal mirror, and if assignment of the diagnosis is based solely on this readily identified clinical sign it seems logical to label the disease process "vocal nodules". However such an approach to classification focuses on organic pathology, often out of context with the individuals' habitual voice use patterns, and does not allow one to differentiate among the predisposing, precipitating and perpetuating factors involved in the etiology. The consequences for effective management are considerable.

A diagnostic classification scheme should be unifying, grouping disorders with common primary causes, yet flexible and expandable, so that individual factors playing etiological roles can be included in descriptions of single patients. The preferred treatment hierarchy may then be implied in a diagnosis. We have attempted to amalgamate a classification system that is comprehensive and promotes the use of diagnostic labels to best reflect all currently recognized patterns of muscle misue associated with dysphonias. Our long-term goal is a data-based descriptive classification scheme that encompasses the most efficacious treatment practices.

Table I. *Classification of muscle misuse voice disorders.*

1. The laryngeal isometric
2. Lateral hyper-adduction states
   a. Glottic
   b. Supra-glottic
3. Supra-glottic anteroposterior contraction
4. Conversion aphonia
5. Psychogenic bowing
6. Adolescent transitional dysphonia

PROBLEMS OF CLASSIFICATION

Although clinical patterns described by different authors may bear resemblances, the assumed underlying pathological processes are often different. In addition, the use of terminology is inconsistent. The same term may be used to infer quite different pathological processes, for example, "plica ventricularis", "ventricular phonation", or "ventricular dysphonia" may designate a degree of adducting movement of the ventricular folds simultaneous with adduction of and phonation with the true vocal folds (1). However, these terms may be employed by others who refer to complete or near complete adduction of, and

* Presented at the symposium: "New Horizons in Laryngology".

phonation with, the ventricular folds in the absence of true vocal fold phonation (2). Conversely, an apparently similar set of processes may be designated by very different terminology by different authors. "Puberphonia", "mutational dysphonia", "falsetto phonation" and "adolescent transitional voice disorder" may all refer to a functional dysphonia seen in teen-age males who are experiencing difficulty using modal register phonation during or following pubertal growth of the larynx and vocal tract.

Finally, the controversy continues as to the interchangeability of the terms "pychogenic" and "functional" when referring to dysphonias not primarily due to organic pathology. Aronson (2) argues for the use of "psychogenic" to refer to the broad group of voice disorders that exist in the absence of organic laryngeal pathology. His argument is based on the assumption that "psychogenic" is broadly synonymous with "functional" in its application to voice disorder classification, but that it more directly implies an inevitable underlying psycho-emotional desequilibrium. Brodnitz (3) in employing the term "psychogenic voice disturbances" has emphasized the importance of the interaction between organic and psychodynamic factors, which he believes belong together "like two sides of the coin", in the formation of all "functional" dysphonias.

Our bias is re-stated here: the terms "functional" and "psychogenic" are not synonymous: "psychogenic" diagnoses should be reserved for those muscle misuse voice disorders that clearly have a primary psycho-emotional etiology, as defined by current standards for psychiatric evaluation (4). Such a conclusion is not reached solely by exclusion of organic pathogeneses, and often requires a formal psychological evaluation.

HISTORY OF CLASSIFICATION

Vocal dysfunction has been classified in many ways. A broad distinction was made formerly between "hyperfunctional" and "hypofunctional" voice disorders (5). Other authors have referred to a diagnostic polarity between "hyperkinesia" and "hypokinesia" (3).

Many authors have agreed that a hyperfunction or hyperkinesia of the laryngeal muscles results in a variety of dysphonia patterns. Further, the secondary organic signs of prolonged misuse of this nature have been highlighted: nodules; polyps; chronic laryngitis; contact ulcers and/or hypofunction of muscles (3, 5–8).

Attempts to classify hypofunctional or hypokinesic voice disorders have resulted in terms like "paretic hoarseness", "lateralis paralysis", "transversus triangle" and "bowing" of the vocal folds (9). While some authors referred to "hypofunctional dysphonia", Jackson (6) employed the term "myasthenia laryngis" to represent the secondary response to hyperfunction, a response he felt accounted for the problems of many professional voice users complaining of voice difficulty. Still other authors have used "phonasthenia" to describe a similar set of signs and symptoms, which were thought to be related to dysfunction of the thyroarytenoid muscles.

In more recent publications, the sub-classes "hyperfunctional" and "hypofunctional" seem to have yielded to a broader classification of musculoskeletal voice disorders (2, 8, 10, 11).

A MUSCULOSKELETAL APPROACH TO CLASSIFICATION OF DYSPHONIAS

Voice disorders can be caused by misuse of the voluntary muscles of phonation including muscles of the larynx, pharynx, jaw, tongue, neck and respiratory system. General postural misalignment is also common. Some dysphonias can be attributed primarily to incorrect vocal techniques such as poor coordination among respiratory, phonatory, resonatory and articulatory gestures; excessive or inadequate laryngeal valving; improper resonance focus; and improper control of pitch and loudness dynamics.

Some of the disorders associated with muscular misuses are not associated with observable organic changes to the vocal folds, while others commonly have associated secondary pathologies, including nodules, polypoidal degeneration, chronic laryngitis or scarring. In some individuals, muscle misuses may be the direct result of psychological stressors, in which case the resulting dysphonia can legitimately be labelled "psychogenic". Psychogenic problems represent failure of an individual to adapt physiologically to a psychological stimulus, usually a conflict based one (12–14). Whatmore & Kohli (15) have described a variety of maladaptive disturbance patterns ("dysponeses") in the signalling system for voluntary muscles which are responses to a variety of psychological states. The dysponetic signals originate in the pre-motor and motor cortices and influence action potentials in descending pathways, side branches, lower motor neurons, skeletal muscles and the various feedback pathways. Others, including Jacobson (16) and Barlow (17) have also focused on misuse of the voluntary muscles as the final common pathway for psychological conflict and dysfunction. The muscle misuse and misalignment patterns associated with symbolic conversion dysphonias or aphonias lead to severe dysfunction that is primarily psychogenic.

Psychological conflict or distress may be an interacting factor with vocal abuse and misuse in the precipitation and perpetuation of dysphonia, thus contributing to pressor responses in the nervous system which in turn create hypertonicity of the voluntary muscles. Psychological distress may also be secondary to dysphonia, being the direct result of a dysfunctional state. The final result is the same: psychological stimuli lead to inappropriate muscle tone, disturbed feedback, and poor coordination of movements in the voluntary muscle system (14).

CLASSES OF MUSCLE MISUSE DYSPHONIA

Type 1: The laryngeal isometric. (Muscular tension dysphonia, (MTD) as described by Morrison et al. (8))

The laryngeal isometric pattern is most commonly seen in untrained occupational and professional voice users, and represents a generalized increase in muscular tension throughout the larynx and paralaryngeal areas. The etiology usually includes a combination of poor vocal technique, extensive and extraordinary voice use demands, and interacting or secondary psychological factors. Anxiety is most commonly identified, and in some cases, the diagnosis of generalized anxiety disorder is made based on criteria listed in the Diagnostic and Statistical Manual of Mental Disorders (DSM-IIIR) (4). Psychological components may be secondary to dysphonia, rather than a primary etiological factor and this implies a perpetuating influence in sign-symptom formation.

A key feature of the isometric pattern of laryngeal and paralaryngeal hypertonicity relates to the characteristics and role of the posterior cricoarytenoid muscle (PCA) in abducting the glottis. The histological structure of the PCA appears to be well adapted to this role. For example it has more type I muscle fibres than all other intrinsic laryngeal muscles (18). Thus when the larynx is in a general hypertonic state, the sustained contraction of the PCA may deflect the arytenoid cartilages down the cricoarytenoid joint and open the posterior commissure, creating a posterior glottal chink (PGC). This hypothesis was supported by a laryngeal muscle pull experiment performed by the authors in 1983 (19). Dissected fresh human cadaver larynges were held in a frame with the intrinsic muscles attached to strings pulled in the direction of the muscle contraction. It was easily seen that when the glottis was closed with firm lateral crico-arytenoid and inter-arytenoid muscle pulls it took only a light traction on the PCA to open the posterior chink in such a way as to produce a glottal shape like that seen in this group of patients. PGC magnitude also may be associated with hypertonicity in supra-hyoid musculature (8).

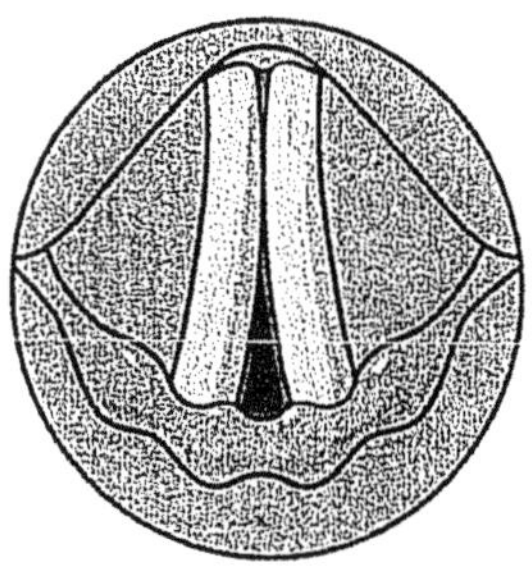

Fig. 1. The laryngeal isometric. Generalized tension in all the laryngeal muscles is often associated with an open posterior glottic chink due to persistent posterior crico-arytenoid muscle pull during phonation. This leads to secondary mucosal vocal fold changes including nodules, chronic laryngitis of polypoidal degeneration.

Studies of clinical populations and normal subjects simulating muscle misuse dysphonias have demonstrated that magnitude of the PGC is directly related to phonatory airflow rate, "whispery/breathy" perceptions, spectral noise, and distinctive intensity profiles in the acoustic spectra (8, 11, 20–22). In clinical populations, the laryngeal isometric may be accompanied by other forms of muscle misuse, such as lateral contraction states, which can confound aerodynamic and acoustic profiles.

Disease of the vocal fold mucosa is often identified as a component of the diagnosis, and generally assumed to be secondary to the specific pattern of muscle misuses associated with the laryngeal isometric posture. Hirano (23) has demonstrated the five-layered vocal fold structure in which the superficial two layers, including mucosa and superficial lamina propria (Reinke's space) make up the cover of the vocal fold and the deeper three layers, namely the middle elastic lamina propria, the deep collagenous lamina propria, and the vocalis muscle itself, make up the body of the vocal cord. The muscles contract during phonation, with the strength of the contraction dependent on various factors discussed above. During phonation, the cover flows around the leading edge of the vocal fold body, producing the so-called "mucosal wave" effect seen on stroboscopy. Looseness in the cover overlying the muscle body is necessary for clear phonation. In cases of tense or very loud phonation particularly in the presence of tense vocal folds, shearing stresses can injure the delicate tissue of the superficial lamina propria leading to edema, haemorrhage or fibrosis. These stresses tend to lead to the development of mid-membranous vocal nodules most commonly identified in premenopausal females and prepubertal children. These are also the clinical sub-groups that demonstrate the largest PGC magnitudes, and widest inter-arytenoid spaces relative to vocal fold length. The posterior margin of the nodules corresponds to the anterior margin of the PGC. This leads one to hypothesize a specific causal relationship between PGC magnitude and bilateral nodules. Perhaps strong adduction forces employed to overcome exaggerated abduction in the posterior glottis lead to greater shearing stresses on the mid-membranous vocal folds at the position where nodules typically develop. Further, lack of adduction posterior to the mid-membraneous vocal folds would inhibit development of the mucosal disease there. Subepithelial edema or polypoidal degeneration is the usual form of secondary organic disease found in postmenopausal females, particularly in those who smoke. There is evidence that PGC magnitude and age in women are inversely related (21, 24). This could provide some explanation for the mucosal disease posterior to the typical nodule site in the older female population. Most adult males will develop a diffuse thickening of the cover that is referred to as "chronic laryngitis".

The laryngeal isometric is frequently associated with palpable increases in suprahyoid muscle tension on phonation particularly in higher pitch ranges during singing, and during high vowels and phoneme transitions in connected speech.

Type 2: Lateral contraction and/or hyperadduction

This dysfunctional pattern is a type of tension fatigue syndrome in which the larynx tends to be squeezed or hyperadducted in a side to side direction. It may exist either at the glottic or supraglottic level, or both. The glottic form is usually related to technical errors, and sometimes acute anxiety states may be identified. Supraglottic squeezing, or "plica ventricularis" on the other hand, is often associated with ongoing psychogenic factors.

Subtype a: Glottic contraction. Simple vocal misues with hyperadduction of the vocal folds produce a tense-sounding voice due to incorrect vocal technique. Phonation is probably associated with high laryngeal resistance forces, which explains why patients complain of "vocal fatigue" and discomfort at the end of a working day. In some situations the problem is triggered by an organic illness such as an upper respiratory infection, but persistent hoarseness remains many weeks after the viral illness has resolved. Koufman has used the term "habituated hoarseness" to note this relationship (10).

The lateral compression in the glottis is generally accompanied by incoordinate breathing such that the larynx functions more like a valve, controlling the rate of expiratory air flow. Proper breath control for speech entails the maintenance of a degree of inspiratory effort during exhalation so that a "push-pull" mechanism exists in the abdominal and thoracic areas to maintain steady flow of air in the trachea. In this situation, the larynx is not required to function as a flow regulator. When speech breathing is incoordinate there may be surges of uncontrolled expiratory air, which must then be valved by the glottis during phonation to allow for continued self-oscillation. An effortful and harsh voice results, with rapid fatigue. With ongoing compression, the voice pitch may drop, and vocal fry register may become prominent suggesting that there may be associated A-P constriction. The fatiguing voice may also be accompanied by general fatigue as well as discomfort or pain in the throat.

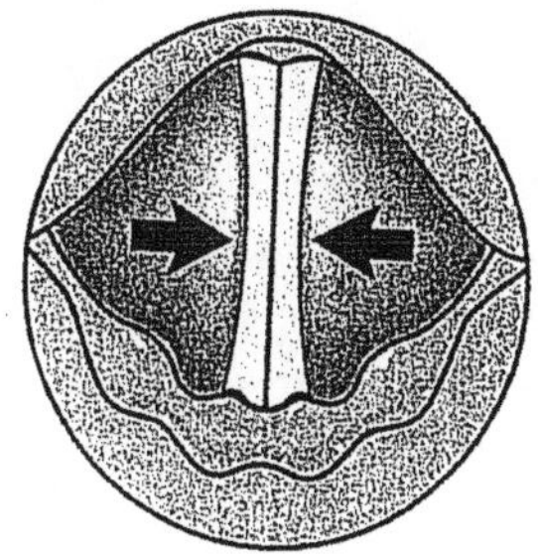

Fig. 2. Lateral hypercontraction at the glottic level. Frequently seen with generalized postural misuses and tension. May be triggered by an infection or chronic reflux.

Laryngoscopy with regular light will generally reveal normal looking structures, although erythema or diffuse thickening of the mucosa may be noted in addition to tight closure of the posterior glottis. Use of the stroboscope will show a prolonged closed phase, reduced vibratory amplitude and suppression of the mucosal wave. Ventricular fold adduction may be seen to a limited degree in association with the glottic level lateral contraction state. In this situation, it is important to differentiate between primary glottic level contraction and primary supra-glottic contraction because relegation of a patient to the supraglottic contraction category carries a much stronger inference of psychogenic etiology.

Subtype b: Supra-glottic adduction. This pattern tends to predominate in psychogenic dysphonia and can exist either with tightly adducted true vocal folds leading to a high-pitched squeaky voice, or with loose partially abducted vocal folds, in which case the voice is breathy or a tense whisper.

When the voice is strident or squeaky it may be difficult to identify whether the sound source is at the level of adducted ventricular folds, i.e. true false fold phonation, from obscured tightly adducted true folds below, or whether the true and false folds are functioning more as a valvular unit to create the voice. The latter two situations are likely more common since in most cases the ventricular bands do not adduct fully to the midline.

It has been our experience that the lateral supraglottic squeeze pattern seen on laryngoscopy in patients with a muscle misuse dysphonia is usually

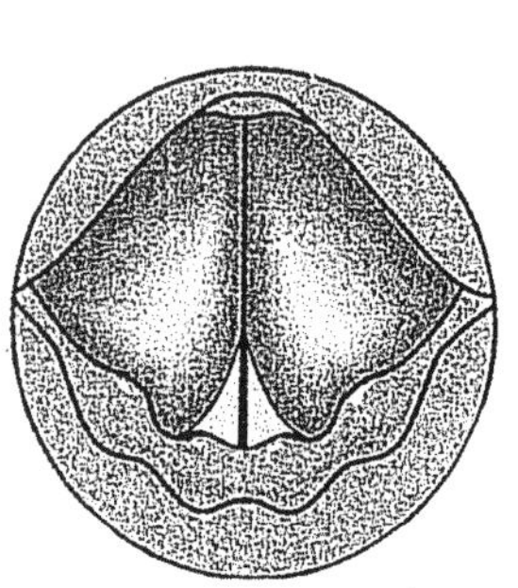

Fig. 3. Supra-glottic lateral contraction, or hyper-adduction of the false vocal folds. Tends to be strongly psychologically based.

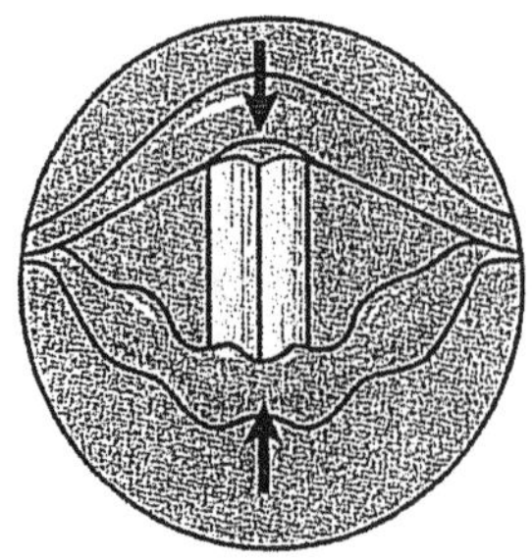

Fig. 4. Antero-posterior supra-glottic contraction. A common technical misuse seen in mild, moderate and severe forms.

associated with unresolved psychological conflict. Therapy approaches must combine correction of specific misuses with a careful evaluation and management of the psychological factors.

Type 3 – Anteroposterior contraction of the supraglottic larynx.

Koufman has presented a voice type labeled "Bogart-Bacall" syndrome (10) in which patients exhibit a tension-fatigue dysphonia with phonation at the very bottom of their vocal dynamic ranges. He describes a contraction pattern which results in reduced space between the epiglottis and the arytenoid prominances in the anteroposterior (AP) direction during phonation. Individuals using this posture complain of effortful voice and rapid fatigue when speaking at a low pitch but are able to talk more clearly and freely at a higher pitch.

This laryngoscopic pattern is not readily seen with mirror examination or with the rigid telescope because the tongue pull may extend the ary-epiglottic length. Transnasal examination during connected speech or song is the most effective way to demonstrate this misuse, which may then be subclassified as mild, moderate or severe.

Type 4. Conversion aphonia

The anxiety that leads to conversion hysteria has produced such mental pain that a physical symptom such as aphonia is much more bearable to the individual (4, 14). The type of psychological stressors and the resulting muscle misuse pattern differs from anxiety related tension misuses associated with type 2a described above. In conversion disorder the misuse may be beyond the awareness of the patient, hence the typical "la belle indifference" facial features. The vocal folds have full movement and can adduct normally for cough or other types of vegetative phonation such as laughter. But they stop short of sufficient adduction for voicing with an attempt to speak. Generalized hypertonicity can be identified in the larynx and when sound does come out it is usually high pitched, squeaky, or breathy.

Type 5. Psychogenic dysphonia with bowed vocal cords

In older patients, presbyphonia is associated with loss of muscular bulk and tone, as well as weakening and fragmentation of elastin and collagen fibres. This so-called "senile" atrophy is not necessarily the principal factor in patients who are seen to have the appearance of bowed vocal folds on indirect laryngoscopy. Occasionally, patients who appear to have a psychogenic functional dysphonia will present with a bowed glottis but may resume normal phonation and laryngoscopic appearance after voice and/or psychotherapy. This may also represent one of the forms of dysphonia in "habituated hoarseness" that follows an upper respiratory tract infection of other organic trigger.

Type 6. Adolescent transitional dysphonia

The normal adolescent voice change during puberty is often accompanied by pitch breaks, register breaks

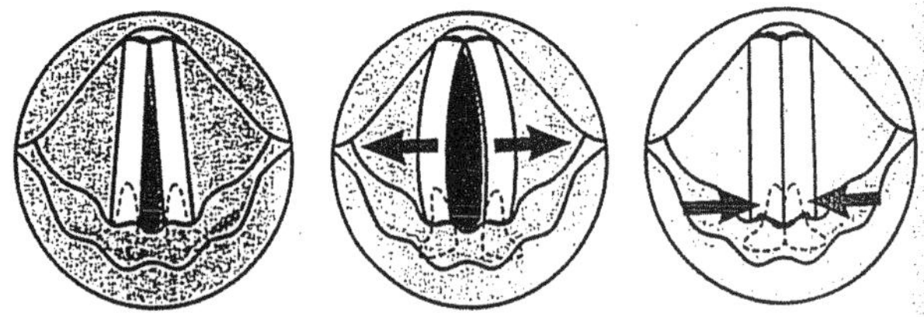

Fig. 5. Less common forms of misuse. (left) Conversion aphonia presents a normal larynx in which the vocal folds are held away from the midline during phonation but function well for other duties such as cough. (middle) Psychogenically based dysphonia is not always associated with hyperadduction, and bowing may be seen even when senile atrophy or sulcus vocalis have been excluded. (right) The voice disorder associated with difficulties making the transition from child to adult male is usually a perpetuated falsetto, and the tension in the posterior glottis is accompanied by a larynx that is held highly and tightly in the neck.

and a degree of embarrassment. Psychological factors may lead to inhibition of the transitional event and establishment of perpetual falsetto phonation. Laryngoscopy reveals a tense glottis and the cartilaginous glottis may be hyperadducted, restricting phonation to the anterior membranous vocal folds. The larynx is generally drawn up tightly into the hyoid bone or base of the tongue. Downward traction on the thyroid cartilages usually results in modal register phonation at a pitch that is more representative of the adult male voice.

DISENTANGLING MULTIPLE ETIOLOGIES IN VOICE DISORDERS

Notwithstanding the principal cause of muscular tension in voice disorders, the severity of the symptoms may fluctuate with changes in physiological shift factors including vocal technique, variable psychological stressors, and altered muscle tone related to chronic gastro-esophageal reflux disease. Figure 6 illustrates this interrelationship. The line represents the operant laryngeal muscle tone without taking into account the changes produced by the shift factors, i.e. due to dystonia or similar processes. This hypothetical trace of muscular tension has many individuals lined up along the abscissa, a point close to which represents normal tone. Since most people are normal this line conceptually extends a great distance to the left. At the far right the muscle tone is very high as it would be in a person suffering from a focal dystonia, and this degree of hypertonicity would produce consistent spasmodic dysphonia. The pathway from the low tension normal level towards the right side likely follows a typical exponential curve.

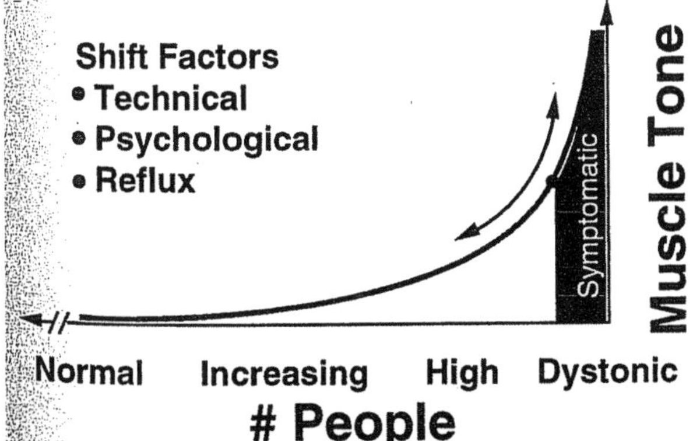

Fig. 6. Shift factors in dysphonia. After the baseline muscle tone, normal, dystonic or otherwise, has been set on the curve. The symptom severity can be shifted up or down by alterable factors including technique, psychological stressors, or reflux.

If a line is dropped from midway up the curve down to the abscissa we may assume that individuals on the right of this point will have muscular tension that will produce symptoms. But once a person's tension level has been set on the curve it can be shifted up or down (left or right) by a number of important alterable shift factors. If the central basal ganglia control and the laryngeal sensori-motor reflexes are relatively constant then the main clinically important shift factors are *i)* technical ability, *ii)* psychological tension, and *iii)* reflux. Each of these factors can be addressed in therapy, regardless of the classification category represented by a patients profile.

REFERENCES

1. Colton RH, Casper JK. Understanding voice problems. A physiological perspective for diagnosis and treatment. Baltimore: Williams and Wilkins, 1990.
2. Aronson AE. Clinical voice disorders: an interdisciplinary approach. 2nd ed. New York: Thieme Medical, 1985.
3. Brodnitz FS. Vocal rehabilitation. Am Acad Ophthal Otolaryngol Monograph. Rochester: Whiting, 1959.
4. Diagnostic and statistical manual of mental disorders, 3rd ed. Washington: American Psychiatric Association, 1987.
5. Froeschels E. Hygiene of the voice. Arch Otolaryngol 1943; 37: 122–30.
6. Jackson C. Myasthenia laryngis. Arch Otolaryngol 1940; 32: 434–63.
7. Greene MCL. The voice and its disorders. Philadelphia: J.B. Lippincott, 1972.
8. Morrison MD, Rammage LA, Belisle GM, Nichol H, Pullan B. Muscular tension dysphonia. J. Otolaryngol 1983; 12: 302–6.
9. Arnold GE. Disorders of laryngeal function. In: Paparella MM, Shumrich DA, eds. Otolaryngology. Vol. 3 Philadelphia: WP Saunders 1980; 2470–88.
10. Koufman JA, Blalock PD. Classification and approach to patients with functional voice disorders. Ann Atol Rhinol Laryngol 1982; 91:372–7.
11. Morrison MD, Nichol H, Rammage LA. Diagnostic criteria in functional dysphonia. Laryngoscope 1986; 96: 1–8.
12. Selye H. The stress of life. New York: McGraw-Hill, 1976.
13. Lazarus RS. Patterns of adjustment. New York: McGraw-Hill, 1976.
14. Rammage LA, Nichol H, Morrison MD. The psychopathology of voice disorders. Hum Commun Canada 1987; 11: 21–5.
15. Whatmore GB, Kohli DR. The physiopathology and treatment of functional disorders. New York: Grune & Stratton, 1974.
16. Jacobson E. Modern treatment of tense patients. Springfield: Charles C. Thomas, 1970.
17. Barlow W. The Alexander principle. London: Jutor Gollancy, 1973.

18. Malmgren L, Gacek R, Etzler C. Muscle fibre types in the human posteroir carcoarytenoid muscle: a correlated histochemical and ultrastructural morphometric study. In: Titze IR, Scherer RC, eds. Vocal fold physiology: biomechanics, acoustics and phonatory control. The Denver Centre for the Performing Arts, 1983: 41–56.
19. Belisle G, Morrison MD. Anatomic correlation for muscle tension dysphonia. J Otolaryngol 1983; 12: 319–21.
20. Rammage LA. Acoustic, aerodynamic and vibratory characteristics of phonation with variable posterior glottis postures. Doctoral dissertation, University of Wisconsin-Madison, 1992.
21. Rammage LA, Peppard RC, Bless, DM. Aerodynamic, laryngoscopic and perceptual-acoustic characteristics in dysphonic females with posterior glottal chinks: a retrospective study. J Voice 1989; 6: 64–78.
22. Milenkovic P, Bless DM, Rammage LA. Acoustic and perceptual characterization of vocal nodules. In: Gauffin J. Hammarberg B, eds. Vocal fold physiology: acoustic, perceptual, and physiological aspects of voice mechanisms. San Diego: Singular Press, 1991: 265–72.
23. Hirano M. Morphological structure of the vocal cord as a vibrator and its variations. Folia Phoniatr 1974; 26: 89–94.
24. Peppard RC. Effects of selected vocal characteristics of female singers and non-singers. Doctoral dissertation, University of Wisconsin-Madison, 1990.

Address for correspondence:
M. D. Morrison
4th floor Willow Pavilion
855 West 12th Ave.
Vancouver B.C.
Canada V5Z 1M9

Commentary

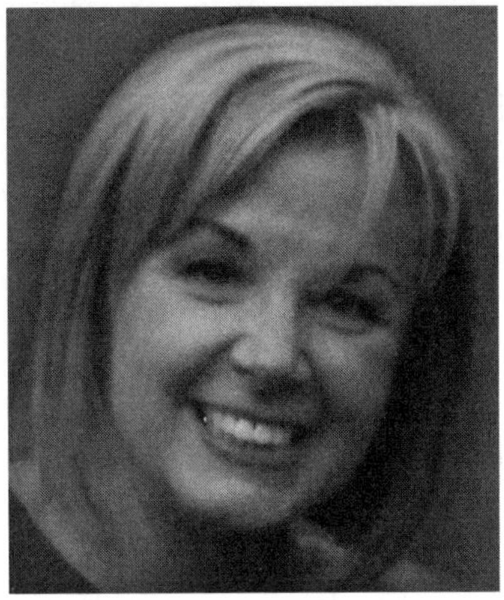

Lorraine O. Ramig, PhD

The LSVT Story

Nearly 90% of the 6 million individuals with Parkinson disease (PD) worldwide have a speech or voice disorder. Neuropharmacologic and neurosurgical treatments for PD, do not make a positive or lasting impact on speech in PD at this time.[1] Given recent neuroscience breakthroughs,[2–3] there are great opportunities in rehabilitation today for speech treatment to be a routine, integral part of disease management in PD. Efficacious speech treatment offers the opportunity to improve quality of life in individuals with PD beyond what neurosurgical and neuropharmacologic treatments offer.

Today LSVT® (Lee Silverman Voice Treatment) is the speech and voice treatment for PD with Level 1 evidence[3–6] and it is being delivered by speech clinicians in over 50 countries around the world. The LSVT differs from previous forms of speech treatment for PD in both the treatment *target* and the *mode* of treatment delivery. The fundamental principles of LSVT are based on the pathological mechanisms hypothesized to underlie voice and speech disorders in people with PD[7]: (1) an overall amplitude scale down of speech motor output (reduced amplitude of neural drive to the muscles of the speech mechanism) that may result in reduced vocal loudness (hypophonia), reduced pitch inflection (hypoprosodia) and reduced range of articulatory movements (hypokinetic articulation),[8–10] and (2) problems in sensory perception of vocal effort and speech movements that prevent a person with PD from accurately regulating (internal cueing/scaling) the optimal amount of effort to produce adequate loudness.[11,12]

LSVT targets amplitude training (increased vocal loudness) as a single motor control parameter. It incorporates: (1) enhancing the voice source, which is consistent with improving the carrier in the classic engineering concept of signal transmission,[13] (2) using vocal loudness as a trigger for distributed system-wide effects across the speech production system; (3) recalibration of vocal loudness and effort so individuals with PD integrate improved loudness into functional communication; and (4) training the individual to rely on his own resources (internal cueing and self-monitoring) to independently control and sustain adequately scaled speech motor output. The result is reduction or elimination of hypophonia, hypoprosodia, and hypokinetic articulation characteristics of the dysarthria associated with PD.[14]

It is critical to recognize that the loudness target in LSVT is a healthy increase in vocal loudness. Patients are not trained to yell or scream or to use pressed voice, rather the speech clinician trains a voice that has improved loudness with healthy voice quality.

On the surface, the simplicity of a single, simple overlearned treatment target for patients "be LOUD" may make it feasible for these individuals with cognitive and learning challenges to successfully improve functional speech production in daily living.[7] Beneath the surface simplicity of the target "be LOUD," the speech clinician is delivering a well-integrated training program that is designed to directly address the complexity underlying the speech problem experienced by patients with PD.[14]

The *mode* of delivery of LSVT also differs from traditional forms of speech treatment. It requires intensive, high-effort speech exercise combined with a simple, redundant, and salient treatment target to facilitate transfer of loudness into functional daily living. The standardized protocol for LSVT embodies many of the fundamental principles of exercise and motor training that have been shown to promote neural plasticity and brain reorganization in animal models of PD.[2] and human stroke-related hemiparesis.[15] Our ability to embrace these principles and integrate them into the mode of delivery of treatment will be essential for advancing rehabilitation science in parallel with neuroscience. Although the standardized protocol for LSVT was developed before these recent neuroscience investigations, it adheres to key principles of neural plasticity (*intensity, complexity, saliency, use it or lose it, and use it and improve it*) which are likely additional explanations for why LSVT has been successful.[16,17]

What Is the Story of LVT? How Did We Get to Where We Are Today?

In 1983, Dr. Wilbur Gould walked into the acoustics lab at the Recording and Research Center of the Denver Center for the Performing Arts and said to me, "Lori, I have a friend who has a Parkinson disease (PD) treatment program and he needs a speech therapist, can you help him?" At the time, I was an Assistant Professor on a tenure track in the Department of Speech, Language and Hearing Science at the University of Colorado-Boulder and the Recording and Research Center in Denver was my primary research lab. I was working diligently to develop a fundable research program which would allow me to study "my current passion": acoustic analysis of voice in aged individuals and those with neurological diseases.

Of course, I followed Dr. Gould's advice and met his friend in Estes Park, Colorado at the location of his PD treatment program. It was here that I had my very first encounter with individuals with PD. Shortly thereafter, during one of my monthly trips to Estes Park, I was introduced to a group of professionals who were developing a PD treatment program in Scottsdale, Arizona. They invited me to visit Scottsdale and to meet the family who was initiating the program in honor of their wife and mother, Mrs. Lee Silverman, who had been diagnosed with PD.

"If only we could hear and understand her" wished Mr. Ray Silverman and his adult children Tom and Carol regarding Mrs. Silverman, when I first met them in Scottsdale. At the time, speech treatment for patients with PD was considered to be unsuccessful. The consensus among the professional communities was "changes in the speech treatment disappear on the way to the parking lot" and while nearly 90% of patients with PD had a speech problem, only 4% received speech treatment.

The Silverman family found their inability to communicate with Mrs. Silverman most difficult. They challenged me to develop a speech treatment to help their mother communicate and invited me to set up a speech treatment program at their newly evolving "Lee Silverman Center for Parkinsons" in Scottsdale. The Lee Silverman Center program was designed to be a month long, daily multidisciplinary program to include medical care, physical therapy, occupational therapy, speech therapy, family support, nutrition, and recreation.

Because the Silverman family was particularly concerned about speech in PD, they agreed to my request to fund a speech research lab within the clinical facility and hired a student of mine (Carolyn Mead Bonitati), a recent graduate of the University of Colorado-Boulder, to be the speech clinician in residence. My role was to design the speech treatment program and collect and analyze once a month pre-, post-, and follow-up speech treatment data.

In 1985, the seeds were sown for what is known today as LSVT. At the time, most speech treatment approaches for PD focused on the classic articulation and rate problems in these patients. However, because I came from the world of voice, my instinct was to treat the voice disorder which included soft volume, monotone, hoarseness, and breathiness. We developed a physiologically based treatment program that we thought (naively at the time) focused primarily on laryngeal function. Our target was vocal fold adduction as an avenue to improve vocal loudness and quality. To motivate patients, we designed the treatment to be a high-effort exercise program that combined voice exercises and generalization in to speech production. The treatment was designed to continuously push patients to new vocal effort levels (eg, "louder, longer"). As a result, patients were highly engaged in physical exercise of their voices for 60 minutes a day within treatment sessions and had daily assignments to use their newly trained louder voice outside of the treatment room. As a part of the Lee Silverman multidisciplinary program, the treatment was delivered at an intense dosage of 4 to 5 hours a week. High-effort physical exercise and intense dosage of delivery remain fundamental elements of what is known as LSVT today.

Our initial approach to speech treatment focused on the motor symptoms underlying the disordered voice in these individuals with PD. However, very soon into the delivery of treatment, we noticed the significant sensory problems that challenged these patients. Soft talking individuals with PD would deny that they were too soft, but claim "my spouse needs a hearing aid." When they were stimulated to increase loudness to a normal level, they would complain, "I feel like I am shouting." Thus, we enhanced the treatment to address these sensory problems. We referred to these sensory retraining activities as "calibration." Today, we recognize that this sensory mismatch together with deficits in internal cueing are two of the most challenging aspects of successfully treating speech in people with PD.

In 1985–1986, I was traveling to Scottsdale once a month clinically evaluating the speech and voice in these patients as well as gathering outcome data. I found the Parkinson treatment work extremely satisfying but I was becoming concerned about the time that I was spending on this project in relation to my goal of establishing a fundable research program in my tenure track position. One day I was discussing this with Ron Scherer, a voice scientist at the Recording and Research Center. I got a significant piece of advice from Ron, "Lori, make the treatment your research!" A light bulb went on and I took this advice to heart!

At that time, speech treatment research was in its infancy. Our field was unaware of the paradigms for scientifically documenting behavioral treatment effects that are well-known today.[18] In 1988, we presented our first treatment outcome research paper (which would today be considered Phase 1 work) and first videotape of two individuals with PD pre to post-treatment to a group of expert researchers and clinicians at the Motor Speech conference in San Diego and received "mixed reviews." One of the pillars in our field said to me, "Well, Lori, you may have stumbled on to something" and another pillar said, "You have clearly measured all the wrong variables." When our idea of intensively teaching patients with PD to increase vocal loudness reached the professional voice community, they universally were certain that we would provoke an outbreak of vocal hyperfunction in the PD community. We, however, remained extremely interested in what we were seeing clinically and our next step was to study it scientifically.

Our first federal research grant was awarded in 1989 by the National Institute of Disability and Rehabilitative Research (NIDRR), followed soon after in 1990 by our first R01 from the National Institutes of Health, National Institutes of Deafness and other Communicative Disorders (NIH-NIDCD). This year, 2007, we were fortunate enough to be awarded our fourth R01 from NIH-NIDCD to continue our studies until the year 2012.

The Recording and Research Center (known from 1994-2000 as the Wilbur James Gould Voice Research Center) and since 2000 as the National Center for Voice and Speech (NCVS) became the home for these studies. New team members were added including speech clinicians Stefanie Countryman and Annette Pawlas as well as otolaryngologist Marshall Smith. Between 1994 and 1995 we collected data at the University of Arizona-Tucson and added Cynthia Fox to the team. Jennifer Spielman (a University of Colorado graduate student at the time) began working with us as well. Shortly thereafter we added speech clinician, Angela Halpern and later speech clinician, Jill Petska. We learned very quickly the value of a team that combines scientific knowledge and passion with 'real world' delivery of treatment and clinical knowledge. Today, we view the ability to span this 'clinical to science' continuum as an essential element in the world of treatment research. Over the years, we have observed consistently that "treatment outcomes can guide basic understanding of neurological condition."

We designed two randomized control trials (RCT), one to study the efficacy of intensive respiratory treatment compared to intensive respiratory and laryngeal treatment and another to evaluate treatment outcomes with an untreated PD and healthy age-matched control groups. We wanted to address three questions: (1) which treatment (respiratory or respiratory and laryngeal) would make the biggest impact in patients with Parkinson disease; (2) would treatment effects be lasting; and (3) what physiologic changes accompany successful treatment. Some of the outcomes of our work have been included in this volume:

Ramig L, Sapir S, Countryman S, et al. Intensive voice treatment (LSVT) for individuals with

Parkinson disease: a two-year follow-up. *J. Neurol Neurosurg Psychiatry.* 2001;71:493–498.

Smith M, Ramig L, Dromey C, Perez K, Samandari R. Intensive voice treatment in Parkinson's disease: laryngostroboscopic findings. *J. Voice.* 1995;9:453–459.

Of particular interest were the videostroboscopic data documenting for the first time the physiologic basis for improved vocal loudness in PD following what was then known as respiratory and laryngeal treatment compared to respiratory treatment alone. We concluded after this series of studies that respiratory and laryngeal treatment had more consistent, significant, and lasting effects on speech production in individuals with PD in the short and long-term than did respiratory treatment alone.

The data published in 2001[19] reported on patients followed for 2 years after 1 month of treatment and have been considered the first Level 1 evidence for a speech treatment for PD.[20] The second RCT[21] reported that respiratory and laryngeal treatment resulted in significant increases in SPL post-treatment and at 6 months follow-up when compared with pretreatment levels. No significant changes were observed over the same period in an untreated PD control group and untreated age-matched healthy control group.

By this time, the Lee Silverman Center for Parkinsons no longer existed. Nevertheless, I asked Mr. Silverman's permission to name the speech treatment in honor of Mrs. Silverman, who by that time had passed away. From that point on the "respiratory and laryngeal" treatment has been known as the Lee Silverman Voice Treatment or LSVT, in honor of Mrs. Silverman.

In 1995 our team wanted to address the underlying mechanism of the laryngeal disorder in PD as well as the neural bases of treatment-related change. We began our collaboration with physiologists Erich Luschei, Shimon Sapir and Kristin Larson Baker as well as the University of Texas San Antonio imaging Center and the group lead by Peter Fox, MD. The outcomes of those studies are been summarized in these publications:

Baker K, Ramig L, Luschei E, Smith, M. Thyroarytenoid muscle activity associated with hypophonia in Parkinson disease and aging. *Neurology.* 1998;51(6):1592–1598.

Luschei E, Ramig L, Baker K, Smith M. Discharge characteristics of laryngeal single motor units during phonation in young and older adults and individuals with Parkinson disease. *J. Neurophysiology.* 1999;81:2131–2139.

Liotti M, Vogel D, Ramig L, New P, et al. Hypophonia in Parkinson disease: neural correlates of voice treatment revealed by PET. *Neurology.* 2003;60:432–440.

Our physiologic findings supported the idea of reduced amplitude in laryngeal muscles of individuals with PD pretreatment when compared with a healthy aged-matched control group and were consistent with our treatment goal of scaling up amplitude to the speech mechanism. Of particular interest were the neural imaging findings. Preliminary studies of PET related changes pre- and post-LSVT documented treatment-dependent functional reorganization in people with PD. These findings included recruitment of the right hemisphere, and activation of central sensorimotor regions in the left hemisphere, such as the thalamus and pre-supplementary motor area.[22] These were the first data to identify the neural bases of treatment-related change following LSVT. A second study[23] has confirmed these findings.

In 1998, I went on a sabbatical to New York City to spend time in the medical world of neurolaryngology. I was based at Mt. Sinai Medical Center and Columbia University. This experience opened my eyes to a bigger world of medical neurology. The perspectives I gained through working with Mitchell Brin, Andy Blitzer, Ira Sanders, and Don Wiesz among others helped us develop new ways of thinking about fundamentals of LSVT at peripheral as well as central levels. It was during this time that I met neuropsychologists Chris Morrison and Joan Borod. Chris helped us understand the value of the simple, redundant nature of LSVT as a feasible way for individuals with Parkinson disease with neuropsychological challenges to actually learn a new behavior.[7] Joan's insight in to facial analysis helped motivate our documentation of the effects of LSVT that went well beyond the larynx.

Although our initial treatment focus was to target vocal loudness through laryngeal function, by 2000 it had become increasingly clear from our research and ongoing clinical experiences, that loudness training, was making a significant impact across the speech production mechanism to positively affect articulation and facial expression as well. In fact, we have now generated pilot data that LSVT effects generalize beyond vocal loudness to make a positive impact on swallowing, articulation, communicative gestures, facial expression, and neural functioning.[14,22,24–26]

Today, we are actively conducting randomized controlled trials (RCT) and are further examining this transfer of effects by (1) evaluating and comparing the system-wide generalized impact of two therapies (voice [LSVT-LOUD] and articulation [LSVT-ENUNCIATE]) on speech articulation, facial expression, swallowing in PD, and the system-wide generalized impact of these two therapies on limb gesture and limb motor functioning in PD. Functional imaging investigations (PET) of these two treatments will be used to identify changes in neural connectivity and functioning and identify any differences associated with these different treatment targets. Results from these studies will further clarify the neural bases for voice and speech disorders in people with PD as well as guide development and modifications for optimal speech treatment approaches for this population. We hypothesize that LSVT LOUD will recruit a wider network of brain regions than is normally seen during speech production, including enhanced basal ganglia function, phylogenetically old brain regions (including the insula and anterior cingulate gyrus) and right (nondominant) hemisphere regions associated with amplitude scaling, emotive vocalization and prosody. In contrast, we hypothesize that LSVT ENUNCIATE will recruit premotor (chiefly of the left [dominant] hemisphere) and primary motor (M1) regions chiefly of the left (dominant) hemisphere in a pattern typical of normal speech production, and will not demonstrate recruitment of nonmotor regions or right-hemispheric regions which are hypothesized for LSVT LOUD. We speculate that these changes will be associated with differential changes in behavior. We are fortunate to have a core team that includes researchers in speech treatment, physiology, swallowing, facial expression, communicative gesture, neuropsychology, neurology and otolaryngology to help us address these issues.

LSVT has evolved over the years through the wisdom of colleagues and collaborators who have enlightened our vision from a laryngeal loudness focus, to address sensory and neuropsychological elements of treatment and to today embrace the realities of neural plasticity. As we learn more, our perspectives on LSVT are further enhanced. Our ongoing research is addressing a range of topics including application of LSVT beyond PD to other adult and pediatric neurological conditions (eg, multiple sclerosis, ataxia, cerebral palsy, and stroke),[27–30] the application of principles of LSVT to physical therapy in PD (LSVT BIG),[31] the hybrid treatment of combined LSVT BIG and LOUD,[32] development of an animal model to evaluate the potential neuroprotective effects of physical and voice exercise,[33] and use of technology to make delivery of intensive treatment dosage feasible globally.[34]

The potential of speech treatment to make an important impact on quality of life in individuals with Parkinson disease and other neurological disorders, while providing insight into the neural bases of these disorders and the underlying mechanism of treatment-related change, is a world that continues to offer humbling challenges and great satisfaction. We continue to be motivated to address this request for patients around the world:

> "if only we could hear and understand her."—family of Mrs. Lee Silverman

Funding Acknowledgments and Disclosures

Dr. Ramig is a Professor at the University of Colorado-Boulder, a Senior Scientist at the National Center for Voice and Speech (Denver), and an Adjunct Professor, Columbia University, New York City. The research reported in this article has been supported in part by funding from NIH-NIDCD R01 DC001150, NIH-NIDCD R21 DC 05583, and NIH-NINDS R21 NS043711.

Dr. Ramig receives a lecturer and travel honorarium from the LSVT Foundation (non-profit organization), a consulting honorarium from the Kinetics Foundation (non-profit organization), receives a lecture honorarium and has intellectual property rights and ownership interest in LSVT Global LLC (for-profit organization that delivers training courses and sells products related to LSVT).

References

1. Schulz GM, Grant MK. Effects of speech therapy and pharmacologic and surgical treatments on voice and speech in Parkinson' disease: a review of the literature. *J Commun Disord.* 2000;33:69–88.
2. Fisher B, Petzinger G, Nixon K, et al. Exercise-induced behavioral recovery and neuroplasticity in the 1-methyl-4-phenyl-1,2,3,6-tetrahydropyridine-lesioned mouse basal ganglia. *J Neurosci Res.* 2004;77:378–390.
3. Tillerson J, Cohen A, Philhower J, Miller G, Zigmond M, Schallert T. Forced limb-use effects on the behavioral

and neurochemical effects of 6-hydroxydopamine. *J Neurosci.* 2001;21(12):4427–4435.

4. Pinto S, Ozsancak C, Tripoliti E, et al. Treatments for dysarthria in Parkinson's disease, *Lancet.* 2004;3:547–556.
5. Trail M, Fox C, Ramig L, Sapir S, Howard J, Lai E. Speech treatment for people with Parkinson's disease. *Neurorehabilitation.* 2005;20:205–221.
6. Yorkston KM, Spencer KA, Duffy JR. Behavioral management of respiratory/phonatory dysfunction from dysarthria: a systematic review of the evidence. *J Med Speech-Lang Pathol.* 2003;11:xiii–xxxviii.
7. Fox CM, Morrison CE, Ramig LO, Sapir S. Current perspectives on the Lee Silverman Voice Treatment (LSVT) for people with idiopathic Parkinson's disease. *Am J Speech Lang Pathol.* 2002;11:111–123.
8. Albin RL, Young AB, Penny JB. The functional anatomy of basal ganglia disorders. *Trends Neurosci.* 1989:12:366–375.
9. Penny JB, Young AB. Speculations on the functional anatomy of basal ganglia disorders, *Ann Rev Neurosci.* 1983;6,73–94.
10. Barbeau A, Sourkes TL, Murphy CF. Les Catecholamines de la Maladie de Parkinson's. In Ajuriaguerra J, ed. *Monoamines et Systeme Nerveux Central.* Geneve, Switzerland: George; 1962:247–262.
11. Demirci M, Grill S, McShane L, Hallet M. Impairment of kinesthesia in Parkinson's disease. *Neurology.* 1995;45:A218.
12. Stelmach GE (1991). Basal ganglia impairment and force control. In Requin E, Stelmach GE, eds. *Tutorial in Motor Neuroscience.* Netherlands: Kluwer Academic Publishers; 2001:147–158.
13. Sapir S, Ramig L, Fox, C. Voice, speech and swallowing disorders. In Factor S, Weiner, W, eds. *Parkinson's Disease: Diagnosis and Clinical Management.* New York, NY: Demos; 2008:77–97.
14. Sapir S, Spielman J, Ramig L, Story B, Fox C. Effects of intensive voice treatment (LSVT®) on vowel articulation in dysarthric individuals with idiopathic Parkinson's disease: acoustic and perceptual findings. *J Speech Lang Hear Res.* 2007;50:899–912.
15. Liepert J, Miltner W, Bauder H, et al. Motor cortex plasticity during constraint-induced movement therapy in stroke patients. *Neurosci Lett.* 1998;250:5–8.
16. Fox C, Ramig L, Ciucci M, Sapir S, McFarland D, Farley B. The science and practice of LSVT® LOUD: neural plasticity-prinicpled approach to treating individuals with Parkinson disease and other neurological disorders. *Sem Speech Lang.* 2006;27:283–299.
17. Farley BG, Fox CM, Ramig LO, McFarland DA. Intensive amplitude-specific therapeutic approaches for Parkinson's disease: toward a neuroplasticity-principled rehabilitation model. *Topics Gerontol Rehab.* 2008;24(2): 92–114.
18. Robey RR, Schultz MC. A model for conducting clinical outcome research: an adaption of the standard protocol for use in aphasiology. *Aphasiology.* 1998;12: 787–810.
19. Ramig L, Sapir S, Countryman S, et al. Intensive voice treatment (LSVT) for individuals with Parkinson disease: a two-year follow-up. *J Neurol Neurosurg Psychiatr.* 2001;7:493–498.
20. Goetz CG. Movement disorders: understanding clinical trials. *Lancet Neurol.* 2005;4(1):5–6.
21. Ramig LO, Sapir S, Fox C, Countryman S. Changes in vocal loudness following intensive voice treatment (LSVT) in individuals with Parkinson's disease: a comparison with untreated patients and normal age-matched controls. *Movement Disord.* 2001;16:79–83.
22. Liotti M, Ramig LO, Vogel D, et al. Hypophonia in Parkinson's disease. Neural correlates of voice treatment revealed by PET. *Neurology,* 2003;60:432–440.
23. Narayana S, Vogel D, Brown S, et al. *Mechanism of action of voice therapy in Parkinson's hypophonia—A PET study.* Poster presented at the 11th Annual Meeting of the Organization for Human Brain Mapping; Toronto, Ontario, Canada; 2005.
24. Duncan S. *Preliminary data on effects of behavioral and levadopa therapies on speech-accompanying gesture in Parkinson's disease.* Presentation at the ICSLP meeting; Denver, Colo; Sept 2002.
25. El Sharkawi A, Ramig LO, Logemann JA, et al. Swallowing and voice effects of Lee Silverman Voice Treatment (LSVT®): a pilot study. *J Neurol Neurosurg Psychiatr.* 2002;71:31–36.
26. Spielman JL, Borod JC, Ramig LO. The effects of intensive voice treatment on facial expression in Parkinson's disease: preliminary data. *Cogn Behav Neurol.* 2003; 16(3):177–188.
27. Sapir S, Spielman J, Countryman S, et al. Phonatory and articulatory changes in ataxic dysarthria following intensive voice therapy with LSVT®: a single subject study. *Am J Speech Lang Pathol.* 2003;12:387–399.
28. Sapir S, Pawlas A, Ramig L, Seeley E, Fox C, Corboy J. Effects of intensive phonatory-respiratory treatment (LSVT®) on voice in two individuals with multiple sclerosis. *J. Speech Lang Pathol.* 2001;9(2):35–45.
29. Fox C, Boliek C, Ramig L. The impact of intensive voice treatment (LSVT) on speech intelligibility in children with spastic cerebral palsy. *Movement Disord.* 2005;20(10):S149.
30. Mahler L. *The effects of intensive voice therapy (LSVT) on motor speech disorder secondary to stroke.* Unpublished dissertation; University of Colorado; 2007.
31. Farley BM, Koshland G. Training BIG to move faster: the application of the speed-amplitude relation as a rehabilitation strategy for people with Parkinson disease. *Exp Brain Res.* 2005;167(3):462–467.

32. Farley B, Fox C, Ramig L, McFarland D. Intensive amplitude-specific therapeutic approaches for Parkinson disease: toward a neuroplasticity-principled rehabilitation model. *Topics Geriatr Rehab.* In press.
33. Ciucci MR, Ma TS, Fox CM, et al. Qualitative changes in ultrasonic vocalization in rats after unilateral dopamine depletion or haloperidol: a preliminary study. *Behav Brain Res.* 2007;182:284–289.
34. Halpern A, Matos C, Ramig L, Petska J, Spielman J, Bennett J. *LSVTC—A PDA supported speech treatment for Parkinson's disease.* Presented at the 9th International Congress of Parkinson's Disease and Movement Disorders; New Orleans, La; 2005.

Comparison of Two Forms of Intensive Speech Treatment for Parkinson Disease

Lorraine Olson Ramig
Department of Communication Disorders and Speech Science University of Colorado-Boulder and The Wilbur James Gould Voice Research Center Denver Center For The Performing Arts

Stefanie Countryman
The Wilbur James Gould Voice Research Center Denver Center For The Performing Arts

Laetitia L. Thompson
Neuropsychology Laboratory University of Colorado School of Medicine

Yoshiyuki Horii
Department of Communication Disorders and Speech Science University of Colorado-Boulder and The Wilbur James Gould Voice Research Center Denver Center For The Performing Arts

This study investigated the effect of two forms of intensive speech treatment, (a) respiration (R) and (b) voice and respiration (Lee Silverman Voice Treatment [LSVT]), on the speech and voice deficits associated with Idiopathic Parkinson disease. Forty-five subjects with Idiopathic Parkinson disease completed extensive pretreatment neurological, otolaryngological, neuropsychological, and speech assessments. All subjects completed 16 sessions of intensive speech treatment, 4 times a week for 1 month. Pre- and post-treatment measures included intensity and maximum duration during sustained vowel phonation. Intensity, habitual fundamental frequency, fundamental frequency variability, and utterance and pause duration were measured during reading of the "Rainbow Passage" and conversational monologue as well. Family and subject self-ratings were completed pre- and post-treatment for the perceptual variables loudness, monotonicity, hoarseness, overall intelligibility, and initiation of conversation. Significant pre- to post-treatment improvements were observed for more variables and were of greater magnitude for the subjects who received the voice and respiration treatment (LSVT). Only subjects who received the LSVT rated a significant decrease post-treatment on the impact of Parkinson disease on their communication. Correlations between descriptive prognostic variables (i.e., stage of disease, speech/voice severity rating, depression, and time since diagnosis) and magnitude of treatment-related change indicated these factors did not significantly predict treatment effectiveness. These findings suggest that intensive voice and respiration (LSVT) treatment, focusing on increased vocal fold adduction and respiration, is more effective than respiration (R) treatment alone for improving vocal intensity and decreasing the impact of Parkinson disease on communication.

KEY WORDS: voice treatment, speech treatment, efficacy, Parkinson disease, intensity

Parkinson disease is a progressive, degenerative neurological disease resulting from nigrostriatal dopamine deficiency (Hornykiewicz, 1966; Hornykiewicz & Kish, 1986). At least 75% of the 1.5 million patients with Parkinson disease have a speech disorder that may limit their ability to function fully in society (Canter, 1965; Hoberman, 1958; Logemann, Fisher, Boshes, & Blonsky, 1978; Oxtoby, 1982; Streifler & Hofman, 1984). The perceptual characteristics of disordered speech and voice in Parkinson disease include reduced loudness, monopitch, monoloudness, imprecise articulation, and disordered rate (Darley, Aronson, & Brown, 1969a, 1969b; Logemann et al., 1978). Traditionally, speech treatment for Parkinson disease has met with limited success (Allan, 1970; Aronson, 1985; Greene, 1980; Sarno, 1968; Weiner & Singer, 1989). Consequently, many Parkinson disease patients do not receive speech treatment (Mutch, Strudwick, Roy, & Downie, 1986; Oxtoby, 1982) and their speech deteriorates as their disease progresses (Logemann et al., 1978; Morley, 1955).

Recently, Ramig and colleagues (Countryman & Ramig, 1993; Countryman, Ramig, & Pawlas, 1994; Ramig, 1995; Ramig, Bonitati, Lemke, & Horii, 1994; Ramig,

Horii, & Bonitati, 1991; Ramig et al., 1988) have reported positive findings following a voice treatment program for Parkinson disease (The Lee Silverman Voice Treatment [LSVT]) that focuses on increasing vocal loudness by increasing phonatory effort. Subjects have been trained to increase vocal fold adduction in maximum phonatory effort tasks and generalize the increased vocal effort to louder speech. Significant increases in maximum duration sustained vowel phonation, maximum fundamental frequency range, habitual fundamental frequency, and fundamental frequency variability in speech have also been documented following this intensive voice treatment (Ramig et al., 1994). Perceptual reports supported corresponding post-treatment increases in vocal loudness and improvements in speech intelligibility and functional communication (Ramig, 1992). The rationale for the Lee Silverman Voice Treatment is summarized in Table 1.

Reduced vocal loudness observed in Parkinson disease has been associated with limited respiratory support (Canter, 1965; Critchley, 1981) as well as reduced vocal fold adduction (Hanson et al., 1984; Smith, Ramig, Dromey, Perez, & Samandari, in press; Perez, Ramig, Smith, & Dromey, in press). Treatment directed toward increasing vocal loudness is dependent upon improving the function of one or both of these systems (Dromey, Ramig, & Johnson, 1995; Ramig, Dromey, Johnson, & Scherer, 1994; Ramig, Fazoli, Scherer, & Bonitati, 1990; Titze & Sundberg, 1992). Although initial studies (Countryman & Ramig, 1993; Ramig, 1992, 1995; Ramig et al., 1988; Ramig et al., 1991; Ramig et al., 1994) have identified phonatory effort and increased loudness (intensity) as key elements in efficacious treatment for Parkinson disease patients, studies have not compared the contributions of the respiratory and laryngeal systems to treatment-related change in intensity.

The interaction of the respiratory and laryngeal systems for control of intensity has been well described in nondisordered speakers (Stathopoulos & Sapienza, 1993a, 1993b). Increases in intensity have been associated with increased subglottal air pressure (Holmberg, Hillman, & Perkell, 1988; Isshiki, 1964) and vocal fold adduction (Colton, 1984; Titze & Sundberg, 1992). Given the significant role of the respiratory system in controlling subglottal air pressure (Hixon, Goldman, & Mead, 1973; Hixon, Mead, & Goldman, 1976; Stathopoulos & Sapienza, 1993a), speech treatment that is designed to improve inspiratory and expiratory respiratory muscle activity should contribute to increased subglottal air pressure and vocal intensity in patients with Parkinson disease. However, given the glottal incompetence frequently observed in patients with Parkinson disease, it is likely that treatment designed to increase vocal fold adduction also would be necessary to generate optimum gains in intensity. For example, Berke et al. (1990) concluded that increasing intensity (in an in vivo canine model) by medial adductory compression was more efficient than by increasing air flow. They reported that increasing air flow alone produced a significantly greater open quotient and vocal fold vibratory excursion. Clarification of the interactive roles of the respiratory and laryngeal systems in treatment-related change will contribute to enhancing the effectiveness of treatment for patients with Parkinson disease.

Identification of patient suitability or prognostic factors for treatment success is another issue of importance in studies of speech treatment efficacy. Previous research has not considered characteristics of Parkinson disease patients such as age, sex, stage of disease, time since diagnosis, and severity of speech disorder in relation to the efficacy of intensive speech treatment. In addition, depression and dementia (cognitive ability or functioning), which are frequently observed in Parkinson disease (Duvoisin, 1984; Gauthier, Dalziel, & Gauthier, 1987; Mayeux, Williams, Stern, & Cote, 1986) and associated with performance limitations (Beatty et al. 1989; Cummings, 1986), should be considered for their potential impact on treatment-related change. Although preliminary work (Mead, Ramig, & Beck, 1989) suggested that moderate dementia is not a limiting factor for speech treatment success, neither cognitive status nor depression has been considered systematically for its impact on the efficacy of speech treatment in Parkinson disease. Clarification of the prognostic role of certain patient characteristics will contribute to maximizing treatment effectiveness.

This study was designed to evaluate the speech and voice characteristics of patients with Parkinson disease following one of two forms of intensive treatment: (a) treatment designed to increase respiratory support for speech (R); and (b) treatment designed to increase vocal fold adduction and respiratory support (LSVT). Pre- to post-treatment changes

TABLE 1. Logic for development and rationale for treatment goals and tasks for the Lee Silverman Voice Treatment.

Perceptual characteristics of speech	Hypothesized laryngeal and/or respiratory physical pathology	Treatment goals and tasks
Reduced loudness	Reduced vocal fold adduction e.g., bowed vocal folds	• Increase vocal fold adduction via isometric effort (pushing, lifting) during phonation • Increase maximum duration vowel phonation at greater vocal intensity
Breathy, weak voice	Reduced respiratory support	• "Think loud/shout"
Hoarseness	Rigidity, hypokinesia, in laryngeal and/or respiratory muscles	• Improve vocal quality during sustained phonation and speaking
Monotone	Rigid cricothyroid muscle	• Increase maximum fundamental frequency range • High/low pitch glides • Sustained phonation at highest and lowest pitches

in intensity and duration characteristics were measured during sustained vowel phonation. Intensity, habitual fundamental frequency and fundamental frequency variability, and utterance and pause duration were measured during reading and conversational speech as well. Utterance and pause duration measurements were included as a secondary measurement of respiration and rate. It was assumed that treatment-related changes in inspiration and expiration would influence these measures because of the relationship previously reported between these respiratory gestures and speech rate (Bellaire, Yorkston, & Beukelman, 1986; Crystal, 1969).

This study was also designed to document treatment-related changes in relation to subject characteristics including: age, sex, stage of disease, time since diagnosis, severity of speech/voice deficits, glottal incompetence, depression, and cognitive functioning.

Method

Subjects

Forty-five patients with idiopathic Parkinson disease volunteered to participate in this study. All subjects were residents of the Denver, Colorado, area. All subjects participated in baseline pretreatment neurological, neuropsychological, otolaryngological, and speech assessments. Subjects were stratified on the variables age, sex, and stage of Parkinson disease (Hoehn & Yahr, 1967), score on the motor examination section (section III) of the Unified Parkinson's Disease Rating Scale (UPDRS) (Fahn, Elton, & members of the UPDRS Development Committee, 1987), time since diagnosis, magnitude of glottal incompetence, and severity of speech disorder. These stratified subjects were randomly assigned to one of two treatment groups: respiration (R) or voice and respiration (LSVT).

An analysis of variance revealed no significant differences between the two groups of subjects at baseline for the variables age, $F(1,43) = .4368$, $p = .51$, stage of disease, $F(1,43) = 2.6113$, $p = .11$, score on the motor examination section of the UPDRS, $F(1,40) = .0309$, $p = .86$, time since diagnosis, $F(1,43) = .6609$, $p = .42$, glottal incompetence, $F(1,19) = 1.8274$, $p = .19$, and severity of speech disorder, $F(1,43) = .6704$, $p = .41$. Lack of subject compliance with pre- and post-treatment assessments and experimental and treatment protocols resulted in unequal group sizes and gender distribution. Difficulty recruiting female patients resulted in a limited female sample ($n = 12$). Descriptive characteristics of the 45 subjects obtained during baseline assessments are summarized in Table 2 and details of the baseline assessments are described below. Subjects initiated no other forms of treatment (e.g., physical therapy, occupational therapy, psychological counseling) while they participated in this study.

Patients were excluded from participation in this study if they had a form of Parkinson disease other than idiopathic or a laryngeal pathology that would contraindicate phonatory effort treatment (e.g., vocal nodules, gastric reflux). Voice treatment efficacy data from patients with non-idiopathic Parkinsonism such as Shy-Drager syndrome, multiple system atrophy, progressive supranuclear palsy and bilateral thalamotomy are summarized elsewhere (Countryman & Ramig, 1993; Countryman et al., 1994).

Baseline Neurology, Neuropsychology, Otolaryngology, and Speech Assessments

Neurological assessment. Routine neurological assessment was carried out on all subjects within 1 month of the initiation of treatment. Stage of Parkinson disease, score on the motor examination section (section III) of the UPDRS, time since diagnosis, and anti-Parkinson medications are summarized in Table 2. Subjects were considered neuropharmacologically stable before and during treatment and did not change medications or dosage during the treatment period.

Neuropsychological assessment. A battery of neuropsychological tests was administered within 1 month of the initiation of treatment to determine status of cognitive functioning in these Parkinson disease subjects. These measures focused on attention and concentration, learning and memory, vocabulary and auditory verbal comprehension, and visual spatial skills. Four subtests from the Wechsler Adult Intelligence Scale–Revised were administered (Vocabulary, Block Design, Object Assembly, Digit Symbol; Wechsler, 1981). In addition, parts A and B of the Trail Making Test (Reitan & Wolfson, 1985), the Digit Vigilance Test (Lewis & Kupke, 1977), Story and Figure Memory Test (Heaton, Chelune, & Lehman, 1978), and the Complex Ideational Material auditory comprehension subtest from the Boston Diagnostic Aphasia Exam (Goodglass & Kaplan, 1972) were included. These measures produced 13 scores, all of which were converted to T scores (mean of 50, standard deviation of 10) that correct for demographic variables of age, education, and sex (Heaton, Grant, & Matthews, 1991). After completion of the cognitive evaluation, subjects were interviewed by the clinical neuropsychologist, who then rated depression using the Montgomery Asberg Depression Rating Scale (MADRS; Montgomery & Asberg, 1979). At this time subjects also completed a self-report depression scale, the Beck Depression Inventory (BDI; Beck, Ward, Mendelson, Mock, & Erbaugh, 1961) as well as the Sickness Impact Profile (SIP; Bergner, Bobbit, Carter, & Gilson, 1981). The SIP instrument assesses the extent to which patients perceive their illness to affect 12 different areas of their lives. For the purposes of this paper, the individual scores for the impact of illness on communication and social interaction were included. Both the BDI and the SIP were completed pretreatment and post-treatment after completion of the last speech treatment session. Pretreatment neuropsychological data for each individual subject as well as group means are summarized in Table 3. Results of analysis of variance revealed no significant differences between treatment groups in cognitive functioning, level of depression, or sickness impact on communication or social interaction at baseline. However, a main effect for gender was revealed for the self-rating of depression, $F(1,41) = 7.368$, $p = .010$, as well as clinical rating of depression, $F(1,41) = 9.971$, $p =$

TABLE 2. Descriptive characteristics of subjects who received the Lee Silverman Voice Treatment (voice and respiration) and subjects who received treatment focusing only on respiration.

Subject	Sex	Age	Years since diagnosis	Hoehn & Yahr stage (1967)	UPDRS Motor exam	Medication* †	Speech/Voice deficits (severity rating)	Glottal incompetence
Subjects who received the Lee Silverman Voice Treatment								
1	F	73	10	4.0	48.0	a, c, f	reduced loudness imprecise articulation (5)	2.25
2	F	52	13	3.0	17.0	a, f, o	reduced loudness rapid rate (3)	1.50
3	F	49	9	2.0	4.0	a, d, g	hoarseness (1)	1.5
4	F	32	1	2.0	UA~	a, j	hoarseness (1)	
5	F	74	1	1.5	12.0	b, c	hoarseness tremor (2)	
Mean (*F*) (*SD*)		56.0 (17.7)	6.8 (5.5)	2.5 (1.0)	20.25 (19.3)		2.4 (1.67)	1.75 (0.4)
6	M	49	1	2.0	13.0	a, b, c	monotone reduced loudness (1)	1.33
7	M	76	1	2.0	20.0	a	hoarseness monotone (2)	
8	M	76	5	3.0	28.0	b, c, l	imprecise articulation reduced loudness (3)	1.75
9	M	62	3	2.0	26.0	a, c	hoarseness reduced loudness (3)	2.0
10	M	71	11	3.5	43.5	j, h	hoarseness reduced loudness (4)	1.75
11	M	50	18	2.0	19.5	a, c, d	reduced loudness monotone (2)	
12	M	68	6	3.0	40.5	a, k	reduced loudness hoarseness (3)	2.0
13	M	75	20	3.5	47.0	b, n	reduced loudness imprecise articulation (4)	1.25
14	M	69	1	3.0	32.0	none	imprecise articulation reduced loudness (2)	
15	M	61	1	2.0	16.0	a, c	reduced loudness imprecise articulation (2)	1.0
16	M	72	5	3.0	30.0	a, c, h	reduced loudness monotone (2)	1.0
17	M	67	8	3.0	16.0	a	reduced loudness imprecise articulation (3)	1.75
18	M	64	7	2.0	26.0	a,	monotone reduced loudness (2)	1.0
19	M	73	10	3.0	27.5	a, h	monotone reduced loudness (3)	
20	M	79	1	3.0	33.0	a, c	monotone imprecise articulation (3)	
21	M	62	4	3.5	35.0	k, n	aphonia hoarseness (4)	

Continued on next page

TABLE 2. ***(Continued)***

Subject	Sex	Age	Years since diagnosis	Hoehn & Yahr stage (1967)	UPDRS Motor exam	Medication* †	Speech/Voice deficits (severity rating)	Glottal incompetence
Subjects who received the Lee Silverman Voice Treatment								
22	M	52	18	3.0	34.0	a, c, d, e	rapid rate reduced loudness (3)	
23	M	75	7	2.0	32.0	a, c	reduced loudness hoarseness (3)	
24	M	61	4	3.0	22.5	a, c, d	imprecise articulation reduced loudness (4)	
25	M	54	15	3.5	45.5	b, i, k	reduced loudness monotone (4)	2.25
26	M	56	7	2.0	2.0	a, c, h	rapid rate reduced loudness (3)	1.0
Mean (*M*)		65.3	8.7	2.7	28.0		2.86	1.5
(*SD*)		(9.3)	(10.1)	(0.6)	(11.3)		(0.85)	(0.5)
Group Mean		63.5	8.3	2.7	26.8		2.77	1.6
(*SD*)		(11.5)	(9.3)	(0.7)	(12.7)		(1.03)	(0.45)
Subjects who received treatment focusing only on respiration								
27	F	64	2	3.0	29.0	a, c, p	hoarseness reduced loudness (1)	1.55
28	F	71	3	1.0	UA~	a	hoarseness tremor (2)	
29	F	68	1	2.0	1.0	a, b, c	reduced loudness (1)	
30	F	68	4	2.0	12.0	a, c	reduced loudness monotone (3)	1.75
31	F	63	3	3.0	42.0	a, c	imprecise articulation slow rate (4)	2.5
32	F	51	4	1.0	16.0	none	reduced loudness (1)	1.75
33	F	83	7	3.0	33.0	a	strained/strangled rapid rate (4)	1.75
Mean (*F*)		66.9	3.4	2.1	23.6		2.29	1.8
(*SD*)		(9.6)	(1.9)	(0.9)	(14.3)		(1.38)	(0.2)
34	M	70	4	3.0	32.0	a, c	reduced loudness monotone (3)	1.0
35	M	71	4	3.0	43.0	a, n	reduced loudness monotone (4)	1.25
36	M	69	1	2.0	27.0	i	monotone reduced loudness (3)	
37	M	65	8	3.0	19.0	none	imprecise articulation rapid rate (2)	1.0
38	M	52	14	2.0	31.0	a, d, e, p	pallilalia rapid rate (3)	1.0
39	M	67	18	3.5	UA	b, c, j	imprecise articulation reduced loudness (4)	
40	M	51	6	1.5	3.0	a, c	rapid rate pallilalia (4)	
41	M	66	12	3.0	41.0	a, c, i	strained/strangled reduced loudness (3)	

TABLE 2. (Continued)

Subject	Sex	Age	Years since diagnosis	Hoehn & Yahr stage (1967)	UPDRS Motor exam	Medication* †	Speech/Voice deficits (severity rating)	Glottal incompetence (2)
Subjects who received treatment focusing only on respiration								
42	M	81	2	2.0	24.5	a, c, n	reduced loudness (2)	1.0
43	M	69	6	2.0	36.0	a, k	reduced loudness monotone (3)	
44	M	64	10	3.0	43.0	a	imprecise articulation monotone (4)	1.5
45	M	54	3	1.0	3.0	b, c, h	reduced loudness monotone (1)	
Mean (*M*)		64.9	7.3	2.4	27.1		3.0	1.1
(*SD*)		(8.7)	(5.2)	(0.8)	(15.0)		(0.95)	(0.2)
Group Mean		65.6	5.9	2.3	25.6		2.74	1.38
(*SD*)		(8.9)	(4.7)	(0.8)	(14.4)		(1.15)	(0.4)

*Parkinson medications
a = sinemet, b = sinemet-cr, c = eldyprel, d = parlodel, e = symmetrel, f = pergolide, g = cogentin, h = artane i = amantadine, j = permax, k = deprenyl, l = parsidol
†Anti-depressants
n = amitriptyline, o = tofranil, p = elavil
~unavailable
Note. Glottal incompetence ratings are on a scale of 1–5. 1 = slight, 3 = moderate, 5 severe.
Higher scores on the UPDRS indicate greater disability. Scores range from 0–108.
Severity ratings of speech and voice deficits are on a scale of 1–5. 1 = mild, 2 = mild/moderate, 3 = moderate, 4 = moderate/severe, 5 = severe.

.003, with the females (n = 12) being more depressed than the males (n = 33).

Otolaryngological assessment. An otolaryngological history and videolaryngostroboscopy examination were obtained on all subjects prior to beginning treatment. Laryngeal imaging and videolaryngostroboscopy examination were conducted utilizing well-described techniques (Bless, Hirano, & Feder, 1987). The nasal passage was topically anesthetized with 4% lidocaine spray. Endoscopic examination was conducted with both an Olympus ENF-P3 fiberscope and Nagashima SFT-1 70-degree rigid telescope. Light sources included both an Olympus halogen constant light source and a Nagashima LS-3A laryngoscope. The subjects were instructed to say /i/ at a comfortable pitch and loudness. Images were recorded with a CCD camera, using a 35-mm lens for the fiberscope and 60-mm lens for the rigid telescope, and a VHS or SVHS tape recorder. The data for pretreatment glottal incompetence ratings were prepared by creating a "master" study videotape that included segments from the laryngostroboscopic videotapes of each subject. The order of the subject videotapes was determined by a computer random number generator. Six subjects' recordings were repeated to assess intrajudge reliability. The audio signal from each subject tape was removed to eliminate auditory perceptual cues. Instead, a "prompter" was overdubbed onto the audio track information that identified the tasks performed during examination of each patient to allow raters to identify them. Glottal incompetence was rated during comfortable pitch, comfortable loudness /i/. Three speech-language pathologists and one otolaryngologist with experience in voice research assessed the recordings. They independently and as a group viewed a practice tape, and met several times to develop standard rating criteria. Ninety-five percent intrarater agreement was achieved on the practice tape. Following the practice procedures, they independently viewed and rated the master tape. Twenty-four percent of the glottal incompetence ratings were reanalyzed to determine reliability. Interexaminer reliability ranged between .78 and .94 whereas intraexaminer reliability ranged between .87 and 1.0. The magnitude of glottal incompetence pretreatment is summarized in Table 2 for 25 of the 45 subjects. Videostroboscopy ratings could not be obtained on 20 subjects due to their inability to tolerate the procedure, excessive involuntary movement, or technical problems. Results of analysis of variance revealed no significant difference between the two treatment groups in glottal incompetence at baseline. Additional details of pretreatment (Perez, Ramig, Smith, & Dromey, in press) and pre- to post-treatment laryngological characteristics (Smith et al., in press) have been previously reported.

Speech assessment. Standard speech and voice assessments were completed at the time of the first pretreatment data collection session. None of the subjects exhibited oral motor and/or speech and voice characteristics uncommon to Parkinson disease. The primary speech and/or voice characteristics and severity of speech disorder rating for each subject determined by clinical observations are presented in Table 2.

In order to provide additional descriptive information on the subjects and to evaluate the relationship between magnitude of speech and voice disorder and severity of Parkinson disease, correlation coefficients were completed

TABLE 3. Neuropsychological characteristics of the Lee Silverman Voice Treatment (voice and respiration) subjects and the respiration-only subjects.

Subject	Cognition (*T* score)	Beck Depression (self-rating)	Depression (clinician's rating)	SIP communication	SIP social interaction
Subjects who received the Lee Silverman Voice Treatment					
1	40.38	10	12	65.24	12.55
2	40.08	11	7	56.41	13.03
3	40.54	20	14	0.00	33.93
4	45.31	20	9	9.66	13.17
5	42.62	14	11	9.66	11.03
Mean (*F*)	41.79	15.0	10.6	28.19	16.74
(*SD*)	(2.21)	(7.28)	(2.70)	(30.21)	(9.65)
6	46.54	6	3	0.00	0.00
7	47.00	5	0	9.66	0.00
8	42.69	0	3	21.10	3.59
9	44.54	2	7	9.66	9.03
10	42.69	6	6	56.00	7.38
11	39.54	3	8	31.31	6.00
12	41.15	4	7	39.17	3.52
13	42.62	13	15	22.48	9.10
14	44.08	4	5	67.86	0.00
15	45.69	1	4	0.00	0.00
16	39.77	12	3	41.79	18.62
17	48.69	12	8	65.24	11.79
18	50.31	3	1	30.24	0.00
19	43.54	16	5	40.41	0.00
20	41.23	4	6	51.86	17.03
21	37.38	12	5	63.03	24.89
22	42.08	12	8	63.86	3.52
23	53.69	15	13	11.45	11.45
24	44.38	8	13	52.41	6.83
25	50.38	10	5	28.97	6.83
26	48.31	11	3	30.76	15.72
Mean (*M*)	44.59	7.57	6.10	35.11	7.40
(*SD*)	(4.08)	(4.87)	(3.86)	(21.75)	(7.11)
Group Mean	44.05	9.0	6.96	33.78	9.19
(*SD*)	(3.92)	(5.62)	(4.05)	(23.07)	(8.33)
Subjects who received treatment focusing only on respiration					
27	53.31	10	9	0.00	0.00
28	39.31	7	7	39.17	6.07
29	48.85	12	0	0.00	0.00
30	50	3	7	18.48	6.48
31	40.54	25	19	73.10	55.17
32	52.77	13	12	0.00	26.76
33	40.54	12	11	55.03	9.10
Mean (*F*)	46.47	11.71	9.29	26.54	14.80
(*SD*)	(6.14)	(6.82)	(5.79)	(29.77)	(19.95)
34	49.38	11	1	0.00	3.52
35	34.46	10	3	32.55	17.59
36	50.69	11	1	9.66	3.52
37	43.85	0	3	40.41	3.52
38	43.54	22	6	52.41	31.38
39	40.31	10	3	66.21	20.41
40	46.08	3	6	9.66	11.45
41	50.08	13	11	63.86	18.69
42	49.23	5	5	9.66	20.48
43	37.54	12	2	31.31	9.59
44	33.91	8	13	52.41	7.10
45	51.92	1	5	0.00	0.00
Mean (*M*)	44.25	8.83	4.92	30.68	12.27
(*SD*)	(6.42)	(6.04)	(3.75)	(24.52)	(9.45)
Group Mean	45.07	9.90	6.53	29.15	13.20
(*SD*)	(6.24)	(6.31)	(4.95)	(25.83)	(13.74)

Note. T scores below 40 are considered impaired. Scores above 9 on self-rating of depression suggest some depression. Scores of 6 or greater on clinician ratings of depression are suggestive of depression. Scores that are larger on the SIP indicate more impact of the sickness in that area. Scores of 0.00 on the SIP indicate no difficulty in that area.

on these baseline data for all 45 subjects. Severity of speech and voice disorder rated on a 1–5 point scale at the time of clinical intake (pre-treatment) were correlated (Pearson product moment) with the variables time since diagnosis (r = .43, p = .003), rating on the motor examination section of the UPDRS (r = .63, p = .001), Parkinson disease stage (r = .62, p = .001), and depression rating (r = .45, p = .004). These findings suggest that subjects who had Parkinson disease longer and were more motorically impaired also had more severe speech and voice deficits.

EXPERIMENT

Instrumentation

In order to measure intensity, frequency, and duration data, sound pressure level (B & K 2230 sound level meter) and microphone (AKG C410) signals were transduced and recorded onto a Sony PC-108M 8-channel digital audiotape recorder (DAT). Forced vital capacity was measured with a Collins wet spirometer (Model RS 2785).

Tasks

Experimental tasks were designed to sample a broad continuum of speech production to address both underlying mechanisms of treatment-related change as well as functional aspects of speech production. Data were collected while subjects performed the following tasks: forced vital capacity, maximum duration sustained vowel phonation, reading of the phonetically balanced "Rainbow Passage" (Fairbanks, 1960) and 25–30 sec of conversational monologue. Because the sound level meter and microphone offer noninvasive signal transduction, measures of intensity, frequency, and duration could be collected from all subjects.

In order to evaluate the subjects' impressions of treatment effectiveness and the impact of treatment on functional communication, perceptual rating scales were completed by all 45 subjects at the time of data collection. Family members from 20 of the 45 subjects completed the perceptual rating scales as well.

Procedures

Pretreatment experimental data were collected within the week before treatment was initiated. Post-treatment data were collected within the week following treatment. For assessment of intrasubject variability and reliability, 58% of the subjects repeated their pretreatment data collection and 36% of the subjects repeated their post-treatment data collection. For experimental data collection, subjects were seated in a medical examining chair located in an IAC sound-treated booth and transducers were positioned and calibrated using standard procedures. The sound level meter was positioned 50 cm from the lips and the microphone was positioned on a head mount 8 cm from the lips. A calibration tone of known intensity was generated at the subjects' lips at the beginning and end of each recording session.

After 2 minutes of tidal breathing, forced vital capacity was measured. Subjects were asked to take their deepest breath and blow out "as hard and fast and long as you can." This task was repeated two or three times at the beginning and end of the recording session and the best performance was taken as maximum forced vital capacity. Because of motor and balance problems of some subjects, all subjects performed the task in a seated position. One subject could not perform the task pre- or post-treatment.

To obtain maximum duration sustained vowel phonation, subjects were instructed to "take a deep breath and sustain 'ah' for as long as you can." A timer with a second hand was within view of the subjects and they were encouraged to monitor their performance and sustain phonation for a longer duration each time. No instructions were given for loudness level. This task was repeated four times at the beginning of the recording session and two times at the end of each recording. For a few subjects, only three of the initial four consecutive maximum duration sustained phonations were possible, due to fatigue. Because of potential instabilities in measures of maximum performance associated with subjects' inconsistent generation of maximum effort (Kent, Kent, & Rosenbek, 1987) as well as the variability in the performance of Parkinson disease patients (Canter, 1965; King, Ramig, Lemke, & Horii, 1994), the experimenter was careful to elicit consistent maximum effort performance from each subject at each recording trial as determined by her clinical decision. The same experimenter collected all the data.

Samples of reading and conversational speech were obtained by asking subjects to read aloud the "Rainbow Passage" at a comfortable rate and loudness and generate a 25–30 sec monologue on a topic of their choice.

A visual analog scale (Kempster, 1984; Schiffman, Reynolds, & Young, 1981) was used to obtain subject self-ratings as well as family member ratings of loudness, monotonicity, hoarseness, overall intelligibility, and the extent to which the subject initiated conversation.

Treatment

Both forms of treatment were designed to be intensive (16 sessions in one month) and high effort (subject was pushed to maximum performance levels throughout the entire duration of each session). Each type of treatment stimulated high effort tasks in repeated drills for half of each 50-minute treatment session and then stimulated carryover of the drilled behavior to speech tasks during the final half of each session. The implementation of high effort, intensive treatment is based on neurology and physical therapy practices (England & Schwab, 1959; Hallet & Khosbin, 1980; McDowell, Lee, & Sweet, 1986) that suggest when pushed to higher effort levels, patients with Parkinson disease can compensate for bradykinesia and improve task performance. The daily training of high effort to increase magnitude of speech motor output is based upon the potentially similar problems in scaling the magnitude of output (e.g., stride length in walking, letter stroke in writing) observed in patients with

Parkinson disease (Brooks, 1986; Grill, Demirchi, Mc Shane, & Hallett, personal communication; Muller & Stelmach, 1991; Stemach, 1991). We speculate that intensive high effort speech treatment teaches patients to rescale the magnitude of speech motor output (Ramig, 1995; Ramig, Bonitati, Lemke, & Horii, 1994) and that daily treatment with intensive practice (Schmidt, 1975, 1988) and feedback (knowledge of results) (Adams, 1971, 1986) facilitates this training.

The respiratory treatment (R) was designed to train increased respiratory muscle activity for inspiration and expiration and sustained expiration to enable subjects to generate increased volumes and subglottal air pressure for speech (Leinonen & Laakso, 1990; McKenzie & Gandevia, 1986; Netsell & Daniel, 1979; Panzarella, 1995; Yorkston, Beukelman, & Bell, 1988). The R treatment trained subjects to increase respiratory effort through tasks such as maximum inhalation and exhalation (Hardy, 1983; Netsell & Rosenbek, 1986), maximum duration of the voiceless continuants /s/ and /f/, and sustained intraoral air pressure (with and without leak tube) (Iowa Oral Performance Instrument [IOPI]; Leith & Bradley, 1976; Robin, Goel, Somodi, & Luschei, 1992). Subjects were stimulated to take deep, frequent breaths during reading and speaking and were given visual feedback (NIMS Respigraph System PN SY03) of the excursion of their rib cage and abdomen during both sustaining of /s/ and /f/ and while reading and speaking. In the respiratory treatment group, no attention was directed toward increasing vocal fold adduction or increasing vocal loudness.

The voice and respiratory treatment (LSVT) focused on increased vocal loudness through increasing vocal fold adduction. Tasks such as pushing the hands together or pushing down or lifting up on the arms of a chair or table while phonating (Aronson, 1990; Froeschels, Kastein, & Weiss, 1955) were used to stimulate increased vocal fold adduction. Drills were carried out on tasks such as maximum duration "ah" phonation and maximum fundamental frequency range. Subjects were encouraged to "think loud" during these tasks and use the same loud, good quality voice generated during sustained phonation during reading and speaking. Attention was directed toward the respiratory system only in the form of encouraging these subjects to take deep breaths frequently and speak "on top of the breath." However, because maximum effort phonatory tasks such as maximum duration of sustained vowel phonation also stimulate respiratory function, the treatment was considered to address both voice and respiration. Feedback for adequate loudness was given using a voice light (lights up at target intensity level) and tape recorder (for self-monitoring of intensity). Training materials for the LSVT approach are summarized elsewhere (Countryman, Ramig, & Pawlas, 1994; Ramig, 1995; Ramig, Bonitati, & Winholtz, 1994; Ramig, Pawlas, & Countryman, 1995).

It is important to point out that the treatment goal of increasing vocal fold adduction in Parkinson disease is designed to maximize the efficiency of the phonatory source. Because of the glottal incompetence frequently observed in patients with Parkinson disease, increased vocal fold adduction may allow patients the ability to generate adequate intensity. It is never the goal of treatment to increase vocal fold adduction so the voice becomes pressed or hyperadducted. The goal is a voice with sufficient loudness, generated with maximum phonatory efficiency (Ramig, 1995).

The treatment intensiveness, daily homework, daily quantification of treatment variables and carryover were all stimulated equally in both treatment groups. Subjects in both treatment groups made progress during treatment as reflected in their daily treatment variables (e.g., maximum durations and ranges). No attention was directed toward improvement of intonation, articulation, or rate in either treatment group. Two clinicians delivered the treatment to all the subjects; both clinicians administered both forms of treatment and were randomly assigned to individual patients. The clinicians worked closely together to ensure consistency and equivalent high effort and motivation across both forms of treatment. A typical treatment session consisted of 25 min of repeated and intensive maximum effort drills and 25 min of high effort speech production tasks moving through a hierarchy of single words, phrases, sentences, reading, and conversation during the 4-week period. Performance feedback (knowledge of results; Adams, 1971, 1986) was provided to subjects using a variety of instruments: tape recorder, stop watch, voice light, respigraph, IOPI, visipitch, and vocal demodulator (Winholtz & Ramig, 1992) depending upon the treatment group.

Data analysis

Sound pressure level (SPL) measures for sustained phonation, reading and the monologue were analyzed using a custom-built software program. The sound level meter signal (Bruel and Kjaer 2230) was preamplified and then digitized at 5000 samples per second into a VAX 4000/200 system computer through a 16-bit resolution DSC-200 A/D converter. The software program displayed the sound level meter signal in decibels (dB). To avoid the inclusion of nonvoiced or pausal segments in the analysis, data points below the noise floor were eliminated from the signal. This was achieved by cursor-marking the first and last negative-going peaks of the signal and then identifying the percentage below which nonvoiced or pausal data points occurred. The percentage was input into the analysis program and the signal was displayed with the percentage cutoff line. This enabled the analyzer to determine if the correct percentage was chosen. After the correct percentage was determined, the program displayed the mean SPL of the signal.

The SPL was measured from five to six maximum duration sustained "ah" vowel phonations and one reading of the "Rainbow Passage" per recording session for all 45 subjects. Due to limited and variable utterance duration, the SPL for conversational monologue was obtained from 29 of the 45 subjects pre- to post-treatment. The average duration of these monologues ranged from 25–30 sec.

Duration of sustained vowel phonation was also calculated by the SPL program using the markings between the first and last negative going peaks. Duration and SPL data were obtained from the same five to six sustained vowel phonations for each subject. After obtaining the mean SPL for each individual /a/, data were averaged across all maximum duration sustained vowel phonations to obtain an overall average mean SPL for sustained phonation.

To obtain measures of mean fundamental frequency and fundamental frequency variability during reading and monologue, the microphone signal was digitized at 5000 samples per second into the same VAX system described above. The files were downloaded onto a 486 computer and then analyzed using CSpeech software (Milenkovic, 1987). The program calculated mean fundamental frequency (F_0) and standard deviation in Hertz. Using standard procedures, the Hertz standard deviation was then converted to express frequency variability in semitones (STSD) (Horii, 1994). Two subjects in the R group had unanalyzable habitual fundamental frequency and fundamental frequency variability data during reading due to severe dysphonia.

Utterance and pause duration data were obtained from both the "Rainbow Passage" and the 25–30 sec monologue. The data of 4 subjects during reading of the "Rainbow Passage" were unanalyzable; thus, 41 passages and 29 monologues were analyzed. The recorded voices were played back, fullwave rectified and smoothed by an RC lowpass filter (Dobkin, 1969). The rectifying and smoothing extracted the intensity envelope in real time. This intensity envelope was digitized by a 12-bit analog-to-digital converter at a rate of 1000 times per second and stored on a 386 microcomputer disk using CSRE (Canadian Speech Research Environment) software.

The digital intensity envelope was subsequently analyzed for utterance and pause durations by software developed by Horii (1983). Given a specification of the maximum amplitude threshold for pause, the minimum duration of pause, and the minimum duration of utterance, the program identified utterances and pauses. The program then printed out means and standard deviations of utterance and pause durations reported here. Standard procedures for analysis of visual analog scales (Boeckstyns & Backer, 1989) were used to obtain perceptual data from the subjects and families.

TABLE 4. Intrasubject (test-retest) reliability for acoustic and perceptual variables expressed in Pearson product-moment correlation coefficients.

Variables	Pre-1 to Pre-2 correlations	Post-1 to Post-2 correlations
SPL		
Sustained phonation	0.78	0.96
Rainbow Passage	0.78	0.97
Monologue	0.82	0.82
Maximum duration	0.83	0.93
STSD		
Rainbow Passage	0.95	0.91
Monologue	0.39	0.43
F_0		
Rainbow Passage	0.98	0.99
Monologue	0.96	0.96
FVC	0.98	0.99
Perceptual-Subject (n = 45)		
Loudness	0.65	0.68
Monotonicity	0.55	0.72
Hoarseness	0.69	0.45
Intelligibility	0.67	0.76
Initiate conversation	0.81	0.83
Perceptual-Family (n = 20)		
Loudness	0.61	0.86
Monotonicity	0.87	0.99
Hoarseness	0.75	0.92
Intelligibility	0.63	0.98
Initiate conversation	0.93	0.71

Note. Correlation coefficients are based upon the following sample sizes: 58% of the 45 subjects repeated the pre-treatment and 36% of the 45 subjects repeated the post-treatment acoustic measures; 100% of the 45 subjects repeated the pre- and post-treatment perceptual self-ratings; 60% of the 20 families repeated the pre-treatment and 20% of the 20 families repeated the post-treatment perceptual ratings.

Results

Reliability

For an assessment of intra-subject reliability, 58% of the subjects completed a second pretreatment voice recording and 36% of the subjects completed a second post-treatment voice recording. One hundred percent of the subjects completed a second set of perceptual self-rating scales pre- and post-treatment. Correlation coefficients reflecting intra-subject reliability for all acoustic and perceptual variables are summarized in Table 4. *T*-tests for related measures were carried out on the acoustic and perceptual variables obtained in the two pre- and the two post-recordings. There were no significant differences among any of these repeated measures. Reliability of perceptual ratings completed by the families are also included in Table 4. Sixty percent of the 20 families completed a second pretreatment visual analog scale and 20% completed a second post-treatment visual analog scale.

Twenty percent of the data were reanalyzed to determine measurement reliability. Correlation coefficients were 0.99 for all measures of SPL, STSD, and F_0 of the "Rainbow Passage," F_0 during conversation, and maximum duration of sustained vowel phonations, and 0.92 for STSD in conversational monologue. Twenty percent of the perceptual data from the subjects' self-ratings as well as the families' perceptual ratings were remeasured to determine measurement reliability. Correlation coefficients were 0.99 for all categories of the visual analog scale.

Acoustic Variables

An analysis of variance carried out to determine pretreatment comparability between the two groups on acoustic and perceptual variables revealed no significant differences. In addition, there were no statistically significant differences on these acoustic and perceptual variables between the two groups of males or the two groups of females at baseline.

A three factor (treatment group × gender × time) repeated measures analysis of variance (ANOVA) was used to evaluate the statistical significance of pre- to post-treatment changes (Campbell & Stanley, 1966). *F* and *p* values for the acoustic variables are reported in Table 5. All means and standard deviations of each acoustic variable for each group and gender pre- to post-treatment are summarized in Table 6.

SPL—Vowels

Statistical analysis of SPL during sustained vowel phonation revealed a significant time (pre- to post-treatment) by treatment group (R or LSVT) by gender interaction [$F(1,41) = 7.37$, $p = .01$] (Table 5). Both the males and females who received the LSVT increased SPL post-treatment (mean increases of 13.96dB [*SD* 5.01] and 9.89dB [*SD* 5.66], respectively) (Table 6 and Figure 1a). Whereas the females who received the R treatment increased on average 1.99 dB (*SD* 6.09), the males who received the R treatment *decreased* on average 3.23 dB (3.83) pre- to post-treatment.

SPL—Reading and Conversation

Statistical analysis for SPL during reading revealed a significant time by treatment group by gender interaction, $F(1,41) = 4.85$, $p = .033$. Both the males and females who received the LSVT increased in SPL pre- to post-treatment (mean increases of 9.13dB [6.05] and 3.39dB [1.91], respectively) (Table 6; Figure 1b). The females who received the R treatment also increased SPL (mean 3.45dB [4.77]); the males who received the R increased on average 1.92dB (2.30).

Statistical analysis for SPL during conversational monologue revealed a significant main effect for time, $F(1,25) = 14.02$, $p = .001$. There were no significant interactions between treatment group or gender (Table 5; Figure 1c). Subjects in both treatment groups significantly improved SPL in conversation from pre- to post-treatment.

Maximum Duration of Sustained Vowel Phonation

Statistical analysis of maximum duration of sustained vowel phonation revealed a statistically significant main effect for time, $F(1,41) = 9.29$, $p = .004$. There were no significant interactions between treatment group or gender (Table 5). Males and females from both treatment groups significantly increased maximum duration of sustained vowel phonation from pre- to post-treatment (Table 6).

Fundamental Frequency (Mean F_0) and Variability (STSD)—Reading and Conversation

Statistical analysis of mean habitual fundamental frequency while reading revealed a significant main effect for time, $F(1,39) = 35.58$, $p = .001$. There were no significant treatment group or gender interactions (Table 5). Males and

TABLE 5. *F* and *p* values for the acoustic variables.

Dependent variables	Between-subject effect									Within-subject effect						
	Group		Gender		Group × Gender		Time			Time × Group		Time × Gender		Time × Group × Gender	
	F	*p*	*F*	*p*	*F*	*p*	*df*	*F*	*p*	*F*	*p*	*F*	*p*	*F*	*p*
SPL																
Sustained phonation	15.55	.000	0.49	.486	0.66	.421	1,41	43.63	.000	53.72	.000	0.11	.738	7.37	.01
Rainbow Passage	4.88	.033	5.30	.027	4.62	.037	1,41	29.41	.000	4.70	.036	1.62	.210	4.85	.033
Monologue	0.39	.537	3.65	.067	1.14	.296	1,25	14.02	.001	3.27	.083	3.67	.067	1.90	.180
Maximum duration	1.68	.202	1.49	.230	.85	.361	1,41	9.29	.004	.63	.431	.51	.480	.48	.493
F_0 Rainbow Passage	6.48	.015	83.64	.000	1.34	.252	1,39	35.58	.000	1.14	.292	1.52	.225	1.61	.212
STSD Rainbow Passage	2.20	.146	1.45	.235	.90	.348	1,39	43.29	.000	1.98	.168	.00	.968	2.40	.129
F_0 Monologue	.88	.358	85.92	.000	1.39	.250	1,25	3.62	.069	2.97	.097	.61	.443	.03	.856
STSD Monologue	.22	.645	.50	.484	.32	.578	1,25	1.02	.321	8.48	.007	.43	.516	.94	.340
Utterance duration																
Rainbow Passage	.07	.786	.60	.442	.90	.350	1,37	19.30	.000	.16	.696	.03	.864	.03	.875
Monologue	1.36	.254	8.90	.006	4.47	.044	1,27	2.23	.147	1.84	.186	.45	.506	.07	.793
Pause duration																
Rainbow Passage	2.97	.093	1.67	.204	4.83	.034	1,37	30.15	.000	6.61	.014	.85	.364	2.79	.103
Monologue	2.02	.167	.29	.593	1.06	.313	1,27	1.87	.183	3.02	.093	.65	.427	3.06	.091
FVC	.70	.408	17.87	.000	.30	.586	1,40	.04	.852	.28	.599	.03	.870	2.15	.151

TABLE 6. Means and standard deviations (in parentheses) for the acoustic variables collected pre- to post-treatment. Means are listed for each group as well as males and females. The *n* is listed for each group, LSVT followed by R.

	LSVT		R only	
Variables	**Pretreatment**	**Post-treatment**	**Pretreatment**	**Post-treatment**
Intensity (dB) (at 50cm)				
Sustained phonation				
Group (*n* = 26;19)	68.20 (4.70)	81.20 (4.65)	69.32 (5.05)	68.01 (4.31)
Males (*n* = 21;12)	68.03 (4.60)	81.99 (3.93)	70.23 (3.75)	66.99 (4.49)
Females (*n* = 5;7)	68.02 (5.70)	77.91 (6.40)	67.76 (6.80)	69.75 (3.64)
Rainbow Passage				
Group (*n* = 26;19)	66.30 (4.02)	74.33 (4.83)	65.68 (2.68)	68.16 (3.33)
Males (*n* = 21;12)	66.56 (4.37)	75.69 (4.06)	66.02 (2.53)	67.94 (3.62)
Females (*n* = 5;7)	65.19 (1.96)	68.58 (3.51)	65.11 (3.05)	68.56 (3.00)
Monologue				
Group (*n* = 16;13)	64.67 (3.37)	69.17 (4.10)	64.66 (2.58)	66.24 (2.11)
Males (*n* = 11;8)	64.94 (3.66)	70.35 (3.61)	65.19 (2.40)	66.70 (2.01)
Females (*n* = 5;5)	63.96 (1.66)	65.34 (3.46)	64.66 (2.58)	65.52 (2.77)
Max duration (sec)				
Sustained phonation				
Group (*n* = 26;19)	21.12 (7.63)	24.84 (10.35)	18.39 (9.65)	21.20 (8.78)
Males (*n* = 21;12)	21.62 (8.17)	24.67 (11.44)	20.67 (11.09)	23.47 (7.93)
Females (*n* = 5;7)	19.00 (4.77)	25.57 (3.79)	14.47 (5.10)	17.32 (9.37)
F_0 (Hz)				
Rainbow Passage				
Males (*n* = 21;12)	124.73 (22.10)	140.78 (23.66)	120.13 (18.72)	125.57 (21.45)
Females (*n* = 5;5)	198.35 (12.13)	214.23 (13.56)	171.47 (11.47)	188.26 (17.58)
F_0 variability (STSD)				
Rainbow Passage				
Group (*n* = 26;17)	1.82 (0.53)	2.38 (0.67)	1.80 (0.41)	2.09 (0.34)
Males (*n* = 21;12)	1.73 (0.42)	2.33 (0.63)	1.82 (0.41)	2.05 (0.30)
Females (*n* = 5;5)	2.22 (0.80)	2.62 (0.87)	1.77 (0.49)	2.19 (0.44)
F_0 (Hz)				
Monologue				
Males (*n* = 12;10)	114.33 (13.19)	120.64 (16.81)	119.80 (21.85)	118.81 (18.62)
Females (*n* = 4;3)	190.52 (20.71)	201.40 (15.34)	179.15 (15.43)	180.99 (25.26)
F_0 variability (STSD)				
Monologue				
Group (*n* = 16;13)	1.68 (0.39)	1.97 (0.58)	2.13 (0.72)	1.95 (0.67)
Males (*n* = 12;10)	1.66 (0.39)	1.90 (0.39)	2.11 (0.73)	1.95 (0.72)
Females (*n* = 4;3)	1.80 (0.61)	2.38 (0.88)	2.18 (0.84)	1.95 (0.59)
Utterance duration (msec)				
Rainbow Passage				
Group (*n* = 24;17)	2665.88 (666.03)	2186.24 (511.62)	2524.08 (530.33)	2132.55 (396.94)
Males (*n* = 19;11)	2671.59 (741.40)	2192.50 (512.17)	2409.05 (421.21)	2040.95 (361.57)
Females (*n* = 5;6)	2644.19 (276.33)	2162.44 (568.97)	2734.97 (680.22)	2300.48 (436.48)
Monologue				
Group (*n* = 18;13)	1943.19 (389.51)	1948.66 (672.05)	2165.12 (851.82)	1872.51 (569.48)
Males (*n* = 13;9)	1883.38 (346.72)	1915.60 (661.21)	1829.16 (582.93)	1604.47 (299.41)
Females (*n* = 5;4)	2098.69 (492.24)	2034.62 (771.47)	2921.04 (946.43)	2475.60 (598.07)
Pause duration (msec)				
Rainbow Passage				
Group (*n* = 24;17)	568.93 (175.95)	720.49 (198.89)	514.67 (138.15)	844.11 (342.80)
Males (*n* = 19;11)	605.95 (178.80)	771.64 (190.17)	536.54 (146.02)	783.43 (268.57)
Females (*n* = 5;6)	428.24 (53.83)	526.13 (71.22)	474.58 (124.09)	955.36 (456.97)
Monologue				
Group (*n* = 18;13)	620.11 (282.66)	753.40 (338.93)	714.79 (297.50)	941.33 (406.46)
Males (*n* = 13;9)	675.24 (292.09)	855.67 (320.08)	721.49 (242.41)	900.16 (332.84)
Females (*n* = 5;4)	440.94 (169.95)	421.03 (101.09)	699.72 (443.71)	1033.89 (590.71)
FVC (ml)				
Males (*n* = 20;12)	3500.00 (720.38)	3535.00 (672.99)	3458.33 (1015.75)	3425.00 (1010.96)
Females (*n* = 5;7)	2580.00 (601.66)	2520.00 (554.08)	2142.86 (506.15)	2228.57 (590.80)

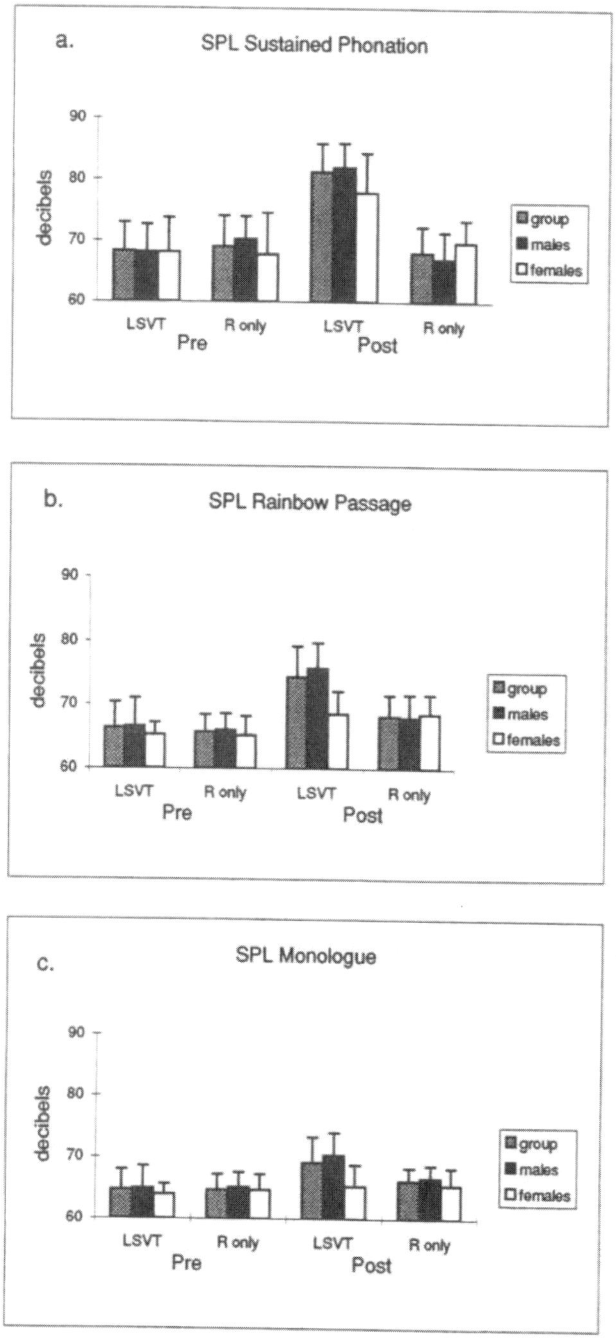

FIGURE 1. Means and standard deviations for sound pressure level (SPL) before and after treatment for the LSVT and R treatment groups, showing male, female, and overall group values. Tasks included: (a) sustained phonation, (b) reading of the Rainbow Passage, and (c) conversational monologue. All measures of SPL were made at a distance of 50cm.

females from both treatment groups significantly increased their fundamental frequency from pre- to post-treatment (Table 6). Statistical analysis of corresponding fundamental frequency variability (STSD) while reading the "Rainbow Passage" revealed a significant main effect for time, $F(1,39) = 43.29$, $p = .001$. Again, there were no significant interactions (Table 5). Male and female subjects from both treatment groups significantly increased STSD from pre- to post-treatment.

Statistical analysis of fundamental frequency during the conversational monologue revealed no significant changes pre- to post-treatment for either gender or treatment group. Statistical analysis of corresponding fundamental frequency variability (STSD) during the monologue revealed a significant time by treatment group interaction, $F(1,25) = 8.48$, $p = .007$, (Table 5). Subjects who received the LSVT significantly increased their STSD during monologue from pre- to post-treatment whereas the subjects who received the R treatment *decreased* their STSD during monologue from pre- to post-treatment. Despite the statistically significant finding, individual variability was apparent in the magnitude of change across treatment groups and in the intrasubject reliability.

Rate

Statistical analysis for utterance duration during reading revealed a significant main effect for time, $F(1,37) = 19.30$, $p = .001$. Both males and females in both treatment groups statistically significantly reduced their utterance duration during reading from pre- to post-treatment (Table 6). Statistical analysis for utterance duration during monologue revealed no significant main effect or interactions pre- to post-treatment (Table 5). Statistical analysis for pause duration during reading of the "Rainbow Passage" revealed a significant time by treatment group interaction, $F(1,37) = 6.61$, $p = .014$. Both groups increased on this measure; however, only subjects who received the R treatment demonstrated a statistically significant pre- to post-treatment increase (Table 5). Statistical analysis for pause duration during the monologue revealed no significant main effect or interactions pre- to post-treatment (Table 5).

Forced Vital Capacity (FVC)

FVC data are summarized in Table 6. Statistical analysis revealed no significant main effect for time or interactions (Table 5).

Perceptual Variables

F and p values for the analysis of variance carried out on the perceptual variables are presented in Table 7. Means and standard deviations for the perceptual variables for subject self-ratings are presented in Table 8.

Statistical analysis for self-ratings of loudness revealed a significant time by treatment group by gender interaction, $F(1,41) = 4.17$, $p = .048$. Males who received the LSVT and females who received the R rated the greatest improvements (mean increases 19.19; SD 17.41 and 26.00; SD 25.24), respectively. Significant main effects for time were measured for the perceptual variables monotonicity, $F(1,41) = 11.82$, $p = .001$, hoarseness, $F(1,41) = 11.64$, $p = .001$, intelligibility, $F(1,41) = 11.92$, $p = .001$, and initiating conversation, $F(1,41) = 10.39$, $p = .002$. Both male and female

TABLE 7. *F* and *p* values for the perceptual variables

	Between-subject effect						Within-subject effect							
	Group		Gender		Group × Gender		Time		Time × Group		Time × Gender		Time × Group × Gender	
Dependent variables	*F*	*p*	*F*	*p*	*F*	*p*	*F*	*p*	*F*	*p*	*F*	*p*	*F*	*p*
Subject self-rating ($n = 45$) ($df = 1{,}41$)														
Loudness	.03	.872	.06	.805	1.51	.226	19.26	.000	.10	.751	.42	.520	4.17	.048
Monotonicity	.01	.922	2.16	.149	2.94	.094	11.82	.001	.17	.686	1.87	.179	1.59	.215
Hoarseness	.22	.645	.51	.481	3.37	.073	11.64	.001	.39	.535	.00	.955	.04	.843
Intelligibility	.00	.978	.15	.697	.67	.416	11.92	.001	.02	.901	.21	.653	.67	.417
Initiate conversation	.07	.791	4.62	.037	.72	.401	10.39	.002	.13	.718	.45	.506	3.98	.053
Family ratings ($n = 20$) ($df = 1{,}16$)														
Loudness	.50	.490	.28	.602	.53	.476	5.73	.029	.09	.773	.03	.867	.20	.660
Monotonicity	.56	.464	2.14	.163	.12	.735	1.50	.239	.15	.707	1.23	.283	.74	.403
Hoarseness	.01	.925	2.27	.151	1.81	.197	.44	.517	.28	.602	.60	.450	1.15	.299
Intelligibility	.40	.538	.87	.366	.62	.442	15.81	.001	6.74	.019	.10	.752	1.56	.230
Initiate conversation	2.80	.114	8.66	.010	.22	.645	1.24	.282	2.62	.125	.07	.791	2.42	.139

subjects from both treatment groups rated statistically significant improvements on these measures from pre- to post-treatment (Table 8).

Family ratings ($n = 20$) of pre- to post-treatment perceptual variables are presented in Table 8. Family ratings of loudness revealed a significant main effect for time, $F(1,16) = 5.73$, $p = .029$ (Table 7). As seen in Table 8, families of subjects from both treatment groups rated statistically significant pre- to post-treatment improvement in loudness. Family ratings of overall intelligibility revealed a significant time by treatment group interaction, $F(1,16) = 6.74, p = .019$. Although families of subjects from both treatment groups rated improvement on overall intelligibility pre- to post-treatment, only the families of the subjects who received the LSVT rated statistically signifi-

TABLE 8. Perceptual variables for the subjects' ($n = 45$) self-ratings by group and gender as well as the families' ratings for both groups. Standard deviations are presented in parentheses.

	LSVT		R Only	
Variables	**Pretreatment**	**Post-treatment**	**Pretreatment**	**Post-treatment**
Loudness				
Group	46.85 (20.23)	64.15 (20.89)	51.37 (29.01)	65.42 (19.88)
Males	43.95 (18.21)	63.14 (18.59)	57.33 (27.83)	64.42 (23.33)
Females	59.00 (25.93)	68.40 (31.17)	41.14 (30.20)	67.14 (13.47)
Family ($n = 20$)	45.50 (22.63)	60.50 (18.47)	49.73 (28.64)	63.12 (21.84)
Monotonicity				
Group	47.00 (22.54)	66.73 (16.28)	57.00 (26.13)	68.05 (20.87)
Males	41.38 (18.45)	64.76 (14.74)	57.42 (29.23)	68.75 (22.48)
Females	70.60 (24.69)	75.00 (21.56)	56.29 (21.91)	66.86 (19.44)
Family ($n = 20$)	52.67 (27.49)	66.75 (19.34)	57.91 (27.03)	68.88 (21.92)
Hoarseness				
Group	55.65 (21.89)	70.11 (16.42)	64.58 (24.14)	75.11 (21.61)
Males	54.52 (23.13)	68.62 (17.66)	70.08 (23.03)	81.00 (23.30)
Females	60.40 (16.92)	76.40 (8.02)	55.14 (24.73)	65.00 (14.75)
Family ($n = 20$)	61.58 (27.10)	66.58 (19.67)	70.45 (18.06)	70.38 (18.75)
Intelligibility				
Group	57.12 (20.30)	71.12 (16.77)	61.63 (20.20)	72.00 (19.99)
Males	54.95 (20.11)	70.52 (15.63)	63.00 (21.17)	72.50 (21.65)
Females	66.20 (20.62)	73.60 (22.96)	59.29 (19.81)	71.14 (18.39)
Family ($n = 20$)	49.50 (17.93)	67.33 (19.59)	57.55 (22.81)	64.63 (17.94)
Initiate conversation				
Group	50.96 (22.37)	66.85 (16.39)	61.26 (22.06)	68.89 (20.83)
Males	45.90 (18.97)	64.90 (15.07)	59.83 (18.17)	64.50 (22.68)
Females	72.20 (25.10)	75.00 (21.00)	63.71 (29.03)	76.43 (15.91)
Family ($n = 20$)	54.67 (20.70)	70.33 (16.70)	67.09 (28.55)	71.50 (18.41)

Note. Perceptual characteristics of loudness, hoarseness, intelligibility, and initiation of conversation are on a scale of 0–100% with 0% the most severe and 100% the least severe.

cant improvement. Family ratings of monotone, hoarseness, and initiating conversation were not statistically significantly different pre- to post-treatment. Families rated that female subjects initiated conversation significantly more often than male subjects, $F(1,16) = 8.66$, $p = .010$.

Neuropsychological Variables of Self-Rated Depression and Sickness Impact

The Beck Depression Inventory (BDI: subject self-rating of depression) and the Sickness Impact Profile on communication and social interaction were completed pre- and post-treatment. The F and p values for the analysis of variance are presented in Table 9. Pre- and post-treatment means and *SD*s are presented in Table 10. Statistical analysis revealed no significant main effect or interactions for the BDI ($n = 35$) pre- to post-treatment. Statistical analysis of the SIP on communication ($n = 35$) revealed a significant time by treatment group interaction, $F(1,31) = 6.86$, $p = .014$. Only subjects who received the LSVT rated a statistically significant reduction in the impact of their sickness on their communication from pre- to post-treatment. Statistical analysis of the SIP on social interaction ($n = 35$) revealed no significant main effect or interactions pre- to post-treatment.

Correlations to Treatment-Related Change

The relationships between magnitude of treatment-related change and patient suitability or prognostic factors for treatment success were examined. Subject pre- and post-treatment change in SPL during reading the "Rainbow Passage" and conversational monologue were correlated (Pearson product moment) with pretreatment age, stage of disease, rating on the motor examination section of the UPDRS, time since diagnosis, severity of speech disorder, glottal incompetence, dementia (cognitive ability), and depression.

All Subjects

There were no significant correlations for the group as a whole between pre- to post-treatment change in SPL and age, stage of disease, rating on the motor examination section of the UPDRS, time since diagnosis, severity of speech disorder, glottal incompetence, cognitive ability, and depression variables or subject ratings of the impact of their disease on communication and social interaction.

All males. No significant correlations were observed for male subjects between prognostic variables and magnitude of treatment-related change in SPL.

All females. No significant correlations were observed for female subjects between prognostic variables and magnitude of treatment-related change in SPL.

LSVT subjects. There was a significant correlation ($r = .56$, $p = .023$) between the magnitude of pre- to post-treatment change in SPL in monologue ($n = 16$) and mean T score pretreatment. Subjects who had greater cognitive ability pretreatment had greater post-treatment increases in SPL in monologue than subjects with lower cognitive abilities. For the males only in the LSVT group there were no significant correlations between magnitude of treatment-related change in SPL and prognostic variables. For the females only ($n = 5$) there was a significant negative correlation ($r = -.88$, $p = .05$) between magnitude of pre- to post-treatment change in SPL on the "Rainbow Passage" and chronological age. Younger female subjects had greater increases in SPL than did older female subjects.

R subjects. No significant correlations were observed for this group as a whole or male or female subjects in this group between prognostic variables and magnitude of treatment-related change in SPL.

Summary

The following pre- to post-treatment changes were statistically significant for all subjects regardless of treatment group: SPL during conversation, mean habitual fundamental frequency and fundamental frequency variability during reading, maximum duration sustained vowel phonation and utterance duration during reading, and perceptual self-ratings of monotonicity, intelligibility, and initiation of conversation, and family ratings of loudness. Only for subjects who received the LSVT were the following pre- to post-treatment changes statistically significant: SPL during vowels, SPL during reading, fundamental frequency variability in monologue, perceptual self-ratings of loudness (males), family ratings of overall intelligibility, and the Sickness Impact Profile for the impact of Parkinson disease on their communication. Only for subjects who received the R treatment were the following pre- to post-treatment changes statistically significant: SPL during read-

TABLE 9. *F* and *p* values for the neuropsychological variables.

	Between-subject effect						Within-subject effect							
	Group		Gender		Group × Gender		Time		Time × Group		Time × Gender		Time × Group × Gender	
Dependent variables	*F*	*p*	*F*	*p*	*F*	*p*	*F*	*p*	*F*	*p*	*F*	*p*	*F*	*p*
($n = 35$) *df* (1,31)														
BDI (self-rating of depression)	.81	.374	9.17	.005	6.64	.015	.45	.508	1.04	.316	.30	.589	.65	.427
SIP Communication	.02	.886	2.19	.149	1.65	.209	10.95	.002	6.86	.014	.04	.839	.11	.741
SIP Social interaction	.14	.711	.08	.776	4.72	.038	2.36	.135	.23	.635	1.20	.282	.40	.533

TABLE 10. Means and SD's (in parentheses) for the neuropsychological variables completed by subjects both pre- and post-treatment.

Scale (n = 35)	LSVT Pre-treatment	LSVT Post-treatment	R Only Pre-treatment	R Only Post-treatment
BDI (self-rating of depression)				
Group	8.3 (6.0)	7.4 (4.6)	8.7 (5.5)	8.9 (5.3)
Male	6.1 (4.4)	5.8 (3.3)	8.5 (6.3)	8.6 (6.2)
Female	16.3 (4.5)	13.3 (3.9)	9.0 (4.1)	9.6 (2.7)
SIP communication				
Group	28.9 (21.8)	11.9 (11.7)	25.6 (25.1)	23.1 (23.6)
Male	29.2 (19.6)	12.4 (11.5)	32.7 (26.1)	29.1 (26.2)
Female	28.2 (30.2)	10.6 (13.8)	11.5 (17.4)	11.1 (12.0)
SIP Social interaction				
Group	9.6 (8.1)	7.9 (4.4)	11.0 (10.4)	9.7 (11.7)
Male	7.2 (6.3)	6.8 (4.4)	12.6 (10.4)	11.8 (13.2)
Female	16.7 (9.6)	11.5 (2.4)	7.9 (11.0)	5.7 (7.5)

ing (females), pause duration during reading and perceptual self-ratings of loudness (females).

Discussion

This study was designed to compare the effects of two forms of intensive speech treatment (respiration [R] and voice and respiration [Lee Silverman Voice Treatment; LSVT]) on the speech and voice deficits of subjects with Idiopathic Parkinson disease. The study also examined the magnitude of treatment-related change relative to subject characteristics including: age, stage of disease, time since diagnosis, severity of speech/voice disorder, glottal incompetence, depression, and cognitive ability.

The data of this study document that intensive speech treatment, particularly the LSVT, made significant short-term improvements in speech and voice characteristics of the subjects studied. Although the R treatment improved some aspects of speech and voice, the subjects who received the LSVT made greater and more consistent post-treatment changes in intensity and fundamental frequency variation. Furthermore, only subjects who received the LSVT reported significant reductions in the impact of Parkinson disease on oral communication following treatment. Given the low vocal loudness reported in patients with Parkinson disease (Aronson, 1985; Blonder, Gur, & Gur, 1989; Boshes, 1966; Critchley, 1981; Darley, Aronson, & Brown, 1969a, 1969b) and its association with reduced speech intelligibility (Ramig, 1992), these findings distinguish these two forms of speech treatment on an important variable.

These findings are logical outcomes when the focus of treatment for each group is considered. The changes in maximum duration sustained phonation and utterance and pause duration are consistent with the goals of the R treatment. It is likely that R treatment contributed to significant post-treatment increases in duration, magnitude, and frequency of inspiration and expiration and the respiratory system control of volume, pressure, and flow (Dromey et al., 1995). However, only following the LSVT were consistent and significant post-treatment increases in intensity observed. It is likely that the improved respiratory support together with the increased vocal fold adduction observed following the LSVT (Brosovic, 1994; Smith et al., in press) resulted in these significant post-treatment increases in intensity. These findings suggest that treatment that trained both increased vocal fold adduction and respiratory support (LSVT) was necessary to generate significant increases in intensity post-treatment in these subjects with idiopathic Parkinson disease. Increasing respiratory support alone was not sufficient to generate significant and consistent increases in intensity in these glottally incompetent subjects.

The intensity changes pre- to post-treatment for the LSVT group were of a perceptually significant magnitude (Pichney, Durlach, & Braida, 1986; Pickett, 1956) for sustained phonation and reading. The pre- to post-treatment increase in intensity for conversational monologue was statistically significant; however, the magnitude was somewhat less than observed in sustained phonation and reading. Given the cognitive disorders and difficulty with complex tasks observed in patients with Parkinson disease (Berardelli, Dick, Rothwell, Day, & Marsden, 1986; Brooks, 1986), this was not surprising. The finding of a statistically significant correlation between cognitive levels and magnitude of pre- to post-treatment changes in intensity in monologue suggests that it is difficult for the more cognitively impaired subjects with IPD to generalize treatment effects. In addition, increased intensity may be more easily achieved and maintained in a task that requires constant vocal fold adduction (e.g., sustained phonation). The reading and monologue tasks require more dynamic abductory and adductory gestures, as well as more attention and concentration, and might therefore have been more difficult for subjects to maintain at a high phonatory effort level.

The changes observed in habitual fundamental frequency and fundamental frequency variability in these subjects are notable given the fact that these variables were not directly trained in treatment. While both treatment groups improved post-treatment, the magnitude and consistency of improvements of the LSVT subjects were greater. Training of adduction and maximum frequency ranges may be the basis for these post-treatment increases in fundamental frequency and fundamental frequency variability. Another explanation may relate to the perception of the LSVT subjects that their communication skills were much less affected by their disease post-treatment. Only the LSVT subjects rated a significant reduction in the impact of their sickness on their communication skills post-treatment. It may be speculated that as the LSVT subjects improved their ability to communicate, their confidence, attitude, and affect improved. This attitude could be reflected in increased pitch and intonation during speech. Higher pitch and increased pitch variability have been associated with descriptive characteristics of happiness, joyfulness, and confidence (Fairbanks & Pronovost, 1939; Scherer, London, & Wolf, 1973). Improvements in confidence, attitude, and affect are also consistent with our subjective observations of the subjects who received the LSVT immediately post-treatment. This finding suggests that improved communication can play an important role in the psychosocial well-being of individuals with Parkinson disease.

Although activities of respiration were the focus of the R treatment and activities of vocal fold adduction and respiration were the focus of the LSVT, it was apparent by clinical observation that post-treatment changes were observed in magnitude and precision of articulatory gestures as well (Ramig, Dromey, Johnson, & Scherer, 1994). These observations were most apparent in subjects who received the LSVT and are consistent with reports of Schulman (1989) who studied articulatory changes following loud speech in nondisordered speakers. These post-treatment changes in untreated articulation have been quantified in a patient with IPD following a course of the LSVT (Dromey et al., 1995). Such findings are in agreement with those of Scott and Caird (1983) who reported that phonation in particular was a prerequisite for intelligible, effective speech in Parkinson disease and as voice production improved other aspects of speech also improved. In addition, they are consistent with those of Rubow and Swift (1985) who reported a positive relationship between improved loudness and articulatory skills in one patient with Parkinson disease. These observations suggest that multiple levels of speech production in patients with Parkinson disease can benefit from a single treatment focus of increased phonatory effort (Ramig et al., 1994). This is useful information since a treatment that is simple is optimal for IPD patients given their known cognitive disorders and difficulty with complex tasks (Beneckel, Rothwell, Dick, Day, & Marsden, 1986; Yanagisawa, Fujimato, & Tamaru, 1989).

The perceptual data presented here were considered as an initial probe of the impact of treatment-related changes on functional communication. Although the ratings of subjects and family members may be biased and less reliable, they represent one important level of assessment of the perceived impact of treatment on functional communication. These findings suggest that both forms of treatment influenced subject and family perceptions of overall communication skills and are consistent with general positive treatment effects across both groups. However, they also suggest that, consistent with acoustic data, subjects who received the LSVT perceived the greatest impact of the treatment on these perceptual variables.

These findings of significant treatment-related change are in contrast to previous reports from Allan (1970), Aronson (1985), Greene (1980), Sarno (1968), and Weiner and Singer (1989) who concluded that speech treatment was not effective for patients with Parkinson disease. The most reasonable explanation for the positive findings reported here is the focus and style of treatment. Previous approaches to treatment for Parkinson disease have focused on articulation and rate and were administered in the classic speech treatment style of once or twice a week. Both treatments studied here were administered 4 days a week for 16 high effort sessions and focused on respiration (R) or voice and respiration (LSVT). Based upon our findings here, we suggest that intensive treatment with the focus on voice and respiration (LSVT) is effective in increasing vocal intensity in patients with Parkinson disease. These findings are consistent with Scott & Caird (1983) and Robertson & Thompson (1984) who also concluded that intensive voice treatment could increase loudness in patients with Parkinson disease.

We suggest that increasing vocal loudness through high phonatory effort (LSVT), teaches patients to rescale the magnitude of their speech motor output. Such interpretation is consistent with amplitude rescaling changes discussed in other motor systems of patients with Parkinson disease (Teulings & Stelmach, 1991). High effort respiratory (R) treatment generated fewer significant changes in the speech of these patients. Therefore, it appears that high effort with the focus on phonation is a critical combination in the successful treatment of patients with Parkinson disease.

Of the 45 subjects in this investigation, prognostic variables of stage of disease, time since diagnosis, severity of speech disorder, glottal incompetence, and depression did not significantly influence post-treatment effects. Age and cognitive status may influence magnitude of treatment-related change (with younger and more cognitively intact subjects improving more on certain measures). This observation must be studied more closely before conclusive statements are made. It should be noted, however, that most of the subjects studied here were in the mild-to-moderate range of their disease. Further research should be carried out in order to examine more severely involved as well as very recently diagnosed subjects to assess the generalizability of treatment across all stages of IPD. Given the heterogeneous nature of Parkinson disease, it is reasonable to assume that all subjects would not respond to treatment in the same way. This variability is clearly reflected in individual subject responses to treatment. It is important to keep in mind that subject heterogeneity may reduce statistically significant group effects despite positive findings for individual subjects. This is an important consideration in evaluating the efficacy of treatment.

The gender differences observed in certain of the pre- to post-treatment data deserve further consideration. The smaller number of females in both treatment groups, the heterogeneity of the females in the LSVT group and the overall higher depression scores for females limit conclusive statements at this time. However, the findings indicate that further study of the effects of intensive speech treatment for female subjects with idiopathic Parkinson disease is essential.

Databased efficacious treatment programs for patients

the pitch characteristics of the voice during expression of emotion. *Speech Monographs, 6,* 87–104.

Froeschels, E., Kastein, S., Weiss, D. (1955) A method of therapy for paralytic conditions of the mechanisms of phonation, respiration and glutination. *Journal of Speech and Hearing Disorders, 20,* 3645–370.

Gauthier, L., Dalziel, S., & Gauthier, S. (1987). The benefits of group occupational therapy for patients with Parkinson's disease. *American Journal of Occupational Therapy, 41,* 360–365.

Goodglass, H., & Kaplan, E. (1972). *The assessment of aphasia and related disorders.* Philadelphia: Lee and Leafebiger.

Greene, H. C. L. (1980). *The voice and its disorders.* London: Pitman Medical.

Hallet, M., & Khosbin, S. (1980). A psychological mechanism of bradykinesia. *Brain, 103,* 301–314.

Hanson, D. G., Gerratt, B. R., & Ward, P. H. (1984). Cinegraphic observations of laryngeal function in Parkinson's disease. *Laryngoscope, 94,* 348–353.

Hardy, J. (1983). *Cerebral palsy.* Englewood Cliffs, NJ: Prentice-Hall.

Heaton, R. K., Chelune, G., & Lehman, R. A. W. (1978). Using neuropsychology and personality tests to assess the likelihood of patient employment. *Journal of Nervous and Mental Disease, 166,* 408–416.

Heaton, R. K., Grant, I., & Mathews, C. G. (1991). *Comprehensive norms for an expanded Halsted-Reitan battery.* Odessa, FL: Psychological Assessment Resources.

Hixon, T. J., Goldman, M. H., & Mead, J. (1976). Dynamics of the chest wall during speech production: Volume displacements of the rib cage, abdomen, and lung. *Journal of Speech and Hearing Research, 16,* 78–115.

Hixon, T. J., Mead, J., & Goldman, M. D. (1976). Dynamics of the chest wall during speech production: Function of the thorax, rib cage, diaphragm, and abdomen. *Journal of Speech and Hearing Research, 19,* 297–356.

Hoberman, S. G. (1958). Speech techniques in aphasia and Parkinsonism. *Journal of the Michigan State Medical Society, 57,* 1720–1723.

Hoehn, M., & Yahr, M. (1967). Parkinsonism: Onset, progression and mortality. *Neurology, 17,* 427.

Holmberg, E. B., Hillman, R. B., & Perkell, J. (1988) Glottal airflow and transglottal air pressure measurements for male and female speakers in soft, normal and loud voice. *Journal of the Acoustical Society of America, 84,* 511–529.

Horii, Y. (1983). An automatic analysis method of utterance and pause lengths and frequencies. *Behavior Research Methods and Instrumentation, 15,* 449–452.

Hornykiewicz, O. (1966). Metabolism of brain dopamine in human Parkinsonism: Neurochemical and clinical aspects. In E. Costa, L. Cote, & M. Yahr (Eds.), *Biochemistry and pharmacology of the basal ganglia* (pp. 171–185). New York: Raven Press.

Hornykiewicz, O., & Kish, S. J. (1986). Biochemical pathophysiology of Parkinson's disease. In M. D. Yahr & K. J. Bergman (Eds.), *Advances in neurology (pp. 19–34). New York: Raven Press.*

Isshiki, N. (1964). Regulatory mechanisms of voice intensity variation. *Journal of Speech and Hearing Research, 7,* 17–29.

Kempster, G. B. (1984). *A multidimensional analysis of vocal quality in two dysphonic groups.* Unpublished doctoral dissertation, Northwestern University, Evanston, IL.

Kent, R. D., Kent, J. F., & Rosenbek, J. C. (1987). Maximum performance tests of speech production. *Journal of Speech and Hearing Disorders, 52,* 367–387.

King, J. B., Ramig, L. O., Lemke, J., & Horii, Y. (1994). Parkinson's disease: Longitudinal variability in acoustic parameters of phonation. *Journal of Medical Speech-Language Pathology, 2,* 29–42.

Leinonen, L., & Laakso, M. (1990) Control of static pressure by expiratory muscles during expiratory effort and phonation. *Journal of Voice, 4*(3), 256–263.

Leith, D., & Bradley, M. (1976) Ventilatory muscle strength and endurance training. *Journal of Applied Physiology, 41*(4), 508–516.

Levin, B. E., Llabre, M. M., & Weiner, W. J. (1989). Cognitive impairments associated with early Parkinson's disease. *Neurology, 39,* 557–561.

Lewis, R., & Kupke, T. (1977). *The Lafayette clinic repeatable neuropsychological test battery: Its development and research applications.* Paper presented at the annual meeting of the Southeastern Psychological Association, Hollywood, FL.

Logemann, J. A., Fisher, H. B., Boshes, B., & Blonsky, E. R. (1978). Frequency and concurrence of vocal tract dysfunctions in the speech of a large sample of Parkinson patients. *Journal of Speech and Hearing Disorders, 42,* 47–57.

Mayeux, R., Williams, J. B. W., Stern, Y., & Cote, L. (1986). Depression and Parkinson's disease. In M. D. Yahr & K. J. Bergmann (Eds.), *Advances in neurology* (pp. 241–250). New York: Raven Press.

McDowell, F. H., Lee, J. E., & Sweet, R. D. (1986). Extrapyramidal disease. In A. B. Baker & R. J. Joynt (Eds.), *Clinical neurology* (pp. 24–26). Philadelphia: Harper and Row.

McKenzie, D., & Gandevia, S. (1986). Strength and endurance of inspiratory, expiratory, and limb muscles in asthma. *American Review of Respiratory Disease, 134,* 999–1004.

Mead, C., Ramig, L. O., & Beck, J. (1989). Parkinson's disease with dementia: Effectiveness of intensive voice therapy. *Asha, 31*(10), 118.

Milenkovic, P. (1987). Least mean square measures of voice perturbation. *Journal of Speech and Hearing Research, 30,* 529–538.

Montgomery, S. A., & Asberg, M. (1979). A new depression scale designed to be sensitive to change. *British Journal of Psychiatry, 134,* 382–389.

Morley, D. E. (1955). The rehabilitation of adults with dysarthric speech. *Journal of Speech and Hearing Disorders, 20,* 58–64.

Muller, F., & Stelmach, G. E. (1991). Scaling problems in Parkinson's disease. In J. Requin & G. E. Stelmach (Eds.), *Tutorials in motor neuroscience* (pp. 161–174). Netherlands: Kluwer Academic Publishers.

Mutch, W. J., Strudwick, A., Roy, S. L., & Downie, A. W. (1986) Parkinson disease: Disability, review and management. *British Medical Journal, 293,* 675–677.

Netsell, R., & Daniel, B. (1979). Dysarthria in adults: Physiologic approach to rehabilitation. *Archives of Physical Medicine and Rehabilitation, 60,* 502–508.

Netsell, R., & Rosenbek, J. (1986). Treating the dysarthrias. In R. Netsell (Ed.), *A neurobiologic view of speech production and the dysarthrias* (pp. 123–152) San Diego: College-Hill Press.

Oxtoby, M. (1982). *Parkinson's disease patients and their social needs.* London: Parkinson's Disease Society.

Panzarella, K. J. (1995). *Expiratory muscle conditioning in speech-impaired children.* Unpublished thesis, State University of New York at Buffalo.

Perez, K., Ramig, L. O., Smith, M., & Dromey, C. (in press). The Parkinson larynx: Tremor and videostroboscopic findings. *Journal of Voice.*

Pichney, M. A., Durlach, N. I., & Braida, L. D. (1986). Speaking clearly for the hard of hearing: II. Acoustic characteristics of clear and conversational speech. *Journal of Speech and Hearing Research, 29,* 434–446.

Pickett, J. M. (1956). Effects of vocal force on the intelligibility of speech sounds. *Journal of the Acoustical Society of America, 28,* 902–905.

Ramig, L. O. (1992). The role of phonation in speech intelligibility: A review and preliminary data from patients with Parkinson's disease. In R. D. Kent (Ed.), *Intelligibility in speech disorders: Theory, measurement and management* (pp. 119–156). Amsterdam: John Benjamin.

Ramig, L. O. (1995). Speech therapy for patients with Parkinson's disease. In W. C. Koller and G. Paulson (Eds.), *Therapy of Parkinson's disease* (pp. 539–548). New York: Marcel Dekker.

Ramig, L. O., Bonitati, C., Lemke, J., & Horii, Y. (1994). Voice treatment for patients with Parkinson disease: Dévelopment of an approach and preliminary efficacy data. *Journal of Medical Speech-Language Pathology, 2,* 191–209.

Ramig, L. O., Bonitati, C., & Winholtz, W. (1994). *Lee Silverman* the pitch characteristics of the voice during expression of emotion. *Speech Monographs, 6,* 87–104.

Froeschels, E., Kastein, S., Weiss, D. (1955) A method of therapy for paralytic conditions of the mechanisms of phonation, respiration and glutination. *Journal of Speech and Hearing Disorders, 20,* 3645-370.

Gauthier, L., Dalziel, S., & Gauthier, S. (1987). The benefits of group occupational therapy for patients with Parkinson's disease. *American Journal of Occupational Therapy, 41,* 360–365.

Goodglass, H., & Kaplan, E. (1972). *The assessment of aphasia and related disorders.* Philadelphia: Lee and Leafebiger.

Greene, H. C. L. (1980). *The voice and its disorders.* London: Pitman Medical.

Hallet, M., & Khosbin, S. (1980). A psychological mechanism of bradykinesia. *Brain, 103,* 301–314.

Hanson, D. G., Gerratt, B. R., & Ward, P. H. (1984). Cinegraphic observations of laryngeal function in Parkinson's disease. *Laryngoscope, 94,* 348–353.

Hardy, J. (1983). *Cerebral palsy.* Englewood Cliffs, NJ: Prentice-Hall.

Heaton, R. K., Chelune, G., & Lehman, R. A. W. (1978). Using neuropsychology and personality tests to assess the likelihood of patient employment. *Journal of Nervous and Mental Disease, 166,* 408–416.

Heaton, R. K., Grant, I., & Mathews, C. G. (1991). *Comprehensive norms for an expanded Halsted-Reitan battery.* Odessa, FL: Psychological Assessment Resources.

Hixon, T. J., Goldman, M. H., & Mead, J. (1976). Dynamics of the chest wall during speech production: Volume displacements of the rib cage, abdomen, and lung. *Journal of Speech and Hearing Research, 16,* 78–115.

Hixon, T. J., Mead, J., & Goldman, M. D. (1976). Dynamics of the chest wall during speech production: Function of the thorax, rib cage, diaphragm, and abdomen. *Journal of Speech and Hearing Research, 19,* 297–356.

Hoberman, S. G. (1958). Speech techniques in aphasia and Parkinsonism. *Journal of the Michigan State Medical Society, 57,* 1720–1723.

Hoehn, M., & Yahr, M. (1967). Parkinsonism: Onset, progression and mortality. *Neurology, 17,* 427.

Holmberg, E. B., Hillman, R. B., & Perkell, J. (1988) Glottal airflow and transglottal air pressure measurements for male and female speakers in soft, normal and loud voice. *Journal of the Acoustical Society of America, 84,* 511–529.

Horii, Y. (1983). An automatic analysis method of utterance and pause lengths and frequencies. *Behavior Research Methods and Instrumentation, 15,* 449–452.

Hornykiewicz, O. (1966). Metabolism of brain dopamine in human Parkinsonism: Neurochemical and clinical aspects. In E. Costa, L. Cote, & M. Yahr (Eds.), *Biochemistry and pharmacology of the basal ganglia* (pp. 171–185). New York: Raven Press.

Hornykiewicz, O., & Kish, S. J. (1986). Biochemical pathophysiology of Parkinson's disease. In M. D. Yahr & K. J. Bergman (Eds.), *Advances in neurology (pp. 19–34). New York: Raven Press.*

Isshiki, N. (1964). Regulatory mechanisms of voice intensity variation. *Journal of Speech and Hearing Research, 7,* 17–29.

Kempster, G. B. (1984). *A multidimensional analysis of vocal quality in two dysphonic groups.* Unpublished doctoral dissertation, Northwestern University, Evanston, IL.

Kent, R. D., Kent, J. F., & Rosenbek, J. C. (1987). Maximum performance tests of speech production. *Journal of Speech and Hearing Disorders, 52,* 367–387.

King, J. B., Ramig, L. O., Lemke, J., & Horii, Y. (1994). Parkinson's disease: Longitudinal variability in acoustic parameters of phonation. *Journal of Medical Speech-Language Pathology, 2,* 29–42.

Leinonen, L., & Laakso, M. (1990) Control of static pressure by expiratory muscles during expiratory effort and phonation. *Journal of Voice, 4*(3), 256–263.

Leith, D., & Bradley, M. (1976) Ventilatory muscle strength and endurance training. *Journal of Applied Physiology, 41*(4), 508–516.

Levin, B. E., Llabre, M. M., & Weiner, W. J. (1989). Cognitive impairments associated with early Parkinson's disease. *Neurology, 39,* 557-561.

Lewis, R., & Kupke, T. (1977). *The Lafayette clinic repeatable neuropsychological test battery: Its development and research applications.* Paper presented at the annual meeting of the Southeastern Psychological Association, Hollywood, FL.

Logemann, J. A., Fisher, H. B., Boshes, B., & Blonsky, E. R. (1978). Frequency and concurrence of vocal tract dysfunctions in the speech of a large sample of Parkinson patients. *Journal of Speech and Hearing Disorders, 42,* 47–57.

Mayeux, R., Williams, J. B. W., Stern, Y., & Cote, L. (1986). Depression and Parkinson's disease. In M. D. Yahr & K. J. Bergmann (Eds.), *Advances in neurology* (pp. 241–250). New York: Raven Press.

McDowell, F. H., Lee, J. E., & Sweet, R. D. (1986). Extrapyramidal disease. In A. B. Baker & R. J. Joynt (Eds.), *Clinical neurology* (pp. 24–26). Philadelphia: Harper and Row.

McKenzie, D., & Gandevia, S. (1986). Strength and endurance of inspiratory, expiratory, and limb muscles in asthma. *American Review of Respiratory Disease, 134,* 999–1004.

Mead, C., Ramig, L. O., & Beck, J. (1989). Parkinson's disease with dementia: Effectiveness of intensive voice therapy. *Asha, 31*(10), 118.

Milenkovic, P. (1987). Least mean square measures of voice perturbation. *Journal of Speech and Hearing Research, 30,* 529–538.

Montgomery, S. A., & Asberg, M. (1979). A new depression scale designed to be sensitive to change. *British Journal of Psychiatry, 134,* 382–389.

Morley, D. E. (1955). The rehabilitation of adults with dysarthric speech. *Journal of Speech and Hearing Disorders, 20,* 58–64.

Muller, F., & Stelmach, G. E. (1991). Scaling problems in Parkinson's disease. In J. Requin & G. E. Stelmach (Eds.), *Tutorials in motor neuroscience* (pp. 161–174). Netherlands: Kluwer Academic Publishers.

Mutch, W. J., Strudwick, A., Roy, S. L., & Downie, A. W. (1986) Parkinson disease: Disability, review and management. *British Medical Journal, 293,* 675–677.

Netsell, R., & Daniel, B. (1979). Dysarthria in adults: Physiologic approach to rehabilitation. *Archives of Physical Medicine and Rehabilitation, 60,* 502–508.

Netsell, R., & Rosenbek, J. (1986). Treating the dysarthrias. In R. Netsell (Ed.), *A neurobiologic view of speech production and the dysarthrias* (pp. 123–152) San Diego: College-Hill Press.

Oxtoby, M. (1982). *Parkinson's disease patients and their social needs.* London: Parkinson's Disease Society.

Panzarella, K. J. (1995). *Expiratory muscle conditioning in speech-impaired children.* Unpublished thesis, State University of New York at Buffalo.

Perez, K., Ramig, L. O., Smith, M., & Dromey, C. (in press). The Parkinson larynx: Tremor and videostroboscopic findings. *Journal of Voice.*

Pichney, M. A., Durlach, N. I., & Braida, L. D. (1986). Speaking clearly for the hard of hearing: II. Acoustic characteristics of clear and conversational speech. *Journal of Speech and Hearing Research, 29,* 434–446.

Pickett, J. M. (1956). Effects of vocal force on the intelligibility of speech sounds. *Journal of the Acoustical Society of America, 28,* 902–905.

Ramig, L. O. (1992). The role of phonation in speech intelligibility: A review and preliminary data from patients with Parkinson's disease. In R. D. Kent (Ed.), *Intelligibility in speech disorders: Theory, measurement and management* (pp. 119–156). Amsterdam: John Benjamin.

Ramig, L. O. (1995). Speech therapy for patients with Parkinson's disease. In W. C. Koller and G. Paulson (Eds.), *Therapy of Parkinson's disease* (pp. 539–548). New York: Marcel Dekker.

Ramig, L. O., Bonitati, C., Lemke, J., & Horii, Y. (1994). Voice treatment for patients with Parkinson disease: Development of an approach and preliminary efficacy data. *Journal of Medical Speech-Language Pathology, 2,* 191–209.

Ramig, L. O., Bonitati, C., & Winholtz, W. (1994). *Lee Silverman*

Voice Treatment. A treatment video tape. Blue Springs, MO: Wintronix, Inc.

Ramig, L. O., Countryman, S., O'Brien, C., & Smith, M. (1995, May). *Efficacy of voice treatment for Parkinson disease.* Paper presented to the annual meeting of the American Academy of Neurology, Seattle, WA.

Ramig, L. O., Dromey, C., Johnson, A., & Scherer, R. (1994, April). *The effects of phonatory, respiratory and articulatory effect treatment on speech and voice in Parkinson's disease.* Paper presented to the Motor Speech Conference, Sedona, AZ.

Ramig, L. O., Fazoli, K., Scherer, R., & Bonitati, C. (1990, January). *Changes in phonation following voice therapy in patients with Parkinson's disease.* Paper presented to the Clinical Dysarthria Conference, San Antonio, TX.

Ramig, L., Horii Y., & Bonitati, C. (1991). The effectiveness of speech therapy for patients with Parkinson's disease. *National Center for Voice and Speech Research Report, 1,* 61–86.

Ramig, L. O., Mead, C., Scherer, R., Horii, Y., Larson, K., & Kohler, D. (1988, February). *Voice therapy and Parkinson's disease: A longitudinal study of efficacy.* Paper presented at the Clinical Dysarthria Conference, San Diego, CA.

Ramig, L. O., Pawlas, A., & Countryman, S. (1995). *The Lee Silverman Voice Treatment (LSVT): A practical guide to treating the voice and speech disorders in Parkinson disease.* Iowa City, IA: University of Iowa, National Center for Voice and Speech.

Reitan, R. M., & Wolfson, D. (1985). *The Halsted-Reitan Neuropsychological Test Battery.* Tucson, AZ: Neuropsychology Press.

Robin, D. A., Goel, A., Somodi, L. B., & Luschei, E. S. (1992). Tongue strength and endurance: Relation to highly skilled movements. *Journal of Speech and Hearing Research, 35,* 1239–1245.

Rubow, R., & Swift, E. (1985). A microcomputer-based wearable biofeedback device to improve transfer of treatment in Parkinsonian dysarthria. *Journal of Speech and Hearing Disorders, 50,* 178–185.

Sarno, M. T. (1968). Speech impairment in Parkinson's disease. *Archives of Physical Medicine and Rehabilitation, 49,* 269–275.

Scherer, K. R., London, H., & Wolf, J. (1973). The voice of confidence: Paralinguistic cues and audience evaluation. *Journal of Research Personality, 7,* 31–44.

Schiffman, S., Reynolds, M. L., & Young, F. W. (1981). *Introduction to multidimensional scaling: Theory, methods and applications.* New York: Academic Press.

Schmidt, R. A. (1975). A schema theory of discrete motor skill learning. *Psychological Review, 82, 225–260.*

Schmidt, R. A. (1988) *Motor control and learning.* Champaign, IL: Human Kinetic Publishers.

Schulman, R. (1989). Articulatory dynamics of loud and normal speech. *Journal of the Acoustical Society of America, 85,* 295–312.

Scott, S., & Caird, F. L. (1983). Speech therapy for Parkinson's disease. *Journal of Neurology, Neurosurgery and Psychiatry, 46,* 140–144.

Smith, M., Ramig, L. O., Dromey, C., Perez, K., & Samandari, R. (in press). Intensive voice treatment in Parkinson's disease: Laryngostroboscopic findings. *Journal of Voice.*

Stathopoulos, E., & Sapienza, C. (1993a). Respiratory and laryngeal function of women and men during vocal intensity variation. *Journal of Speech and Hearing Research, 36,* 64–75.

Stathopoulos, E., & Sapienza, C. (1993b). Respiratory and laryngeal measures of children during vocal intensity variation. *Journal of the Acoustical Society of America, 94,* 2531–2543.

Stelmach, G. E. (1991). Basal ganglia impairment and force control. In J. Requin & G. E. Stelmach (Eds.), *Tutorials in motor neuroscience* (pp. 137–148). Netherlands: Kluwer Academic Publishers.

Streifler, M., & Hofman, S. (1984). Disorders of verbal expression in Parkinsonism. In R. G. Hassler & J. F. Christ (Eds.), *Advances in neurology* (pp. 385-393). New York: Raven Press.

Teulings, H.-L., & Stelmach, G. E. (1991). Control of stroke size, peak acceleration, and stroke duration in parkinson handwriting. *Human Movement Science, 10,* 315–334.

Titze, I. R., & Sundberg, J. (1992). Vocal intensity in speakers and singers. *Journal of the Acoustical Society of America, 91,* 2936–2946.

Wechsler, D. (1981). *WAIS—R manual.* New York: The Psychological Corporation.

Weiner, W. J., & Singer, C. (1989). Parkinson's disease and nonpharmacologic treatment programs. *Journal of the American Geriatrics Society, 37,* 359–363.

Winholtz, W. S., & Ramig, L. (1992). Vocal tremor analysis with the vocal demodulator. *Journal of Speech and Hearing Research, 35,* 562–573.

Yanagisawa, N., Fujimato, S., & Tamaru, F. (1989). Bradykinesia in Parkinson's disease: Disorders of onset and execution of fast movement. *European Neurology, 29* (Suppl.), 19–28.

Yorkston, K., Buekelman, D., and Bell, K. (1988). *Clinical management of dysarthria speech.* Boston: College Hill.

Received November 18, 1994
Accepted April 28, 1995

Contact author: Lorraine Olson Ramig, PhD, Department of Communication Disorders and Speech Science, University of Colorado, Campus Box 409, Boulder, CO 80309-0409. E-mail: ramig@spot.colorado.edu

Frequency and Effects of Teachers' Voice Problems

Elaine Smith, *Steven D. Gray, *Heather Dove, Lester Kirchner, and †Heidi Heras

*Department of Preventive Medicine, College of Medicine, University of Iowa, Iowa City, Iowa; *Division of Otolaryngology, Department of Surgery, College of Medicine, University of Utah, Salt Lake City, Utah; and †Department of Otolaryngology, College of Medicine, Albany Medical Center, Albany, New York, U.S.A.*

Summary: This study compared the frequency and effects of voice symptoms in teachers to a group of individuals employed in other occupations. Teachers were more likely to report having a voice problem (15 vs. 6%), having 10 specific voice symptoms, and having 5 symptoms of physical discomfort. They averaged almost 2 symptoms compared with none for nonteachers. Likewise, teachers were more likely to perceive that a voice problem would adversely affect their future career options, had done so in the past, and was limiting their current job performance. Over 20% of teachers but none of the nonteachers had missed any days of work due to a voice problem. These findings suggest that teaching is a high-risk occupation for voice disorders and that this health problem may have significant work-related and economic effects. **Key Words:** Epidemiology—Voice disorder—Occupational disease.

Despite the devastating effects of voice problems, there are no reliable data on the prevalence of voice disorders in the adult population, and there is little information about voice problems in potentially high-risk occupational groups. Prevalence estimates of voice disorders are based on decade-old U.S.-National Center for Health Statistics National Health Interview Surveys, and their emphasis is on speech and language impairment rather than on voice disorders, and on children rather than on adults (1,2). Accurate prevalence and incidence data are important in elucidating the causes of voice disorders, describing the frequency with which new disease develops in a population, identifying the characteristics that increase the risk, and developing early screening or disease prevention programs to protect against further deterioration of the larynx and related structures.

Accepted January 30, 1996.

Address correspondence and reprint requests to Dr. E. Smith, Department of Preventive Medicine, College of Medicine, University of Iowa, Iowa City, IA 52242, U.S.A.

The results of this study were presented at the 24th annual Voice Foundation meeting, Philadelphia, 1995.

Several studies have linked potentially vocally demanding vocations to high risk of voice disorders (3–8). Teachers are considered to be at high risk of developing voice disorders due to their professional activities and to their exposure to children who frequently develop upper respiratory infections (URIs). In a study by Gotaas and Starr (7), 80% of teachers who participated in their study indicated that they had experienced problems with fatigue. This symptom was particularly prevalent among teachers who spent more time in activities that were vocally demanding and anxiety producing. In a large study of 237 female teachers (8), the average number of symptoms associated with vocal attrition was four. Those reporting multiple vocal problems were more likely to report that their symptoms adversely affected their work effectiveness and that their voice was a source of continual stress.

Teaching was the most frequent occupation identified in our two university hospital voice clinic populations, comprising 16.4% of those diagnosed with a voice disorder. Yet teachers comprise only 2% of the working population. This is a large professional group in which identification of voice disorders could have wide-reaching implications for all kinds of teachers. Teachers with voice disorders may also be representative of those in other professional groups who use the voice extensively for employment or communication. Some voice disorders identified in this professional group may be amenable to known treatment that they do not currently use; other identified voice disorders may need further research concerning early identification, treatment, or prevention.

The purpose of this preliminary study was to determine the frequency and kinds of vocal problems in a group of teachers and to include a comparison group of nonteaching occupations. An employed comparison group was included to determine whether the frequency and severity of voice symptoms was higher among teachers than in a cross-section of employed adults. Effects of voice problems on past, current, and future employment or career plans were compared between the two groups. Finally, differences in specific communication problems and in the association between number of symptoms and by age were examined.

METHODS

Study population

Participants included employed primary and secondary teachers selected from a northeastern Nevada and a northern Utah school. The self-administered questionnaires were collected from 242 teachers between November 1993 and February 1994. The forms were anonymously completed and returned to one of the research staff (H.H.). Approximately 5% were not collected due to absence from school on the day of administration. The nonteacher comparison group included a random sample of 178 employed adults solicited from 1993 to 1995 who accompanied patients to the Otolaryngology clinic or who were seeking care at the University of Utah Medical Hospital and Dental Clinic for non–voice-related conditions, or who lived in Utah and were solicited from the community. Teachers were excluded from the comparison group. The questionnaires were returned to the speech pathology staff (H.D.) who worked in the voice clinics. Only those between ages 20 and 65 were included in the comparison with teachers. All participants received an approved IRB Human Subjects Consent form before agreeing to complete the questionnaire. The nonteacher group completed the same questionnaire as the teachers and were included in the study to compare the two groups in frequency of voice conditions and the conditions' impact on lifestyle.

Questionnaire

The questionnaire administered to the teacher and comparison groups was designed to elicit information about: (a) the frequency of 10 specific current or past voice symptoms typically associated with voice disorders and the identification of other vocal problems they were experiencing; (b) the degree of physical discomfort associated with those symptoms; (c) current occupation and job changes due to voice symptoms; (d) functional impact of voice problems on work, and communication problems; and (e) social and demographic characteristics of the study population that may represent confounding or biologic risk factors. Instructions requested participants not to limit symptoms they believed were due to work activities because of concern over whether teachers might be more likely than other occupational groups to recall voice problems they thought were related to work activities. Because teachers and those working in other selected occupations may be at high risk of exposure to URIs, potentially URI-related voice symptoms were not excluded.

The functional impact of voice conditions was assessed using questions designed to cover issues that otolaryngologists and speech pathologists commonly experience in their clinical practice with patients presenting with voice symptoms. These questions were asked to determine how frequently participants had experienced adverse work-related effects due to a voice problem and which symptoms were most often reported to produce these adverse effects. They also were asked to identify the impact of their voice on their work activities. The five work-related issues evaluated in association with voice problems were: (a) past job/career decisions, (b) recent job/career decisions, (c) current job performance limitations, (d) job/career change needed, and (e) future limitations in job/career options. These questions were designed to elicit perceived effects on the participant's career or employment rather than in reference to their current job. A second set of questions examined various communication problems due to the voice symptom: (a) overall trouble being understood, (b) problems being understood on the phone, (c) the necessity of repeating statements that were not clearly understood, (d) inability to express oneself, and (e) inability to be understood in background noise.

Statistical analyses

To evaluate the frequency of adverse effects of a voice condition on life-style, responses to these questions were categorized in a Likert-type scale, combining responses of Not At All/Very Little (defined as "no" problem) versus Moderately/Very Much/Extremely (defined as "Yes," a problem); these two groupings were used in the multivariate analyses as well. The Mantel-Haenszel chi-square test was employed to examine the univariate analyses, and the Wilcoxon nonparametric test to report the difference in ordinal means. Odds ratios (ORs) and 95% confidence intervals (CIs) were determined from these procedures (4). ORs designate the risk of voice symptoms or other outcome in the high-risk group (teachers) compared to the risk of the outcome in the unexposed (comparison) group. CIs that do not include unity (1.0) are statistically significant, regardless of whether the range is greater or less than 1.0. CI also provides information about the power of a study to truly detect a difference based on the sample size in the study. Multivariate analyses were used to examine the association between symptomatology and occupational status (teacher/nonteacher) controlling for the potential confounding effects of age, gender, and duration of employment.

RESULTS

Demographic and employment characteristics

Table 1 shows demographic characteristics of the teachers and the comparison group. As is characteristic of primary and secondary teachers, a large proportion were women. Most (93%) participants were non-Hispanic whites (data not shown). The largest percentage of teachers were in their forties, in contrast with the comparison group, who, having a higher proportion of younger individuals, also had a greater portion with fewer years in their current occupation. Among the teachers, the average number of years taught was about 10, but 20% had taught 20 years or more. No specific occupations were frequently reported in the nonteacher group, but titles included salespeople; clerical staff; health care providers; and technicians, craftspersons, and laborers.

Voice symptoms and physical discomfort

When asked whether they thought they currently had a voice problem, 14.6% of teachers and 5.6% of the comparison group responded "Yes" ($p < .0001$). An even larger number of individuals in both groups responded that they currently had experienced a variety of voice symptoms that are associated with voice disorders. Table 2 shows voice symptoms and physical discomfort in order of frequency cited by the teacher and comparison groups. The order of symptom frequency is similar between the two study groups.

TABLE 1. *Characteristics of the teacher and comparison groups*

Characteristic	Teacher %	Teacher (N)	Comparison %	Comparison (N)
Gender				
Female	79.6	(191)	71.3	(127)
Male	20.4	(49)	28.7	(51)
Age (yr)				
20–29	13.1	(31)	32.0	(57)
30–39	26.6	(63)	24.7	(44)
40–49	35.0	(83)	18.0	(32)
≥50	25.3	(60)	25.3	(45)
Years in occupation				
≤5	25.4	(61)	44.9	(71)
6–10	21.3	(51)	20.9	(33)
11–20	33.8	(45)	21.5	(34)
≥21	19.6	(47)	12.7	(20)

Teachers were significantly more likely to report 6 of the 10 voice symptoms about which patients with voice problems commonly are asked by clinicians, and had a higher frequency for each symptom (Table 2). The most common voice symptom currently experienced among teachers was hoarseness. Although this also was true for the comparison group, teachers were more than twice as likely to report this condition. Difficulty with high note singing was reported by over a third of the teaching population. This symptom was reported more than twice as often as in the comparison group. Other voice problems that were significantly more likely to be noted in the teacher group were tired voice, weak voice, effortful voice, and difficulty speaking in low tones.

Specific physical discomfort symptoms were significantly more likely to be reported by teachers as well (Table 2). The frequency reported for discomfort associated with each symptom was fairly similar (9–12%) in teachers. The most common severe problems reported by teachers were a tired and an effortful voice. In contrast, the comparison group reported severity only a third or half as often as the teacher group.

When the two occupational groups were examined for number of symptoms experienced (Table

TABLE 2. *Frequency of voice symptoms and physical discomfort in the teacher and comparison groups*

Voice symptom	Teacher %	Teacher (N)	Comparison %	Comparison (N)
Hoarseness	47.5	(114)	21.3	(38)[a]
H-notes difficult	34.6	(83)	16.9	(30)[a]
Tired voice	19.5	(47)	9.0	(16)[a]
L-speaking voice	18.7	(45)	11.2	(20)[a]
Weak voice	11.6	(28)	4.5	(8)[a]
Effortful	10.4	(25)	3.9	(7)[a]
L-notes difficult	8.3	(20)	5.6	(10)
Breathy	5.4	(13)	2.8	(5)
Voice spasms	2.9	(7)	1.7	(3)
H-speaking voice	3.7	(9)	1.7	(3)
Physical discomfort				
Tiring	11.6	(28)	3.9	(7)[a]
Effortful	11.3	(27)	3.4	(6)[a]
Scratchy	10.5	(25)	6.7	(12)
Ache	9.5	(23)	2.8	(5)[a]
Uncomfortable	9.3	(20)	2.2	(4)[a]
Rough	9.2	(22)	3.4	(6)[a]
No. symptoms[a]				
0	31.8	(77)	64.6	(115)
1	25.6	(62)	16.9	(30)
≥2	42.6	(103)	18.5	(33)
No. physical discomfort symptoms[a]				
0	79.8	(193)	89.3	(159)
1	8.3	(20)	6.2	(11)
≥2	12.0	(29)	4.5	(8)

[a] $p < .05$.

2), teachers reported an average of twice as many symptoms as nonteachers: 2.0 vs. 1.0 ($p < .0001$). Likewise, teachers were twice as likely to report symptoms of physical discomfort: 1.0 vs. 0.0 ($p < .001$). There were no differences between men and women in reported number of symptoms, regardless of occupational group. However, female teachers were more likely than female nonteachers to report two or more symptoms (45.6 vs. 22.1%; $p < .0001$) as were male teachers versus nonteachers (30.6 vs. 15.7%; $p < .001$). The same finding was identified with number of symptoms of physical discomfort for females (20.4 vs. 8.7%; $p < .01$) but not for males (18.4 vs. 15.7%).

Lifestyle effects

Next, the work-related effects of having voice problems were evaluated (Table 3). Teachers were almost twice as likely as nonteachers to identify their voice as a problem in their future vocation. The most adverse work-related effect of having a voice problem in both groups was related to options for a future career. The next most highly rated adverse effect of a voice condition was its effect on their career in the past. Here, the teaching population was three times as likely to have had vocal symptoms that significantly interfered with their performance as a teacher. Even the current job was adversely affected by having a voice condition. The most significant effect among teachers was with limitations the voice problem placed on their current job performance. Teachers were also much more likely to associate their voice problems with limiting their current job decisions and their ability to change their career ($p = .07$, each response).

TABLE 3. *Frequency of adverse effects of work-related voice disorders on work life among teacher and comparison groups*

Effect	Teacher %	Teacher (N)	Comparison %	Comparison (N)
Work				
Past job/career	12.2	(29)	4.0	(7)[a]
Current: limit job decisions	5.0	(12)	1.7	(3)
Current: limit job performance	9.2	(21)	1.2	(2)[a]
Current: change job/career	4.2	(10)	1.2	(2)
Future job/career options	39.7	(74)	26.5	(45)[a]
Communication				
Background noise	9.2	(22)	6.7	(12)
Can't express self	6.6	(16)	4.0	(7)
Repeat statements	6.2	(15)	4.5	(8)
Trouble being understood	4.6	(11)	4.5	(8)
Telephone problems	4.2	(10)	4.5	(8)

[a] $p < .05$.

These work-related responses are in sharp contrast to those reported in the comparison group who rarely noted any past or current effects. Despite these differences in the effects of the voice on their occupation, teachers were not more likely than nonteachers to have changed (0.0 vs. 0.5%) their current occupation as a result of having a voice problem. Most significantly, when asked how many days they had missed from work due to their voice problem during the past year, >20% of teachers but none of the nonteachers had missed any workdays due to a voice problem.

Although there were no significant differences in frequency of reporting communication difficulties between teachers and other occupational groups (Table 3), the most common communication problem was talking over background noise, an everyday situation among teachers today. Teachers also were more likely to be unable to express themselves or were asked more frequently to repeat their statements than were nonteachers.

Association between number of voice problems and age and duration in employment

Table 4 shows differences between number of voice symptoms and number of physical discomfort symptoms by age and years of employment. Because of the difference in age frequency and years of employment between the teacher and nonteacher groups, we evaluated whether these two factors might influence the frequency of reporting a voice disorder. Table 4 shows the results of the stratified assessments. The likelihood of reporting two or more symptoms or one or more symptoms of physical discomfort was greater in the teacher group than in the comparison group for each age and each years of employment category. The number of symptoms and physical discomfort symptoms increased with age in the teacher group, whereas in the comparison group there were no age-related effects. Likewise, with increasing years of employment, the teacher group but not the comparison group reported a greater number of voice symptoms and symptoms of physical discomfort. Female teachers were more likely than male teachers to cite two or more symptoms (45.6 vs. 30.6%) but not more symptoms of physical discomfort (12.0 vs. 10.2%; data not shown).

When risk of reporting vocal symptoms was compared by occupational group, teachers were at greater risk of having voice symptoms (OR = 3.5, 95% CI: 2.3–5.4) and symptoms of physical discomfort (OR = 2.06, CI: 1.14–3.74). Thus, teachers incurred a 3½-fold greater likelihood of vocal symptomatology and a two-fold increase of reporting symptoms of physical discomfort associated with vocal disorders compared with nonteachers. The risk factors gender, age, or years of employment did not significantly change the association between being a teacher and reporting greater risk of having voice symptoms and physical discomfort; nor were they significant independent risk factors of symptomatology.

DISCUSSION

The results of this preliminary investigation suggest that teachers are at high risk of voice symptoms compared with others in the working popula-

TABLE 4. *Voice symptoms and physical discomfort associated with age and years of employment among teacher and comparison groups*

	No. symptoms[a]			No. physical discomfort symptoms[a]	
	0	1	≥2	0	≥1
Characteristic	Teacher/comparison	Teacher/comparison	Teacher/comparison	Teacher/comparison	Teacher/comparison
Age (yr)					
20–29	19.4 (6) 64.9 (37)	41.9 (13) 21.1 (12)	38.7 (12) 14.0 (8)	87.1 (27) 89.5 (51)	12.9 (4) 10.5 (6)
30–39	34.9 (22) 69.2 (18)	25.4 (16) 15.4 (4)	39.7 (25) 15.4 (4)	81.0 (51) 90.9 (40)	19.1 (12) 9.1 (4)
40–49	34.9 (22) 66.7 (16)	21.7 (18) 12.5 (3)	43.4 (36) 20.8 (5)	79.5 (66) 87.5 (28)	20.5 (17) 12.5 (4)
≥50	31.7 (15) 66.7 (28)	23.3 (14) 16.7 (7)	45.0 (27) 16.7 (7)	75.0 (45) 88.9 (40)	25.0 (15) 11.1 (5)
Years in occupation					
≤5	29.5 (18) 64.8 (46)	31.2 (19) 18.3 (13)	39.3 (24) 16.9 (12)	83.6 (51) 85.9 (61)	16.4 (10) 14.1 (10)
6–10	27.5 (14) 57.6 (19)	27.5 (14) 12.1 (4)	45.1 (23) 30.3 (12)	78.4 (40) 93.9 (31)	21.6 (11) 6.1 (2)
11–20	35.8 (29) 58.8 (20)	23.5 (19) 26.5 (9)	40.7 (33) 14.7 (5)	82.7 (67) 88.2 (30)	17.3 (14) 11.8 (4)
≥21	31.3 (15) 80.0 (16)	20.8 (10) 5.0 (1)	47.9 (23) 15.0 (3)	72.3 (34) 95.0 (19)	27.7 (13) 5.0 (1)

[a] Percent positive response.

tion. The findings also indicate that these adverse health conditions have or could have adverse work-related effects on employment among teachers. This is one of the first studies to confirm clinical impressions that teachers are more likely than those in other occupations to have a significantly higher frequency of specific voice symptoms and physical discomfort associated with those symptoms, and to have work-related problems as a result of these voice conditions. Although it is likely that other occupational groups also suffer a higher frequency of voice conditions (e.g., trial lawyers, telephone operators, or ministers), these groups are not as commonly seen in our voice clinics. However, these occupations also comprise a smaller percentage of the working population than do teachers.

Over one-fifth of the teacher population reported missing work as a result of a voice problem. Although only a small percentage of teachers (4.2%) in this study reported thinking about changing their current job because of their voice problems, and none had reported doing so in the past, it is unclear what percentage may have taken early retirement as a result of their health problem and thus were not available for interview. In 1993 alone, 20% of the teaching population in the U.S. retired due to a health problem, while another 8% stopped teaching to pursue a different career (9). These are large percentages for a single occupation that does not require severe physical exertion as in other jobs. Unfortunately, neither workers' compensation nor occupational medicine specialists yet recognize voice problems as work-related risks. In support of these national statistics, we found an association between duration of employment as a teacher and increasing symptomatology and physical discomfort, suggesting that those who feel increasing difficulty in teaching due to their voice problems may change their career or retire. In contrast, neither age nor years of employment were associated with symptomatology or physical discomfort in the comparison group. The higher frequency of vocal symptoms experienced by teachers (67%) compared with nonteachers (33%), regardless of age, suggests that this profession is at high risk and needs to be taught how to compensate for the voice demands of their vocation. Teachers clearly have high demands on their vocal mechanism because they not only have to use their voices for a long duration, but also speak over loud background noise and are continually exposed to URIs that adversely affect their vocal apparatus.

One of the NIDCD research priorities is to characterize the prevalence of voice disorders in high-risk adult populations; another priority is to assess the economic and work-related impact of voice disorders. People who have these conditions are often unable to function in work activities, and careers may be lost. To date, however, only a few studies have described the frequency of voice disorders in adult populations; and these focus on a narrow range of disorders. Existing studies are based primarily on clinical (nonrandom/biased) patients, utilize small sample sizes, or do not include a comparison group. Investigations have not evaluated the range of voice disorders that may occur in a high-risk occupational group. Nor have studies collected data or statistically analyzed populations by gender, race, or other potential exposures for risks of voice dysfunction. Research of this nature typically requires an epidemiologic approach and large sample sizes before results are forthcoming.

Our study provides preliminary data of a potentially high-risk occupation using a nonclinical setting and including a comparison group. Further research needs to confirm if teachers are at greater risk of vocal disorders, to determine if changes in their employment are due to voice problems, and to clarify which voice-related problems occur as a result of specific teaching activities. In addition to controlling for the confounding effects of disease-related risks (URIs) in this occupation, details regarding work activities that may differentiate those teachers with voice problems from those without them need further exploration. This information subsequently should be used to develop health education programs targeted for this high-risk occupation, to initiate research in disease prevention, and to identify the burden of health care provider services that will be needed to resolve these unmet needs. Vocal hygiene intervention over the course of the school year may be useful in reducing vocal fatigue, hoarseness, and other symptoms associated with teaching, and may need to be incorporated into the training and retention of teachers.

Acknowledgment: This research was supported by NIH NIDCD R55 DC02285-01 (E.M.S., L.K.), NIH NIDR P50 DE10758-0281 (E.M.S., L.K.), and NIH NIDCD P60 DC00976-04 (S.D.G., H.D.).

REFERENCES

1. The prevalence of speech and language impairments. *ASHA* 1983;25:37.

2. Leske MC. Prevalence estimates of communicative disorders in the U.S. Speech disorders. *ASHA* 1981;23:217–24.
3. Reich A, McHenry M, Keaton A. A survey of dysphonic episodes in high-school cheerleaders. *Lang Speech Hear Sev Sch* 1986;17:63–71.
4. Sapir S. Vocal attrition in voice students: survey findings. *J Voice* 1993;7:69–74.
5. Sapir S, Attias J, Sharar A. Symptoms of vocal attrition in women army instructors and new recruits: results from a survey. *Laryngoscope* 1990;100:991–4.
6. Peppard R, Bless D, Milenkovic P. Comparison of young adult singers and nonsingers with vocal nodules. *J Voice* 1988;2:250–60.
7. Gotaas C, Starr CD. Vocal fatigue among teachers. *Folia Phoniatr Logop* 1993;45:120–9.
8. Sapir S, Keidar A, Mathers-Schmidt B. Vocal attrition in teachers: survey findings. *Eur J Disord Comm* 1993;28:177–85.
9. Crispnell D. American Demographics 1994. *Wall Street Journal* July 29, 1994:B1.

5

Laryngopharyngeal Reflux and Its Sequelae

Introduction

Papers on laryngopharyngeal reflux (LPR) are among the most often cited in laryngology. In fact, Koufman's Triologic thesis on the topic, reproduced here in its entirety, is the most frequently cited single paper in this collection. This is a clear reflection of a sea change in the perception of the role of LPR in the pathogenesis of laryngeal injury—from irrelevant to fundamental, as much as smoking and phonotrauma are. The number of citations is also without a doubt a reflection of controversy. For a period of several years, hardly an issue of our major professional journals seemed to be without at least one, and often multiple works dealing with the subject. These were just as likely to be contradictory as confirmatory, and debate raged about various aspects of LPR. The furor has yet to dwindle.

The controversy has yielded an interesting clinical paradox: LPR may have become at once the most underdiagnosed and the most overdiagnosed clinical entity in laryngology (although vocal fold paresis may yet challenge it in both categories). Many patients with a variety of laryngeal complaints—especially laryngospasm, cough, throat discomfort, or even pain—have not been investigated or treated for reflux, despite having seen multiple physicians. At the same time, many patients present to the laryngologist with laryngeal lesions and disorders—some of them subtle, some of them less so—whose complaints have been attributed entirely to LPR. Sadly, LPR now seems to occupy the place once held by "allergies," "postnasal drip," and "voice abuse," a diagnosis not of exclusion but of dismissal. LPR has come to be regarded by some as so ubiquitous that they consider it an adequate explanation for hoarseness that should be further investigated. Both aspects of this situation are a product of confusion. The unreliability of clinical signs for diagnosis, the vast differences in the conception of the disease across specialties (principally otolaryngology and gastroenterology/internal medicine), disagreement about the utility and type of diagnostic testing, and about what constitutes adequate treatment have all led to an ambiguous clinical picture that has caused some to attribute virtually every laryngeal complaint to LPR, at the same time that others have found it so bewildering as to ignore it or turn indiscriminately skeptical.

The story of LPR in laryngology is not an entirely new one. The first chapter was written well before LPR was distinguished from gastroesophageal reflux disease, when reflux was solidly established as a major cause in the formation of laryngeal contact ulcer and granuloma. These papers are cited in the following roster, and one is presented in full. In his accompanying commentary, Dr. Cherry recalls the inspirations and the circumstances surrounding his work. Subsequently, the importance of LPR was gradually appreciated, first in subglottic stenosis and laryngospasm, and then in other benign laryngeal pathologies. This important evolution is recounted from a personal perspective by Dr. Toohill. Dr. Koufman has devoted much of her career to a determined investigation of reflux-related laryngeal injury. From her Triologic thesis until today, she has been a vocal advocate of the need for aggressive treatment of LPR in a number of laryngeal diseases. Her commentary acknowledges that LPR remains contentious, and offers an important insight into recent developments in thinking in this field that may explain some of the discrepancies and apparent contradictions. Finally, the position statement issued by the Speech, Voice & Swallowing Committee of the AAO-HNS presents a snapshot of where the consensus on the subject stood in 2002.

Much more remains to be written before the place of LPR in the spectrum of laryngeal disease can be accurately assessed. There is no doubt, though, that the field has experienced a crucial awakening, reflected in the classic papers presented in this section.

Classic Articles

●Reprint of article included in this chapter.
♦Commentary on this article.

●♦Cherry J, Margulies SI. Contact ulcer of the larynx. *Laryngoscope.* 1968;78(11):1937–1940.

Delahunty JE, Cherry J. Experimentally produced vocal cord granulomas. *Laryngoscope.* 1968;78(11):1941–1947.

Kambic V, Radsel Z. Acid posterior laryngitis. Aetiology, histology, diagnosis and treatment. *J Laryngol Otol.* 1984;98(12):1237–1240.

Little FB, Koufman JA, Kohut RI, Marshall RB. Effect of gastric acid on the pathogenesis of subglottic stenosis. *Ann Otol Rhinol Laryngol.* 1985;94(5 pt 1):516–519.

Gaynor EB. Gastroesophageal reflux as an etiologic factor in laryngeal complications of intubation. *Laryngoscope.* 1988;98(9):972–979.

Wilson JA, White A, Heading RC, Von Haacke NP, Pryde A. Maran AGD, Piris J. Gastroesophageal reflux and posterior laryngitis. *Ann Otol Rhinol Laryngol.* 1989; 98(6):405–410.

Weiner GJ, Koufman JA, Wu WC, Cooper JB, Richter JE, Castell DO. Chronic hoarseness secondary to gastroesophageal reflux disease: documentation with 24-H ambulatory pH monitoring. *Am J Gastroenterol.* 1989; 84(12):503–1508.

●♦Koufman JA. The otolaryngologic manifestations of gastroesophageal reflux disease (GERD): a clinical investigation of 225 patients using ambulatory 24-hour pH monitoring and an experimental investigation of the role of acid and pepsin in the development of laryngeal injury. *Laryngoscope.* 1991;101(4 pt 2, suppl 53):1–64.

Gaynor EB. Otolaryngologic manifestations of gastroesophageal reflux. *Am J Gastroenterol.* 1991;86(7):801–808.

Wetmore RF. Effects of acid on the larynx of the maturing rabbit and their possible significance to the sudden infant death syndrome. *Laryngoscope.* 1993;103(11 pt 1): 1242–1254.

Hanson DG, Kamel PL, Kahrilas PJ. Outcomes of antireflux therapy for the treatment of chronic laryngitis. *Ann Otol Rhinol Laryngol.* 1995;104(7):550–555.

Loughlin CJ, Koufman JA. Paroxysmal laryngospasm secondary to gastroesophageal reflux. *Laryngoscope.* 1996;106(12 pt 1):1502–1505.

Koufman J, Sataloff RT, Toohill R. Laryngopharyngeal reflux: consensus conference report. *J Voice.* 1996; 10(3):215–216.

●♦Toohill RJ, Kuhn JC. Role of refluxed acid in pathogenesis of laryngeal disorders. *Am J Med.* 1997;103(5A): 100S–106S.

Wo JM, Grist WJ, Gussack G, Delgaudio JM, Waring JP. Empiric trial of high-dose omeprazole in patients with posterior laryngitis: a prospective study. *Am J of Gastroenterol.* 1997;92(12):2160–2165.

Kuhn J, Toohill RJ, Ulualp SO, Kulpa J, Hofmann C, Arndorfer R, Shaker R. Pharyngeal acid reflux events in patients with vocal cord nodules. *Laryngoscope.* 1998;108(8 pt 1):1146–1149.

Halstead LA. Role of gastroesophageal reflux in pediatric upper airway disorders. *Otolaryngol Head Neck Surg.* 1999;120(2):208–214.

Ulualp SO, Toohill RJ, Hoffmann R, Shaker R. Pharyngeal pH monitoring in patients with posterior laryngitis. *Otolaryngol Head Neck Surg.* 1999;120(5):672–677.

●♦Koufman JA, Aviv JE, Casiano RR, Shaw GY. Laryngopharyngeal reflux: position statement of the Committee on Speech, Voice, and Swallowing Disorders of the American Academy of Otolaryngology-Head and Neck Surgery. *Otolaryngol Head Neck Surg.* 2000; 127(1):32–35.

Koufman JA, Amin MR, Panetti M. Prevalence of reflux in 113 consecutive patients with laryngeal and voice disorders. *Otolaryngol Head Neck Surg.* 2000;123(4): 385–388.

Wong RKH, Hanson DG, Waring PJ, Shaw G. ENT manifestations of gastroesophageal reflux. *Am J Gastroenterol.* 2000;95(8 suppl):S15–S22.

Belafsky PC, Postma GN, Koufman JA. Laryngopharyngeal reflux symptoms improve before changes in physical findings. *Laryngoscope.* 2001;111(6):979–981.

Belafsky PC, Postma GN, Koufman JA. The validity and teliability of the Reflux Finding Score (RFS). *Laryngoscope.* 2001;111(8):1313–1317.

Belafsky PC, Postma GN, Koufman JA. Validity and reliability of the reflux symptom index (RSI). *J Voice.* 2002;16(2):274–277.

Jaspersen D, Kulig M, Labenz J, Leodolter A, Lind T, Meyer-Sabellek W, et al. Prevalence of extra-oesophageal manifestations in gastro-oesophageal reflux disease: an analysis based on the ProGERD Study. *Alimentary Pharmacol Therapeut.* 2003;17(12):1515–1520.

Richter JE. Extraesophageal presentations of gastroesophageal reflux disease. *Sem Gastrointest Dis.* 2007; 8(2):75–89.

Commentary

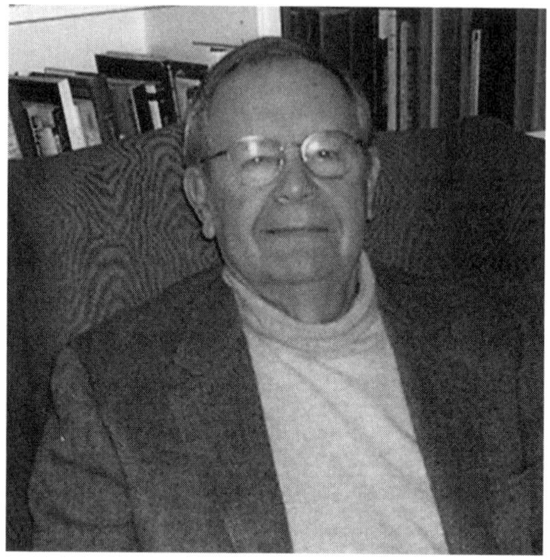

Jerrie Cherry, MD

In the mid-1960s, there was interest in the frequency and extent of gastroesophageal reflux. At John's Hopkin's Hospital there was a medical scientific club that met regularly where various investigators reported on their work in progress. Dr. Martin Donner, professor of radiology, reported on his work on seniesophagrams and acid barium meals in which he showed that gastric reflux was quite frequent and I noticed that extended up to and possibly into the pharynx. This led me to study the effects of gastric juices in the larynx. We had cases of contact ulcers of the larynx not made better by standard therapies such as antacids, there was no Prilosec then, but they were helped on the old antacid regimens and small meals, etc. Then we tried to make contact ulcers in dogs by painting their vocal cords with their gastric aspirate over a period of time. We thought that when we showed that gastric juices went into the larynx and caused lesions we felt that longstanding reflux could cause other lesions in the larynx possibly even leading to cancer and that lesions of the lungs such as bronchitis or bronchiectasis might be influenced by this longstanding repeated gastrolaryngeal and respiratory reflux.

So much of what a young investigator does is influenced by his environment; Hopkins in the 1960s was a smallish workplace with open labs and very free exchange of ideas where a young assistant professor could talk with the professor of various disciplines in great ease and the professor would listen and encourage you. We hoped and even half-expected that some of our work would stand out. In late 1968, I went to Vanderbilt Medical School as chairman of Otolaryngology and Head and Neck Surgery and published only one more paper on reflux and the pharyngolarynx in 1970. However, the wave of interest in gastroesophageal reflux has continued and, as we hoped, many others have expanded this work into the larynx and respiratory tract during the past 40 years, further demonstrating the relationship of faulty deglutition and respiratory problems and laryngeal lesions.

CONTACT ULCER OF THE LARYNX.

JERRIE CHERRY, M.D.,
and
STANLEY I. MARGULIES, M.D.,
Baltimore, Md.

The contact ulcer of the larynx, a benign lesion found on the posterior portion of the vocal cords, can be a most difficult problem as it is often refractory to the standard types of therapy.

Vocal abuse is the accepted causative factor. It is postulated that repeated trauma from vocal abuse causes the mucosa over the vocalis process to be denuded with the resultant growth of granulation tissue. Hoarseness develops when complete closure of the glottis is prevented by this mass of granulation tissue.

The recommended therapy has been both vocal rehabilitation and local removal of the excessive granulations; but often little benefit results from this form of therapy. Because of the poor results from this accepted form of therapy, the possibility that other factors might be involved in the production of the contact ulcer was explored.

The development of more sophisticated radiographic techniques allowed a more careful study of the laryngopharynx and esophagus during deglutition by the combined use of image intensified fluoroscopy and radiography. The supplemental use of the "acid barium" meal makes possible the diagnosis of reflux peptic esophagitis and by combining these techniques esophagopharyngeal reflux can be visualized.

Three patients with persistent contact ulcers of the larynx refractory to the accepted treatment were studied, using the cine esophagram pharyngography with an acid barium meal.

Editor's Note: This manuscript received in THE LARYNGOSCOPE Office and accepted for publication November 27, 1967.

Request for reprints should be sent to Jerrie Cherry, M.D., Division of Otolaryngology, Vanderbilt University, Nashville, Tenn. 37203.

All three patients showed reflux peptic esophagitis, and when the esophageal motility disturbances occurred, showed reflux from the esophagus through the cricopharyngeus muscle into the pharynx.

None of these patients volunteered symptoms suggestive of peptic esophagitis, but on careful questioning each patient had typical symptoms of reflux peptic esophagitis.

CASE REPORTS.

Case 1. P. M., a 62-year-old white business executive, a non-smoker, was first seen in July, 1965, with the chief complaint of tightness in his throat and hoarseness of eight months' duration. He related the onset of his hoarseness to excessive vocal abuse during an Army-Navy football game in November, 1964. His hoarseness was painless in nature and was intermittent in character. During the eight months prior to his visit, his symptoms had gradually increased to paroxysms of coughing and an almost continual sensation of a "lump in my throat" which necessitated frequent efforts to clear his throat. His voice was so weak that he could not carry on his usual business conferences.

He spoke with a breathy quality, and his voice had a limited volume. The larynx showed a granular red-gray mass on the posterior surface of the left true vocal cord abutting on the arytenoid process and overhanging the free edge. Biopsy of this material showed granulation tissue confirming the diagnosis.

The patient was then treated with voice rest, vocal rehabilitation, antibiotics and steroids without significant change in his larynx or voice. In the Winter of 1965, the ulceration of the left cord diminished, but bilateral diffuse redness of the endolarynx persisted. He continued his voice therapy throughout the Winter of 1966, yet his hoarseness grew worse as did the sensation of a lump in his throat. At this time indirect laryngoscopy revealed an enlarged granular lesion on the posterior surface of the left vocal cord.

Because of the nocturnal paroxysms of coughing associated with shortness of breath and a sour taste in his mouth, his digestive history was carefully reviewed. He had typical symptoms of reflux peptic esophagitis. On the basis of this information a cine esophagram with an acid barium meal was performed. Clear evidence of acid induced esophageal motility disturbance was found, and gastro-esophageal reflux and esophagopharyngeal reflux was demonstrated. The patient was started on a regimen for peptic esophagitis, consisting of liquid antacids after meals and at bedtime, elevation of the head of the bed eight inches and no food for three hours before bedtime.

On this regimen alone, he showed improvement in two months and in six months his larynx and voice were normal; furthermore, his indigestion had been completely relieved.

Case 2. A. M. This 53-year-old white male business man and preacher was first seen in December, 1965, with a history of hoarseness of two years' duration. His hoarseness was intermittent for many months becoming constant during the Spring of 1965. Although he was aware of a sensation of something in his throat which necessitated coughing and frequent efforts to clear his throat, he had no pain whatsoever.

In December, 1965, a direct laryngoscopy was done, and the biopsy of the laryngeal mass was reported as benign granulation tissue; however, the patient's symptoms persisted, and he sought other medical help. When we first saw the patient there were granular lesions on the posterior aspects of both vocal cords, more pronounced on the left. Biopsy again revealed granulation tissue confirming the diagnosis of contact ulcer of the larynx. The patient was initially treated with voice rest, then speech therapy for several months and finally with two courses of antibiotics and steroids. His voice remained hoarse, and his larynx was diffusely red with granular raised lesions on the posterior aspect of each vocal cord.

In January, 1967, careful questioning of the patient's digestive history revealed symptoms of acid peptic disease and reflux esophagitis. A cine esophagram with an acid barium meal showed peptic esophagitis and both gastroesophageal and esophagopharyngeal reflux. The patient was started on a regimen of antacids between meals and after meals, elevation of the head of his bed eight inches and restriction of food for three hours prior to bedtime.

In two months his larynx improved, there being no redness and only a small amount of granulation tissue. His voice was normal, and his throat symptoms had disappeared. After six months of therapy his larynx was normal and no symptoms of esophagitis remained.

Case 3. A. C. This 51-year-old white non-smoking, business man was first seen in September, 1966, with a five-month history of tightness in his throat and painless hoarseness. On indirect laryngoscopy, one could see a granular raised lesion on the posterior superior surface of the right true vocal cord with some overhang into the glottic lumen. A direct laryngoscopy with biopsy confirmed the diagnosis of contact ulcer of the larynx. The patient was treated with voice rest and vocal rehabilitation by speech therapy without improvement of his larynx or voice. Two courses of antibiotics and steroids were then employed without objective or subjective improvement.

Approximately five months after this patient was first seen questions regarding his digestive history indicated symptoms of esophagitis. A cine esophagram with an acid barium meal confirmed peptic esophagitis and showed gastroesophageal reflux and esophagopharyngeal reflux. This patient was started on a similar regimen for peptic esophagitis. In three months his larynx and voice were virtually normal, there remaining only a small raised lesion on the right vocal cord. Two months later his larynx was normal.

DISCUSSION.

Since Chevalier Jackson described the contact ulcer in 1928, the etiology has been thought to be only vocal abuse. It has been stated that, as the anterior tip of one vocalis process meets the anterior tip of the opposite vocalis process, their mucosal surfaces may be injured, allowing granulation tissue to develop, thus forming a contact ulcer. While some patients are cured merely by vocal rehabilitation which is directed towards this etiology, others are resistant to this standard means of therapy. It is in this group that additional etiological factors must be sought.

We, therefore, suggest that an additional factor may be involved in the development of contact ulcers of the larynx. Pharyngolaryngeal reflux of gastric material bathes the larynx with acidic material causing inflammation of the vocal cord mucosa thus enhancing its breakdown while stimulating the formation of granulation tissue.

The three patients described in this report were first treated by voice rest, voice rehabilitation, antibiotics and steroids but failed to show significant improvement; however, intensive treatment of their peptic esophagitis resulted in prompt and apparently permanent objective and subjective cures.

Esophagopharyngeal reflux may well be a factor in causing other laryngopharyngeal problems, for the possible relationship of gastric reflux to contact ulcers of the larynx adds a new dimension in the evaluation of laryngeal pathology; therefore, additional information may be forthcoming in other laryngeal lesions by a more wide spread use of the cine esophagram with an acid barium meal.

BIBLIOGRAPHY.

1. DONNER, M. W.; SILBIGER, M. L.; HOOKMAN, P., and HENDRIX, T. R.: Acid Barium Swallows in the Radiographic Evaluation of Clinical Esophagitis. *Radiol.*, 87:220-225, Aug., 1966.

2. HOLINGER, P. H., and JOHNSTON, K. C.: Contact Ulcer of the Larynx. *Jour. A.M.A.*, 172:511-515, Feb., 1960.

3. JACKSON, C.: Contact Ulcer of Larynx. *Arch. Otol.*, 22:1, July, 1935.

4. JACKSON, C.: Contact Ulcer of the Larynx. *Ann. Otol.*, 37:227-230, March, 1928.

5. NEW, G. B., and DEVINE, K. D.: Contact Ulcer Granuloma. *Ann. Otol.*, 58:548-558, June, 1949.

6. PEACHER, G. M.: Vocal Therapy for Contact Ulcer of the Larynx. THE LARYNGOSCOPE, 71:37-47, Jan., 1961.

7. VON LEDEN, H., and MOORE, P.: Contact Ulcer of the Larynx. *Arch. Otol.*, 72:746-752, Dec., 1960.

Commentary

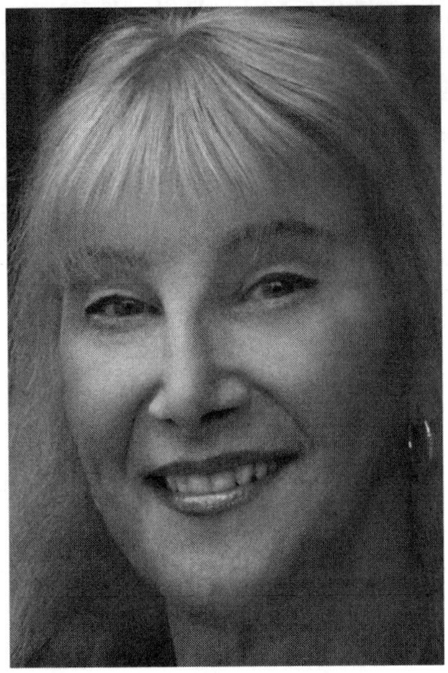

Jamie Koufman, MD, FACS

I have been interested in laryngology for 35 years; but 1981 was a watershed year for me. That's when I stopped doing the *oto* and *rhino* parts of *otorhinolaryngology*. That same year, I first became aware of *gastroesophageal reflux disease* (GERD) that affected the larynx. Ever since, I have specialized in laryngology and *laryngopharyngeal reflux* (LPR) has been the main focus of my research. From a personal perspective, the early years of LPR weren't easy. For at least a decade people were very skeptical, even laughed, when I spoke about LPR at national meetings. The apparent joke was that I was delusional, that I was so preoccupied with LPR that reason and good judgment had abandoned me. That LPR remains so controversial is surprising as there is now credible science; and I believe that clinical observations that I had in the 1980s, expressed in my Triological thesis[1] will stand the test of time.

Some people who deserve credit for seminal thinking in LPR and who most influenced me were Nels Olson, Paul Ward, Paul Chodosh, and Bob Toohill. I remember Dr. Olson warning me that LPR was contentious. He told me that some of his academic contemporaries had tried to discredit him because of his beliefs that LPR was ubiquitous and caused a myriad of airway diseases. Of course when Dr. Olson talked about reflux, it was GERD. It wasn't until 1991 that I coined the term *laryngopharyngeal reflux*, the same year as the publication of my thesis.[1] I felt that we needed a new term to for the type of "silent" reflux disease that our patients demonstrated. I chose the term laryngopharyngeal reflux to call attention to the fact that the symptoms and manifestations were laryngeal and pharyngeal, that is, not esophageal. I also believed that the diagnosis and treatment of LPR were different than those for GERD.

The idea was to intentionally create a nosological schism between the specialties so that otolaryngologists would consider new ideas that were not yet acknowledged by gastrointestinal (GI) colleagues. Incidentally, the term *silent reflux* was coined by Dr. Walter Bo, chair of the anatomy department at Wake Forest University. Walter was my patient in 1988, and he had LPR. After I had explained how one could have reflux without heartburn, Dr. Bo rolled his eyes and then announced, "I see; I have the silent kind of reflux."

Early on I recognized that LPR was controversial, because for almost 5 years I couldn't get anything published on the subject. Papers on the laryngeal findings, prevalence of LPR, as well as papers about the possible relationship between LPR and laryngeal cancer were rejected outright. Perhaps intended as a warning, the comments of one anonymous reviewer for a prestigious journal were forwarded to me, "Something has to be done about Koufman's preoccupation with GERD"; and the reviewer went on to actually suggest that I was on the payroll of one of the big pharmaceutical companies. This was certainly untrue! I was surprised and disappointed by that communication and its implications; it wasn't exactly a positive testimonial for peer review.

Even before publication of my thesis,[1] it was apparent that resolution of the controversies about the diagnosis and treatment of LPR, as well as its causal relationship to airway disease, would require credible bench research, that is, more than pH-monitoring data. Table 5–1 summarizes many of the types of research that have helped establish LPR entity.[1–46] Twenty years later, the cell biology of LPR is beginning to yield some answers about epithelial defenses of the larynx, the mechanisms of reflux-related inflammation and tissue injury, and the causal relationship between LPR and many laryngeal diseases.[30-37,46]

LPR Is Different Than GERD

In part, I became interested in LPR because I felt there were missing clinical pieces, confounding questions. Even the clinical basics were difficult to understand. For one thing, many LPR patients stated unequivocally that they didn't have reflux. People generally equate reflux with heartburn; thus, no heartburn, no reflux. It was sometimes difficult trying to explain "silent reflux" to patients with LPR because it is fundamentally counterintuitive. Then there were also questions like: Why did patients who didn't use tobacco get laryngeal cancer? Why did vocal process granulomas recur so frequently after surgical removal; or for that matter, why did they arise following endotracheal intubation? What was the cause of sulcus (striking-zone scarring), subglottic stenosis, and arytenoid fixation? Why did patients without apparent lung disease have chronic cough? Many of these questions remain unanswered.

By 1989, we already understood that the mechanisms and patterns of reflux in LPR were different than those of GERD.[1,3–5] Most GERD patients had heartburn,

Table 5–1. Levels and types of LPR Research (and References)

	References
Manifestations and Epidemiology	
Symptoms and manifestations of LPR	1–20, 40
Association data (eg, 92% of subglottic stenosis patients have LPR	1,3–14
Prevalence data (eg, 57% of patients with voice disorders have LPR	15
Laryngeal findings observational data (eg, the reflux finding score	1,14–17, 39, 41, 45
Normative control data (eg, normals have LPR between pH 4-5	25,44
Patterns and Mechanisms of LPR (How LPR differs from GERD)	
Pattern of reflux (eg, LPR patients have upright (daytime reflux)	1,3–5,7,10,19
Lack of esophagitis in LPR (eg, 12% esophagitis, 7% Barrett's esophagus	1,22,39
Studies of the refluxate, including stability and activation of pepsins	1,23–25
Studies of vagal reflexes (eg, acid-induced laryngospasm)	8,13,26,27
Diagnosis and diagnostics for LPR	1,3–5,7,10–18,30–36
Treatment	1,5,7,20,29,30,45
Cell Biology and Beyond	
Impact of acid and pepsin on laryngeal epithelim	30,31,33,34,37,46
Comparative studies of laryngeal and esophageal injury thresholds	32
Characterization of the internal environment	21,23,34,30–37,45
Characterization of pepsin binding sites and protein cascade	30,31,33,34
Effects of refluxate on scar formation and carcinogenesis	1–3,6,10,11,31

esophagitis, dysmotility, and a supine (nocturnal) reflux pattern with prolonged periods of acid/pepsin exposure. Conversely, LPR, patients usually did not have heartburn or esophagitis, and an upright (daytime) reflux pattern predominated. A summary of the typical differences between LPR and GERD is shown in Table 5–2.

One of the key differences between GERD and LPR is that the thresholds for esophageal and laryngeal damage are quite different.[1] Based on normative pH monitoring data, one can have up to 50 esophageal reflux (pH <4.0) events, occurring mostly after meals, and that is considered normal; in the larynx, as few as three episodes a week may be too many.[1] In addition, pepsin and not acid is the primary injurious component of the refluxate.[1,2,23-25,30,31] From animal (mostly esophageal) experiments, we knew that acid and pepsin in combination (i.e., activated pepsin) produced more tissue damage than any other combination of enzymes; adding bile salts to the mix, for example, reduced the potency of the refluxate.[1,23,24]

Table 5–2. Typical Differences Between LPR and GERD (*PPIs = Proton Pump Inhibitors)

	GERD	LPR
Symptoms		
Heartburn and/or regurgitation	++++	+
Hoarseness, cough, dysphagia, globus	+	++++
Findings		
Esophagitis	+++	+
Laryngeal inflammation	+	++++
Test Results		
Erosive esophagitis or Barrett's	+++	+
Abnormal esophageal pH monitoring	++++	++
Abnormal pharyngeal pH monitoring	+	++++
Esophageal dysmotility	+++	+
Pattern of Reflux		
Supine (nocturnal) reflux)	++++	+
Upright (daytime) reflux	+	++++
Both (abnormal upright and supine reflux)	+	+++
Response to Treatment		
Effectiveness of dietary and lifestyle modifications	++	+
Successful treatment with single-dose PPIs	+++	+
Successful treatment with twice-daily PPIs	++++	+++

Most of the animal experiments used perfusion models and intact epithelium. In designing animal experiments for my thesis, I wanted to mimic the conditions that presumably led to granuloma formation. In a 1985 study, we had already reported that subglottic stenosis could be recreated in a canine model by the combination of repeated epithelial trauma and experimental reflux.[2] For my thesis, the idea was to create controlled intracricoid epithelial abrasions in animals followed by the intermittent (every other day) application of (a) control substances (such as saline); (b) HCl acid alone at pH 1.5, 2.0, and 4.0; or (c) acid and pepsin in physiologic proportions also at pH 1.5, 2.0, and 4.0.[1] After the initial mucosal injury, painting of the test substances was done six times over a 2-week period (M, W, F, M, W, F). The next week, the animals were sacrificed, the larynges harvested, and microscopic examinations were performed by a blinded pathologist who scored each for inflammation and tissue damage.

The results showed that control and acid-alone groups were no different and that most of those larynges showed healing and reepithelization. On the other hand, the acid and pepsin painted specimens showed tissue damage that was statistically significantly worse than the other groups; and half of the acid/pepsin painted larynges showed mucosal ulceration.[1] The data confirmed that it was pepsin and not acid that produced laryngeal tissue damage. The most surprising finding was that there appeared to be comparable damage at pH 1.5, 2.0, and 4.0.[1] The previous GI literature that suggested that pepsin was virtually inactive above pH 4.0 was incorrect. On the basis of this laboratory experience, I began further investigations of the biology of human pepsin, its tissue effects, and its possible uses as a diagnostic marker.[32,35,36,37]

A Diagnostic Dilemma

In 1982, when I first approached my gastroenterology colleagues to ask about the effects of reflux on the larynx and how to make the diagnosis of "reflux laryngitis," I was initially rebuffed. Laryngeal symptoms, I was told, occurred as a result of vagally-mediated reflexes, not because of the actual backflow of gastric contents into the throat. However, the GI department was doing ambulatory 24-hour esophageal pH monitoring; so I sought out a collaborator to test the hypothesis that patients with hoarseness might actually have acid in their throats. I wanted to investigate my patients with two separate pH-monitoring devices, one in the esophagus and another in the pharynx. Thus, ambulatory 24-hour double-probe (simultaneous esophageal and pharyngeal) pH monitoring was born.[3] The first patients studied using ambulatory 24-hour double-probe (simultaneous esophageal and pharyngeal) pH monitoring had unexplained hoarseness and laryngeal inflammation.[3,5]

About 1990, the reflux symptom index (RSI) and the *reflux finding score* (RFS) became codified and formalized in my practice, but they were not individually reported as validated outcomes instruments until a decade later.[16–18,28,41] These indices are very useful for following the response to treatment over time. For the RSI, there is not an absolute number that is diagnostic of LPR; although from my perspective, it is very uncommon that a patient with a RSI of 20 or more doesn't actually turn out to have LPR. For the RFS, the comparable "magic number" is 10. It is worth noting that the combination of pseudosulcus and ventricular obliteration are virtually diagnostic of LPR; whereas, posterior commissure erythema and parchydermia (posterior commissure hypertrophy) are not as useful diagnostically.

After many years and in spite of considerable experience, I still did not always know the best way to diagnose LPR. pH monitoring sufficed when it was positive; and our normative data suggested that even a single pharyngeal reflux event pH <4.0 was diagnostic of LPR. But even in those early years, that criterion seemed too narrow. What about a patient who had a lot of reflux at pH 4.1? Was that normal? About two-thirds of the patients whom I believed had LPR on clinical grounds had positive pharyngeal pH studies. Most of the apparent false-negative pH study patients were treated with antireflux medication (as well as dietary and lifestyle modifications) anyway; most got well. Consequently, for the difficult to diagnose patient, a therapeutic trial became an important diagnostic. From my point of view, the laryngeal findings had to improve as well as the symptoms for antireflux therapy to be considered a success.

In the 1980s, having already rejected radiographic and radionuclide imaging and esophagoscopy because they were insensitive and nonspecific for LPR, I began to look at new pH monitoring criteria as well as for other diagnostics. Since there was evidence that there was at least 70% of peptic activity at pH 4.5 and perhaps as much as 40% activity at pH 5.0,[1] in 1991 our pH monitoring laboratory began to report the number of pharyngeal reflux events at pH <5.0 as well as at pH <4.0. We recently reported normative pharyngeal pH monitoring results in 20 carefully selected normal controls[21]; 15% (3/20) had pharyngeal reflux episodes pH <4.0, and 90% (18/20) had pharyngeal reflux between pH 4.0–5.0, with a mean number of 2.5 such episodes.[21]

Even though the symptoms and laryngeal findings of LPR have been well-described, even using expanded threshold criteria for positive pH monitoring, and even using therapeutic trials, it is still sometimes difficult to diagnose LPR with certainty. There are so many clinical variables, not the least of which is intermittency. As a gold standard, pH monitoring has had it limits, yet it is the still one of the best diagnostics as of this writing as long as there is a pH sensor in the pharynx; pH monitoring without pharyngeal data is virtually meaningless in LPR. In one study, we showed that the positive predictive value of a single esophageal pH probe for the diagnosis of LPR was 49%. For 25 years I have remained uncomfortable with "threshold pH level" LPR diagnosis. The idea that reflux events below a certain pH-level are diagnostic of disease didn't make sense in the light of what we know about peptic injury.[31,37] For example, there was no way to compare the potential tissue impact of LPR episodes lasting a few minutes at pH 2 with hours at pH 5.

It is useful to reflect on why Johnson and DeMeester originally selected pH <4.0 as the threshold for determination of an acid-reflux event for esophageal pH monitoring.[25] It was relatively arbitrary; however, pH <4.0 was selected for two reasons. First, at the time it was believed that there was little or no peptic activity above pH 4.0; and second, when GI patients with heartburn and GERD were pH-tested, it seemed that the symptom heartburn was associated with pH <4.0 events.[25] As it turns out, it has been shown that esophageal damage occurs at pH <4.0 and laryngeal damage at pH <5.0.[31,37] However, human pepsin (primarily pepsin 3b) has proteolytic activity across a wide pH-range. Peptic activity is a function of pH, and even at pH 6, there is still 10% peptic activity. In addition, human pepsin is stable at pH 7, and it is likely that it can be reactivated by hydrogen ions from any source, for example, a sip of soda pop.[37]

Recently, we began to reexamine pH monitoring data by looking at the entire "area under the curve," that is, the acid exposures at all pH levels (from 1–7), using the pepsin activity curve to modify the relative risk of tissue damage at each pH level. A new system for interpreting pharyngeal pH monitoring data is currently under investigation, as outlined below.

Because of limitations using a pH threshold level, we derived the pepsin injury coefficient (PIC) for each pH level (Table 5–3) using 1.00 (ie, 100%) for peak peptic

Table 5–3. Method of Calculation of the Reflux Injury Profile (RIP), the Reflux Injury Score (RIS), and Case Illustrations

A. Normal

pH	>1	>2	>3	>4	>5	>6	>6	
PIC*	0.80	1.00	0.70	0.55	0.40	0.10	0.00	
Min	0	0	0	0	20	400	1020	
RIP	0	0	0	0	8	40	0	*RIS = 48*

B. Abnormal

pH	>1	>2	>3	>4	>5	>6	>6	
PIC*	0.80	1.00	0,70	0.55	0.40	0.10	0.00	
Min	0	10	30	100	200	100	100	
RIP	0	10	21	55	80	10	0	*RIS = 176*

C. Abnormal

pH	>1	>2	>3	>4	>5	>6	>6	
PIC*	0.80	1.00	0.70	0.55	0.40	0.10	0.00	
Min	10	30	100	200	400	500	200	
RIP	8	30	70	110	160	50	0	*RIS = 440*

D. Abnormal

pH	>1	>2	>3	>4	>5	>6	>6	
PIC*	0.80	1.00	0.70	0.55	0.40	0.10	0.00	
Min	0	0	0	0	1000	400	40	
RIP	0	0	0	0	400	40	0	*RIS = 440*

*PIC = Pepsin injury coefficient based on the pepsin activity curve (Fig 5–1).

activity at pH 2.0. Then, the number of minutes of pharyngeal exposure in each pH range (intervals were 0.0–1.0, 1.1–2.0, 2.1–3.0, etc) was multiplied by its corresponding PIC, corrected for a complete 24-hour study (1440 minutes). This produced a *r*eflux *i*njury *p*rofile (RIP), an injury score for each pH level (Table 5–3); and the sum of RIP scores was then reported as the reflux injury score (RIS).

In Table 5–3, there are four case illustrations, one normal (A) and three abnormal (B–D). In the normal example, the % time pH <5.0 is only 1% and the RIS is 48. In abnormal case example 3B, the % time pH <4.0 is 10%; the % time pH <5.0 is 17%; and the RIS is 176. It is instructive to compare case examples 3C and 3D. By traditional pH criteria, study C would have been considered to be profoundly abnormal and study D would

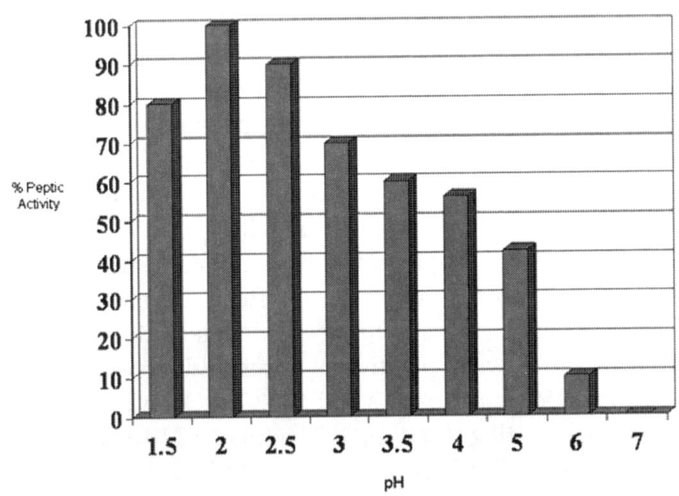

Figure 5–1. Human Pepsin Activity Curve

have been considered normal. For 3C and 3D, the % time pH <4.0 are 27% and 0% respectively, but for % time pH <5.0, they are 51% and 69% respectively. For 3C, the RIS is 428 and it is 440 for 3D.

Using the RIP/RIS scoring method, it appears that prolonged pharyngeal exposure at weakly acidic pH may be more damaging than a shorter period of exposure at low pH. It is important to remember that RIP/RIS scoring is designed for interpretation of pharyngeal reflux testing. The RIP/RIS are based upon the observation that the esophagus is more robust than the larynx when it comes to mucosal resistance to weakly acidic reflux.[1,31] The concept of looking at the entire pH test profile is appealing, because it avoids the "which pH threshold?" question. Time will tell whether or not the RIP and RIS prove to be good clinical measures.

Implications of Detection of Pepsin in Airway Secretions

In the early 1990s, we performed an experiment (unreported data) designed to test the hypothesis that pepsin as a relatively large and stable molecule might be a good marker for LPR. Porcine pepsin was sprayed in the throat of rats, which were subsequently sacrificed at intervals from 0 to 5 hours after spraying. At sacrifice, the laryngopharynx of each animal was lavaged with saline and then the samples were assayed for pepsin using a hemolytic (modified Anson) method. As expected, there was a large peak within 15 minutes of spraying of the pepsin. Notably, there was a moderate amount of pepsin detected 5 hours later (and not in the controls).

We subsequently developed a sandwich immunoassay (ELISA) for human pepsin with a sensitivity of 0.1ng/ml and 100% specificity.[35,36,43] It did not cross-react with pepsinogen, gastricin, or porcine pepsin. The purpose of the assay was to detect pepsin in saliva and airway secretions. Essentially, we developed a spit-in-a-cup test for gastric reflux, especially LPR. Recently, we tested otolaryngology patients with pH-documented LPR, a group of GI patients with biopsy-proven esophagitis, and normal controls.[36] Fifteen percent (3/20) of the control subjects had pepsin detected; although two of those were positive at threshold pepsin levels (~3 ng/ml); the third had silent GERD and Barrett's esophagitis, diagnosed by subsequent pH testing and esophagoscopy.[36] Pepsin was detected in the expectorated samples of 75% (69/92) of the LPR patients and 64% (23/36) of the esophagitis/GERD group.[36] The latter finding was unexpected; but it part, it may help explain why LPR remains so enigmatic: If pepsin is recovered from expectorated samples of GERD patients who do not have LPR symptoms, then possibly local epithelial resistance may play an important role in preventing LPR disease.

Cell Biology of LPR and Laryngeal Carcinogenesis

By 1991, I was hungry for basic science research, but it wasn't until 1995 that I began doing bench research at Wake Forest University in a dedicated laboratory. In 1998, we organized several multidisciplinary LPR meetings in the United Kingdom, including the 1st International Symposium on Human Pepsin (1999), held at the University of York in England. One of my colleagues on the planning committee suggested that we didn't know enough about pepsin to use such a title. I proposed to get U.K. scientists interested in LPR, especially the cell biology of peptic injury. I may have been the only person who mentioned pepsin that first year. However, out of that meeting and similar ones that followed emerged an international reflux research network. Our first article on the cell biology of LPR was published in 2001.[30] And not long after that, Dr. Nikki Johnston came to work as a molecular biologist in my laboratory at Wake Forest.

We studied pepsin, carbonic anhydrase and E-cadherin and then the stress proteins in LPR patients and controls as well as in animal and in vitro models. The cell biology of reflux is marvelous and it has yielded some expected findings. For one thing, it revealed that the esophagus was far better defended than the larynx against peptic tissue damage; and even within the larynx, there were differences in the cellular response to acid and pepsin.[30–37]

Even before our first scientific experiment, we sensed that the larynx had at least two biologic compartments in terms of its response to LPR; at least the posterior commissure was different than the rest. Here's why. Only once in my career had I seen a primary squamous cell carcinoma arise in the posterior commissure and that was in a lifetime nonsmoker. Furthermore, granulomas and other growths did not seem to arise there. The only pathology of the posterior commissure mucosa was posterior commissure hypertrophy ("parchydermia") due to LPR. Hence, we reasoned that the posterior commissure was defended differently than of the rest of the larynx; we felt that it was more resistant to reflux and carcinogenesis. Perhaps it had evolved to be more resistant because as a posterior hypopharyngeal structure; it was more directly in the path of LPR than any other part. So from the beginning, as we investigated the biology of LPR, we looked at both vocal fold and posterior commissure epithelia as though they might be different. As it turns out, they are, and those differences have clinical and research implications.

The enzyme carbonic anhydrase (CA), ubiquitous in all mammalian cells. It hydrolyzes CO_2 to form bicarbonate, and it is believed to be important in maintaining intracellular acid-base balance. Interestingly, with (GERD) esophagitis, the esophageal epithelium actually secretes bicarbonate, not so with the larynx. Not only does the larynx not have a comparable defense, CA in vocal fold epithelium depletes in response to LPR, especially to pepsin.[30–33] At the same time, CA increases in the posterior commissure mucosa in response to LPR. So, as CA depletes on the vocal fold, it increases in the posterior commissure. Furthermore, the amount of CA found in posterior commissure epithelium correlates with the reflux symptom index; the higher the RSI score, the more the CA. Does CA have a role in preventing laryngeal carcinoma? Perhaps.

CA is not the only protein in vocal fold epithelium that depletes with LPR.[30–34] So too does E-cadherin that makes up the tight junctions (intercellular bridges) between squamous epithelial cells and most of the stress proteins (previously known as "heat shock" proteins). Using our pepsin peptide antibodies, we have performed Western blot analysis of laryngeal tissue from LPR patients and controls. Most LPR patients have tissue-bound pepsin and most controls do not. Furthermore, the finding of pepsin by Western blot is associated with depletion of the protective proteins. The tissue profile of LPR and laryngeal carcinoma is similar (Table 5–4). The notable difference is stress protein HSP70; it appears to be depleted in carcinoma but not in LPR.

As a clinician, I have observed that LPR findings are virtually always present in patients with vocal fold carcinoma. In the past, clinicians have assumed that those inflammatory findings were due to tobacco use and not reflux. In a paper entitled, "Reflux and early laryngeal carcinoma," we presented a prospective series of 50 consecutive patients with T_1 laryngeal carcinoma, all of whom had biopsy-proven vocal fold disease and reflux testing.[45] Of the study population, 44% (22/50) were smokers, 42% (21/50) were ex-smokers (with a median duration of smoking cessation of 8 years), and

Table 5–4. Tissue Profile of LPR, Carcinoma, and Controls

	Controls	LPR	Cancer
Pepsin	None	+	+
CAIII	?	?	?
E-Cahedrin	?	?	?
SEP70	?	?	?
SEP53	?	?	?
HSP70	?	?	?

+ = Positive (present); ? = Normal (baseline level; ? = Decreased compared to normal controls.

14% (7/50) were lifetime nonsmokers. Seventy-six percent (38/50) had reflux.[45]

In my thesis,[1] I presented some interesting cases; six patients with recurrent leukoplakia that vanished with antireflux treatment, and six nonsmokers were felt to have reflux-related carcinoma. One exemplary case was that of a real estate agent from Statesville NC (case example 1 in my thesis) is exemplary. He presented with a 3-mm granulomalike lesion of the left vocal fold that turned out to be a microinvasive carcinoma. He was a lifetime nonsmoker and nondrinker. I did a local endoscopic laser excision, but it granulated for months without healing. Then I biopsied the granulation and it took another 2 months before it healed. Over the course of 6 years (1980–1986), he developed three small vocal fold carcinomas, each of which was excised with subsequent granulation for months. After the third lesion, he had a positive pH study and underwent fundoplication. At follow-up 10 years later, he had a normal laryngeal examination. This case (and the data below) suggests that laryngeal papillomas and LPR may be related to laryngeal carcinogenesis.

In another unpublished paper, "Papilloma-carcinoma and its possible relationship to gastroesophageal reflux," we reviewed the data of 88 adult-onset papillomas patients followed for 10 years, 16% (14/88) of whom had developed squamous cell carcinoma of the lung or laryngopharynx. All 14 had pH-documented LPR; and in addition, 6 were cigarette smokers. Of the remaining 74 patients, there were 14 with LPR, all on antireflux treatment. Thus, treatment of LPR and smoking cessation are important interventions in adult patients with papillomas.

One might hypothesize that part of the common pathway of LPR and carcinogenesis might be as follows:

On the mucosal surface, acid and pepsin break down the mucus barrier; then pepsin binds to epithelial cell membranes. In addition, destruction of E-cadherin (the cell-cell mortar between squamous epithelial cells) allows the pepsin to get between the surface layers and down to the active basal levels of the epithelium. Tissue-bound pepsin is then endocytosed. Once intracellular, it damages protective proteins (eg, stress proteins) and DNA. A specific effect of carbonic anhydrase depletion may be to further alter acid-base imbalance and lower pH, which could accelerate the cascade of adverse protein consequences. These relationships, including the effects of LPR on immumological status of laryngeal epithelium, remain to be elucidated.[46]

LPR and the Internal Environment

If almost everyone in Chernobyl develops cancer, is cancer normal? LPR remains enigmatic because there still are confounding factors related to its diagnosis and treatment and because LPR begs the question of what is normal. The finding of pepsin in the secretions of 64% GERD patients[36] suggests the possibility that LPR-related diseases may depend more on local epithelial defenses than on the effluence In other words, people have who do have LPR symptoms (disease) but who have some LPR may have robustly defended laryngopharyngeal epithelium; and he difference between health and disease may depend upon whether or not pepsin is tissue-bound.

The external environment has gotten a lot of attention in the past two decades; however, it is but one component of *the internal environment*. Table 5–5 summarizes some of the elements of the internal environment. These humoral and cellular elements are under the influence of neuromuscular, hormonal, vascular and genetic control, and they are also interdependent. The internal environment is the aerodigestive tract conceptualized as an integrated, multicomponent, multifunction biologic system. That is in balance in health seems reasonable; however, surprisingly little is known about how all the elements interact, and specifically which factors and sequences cause decompensation and disease. It seems likely, for example, that LPR predisposes to upper respiratory infection (URI) and *visa versa*. In 2006, I reviewed a series LPR patients diagnosed by pH-monitoring; 26% (15/57) had the onset of their symptoms with a URI [unreported data]. In addition, seemingly important relationships between LPR and reactive airway diseases remain to be elucidated.

Table 5–5. Components of the Internal Environment

Cells
Saliva
Acid and pepsin
Inflammatory mediators (eg, kinens)
Food and drink (that which is ingested)
Mucus and mucus breakdown products
Gastricin, bile, and other digestive enzymes
The external environment (that which is inhaled/breathed)

The concept of LPR as an uncomplicated all-or-nothing ("threshold") disease should be abandoned. Within this context, any single pH threshold diagnostic measure seems woefully inadequate. As of this writing, poorly conceived clinical studies (e.g., pH monitoring and treatment studies) have only further fueled a confusing and anachronistic model.

The challenge for future clinicians and researchers will be to integrate the whole that has been fragmented; however, cell biology holds the key. And multidisciplinary translational research is going to unravel the LPR conundrum. Meanwhile, internal environment concept will spawn development of new diagnostics and therapeutics. In the future, examination of the expectorate for mucus breakdown products, kinins, and immunoglobulins, in addition to pepsin, may make the diagnosis of LPR noninvasive and definitive. As treatment alternatives to acid-suppression, anti-pepsin therapeutics will be possible by: (1) suppression of production or secretion, (2) suppression of secretion, (3) prevention of activation of pepsinogen, (4) inactivation of pepsin, and/or (5) prevention of binding of pepsin to tissue.

References

1. Koufman JA. The otolaryngologic manifestations of gastroesophageal reflux disease (GERD): a clinical investigation of 225 patients using ambulatory 24- hour pH monitoring and an experimental investigation of the role of acid and pepsin in the development of laryngeal injury. *Laryngoscope*. 1991;101(Suppl 53):1–78.
2. Little FB, Koufman JA, Kohut RI, et al. Effect of gastric acid on the pathogenesis of subglottic stenosis. *Ann of Otol Rhinol Laryngol*. 1985;94:516–519.

3. Wiener GJ, Copper JB, Wu WC, et al. Is hoarseness an atypical manifestation of gastroesophageal reflux (GER)? An ambulatory 24 hour pH study. *Gastroenterology.* 1986;90:A1691.
4. Ossakow SJ, Elta G, Colturi T, et al. Esophageal reflux and dysmotility as the basis for persistent cervical symptoms. *Ann Otol Rhinol Laryngol.* 1987;96:387–392.
5. Koufman JA, Wiener GJ, Wu WC, Castell DO. Reflux laryngitis and its sequelae: the diagnostic role of 24-hour pH monitoring. *J Voice.* 1988;2:78–89.
6. Ward PH, & Hanson DG. Reflux as an etiological factor of carcinoma of the laryngopharynx. *Laryngoscope.* 1988;98:1195–1199.
7. Wiener GJ, Koufman JA, Wu W, et al. Chronic hoarseness secondary to gastroesophageal reflux disease: documentation with 24-h ambulatory pH monitoring. *Am J Gastroenterol.* 1989;84:1503–1508.
8. Loughlin CJ, Koufman JA. Paroxysmal laryngospasm secondary to gastroesophageal reflux. *Laryngoscope.* 1996;106:1502–1505.
9. Toohill RJ, & Kuhn JC. Role of refluxed acid in pathogenesis of laryngeal disorders. *Am J Med.* 1997;103: 100S–106S.
10. Little JP, Matthews BL, Glock MS, et al. Extraesophageal pediatric reflux: 24-hour double-probe pH monitoring of 222 children. *Ann Otol Rhinol Laryngol.* 1997; (Suppl 169):1–16.
11. Geterud A, Bove M, & Ruth M. Hypopharyngeal acid exposure: an independent risk factor for laryngeal cancer? *Laryngoscope.* 2003:113:2201–2205.
12. Wise SK, Wise JC, & DelGaudio JM. Association of nasopharyngeal and laryngopharyngeal reflux with postnasal drip symptomatology in patients with and without rhinosinusitis. *Am J Rhinol.* 2006:20:283–289.
13. Murry T, Tabaee A, Owczarzak V, & Aviv JE. Respiratory retraining therapy and management of laryngopharyngeal reflux in the treatment of patients with cough and paradoxical vocal fold movement disorder. *Ann Otol Rhinol Laryngol.* 2006:115:754–758.
14. Payne RJ, Kost KM, Frenkiel S, et al. Laryngeal inflammation assessed using the reflux finding score in obstructive sleep apnea. *Otolaryngol Head Neck Surg.* 2006:134:836–842.
15. Koufman JA, Amin M, & Panetti M. Prevalence of reflux in 113 consecutive patients with laryngeal and voice disorders. *Otolaryngol Head Neck Surg.* 2000;123: 385–388.
16. Belafsky PC, Postma GN, & Koufman JA. The validity and reliability of the reflux finding score (RFS). *Laryngoscope.* 2001;111:1313–1317.
17. Belafsky PC, Postma GN, & Koufman JA. Validity and reliability of the reflux symptom index (RSI). *J Voice.* 2002;16:274–277.
18. Carrau R, Khidr A, Gold K, et al. Validation of a quality-of-life instrument for laryngopharyngeal reflux. *Arch Otol Head Neck Surg.* 2005;131:315–320.
19. Postma GN, Tomek MS, Belafsky PC, & Koufman JA. Esophageal motor function in laryngopharyngeal reflux is superior to that of classic gastroesophageal reflux disease. *Ann Otol Rhinol Laryngol.* 2001;110:1114–1116.
20. Koufman JA, Aviv JE, Casiano RR, & Shaw GY. Position statement of the American Academy of Otolaryngology-Head and Neck Surgery on laryngopharyngeal reflux. *Otolaryngol Head Neck Surg.* 2002;127:32–35.
21. Koufman JA, Wright SC, Lively MO, Johnston WC, Johnston N, Bishwokarma B, & Postma GN. *Normal values for pharyngeal pH monitoring.* Presented at the annual meeting of the American Broncho-Esophagological Association; Orlando Fla; May 1, 2008
22. Koufman JA, Belafsky PC, Daniel E, et al. Prevalence of esophagitis in patients with pH-documented laryngopharyngeal reflux. *Laryngoscope.* 2002;112:1606–1609.
23. Lillemoe KD, Johnson LF, & Harmon JW. Role of the components of the gastroduodenal contents in experimental acid esophagitis. *Surgery.* 1982,92:276–284.
24. Johnson LF, & Harmon JW. Experimental esophagitis in a rabbit model: clinical relevance. *J Clin Gastroenterol.* 1986, 8(Suppl 1):26–44.
25. Johnson LF. Personal communication. 2000–01.
26. Loughlin CJ, Koufman JA, Averill DB, et al. Acid-induced laryngospasm in a canine model. *Laryngoscope.* 1996; 106:1506–1509.
27. Duke SG, Postma GN, McGuirt Jr. WF, et al. Laryngospasm and diaphragmatic arrest in the immature canine after laryngeal acid exposure: a possible model for sudden infant death syndrome (SIDS). *Ann Otol Rhinol Laryngol.* 2001;110:729–733.
28. Belafsky PC, Postma GN, & Koufman KA. Laryngopharyngeal reflux symptoms improve before changes in physical findings. *Laryngoscope.* 2001;111:979–981.
29. Amin MR, Postma GN, Johnson P, et al. Proton pump inhibitor resistance in the treatment of laryngopharyngeal reflux. *Otolaryngol Head Neck Surg.* 2001;125:374–378.
30. Axford SE, Sharp N, Ross PE, Pearson JP, Dettmar PW, Pannetti M, & Koufman JA. Cell biology of laryngeal epithelial defenses in health and disease: preliminary studies. *Ann Otol Rhinol Laryngol.* 2001;110:1099–1108.
31. Johnston N, Bulmer D, Gill GA, et al. Cell biology of laryngeal epithelial defenses in health and disease: further studies. *Ann Otol Rhinol Laryngol.* 2003;112:481–491.
32. Johnston N, Knight J, Dettmar PW, Lively MO, Koufman J. Pepsin and carbonic anhydrase isoenzyme III as diagnostic markers for laryngopharyngeal reflux disease. *Laryngoscope.* 2004;114:2129–2134.
33. Gill GA, Johnston N, Buda A, Pignatelli M, Pearson J, Dettmar PW, & Koufman J. Laryngeal epithelial defenses

against laryngopharyngeal reflux (LPR): investigations of pepsin, carbonic anhydrase III, pepsin, and the inflammatory response. *Ann Otol Rhinol Laryngol.* 2005;114:913–921.

34. Johnston N, Dettmar PW, Lively MO, & Koufman J. Effect of pepsin on laryngeal stress protein (Sep70, Sep53, and Hsp70) response: Role in laryngopharyngeal reflux disease. *Ann Otol Rhinol Laryngol.* 2006;115:47–58.
35. Knight J, Lively MO, Johnston N, Dettmar PW, & Koufman J. Sensitive pepsin immunoassay for detection of laryngopharyngeal reflux. *Laryngoscope.* 2005;115: 1473–1478.
36. Koufman JA, Lively MO, Rubin M, et al. *Use of a sensitive ELISA for the detection of pepsin in the airway secretions of patients with laryngopharyngeal reflux (LPR), gastroesophageal reflux disease (GERD), and healthy controls.* Presented at the annual meeting of the American Laryngological Association; Orlando Fla; May 1, 2008.
37. Johnston N, Dettmar PW, Bishwokarma B, Koufman JA, & Lively MO. Activity/stability of human pepsin: implications for reflux attributed laryngeal disease. *Laryngoscope.* 2007;117:1036–1039.
38. DeMeester TR, Johnson LF, Joseph GJ, Toscano MS, Hall AW, & Skinner DB. Patterns of gastroesophageal reflux in health and disease. *Ann Surg.* 1976;184:459–470.
39. Hill RK, Simpson CB, Velazquez R, & Larson N. Pachydermia is not diagnostic of active laryngopharyngeal reflux disease. *Laryngoscope.* 2004:114:1557–1561.
40. Koufman JA, & Burke AJ. The etiology and pathogenesis of laryngeal carcinoma. *Otolaryngol Clin North Am.* 1997;30:1–19.
41. Koufman JA. Methods and compositions for the diagnosis of extraesophageal reflux. United States Patent 1996; 5,879,897.
42. Reulbach TR, Belafsky PC, Blalock PD, Koufman JA, & Postma GN. Occult laryngeal pathology in a community-based cohort. *Otolaryngol Head Neck Surg.* 2001;124: 448–450.
43. Westcott CJ, Hopkins MB, Bach KK, et al. Fundoplication for laryngopharyngeal reflux. *J Am Coll Surgeons.* 2004;199:23–30.
44. Wetmore RF. Effects of acid on the larynx of the maturing rabbit and their possible significance to the sudden infant death syndrome. *Laryngoscope.* 1993;103:1242–1254.
45. Koufman JA, & Cummins MM. *Reflux and early laryngeal carcinoma.* Presented at the annual meeting of the Southern Section of the Triological Society; Key West, Fla; January 6, 1995.
46. Rees LEN, Pazmany L, Gutowska-Owsiak D, et al. *The mucosal immune response to laryngopharyngeal reflux.* Presented at the annual meeting of the American Broncho-Esophagological Association; Orlando, Fla; May 1, 2008).

The Otolaryngologic Manifestations of Gastroesophageal Reflux Disease (GERD): A Clinical Investigation of 225 Patients Using Ambulatory 24-Hour pH Monitoring and an Experimental Investigation of the Role of Acid and Pepsin in the Development of Laryngeal Injury

JAMES A. KOUFMAN, MD

All laryngologists are familiar with the many throat conditions which appear as salient features of underlying systemic states, and yet in the overswing towards localism [specialization], general pathologic data, systemic therapeutics and hygienic aids are not always utilized to the utmost. The laryngologist should continue to be, first of all, a good physician, and after that, something more—a specialist.

William E. Casselberry[1]
President's Address, May 22, 1899
American Laryngological Association

ABSTRACT

Occult (silent) gastroesophageal reflux disease (GER, GERD) is believed to be an important etiologic factor in the development of many inflammatory and neoplastic disorders of the upper aerodigestive tract. In order to test this hypothesis, a human study and an animal study were performed. The human study consisted primarily of applying a new diagnostic technique (double-probe pH monitoring) to a population of otolaryngology patients with GERD to determine the incidence of overt and occult GERD. The animal study consisted of experiments to evaluate the potential damaging effects of intermittent GER on the larynx.

Two hundred twenty-five consecutive patients with otolaryngologic disorders having suspected GERD evaluated from 1985 through 1988 are reported. Ambulatory 24-hour intraesophageal pH monitoring was performed in 197; of those, 81% underwent double-probe pH monitoring, with the second pH probe being placed in the hypopharynx at the laryngeal inlet. Seventy percent of the patients also underwent barium esophagography with videofluoroscopy.

The patient population was divided into seven diagnostic subgroups: carcinoma of the larynx (n = 31), laryngeal and tracheal stenosis (n = 33), reflux laryngitis (n = 61), globus pharyngeus (n = 27), dysphagia (n = 25), chronic cough (n = 30), and a group with miscellaneous disorders (n = 18).

The most common symptoms were hoarseness (71%), cough (51%), globus (47%), and throat clearing (42%). Only 43% of the patients had gastrointestinal symptoms (heartburn or acid regurgitation). Thus, by traditional symptomatology, GER was occult or silent in the majority of the study population.

Twenty-eight patients (12%) refused or could not tolerate pH monitoring. Of the patients undergoing diagnostic pH monitoring, 62% had abnormal esophageal pH studies, and 30% demonstrated reflux into the pharynx. The results of diagnostic pH monitoring for each of the subgroups were as follows (percentage with abnormal studies): carcinoma (71%), stenosis (78%), reflux laryngitis (60%), globus (58%), dysphagia (45%), chronic cough (52%), and miscellaneous (13%). The highest yield of abnormal pharngeal reflux was in the carcinoma group and the stenosis group (58% and 56%, respectively).

By comparison, the diagnostic barium esophagogram with videofluoroscopy was frequently negative. The results were as follows: esophagitis (18%), reflux (9%), esophageal dysmotility (12%), and stricture (3%).

Presented as a Candidate's Thesis to the American Laryngological, Rhinological and Otological Society, September 1989 (Honorable Mention).

From the Department of Otolaryngology, The Bowman Gray School of Medicine of Wake Forest University, Winston-Salem, NC.

Supported in part by NIH Grant RR-05404. The laboratory (animal) investigation portion of this study was performed in accordance with a protocol approved by the Medical Center Institutional Animal Care and Use Committee.

Publication of this supplement was made possible through a grant from Merck Sharp & Dohme.

Send Reprint Requests to James A. Koufman, MD, Department of Otolaryngology, 300 South Hawthorne Road, Winston-Salem, NC 27103.

All of the study patients were treated with antireflux therapy. Follow-up was available on 68% of the patients and the mean follow-up period was 11.6 ± 12.7 months. After 6 months of treatment, symptoms had resolved in 85% and medical therapy had failed in 15%. Subsequently, an additional 20% experienced medical treatment failure. Fifteen percent of patients underwent Nissen fundoplication, and all subsequently had resolution of symptoms.

To further investigate the role of gastroesophageal reflux in the development of laryngeal damage, experiments mimicking the effects of intermittent reflux (of acid and pepsin) on the canine larynx were performed. The results of these experiments revealed: *1.* Intermittent reflux (three episodes per week) can result in severe laryngeal damage if there is prior mucosal injury; *2.* pepsin, and not hydrochloric acid, is the principal injurious agent of the refluxate; and, *3.* severe laryngeal damage can occur even when the pH of the refluxate is 4.0.

The manuscript describes the limitations and advantages of standard diagnostic procedures and of 24-hour pH monitoring. The differences between gastroenterology and otolaryngology patients with GERD are emphasized and specific new diagnostic and therapeutic recommendations are made.

INTRODUCTION

Although it has been estimated that 10% of Americans have symptoms of heartburn and regurgitation on a daily basis, and 30% to 50% less frequently,[2] the epidemiology and the natural history of gastroesophageal reflux disease (GER, GERD) remain incompletely understood. It is often assumed by gastroenterologists and otolaryngologists alike that clinically manifest GERD should be associated with typical gastrointestinal symptoms such as heartburn and regurgitation. However, what if otolaryngology patients with GERD were atypical? What if the standard GER diagnostic methods were insensitive and inaccurate? What if symptoms and complications of GER could result from intermittent reflux? What if occult (silent) GER produced a broad constellation of upper aerodigestive symptoms and sequelae in otolaryngology patients? It is the purpose of this thesis to address these questions.

Case Example

In 1981, a 55-year-old clergyman presented with a recurrent granuloma on the laryngeal surface of the epiglottis (Fig. 1-A). The patient was otherwise healthy and his only symptoms were a sensation of a lump in the throat, chronic throat clearing, cough, and hoarseness. He denied heartburn, regurgitation, or sour taste on eructation.

Three and six months earlier, he had undergone endoscopic (cold knife) removal of the lesion, but it recurred. Histologically, pyogenic granuloma had been found on both occasions. A third endoscopic excision with the carbon dioxide laser was performed. The histologic specimen again demonstrated pyogenic granuloma, and, again, the lesion recurred. An endoscopic epiglottectomy was then performed; however, within 1 week of operation, granulation tissue was forming in the base of the tongue at the surgical site.

A barium swallow esophagogram was obtained and was normal. Nevertheless, because of the intractability of disease and the remote possibility of GER contributing to the disorder, the patient was started on an antireflux regimen, including cimetidine (300 mg q.i.d.). Within 3 weeks (1 year his after initial presentation), the lesion had healed.

For years, otolaryngologists have realized the limitations of the diagnostic tests for GERD and have relied, as in this patient, primarily upon clinical diagnosis. Although the specificity of many of the standard tests for GERD is reasonably good, the sensitivity is often poor. Ambulatory 24-hour pH monitoring (pH manometry; pH-metry) is by far the most sensitive and specific test for GERD currently available.[3–8] At this time, there are scant pH-metry data available in otolaryngology patients with GER-related conditions.

Some GERD syndromes have been well described, including the vocal process granuloma[9–15] and posterior laryngitis (red arytenoids and piled-up interarytenoid mucosa).[16–19] Even with this information, there is some disagreement. Posterior laryngitis, for instance, which is considered by many clinicians to be virtually pathognomonic for GER, has been found by some investigators not to be invariably associated.[20]

In spite of the diagnostic limitations, GER has been postulated to be associated with or responsible for an array of upper aerodigestive conditions, including laryngeal carcinoma[14,21,22] and subglottic stenosis.[23,24] However, none of the previous reports have suggested that GER-related upper aerodigestive tract conditions may result from occult or intermittent GERD.

HYPOTHESIS

Occult (silent), and sometimes intermittent, gastroesophageal reflux disease is associated with the development of inflammatory and neoplastic disorders of the upper aerodigestive tract.

OBJECTIVES

1. To report the findings (including the incidence of occult and intermittent GER) of 225 otolaryngology patients with GERD-related upper aerodigestive conditions.

2. To describe and contrast the patterns of GERD in otolaryngology patients with those of gastroenterology (esophagitis) patients.

3. To describe the results of ambulatory 24-hour intraesophageal pH monitoring in otolaryngology patients with GERD.

4. To evaluate and report the usefulness of pha-

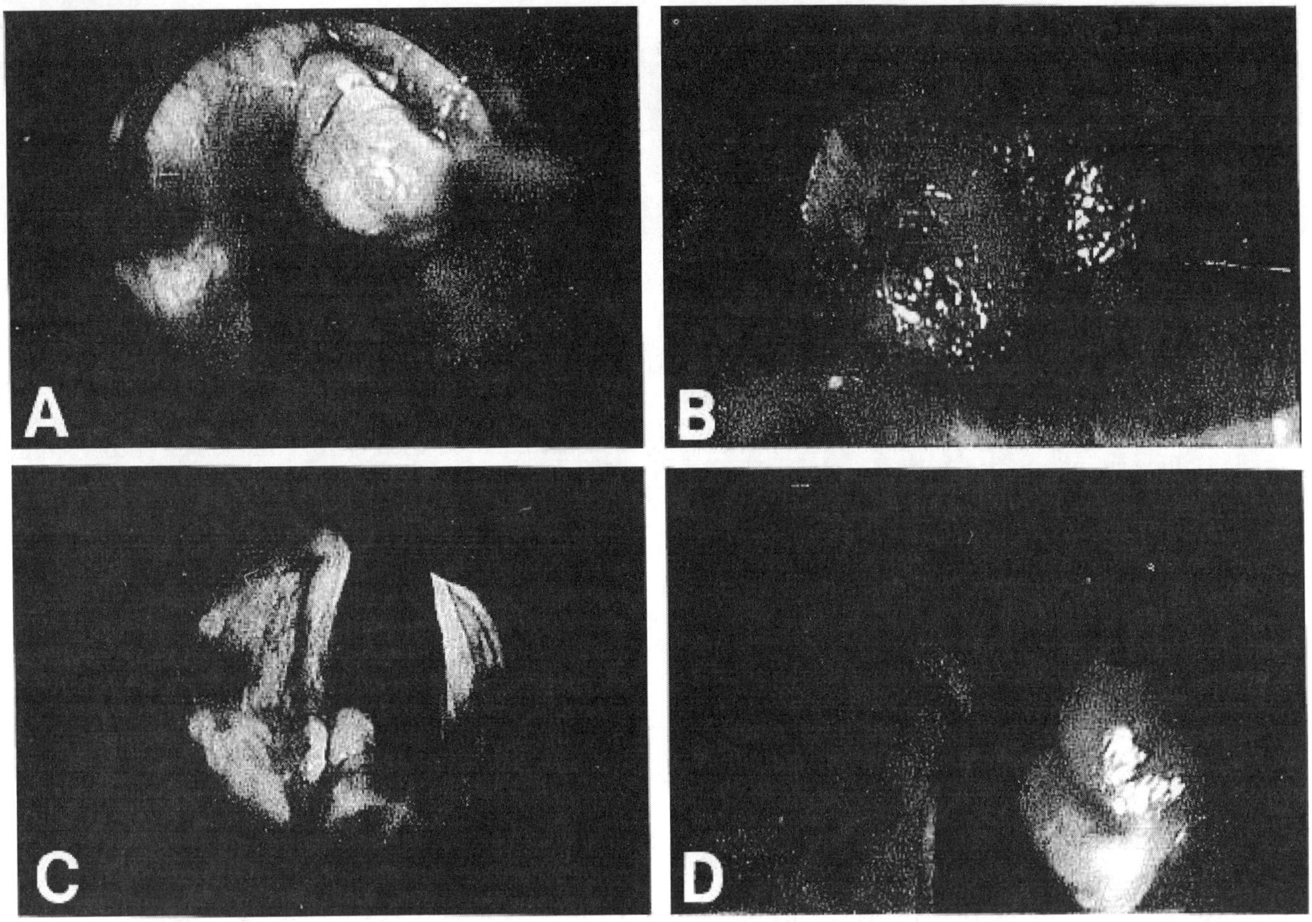

Fig. 1. Laryngeal granulomas caused by GERD. **A.** Granuloma laryngeal surface of the epiglottis; **B.** bilateral obstructing vocal process granulomas; **C.** "intubation granuloma" of the vocal process; **D.** unilateral sessile vocal process granuloma.

ryngeal pH monitoring in determining the incidence of "high" laryngopharyngeal reflux.

5. To determine and report the incidence of GER and its symptoms in six consecutive series of patients, each constituting a separate diagnostic study group: (A) carcinoma of the larynx (n = 31); (B) subglottic and tracheal stenosis (n = 33); (C) reflux laryngitis (n = 61); (D) globus pharyngeus (n = 27); (E) dysphagia (n = 25); and (F) chronic cough (n = 30).

6. To establish an animal model to investigate the threshold for laryngeal injury with "intermittent reflux."

7. To investigate the relative role of acid and pepsin in the development of tissue damage.

8. To identify new principles of diagnosis and treatment derived from these studies.

9. To test these new principles against traditional methods of diagnosis and treatment.

10. To identify the needs for evaluation and treatment of patients with GER-related otolaryngologic conditions.

11. To make recommendations for future studies of otolaryngologic GERD.

APPLICATION OF FINDINGS

The results of these studies suggest that the successful treatment of otolaryngologic patients with GER-related conditions depends upon:

1. Accurate diagnosis, including differentiation between upright and supine nocturnal reflux.

2. Identification of the specific underlying factors responsible for GER in each patient.

3. Modification of the duration, intensity, and focus of antireflux therapy to conform to the needs (reflux pattern) of each patient.

New criteria are proposed for:

1. Identification of the GER patient by:

a. history,

b. physical examination,

c. conventional diagnostic methods, and

d. diagnostic pH-metry.

2. Medical treatment failure.

The data from these studies suggest that:

1. There is a high degree of association between GERD and carcinoma of the larynx, upper airway stenosis, and globus pharyngeus.

2. There is a moderately high degree of association between GERD and chronic laryngitis, dysphagia, and cough.

3. GERD in otolaryngology patients has different manifestations than GERD in gastroenterology patients with esophagitis.

4. Some of the sequelae due to GER, such as laryngeal and tracheal stenosis, may be preventable through early recognition and treatment.

5. Collaborative studies between otolaryngologists and gastroenterologists and those in other disciplines will further expand our knowledge of the pathophysiology of GERD.

LITERATURE REVIEW

HISTORICAL PERSPECTIVE

It is likely that gastroesophageal reflux disease (GER, GERD) was recognized in antiquity. In 1618, Fabricius described the gastroesophageal junction and attributed its name "cardia" to Galen (c. 129 to c. 200 A.D.), who had coined the term because symptoms arising from the gastroesophageal junction were similar to those arising from the heart.[25] It was not until the 20th century, however, that the relationship between the symptoms and GER was established.[26,27]

In 1890, Chevalier Jackson introduced the esophagoscope[25] and the modern era of esophagology began. Nine years later, using a crude manometric system, Meltzer (1899) described esophageal peristalsis.[28] Although Tileston (1906),[29] Mosher (1921),[30] and Jackson (1922)[31] described the anatomic, endoscopic, and pathological findings of stricture and "peptic ulcer" of the esophagus, they did not consider the cause to be related to reflux of the gastric contents.

Mosher[30] commented:

> I feel that narrowing of the liver tunnel due to an inflammatory involvement of the lesser omentum will be found in the future to play a large part . . . in producing these strictures. . . . This shares in the inflammations, acute and chronic, of the rest of the peritoneal tissue of the abdominal cavity.

He attributed such inflammation to gallbladder disease, stomach causes, or foreign body.

In a landmark article in JAMA, Winkelstein (1935)[27] reported "peptic esophagitis: a new clinical entity." He reviewed the prevailing beliefs of his time that the causes of esophagitis were: *1.* irritative (mechanical, thermal, and chemical irritants, including alcohol and tobacco); *2.* specific (syphilis, tuberculosis, actinomycosis); and *3.* secondary to *a.* cardiospasm, *b.* diverticula, or *c.* neoplasm). He described in detail five patients with heartburn, dysphagia, esophagitis, stricture and esophageal spasm, and stated, "the type of substernal pain, heartburn, sour regurgitations and the hyperchlorhydria in all recall the clinical features of peptic ulcer of the esophagus." Indeed, in three of his patients there was a history of a preexisting peptic ulcer. Winkelstein's patients all responded to antireflux treatment, although four had periodic relapses and one required a gastrectomy. In addition to reviewing the symptom complex in his patients, Winkelstein reported the endoscopic and radiographic findings.

Throughout the 1940s and 1950s, hiatal hernia became equated with GERD and surgical correction of "symptomatic sliding hiatal hernia" became the focus of treatment.[32] The belief that the sphincteric function of the lower esophageal sphincter was created by mechanical factors was supported by the failure of anatomists and operating surgeons to demonstrate a separate anatomic muscle at the gastroesophageal junction.[25,32]

In 1950, Berenberg and Neuhauser[26] reported "cardio-esophageal relaxation (chalasia) as a cause of vomiting in infants." They made the following observations:

> *1.* "We have observed 24 patients . . . with repeated vomiting apparently due to persistent relaxation of the hiatal portion of the esophagus with failure of the gastric cardia to perform its usual 'sphincter' action."
>
> *2.* "The normal hiatus esophagus does not gape, but, as Jackson states, is closed by a pinchcock-like action of the diaphragm."
>
> *3.* "In normal deglutition this muscular sphincter relaxes to allow the passage of food into the stomach. If it fails to close, gastric contents will reflux into the esophagus, resulting in regurgitation."
>
> *4.* "The vomiting seems effortless and rarely is forceful or projectile. It is more apt to take place . . . when the baby is put back in his crib in the supine or decubitus position. . . . In a few instances, there have been pulmonary changes due to aspiration pneumonitis."
>
> *5.* "Relief of symptoms has been achieved . . . only by empiric measures [including keeping the infant upright during and after the feeding, and thickening of the feeding formula]."
>
> *6.* "From the nature of the syndrome and its self-limiting course in most instances it would appear likely that it is most often produced by temporary neuromuscular dysfunction."

The description of GERD by Berenberg and Neuhauser was the most accurate and comprehensive after Winkelstein's. Dysfunction (low resting pressure) of the lower esophageal sphincter was believed to be the sole factor responsible for reflux. However, despite the insight afforded by their study, knowledge about the physiology of esophagogastric function and

TABLE I.
Historical Landmarks in GERD.

Landmark	Reference	Date
Gastroesophageal (GE) junction named "cardia"	Galen[47]	c. 129 to c. 200 A.D.
Description of GE junction	Fabricius[47]	1618
Upper esophageal sphincter (UES) named "crico-pharyngeus"	A. Valsalva[48]	1717
Invention of esophagoscope	C. Jackson[49]	1890
Description of esophageal peristalsis	S. Meltzer[28]	1899
Description of "peptic ulcer" of the esophagus	W. Tileston[29]	1906
Description of crico-pharyngeus	G. Killian[50]	1907
Description of esophageal stricture	H. Mosher[30]	1921
Anatomic and endoscopic description of GE junction	C. Jackson[31]	1922
Clinical description of "peptic esophagitis" in 5 adults	A. Winkelstein[27]	1935
Description of heterotopic columnar ("gastric") mucosa	C. Jackson[51] N. Barrett[52]	1929 1950
Modern manometry	F. Ingelfinger[53]	1940
Clinical and radiographic description of GERD in 24 children	W. Berenberg[26]	1950
Surgical repair of "sliding hiatal hernia"	P. Allison[32]	1951
Manometric description of the lower esophageal sphincter (LES)	F. Fyke[33]	1956
Acid perfusion test	L. Bernstein[38]	1958
"Fundoplication" reported	R. Nissen[54]	1961
Introduction of flexible fiberoptic esophagoscope	P. LoPresti[35] W. Burnett[37]	1962 1962
Prolonged pH monitoring	F. Miller[39] J. Spencer[40]	1964 1969

TABLE II.
Cited References in the English Language: Hiatal Hernia (HH), Gastroesophageal Reflux (GERD), and Peptic or Reflux Esophagitis (ESOPH) (Medline Search) 1966 through 1988.

Year	HH	GERD	ESOPH	Total
1966	49	75	56	180
1967	63	78	37	178
1968	68	114	51	233
1969	60	126	54	240
1970	53	126	43	222
1971	49	138	36	223
1972	46	150	57	253
1973	56	177	45	278
1974	83	177	61	321
1975	115	165	81	361
1976	129	156	66	351
1977	119	197	102	418
1978	123	178	143	444
1979	130	186	102	418
1980	113	187	119	419
1981	84	199	125	408
1982	106	226	127	459
1983	88	252	117	457
1984	105	269	125	499
1985	85	288	147	520
1986	52	282	139	473
1987	71	337	142	550
1988	57	273	134	464
Total	1904	4356	2109	8369

the mechanisms of GERD was still limited.

With the introduction of modern manometry, Fyke, *et al.*[33] (1956) and Ingelfinger[34] (1958) began to unravel the complex neurophysiologic events associated with swallowing and with the pathogenesis of GERD. The lower esophageal sphincter remained the primary focus of reference, but esophageal motility and dysmotility also became recognized as factors in GERD.

The presupposition of the 1940s that hiatal hernia caused reflux gave way in the 1950s to the concept of lower esophageal sphincteric incompetence as the sole cause. However, as esophageal physiology was further elucidated, a multifactorial model of the pathogenesis of GER began to emerge.

With the introduction of the flexible fiberoptic esophagoscope in 1962,[35–37] some aspects of diagnostic esophagology moved out of the operating theater and into the gastroenterologist's laboratory. However, despite advances in diagnosis, GER research remained almost exclusively focused on the problem of esophagitis.

In 1958, Bernstein and Baker[38] introduced the acid perfusion test, which proved to be more sensitive than contrast radiography for the diagnosis of reflux esophagitis. These and most other diagnostic tests were for the consequences and complications of esophagitis.[6]

In the 1960s, prolonged pH monitoring was introduced.[39,40] It readily became apparent that pH manometry was both highly sensitive and specific *for the reflux event itself*. Within the last 20 years, this test has resulted in new insights into the pathophysiology of GERD[41–46] (Table I).

Perhaps because of esophageal manometry, fiberoptic esophagoscopy, and pH-metry, the body of literature on GERD since the 1960s is primarily within the specialty of gastroenterology. Since 1966 there have been over 8000 general references in the English language alone; every decade since has seen an escalation of interest in GERD (Table II). (To set this tremendous volume of literature in perspective, consider that in 1988 there were 464 Medline citations for GERD, 263 for gallbladder disease, 189 for vertigo, and 34 for subglottic stenosis.)

The most common pattern of GERD in the gastroenterology patient is typically heartburn associated with esophagitis.[45] Many of the otolaryngologic upper aerodigestive tract manifestations of GERD are considered "atypical" by the gastroenterologist because they are not the focus of attention of a gastroen-

TABLE III.
"First" Reports in the Otolaryngology Literature
In Which Gastroesophageal Reflux is Attributed an Etiologic Role.

Condition	Reference	Year
Contact ulcer and granuloma	J. Cherry[9]	1968
Globus pharyngeus	K. Malcomson[59]	1968
	J. Delahunty[60]	1970
Zenker's diverticulum	J. Delahunty[61]	1971
Posterior laryngitis ("pachydermia")	J. Delahunty[16]	1972
Multiple symptoms:	P. Chodosh[62]	1977
Hoarseness, dysphagia, otalgia, chronic cough and laryngospasm	P. Ward[19]	1982
Aspiration pneumonia	B. Fearon[94]	1981
Intubation granuloma	N. Olson[14]	1983
Laryngeal carcinoma	H. Glanz[64]	1976
	N. Olson[14]	1983
	P. Ward[22]	1988
	M. Morrison[21]	1988
Laryngeal stenosis	R. Bogdasarian[65]	1980
	W. Bain[23]	1983
	F. Little[24]	1985

terologic practice, and often they may be unassociated with heartburn or esophagitis.[55–58] What is an "atypical" GERD patient for the gastroenterologist may be a "typical" patient for the otolaryngologist. Manifestations of GERD may involve any portion of the upper aerodigestive tract.

The otolaryngologic upper aerodigestive tract manifestations of "atypical" GERD include contact ulcer and granuloma, pachyderma laryngitis, chronic cough, subglottic stenosis, and laryngeal carcinoma; Table III lists some of the landmark reports in the otolaryngology literature. Many of these GER-related conditions appear to have been "discovered" only recently.

OVERVIEW

The orderly transit of a bolus from the oral cavity to the stomach requires the interaction of complex neurophysiologic events,[66] and a host of factors mediate the homostatic process that prevents backflow into the esophagus.[67] Since each component of the deglutitory mechanism is interrelated, daily alterations in dietary behavior tend to create a state of dynamic dysequilibrium in which each physiologic parameter (*e.g.*, salivary flow, peristaltic amplitude, lower esophageal sphincteric pressure, gastric emptying, *etc.*) has a broad dynamic range in health and in GERD.[7,34,68–79]

There are three principal physiologic defense mechanisms against esophageal injury due to reflux of the gastric contents.[2,6] These are:

1. the lower esophageal sphincter (LES);

2. esophageal motor function with acid clearance; and

3. esophageal mucosal (tissue) resistance.

These mechanisms form the lines of defense against GERD; when the first line is penetrated, the other defenses become important.

In terms of protecting the upper aerodigestive tract and preventing aspiration of gastric contents into the tracheobronchial tree, the upper esophageal sphincter (UES) may provide a final (fourth) line of defense.[80–82] Nevertheless, LES and esophageal motor function are usually considered to determine the degree and consequences of reflux.[43,83,84]

Within his important article on esophageal motility, Franz Ingelfinger[34] (1958) stated:

> The function of the esophagus is to convey material from pharynx to stomach, and sometimes vice versa. Between swallows and regurgitations, mechanisms at either end of the tube prevent easy access of air from above and gastric contents from below, but these barriers are rather easily inhibited or forced under various circumstances. The essentials of esophageal function are thus very simple; in detail, however, they are both complex and controversial.

Physiologic and Pathologic Reflux

Gastroesophageal reflux (GER) is the retrograde flow of the gastric contents back into the esophagus. The term "reflux" itself literally means "backflow" from the Latin *Re-*, back, and *fluere*, to flow. In the awake state, *all* individuals experience some degree of reflux without the development of symptoms or complications; this is called "physiologic reflux."[6,38,85] Physiologic reflux is predominantly postcibal (occurring after the consumption of food).[6] (Postprandial is sometimes used as a synonym for postcibal; postprandial means "after dinner," from the Latin word *prandium*, dinner.)

Whether or not esophageal injury occurs depends upon the potency of the refluxate and the duration of mucosal exposure.[46,86] GER that causes symptoms or complications is known as "pathologic reflux," or "gastroesophageal reflux disease" (GERD). GERD encompasses "reflux esophagitis," which implies unequivocal histologic change in the lining mucosa.[2,6]

Symptoms and complications determine the difference between physiologic and pathologic GER. It is therefore not surprising that some patients with physiologic reflux may develop pathologic reflux, either intermittently or chronically, and that some patients with pathologic reflux may revert to normal.[87–90]

The Natural History of Gastroesophageal Reflux Disease

Although the natural history of GERD remains to a great extent unknown, five longitudinal studies have been reported,[87–91] the results of which are summarized in Tables IV and V. Although the studies have dissimilar limitations of method, the results are surprisingly similar.

TABLE IV.
Longitudinal Studies of GERD: Outcome (Medical Treatment Only).

Reference	Year	Duration of Study (years)	N	Improved or Well (%)	Same or Worse (%)	Esophageal Stricture (%)
Flood and Hennig[87]	1958	4	100	53	47	10
Rex, *et al.*[90]	1961	10	365	58	42	10
Palmer[89]	1968	5	142	52	48	11
Behar, *et al.*[91]	1975	2	83	19	81	—
Lieberman[88]	1987	2	25	55	45	0

GERD = gastroesophageal reflux disease.

TABLE V.
Longitudinal Studies of GERD: Outcome at the Extremes of Wellness and Intractability (Medical Treatment Only).

Reference	Year	N	Complete Remission (%)	Intractable Disease (%)
Flood and Hennig[87]	1958	100	27	13
Rex, *et al.*[90]	1961	365	—	10
Palmer[89]	1968	142	35	—
Lieberman[88]	1987	25	40	20

GERD = gastroesophageal reflux disease.

Flood and Hennig[87] followed 100 patients with "symptomatic hiatus hernia" treated medically for an average of 4 years (range of 6 months to 10 years). They found that symptoms, with time, became mild in 26%, and 27% had no symptoms whatsoever. (After 1 year of treatment, one third of the patients were well, one third of the patients were improved, and the remaining one third were worse or unchanged.)

Twenty percent of the patients had had ulceration of the stomach or duodenum, 18% upper gastrointestinal bleeding, and 10% stricture. Thirteen percent of the patients were considered to have intractable esophageal disease; the prognosis in the patients with ulceration of the stomach or duodenum was relatively poor. However, analysis of a number of other factors, including the duration of symptoms and the size of the hernia, did not establish a relationship between these factors and prognosis.

In 1961, Rex, *et al.*[90] reported a follow-up study of medically treated esophageal hiatal hernia. Three hundred sixty-five of the 873 patients seen at the Mayo Clinic for "symptomatic sliding hiatal hernia" in 1949 had responded to a follow-up letter 10 years later. Fifty-eight percent of the patients claimed to be symptomatically improved. Ninety-nine of the 365 patients underwent a follow-up endoscopy. Of those, 48% had endoscopic evidence of improvement, 21% had normal examinations, and 10% had esophageal stricture. Over the 10-year period, the mortality related to the esophageal disease (esophageal rupture or carcinoma) was less than 1%.

Palmer[89] studied the interrelationship between hiatal hernia (n = 786), esophagitis (n = 413), and stricture (n = 45) over 1 to 20 years. More than one half of the patients were initially asymptomatic and had had hiatal hernia or esophagitis demonstrated by chance. Of patients with hiatal hernia, 24% had esophagitis. However, of all the patients with esophagitis, only 45% had a hiatal hernia.

One hundred forty-two of the esophagitis patients in Palmer's study who received medical management underwent esophagoscopy on at least two occasions. The span between the first and final examination averaged 4.5 years. The final examination revealed the development of esophagitis in 13%, worsening of preexisting esophagitis in 15%, no change in 20%, improvement in 17%, and no esophagitis in 35%. (Fifty-two percent of the patients improved or the esophagitis disappeared.) Complications consisted of upper gastrointestinal bleeding in 24% and esophageal stricture in 11%.

Lieberman[88] followed 25 patients with long-standing reflux esophagitis for over 2 years (average duration of symptoms at presentation: 13 years). Diagnosis was by symptoms, endoscopy, and biopsy. The patients then received intensive antireflux therapy for 9 months (cimetidine, metoclopramide, and lifestyle modification). Eighty percent (20/25) had remission; 20% (5/25) had persistent symptoms. Of those that had remission, 45% (9/20) experienced immediate relapse when treatment was discontinued, 15% (3/20) experienced relapse after 2 years, and eight (40%) remained in remission at 26 months. (These patients clearly received the most aggressive antireflux treatment of the above series and yet it appears that the outcome was similar to that in all the other studies.)

Behar, *et al.*[91] reported on the medical and surgical management of reflux esophagitis: a 38-month report on a prospective clinical trial. They compared the surgical and medical management of biopsy-proven cases of reflux esophagitis by randomly assigning patients to surgical (15 patients) and medical (16 patients) groups. In addition, a third nonrandomized medical treatment group (20 patients) was studied. The groups were similar in age and symptoms, and each patient had endoscopy with biopsy, a Bernstein acid perfusion test, and intraesophageal pH-metry prior to inclusion in the study. Surgical management consisted of Belsey fundoplication, and medical management consisted of elevation of the head of the bed, bland diet with small meals, weight reduction, and liquid antacids. H_2 antagonists were not employed.

Seventy-three percent of the surgical group and 19% of the medical group had an excellent-to-good response at 3 years. Fair-to-poor results were observed in 81% of the medical patients and 27% of the surgical patients. Despite the "minimal" medical antireflux therapy, the relapse (recurrence) rates compare with those in a recent study by Hetzel, *et al.*[92] of patients treated with omeprazole (a hydrogen ion

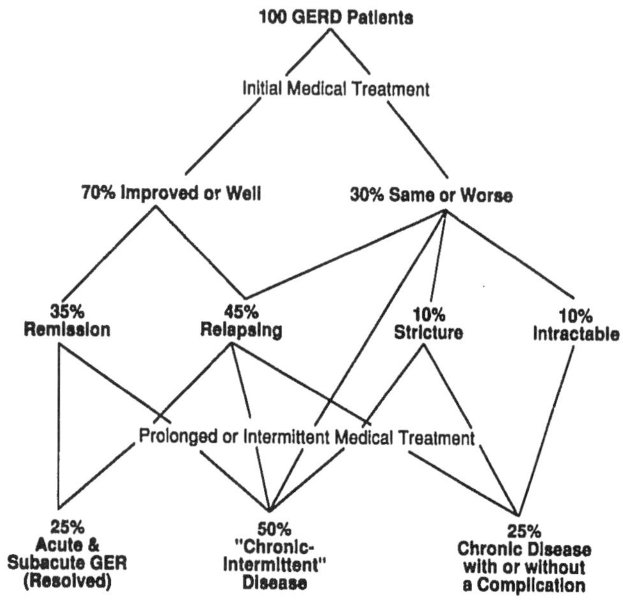

Fig. 2. Summary estimate of the natural history of 100 patients with gastroesophageal reflux disease.

blocker that totally suppresses acid production). Hetzel, *et al.*[92] studied 196 reflux esophagitis patients using various dosing schedules of omeprazole. Patients receiving 40 mg daily demonstrated healing at 4 weeks in 97% with moderate esophagitis, 88% with severe esophagitis, and 44% with Barrett's ulceration. However, the rate of endoscopic relapse in 107 patients with severe esophagitis was 82% by 6 months, similar to Behar's "minimal" medical antireflux therapy.

Considering the above studies, it would appear that GERD covers a wide spectrum of severity, which may be acute and self-limited, intermittent, or intractable. Many patients who initially respond to therapy may suffer relapses either when treatment is discontinued or at a later date. Based upon the limited data of these studies, Figure 2 represents a "summary estimate" of the natural history of GERD.

Manifestations of Gastroesophageal Reflux Disease: Typical and Atypical

The distinction between a typical and an atypical designation in GERD is based upon different symptom complexes. Heartburn and regurgitation are the principal symptoms of esophagitis, which is the most common disorder associated with GERD, and are considered *typical*.[6,93] The *atypical* group have pulmonary, laryngeal, pharyngeal, and cervical symptoms attributable to GERD. Otolaryngologic patients and pediatric patients usually have the atypical form, commonly without heartburn, which is the single most common symptom in the esophagitis patient of the typical group.[58,94,95] Table VI compares the reported GER symptoms of three groups of patients, typical gastroenterology patients, atypical otolaryngology patients, and pediatric patients.

TABLE VI.
A Comparison of the GER Symptoms of the Typical Esophagitis Patient, the "Atypical" Otolaryngology Patient, and the Pediatric Patient.

Symptom	Typical* (%)	Atypical† (%)	Pediatric‡ (%)
Heartburn	83	20	16
Regurgitation	23	—	68
Dysphagia	40	12	30
Cough	47	26	—
Pulmonary infection	16	—	36
Hoarseness	12	44	—
Throat irritation (soreness, clearing)	3	87	—

*Urschel[95] (n = 636).
†Toohill[58] (n = 207).
‡Fearon[94] (n = 56).

Stiegmann, *et al.*[55] reported the incidence of upper aerodigestive symptoms, including hoarseness and cervical dysphagia during a 5-year period in which 376 gastroenterology patients were evaluated endoscopically for GER. Twenty-two (6%) had predominantly upper aerodigestive complaints; of that group only 23% had heartburn. Thus, 6% were considered to have atypical GERD. Ward, *et al.*[96] have suggested that the true incidence of many of these so-called atypical conditions remains unknown, since it seems likely that many of these patients had been underdiagnosed in the past.

Even patients with esophagitis may lack typical symptoms on occasion. Helm, *et al.*[97] reported a series of patients with esophageal stricture, one half of whom did not have heartburn. Furthermore, heartburn in those patients could not be provoked, even with acid perfusion of the distal esophagus.

In a recent review in the American Journal of Gastroenterology,[56] Deschner and Benjamin concluded:

> Whereas the esophagus is the primary target of injury in GER, any contiguous structure can be affected due to the direct contact of gastric irritants or due to neurally mediated mechanisms. Reflux may result in chronic cough, aspiration pneumonia, and perhaps chronic interstitial lung disease. It may also produce disease of the head and neck, presumably by bathing these structures with gastric contents. However, it appears that some manifestations of GER, most notably bradycardia and asthma, may be reflex mediated through some specific esophageal receptors. The expanding use of new diagnostic technologies should provide future clarification of pathophysiology and, perhaps, direct successful therapy. In an individual with unexplained symptoms in areas proximal to the esophagus, gastroesophageal reflux should be considered, even if 'classic' symptoms of reflux are not present.

THE ANTIREFLUX BARRIER

In its elemental form, the antireflux barrier con-

TABLE VII.
Components of the Antireflux Barrier.

A. Lower Esophageal Sphincter Tone
  1. Anatomic factors
    a. Diaphragmatic pinchcock
    b. Esophagogastric "cardiac" angle
    c. Intra-abdominal esophagus
    d. Phrenoesophageal ligament
  2. Neural innervation
  3. Hormonal influences
    a. Gastrin
    b. Gastric alkalinization
B. Esophageal Acid Clearance
  1. Volume clearance (peristalsis)
  2. Acid neutralization
    a. Secondary peristalsis
    b. Salivary bicarbonate
C. Esophageal Epithelial Resistance
  1. Preepithelial
    a. Mucus
    b. Unstirred water layer
    c. Surface bicarbonate
  2. Epithelial (cell membrane)
  3. Postepithelial (metabolic buffering)
  4. Gastroduodenal influences
    a. Potency of the refluxate
    b. Volume of the refluxate
D. Upper Esophageal Sphincter Tone
  1. Diurnal variation
  2. Esophageal volume
  3. Esophageal acidity (pH)

sists of four lines of defense (Table VII). In addition, salivary[46,68,97–99] and gastroduodenal[78,79,100] functions substantially influence antireflux mechanisms. Thus, the integrity of the antireflux barrier is inexorably tied to the processes of deglutition and digestion. The components of the deglutitory mechanism are shown in Table VIII.

Normal Deglutition

Even before the consumption of food, thoughts of food stimulate salivary and gastric secretion (cephalic phase).[101] Therefore, the digestive process actually begins before the consumption of food.

The oral preparatory phase is the first phase of deglutition. Its purpose is to break down food into a consistency suitable for bolus formation and swallowing. This is facilitated by mixing the food with saliva and mastication. Once the bolus is formed, swallowing is initiated in the brain stem as the tongue moves upward and backward, thrusting the bolus into the oropharynx. From this point on, swallowing is a reflex action.

The pharyngeal phase is characterized by reflex inhibition of respiration, velopharyngeal closure, glottic closure (true cords, false cords, and aryepiglottic folds), and laryngeal elevation and anterior displacement; only then does pharyngeal contraction propel the bolus into the hypopharynx, at which point the

TABLE VIII.
Components of the Normal Swallowing Mechanism.

A. Oral Phase
  1. Oral preparation
    a. Mastication
    b. Salivation
    c. Bolus formation
  2. Initiation of the swallowing reflex
    a. Central recognition (brain stem)
    b. Bolus propulsion (tongue thrust)
B. Pharyngeal Phase
  1. Reflex inhibition of respiration
  2. Velopharyngeal closure
  3. Laryngeal closure and elevation
  4. Pharyngeal contraction ("peristalsis")
  5. Relaxation of the cricopharyngeus and opening of the upper esophageal sphincter
C. Esophageal Phase
  1. Primary peristalsis
  2. Relaxation and opening of the lower esophageal sphincter
  3. Secondary peristalsis

cricopharyngeus relaxes, opening the upper esophageal sphincter for passage of the bolus into the esophagus.[66]

The traditional view of the pharyngeal phase has come under scrutiny recently and the mechanics of this phase have become somewhat controversial. McConnel,[102] using solid-state computer-analyzed manofluorographic swallowing analysis (modern manometry with simultaneous cinefluorography), has suggested that peristaltic activity does not occur in the pharynx, but rather bolus transit is accomplished by tongue thrust (piston-like action) and secondary suction-pump action of the hypopharynx. (However, the acceptance or rejection of this viewpoint does not alter the swallowing sequence or the normal physiology of the pharyngeal phase.)

The pharynx generates pressures of 200 to 400 mm Hg at rates up to 4000 mm Hg/s. Cricopharyngeal relaxation must be complete and synchronous with arrival of the bolus; otherwise, cervical dysphagia or aspiration may result.[74,102–109] Once the bolus enters the upper esophagus the speed of the pharyngeal waves (9 to 25 cm/s) is maintained in the upper half of the esophagus until the lower portion of the esophageal body is reached, at which point the striated muscle, which is contiguous with the pharynx, changes to smooth muscle. In the lower half of the esophagus, the rate of peristalsis is 4 cm/s. (In actuality, the speed of esophageal transit varies with consumption of solids and liquids; transit time is slower for solids.)[102]

When the primary peristaltic wave arrives at the gastroesophageal junction, reflex relaxation and opening of the lower esophageal sphincter occur. Subsequently, under normal conditions, additional swallows and secondary peristaltic waves continue approximately once each minute.[46]

Lower Esophageal Sphincter (LES)

Although difficult to identify anatomically, a functioning LES can be demonstrated easily both radiographically and manometrically.[25] The primary functions of the LES are *1.* relaxation from the usual tonic state during swallowing to allow free passage of ingested material from the esophagus into the stomach, and *2.* maintenance of an effective high-pressure zone to prevent reflux of the gastric contents back into the esophagus.[71] LES competence and LES pressure are determined by anatomic, neural, hormonal, and life-style related factors.[17,33,71,72,110–114]

Anatomic Factors

The relation of the diaphragm to the lower esophagus varies widely; however, most commonly, the right crus dominates in the formation of a hiatus, creating a muscular sling.[25,31] Using a dog model, Radmark and Pettersson[114] demonstrated that excision of half of the diaphragm lowered manometrically measured LES pressure from an initial mean of 20 cm H_2O to 15 cm H_2O. In the preoperative state, "spontaneous" (provoked) reflux occurred when a gastric volume of 3200 ml was reached, whereas the volume necessary to create such reflux after removal of the diaphragm was only 1400 ml. Thus, the diaphragm may be considered to contribute up to 25% of LES competence.

Also believed to be important in maintaining LES competence is the "cardiac angle" (*i.e.*, the angle of entry of the esophagus into the stomach).[25,30] It is believed that the acute angle of entry helps create a valve-effect; however, there is a great variability in the angle in normal people, ranging from 7 to 60 degrees with a mean angle of 21 degrees.[6]

A third anatomic factor thought to contribute to LES competence is the intra-abdominal segment of esophagus. This portion of esophagus is exposed to the same pressures as the rest of the abdominal cavity; therefore, increased intra-abdominal pressure will tend to be transmitted to the lower esophagus as well as to the gastric cavity, tending to force the esophagus closed.[6,25]

Bonavina, *et al.*[110] demonstrated that the length of the intra-abdominal segment seemed to correlate well with LES pressure. They found that the longer the intra-abdominal segment, the lower the pressure required to act as a barrier to reflux.

Finally, the phrenoesophageal ligament is a fibroelastic membrane that arises as a condensation of the abdominal fascia. Allison[32] believed that this ligament was an important anatomic structure, which, when defective, gave rise to hiatal hernia. While there is no question that the phrenoesophageal ligament is a definable anatomic structure that inserts in the lower esophagus, the role of the ligament in promoting LES competence has not been definitively demonstrated.[6]

Neural Innervation

Full details of the neural control of LES function remain to be elucidated. It is clear, however, that vagotomy, whether intra-abdominal or cervical, does not result in a change of resting LES pressure.[71] Although this observation suggests that parasympathetic innervation of the LES may not be important, pharmacologic doses of cholinergic or anticholinergic substances markedly raise and lower LES pressure. Observations from animal models suggest that non-adrenergic inhibitory fibers may be responsible for normal relaxation of the LES during swallowing.[71]

Hormonal Factors

In 1970, Castell and Harris demonstrated that gastrin increases LES pressure.[72] It is now clear, however, that a host of hormones have a marked influence on the LES. In addition to gastrin, those that increase LES tone are Pitressin®, angiotensin II, and motilin. Those that decrease LES pressure are secretin, cholecystokinin, glucagon, and vasoactive intestinal peptide.[113]

LES pressure increases with gastric alkalinization.[115] However, the relationship is now believed to be more complicated than simply a response to serum gastrin. Even though the pharmacologic hormonal interrelationships have not been fully elucidated, this mechanism appears to be important in preventing postcibal reflux.[71,115]

Esophageal Acid Clearance

Helm, *et al.*[99] demonstrated that when a 15-ml bolus of acid is instilled into the distal esophagus, a single peristaltic wave normally clears virtually all the volume of the bolus. The intraluminal pH, however, does not begin to rise until subsequent swallows of saliva, with its buffering capacity due to its high bicarbonate content. Indeed, following instillation of the acid bolus, spontaneous swallowing occurs approximately every 30 to 60 seconds. With each swallow, there is an increase in pH back to a neutral pH of 7. In subjects swallowing once every 30 seconds, pH returns to normal within 3 minutes. (This forms the basis of the "standard acid clearance test.")[46,99]

To demonstrate the importance of salivary bicarbonate, additional experiments were performed, with aspiration (removal) of all the saliva from the oral cavity. When this was done, the intra-esophageal pH remained below 4 despite secondary esophageal activity. Finally, using a third variation, the experiments were repeated in patients with impaired esophageal motility (whose primary peristalsis was defective). The authors found that it was not until volume clearance of the acid was achieved that the buffering capacity of salivary bicarbonate became effective in restoring neutral intraluminal pH.[99]

Helm, *et al.*[68] also have demonstrated that normal subjects with a salivary flow of 1.2 ml/min produce enough saliva in 5 minutes to titrate 1.0 ml of 0.1 normal hydrochloric acid from a pH of 1.2 to a pH of 4.0. In addition, they have found that the concentration of bicarbonate in the saliva increases with salivary stimulation caused by instilling acid into the distal esophagus. The reflex pathways responsible for increasing the bicarbonate content have been postulated to be parasympathetic, but the exact mechanism remains unproven.

Following a spontaneous "physiologic" reflux episode, it is postulated that peristalsis (following a single swallow) clears acid volume from the distal esophagus; thereafter, salivary bicarbonate neutralizes the remaining intraluminal acid. These observations are supported by pH-metry results in normal subjects, which reveal that when spontaneous reflux events occur, pH is restored to pH greater than 4 in less than 5 minutes.[8] As a corollary, patients with abnormal esophageal motility and/or xerostomia are more likely to develop gastroesophageal reflux disease than normal subjects, even if LES function is normal.[116]

Esophageal Epithelial Resistance

The third determinant of the degree to which esophageal injury may occur is referred to as "epithelial (tissue) resistance." Tissue resistance is not a single factor, but represents a number of layered "structures" and functions that interact to form a dynamic barrier[86] (Table VII).

Mucus, with its viscoelastic and gel properties, forms an excellent barrier to the penetration of large molecules, such as pepsin. Mucus, however, does not block penetration of the hydrogen ion (acid).[86] The layer below does that.

The outermost layer of protection is the mucus layer, below which is the "unstirred water layer." This layer has a relatively high bicarbonate content, which is probably derived from saliva, mucosal secretions, serum, or is transported from epithelial cells. This unstirred water layer produces a buffering sink by creating an alkaline environment adjacent to the cell surface.[86]

At the epithelial level, both the cell membrane and the intracellular bridges form a barrier to penetration of both acid and pepsin. Finally, the post-epithelial defenses are composed of the buffering capacity of the outer layers of the epithelium and the subepithelial blood flow. The latter removes toxic by-products, thereby providing local tissue buffering once injury has occurred. Furthermore, when esophageal mucosal injury occurs, blood flow in the esophageal wall increases to provide additional buffering by delivering nutrients and bicarbonate to reestablish tissue acid-base balance.[86]

Upper Esophageal Sphincter (UES)

The upper esophageal sphincter, or cricopharyngeus, was first described in 1717 by Valsalva.[48] Valsalva distinguished the cricopharyngeal muscle as a separate entity from the inferior constrictor. Killian (1907)[50] subdivided the cricopharyngeus muscle anatomically into two portions: the upper, pars obliquus, and the lower, pars fundiformis. The superior fibers of the inferior pharyngeal constrictor pass obliquely from the origin in the thyroid cartilage to be inserted on the median raphe, whereas the inferior-most fibers from the cricoid cartilage pass without interruption in a horizontal direction encircling the cricoid. The cricopharyngeus has no midline raphe. It is still controversial whether the cricopharyngeus is wholly distinct from the inferior constrictor.[117] However, among surgeons and anatomists there seems to be at least a consensus that the lower horizontal portion is discrete.

There are two areas of relative weakness. The first, between the two groups of muscle, the oblique and horizontal, is the area known as Killian's area, which is believed to be the exit point for Zenker's diverticula. The second is Laimer's triangle, which is situated posteriorly between the cricopharyngeus and the uppermost fibers of the esophagus. The terms "cricopharyngeus" and "upper esophageal sphincter" (UES) are used interchangeably.

The cricopharyngeus is innervated by the pharyngeal plexus, vagus, and glossopharyngeal nerves. The parasympathetic function is probably entirely vagal and the sensory function is probably entirely glossopharyngeal. Sympathetic fibers arise from the superior cervical ganglia and also join the pharyngeal plexus. In its normal resting state, the cricopharyngeal muscle is in a state of tonic contraction. Vagal stimulation produces relaxation.

Kirchner[48] demonstrated that sectioning the vagus nerves bilaterally (in dogs) abolished the relaxation phase and produced severe dysphagia. Electrical stimulation of the superior cervical sympathetic ganglion produced an increase in the UES pressure. Conversely, electrical stimulation of the cut vagi produced full relaxation.

Thus, in contradistinction to the LES, the UES is a clearly defined anatomic entity and its innervation has been well defined. On the other hand, cricopharyngeal physiology is poorly understood because the development of solid-state pressure transducers (not dependent upon pull-through or water perfusion systems) has been recent. Furthermore, because of the anatomic configuration of the cricopharyngeus and its relationship to the cricoid with deglutition, manometric pressures recorded in anteroposterior diameter may be considerably higher than those measured from side to side. Gerhardt, *et al.*,[73] using a pull-through technique, found a differential in pressure, depending upon how the recording device was oriented. In the posterior direction the mean was 109 ± 4 mm Hg; anteriorly it was 88 ± 4

TABLE IX.
Etiologic Factors Associated with GERD.

A. Decreased Lower Esophageal Sphincter Pressure (LESP)	
1. Hiatal hernia	3. Tobacco
2. Diet	4. Ethanol
a. Fat	5. Drugs
b. Chocolate	6. GERD
c. Mints	
B. Abnormal Esophageal Motility	
1. Neuromuscular disease	3. Ethanol
2. Laryngectomy	4. GERD
C. Abnormal or Reduced Mucosal Resistance	
1. Xerostomia	2. Tobacco
a. Sicca syndrome	3. Ethanol
b. Oral cavity XRT	4. Drugs
c. Esophageal XRT	5. GERD
D. Delayed Gastric Emptying	
1. Outlet obstruction	2. Diet (fat)
a. Ulcer	3. Tobacco
b. Neoplasm	4. Ethanol
c. Neurogenic	
E. Increased Intra-abdominal Pressure	
1. Tight clothing (corsets, belts, etc)	3. Obesity
	4. Pregnancy
2. Diet	5. Occupation
a. Overeating	6. Exercise
b. Carbonated beverages	
F. Gastric Hypersecretion (of acid and/or pepsin)	
1. Stress	2. Tobacco
a. Trauma	3. Ethanol
b. Surgery	4. Drugs
c. Life-style	5. Diet

GERD = gastroesophageal reflux disease; XRT = radiation (x-ray) therapy.

mm Hg; to the left, 48 ± 2 mm Hg; and to the right, 45 ± 2 mm Hg.

In spite of the limitations of these techniques, significant physiologic events and responses of the UES have been described. Gerhardt, *et al.*[73] demonstrated that intraesophageal infusion of 0.1 normal hydrochloric acid produced significant UES pressure increases, and that increases in UES pressure occurred in response to volume, rate of infusion, and pH. (Increases in infusion volume, increases in rate of infusion, and decreases in pH each produced increased UES pressure.)

Like the LES, the UES has its own diurnal cycle. The resting pressure of the cricopharyngeus has been found to decrease significantly during sleep. In a study of eight healthy volunteers,[81] the mean resting pressure during wakefulness was 40 ± 17 mm Hg; during light sleep, 20 ± 17 mm Hg; and during deep sleep, 8 ± 3 mm Hg.[81] It was also noted that: *1.* UES pressure increased transiently with each inspiration during both wakefulness and sleep; and *2.* UES pressure after a meal was no different from than before a meal.

Within the last few years, improved technology has been developed to evaluate UES function.[102,118] As a consequence, a range of normal UES pressures has been established, but there is still significant variation from laboratory to laboratory. Kahrilas, *et al.*[81] found mean resting UES pressures in normal subjects to be 40 ± 17 SD mm Hg. Green, *et al.*[118] found values of 67 ± 5.4 mm Hg with a round catheter and 64.4 ± 8.3 mm Hg with an oval catheter.

In summary, the UES is believed to have two physiologic functions:[66,73,81]

1. To prevent aerophagia (air swallowing) during respiration; and

2. To act as an upper esophageal barrier to reflux and thereby prevent regurgitation of gastric contents into the upper aerodigestive tract and lungs.

PATHOGENESIS OF GASTROESOPHAGEAL REFLUX DISEASE

No review of the factors associated with the development of GERD can consider every variable. Many of the known or postulated etiologic factors are listed in Table IX. Within this listing are factors that alone can lead to GERD, such as esophageal dysmotility, gastric outlet obstruction, and xerostomia; however, more often than not, the etiology is multifactorial and related to diet, ingested substances, and lifestyle, as well as to constitutional factors. Furthermore, many factors, such as smoking and drinking of ethanol, have a simultaneous adverse effect on several of the anti-reflux mechanisms.

Decreased Lower Esophageal Sphincter (LES) Pressure

Hiatal Hernia

The relationship between hiatal hernia and GERD remains somewhat controversial. In 1951, Allison[32] equated reflux esophagitis with "sliding hiatus hernia." For the next two decades, the terms were used virtually interchangeably.

Cohen and Harris (1971)[75] performed esophageal manometry in four groups of patients:

1. patients with esophagitis, without hiatal hernia;

2. patients with esophagitis and hiatal hernia;

3. patients without esophagitis, with hiatal hernia;

4. patients without esophagitis and without hiatal hernia.

They found that patients without symptoms of esophagitis (with or without a hiatal hernia) had a mean LES pressure of 19.6 ± 1.2 mm Hg, and patients with esophagitis (with or without a hiatal hernia) had mean LES pressures of 3.0 ± 1.3 mm Hg (hernia group) and 3.8 ± 1.2 mm Hg (nonhernia group).

They commented, "It somehow seems unreasonable—even irritating—that this study turned out as it did. It had seemed logical to expect that a hiatus hernia would inevitably make the LES weaker. Logical or not, the data no longer allow this reasonable expectation." They concluded that hiatal hernia does not predispose to GER.

The clinical significance of hiatal hernia is further downgraded by the observation that, within a certain population, the technique of radiographic examination is probably more important in determining the incidence of hiatal hernia than any other factor. Schatzki,[119] for example, found the incidence of hiatal hernia to be 73.3%. To obtain this high percentage, he increased the intra-abdominal pressure in 30 elderly people by inflating their colons with air. Wolf, *et al.* (1959)[120] found that hiatal hernia increased with age. In the fifth decade, the incidence was 32%; in the sixth, 44%; in the seventh, 59%; and in the eighth, 76%.

Dyer and Pridie [121] carried out barium studies in 95 asymptomatic volunteers. They examined patients lying prone over a bolster with hiatal hernia being defined as gastric folds appearing above the diaphragm. This was observed in 43% of the patients.

Conway-Hughes[122] analyzed 453 consecutive barium esophagograms and showed barium reflux in 24 (6%) of 421 patients in whom no hiatal hernia was demonstrable, and reflux in 30 (94%) of 32 patients who had hiatal hernia. It was not clear, however, if any of these patients had GERD.

Finally, Wright and Hurwitz[123] established a statistical relationship between the endoscopic finding of esophagitis and hiatal hernia. They studied 293 patients with esophageal symptoms. Of these, 64 had hiatal hernia, of whom 32 (50%) had esophagitis. In 229 of the patients in whom no hernia was found, only 6 patients (3%) had endoscopic esophagitis. Wright and Hurwitz therefore concluded that if the patient did not have a hiatal hernia, there was only a 3% chance of finding endoscopic evidence of esophagitis; if hiatal hernia was present, there was a 50% chance of finding esophagitis.

In summary, hiatal hernia may or may not be associated with LES incompetence, even though in some groups of patients there is a statistical association between hiatal hernia and GERD. The finding of a hiatal hernia, however, does not make the diagnosis of GERD, nor does the lack of a demonstrable hiatal hernia rule it out.

Dietary Factors

Becker, *et al.*[124] studied the effect of fatty foods on gastroesophageal reflux. They used ambulatory 24-hour pH monitoring to assess GER in 10 normal subjects following low-fat and high-fat meals, eaten in two body positions on two consecutive days. The low-fat meal (16% fat) consisted of McDonald's skim milk and hot cakes with butter and syrup. The high-fat meal (61% fat) consisted of McDonald's sausage biscuit with egg and water. The meals had nearly identical protein content, volume, and calories. On successive days, patients ingested one of the meals twice, followed by random assignment of 3 hours upright or 3 hours supine. Acid exposure for each hour was assessed as the percentage time pH was less than 4.0.

Following the low-fat meal, the percentage of time pH was less than 4 for the first hour was 1.8 ± 0.8%; for the second hour, 2.1 ± 1.1%; and for the third hour, 0.5 ± 0.2%. Following the high-fat meal, the results were: for the first hour 7.4 ± 3.6%; the second hour, 8.1 ± 2.9%; and the third hour, 2.9 ± 1.2%. The differences were statistically significant.

In addition to fat, Murphy and Castell[125] investigated the relationship between chocolate and GER, attempting to control for fat content. They found that chocolate ingested postcibally resulted in a significant increase in GER.

Other foods have been found to predispose to GER (Table X-A). Ingestion of cola or mints (peppermint, spearmint) has also been shown to decrease LES pressure. However, of the foods that unequivocally decrease LES pressure, the most commonly consumed in contemporary society are fat and ethanol.

Sphincter Incompetence

Since 1970, LES pressures have been measured in hundreds of GERD patients and hundreds of normal subjects. In a study comparing patients with Barrett's esophagus (the most severe form of ulcerative reflux esophagitis) with "ordinary" reflux patients and controls, it was found that the reflux patients had lower mean resting LES pressures than the controls, and that the Barrett's group had significantly lower mean resting pressures than both groups.[2,126] These data seemed to indicate that LES pressure might be a predictor of severity of disease[2] and that very low LES pressures simply reflect sphincteric incompetence. Although there may be a "significant value" below which LES incompetence is a certainty, it has not been clearly established.[67] It has been demonstrated that reflux events rarely occur unless the LES pressure falls below 3 mm Hg.[83] However, there are very few patients with a resting LES pressure of 3 mm Hg or below.[67,75]

Mechanisms of Reflux

Dodds, *et al.*[44] found the mean LES pressure of reflux patients to be 14 ± 8 mm Hg, that of normal controls to be 29.9 mm Hg ($P < .001$). Reflux events could be characterized in terms of three mechanisms. Sixty-five percent were accompanied by transient LES relaxation; 17% were accompanied by a transient increase in the intra-abdominal pressure; and 18% occurred spontaneously. Complete LES relaxation alone, however, was not necessarily associated with an event of gastroesophageal reflux because many transient complete LES relaxations were not accompanied by detectable reflux. They postulated that, "other factors appear to be operative, such as body position, intragastric pressure, relaxation of the diaphragmatic hiatus, and perhaps longitudinal esophageal shortening." In this study, some GERD patients had normal LES resting pressures while some of the normal subjects had relatively low pressures overlapping those of GERD patients with esophagitis. This study and others[43,83,127] confirm that LES pressure alone is not an absolute predictor of reflux or of its severity.

Mittal and McCallum[128] studied patients with both subjective and objective evidence of GERD, and a normal control group by simultaneously performing esophageal manometry and pH studies. In normal subjects, transient relaxation of the LES was the only mechanism of acid reflux observed, and reflux occurred with less than one-third of such transient relaxations. In patients with esophagitis, however, when transient LES relaxation occurred, reflux episodes occurred 65% of the time (and transient LES relaxation was the mechanism in 73% of the reflux episodes).

Dent, *et al.*[43] studied the patterns of LES dysfunction associated with GERD and found LES relaxation was the prevalent mechanism, accounting for 82% of reflux episodes. They noted that the timing of most (69%) LES relaxations associated with reflux was not triggered by swallowing. Absent basal LES pressure was also found to be a mechanism of GER, accounting for 23% of episodes, mostly in patients with severe esophagitis.

Reflux as a Cause of Gastroesophageal Reflux Disease

One of the most intriguing and controversial mechanisms postulated in the pathogenesis of GERD is that reflux itself impairs LES pressure. Eastwood, *et al.*[129] studied the effect of esophageal inflammation on LES pressure in cats. LES pressure measurements and esophageal biopsies were obtained before, during, and after the development of experimental esophagitis, as well as after a 3-week recovery period. Perfusion of the esophagus with 0.1 normal HCl for either 1 or one-half hour per day for 4 days produced inflammatory changes confirmed by mucosal biopsy that were associated with a marked decline in LES pressure. (LES pressure began to drop by the second day.) After 3½ weeks of healing, the LES pressure returned to normal.

Baldi, *et al.*[130] measured LES pressure in 11 patients with severe erosive esophagitis before and after treatment, and found that antireflux treatment resulted in a mean LES pressure increase (3.5 ± 0.5 mm Hg pretreatment, to 12.5 mm Hg post-treatment).

Katz, *et al.*[131] investigated 13 patients with GERD who underwent esophageal manometric evaluation during acute exacerbations of disease and during remissions to determine whether LES pressure and esophageal peristaltic pressure responded to treatment. Contrary to the findings of Baldi, *et al.*,[130] no change was noted in the post-treatment LES or the peristaltic pressures. However, both LES pressure and distal esophageal amplitude were lower in the GERD patients than in the controls ($P < .05$).

TABLE X.
Foods, Drugs, Substances, and Hormones That Alter (Increase or Decrease) Lower Esophageal Sphincter Pressure.

Decrease	Increase
A. Foods	
Fat	Protein
Ethanol	
Chocolate	
Cola	
Mint	
B. Drugs and Substances	
Caffeine	Cholinergic agents (bethanechol)
Tobacco	Metoclopramide
Theophylline	Cisapride
Nitrates	Anticholinesterases (edrophonium)
Anticholinergics (atropine)	Indomethacin
Dopamine	Histamine
Morphine	Antacids
Meperidine	
Nitroprusside	
Lidocaine	
Diazepam	
Calcium-channel blockers	
Beta-adrenergic agents (isoproterenol)	
Alpha-adrenergic antagonists (phentolamine)	
Birth control pills (progesterone)	
C. Hormones	
Secretin	Gastrin
Cholecystokinin	Pitressin
Glucagon	Angiotensin
Gastric inhibiting peptide (GIP)	Bombesin
Vasoactive intestine peptide (VIP)	Substance P
Progesterone	Motilin
Neurotensin	
Hypothyroidism	

The disparity between these studies does not negate the possibility that LES tone may be adversely altered by GERD. Furthermore, in some patients, long-standing GERD may result in irreversible damage to the LES. The issue remains unresolved.

Other Factors

Gudmundsson, *et al.*[132] demonstrated significant diurnal variation in basal LES pressure. They studied 220 patients with GERD and recorded LES pressures at 8 AM, noon, and 4 PM. The median pressure at 8 AM was 13.4 mm Hg, at noon (11.5 mm Hg), and at 4

PM (8.5 mm Hg). The pressure was significantly decreased at 4 PM ($P < .05$). On pH-metry in the same patients, the greatest amount of reflux was observed during the evening period.

Many drugs and other substances have been implicated in decreasing LES pressure (Table X-B), and the list grows every year. Furthermore, as the hormonal regulation of the digestive process is further elucidated, it appears that many hormones (or their absence) may influence LES pressure (Table X-C). The mechanisms of action and the importance of these hormones in GERD remain primarily speculative.

Abnormal Esophageal Motility

The role of abnormal esophageal acid clearance is an important factor in the pathogenesis of GERD. In the previous section on the antireflux barrier, it was shown that esophageal acid clearance is a two-step process.[46] Following an episode of "physiologic" reflux, the first step, peristaltic volume clearance of the esophagus (a single swallow in normal subjects), is a prerequisite for the second step, neutralization of residual intraluminal acid by salivary bicarbonate.[46] Not surprisingly, esophageal dysmotility is common in GERD; both primary and secondary peristalsis are often impaired, as measured by peristaltic amplitude.[25,131]

Ferguson, *et al.*[84] studied esophageal acid bolus emptying in 250 GER patients, and found that delayed esophageal emptying was the predominant component of abnormal acid clearance. Decreased amplitude of peristaltic waves was believed to be the defect. Arana, *et al.*[133] also studied esophageal motility in GERD patients and found that tertiary (nonpropulsive) esophageal waves accounted for an average of 75% of all peristaltic activity in the basal state and, with instillation of acid into the esophagus, the percentage increased to 80%.

Siegel and Hendrix[76] studied 25 GERD patients and 25 controls with simultaneous esophageal manometry and a Bernstein acid perfusion test. Sixteen percent (4 of 25) of the controls and 100% (25 of 25) of the GERD patients were shown to have esophageal motor abnormalities. These consisted of three types: *1.* nonprogressive (tertiary) esophageal contraction; *2.* increased amplitude and duration of contractions ("nutcracker esophagus"); and *3.* increased esophageal tone.

Kahrilas, *et al.*[134] studied esophageal volume clearance in GERD patients by simultaneously performing esophageal manometry and videofluoroscopy. The minimal effective contractile strength for emptying the distal esophagus was 20 mm Hg, whereas, in the proximal esophagus, virtually any propagated contraction was effective. Peristaltic amplitudes of 16 mm Hg in the proximal esophagus and 30 to 40 mm Hg in the distal esophagus were required for invariable bolus clearance.

Gerhardt, *et al.*[135] compared esophageal motility in three groups: normal subjects, GERD patients with heartburn, and GERD patients with regurgitation. They found that the peristaltic amplitude in the regurgitation group was significantly less than in the other two groups.

Esophageal Motor Abnormalities in GERD: Cause or Effect?

Primary motor abnormalities in GERD are extremely common; nevertheless, there is considerable evidence to support the possibility that GER itself causes secondary esophageal dysmotility. Pre-treatment and post-treatment esophageal motility studies reveal that the motor abnormalities observed in GERD may be reversible.

Gill, *et al.*[136] performed esophageal manometry in 32 patients with GERD, both before and after fundoplication, and in 18 healthy normal subjects. Preoperatively, the patients with GERD had mean peristaltic amplitudes that were significantly lower than those in controls ($P < .001$). After antireflux surgery, the mean amplitudes of peristaltic contractions increased significantly ($P < .01$) at all levels of the esophagus, and were not significantly different from normal values. In further support of the concept of reversible dysmotility, Moses[137] reported a case of "reversible aperistalsis" as a complication of GERD. Arana, *et al.*,[133] in a study similar in design to that of Gill, *et al.*,[136] demonstrated improved esophageal motility in a postoperative fundoplication group; however, the improvement was not statistically significant.

Eckardt[138] performed manometry on 18 patients with erosive esophagitis preoperatively and postoperatively, and followed these patients for an average of 3 years. Preoperatively, the patients all had significantly lower contraction amplitudes and lower LES pressures compared to controls. Postoperatively, all the patients remained asymptomatic; however, no improvement in esophageal motor function was observed.

Although it is still unclear whether esophageal dysmotility is a major cause of GERD or vice versa, it is likely that there are some patients with primary dysmotility leading to GERD and some patients with secondary dysmotility as a result of GER. Thus, reflux may contribute to a vicious cycle in which reflux causes abnormalities in LES pressure and esophageal clearance that lead to further reflux.

Decreased Mucosal Resistance

As the keratin layer is protective of the skin, the mucous layer is protective of the lining of the aerodigestive tract. The potency of the refluxate and its contact time with the esophageal lining are the primary determinants of mucosal injury; however, conditions associated with decreased salivation, mu-

TABLE XI.
Causes of Xerostomia.

A. Autoimmune disease
Acquired autoimmune disease (AIDS)
Collagen vascular disease
Sjogren's syndrome
Sicca syndrome
Scleroderma
B. Drugs
Anticholinergics (atropine, scopolamine, propantheline, dicyclomine, phenothiazines, belladonna, amitriptyline, chlorpromazine, clonidine)
Alpha-adrenergic antagonists (Dibenamine®, phentolamine, ergotamine, chlorpromazine, propranolol, fenfluramine)
Ganglion blocking agents (pentolinium, hexamenthonium)
CNS inhibitors (benzodiazepines, diphenhydramine, general anesthetics)
Other (analgesics, antiemetics, anticonvulsants, antinauseants, antipsychotics, antidepressants, diuretics, MAO inhibitors, antihistamines, antihypertensives, muscle relaxants (diazepam), cardiac antiarrhythmics, appetite suppressants)
C. Miscellaneous
Radiation therapy (oral cavity)
Cystic fibrosis
Ethanol
Tobacco

cus production, or both may significantly reduce the effectiveness of the mucosal barrier. If the mucus, the unstirred water layer, or both, which together provide the primary barrier to epithelial penetration, are altered, mucosal damage is likely.[86]

There is little information available on the effect of xerostomia (decreased mucus and saliva) as a primary factor in the pathogenesis of GERD. However, Rosman, *et al.*[116] reported esophageal acid clearance abnormalities in seven patients with xerostomia secondary to radiation therapy for head and neck malignancy. Basal salivary flows in the seven patients were less than 0.1 ml per minute and stimulated flows were less than 0.8 ml per minute. No patient had a history of esophageal symptoms, and all underwent esophageal manometry, acid clearance studies, and ambulatory 24-hour pH monitoring. Also evaluated were eight age-matched controls with comparable histories of alcohol intake.

There were no abnormalities of esophageal motility or LES pressure in any of the patients, but six of seven had impaired esophageal acid clearance tests and 24-hour pH-metry. Compared to controls, the mean number of reflux episodes increased from 7.0 ± 2.3 to 82.4 ± 22.8 ($P < .01$), and the total percentage of time that pH was less than 4 increased from 0.77 ± 0.23% in controls to 9.6 ± 3.1% in the patients with xerostomia ($P < .001$).

The degree of abnormality on the esophageal acid clearance test correlated well with the pH-metry data; however, the patients with xerostomia had impaired acid clearance and abnormal indices of esophageal pH, despite normal esophageal motility and LES pressures. Rosman, *et al.* concluded, "These results confirm that saliva plays an important role in maintaining normal esophageal pH and that patients with xerostomia may benefit from medical anti-reflux therapy." The causes of xerostomia are summarized in Table XI.

Autoimmune diseases, including Sjögren's syndrome and scleroderma, not only decrease salivary output and mucus production, but may also alter esophageal motility.[139] A high incidence of GERD has also been found in association with cystic fibrosis,[140,141] progressive systemic sclerosis,[142,143] and scleroderma.[141]

Finally, acid and pepsin in the refluxate may significantly alter mucosal defenses. Reflux produces inflammation, erosion, ulceration, and even metaplasia to columnar (gastric) mucosa, and malignant transformation. Metaplasia to columnar ("gastric") mucosa is a bizarre form of mucosal defense, the incidence of which increases with age in severe GERD but is reversible with adequate GERD treatment.[144,145]

Delayed Gastric Emptying

The volume of the intragastric contents reflects a balance between input and output. The input results from swallowing food or saliva and from gastric secretion, and the output corresponds to gastric emptying. Experimentally, acid has been shown to flow back into the esophagus after intragastric injection of volumes of greater than 140 ml of 0.1 normal HCl when LES pressure was 7.5 mm Hg or less. In contrast, volumes of greater than 308 ml were necessary to produce reflux when LES pressure was 13.8 ml or greater.[146]

In children, Sutphen and Dillard,[147] using pH-metry, demonstrated that the volume of feedings in patients with gastroesophageal reflux disease was an important determinant of reflux. The total time of acid exposure was doubled in the postcibal period when the feeding volume was increased from 9 ml to 18 ml per kilogram.

It has been demonstrated that fat or a fatty meal delays gastric emptying.[2,148] Little, *et al.*[148] found that patients with reflux esophagitis who were over 50 years of age often had delayed gastric emptying. Alcohol and tobacco have been shown to delay gastric emptying.[6,149,150] On occasion, gastric outlet obstruction by a duodenal ulcer, neoplasm, or neurogenic cause may precipitate GERD.[151]

Increased Intra-abdominal Pressure

Intragastric pressure is increased indirectly by increases in intra-abdominal pressure or directly by gastric distension. The Valsalva maneuver, tight clothing, overeating, consumption of carbonated beverages, a variety of strenuous activities, and obesity increase intragastric pressure. Hagen, *et al.*[152] performed barium esophagography, esophagoscopy, and manometry on 55 massively obese patients (weighing more than twice their ideal weight), 73% of whom had GERD symptoms. Radiographically, spontaneous reflux was demonstrated in 16% and endoscopic esophagitis in 31%; almost half the patients had subnormal LES pressures. Patients over age 35 years had significantly lower LES pressures and a higher incidence of reflux symptoms than those who were younger.

Nebel, *et al.*[153] found the incidence of daily heartburn in pregnancy to be 25%. Motil, *et al.*[154] reported exercise-induced gastroesophageal reflux with strenuous physical activity. Any exertional activity may increase intra-abdominal pressure and thus may predispose to GERD.

Gastric Hypersecretion

The normal human stomach contains approximately one billion parietal cells, which are located in the walls of the oxyntic glands, the secretory unit of the gastric mucosa. The regulatory processes for gastric secretion of acid involve three distinctly different phases: cephalic, gastric, and intestinal. A fourth phase, interdigestive or basal, is probably of great significance in GERD.

The cephalic phase of gastric acid secretion is activated by the thought, sight, smell, or taste of appetizing food.[101] The gastric phase is stimulated by both chemical and physical factors related to gastric distension, with stimulation of stretch receptors in the stomach wall and also of vagovagal pathways (vagotomy decreases the acid response to distension by more than 80%).[155] During the gastric phase, buffering by ingested food increases the intraluminal pH to 3.0 to 3.5, and gastrin release and acid secretion are enhanced. After the meal (*i.e.*, the intestinal phase), the secretion of acid is modulated by a negative feedback mechanism, which inhibits further acidification by inhibiting further release of gastrin.

Gastric secretion can be influenced by a person's emotional state, and basal acid and pepsin secretion increases with stress.[155–157] Basal acid secretion also appears to follow a diurnal rhythm, reaching its peak around midnight and its nadir at approximately 7 AM.[112] White wine and 5% ethanol have been shown to be potent stimulants of gastric acid secretion in humans.[158] Total 3-hour responses to white wine and ethanol were 5 and 4.5 times greater, respectively, than those to water.

There is a relative paucity of data on gastric hypersecretion in GERD; however, Aylwin[159] compared the pH and pepsin concentrations of the basal intragastric contents of three groups of patients, those with: *1.* no esophagitis; *2.* minimal esophagitis; and *3.* severe erosive esophagitis with strictures.

TABLE XII.
Sensitivity and Specificity of Diagnostic Tests for Esophagitis and for GER.*

Tests	Sensitivity (Abnormality in Disease)	Specificity (Normalcy in Health)
For Esophagitis		
Barium esophagography	++	++
Acid perfusion test ("Bernstein" test)	+++	++
Acid barium test	++	++
Esophagoscopy	++	+++
Mucosal biopsy	+++	+++
Demonstrating or Measuring GER		
Barium esophagography (Cinefluoroscopy)	+	++
Radionuclide scanning	++	+++
Lipid-laden macrophage test (Tracheobronchial sampling)	+++	unknown
Standard acid reflux test	+++	+++
Prolonged pH manometry	++++	++++

*Adapted from Jamieson and Duranceau.[6]
++++ = excellent; +++ = good; ++ = fair; + = poor.

Overnight, the gastric contents were aspirated and then assayed. The basal pepsin output in patients without esophagitis was very low, but pepsin concentration increased as the severity of the esophagitis increased. In addition, the pH was lower in patients with ulcerative esophagitis and stricture. Thus, in this study, the potency of the refluxate was demonstrated to correlate well with the severity of the injury. (This topic will be discussed further in "Experimental Investigations.")

DIAGNOSTIC TESTS

Most of the diagnostic methods used in GERD either test for consequences of reflux, such as esophagitis, or qualitatively or quantitatively test for reflux itself. These methods each have advantages and disadvantages and none offer 100% accuracy. The most commonly performed tests, as well as their relative sensitivities and specificities, are listed in Table XII.

Tests for Esophagitis

Barium Esophagography

Barium radiography is the oldest of the diagnostic tests. It was originally used in the 1930s and 1940s to demonstrate a "sliding hiatal hernia." The association between hiatal hernia and GERD is no longer considered clinically important, since 40% to 60% of asymptomatic adults have easily demonstrable hiatal hernias.[2]

Barium esophagography with cinefluoroscopy has been used to demonstrate GER. However, in a recent review,[2] the sensitivity of radiographic examination for reflux was only 33%, and Ott, *et al.*[160] found radiographic reflux in only 25% of 40 patients with endoscopic esophagitis and in 20% of 35 normal controls.

Acid Perfusion ("Bernstein") Test

In 1958, Bernstein and Baker[38] introduced the acid perfusion test for esophagitis. The test is performed by placing a nasogastric tube in the distal esophagus and infusing normal saline for 15 minutes followed by 0.1 normal HCl at a rate of 6 ml per minute, until either symptoms are produced or 45 minutes have elapsed. They reported both the sensitivity and the specificity of the test to be 95%.

Battle, *et al.*[161] found the sensitivity of the acid perfusion test to be 32%, and Krejs, *et al.*[162] found it to be 54%. Sonnenberg, *et al.*[163] found the sensitivity to be 80% but the specificity to be only 59%.

The acid perfusion test is not specific for esophagitis or reflux. Patients with motor disorders often have a positive study even when there is no evidence of GERD.[164] Thus, it would appear that a positive acid perfusion test indicates only a likelihood that the symptoms mimicked are primarily esophageal.

Acid Barium Test

Donner, *et al.*[165] introduced the acid barium test. (Standard barium sulfate (100 ml) is mixed with hydrochloric acid, producing a mixture with a pH of 1.7.) Ten patients with esophagitis and 10 controls were studied. None of the controls showed any abnormality, but all 10 of the patients showed cessation of peristaltic activity and segmental nonpropulsive tertiary contractions. Benz, *et al.*[3] carried out this radiologic assessment in a blinded fashion and found a sensitivity of 83%, but a specificity of only 50%.

Esophagoscopy and Biopsy

Subjective evaluation of the esophageal lining is useful when esophagitis is present. Many grading systems have been proposed, but many contemporary gastroenterologists use a very simple scoring system: grade I, erythema; grade II, ulceration; grade III, stricture.[6]

The endoscopic diagnosis of esophagitis does not tally with either the histologic assessment or the patient's symptoms.[6] Endoscopic esophagitis has been confirmed histologically in 33% to 72% of GERD patients.[6] Clearly, when esophagitis is likely, endoscopy with biopsy is a reasonably sensitive diagnostic option.

Tests Demonstrating or Measuring Reflux

Radionuclide Scanning

Radionuclide scanning was introduced by Fisher, *et al.*[166] (Three hundred milliliters of saline with technetium are swallowed by the patient, who is then placed supine under the gamma camera and abdominal pressure is applied.) Fisher, *et al.* devised a scoring system to semiquantitate the amount of reflux observed. However, Ott, *et al.* reported the sensitivity of this test to average 68%, with a range of 14% to 90%.[167] The reported sensitivity of radionuclide scanning in otolaryngology patients with GERD was recently reported to be only 11%.[168]

Lipid-Laden Macrophage Test

The presence of lipoid intracellular inclusions in the macrophage has been postulated to be due to GERD. Nussbaum, *et al.*[169] and Corwin and Irwin[170] have shown an increase in lipid-laden macrophages in children with pulmonary complications of GERD. The potential advantage of the lipid-laden macrophage test is that lipid-laden macrophages may remain for days after a reflux episode has occurred, so that the test potentially offers the clinician an opportunity to "track" GERD days after the fact. Unfortunately, the test requires tracheobronchial sampling (*e.g.*, suction aspiration), and the specificity of the test is completely unknown.

Short-term pH Assessment

Several different techniques have been employed for short-term pH monitoring in assessment of GERD. The "standard acid reflux test"[171] is the most widely used. The test is performed by placing a pH catheter into the stomach and instilling 300 ml of 0.1 normal HCl. The pH electrode is then withdrawn to a point 5 cm above the lower esophageal sphincter and the patient performs a variety of maneuvers designed to stimulate reflux (*i.e.*, deep breath, Valsalva's maneuver, cough). A fall in pH to less than 4 is positive evidence for reflux. The test is graded in a standard fashion. The average reported sensitivity of the test is 80%, with a range from 54% to 100%, and the average specificity is 84%, with a range from 70% to 95%.[6]

Prolonged pH Monitoring

Since its introduction by Miller, *et al.*[39] and Spencer,[40] prolonged pH monitoring has been used simultaneously as a research tool and as a clinical test. Whereas the previous diagnostic methods have relied on *1.* demonstration of esophagitis (*e.g.*, barium esophagogram, endoscopy); *2.* reproduction of symptoms by provocative testing (*e.g.*, acid perfusion test); *3.* demonstration of abnormal esophageal function (*e.g.*, esophageal clearance test); and *4.* nonquantitative demonstration of reflux or dysmotility (*e.g.*, radionuclide scanning, acid barium swallow study), prolonged pH manometry quantitates the event of gastroesophageal reflux itself.

Much of the credit for pioneering work in pH manometry to establish standards and to popularize the technique as a clinical tool belongs to DeMeester and Johnson.[7,8,42,172–174] Johnson[8] defined a reflux event with pH manometry as a drop in pH to less than 4.0. This value was chosen because Tuttle, *et al.*[175]

TABLE XIII.
Normal Values for Ambulatory 24-Hour pH Manometry (Percentage of Time pH < 4.0, Upright, Supine, and Total).

Reference	Year	N	Average Age (years)	Percent Time pH < 4.0*		
				Upright	Supine	Total
Johnson and DeMeester[173]	1974	15	—	6.27	1.22	4.23
Boesby[176]	1975	26	49	—	—	2.00
Fink and McCallum[178]	1984	8	—	2.80	—	1.90
Weiner, *et al.*[57]	1986	20	—	2.70	0.70	2.10
Bianchi Porro and Pace[4]	1988	20	46	—	—	8.30
Johnsson and Joelsson[180]	1988	15	41	4.60	3.20	3.80
Pujol, *et al.*[181]	1988	15	49	5.00	0.60	2.70
Mattioli, *et al.*[85]	1989	20	43	7.62	2.28	4.99
Smout, *et al.*[182]	1989	16	<45	4.38	1.70	3.22
		16	>45	12.12	3.67	8.63
Average Values				5.68	1.91	4.19

*All values expressed are the upper limit of normal (mean plus two standard deviations).

had shown that heartburn occurs at pH of less than 4 and because it was believed that there is minimal peptic activity at pH above 4.0.

Boesby[176] performed 12-hour pH monitoring on 26 normal subjects. There were 31 reflux episodes, and the percentage of time pH was less than 2.3 was 0.08%; pH less than 3, 0.18%; pH less than 4, 0.46%; and pH less than 5, 1.02%. Thus, there was a direct relationship between percentage of time and pH.

Many parameters have been investigated and reported, including: percentage of time pH is less than 4 (usually reported in terms of percentage of time upright, percentage of time supine, and total time); number of reflux episodes; duration of longest reflux episode; episodes lasting longer than 5 minutes per hour; and episodes per hour supine, upright, and total.[177] In terms of reporting pH-metry results, percentage of times pH is less than 4 supine, upright, and total have become relatively common, and these parameters are considered the most reliable and reproducible.[4,85–173,176–182]

Many laboratories have established normal standards; Table XIII lists the upper limit of normal for nine studies (of normals) for pH time less than 4.0 in both positions and total. All values are expressed as the mean plus two standard deviations. For these studies, the average value for upright reflux was 5.68%; supine, 1.91%; and total, 4.19%.

Recently, Smout, *et al.*[182] studied 16 "normals" under 45 years of age and 16 "normals" over 45 years of age, and found a significant increase in all three values in the over 45 age group. On the other hand, Boesby[176] examined a similar-aged population and found the value for total time pH was less than 4 to be significantly lower than the mean in Table XIII.

It also appears that there may be significant variation in pH-metry in the normal neonatal and infant population. Euler and Byrne[183] reported the results of 22 children (average age about 1 year); upright (2.48%), supine (1.79%), and total (3.19%). Sondheimer and Haase,[184] studying a slightly younger population, found the mean value for total time to be 4.8%.

Vandenplas and Sacré-Smits[185] studied pH in 285 infants ranging in age from 5 days to 16 months. The values that follow are percentage of total time that pH was less than 4.0:

5 to 15 days (n = 92)	3.02%
24 to 37 days (n = 28)	4.49%
7 to 8 weeks (n = 44)	7.02%
3.5 to 4.5 months (n = 52)	9.38%
5.5 to 6.5 months (n = 30)	9.27%
7.5 to 8.5 months (n = 24)	11.37%
14 to 16 months (n = 15)	6.45%

Although this study has not been duplicated, it would appear that GER in asymptomatic normal infants may not have one standard but several, and that total acid exposure time in the distal esophagus may be the greatest at around 8 months of age.

Although the issue of relating "normal" values to various age groups has not been fully resolved, it would appear that the results in older children and adults are roughly similar. Of concern in establishing normal values is the possibility that "abnormals" are being considered "normals." In no study has routine esophagoscopy with biopsy been carried out before inclusion of a subject as a "normal control."

The reported sensitivity of 24-hour pH manometry varies from 81% to 96%, and specificity varies from 93% to 100% (Table XIV). The average for five studies is 90% sensitivity and 98% specificity.

Mattioli, *et al.*[85] found that 5.3% of patients would not tolerate pH manometry due to its invasiveness and 14.7% markedly attenuated or altered their

TABLE XIV.
Reported Sensitivity and Specificity of Ambulatory 24-Hour pH Manometry.

References	Year	Sample Size: Normal Controls	Sample Size: Patients with GERD	Sensitivity (Abnormality in Disease) (%)	Specificity (Normalcy in Health) (%)
Fuchs, *et al.*[5]	1987	45	45	96	96
Schindlbeck, *et al.*[186]	1987	42	45	93	93
Bianchi Porro and Pace[4]	1988	20	20	81	100
Pujol, *et al.*[181]	1988	15	47	94	100
Mattioli, *et al.*[85]	1989	20	68	85	100
Average				90	98

life-style. In a group of 34 pediatric patients, Sondheimer and Haase[184] found that probe dislodgement occurred in three patients, and either the probe failed or there was an inadequate poststudy standardization in another four, thereby invalidating almost 20% of the tests. In adults, technical failure of a pH probe probably accounts for 1% to 3% of cases.[71]

Attempts have been made to determine whether a shorter duration of study provides adequate sampling and accurate reflux data. Bianchi Porro and Pace[4] studied 20 patients and 20 controls with 12-hour, 10-hour "postprandial," and 24-hour pH monitoring. The 10-hour postprandial test included the daytime hours; the 12-hour test, the nighttime hours; and the 24-hour test, both. The relative sensitivities of the three tests were 50% (12-hour), 70% (10-hour postprandial), and 81% (24-hour). The overnight sampling method (12-hour test) is more prone to false-negative error, because supine nocturnal reflux occurs less commonly than upright or combined (supine and upright) reflux. Thus, it appeared that as the sampling time is decreased, the sensitivity of the test also decreases.

Johnson[7] studied 100 patients with GERD and found 9% had abnormal supine reflux, 37% had abnormal upright reflux, and 54% had both abnormal supine and upright reflux. He also reported that combined refluxers had esophagitis 60% of the time; supine refluxers, 50% of the time; and upright refluxers, only 15% of the time.

One of the advantages of ambulatory pH monitoring as a diagnostic test is that the patient can continue his or her life-style in an uninterrupted fashion; however, standardization of the test often prohibits consumption of foods with pH less than 4.0. These include Coca-Cola™ and Pepsi-Cola™ (pH 2.3), Seven-Up™ (pH 3.2), and orange juice (pH 3.7). Usually, those beverages are allowed only at mealtime or not at all during pH monitoring.[6]

The reproducibility of GER findings with pH manometry has recently come under investigation. Johnsson and Joelsson[180] performed 24-hour pH monitoring on 20 GERD patients on two consecutive days and found an overall concordance of 77%: 83% for the upright position, and 62% when supine. To investigate the possibility of false-negative results in pH probing, Murphy, *et al.*[187] simultaneously placed two separate pH electrodes in 10 patients. They found that the amount of acid exposure differed greatly in some instances, and that these differences could not be attributed to probe performance, although the reason for the discrepancy was not apparent. They concluded that false-negative pH-metry could occur in up to 20% of patients.

In a companion study, Murphy, *et al.*[188] placed two side-by-side probes in the distal esophagus of dogs, then irrigated the esophagus from below with acid, using a perfusion catheter placed through a gastrostomy with its tip up through the gastroesophageal junction. In four of the nine trials, infusions of acid did not cause a drop in pH as recorded by either electrode, despite total infusions of 15, 13, 8, and 5.5 ml. The authors pointed out, however, that the supine dogs were absolutely immobile. They postulated that there may have been pooling of secretions around the probe tip, mucosal abutment (preventing access of the "refluxate"), or location of the intraesophageal electrodes above an air-fluid level.

In summary, false-negative pH-metry results can occur for three reasons: *1.* technical probe failure; *2.* inappropriate sampling; and *3.* inappropriate definition of normal. In spite of the work by Murphy, *et al.*,[187,188] the false-negative rate in clinical practice is low and the specificity is high (Table XIV). Although there are still some questions about the definition of normal time pH is less than 4 in the aged and the very young, standards are now generally accepted to be approximately 6.3% upright, 1.2% supine, and 4.2% total.[189] Twenty-four-hour pH manometry has become the "gold standard" in the diagnostic evaluation of GERD. pH manometry as a clinical test in otolaryngology patients will be discussed subsequently.

CLINICAL OBSERVATIONS

Gastroenterologic Manifestations

Americans, as a population, are relatively overweight, are sedentary, and consume a high-fat diet. It is therefore not surprising that GERD may affect 25 to 75 million people in the United States (10% to 30%).[190] Table XV lists reported GER-related conditions. Clearly, the manifestations and complications of reflux are most commonly esophageal; however, even among "typical" patient populations, there is considerable variation in the symptoms and sequelae of GERD.

Esophagitis can be found on endoscopy and biopsy in only 60% to 70% of patients who complain of heartburn; conversely, as few as 50% of patients with esophagitis may have heartburn.[198,268,277] In 1966, Belsey reported his experience with 824 cases of esophageal dysfunction.[289] Seventy-six percent were cases of incompetence of the LES (GERD), but 26% were related to other problems.

Although the extrinsic innervation of the esophagus is known, pain receptors in the esophagus have not been clearly identified. As a consequence, the mechanisms of esophageal chest pain are unknown. Patients with heartburn clearly reflux more often than normal subjects, but heartburn occurs with only a small percentage of reflux events.[290] It is believed that mucosal disruption with inflammation may be contributory, but patients with heartburn do not necessarily have esophagitis.[291] Symptoms of heartburn can be reproduced in patients with esophagitis with infusion of solutions of pH 1 and 1.5, but only in half of patients with solutions of pH 2.5 to 6.[93] The variability in symptoms is further substantiated by the observatrion that up to 50% of patients with Barrett's esophagus (the most severe form of esophagitis) deny heartburn.[97]

Symptoms aside, there is clearly a relationship between the degree of esophageal dysmotility and the severity of esophageal symptoms of GERD. In addition to heartburn and regurgitation, patients with GERD may have a variety of symptoms of "dysmotility." (Esophagitis has been covered previously; attention will now be focused upon "esophageal angina," lower esophageal ring, stricture, and "Barrett's esophagus.")

TABLE XV.
Reported GER-Related Conditions.

	Reference(s)
A. ESOPHAGUS	
Esophagitis	44,45,67,100,191–195
Dysmotility	46,70,76,130,131,134–138, 164,196–199
Lower esophageal ring	6,200
Barrett's epithelium	51,52,144,145,201–208
Carcinoma	145,204–209
Stricture	6,200,203,210
Achalasia	211
B. PULMONARY	
Bronchopulmonary dysplasia	56,212,213
Aspiration pneumonia	56,214–226
Chronic bronchitis	217,223–226
Pulmonary fibrosis	227–229
Chronic cough	19,217,230–232
Asthma	217,233–245
Cystic fibrosis	140,141
C. LARYNX	
Carcinoma	14,21,22,64,249
Subglottic stenosis	23,24,65,246,247
Chronic hoarseness	17,20,57,58,248–251
Contact ulcer	13,15
Vocal cord granuloma	11,13,15
Cricoarytenoid fixation	14
Intubation granuloma	14
Laryngomalacia	252
Pachydermia	19,58
Laryngospasm	58,221,253–255
D. PHARYNX & CERVICAL ESOPHAGUS	
Chronic pharyngitis	15,19,58
Dysphagia	58,74,143,248,251,256–259
Globus	58,60,179,251,260–270
Zenker's diverticulum	61,257,271
E. MISCELLANEOUS	
SIDS	272–274
Noncardiac chest pain	164,268,275–281
Torticollis	282
Dental erosions	283,284
Reflex bradycardia	285–287
Scleroderma	139,288

"Esophageal Angina"

Over 600,000 new patients each year undergo cardiac catheterization in the United States; and normal coronary arteries are found in as many as 30% of patients with anginal syndromes. Of those, up to 50% have demonstrable esophageal abnormalities.[268] Davies, *et al.*[278] followed 100 consecutive medical emergency patients with anterior chest pain to their final diagnosis. Although the pain was anginal in character in the majority of cases, 16% were found to have an esophageal disorder and half of those patients had their symptoms reproduced by an acid perfusion study.

DiPalma and Meyer[198] reported that, frequently, angina-like esophageal pain could be differentiated from cardiac pain by history. With chest pain of esophageal origin, attacks occurred spontaneously without exertion; or the pain could begin as long as 10 minutes after exercise had stopped. Pain could be provoked by swallowing or stooping; and antacids often relieved the pain. In contrast, coronary pain was often associated with peripheral pain radiation and, infrequently, it occurred spontaneously as a nonexertional attack.

Angina-like pain has been reported to be associated with esophagitis, high amplitude peristalsis ("nutcracker esophagus"), hypertensive LES, and with other esophageal motor disorders.[70,275,277] The differentiation between cardiac and esophageal pain frequently requires both a cardiac and an esophageal evaluation.[275–277,280]

Lower Esophageal Ring and Esophageal Stricture

Chen, *et al.* (1987)[200] have reported the progression from normal esophagus to lower esophageal ring to esophageal stricture in association with reflux esophagitis in 22 patients. In two cases, lower esophageal ring developed from a normal esophagus. In three patients, there was increasing stenosis of the lower esophageal mucosal ring; in eight patients, the ring was transformed into an esophageal stricture; and in nine patients there was no change. Of the last nine patients, only one had active esophagitis. Thus, lower esophageal ring was considered an early stage of stricture formation.

Esophageal strictures are the consequence of recurrent ulceration of the esophageal mucosa in the presence of ongoing GER. Fibrosis is usually limited to the submucosa, but with recurrent or persistent ulceration, even more extensive fibrosis can occur, involving the muscular layers of the esophageal wall. Fibrosis of the circular muscle layer results in stenosis, whereas fibrosis of the longitudinal muscle layer results in esophageal shortening.[6]

The majority of peptic strictures are short and located near the squamocolumnar (gastroesophageal) junction. In general, higher strictures are usually associated with Barett's esophagus. Patients with strictures usually have a long-standing history of heartburn and regurgitation, which become associated with progressive dysphagia. Dysphagia is usually primarily for solids, but it can progress to involve liquids as well.[6] The patient's localization of symptoms is often inaccurate and the obstruction may be referred to as a sensation of discomfort in the neck.[6] Barium esophagography is extremely useful in the demonstration of strictures, which have an incidence of about 10% in patients with GERD.[87,89,90]

The medical management of GERD in association with esophageal dilation is sufficient in most cases, but severe cases may require surgical treatment.[6]

Barrett's Esophagus

Metaplasia of the esophageal stratified squamous epithelium to columnar epithelium resembling that of the stomach and intestines is known as Barrett's esophagus.[52,201,203–207] Early controversy regarding the pathogenesis of Barrett's epithelium focused on whether the aberrant mucosa was congenital or acquired. The evidence at present is overwhelmingly in favor of metaplasia (acquired), as a result of GERD.

Gastroesophageal reflux produces esophagitis with destruction of squamous epithelium and ulceration; the ulcers reepithelialize by multipotential undifferentiated stem cells and in the abnormal milieu of ongoing GER, these immature cells differentiate into a variety of cells characteristic of Barrett's epithelium.[206] Gillen, *et al.*[144] have reported producing reversible Barrett's esophagus in dogs. They found that the cell of origin of Barrett's epithelium is located in the esophageal gland ducts, and demonstrated the metaplastic sequence.

The reported rates of esophageal adenocarcinoma arising in Barrett's esophagus range from 0% to 46.5%, with an average rate of 10%.[145,205–208] Naef, *et al.*[204] analyzed a series of 1225 cases of reflux esophagitis and found a 10% incidence of adenocarcinomas in 140 cases of Barrett's esophagus. Radigan, *et al.*[145] reported a 26.3% incidence of adenocarcinoma in Barrett's esophagus. The majority of the patients in that series presented with obstructive dysphagia and almost half had stricture in association with Barrett's epithelium.

Lee and Isaacs[203] treated 28 patients with "Barrett's ulcer" of the esophagus with *1.* standard-dose ranitidine, *2.* high-dose ranitidine, and *3.* omeprazole. In 17 (60%), standard measures and ranitidine, 300 mg daily, resulted in healing; two other patients underwent surgical treatment. Nine patients in whom healing failed to occur were treated with high-dose ranitidine, and five had complete healing after 8 weeks. Three patients with unhealed ulcers after high-dose ranitidine were treated with omeprazole, 40 mg q.i.d: After 8 weeks, two were healed and the third was substantially improved. The authors noted that, despite healing of the Barrett's esophagus, most of the patients had persistent reflux symptoms. Zaninotto, *et al.*[69] demonstrated that patients with Barrett's esophagus had both esophageal dysmotility and poor LES function; Nissen fundoplication provided relief of dysphagia in 86%. Other authors[104,206] have reported excellent results with surgical treatment.

In summary, Barrett's epithelium is caused by GER, can be produced experimentally in the dog, and is entirely reversible with appropriate therapy.[144] In addition, Barrett's epithelium increases as the age of the GERD patient increases, and the incidence of carcinoma of the esophagus developing in Barrett's esophagus also increases with age.[202]

Otolaryngologic Manifestations

Carcinoma of the Larynx

The most common site of squamous cell carcinoma (SCC) of the head and neck is the larynx.[292] Ninety-six percent of laryngeal cancer is of the squamous cell type, and accounts for 26% of head and neck SCC. Oral cavity and esophageal cancer are next in frequency with 16% each, followed by tongue, 12%, and pharynx, 8%.[292]

It has been estimated that the greatest single risk factor for development of SCC of the larynx is cigarette smoking. Ethanol (alcohol) is also (by itself) associated with an increased incidence of laryngeal carcinoma.[293] However, tobacco and alcohol interact to elevate the risk for developing laryngeal carcinoma above that which would be expected if these risks were solely additive effects.[292,293] This synergistic interaction is manifest both in the incidence of laryngeal cancer in heavy smokers/drinkers, and a propensity for synchronous multiple tumor site presentations (*i.e.*, field cancerization). Second synchronous primary SCC tumors occur in approximately 20% of head and neck cancer patients with a reported range of 6.5% to 35%.[294] The esophagus is the most common second site and may account for up to 40% of synchronous second primaries (the reported range is 11% to 43%).[295]

In a large series of patients with GERD, 92% were found to be smokers.[296] Dennish and Castell[297] found that smoking led to a fall of LES pressure in normal people. Stanciu and Bennett,[296] using pH manometry in 25 chronic smokers, found that the mean basal LES pressure of 10.8 ± 3.7 cm H_2O fell to 6.4 ± 2.9 cm H_2O during smoking ($P < .01$). Sphincter pressure began to fall within 1 to 4 minutes of initiation of smoking and reflux episodes occurred with two thirds of cigarettes smoked. Miller, *et al.* found that smoking delayed gastric emptying, but that nicotine chewing gum did not produce the same effect.[149]

Vitale, *et al.*[150] studied the effects of alcohol consumption on supine nocturnal reflux. Seventeen healthy volunteers were studied using pH manometry on two consecutive evenings. Three hours after dinner, each subject ingested 4 ounces of Scotch on one occasion and an equal volume of water on the alternate night. Supine nocturnal reflux occurred more frequently with the alcohol consumption ($P < .02$), and the effective alcohol peak during the third hour corresponded to the time when most of the reflux events occurred.

Tobacco and alcohol are also major risk factors for the development of GERD (Table IX). Tobacco has been demonstrated to decrease LES pressure, reduce mucosal resistance, delay gastric emptying, and stimulate gastric hypersecretion. Ethanol has been shown to decrease LES pressure, promote esophageal dysmotility, impair mucosal resistance, delay gastric emptying, and stimulate gastric hypersecretion. Thus, tobacco and alcohol adversely modify almost all the physiologic defenses against GERD.

The high incidence of squamous cell carcinoma of the larynx and the esophagus in heavy drinkers/smokers and the high association between alcohol and tobacco usage with GERD suggest the possibility that GERD may be an important cofactor in the development of upper aerodigestive carcinoma, particularly laryngeal carcinoma.

Gabriel and Jones[298] were the first to report a series of patients in which they believed "chronic laryngitis" had led to the development of carcinoma. Over a 5-year period (1954 through 1958), they found 21 patients with laryngeal cancer, 10 of whom had a documented history of preceding chronic laryngitis and pharyngitis. Although the authors did not postulate GER as a cause, the findings on physical examination were often characteristic of the findings that have come to be associated with GERD. The possibility of chronic laryngitis leading to cancer has been raised by Glanz and Kleinsasser,[64] Weiner, *et al.*,[249] Morrison,[21] Ward and Hanson,[22] and Olson.[14]

In 1983, Olson[14] reported five cases of vocal process SCC that resembled contact ulcer with granuloma on physical examination. All five of the patients were smokers. No information relative to the methods of diagnosing GERD was provided other than the history and the examination.

Some investigators have reasoned that, by removing the variable of tobacco, the role of GER in the development of laryngeal carcinoma might be explored. Morrison[21] reported six lifetime nonsmokers with T1 SCC in the anterior two thirds of the vocal cord. All five of the patients having barium esophagography had abnormal results (sliding hiatal hernia, 4; reflux, 4). On reviewing 20-year tumor records, Morrison was able to find an additional 21 patients with SCC of the larynx who were nonsmokers; 48% had a positive reflux history.

Ward and Hanson[22] reported 19 cases of carcinoma of the larynx in lifetime nonsmokers. There was no pattern or prevalence for the location of the lesions; half were anterior and half were posterior. In three patients, benign lesions documented in 1980 evolved into carcinoma 5, 5, and 8 years later. In those patients, the diagnosis of GERD was made by history and by barium esophagography.

In 1987, Wiener, *et al.*[249] reported the 24-hour esophageal pH manometry results of 16 patients with laryngeal carcinoma; 56% had abnormal studies. Abnormal upright reflux occurred 2½ times more frequently than supine nocturnal reflux. Previously, Wiener, *et al.*[57] had studied 14 patients with hoarseness and had found that 78% had abnormal pH manometry. Those patients had also undergone esophageal manometry (100% normal), fiberoptic esophagoscopy (72% normal), Bernstein acid perfusion test (66% negative), and barium esophagography (66% normal).

The results of that study suggested that GERD was common in patients with hoarseness and that those patients often had neither esophagitis nor dysmotility. The data supported the postulate that smoking (and drinking) were related to the development of both GERD and carcinoma. Thus, there is an established association between smoking and cancer, between smoking and GERD, and between GERD and cancer.

Laryngeal and Tracheal Stenosis

Acquired laryngeal and tracheal stenosis may be associated with blunt and penetrating trauma, but more often occur as a complication of endotracheal intubation. For the purposes of this thesis, the traumatic causes of upper airway stenosis are not relevant.

TABLE XVI.
Factors Responsible for the Development of Laryngeal and Tracheal Damage With Endotracheal Intubation.

Causative Factor	Reference(s)
1. Anatomy (configuration) of the upper airway	305,306
2. Traumatic intubation	307,308
3. Multiple intubations (≥3)	309
4. Endotracheal tube size	306,310
5. Excessive tube mobility	299
6. Duration of intubation	306,309,311
7. Tube composition	306,307
8. Tube cuff	
a. Location (too high)	299,308
b. Excessive pressure	200,308
9. Mucosal drying	308
10. Systemic factors	
a. Hypotension	312
b. Sepsis/infection	312,313
c. Corticosteroids	299
11. Subsequent tracheotomy	308,313,314
12. Gastroesophageal reflux	23,24,247

Endotracheal intubation had been performed before the turn of the century; however, it was not commonly employed until the 1950s and 1960s, when it became the preferred method of long-term air support over tracheotomy.[299] The incidence of subglottic stenosis in intubated patients has been reported to range from 1% to 11%.[300–304] Numerous mechanisms have been proposed as being responsible for the development of upper airway stenosis (Table XVI).

The anatomic configuration of the upper airway is not compatible with the shape and curve of the conventional endotracheal tube, and so the vocal process of the arytenoid and the posterior cricoid are frequently injured.[305–307,311] Traumatic intubation and multiple intubations (reintubation) have been associated with an increased incidence of stenosis.[307–309] Endotracheal tube size,[306,310] excessive mobility of the tube creating a piston-like effect within the larynx,[299] tube composition,[306,307] cuff too high,[299,308] excessive cuff pressure,[308,311] and mucosal drying,[308] as well as systemic factors, such as hypotension, sepsis/infection, corticosteroid administration,[299,312,313] and subsequent tracheotomy,[308,313,314] have all been suggested as playing a role in the development of stenosis.

Of all the factors, duration of intubation is the most controversial and unresolved. Donnelly[311] examined 99 postintubation laryngeal specimens at autopsy, and correlated his findings with the duration of intubation. Patients intubated less than 12 hours demonstrated pale, oval areas on the mucosa of the local processes and the posterior cricoid directly below. Microscopic examination of these areas revealed complete or focal loss of surface epithelium. Patients intubated 12 to 48 hours demonstrated mucosal ulcers of the vocal process and in the posterior subglottis. Ulceration was more severe in female than in male specimens. After 48 hours, vocal process and subglottic ulcers were broader and deeper. Beyond 72 hours, the ulcers were confluent and extended across the posterior midline. Perichondrium of the vocal process and of the cricoid was exposed. After 96 hours of intubation, the ulcers were deeper in the perichondrium of both the vocal process and the cricoid lamina. Similar findings have been reported by McGovern, *et al.*[308] and Hilding.[307] In addition to describing the sequential changes in the larynx, Donnelly[311] noted that the incidence and severity of damage in female patients was significantly greater than in male patients, and he postulated that this was due to the smaller female laryngeal anatomy relative to standard recommended endotracheal tube sizes.

Whited[313] followed a series of 200 patients in a prospective study of the sequelae associated with intubation. Fifty patients were intubated for 2 to 5 days (group I), 100 patients for 6 to 10 days (group II), and 50 patients for 11 to 24 days (group III). All patients were followed for at least 6 months after removal of the endotracheal tube. In group I, 3 patients experienced transient postintubation stridor; in group II, 2 patients had postintubation stridor, 16 had required a tracheotomy, and 5 (31%) of 16 subsequently developed laryngeal stenosis; in group III, 3 patients had postextubation stridor, and none had required a tracheotomy. In group III, mucosal ulcerations were found on fiberoptic laryngoscopy after extubation in 22 of 32 patients, and impaired vocal cord mobility was noted in 5; however, all complications resolved uneventfully by 3 weeks, except in one patient who developed posterior glottic stenosis.

McGovern, *et al.*[308] reviewed the records of 366 patients who had been intubated in the intensive care unit. They also carried out postmortem examinations and found that 70% of the patients with severe damage had had endotracheal tubes in place for more than 48 hours, and 80% of those having minimal damage had had endotracheal tubes in position for less than 48 hours. They noted, however, that a few of the surviving patients had developed laryngeal stenosis, but that the necessity of placing the tracheotomy after endotracheal intubation had doubled the incidence of stenosis.

Burns, *et al.*[299] followed 117 patients who had been extubated successfully in the respiratory care unit and examined the autopsy reports of an additional 68 patients who had failed to survive in the same respiratory unit. Patients were intubated for periods of 1 to 13 days. The postintubation incidence of hoarseness was 73%; that of dyspnea, 15%; that of dysphagia, 14%; and that of aspiration, 4%. One third of the patients had glottic loss of mucosal surface, and 10% had subglottic mucosal loss. The authors concluded that the lowest incidence of laryngeal damage was observed in patients intubated for less than 48 hours. They also found that injuries had resolved uneventfully in almost all of the 57 patients available for follow-up.

In several reviews of the problem of subglottic stenosis,[300–304] many of the factors listed in Table XVI are mentioned, but GERD as a potential factor in the pathogenesis of stenosis is not. In a 1980 article on posterior glottic stenosis, Bogdasarian and Olson[65] did mention in passing that, in addition to the usual factors, the presence of gastric acid reflux should be ruled out.

In 1983, Bain, *et al.*[23] reported a case of subglottic stenosis in a 57-year-old woman, which was unassociated with previous intubation, trauma, or surgery. The patient underwent a Nissen fundoplication and endoscopic laryngeal repair. What had been a "pencil eraser size" subglottic opening before fundoplication and surgical repair was reportedly normal 5 months after treatment. In 1985, Little, *et al.*[24] reported the case of a 12-year-old girl with recalcitrant subglottic stenosis who continued to produce exuberant granulation tissue for a period of years. During one endoscopic procedure, it was noted that she had gastroesophageal contents in the hypopharynx. She was subsequently treated for reflux, with resolution of her chronic persistent granulation, and subsequent tracheotomy decannulation. In 1987, Gray, *et al.*[315] published a paper entitled "Adjunctive Measures for Successful Laryngotracheal Reconstruction." They commented:

> Gastroesophageal reflux is a condition that is frequently overlooked. It has been our impression that patients with uncontrolled GER have a higher rate of failure in laryngotracheal reconstruction and also require more postoperative procedures, especially if a laryngeal stent is present. When GER occurs with a stent in place, prime conditions exist for formation of excessive granulation tissue and scarring.

They went on to note:

> Several infants have failed decannulation following an apparently successful laryngotracheal reconstruction because of apnea and laryngospasm associated with GER. Correction of the GER subsequently allowed decannulation.

The authors recommended that every patient undergoing laryngeal reconstruction be examined for GER. All methods of repair, whether endoscopic,[316,317] or open[302,318–320] are doomed to failure in the presence of GER and/or local wound sepsis.

Borowiecki and Croft[321] demonstrated, in a canine model of subglottic stenosis, that lesions confined to the subglottic mucosa healed uneventfully, whereas stenosis developed at the site of cricoid lesions that extended into the cartilage. In a variation of the model created by Borowiecki and Croft, Little, *et al.*[24] created subglottic stenosis in dogs by painting the subglottic region with gastric juices every other day.

Using a canine model, Klainer, *et al.*[322] intubated dogs for 2 hours with a minimally occlusive low-pressure cuff, and subsequently examined the tracheal mucosa. After 2 hours of intubation, there was complete ciliary denudation, especially over the tracheal rings. They also examined the tracheae of previously intubated patients and found the area of the cuff site to be metaplastic; the respiratory epithelium had changed to squamous epithelium.

Wynne, *et al.*,[323] using a mouse model, examined the effect of tracheobronchial tree aspiration of minute quantities (0.1 ml) of saline (group I), hydrochloric acid pH 1.5 (group II), gastric juice pH 1.5 (group III), and gastric juice pH 5.9 (group IV). The animals that aspirated the gastric juices demonstrated widespread tracheal desquamation. The group III animals (acid and pepsin at pH 1.5) had very delayed regeneration, none showing signs of regeneration at 72 hours. The authors concluded that, ". . . *1.* gastric contents cause marked damage to the tracheal mucosa, even when the amount aspirated is too small to induce a clinically significant pneumonia, *2.* damage is more severe when the pH of the gastric content is low, and *3.* gastric juice may contain substances that delay healing."

Gaynor[247] used a rabbit perfusion model in which the larynx was isolated (by placing a cuffed tube below) and irrigated with acid, pepsin, or acid and pepsin, at pH 1.4 or 4.0. Irrigations were carried out from 1 to 4 hours. Control animals irrigated with saline demonstrated no significant mucosal changes. At a pH of 4.0 with pepsin, the inflammatory response involved the submucosa and muscle, and the degree of damage was greater as the period of irrigation lengthened. When a pH of 1.4 with pepsin was used, severe mucosal ulceration and submucosal and deeper hemorrhage with marked inflammatory response, as well as necrosis, were noted. The extent of tissue damage correlated with the duration of acid irrigation.

Gaynor also placed pH electrodes overnight in the hypopharynx of 20 patients in the intensive care unit (ICU) and found that 8 (40%) exhibited episodes of reflux to pH levels of less than 4.0. Kuriloff[324] has pointed out, however, that the role of GER in producing laryngeal injury in intubated ICU patients is multifactorial, and that the exact mechanism of and threshold for laryngeal injury in such patients has not yet been established.

In summary, it has been demonstrated that patients who were intubated in an intensive care unit setting had a high incidence of pharyngeal reflux, that perfusion of the rabbit larynx with acid and pepsin produces severe inflammation, and that intermittent application of the gastric contents to the larynx in a dog model produces subglottic stenosis if a prior mucosal injury exists. However, the clinical relationship between subglottic stenosis and gastroesophageal reflux disease has not yet been established convincingly.

Reflux Laryngitis

In 1858, Rudolf Virchow described "pachydermia

laryngis" and in 1880, Morel Mackenzie described "erosions or very fine ulcerations which extend no deeper than the epithelial layer. . . . Their most frequent seat is between the arytenoid cartilages."[325] Thus, vocal cord ulcers and granulomas were described more than 100 years ago.

At the American Laryngological Association meeting of 1903, Dr. L. A. Coffin[326] presented a paper entitled, "The Relations of the Upper Air Passages to Diseases of the Gastrointestinal Tract." Expressing an insight far ahead of its time, Dr. Coffin noted that he

> . . . had been struck by the large number of his clinic patients who complained only of post-nasal catarrh . . . As the anterior nares frequently escaped the disease altogether, it was evident that one must look elsewhere than to the inspired air. . . . The chief cause . . . was the irritation resulting from the eructations of gases from the stomach. . . .

In the conclusion of his paper, Dr. Coffin stated:

> Hyperacidity was a most common cause, and the reason it was overlooked was that the great majority of these persons gave no symptoms pointing to gastric disorder.

In the discussion that followed, Dr. Joseph White commented that ". . . rheumatism was the basis of many of these affections of the upper air passages, and then, in turn, disorders in women, and smoking and drinking in men. . . ." Dr. MacCuen Smith commented, ". . . so-called 'billous spells' were often associated with coryza and hoarseness and more or less pain, and the patient at the same time became weak from intestinal intoxication. . . ." Dr. J. A. Thompson added that he had seen ". . . cases of marked laryngitis which had proved absolutely rebellious to treatment until hyperacidity of the stomach had been diagnosed and properly treated." He also added that, "The regurgitation of irritating secretion during sleep was often responsible for pharyngitis and rhinitis."

Not surprisingly, there was considerable disagreement among the otolaryngologists in attendance: some completely rejected the notion of reflux-related laryngeal and pharyngeal disorders, while others granted its possibility but noted that the relationship was conjectural. Dr. C. F. Thieson closed the meeting by emphasizing "the need for great general knowledge among specialists" and quoted Virchow's comparison of the specialties to offshoots of the tree, the trunk being general medicine.

In 1928, Chevalier Jackson[327] coined the term "contact ulcer."

> Contact ulcer is the name I have given to superficial ulceration occurring on one or both sides of the larynx posteriorly, the ulcerated surface coming in contact on phonation with that of its fellow of the opposite side, the latter being ulcerated or not, according to whether the ulcer is monolateral or bilateral.

He described many of the patients as complaining of choking episodes at night and suggested that "leakage into the larynx of oral secretions that should drain away downward into the esophagus" was the cause of contact ulcer. For treatment, Jackson recommended absolute silence. Jackson also noted that the lesion was not a common one, "inasmuch as I have seen only 127 cases in forty years."

For the next 40 years, various authors[325,328–330] modified and debated Jackson's recommendation for treatment. The consensus was that surgical treatment should be reserved for cases with airway obstruction and that in lieu of voice rest "vocal re-education" should be employed. In spite of these recommendations, most authors of the time recognized the poor prognosis of contact ulcer and granuloma of the vocal cords.

In 1968, Cherry and Margulies[9] reported three patients with contact ulcers of the larynx related to reflux "peptic" esophagitis. The authors noted that none of the patients volunteered symptoms suggestive of peptic esophagitis, but all three had resolution with antireflux treatment consisting of antacids, dietary modification, and elevation of the head of the bed. The authors pointed out that "more sophisticated radiographic techniques (acid barium meal) had made the diagnosis possible." In the same year, Delahunty and Cherry[10] experimentally produced vocal process granulomas in two dogs by applying a cotton ball soaked in the gastric juices to the laryngeal mucosa for 20 minutes 5 days a week for several weeks. They noted that by the fourth day

> . . . the posterior half of the left true vocal cord was exhibiting injection and slight edema. . . . The edema and inflammation slowly progressed with further applications. . . . When seen, on the fourth week the left vocal cord of each dog was markedly inflamed, thickened and irregular in the posterior half. Epithelial slough became apparent at the site of application on day 29 in dog 1 and day 32 in dog 2.

A control larynx painted with saliva did not develop ulceration or granulation.

In 1972, Delahunty[16] described nine patients with "intractable, unexplained posterior laryngitis." The findings were characteristically ". . . interarytenoid heaping of mucosa with chronic inflammation of the posterior third of the true vocal cords." Of the nine patients presented, five had gastrointestinal symptoms suggesting reflux, and three had a globus sensation. All had positive acid barium swallows, and reflux into the pharynx was noted in two. Treatment with antireflux measures usually provided significant improvement in 6 to 8 weeks.

Ward, *et al.*[15] reported 28 patients with contact granulomas and demonstrated hiatal hernia in 72%. The authors concluded that, although vocal abuse and chronic throat clearing may perpetuate the lesion, chronic irritation due to "acid's regurgitation secondary to hiatal hernia" is usually causal.

In 1948, Hill[331] described granuloma of the larynx following endotracheal anesthesia. Feder and Michell[11] reported 27 patients with vocal process granuloma in a paper entitled "Hyperfunctional, hyperacidic, and intubation granulomas." They concluded that 5 of the 27 cases in their series were due to gastroesophageal reflux, 5 were due to intubation, and 17 were hyperfunctional (due to vocal abuse). They believed that vocal process granulomas had three separate causes: vocal abuse, reflux, and intubation. However, Olson[14] has also reported an intubation granuloma due to GERD.

The first series of patients with contact ulcers evaluated by modern diagnostic methods was reported in 1983. Öhman, *et al.*[13] investigated 43 men with "previous or present" contact ulcers (three quarters of the patients did not have contact ulcers at the time of examination and one quarter did). The patients underwent diagnostic barium esophagography, esophageal manometry, pH manometry, acid perfusion (Bernstein) testing, and esophageal acid clearance testing. Fifty-one percent of the patients had abnormal GER on pH manometry, 37% had abnormal esophageal acid clearance, 23% had esophageal dysmotility, and 7% had a positive acid perfusion test. Although only 25% of the patients in the series had active laryngeal lesions at the time of the study, 74% had abnormal studies. In other words, three times as many patients in the group had abnormal GER as patients with active vocal cord lesions.

Ossakow, *et al.*[251] studied 63 otolaryngology patients with "cervical symptoms" (cough, hoarseness, chronic throat clearing, globus sensation, sore throat, and dysphagia), as well as 36 esophagitis patients with "typical" GERD, and 10 controls. Study patients underwent *1.* head and neck examination, *2.* barium esophagography, *3.* esophagoscopy and biopsy, *4.* esophageal manometry, *5.* standard acid reflux testing, *6.* acid perfusion testing, and *7.* esophageal acid clearance testing. The mean age of the population was 51 years, with a range of 17 to 81 years. Only 6% of the otolaryngology patients had heartburn or regurgitation, whereas 89% of the esophagitis patients had those symptoms. Thus, with regard to gastrointestinal symptoms, GER was largely occult (silent) in the otolaryngology patients.

All the esophagitis patients had normal head and neck examinations, as did half of the otolaryngology group. The other half was equally divided between those with laryngeal ulcers and granulomas (25%) and those with laryngeal erythema alone (25%). One hundred percent of the typical GERD patients demonstrated reflux on the standard acid reflux test, as did 68% of the otolaryngology patients. (All controls had normal findings with the exception that 10% had positive acid perfusion (Bernstein) tests.) Sixty percent of the otolaryngology patients had esophageal dysmotility and 78% had abnormal acid clearance tests. The findings of Ossakow, *et al.*[251] are similar to those of Öhman, *et al.*,[13] with the exceptions that Ossakow's group found that twice as many of their patients had abnormal esophageal acid clearance and dysmotility. Their patients with "cervical" dysphagia and esophagitis are summarized in Table XVII.

TABLE XVII.
Comparison of History, Laryngeal Examination, and Diagnostic Testing in Otolaryngology Patients With "Cervical Symptoms" (n = 63) or Esophagitis (n = 36), and in Controls (n = 10).*

	Otolaryngology Patients	Esophagitis Patients
A. Symptoms		
Heartburn and/or regurgitation	6%†	89%
Hoarseness, dysphagia, globus, throat clearing and cough	100%†	0%
B. Laryngeal Examination		
Normal	50%†	100%
Erythema	25%†	0%
Contact ulcer or granulation	25%†	0%
C. Diagnostic Studies		
Upper esophageal sphincter pressure (mm Hg)	144 ± 121	71 ± 40
Positive standard acid reflux test	68%	100%
Positive Bernstein acid perfusion test	5%†	89%
Abnormal esophageal manometry	10%	8%
Esophageal dysmotility	60%†	10%
Abnormal esophageal acid clearance	78%	80%

All control subjects had normal studies, except for 10% who had positive Bernstein acid perfusion tests.

*Derived from Ossakow, *et al.*[251]

†Statistically significant difference.

Even with the advent of new diagnostic technology, the significance of interarytenoid mucosal thickening and posterior erythema (posterior laryngitis) remains somewhat uncertain. Kambic and Radsel[17] reported 44 patients with posterior laryngitis, all of whom underwent biopsy and evaluation by a gastroenterologist. The biopsies showed hyperplasia of the prickle cell layer, keratinization, lymphocytic and plasma cell infiltration, and fibrosis. The method of diagnosis was not reported, but the authors stated that 42 of 44 patients undergoing gastroenterologic evaluation had GER.

Wilson, *et al.*[20] reported a negative association between GER and posterior laryngitis in 96 patients with posterior laryngitis and 54 controls. Biopsies of the posterior larynx were performed, and subjects underwent 24-hour pH manometry. "Posterior laryngitis" in association with documented prolonged acid exposure time (by pH manometry) was demonstrated in only 17.5%.

In summary, the relationship between GERD and laryngeal disease remains, to some extent, unproven. Furthermore, the effect of intermittent GER is essentially unknown. Nevertheless, the available data indicate that GERD is usually the cause of contact ulcers and vocal process granulomas, and that throat clearing (because of a foreign body sensation) may help to perpetuate the lesion, although vocal abuse is no longer considered causative. The findings of mucosal thickening and erythema in the posterior larynx remain controversial, in part, because the reported descriptions of the physical findings vary. (Four reflux-related granulomas are shown in Figure 1. Only examples **B** and **D** are typical; the intubation granuloma **(C)** and the epiglottic granuloma **(A)** were also due to GER. Thus, even the appearance of GER-related granulomas may vary.) The granuloma is clearly distinguishable by histology and appearance, but the thickness, color, and general appearance of the interarytenoid region vary considerably in a normal population, as well as in those with disease.[20]

Globus Pharyngeus

"Globus hystericus" was described by Hippocrates. The term is derived from the Latin *globus*, ball, sphere; and the Greek *hystericus*, the uterus, womb. Two thousand years ago it was believed that the womb was a floating organ that moved freely around the woman's body, and hence the lump-in-the-throat symptom was caused by this organ rising into the neck.[332] The term came to be applied to the sensation of a lump in the throat due to hysteria (emotional excitability or anxiety).[332] (In this manuscript, the term hystericus will henceforth be dropped and the symptom in the throat will be referred to as "globus," "the globus symptom," or "globus pharyngeus.") The incidence of a globus symptom has been estimated to account for between 0.7% and 4.1% of all patients seeking the medical attention of an otolaryngologist.[59,264,265,267]

In 1968, Malcomson[59] presented the diagnostic and therapeutic data of 370 globus patients. Almost all the patients described a foreign body sensation in the throat, which was independent of swallowing. All patients underwent barium study and otolaryngologic examination: 30% were found to have lesions directly related to the site of complaint in the neck, including cervical osteophytes, hyperplastic tonsils, goiter, postcricoid web, etc., and 48% were found to have a hiatal hernia, duodenal or gastric ulcer, or some other esophageal or intra-abdominal lesion. Twenty-two percent remained without diagnosis.

In the early 1970s, Delahunty and Ardran,[60] Cherry, *et al.*[333] and Freeland, *et al.*[264] all studied globus patients using the acid barium meal. Abnormalities were found in 88%, 92%, and 77% of patients, respectively. These authors reported excellent responses to antacid treatment. On the other hand, Mair, *et al.*[266] found only 13% of 77 globus patients to have esophagitis or reflux on barium swallow and only 18% to have a positive acid barium test; overall, these authors believed that esophagitis occurred in no more than 45% of their patients.

Caldarelli, *et al.*[262] and Watson and Sullivan[269] each carried out UES manometry in normal subjects and in patients with globus. Caldarelli, *et al.* found no difference in the resting UES pressures of the two groups. The results of Watson and Sullivan were completely the opposite. The globus patients (n = 9) had a mean resting UES pressure of 175.6 ± 22 mm Hg (range, 140 to 210 mm Hg), whereas, in the controls (n = 22), it was 96 ± 15.6 mm Hg (range, 70 to 140 mm Hg). There was no overlap whatsoever. Wallin, *et al.*[334] demonstrated in normal subjects that esophageal perfusion with hydrochloric acid produced roughly a 33% increase in UES pressure within one minute of instituting perfusion. The difference was statistically significant ($P < .05$).

Pratt, *et al.*[332] performed psychologic testing (Minnesota Multiphasic Personality Inventory (MMPI)) on 49 patients with a globus symptom (23 male and 26 female). The patients had higher than average scores for depression and hypochondriasis. Psychiatric referral was recommended for approximately half the patients.

During the 1980s, conflicting reports about the relationship of GERD and globus continued.[179,256,260,261,263,265,335] Moloy and Charter[267] studied 4330 consecutive otolaryngology patients over a 15-month period and found the incidence of globus symptoms to be 4.1%. Of those 178 patients, 38% had reflux symptoms and 1% underwent barium swallow esophagoscopy. In 8 (20%) of 40 patients, the barium swallow was abnormal. Eighty percent of the population responded to treatment; however, reassurance was the primary treatment for 75% of the patients. These authors noted that in patients under 50 years of age, the globus symptom occurred with a female:male predominance of 3:1. For patients over 50 years of age, that ratio was 1:1.

Wilson, *et al.*[270] performed esophageal monitoring and 24-hour pH manometry in 47 patients with globus, 48 controls, and 28 patients with documented esophagitis. Manometry was normal in 38 of the 47 globus patients (81%). Thirteen percent had distal esophagitis on biopsy and only 15% had abnormal pH studies.

Flores, *et al.*[263] performed esophageal manometry in 12 patients with globus and found UES pressure to be normal; however, 10 of the 12 patients had high esophageal body-resting pressures and 9 of the patients had dysmotility.

Finally, Batch[260] studied 136 globus patients (one-third male, two-thirds female), with a mean age of 45 years. Symptoms were carefully elicited: dysphagia (60%), hoarseness (52%), heartburn (51%), and regurgitation (36%). The results of investigative studies revealed reflux and/or esophagitis: barium swallow (15%), endoscopy and biopsy (73%), Bernstein acid perfusion test (60%), and pH manometry (65%). Every patient had one or more of these symptoms, but UES studies and esophageal motility studies were usually normal. Patients were treated with antireflux treatment, including the use of prokinetic agents such as metaclopramide, and of H_2 blockers such as cimetidine. Seventy percent of the patients responded to treatment and 30% did not.

In summary, a globus sensation rarely seems to be due to a psychogenic cause (hysteria). Local, inflammatory, and neoplastic conditions, as well as GERD, account for the diagnosis in most patients; barium study and otolaryngologic examination are useful screening tools. A substantial proportion of patients with globus have GERD, but it is not clear whether the symptoms represent referred discomfort from esophagitis, esophageal dysmotility, or cricopharyngeal hypertension, or whether they result directly from acid irritation of laryngopharyngeal structures.

Dysphagia

Throat pain and dysphagia are complaints that may result from infectious, neoplastic, myopathic, neurologic, traumatic, inflammatory, or idiopathic causes. It is beyond the scope of this paper to review all the causes of dysphagia. Rather, the focus will be on GERD as a cause of chronic throat pain and dysphagia.

As was the case with globus pharyngeus, there are three possible mechanisms of symptom production, which may be associated with GERD: *1.* direct irritation of laryngopharyngeal structures by reflux; *2.* referred discomfort to the cervical region, secondary to esophageal dysfunction (esophagitis and/or dysmotility); and *3.* upper esophageal sphincter (UES) dysfunction. UES dysfunction may be related to changes in resting tone and/or disorders of sphincter relaxation (premature, delayed, or incomplete).

Resting UES pressure has been measured in patients with Zenker's diverticulum and values in general are reported to be normal or below normal.[106,259,336] However, UES measurements (*cf.* previous sections) are subject to tremendous variations based upon differences in technique and technical difficulties inherent in measuring sphincter function.[50] Nevertheless, there have been several reports of the relationship between GERD and Zenker's diverticulum.[61,257,259,271,336,337] Ellis and Crozier[336] reported 10 patients with Zenker's diverticulum, only four of whom had elevated UES pressures; however, all 10 patients had UES dysfunction characterized by premature relaxation and contraction. Although true cricopharyngeal achalasia (failure to open) has been reported,[106,338] it is very uncommon.

Hurwitz, *et al.*[259] reported findings in 14 patients with oropharyngeal dysphagia. Unfortunately, the patient population was heterogeneous, including one patient who had had radical neck surgery, two patients with Parkinson's disease, two patients with Zenker's diverticulum, one patient each with amyotrophic lateral sclerosis, mononeuritis multiplex, ocular pharyngeal dystrophy, polio, and hypertrophic cervical osteoarthritis, and five patients with idiopathic disease. Failure of the UES to relax completely, uncoordinated UES relaxation, and poor initiation of swallowing were noted.

Although the report of Ossakow, *et al.*[251] provides good information about otolaryngology patients with a variety of "cervical" symptoms, patients with sore throat and dysphagia were not specifically subgrouped, and no specific information can be drawn about that group from their report. However, there seemed to be a high incidence of esophageal dysmotility. Mean UES pressures were higher in patients with cervical symptoms (144 ± 121 mm Hg), but were not significantly different from those in patients with GER (71 ± 40 mm Hg) and controls (58 ± 20 mm Hg).

Henderson, *et al.*[258] reported pharyngoesophageal dysphagia occurring in 51.3% of 1000 consecutive patients with gastroesophageal disease. Aspiration occurred in 30% of these patients and some developed significant secondary respiratory symptoms. Upper esophageal and pharyngeal manometry was carried out in 52 patients and 20 demonstrated cricopharyngeal incoordination. Surgical correction of GER in patients with intractable symptoms was effective in relieving the dysphagia in all but a few.

In Toohill's report of 207 patients with GERD seen in otolaryngologic practice, dysphagia occurred as a primary symptom in 24 (12%).[58] The results of therapy for that specific subgroup were not provided.

There is no question that regurgitation of gastric contents into the laryngopharynx and oral cavity can occur. The use of double-probe pH manometry[250] and four-channel probes[339] has documented such events. However, pharyngolaryngeal reflux events occur with only a small proportion of esophageal reflux episodes.[184,339] Falor, *et al.*,[339] using a four-channel recording device with the upper channel in the pharynx, reported the case of a man with recurrent staphylococcal pneumonia and lung abscess caused by regurgitation and aspiration. In addition to the above symptoms, he had an incompetent LES and a hyperfunctioning cricopharyngeus. Cricopharyngeal myotomy had been proposed, but four-channel pH manometry used to assess the time over which pH was less than 4.0 yielded: lower esophagus (56.37%), mid esophagus (43.59%), upper esophagus (25.50%), and pharynx (31.91%). Thus, acid refluxing into the pharynx had caused his symptoms; the treatment prescribed was antireflux therapy.

In summary, there is little strong documentation of the relationship between GER and dysphagia—perhaps because multiple-probe pH manometry has not been applied to the investigation of these patient groups, but more likely because patients with dysphagia represent a heterogeneous group in terms of causality. In some patients, however, GERD may cause dysphagia, which may be the primary symptom.

Chronic Cough

As with the dysphagia group, chronic cough is a symptom and not a diagnosis, but some patients with GERD have chronic cough as their primary complaint. Irwin, *et al.*[232] found that 49 (10.3%) of 474 patients referred to the pulmonary clinic were treated for chronic cough. Of that group, 10% (5 of 49) had GERD as their primary diagnosis.

Stiegmann, *et al.*[55] reported 22 patients with predominantly upper aerodigestive tract manifestations of GERD. This represented 5.8% of patients evaluated in a gastroenterology practice for GERD. Sixteen of the 22 patients (73%) had no typical GERD symptoms. Urschel and Paulson[95] reported the complications of GERD in 636 patients, including children and adults. Respiratory symptoms and complications were common: cough (47%), bronchitis (35%), asthma (16%), and pneumonitis (16%).

Kennedy (1962)[340] reported 25 patients with pulmonary infection as a complication of GERD; the GERD was relieved by surgery alone in nine. Pearson and Wilson[229] reported a 4% incidence of pulmonary fibrosis related to GERD, and Iverson, *et al.*[226] reported a 40% incidence of pulmonary complications in GERD, with a 56% incidence in patients with GERD and esophageal stricture. The complications, in descending order of frequency, were pneumonia, bronchitis, chronic cough, bronchiectasis, lung abscess, and tracheomalacia.

Ducolone, *et al.*[341] studied 30 patients with chronic bronchitis, 29 of whom were smokers averaging 34 pack-years. Patients underwent radionuclide scan and pH monitoring. Seventeen of the patients (57%) were found to have abnormal reflux and 13 (43%) were not.

Fitzgerald, *et al.*[231] reported 20 patients with chronic cough of unknown etiology. Fifteen had heartburn and/or regurgitation, and six of those had reflux demonstrated on barium esophagoscopy; 14 had resolution of reflux with medical antireflux therapy, and 5 were referred for fundoplication.

Kelly, *et al.*[342] evaluated 20 patients with recurrent pneumonia using double-probe pH manometry, the second probe being placed in the hypopharynx. The dual-probe pH manometry was abnormal in 18 of 20 patients. The authors concluded that dual-probe pH monitoring substantially increases the recognition of patients with reflux-related pulmonary symptoms compared to standard pH criteria or barium studies.

The relationship between GERD and asthma has been established both in adults[238,239,341,343,344] and in children.[221,240,244] Mays[343] reported 28 patients with severe asthma examined with barium esophagography, 13 (46%) of whom had had demonstrable GER. Mitsuhashi, *et al.*[243] studied 15 asthmatic children with pH-metry and found that episodes of asthmatic attacks after overeating were closely correlated with both decreased LES pressure and GERD. Goodall, *et al.*[238] studied 25 patients with bronchial asthma and GERD. Both the severity of the reflux and the severity of the asthma were graded and the patients were entered into a double-blind crossover study in which cimetidine was used. Significant improvement in both the reflux and the asthma was seen after treatment. Harper, *et al.*[239] reported beneficial results of antireflux therapy in a nonrandomized study of 15 patients with nonallergic asthma and GERD.

In eight patients with esophagitis and bronchial asthma, Andersen, *et al.*[233] performed the Bernstein acid perfusion test with simultaneous monitoring of pulmonary function, including total lung capacity, airway resistance, residual volume, and peak expiratory flow. The pulmonary variables were measured five times during a single trial before and after instillation of 50 ml of 0.1 normal HCl. A significant decrease in the peak expiratory flow and increase in the airway resistance followed instillation of the HCl ($P < .002$). Three days later, six of the eight patients underwent another trial, this time having been pretreated with atropine 0.01 mg/kg twice daily for 3 days. Instillation of the acid following pretreatment did not produce any change in peak expiratory flow or airway resistance. Thus, a vagally mediated reflux pathway for GER-induced bronchoconstriction was postulated.

In 1978, Mansfield and Stein[241,344] also postulated a vagally mediated reflux pathway in a subset of asthmatic patients with gastroesophageal reflux disease, and direct acid irritation of the tracheobronchial tree was postulated in another subset.

The problem of asthma and GERD is compounded by the increased intra-abdominal pressure associated with airway distress and coughing, and asthmatics are frequently treated with theophylline, which has an adverse effect upon LES pressure.[345,346]

Sontag, *et al.*[244] performed antireflux surgery in 13 adults with both GERD and asthma. Postoperative follow-up ranged from 13 months to 5 years. Six patients were completely free of asthma, six patients were improved, and one patient was unchanged.

In addition to chronic lung infection, pulmonary fibrosis, and asthma, GERD has been implicated in neonatal bronchopulmonary dysplasia,[56,212,213] cystic fibrosis,[140,141] sudden infant death syndrome (SIDS),[272–274] and reflex bradycardia.[285–287] In addition, it would appear that in patients with chronic cough of unknown etiology, or in patients with chronic bronchitis (even those who are smokers), GERD may also be a significant cofactor.

TREATMENT

Medical

At the turn of the century, "billous spells" were treated with calomel, chlorate of potash, mercury, chalk, colonic irrigations, and bicarbonate of soda.[326] For most of this century, life-style modification and antacids have been the mainstay of treatment for symptomatic GERD.

The amount of antacid needed to relieve symptoms is apparently less than that needed to neutralize acid. Thus, the effect of antacid in GERD is probably that it acts to coat the esophagus.[6] In addition, it has also been shown that when antacid is given 1 hour after meals, it appears to depress gastric acidity for almost 3 hours.[347] This may, in part, be due to the fact that gastric alkalinization modifies the pepsin response. Furthermore, antacids also seem to increase LES pressure. (Alginic acid-containing compounds, such as Gaviscon®, do not appear to be any more beneficial than antacids.[348,349])

Dietary modification is an important part of antireflux therapy. Protein increases LES pressure, whereas fat decreases LES pressure and delays gastric emptying. Therefore, a low-fat, high-protein diet is recommended for patients with GERD.[113] Consumption of alcohol and use of tobacco are both discouraged in the patient with GERD, because these agents adversely influence several pathophysiologic GER mechanisms.

Elevation of the head of the bed or sleeping on a wedge has been shown to improve acid clearance time in two thirds of patients, although the number of reflux episodes does not change.[350] GERD patients are also instructed to avoid wearing corsets, tight belts, and tight-fitting clothing, which increase the abdominal pressure. A host of other foods and drugs associated with the promotion of GERD are listed in Table X.

Treatment of GERD in three phases is recommended by most gastroenterologists.[351] The components of three-phase therapy are shown in Table XVIII; Table XIX shows many of the more commonly employed antireflux drugs and some of the newer drugs (and the year they were introduced).

Phase I therapy consists of dietary and life-style modification, with the use of antacids. Depending upon the severity of the patient's symptoms, this therapy may suffice. This treatment alone, however, is not adequate for patients with severe disease or those with complications.[352]

H_2 blockers (cimetidine, ranitidine, famotidine) effectively and safely depress acid secretion and are considered phase II treatment. These agents selectively inhibit the stimulation of the parietal cell by histamine at the H_2 receptor site. Because of the interdependency among the pathways involved in hydrogen ion production, they effectively reduce the secretion of acid stimulation by gastrin, cholinergic stimulation, and food. Unfortunately, other secretory pathways are not inhibited by H_2 blockers so that total acid suppression is not achieved with these agents.[153]

TABLE XVIII.
Antireflux Therapy (ART).

Phase I
A. Dietary modification
1. Avoidance of fat, chocolate, mints, carbonated beverages, caffeine
2. Avoidance of ethanol
3. Avoidance of overeating
4. No food or drink within 3 hours of recumbency
B. Life-style modification
1. Cessation of tobacco usage
2. Elevation of the head of the bed (6")
3. Avoidance of tight-fitting clothing
4. Weight reduction (for obesity)
C. Medication(s)
1. Liquid antacids (one tablespoon 1 hour after each meal, and two tablespoons before bed)
2. Avoidance of the refluxogenic medications (*cf.* Tables X and XI)
Phase II
A. Medication(s)
1. H_2 blockers
Cimetidine
Ranitidine
Famotidine
2. Prokinetic agents
Bethanecol
Metoclopramide
Cisapride
3. Mucosal cytoprotectants
Sucralfate
Phase III
A. Medication
1. Hydrogen ion blockers
B. Surgery
1. Angelchik™ prosthesis
2. Fundoplication

Before the development of the H_2 blockers, antimuscarinic agents such as bethanechol were the only drugs available that effectively reduced gastric output after stimulation; however, the reduction in acid output was modest (30%).[155,353] When an anticholinergic drug was combined with an H_2 blocker (*e.g.*, cimetidine and propantheline), the combined effect in terms of inhibiting acid secretion was potentiated and synergistic.[353] Lieberman and Keeffe[194] studied 25 patients with chronic reflux esophagitis refractory to cimetidine treatment alone, and found that 9 of 12 patients receiving cimetidine and metoclopramide had significant symptomatic and endoscopic improvement at the end of 8 weeks.

The healing and relapse rate of reflux esophagitis during treatment with ranitidine was studied in 108 patients with severe reflux esophagitis.[354] Patients

TABLE XIX.
Representative Drugs Used in the Treatment of GERD.

Pharmacologic Class	Generic Name	Trade Name	Manufacturer	Year Introduced
A. Antacids	Magnesium and aluminum hydroxide	Maalox®	Rorer	1950
B. Parasympathomimetics	Bethanechol	Urecholine®	MSD	1953
	Metoclopramide	Reglan®	A.H. Robins	1979
	Cisapride	—	Janssen	Investigational
C. H_2 Antagonists	Cimetidine	Tagamet®	SKF	1977
	Ranitidine	Zantac®	Glaxo	1983
	Famotidine	Pepcid®	MSD	1986
D. H^+ Pump Blockers	Omeprazole	Prilosec®	MSD	1989
	SKF96022	—	SKF	Investigational
	SKF96067	—	SKF	Investigational
E. Cytoprotectants	Sucralfate	Carafate®	Marion	1981

with isolated erosions had a 6-week healing rate of 78%; the healing rate was 36% in patients with confluent lesions and 23% in those with circumferential erosions of the distal esophagus. Thus, in more severe disease, H_2 blockers seemed to be less effective.[354]

Multiple, randomized control double-blind studies have demonstrated the efficacy of H_2 blockers.[354–356] Generally, improvement was found in 70% of patients and complete healing in 50%.[356,357] Ranitidine has even been shown to be effective in healing Barrett's esophagus. Lee and Isaacs[203] reported 28 patients with Barrett's epithelium, 60% of whom healed at 8 weeks of therapy. However, improvement in patients who need long-term maintenance seems to reach a plateau by 6 months. Thereafter, relapses, even with therapy, are not uncommon.[358] Surprisingly, Sontag, *et al.*,[356] in a large double-blind trial, found patients taking ranitidine to be symptomatically improved, but found no differences between the control and treatment groups in respect to esophageal mucosal sensitivity to acid perfusion or histologic grading of esophageal mucosal biopsy specimens following treatment. The authors were forced to conclude that "ranitidine therapy, 150 mg twice daily, markedly reduced the heartburn symptoms of reflux disease and improved the endoscopic appearance of the esophageal mucosa."

In recent controlled studies, response rates of severe esophagitis, that is, with confluent ulcerations and/or Barrett's epithelium, even to potent H_2 blockers, were lower than expected.[192,358–360] These studies represent the selection of recalcitrant cases; nevertheless, medical treatment in these populations is associated with high failure and recurrence rates.

Ranitidine is six to eight times more potent than cimetidine as an inhibitor of gastric secretion, and it also causes greater reduction in the basal resting output. The half-life of cimetidine is 1.7 to 2.1 hours, and that of ranitidine, 2.1 to 3.1 hours. Thus, ranitidine is usually preferred over cimetidine for the majority of cases treated with H_2 blockers.[361]

Cisapride, a new cholinergic agent, has several beneficial effects. It has been shown to increase LES pressure, to increase the amplitude of esophageal peristalsis, and to promote gastric emptying. It does not appear to increase gastric acidity.[362] In addition, cisapride seems devoid of the antidopaminergic and muscarinic activity of the older agents (dry mouth, blurred vision, *etc.*). Baldi, *et al.*[362] compared the effect of cisapride (10 mg q.i.d.) with a placebo in 63 patients. Only one patient in the cisapride group was not improved symptomatically at 6 weeks, and by 12 weeks of therapy, 63% of the cisapride patients and only 12% of the placebo patients were healed. Drugs such as cisapride are known as prokinetic agents because of their ability to improve gastrointestinal tract motility. The side effects of the prokinetic drugs, at least until cisapride, have made H_2 blockers the mainstay of phase II treatment, and prokinetic agents have been added to the treatment of patients who fail on H_2 blockers.

Phase III antireflux treatment has traditionally consisted of surgical repair of hiatal hernia with the reestablishment of a functioning LES. The most exciting new treatment option is the H^+K^+-ATPase inhibitors (hydrogen ion blocker).[92,155,192,203,359,360,363–365] The last stage of hydrogen ion production in the acid-secreting pathway within the parietal cell is a hydrogen ion pump in which potassium is exchanged for hydrogen. This step is carried out by the H^+K^+-ATPase.[155,365] Omeprazole acts on this final step in the stimulatory process of acid secretion and totally inhibits both stimulated and basal acid secretion, whether stimulated by histamine, acetylcholine, gastrin, or food.[155] In addition, this drug acts within 24 hours to abolish all acid secretion.[155]

Sandmark, *et al.*[359] studied 152 patients with endoscopically verified ulcerative esophagitis in a double-blind randomized study, comparing 20 mg of omeprazole given once daily, and 150 mg of ranitidine, given twice daily. At 4 weeks the healing rate was 67% in the omeprazole group and 31% in the ranitidine group, and at 8 weeks, 85% and 50%, respectively. The higher healing rate with omeprazole was also accompanied by significantly faster and more substantial improvement in reflux symptoms. Both drugs were well tolerated. Klinkenberg-Knol, *et al.*,[363] in a similar double-blind randomized study using a larger dose of omeprazole (60 mg per day), found 88% of their 51 patients to be healed at 8 weeks with omeprazole and 38% to be healed with ranitidine. Brunner, *et al.*[192] followed up 28 patients with resistant ulcerative esophagitis, all being treated with 20 to 60 mg of omeprazole per day. Eighty-six percent were healed by 4 weeks and all by 12 weeks. Maintenance therapy with 40 mg of omeprazole has been continued for up to 4 years without any adverse effects. Hetzel, *et al.*[92] demonstrated healing within 4 weeks of ulcerative esophagitis in 88% of patients, and in 48% of patients with Barrett's esophagus. Following cessation of therapy, 82% of the patients relapsed within 6 months.

Complete abolition of acid secretion by omeprazole does not result in malabsorption, because malabsorption syndromes are the result of two other conditions.[155] The first is pernicious anemia, an autoimmune disease in which there are auto-antibodies to an intrinsic factor, and the second occurs in the achlorhydric patient in whom there is bacterial overgrowth of the small intestine. No malabsorption, anemia, or any abnormalities of liver enzymes have been found in any of the patients treated with long-term omeprazole. Omeprazole does, however, lead to hypertrophy of the gastrin-producing cells in the secretory unit, and long-term, high-dose administration in rats has led to the development of carcinoid tumors of the stomach wall.[155]

Omeprazole has been shown to inhibit acid secretion for more than 24 hours after a single dose and, as a consequence, patient compliance, as well as effectiveness of therapy, may make this drug the treatment of choice for GERD in the future.[155,364,365] Furthermore, pulsed or intermittent therapy may eventually be employed.[366] Omeprazole has demonstrated therapeutic results superior to any other previous medical treatment.[92,192,203,359,360,363]

Another new drug, which enhances the effectiveness of the mucosal barrier, is also available.[366–368] Sucralfate is the polysulfated salt of sucrose, and it binds selectively to areas of injured gastrointestinal tract mucosa to form a protective layer. It is a barrier both to acid and to pepsin.[366,368] Sucralfate was used in an experimental model of peptic esophagitis in the rabbit[367] and led to significantly diminished esophagitis. A similar study was carried out in cats, and sucralfate given before acid perfusion consistently prevented any acid-induced lesions from developing.[369]

In summary, the severity of GERD indicates the necessity for prolonged and often multiple-modality treatment. New therapeutic options, which are likely to improve substantially the results of medical antireflux treatment, are currently being explored.

Surgical

In the only randomized study comparing medical and surgical treatment of erosive esophagitis, surgery was found to be highly effective in 73%; medical treatment in only 19%.[91] A discussion of surgical technique is beyond the scope of this paper; however, modifications of the Hill and Belsey techniques, as well as the Nissen fundoplication, are all being employed in the surgical treatment for GERD.[69,95,370–378]

The goals of surgical therapy are to lengthen the intra-abdominal esophageal segment, to recreate an acute esophagogastric angle, and to establish a higher resting LES pressure. Postoperative follow-up at 1 to 5 years in large series of patients demonstrates that surgery is effective therapy with relatively low recurrence rates, morbidity, and mortality.

Csendes, *et al.*[377] evaluated 150 patients 5 years or more after operation. The authors used a modification of the Hill operation and found, on follow-up endoscopy, that 83% had healed completely and 93% were improved. They also found a significant increase in LES pressure and esophageal clearance. The standard acid reflux test, which was positive in 100% of patients preoperatively, was positive in only 16% at follow-up. The final results after 5 years of surgery were: excellent or good results (85% of the patients); failure or reoperation (8%).

Stirling and Orringer[373] performed follow-up evaluations of 353 patients who had undergone Nissen fundoplication at least 1 year earlier. Intraesophageal pH studies showed good reflux control in 91% and poor reflux control in 9%. Ten percent required reoperation for recurrent reflux or dysphagia. Johnsson, *et al.*[378] evaluated at 6 months 40 patients who had undergone 360° Nissen fundoplication and compared them with 50 normal volunteers. They found the amount of reflux in the operative patients to be less than that in the controls and the LES pressure to be similar in both groups.

Low, *et al.*[371] evaluated the experience with 1600 Nissen fundoplications. Approximately 18% required reoperation, most commonly (48%) for "slipped Nissen." Of patients undergoing reoperation, complaints included recurrent reflux (86%), dysphagia (60%), and gastric perforation or fistulization (5%). Turnage, *et al.*[375] evaluated the effect of fundoplication on gastroesophageal reflux in infants and children. Seventy-four percent had no symptoms, 14% had mild symptoms, and 11.5% had symptomatic recurrence of GERD, necessitating reoperation.

Because of the technical difficulties in performing surgery at the gastric cardia, a prosthesis (Angelchik™) has been introduced as an option. In a prospective randomized clinical trial comparing the Nissen fundoplication with the Angelchik prosthesis (mean follow-up 38 months),[374] reflux had resolved in 77% of the Angelchik group, and in 94% of the Nissen group. This assessment included 24-hour pH monitoring and manometry. Patients with grade III esophagitis did poorly in the Angelchik group. Furthermore, the prosthesis migrated in 10% of patients. Migration of the Angelchik™ prosthesis has been reported in other series, and the use of this prosthesis is not widespread.[374,379,380]

At present, the Nissen fundoplication (360° wrap) is the most commonly performed operation in the United States. It has a mortality of 0.4% and a complication rate of 5% to 20%; approximately 8% to 18% of patients require reoperation subsequently for recurrent GER or dysphagia.[370,371,374,375,381–384]

In summary, reported indications for GER surgery are: *1.* when reflux-related symptoms are intolerably severe and/or persistent despite compliance with medical antireflux therapy, and *2.* when complications develop, which demand effective and prompt remedial therapy.

EXPERIMENTAL INVESTIGATIONS

The difference between physiologic reflux and GERD is that the latter represents a form of self-digestion. The word pepsin (peptic) is from the Greek word *pepsis,* digestion. The role of pepsin in GERD has been somewhat underplayed for two reasons: first, measurement of acid by pH-metry is relatively inexpensive, foolproof, and widely available, whereas pepsin or pepsinogen assays are complex, rarely available, and potentially fraught with error;[385] and second, both acid and pepsin are always present in the gastric juices, and the activity of pepsin is pH dependent.

Animal models clearly demonstrate that pepsin produces more extensive damage than acid. Almost all experiments using animal models to produce esophagitis have used a perfusion technique in the rabbit, dog, or cat. Lillemoe, *et al.*,[386] using the cat, perfused the esophagus with HCl alone, HCl with pepsin, HCl with bile, and HCl with trypsin (all at pH 2). Pepsin with acid caused significantly more esophageal injury than bile with acid, trypsin with acid, or acid alone ($P < .005$).

In similar experiments, Johnson and Harmon[387] assessed the effect of acid and combinations of gastroduodenal enzymes. Pepsin (and acid) caused significantly more esophageal injury by gross and microscopic criteria than bile and acid, trypsin and acid, or acid alone ($P < .005$). When the pepsin concentration was increased, the extent of injury increased in a dose-dependent manner ($P < .005$). Neither bile nor trypsin resulted in more esophageal injury than acid alone. Pepsin injury was characterized by mucosal ulceration, erosion, and extensive submucosal hemorrhage. In contrast, the effect of acid, bile, and trypsin was limited in most cases to submucosal edema without mucosal disruption. When pepsin and bile were combined, the effect was to reduce, rather than to increase, the damaging effect of pepsin. Bile (taurodeoxycholate, TDC) produced injury only when in an alkaline environment.

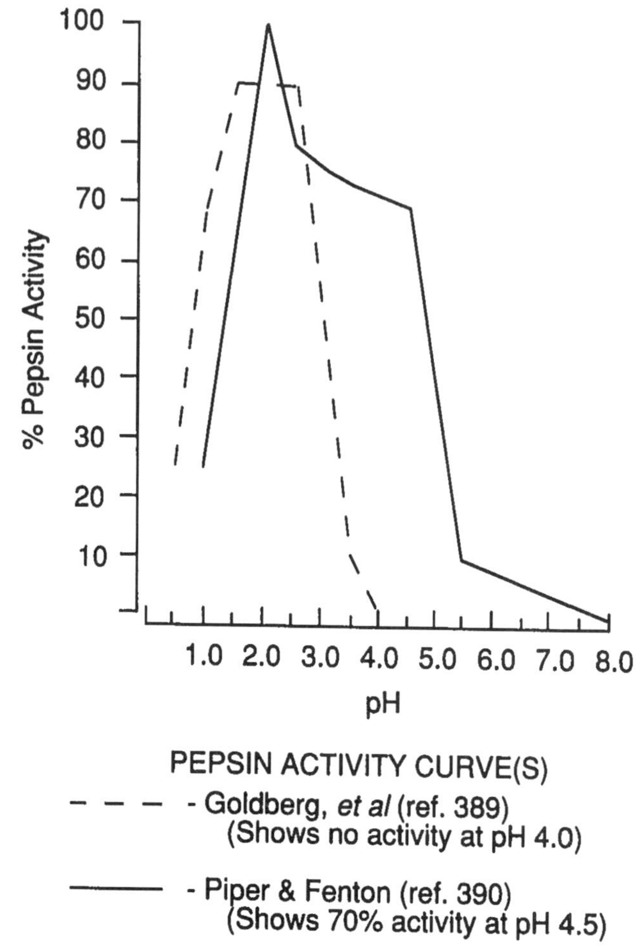

Fig. 3. Pepsin activity as a function of pH (in vitro).

Clinical studies of patients with GERD and normal controls using aspiration techniques with simultaneous pH monitoring have demonstrated minimal concentrations of bile in the refluxate. Penagini, *et al.*,[388] using simultaneous 24-hour pH manometry and intragastric aspiration, studied 22 patients with GER, including seven patients who had had previous partial gastrectomy. Intragastric pH greater than 7 was recorded only in patients who had previously undergone partial gastrectomy. The authors concluded that alkaline reflux is unlikely to be the cause of esophagitis, except following gastric surgery.

It is generally believed that pepsin activity is absent or minimal at pH of 4 or above. Goldberg, *et al.*,[389] using a porcine pepsin solution (0.05 mg/ml) and acid in a perfusion study, demonstrated maximal esophageal injury at pH 1.3 to 2.5. The in vitro pepsin activity curve from the report of Goldberg, *et al.* is reproduced in Figure 3 (dotted line). It shows virtually no pepsin activity at pH 3.5 to 4.

Piper and Fenton,[390] using human pepsin, demonstrated that 70% of maximal peptic activity was still present at pH 4.5 and that complete inactivation of pepsin did not occur until pH 8 (Figure 3, solid line). It is not clear whether the disparity between the results of these two studies was due to the method (technique) or to the type of pepsin. Nevertheless, contrary to current consensus, pepsin is probably still biologically active at pH 4.5.[385]

Gaynor[247] used a perfusion rabbit model to evaluate the effect of acid and pepsin on the larynx. At pH 1.4, severe mucosal ulceration, submucosal hemorrhage with marked inflammatory response, and necrosis were observed. The extent of tissue damage correlated with the duration of acid irrigation.

Little, *et al.*[24] studied the effects of intermittent application of the gastric contents on the subglottis in dogs who had undergone either removal of mucosa in the intercricoid area or removal of mucosa and perichondrium. On alternate days, the subglottic regions of the experimental animals were painted with gastric contents and those of the controls were painted with saline. All animals with perichondrial lesions and those with mucosal injuries only developed stenosis to varying degrees. (In the mucosal injury only group, the average pH was 1.6.) Control animals healed uneventfully without stenosis, and a single animal treated with ranitidine during the experimental period developed an intermediate degree of stenosis between that of the experimental group and that of the controls (pH 2.9). Thus, Little, *et al.*[24] demonstrated that intermittent application of the gastric contents could produce subglottic stenosis, but they did not evaluate the relative roles of acid, pepsin, and pH.

Pepsinogen I and II, the precursors to pepsin, can be assayed in serum and urine. Pepsinogen I is the predominant pepsinogen in most people and it operates at a lower pH than pepsinogen II. Pepsinogen stimulation may occur by cholinergic stimulation (vagal) or by a variety of other neural and humoral stimuli, including histamine, gastrin, and secretin. The principal stimulus is, however, cholinergic.

There is considerable evidence that duodenal ulcer disease may be genetically transmitted disorder. More than 50% of patients with duodenal ulcer have high pepsinogen I levels, and first-order relatives of duodenal ulcer patients also have been shown to have elevated pepsinogen I and a three-fold increase in the likelihood of developing duodenal ulcer disease.[385]

In summary, pepsin is the major injurious component of the refluxate and 70% of its maximal activity is present at pH 4.5. Other combinations of acid and gastroduodenal enzymes produce less injury than acid with pepsin. Bile (alkaline) reflux is not a clinical problem except in patients who have previously undergone gastric resection (usually for ulcer disease). Pepsinogen and pepsin assays (gastric analysis) may, in the future, reveal a genetic predisposition and provide a diagnostic marker for GERD.

TABLE XX.
Clinical Study Selection Criteria by Diagnostic Subgroup.

Group I. Carcinoma of the Larynx
- A. *All cases* of in situ, T1, or T2 squamous cell carcinoma of the larynx
- B. *All cases* of squamous cell carcinoma of the larynx in *non-tobacco users* (unless pH manometry was contraindicated due to risk of hemorrhage or airway obstruction)
- C. Any case with excessive granulation or stenosis following initial treatment of glottic carcinoma

Group II. Laryngeal Stenosis
- A. *All cases* of acquired stenosis *excluding* laryngeal trauma patients
- B. Any case of recurrent stenosis following initial successful treatment

Group III. Reflux Laryngitis
- A. *All cases* of posterior laryngitis (arytenoid erythema and piled up intra-arytenoid mucosa)
- B. *All cases* of diffuse laryngeal erythema and edema with or without mucosal ulceration
- C. *All cases* of vocal process or other laryngeal granulomas
- D. Any patient with bouts of hoarseness related to symptoms of gastroesophageal reflux
- E. Any patient with hoarseness of unexplained origin associated with throat clearing, globus, dysphagia, and/or cough

Group IV. Globus

All patients with a sensation of a lump in the throat (unassociated with a mass lesion or thyromegaly; head and neck examination, transnasal fiberoptic laryngoscopy, and barium swallow all negative)

Group V. Dysphagia

All patients with chronic throat pain or difficulty in swallowing of unexplained origin with associated symptoms of hoarseness, throat clearing, globus or cough; or with findings on laryngeal examination similar to those in group III

Group VI. Chronic Cough
- A. *All patients* with chronic cough and a history of GER
- B. *All patients* with nocturnal choking episodes, suggestive of regurgitation and aspiration by history
- C. *Any patient* with chronic cough of unexplained origin with a complete negative work-up in the pulmonary department

Group VII. Miscellaneous

(*cf.* text and Table XXII)

CLINICAL STUDY

MATERIALS AND METHODS

In order to test the hypothesis that occult and/or intermittent gastroesophageal reflux disease (GER, GERD) is associated with the development of upper aerodigestive tract conditions, 225 consecutive otolaryngology patients with suspected GER-related upper aerodigestive tract conditions were evaluated over a 4-year period (January 1, 1985 through December 31, 1988). Each patient was assigned to one of seven diagnostic subgroups, based upon the criteria in Table XX. The diagnostic subgroups were:

1. carcinoma of the larynx (n = 31),

TABLE XXI.
Study Population by Diagnostic Subgroup (Number of Patients).

Subgroup	Unable to Tolerate or Refused pH-Metry	Diagnostic pH Studies	Total
Carcinoma	0	31	31
Stenosis	1	32	33
Laryngitis	13	48	61
Globus	3	24	27
Dysphagia	3	22	25
Cough	5	25	30
Miscellanous	3	15	18
Total	28	197	225

TABLE XXII.
Breakdown of Miscellaneous Patients (Group VII) Undergoing pH Monitoring by Diagnosis.

Vocal cord polyps	3
Asthma	3
Spastic dysphonia	2
Burning mouth/throat	2
Laryngeal papillomas	1
Laryngeal cyst	1
Sleep apnea syndrome	1
S/P fundoplication	1
Kawasaki disease	1

2. laryngeal and/or tracheal stenosis (n = 33),
3. reflux laryngitis (n = 61),
4. globus (n = 27),
5. dysphagia (n = 25),
6. chronic cough (n = 30),
7. miscellaneous (n = 18).

Each subgroup represented a consecutive series of patients, with the exception of the miscellaneous group, in which consecutiveness was lost because of the heterogeneity of the group. All patients in the study were referred to the Department of Gastroenterology for ambulatory 24-hour pH monitoring (pH manometry, pH-metry). Twenty-eight patients (12%) either refused to undergo pH-metry or were unable to tolerate it. The entire study population is shown in Table XXI.

Fifteen of the patients in the miscellaneous group had pH-metry performed to rule out the possibility of GERD, even though the medical conditions in this group, as shown in Table XXII, are not usually associated with GERD. Furthermore, none of the patients had findings typically associated with "reflux laryngitis." Thirteen of the 15 patients had normal pH studies; one patient with polypoid degeneration of the vocal cords and one with spastic dysphonia had abnormal studies. The data are included to show the nonrelationship of the underlying conditions to GERD (the raw data for the group can be found in Appendix B.) The miscellaneous group was not, therefore, included in the data analysis of the pH monitoring results, nor will this group be discussed further.

Of the 182 remaining patients who underwent diagnostic pH-metry, 148 (81%) underwent diagnostic pH-metry before any form of antireflux therapy had been instituted.

TABLE XXIII.
Study Population by Diagnostic Subgroup and Timing of pH Study (ART *vs.* No ART) (excluding the miscellaneous group).

Subgroup	ART*	No ART†	Total
Carcinoma	6	25	31
Stenosis	7	25	32
Laryngitis	12	36	48
Globus	2	22	24
Dysphagia	2	20	22
Cough	5	20	25
Total	34	148	182

ART = antireflux therapy.

*Started on antireflux therapy before pH manometry. (Nineteen percent (34/182) of the subjects had been on antireflux therapy for between 3 weeks and 3 months at the time pH manometry was performed.)

†*No* antireflux treatment was started before pH manometry. (Eighty-one percent (148/182) of the subjects underwent "clean" diagnostic tests; no form of antireflux treatment had been instituted before diagnostic pH manometry.)

TABLE XXIV.
Age Distribution of the Study Population (Years).

Subgroup	N	Mean Age	SD
Carcinoma	31	58.9	11.2
Stenosis	32	30.6	23.2
Laryngitis	48	49.1	13.2
Globus	24	49.0	15.0
Dysphagia	22	47.0	18.5
Cough	25	49.5	17.8
Miscellaneous	15	54.9	12.6
Total	197	47.9	18.4

Thirty-four patients (19%) had been on antireflux therapy for between 3 weeks and 3 months at the time pH-metry was performed. For patients on antireflux treatment, the antireflux medications were discontinued for a 24-hour period before and during the pH monitoring period.

Patients were started on antireflux therapy before diagnostic pH-metry because of one or more of the following reasons: *1.* scheduling or equipment difficulties in the gastroenterology laboratory; *2.* urgency in initiating treatment due to the severity of GERD and/or its accompanying complication(s); *3.* initial patient refusal to undergo pH-metry (but subsequent consent); and *4.* patient initially too sick to undergo testing, or patient intubated. The study population (excluding the miscellaneous group) is shown in Table XXIII.

Although all of the study subjects underwent intraesophageal pH monitoring, 147 of the subjects (81%) underwent double-probe pH-metry with a second probe being placed in the hypopharynx 2 cm above the cricopharyngeus at the laryngeal inlet (Fig. 4). The double-probe technique was introduced in adults in March 1986 and became routine in January 1987. Double-probe studies were not performed in children before July 1988.

Of the study population, 46% were female and 54% were male. There was no preponderance of either sex in any group except for the carcinoma of the larynx group (23 men; 8 women). The mean age of the study population was 47.9 ± 18.4 years (Table XXIV). The oldest patients were those with

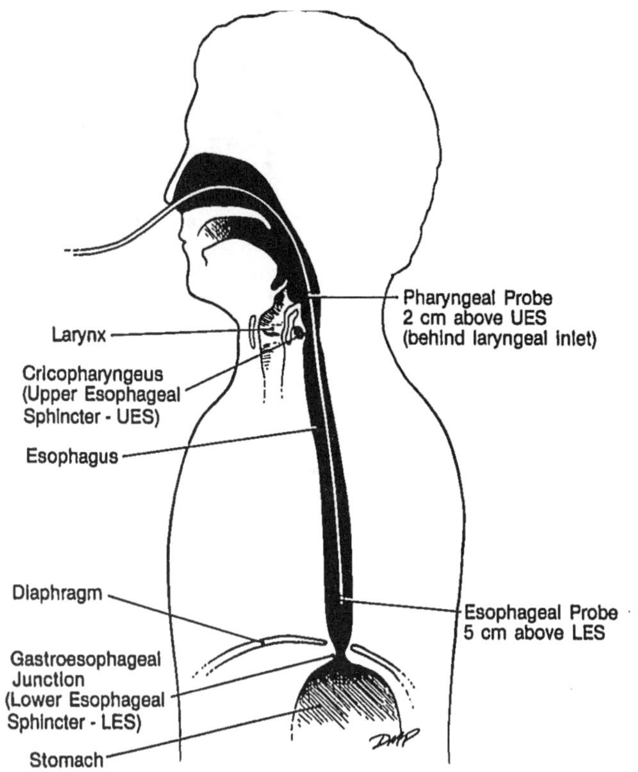

Fig. 4. Technique of double-probe ambulatory intraesophageal and pharyngeal pH monitoring.

carcinoma of the larynx and the youngest were those with laryngeal stenosis.

The laryngeal stenosis group included 11 pediatric patients (under age of 16 years) and 21 adults. Sixty-six percent of the patients had prior intubation, and 34% had not been intubated before the development of stenosis. All of the pediatric patients had subglottic stenosis, as did most of the adult patients; three adult patients had tracheal stenosis only and four had combined stenosis of the trachea and subglottic regions. The breakdown by type of stenosis, age group, and incidence of prior endotracheal intubation in the stenosis group is shown in Table XXV.

TABLE XXV.
Stenosis Group: Breakdown by Type of Stenosis, Age Group, and Incidence of Prior Endotracheal Intubation (Number Intubated in Parentheses).

	Pediatric	Adult	Total
Subglottic stenosis	11(9)	14(8)	25(17)
Tracheal stenosis		3(2)	3(2)
Combined stenosis		4(2)	4(2)
Total	11(9)	21(12)	32(21)*

*Thirty-four percent of the group (9 adults and 2 children) had not been intubated before the development of stenosis.

History

At the time of initial interview for the patients meeting the entrance criteria of the study, the first half of a data flow sheet was completed (Appendix A). This included information relevant to the chief complaint, present illness, medical history, review of systems, physical examination, and provisional diagnosis. Also recorded were the patient's age, sex, race, tobacco and alcohol history, and peptic ulcer and dietary history.

Gastrointestinal symptoms were elicited in terms of frequency of heartburn or regurgitation. Heartburn and/or regurgitation one to four times per week were considered "mild" gastrointestinal (GI) symptoms; those symptoms daily were considered "moderate"; and those symptoms "most of the time" were considered "severe." The presence of hoarseness (chronic or intermittent), globus (a sensation of a lump in the throat), dysphagia (difficulty swallowing), throat clearing, and cough was also noted. Each patient was also asked about the use of medicines, including antacids and any other drugs affecting the gastrointestinal tract.

The height, weight, and laryngeal findings were also recorded. When the data became available, the barium esophagographic, manometric, and pH-metry results, as well as the treatment prescribed and the outcome of treatment, were recorded on the data flow sheet.

Manometric and pH Studies

After an overnight fast, each patient underwent esophageal manometry in the gastroenterology laboratory with a low compliance pneumohydraulic perfusion system.[391] LES position and pressure were established using slow pull-through technique. When patients underwent single-probe pH monitoring, the probe was placed 5 cm above the LES. The probe tip was passed transnasally and located manometrically. The presence of gastric acid was documented by advancing the probe until pH readings were less than 2.5; the probe was then withdrawn to the monitoring position.

For double-probe (pharyngeal) pH monitoring early in the study, a second pH probe was piggybacked onto the esophageal probe and connected using small dental rubber bands. The lower probe was again placed 5 cm above the LES, and the pharyngeal probe was placed in the hypopharynx 2 cm above the cricopharyngeus (Fig. 4). The Sandhill RMS, the Oxford Medilog 100, and the Delmar 705 probes, as well as the Sandhill P-32 Konigsberg antimony pH probe and the Microelectrode MI-506 pH probe, were used for tests done earlier than 1988.

By January 1988, two separate contiguous probes were no longer being used, but had been replaced by a Synectics monocrystant special pH catheter, which had two sensing devices. These are available with the dual probes 18, 20, 22, 24, and 26 cm apart. The upper probe was therefore placed 2 cm above the UES and the lower probe was located in the distal esophagus, 4 to 5 cm above the LES.

Patients were instructed to abstain from all nonessential drugs and drugs known to modify the LES pressure or gastric secretion for at least 24 hours before and during the test. Specifically, antacids and H_2 antagonists were stopped. Patients were asked to follow a diet consisting principally of foods with a pH greater than 5; carbonated beverages, milk, coffee, and tea were restricted to meal times. Using an event marker, the patient recorded on the monitoring apparatus the meal times, bed and rising times, and any reflux, laryngeal, or respiratory symptoms that occurred.

A drop in pH to less than 4.0 was considered evidence of GER.[8] The pH variables studied were the percentage of time when the esophageal pH was less than 4.0 in the supine position, in the upright position, and over the total time. All tracings were inspected by a gastroenterologist to confirm the computerized calculations and to ensure the quality of recordings.

The pH study was considered abnormal if the pH variables exceeded two standard deviations from the mean derived from 32 asymptomatic normal subjects studied in our laboratory. These values were 5.85% upright, 1.81% supine, and 4.39% total. These normal values are comparable to those derived in other laboratories (Table XIII). Twelve normal volunteers also underwent pharyngeal probing (double-probe pH manometry).

In patients undergoing pharyngeal probe monitoring, even a single pH drop below 4 recorded by the pharyngeal probe was considered to be positive evidence for pharyngeal reflux if it was preceded by an esophageal pH drop of similar magnitude.

Barium Esophagography with Videofluoroscopy

Seventy percent of the patients (128 of 182) also underwent barium esophagography with videofluoroscopy as part of their evaluation. Thirty percent of the patients did not have barium studies because barium esophagography was not routinely performed during the first year of the study and because of scheduling difficulties for some of the out-of-town patients. (Barium examinations cannot be carried out with pH probes in place.)

The barium examination was done with patients sitting, then lying prone. Neither a bolster nor any other provocative test such as abdominal pressure was used. Evaluations were made for free reflux and for esophagitis, which was defined by thickened, longitudinal folds (mild), ulcerated mucosa (moderate), or eroded esophageal mucosa (severe).

Treatment

All 182 patients had abnormal pH-metry, barium studies, and/or clinical GERD evidenced by gastrointestinal symptoms or laryngeal findings; thus, all received treatment for GERD. Each patient was given an information sheet that provided background information about GER-related disorders and also explained the antireflux regimen: *a.* no eating or drinking within 3 hours of recumbency; *b.* small, frequent feedings; *c.* avoidance of refluxogenic foods and beverages, especially carbonated beverages, alcohol, chocolate, mints, and fatty or fried foods; *d.* 1 tablespoon of a liquid antacid 1 hour after meals and 2 tablespoons before bed; *e.* elevation of the head of the bed 6 inches; *f.* prohibition of tight-fitting clothing; and *g.* an H_2 blocker, ranitidine acid, 150 mg given twice daily. Patients were instructed to take the first ranitidine at breakfast time and the second at dinner time. Patients were not treated with prokinetic agents such as bethanechol or metoclopramide.

After initiation of therapy, patients were seen for initial follow-up evaluation in 6 to 8 weeks. If the presenting symptoms and findings had not improved, the dose of ranitidine was increased to 300 mg b.i.d. and the patient was seen again 6 to 8 weeks later. If symptoms and findings still had not improved, the dose of ranitidine was increased to 300 mg t.i.d., or famotidine (40 mg b.i.d.) was prescribed instead.

The success of antireflux therapy (improvement or no improvement) was individually defined for each patient based upon both subjective and objective criteria. For patients with specific symptoms, such as hoarseness, dysphagia, throat clearing, cough, heartburn, and regurgitation, symptomatic improvement was considered as evidence of a response to treatment. For patients with inflammatory changes of the larynx, such as posterior laryngitis or granulation tissue, resolution (response to treatment) was judged by normal findings on physical examination. For patients in the carcinoma and stenosis groups, objective criteria for improvement were *a.* resolution of any laryngeal edema, erythema, and granulation, or *b.* resolution of any associated symptoms. A successful (uncomplicated) treatment outcome of the principal diagnosis was also considered as evidence of antireflux treatment success.

Antireflux therapy was continued for at least 6 months. Patients who failed to improve on the antireflux regimen at 6 months of treatment underwent repeat pH-metry while continuing on the antireflux regimen. If the repeat pH-metry was abnormal, these patients were referred for Nissen fundoplication. All of the Nissen fundoplications in the series were carried out by two experienced surgeons.

Any patient whose symptoms and/or laryngeal lesions had resolved at 6 months was taken off the H_2 antagonist and antacid regimen, as well as all other therapeutic measures. The patient was then seen again in 4 to 6 weeks for reevaluation. If symptoms and/or laryngeal findings had reappeared, the patient was either started again on antireflux therapy or referred for fundoplication.

Follow-up

Follow-up was available on 123 (68%) of the 182 patients treated for GERD. Fifty-nine patients were lost to follow-up. These patients were primarily among those who were referred to the author for diagnostic evaluation and initiation of therapy, but who received continuing treatment and follow-up by the referring physician. The mean duration of follow-up was 11.6 ± 12.7 months. Patients who were followed by the author were interviewed and examined every 4 to 16 weeks during the study.

RESULTS

Normative Data

The 32 normal subjects had experienced some GER (% of time upright, 1.71 ± 2.07; supine, 0.35 ± 0.73; and total, 1.27 ± 1.56). The upper limits of normal as determined by the mean value plus the standard deviation were: 5.85% upright, 1.81% supine, and 4.39% total. These values are similar to those that had been reported previously for normal subjects in other series (Table XIII). (Indeed, the mean "upper limit of normal" values for the nine studies reported—5.68% upright, 1.91% supine, 4.19% total—were almost identical to our values.) Twelve additional normal subjects underwent double-probe pH monitoring; none had any evidence of pharyngeal reflux.

Symptoms

Of the study group, only 43% of the patients had

TABLE XXVI.
Incidence and Severity of Gastrointestinal Symptoms* in the Study Population by Diagnostic Subgroup (n=182).

Subgroup	Gastrointestinal Symptoms None	Mild	Moderate	Severe
Carcinoma	20 (65%)	3 (10%)	6 (19%)	2 (6%)
Stenosis	27 (85%)	2 (6%)	1 (3%)	2 (6%)
Laryngitis	24 (50%)	6 (13%)	13 (27%)	5 (10%)
Globus	11 (46%)	6 (25%)	6 (25%)	1 (4%)
Dysphagia	7 (32%)	9 (41%)	5 (23%)	1 (4%)
Cough	15 (60%)	6 (24%)	2 (8%)	2 (8%)
Total (Mean %)	104 (57%)	32 (18%)	33 (18%)	13 (7%)

*Heartburn and/or regurgitation.

TABLE XXVIII.
Tobacco Consumption Profile of the Study Population by Diagnostic Subgroup (N = 182).

Subgroup	Cigarettes	Other Tobacco*	Ex-Smoker	Never Smoked
Carcinoma	16 (52%)	2 (6%)	7 (23%)	6 (19%)
Stenosis	3 (9%)	0 (0%)	3 (9%)	26 (81%)
Laryngitis	9 (19%)	2 (4%)	5 (10%)	32 (67%)
Globus	5 (21%)	0 (0%)	3 (12%)	16 (67%)
Dysphagia	7 (32%)	0 (0%)	5 (23%)	10 (45%)
Cough	3 (12%)	1 (4%)	1 (4%)	20 (80%)
Total (Mean %)	43 (23%)	5 (3%)	24 (13%)	110 (60%)

*Cigar, pipe, smokeless, snuff.

gastrointestinal (GI) symptoms of heartburn and/or regurgitation; 57% had no GI symptoms. Eighteen percent had mild GI symptoms, 18% had moderate symptoms, and 7% had severe symptoms. Of the study patients with upper aerodigestive tract disorders, when the subgroups are ranked by the percentage of patients with GI symptoms, the dysphagia group had the largest proportion (68%), followed by the globus (54%), laryngitis (50%), cough (40%), carcinoma (35%), and stenosis (15%) groups.

When ranked by severity of symptoms, the reflux laryngitis group had the highest percent of patients with moderate to severe gastrointestinal symptoms (37%) and the stenosis group had the lowest (91%). The incidence of gastrointestional symptoms experienced by the study population and broken down by severity of symptoms and diagnostic subgroup is shown in Table XXVI.

Of other symptoms associated with GERD in the study population, hoarseness was the most common (71%), followed by chronic cough (51%), globus (47%), chronic throat clearing (42%), and dysphagia (35%). The highest incidence of hoarseness occurred in the carcinoma and the reflux laryngitis groups (97% and 92%, respectively), and the lowest incidence occurred in the globus group (50%).

The incidence of globus as an associated symptom was high in the dysphagia and chronic cough groups (64% and 60%, respectively); chronic throat clearing was most common in the chronic cough group (56%). The globus group and the stenosis group both had relatively high incidences of chronic cough (54% and 53%, respectively). The frequency of associated symptoms by diagnostic subgroup is shown in Table XXVII.

Tobacco Usage

At the time of inclusion in the study, 43 patients (23%) were smoking cigarettes, and another 5 patients (3%) were using some other form of tobacco. Another 24 patients (13%) were ex-smokers and 110 patients (60%) were nontobacco users who had never been tobacco users.

In the carcinoma of the larynx group, 16 (52%) of 31 patients were actively smoking; 2 (6%) of 31 were using some other form of tobacco; 7 (23%) of 31 were ex-smokers; and 6 (19%) of 31 were lifetime nonsmokers. Of the ex-smokers, the mean duration since quitting smoking was 7.3 years, with a median of 5 years and a range of 1 to 23 years. Excluding the carcinoma of the larynx group, only 20% of the study population was using tobacco at the time of study. The tobacco consumption profile of the study population is shown in Table XXVIII.

Laryngeal Findings

Sixty percent (105 of 175) of the study population

TABLE XXVII.
Frequency of Symptoms by Diagnostic Subgroup (N = 182).

Subgroup	Symptom GI*	Hoarseness	Globus	Dysphagia	Throat Clearing	Cough
Carcinoma	11 (35%)	30 (97%)	9 (29%)	6 (19%)	12 (39%)	12 (39%)
Stenosis	5 (16%)	16 (50%)	8 (25%)	4 (12%)	6 (19%)	17 (53%)
Laryngitis	24 (50%)	44 (92%)	16 (33%)	13 (27%)	24 (50%)	21 (44%)
Globus	13 (54%)	12 (50%)	24 (100%)	10 (42%)	12 (50%)	13 (54%)
Dysphagia	15 (68%)	13 (59%)	14 (64%)	19 (86%)	9 (41%)	4 (18%)
Cough	10 (40%)	15 (60%)	15 (60%)	11 (44%)	14 (56%)	25 (100%)
Total (Mean %)	78 (43%)	130 (71%)	86 (47%)	63 (35%)	77 (42%)	92 (51%)

*Heartburn and/or regurgitation.

TABLE XXIX.
Laryngeal Findings by Diagnostic Subgroup (N = 175*).

Subgroup	(N)	Abnormal Examination (Total)	Edema			Erythema		Ulceration	Granuloma/ Granulation
			Mild	Moderate	Severe	Diffuse	Posterior		
Carcinoma	31	31 (100%)	2 (6%)	7 (23%)	2 (6%)	8 (26%)	1 (3%)	1 (3%)	8 (26%)
Stenosis	30	30 (100%)	0 (0%)	4 (13%)	3 (10%)	3 (10%)	3 (10%)	0 (0%)	20 (67%)
Laryngitis	46	46 (100%)	11 (24%)	28 (61%)	2 (4%)	6 (13%)	34 (74%)	1 (2%)	9 (19%)
Globus	22	17 (77%)	6 (29%)	8 (36%)	1 (5%)	3 (14%)	14 (64%)	0 (0%)	1 (5%)
Dysphagia	21	18 (86%)	5 (24%)	10 (48%)	1 (5%)	4 (19%)	14 (67%)	2 (10%)	0 (0%)
Cough	25	22 (88%)	5 (20%)	10 (40%)	0 (0%)	4 (16%)	15 (60%)	0 (0%)	0 (0%)
Total (Mean %)	175	164 (94%)	29 (17%)	67 (38%)	9 (5%)	28 (16%)	81 (46%)	4 (2%)	38 (22%)

*Data missing for seven subjects.

had laryngeal edema, and 60% had laryngeal erythema. (For the laryngeal findings, n = 175 instead of 182 because of missing data on seven patients.) Forty-six percent (81 of 175) had posterior laryngitis; 2% (4 of 175) had ulceration; and 22% (38 of 175) had granulation. The highest incidence of posterior laryngitis was seen in the reflux laryngitis group (74%), and the lowest incidence was seen in the carcinoma of the larynx group (3%).

Granulation tissue was present in 26% of the carcinoma of the larynx group, 19% of the reflux laryngitis group, and 5% of globus patients; these were almost all vocal process granulomas. Sixty-seven percent (20/30) of the stenosis group had active granulation tissue. In distinction to the above groups, these patients with stenosis did not have solitary vocal process (pyogenic) granulomas, but rather, exuberant subglottic and/or tracheal granulation tissue.

Only 11 patients in the study population (6%) had normal laryngeal examinations, and these patients were in the globus, the dysphagia, and the chronic cough groups. The laryngeal findings by subgroup are displayed in Table XXIX.

Ambulatory 24-Hour pH Monitoring

On the basis of the normative values established in our laboratory (upper limit upright (5.85%), supine (1.81%), and total (4.39%)), a total of 113 (62%) of 182 patients had abnormal studies. The abnormalities on esophageal monitoring were equally divided between patients with upright reflux and patients with supine reflux (40%). When abnormal pH-metry results were tallied for each diagnostic subgroup, the highest total pH manometry rate of abnormality was seen in the stenosis group (78%), followed by the group categories of carcinoma (71%), reflux laryngitis (60%), globus (58%), dysphagia (45%), and chronic cough (52%). The breakdown of the abnormal esophageal and pharyngeal studies is shown in Table XXX-A.

Of patients with abnormal esophageal studies, 25% (28/113) were upright refluxers alone, 27% (30/113) were supine refluxers alone, 38% (43/113) were combined (upright and supine) refluxers. Eleven percent (12/113) had normal esophageal pH manometry but were found to have abnormal pharyngeal reflux alone (In those cases, pharyngeal reflux was recorded; however, the total time of esophageal reflux in both upright and supine positions was within normal limits) (Table XXX-B).

Looking just at patients with abnormal pH studies by diagnostic subgroup (Table XXX-C), it can be seen that the highest incidences of upright reflux with the esophageal probe were seen in the globus, carcinoma, and stenosis groups (78%, 77%, and 72%, respectively), and the lowest percentage of upright

TABLE XXX-A.
Results of Diagnostic Ambulatory 24-Hour pH Manometry by Subgroup (N = 182).

Subgroup	Esophageal Probe		Pharyngeal Probe		Total Abnormal*	
	Abnormal Upright	Abnormal Supine	(N)	Abnormal	(N)	Abnormal
Carcinoma	17 (53%)	12 (39%)	26	15 (58%)	31	22 (71%)
Stenosis	18 (56%)	15 (47%)	18	10 (56%)	32	25 (78%)
Laryngitis	14 (29%)	21 (44%)	42	7 (17%)	48	29 (60%)
Globus	11 (46%)	12 (50%)	18	5 (28%)	24	14 (58%)
Dysphagia	6 (27%)	7 (32%)	20	2 (10%)	22	10 (45%)
Cough	7 (28%)	6 (24%)	23	5 (22%)	25	13 (52%)
Total (Mean %)	73 (40%)	73 (40%)	147	44 (30%)	182	113 (62%)

*Esophageal and/or pharyngeal probe.

TABLE XXX-B.
Breakdown of Abnormal pH Studies (N = 113): Only Upright Abnormal, Only Supine Abnormal, Both Upright and Supine Abnormal, Only Pharyngeal Abnormal.

Subgroup	Only Upright Abnormal	Only Supine Abnormal	Both Upright and Supine Abnormal	Only Pharyngeal Abnormal	Total Abnormal
Carcinoma	7 (32%)	2 (9%)	10 (45%)	3 (14%)	22 (100%)
Stenosis	7 (28%)	4 (16%)	11 (44%)	3 (12%)	25 (100%)
Laryngitis	6 (21%)	15 (51%)	6 (21%)	2 (7%)	29 (100%)
Globus	1 (7%)	2 (14%)	10 (72%)	1 (7%)	14 (100%)
Dysphagia	3 (30%)	4 (40%)	3 (30%)	0 (0%)	10 (100%)
Cough	4 (31%)	3 (23%)	3 (23%)	3 (23%)	13 (100%)
Total (Mean %)	28 (25%)	30 (27%)	43 (38%)	12 (11%)	113 (100%)

reflux was seen in the reflux laryngitis group (48%) (Table XXX-C). The highest percentages of supine reflux were seen in the globus, reflux laryngitis, and dysphagia groups (86%, 72% and 70%, respectively) and the lowest were seen in the carcinoma and cough groups (55% and 46%, respectively). The highest percentages of pharyngeal reflux were seen in the carcinoma and stenosis groups (88% and 67%, respectively), and the lowest percentages were seen in the reflux laryngitis and dysphagia groups (27% and 25%, respectively) (Table XXX-C).

When the study population was evaluated by comparing patients who were already on antireflux therapy at the time of study with those who underwent pH-metry without having received any treatment, the pH manometry results appeared dramatically different (Table XXX-D). In patients who had not been on any treatment, the overall rate of abnormality was 68%, whereas in those who had been on antireflux treatment before pH evaluation, it was only 35%. This was true for almost every diagnostic subgroup. The highest rate of abnormality in patients on no antireflux therapy (no ART) was seen in the stenosis group (92%), followed by the group categories of carcinoma (84%), laryngitis (67%), globus (64%), cough (55%), and dysphagia (40%). Similar findings were noted for double-probe monitoring. The pharyngeal probe positivity in patients who had not been treated was observed to be twice as frequent as that in treated patients (33% and 17%, respectively).

When the pH manometry results of smokers and nonsmokers with abnormal pH studies were compared, there was no significant difference.

Barium Esophagography

Seventy percent (128/182) of the study patients underwent barium esophagography with videofluoroscopy. Thirty patients (23%) had completely normal studies. Abnormalities noted were hiatal hernia (69%), esophagitis (18%), dysmotility (12%), lower esophageal ring (14%), spontaneous GER (9%), and stricture (3%). The results of the barium studies by finding and diagnostic subgroup are displayed in Table XXXI.

Results of Treatment

All patients were placed on antireflux therapy for 6 months and reevaluated at the end of that period. Follow-up was available on 68% (123/182). There were four deaths in the series, all in the carcinoma of the larynx group (two related to carcinoma, two unrelated).

After six months of antireflux treatment, 85% (104/123) of the patients had resolution of their symptoms; the remaining 15% (19/123) had recalcitrant symptoms. Over the five years of the study, nearly half (51/104) of the patients who initially responded to antireflux therapy experienced relapses. Once a relapse occurred, the chance of subsequent medical treatment failure was more likely than that of primary (initial) treatment failure. Table XXXII summarizes the response to initial medical antireflux treatment and the medical treatment failure rates in patients experiencing relapses.

Medical treatment failure was documented by repeat pH-metry with the patient still on the therapeutic regimen. Patients who failed medical treatment were referred to a surgeon for Nissen fundoplication. Thus, a total of 35% of the patients failed medical treatment, 15% during the first six months of treatment and another 20% subsequently. Notably, the stenosis group had a 55% medical treatment failure rate. The total medical treatment failure rates and fundoplication rates by subgroup are shown in Table XXXIII.

TABLE XXX-C.
Breakdown of Abnormal pH Studies by Total Percentage of Upright, Supine and/or Pharyngeal Abnormal Results.

Subgroup	Abnormal Results: Upright	Supine	Pharyngeal
Carcinoma	17/22 (77%)	12/22 (55%)	15/17 (88%)
Stenosis	18/25 (72%)	15/25 (60%)	10/15 (67%)
Laryngitis	14/29 (48%)	21/29 (72%)	7/26 (27%)
Globus	11/14 (78%)	12/14 (86%)	5/11 (45%)
Dysphagia	6/10 (60%)	7/10 (70%)	2/8 (25%)
Cough	7/13 (54%)	6/13 (46%)	5/11 (45%)
Mean Percent	73/113 (65%)	73/113 (65%)	44/88* (50%)

*Of patients with abnormal pH manometry, 88 (78%) of 113 had double-probe studies performed.

TABLE XXX-D.
Results of Ambulatory 24-Hour pH Manometry (N = 182): Comparison of No ART and ART Groups.

	Esophageal Probe		Pharyngeal Probe		Total Esophageal and/or Pharyngeal Probe	
	Abnormal Upright	Abnormal Supine	(N)	Abnormal	(N)	Abnormal
NO ART*						
Carcinoma	16 (64%)	12 (48%)	20	14 (70%)	25	21 (84%)
Stenosis	16 (64%)	14 (56%)	14	10 (71%)	25	23 (92%)
Laryngitis	13 (36%)	18 (50%)	31	6 (19%)	36	24 (67%)
Globus	11 (50%)	12 (55%)	16	5 (24%)	22	14 (64%)
Dysphagia	4 (20%)	5 (25%)	18	1 (6%)	20	8 (40%)
Cough	7 (35%)	5 (25%)	18	3 (17%)	20	11 (55%)
Total (Mean %)	67 (45%)	66 (45%)	117	39 (33%)	148	101 (68%)
ART†						
Carcinoma	1 (17%)	0 (0%)	6	1 (17%)	6	1 (17%)
Stenosis	2 (29%)	1 (14%)	4	0 (0%)	7	2 (29%)
Laryngitis	1 (8%)	3 (25%)	11	1 (9%)	12	5 (42%)
Globus	0 (0%)	0 (0%)	2	0 (0%)	2	0 (0%)
Dysphagia	2 (100%)	2 (100%)	2	1 (50%)	2	2 (100%)
Cough	0 (0%)	1 (20%)	5	2 (40%)	5	2 (40%)
Total (Mean %)	6 (18%)	7 (21%)	30	5 (17%)	34	12 (35%)

*No antireflux treatment before pH manometry.
†Antireflux treatment (3 weeks to 3 months) before pH manometry.

DISCUSSION

The clinical data herein presented confirm the relationship (association) between GERD and many upper aerodigestive (otolaryngologic) conditions. Clinicians have previously presumed these conditions to be related to GERD, but that relationship has not previously been documented convincingly. The data reported are among the first using ambulatory 24-hour pH manometry in a large series of otolaryngology patients.

Occult Reflux

Only 43% (78/182) of the entire study population had gastrointestinal symptoms of heartburn or regurgitation. The incidence of gastrointestinal symptoms in patients with abnormal pH manometry studies was 45% (51/113) and the incidence in patients with normal pH studies was 39% (27/69). (This difference is not significant, $P = .07$.) Thus, the majority of patients with abnormal pH studies were documented to have occult (silent) GER, absent heartburn, and regurgitation.

Intermittent Reflux

When the barium esophagography data of patients with abnormal and with normal pH monitoring were compared, both groups appeared similar. The findings were as follows (abnormal pH-metry group *vs.* normal pH-metry group): hiatal hernia (67% *vs.* 73%), stricture (3% *vs.* 4%), free reflux (13% *vs.* 5%), esophagitis (15% *vs.* 22%), dysmotility (11% *vs.* 13%), and lower esophageal ring (18% *vs.* 9%) (Table XXXIV-A). Of note, 27% (15/55) of the patients who had normal pH manometry demonstrated free reflux and/or esophagitis on barium esophagography. Thus, a diagnosis of reflux was made on objective radiographic grounds in these 15 patients despite their

TABLE XXXI.
Results of Barium Esophagography by Finding and Diagnostic Subgroup (N = 128).

Subgroup	(N)	Normal	Hiatal Hernia	Esophagitis	Dysmotility	Ring	Free Reflux	Stricture
Carcinoma	21	2 (10%)	18 (86%)	3 (14%)	5 (24%)	3 (14%)	3 (14%)	1 (5%)
Stenosis	15	5 (33%)	9 (60%)	0 (0%)	0 (0%)	0 (0%)	4 (27%)	0 (0%)
Laryngitis	36	10 (28%)	22 (61%)	7 (19%)	4 (11%)	4 (11%)	1 (3%)	1 (3%)
Globus	20	5 (25%)	13 (65%)	6 (30%)	2 (10%)	2 (10%)	2 (10%)	1 (5%)
Dysphagia	21	3 (14%)	17 (81%)	4 (19%)	2 (10%)	8 (38%)	1 (5%)	1 (5%)
Cough	15	5 (33%)	9 (60%)	3 (20%)	2 (13%)	1 (7%)	1 (7%)	0 (0%)
Total (Mean %)	128	30 (23%)	88 (69%)	23 (18%)	15 (12%)	18 (14%)	12 (9%)	4 (3%)

TABLE XXXII.
Response to Medical Antireflux Treatment of the Signs and Symptoms of Gastroesophageal Reflux.

A. On Therapy (at 6 Months)

Subgroup	Resolved	Failed
Carcinoma	26/26 (100%)	0/26 (0%)
Stenosis	13/22 (59%)	9/22 (41%)
Laryngitis	28/33 (85%)	5/33 (15%)
Globus	15/17 (88%)	2/17 (12%)
Dysphagia	7/7 (100%)	0/7 (0%)
Cough	15/18 (83%)	3/18 (17%)
Total	104/123 (85%)	19/123 (15%)

B. Subsequent Medical Treatment Failure Rates of Patients Relapsing (After Initial Medical Treatment Success)*

Subgroup	Failed	Subgroup	Failed
Carcinoma	6/26 (23%)	Dysphagia	2/7 (29%)
Stenosis	3/13 (23%)	Cough	2/15 (13%)
Laryngitis	6/28 (21%)	Total	24/104 (23%)
Globus	5/15 (33%)		

*Forty-nine percent (51/104) of the patients experiencing initially successful medical treatment, experienced relapses of GERD months or years after initial treatment.

TABLE XXXIII.
Response to Medical Antireflux Treatment of the Signs and Symptoms of Gastroesophageal Reflux.

Subgroup	Medical Treatment Failure*	Fundoplication
Carcinoma	6/26 (23%)	5/26 (19%)
Stenosis	12/22 (55%)	9/22 (41%)
Laryngitis	11/33 (33%)	2/33 (6%)
Globus	7/17 (41%)	1/17 (6%)
Dysphagia	2/7 (29%)	0/7 (0%)
Cough	5/18 (28%)	2/18 (11%)
Total	43/123 (35%)	19/123 (15%)

*Initial failure plus relapse failure groups.

negative pH manometry. These patients are likely to have had false-negative pH-metry studies because of intermittent GER.

The symptom profile of the patients with abnormal and normal pH studies, as well as the laryngeal findings, were also similar (Tables XXXIV-B, C). Of the 16 patients who had pyogenic granulomas, 9 had abnormal pH studies and 7 had normal pH studies. From a clinical point of view, both populations were indistinguishable and responded equally to antireflux therapy.

Six patients with initially negative pH manometry studies underwent second studies, which were positive (abnormal). In these cases, patients were instructed to return to have a second study performed when symptoms (*e.g.*, hoarseness, chronic cough, etc.) recurred or worsened. Therefore, in these patients, who represent 3.3% of the study population, intermittent reflux was unequivocally documented.

In addition, 12 patients (6.6%) had normal esophageal studies but positive pharyngeal reflux. In consideration of the fact that these patients would have been designated as "normal" with esophageal monitoring alone, the esophageal pH study may be considered to have been falsely negative.

TABLE XXXIV.
Comparison of the Barium Esophagography, Symptoms, and Laryngeal Findings in Patients with Abnormal and Normal pH Manometry.

Findings	Abnormal pH-Metry	Normal pH-Metry	*P* Value
A. Barium Esophagography	(N = 72)	(N = 55)	
Hiatal hernia	48 (67%)	40 (73%)	0.63
Esophageal stricture	2 (3%)	2 (4%)	0.87
Free reflux	9 (13%)	3 (5%)	0.97
Esophagitis	11 (15%)	12 (22%)	0.76
Dysmotility	8 (11%)	7 (13%)	0.59
Lower esophageal ring	13 (18%)	5 (9%)	0.13
B. Symptoms	(N = 113)	(N = 69)	
Heartburn	51 (45%)	27 (39%)	0.07
Hoarseness	85 (75%)	45 (65%)	0.15
Globus sensation	49 (43%)	36 (52%)	0.25
Dysphagia	40 (35%)	23 (33%)	0.78
Throat clearing	45 (40%)	32 (46%)	0.70
Cough	59 (52%)	31 (45%)	0.34
C. Laryngeal Findings	(N = 108)	(N = 67)	
Mild edema	15 (14%)	11 (21%)	0.23
Moderate edema	40 (37%)	27 (40%)	0.67
Severe edema	8 (7%)	1 (1%)	0.16
Posterior erythema	43 (40%)	38 (57%)	0.03
Pyogenic granuloma	9 (8%)	7 (10%)	0.64

In summary, of the 38% (69/182) of patients who had normal esophageal pH studies, 15 patients had radiographically diagnosed GERD; 7 patients had granulomas (findings strongly suggestive of GER); and an additional 12 patients had pharyngeal positive studies with normal esophageal pH manometry. Thus, almost half (34/69) of the patients with negative (normal) intraesophageal pH studies had evidence of GERD based upon other objective diagnostic criteria. By far, the most likely explanation for this finding is intermittent reflux (*i.e.*, the pH-metry was falsely negative due to intermittency). In addition, the degree of upper aerodigestive dysfunction in this series did not uniformly correlate with the severity of GER as measured by pH manometry. Therefore, the clinical data suggest that the incidence of intermittent reflux in otolaryngology patients with GERD may be between 19% (34/182) and 38% (69/182).

Advantages of Ambulatory 24-Hour pH Monitoring

Compared to other diagnostic tests, pH manometry is highly quantitative for GER.[2,5,189] Furthermore, it is sensitive for the reflux event itself and measures actual acidity (pH) rather than quantitating the effects of reflux (*e.g.*, esophagitis, etc.). pH manometry not only provides overall quantitative data (percentage of time pH less than 4), but also

TABLE XXXV.
Advantages and Disadvantages of Diagnostic Ambulatory 24-Hour Intraesophageal pH Monitoring.

A. Advantages
   1. Ambulatory (outpatient) test
   2. Quantitatively measures GERD
   3. Records pattern of GERD (upright, supine, postcibal)
   4. Can be used to estimate esophageal acid clearance
   5. High degree of sensitivity
   6. High degree of specificity
B. Disadvantages
   1. Definition of normal
   2. False-negative results
      a. Technical failure
      b. Alkaline reflux
      c. Betterment of the subject's life-style during the test
      d. Partial response to treatment
      e. Intermittent reflux
   3. Invasiveness of the test (poor patient acceptance)
   4. Limited availability
   5. Cost

provides information as to the actual reflux pattern (upright, supine, postcibal). This affords the clinician the opportunity to individualize the treatment plan of each patient in accordance with the reflux profile.

The test can be performed on an outpatient ambulatory basis, which simultaneously reduces its costs and enables the clinician to evaluate the subject in his or her own home setting. This increases the likelihood that the test will reflect the life-style habits of test subjects.

Although not used in this study for the purpose of evaluating esophageal acid clearance, pH manometry can provide such information. If the strip recordings are analyzed for the duration of decreased pH, acid clearance can be estimated. Parameters analyzed for this purpose are: *1.* longest episode pH less than 4, supine and upright; *2.* mean duration of pH decrease episodes, supine and upright; *3.* number of episodes that pH decrease lasts for longer than 5 minutes; and *4.* number of episodes per hour that pH decreases last for longer than 5 minutes per hour, supine, upright, and total. Thus, using pH manometry, data can be gathered about the effectiveness of esophageal acid clearance once a reflux event has occurred.

Finally, the test is highly specific (approaching 100%) and its sensitivity, although not 100%, is probably higher than that of any other available diagnostic test. The advantages (and disadvantages) of pH manometry are shown in Table XXXV.

Disadvantages and Limitations of Ambulatory 24-Hour pH Manometry

If one were to assume that all 182 patients in this study had GERD, then the finding of only 62% with positive (abnormal) studies would suggest that the rate of false-negatives in this population was 38%. Since 24-hour pH manometry is considered the gold standard, it is difficult to draw that conclusion—however, it is possible. Five reasons have been postulated to account for false-negative pH manometry.

Technical Failure

Although the incidence of technical (probe) failure has been reported to be as high as 10%,[184] in this study esophageal probe failure occurred in only 1.6%, and those patients had repeat studies. Pharyngeal probe "failure" occurred somewhat more frequently, due to drying out of the pharyngeal probe (mucus drying over the probe tip). The incidence of this failure, however, cannot be reported with certainty.

Alkaline Reflux

One patient in this series had alkaline reflux (Case Report 5, Appendix C). He had previously undergone gastric surgery for ulcer disease. The available data on GERD suggest that alkaline reflux is extremely uncommon except in such patients;[388] nevertheless, alkaline reflux is not diagnosed by 24-hour pH manometry. When alkaline reflux is considered in the differential diagnosis, endoscopy with aspiration and analysis of the refluxate may be indicated.

Betterment of the Subject's Life-style During the Study Period

Following 24-hour pH manometry, occasionally a patient would state that he or she "ate virtually nothing during the study period." This is, in part, due to the variable difficulty in tolerating the pH probes. The diagnostic validity of a test done during fasting may be in question. Furthermore, dietary modifications, which may remove refluxogenic behaviors, are routinely imposed during the study period. Specifically, consumption of carbonated beverages and orange juice is limited, because of the low pH of these beverages (Coca-Cola™, and Pepsi-Cola™, pH approximately 2.3; Seven-Up™, pH approximately 3.2; orange juice, pH approximately 3.7[6]). Coffee and tea are also limited to meal times.

As a consequence, in some patients, the life-style modifications imposed by the test situation may give test results that do not reflect the usual condition. In the future, it may be appropriate to consider doing pH manometry without any such restrictions; however, for the data so derived to be meaningful, the patient will need to be able to indicate, using an event marker, the times food was consumed and to identify the food or other substance(s) being consumed.

Early Response to Treatment

Thirty-four patients in this series had been on antireflux therapy for 3 weeks to 3 months before pH manometry was carried out. The rates of abnormality both with esophageal and pharyngeal probes were approximately half those of patients who underwent diagnostic pH-metry before any antireflux treatment. The patients receiving antireflux therapy were taken off that regimen for 24 hours before and during the test period. However, it seems possible that the considerably lower rates of positivity may reflect an early response to treatment in patients with the ability to reconstitute antireflux mechanisms.

The significance of this observation remains uncertain; however, one could postulate that approximately half of otolaryngology patients with GERD may have a response to treatment early on. The only method that could be used to answer the question of response to treatment (reversibility of disease with antireflux therapy) would be longitudinal (continuous, interval, or repeated) pH manometry in a population of patients before, during, and after therapy. When, in other studies, esophagitis patients have been evaluated with pH manometry before and after treatment, the available data suggest that recurrence of reflux is prompt in the majority following cessation of therapy.[88,92,193] Whether or not discontinuance of medicine for 1 day constitutes a cessation of therapy is debatable.

Intermittent Reflux

The possibility of intermittent reflux as a frequent pattern in otolaryngology patients with GERD remains a troubling possibility. Even the best diagnostic tests are limited unless the test period coincides with a period of reflux.

The development of longitudinal pH studies, even extended telemetric pH monitoring (over a period of days, weeks, or months), may be possible with future technology. Such studies, and only such studies, may clearly elucidate the day-to-day patterns and natural history of GERD.

Invasiveness of pH Manometry and Patient Acceptance

In this series, 12% of the patients either refused to undergo or could not tolerate pH manometry. This rate of refusal/intolerance is similar to that reported in other series.[184,189,392]

Of considerable influence on pH monitoring itself is the use of prior conventional manometry to locate the esophageal sphincters. Furthermore, the technique of insertion of these instruments probably could be improved to increase patient acceptance. This might include anesthetizing the nose before manipulation and the use of smaller, softer, even fiberoptic guided instrumentation.

With the exception of Gaynor,[247] who placed probes in the pharynges of intubated ICU patients overnight, the use of a single pharyngeal or upper esophageal probe as a screening test for GERD in otolaryngology patients has not been reported. Presumably, such a probe could be placed in the clinic under direct vision with minimal patient discomfort. Although manometric data would not be available with such a technique, patient acceptance would probably be much higher than is currently the case. Thus, as a screening test, it could provide more information than those tests now employed (*e.g.*, barium swallow), but less information than is gained from standard manometry and pH manometry.

Cost and Limited Availability

At this time, 24-hour pH manometry requires expensive manometric sphincter location and pH monitoring instrumentation. Unfortunately, the cost for such equipment is several thousand dollars. In addition, the pH probes in current use have a limited lifespan. In our institution, probes costing approximately $250 are used approximately 10 times before being discarded. The cost of these probes per use, therefore, is approximately $25. pH manometry has been used principally in academic centers with gastroenterology research facilities. As a consequence, the technology is not yet widely available.

The Significance of Pharyngeal Positivity in Double-Probe Monitoring

It is presumed by investigators using double-probe pH monitoring that laryngopharyngeal reflux does not occur in normal subjects except very rarely and under extraordinary circumstances.[184,392,393] In this clinical study of patients who had abnormal esophageal pH studies with a double-probe in place, 50% had documented pharyngeal reflux (Table XXX-C). The incidence of pharyngeal probe positivity was very high in the carcinoma of the larynx and stenosis groups. Furthermore, 11% of the patients with abnormal pharyngeal pH had normal esophageal pH-metry. Although at first glance this appears to be a relatively small proportion of the patients, the significance of this finding cannot be overemphasized. Were it not for the pharyngeal probe, these patients would have been assumed to be normal. Thus, the pharyngeal probe is an important part of pH-metry with which to identify and document pharyngeal reflux in patients with aerodigestive tract disorders.

Until such time as further data become available from double-probe monitoring in large populations of patients, it must be assumed that a single episode of documented pharyngeal reflux has clinical significance in patients with upper aerodigestive tract disorders such as those herein reported. It also appears that the pharyngeal component of the pH-metry may be particularly important in identifying the intermittent refluxer, since a single positive event may outweigh other negative findings.

Clinical Implications (by Diagnostic Subgroup)

Group I: Carcinoma of the Larynx

The high degree of association between GER and

carcinoma of the larynx suggests the possibility that GERD may be a major cofactor in the development of such neoplasia. Overall, 71% of the patients with carcinoma of the larynx had abnormal studies and 58% had documented pharyngeal reflux. Three other patients had reflux and/or esophagitis on barium esophagography, although the pH manometry was normal. Thus, if these cases are included, 81% of the patients with carcinoma had documented reflux; if only patients who had not been on antireflux therapy (No ART group: Table XXX-D) are considered, reflux was documented in 22 (88%) of 25 patients. In addition, of the six lifetime nonsmokers in this group, all had documented reflux. (These case histories are summarized in Appendix C.)

The major risk factors for the development of carcinoma of the larynx are believed to be tobacco and ethanol, agents that appear to act synergistically. These same agents also seem to act synergistically to enhance GER by abnormally influencing most of the antireflux defenses. Tobacco and alcohol are therefore simultaneously major risk factors for carcinoma and for GERD. Although it remains conjectural at this point, one could postulate that smoking is associated with GER and that GER (namely, of pepsin) "digests" the protective covering of the laryngeal mucosa, rendering it more susceptible to carcinogenic influences. These "influences" may be contained within tobacco smoke itself, may be viral, or may even possibly be related to the refluxate, as in carcinoma of the esophagus in Barrett's epithelium.[145,204]

Group II: Laryngeal and Tracheal Stenosis

The highest rate of abnormal pH manometry was found in the stenosis group (78%). If the patients on antireflux treatment at the time of pH-metry are excluded, reflux was found in 23 (92%) of 25, with a 71% incidence of positive pharyngeal reflux. These findings have profound implications for the diagnosis and treatment of patients with airway stenosis.

Two thirds of the stenosis patients presented with obstructing inflammatory (granulation) tissue. The other one third had either massive soft-tissue edema producing a "malacia-like" stenosis or firm mature scar with relatively normal overlying epithelium. These findings are relevant to an understanding of the pathophysiology of acquired upper aerodigestive tract stenosis, including supraglottic stenosis, laryngeal web, and subglottic and tracheal stenosis. Such stenoses are most commonly due to the combination of endotracheal intubation and GERD.

The pathophysiology of subglottic stenosis. The pathophysiology of subglottic stenosis is multifactorial. Excluding blunt trauma (cricoid cartilage disruption), two other mechanisms have been proposed: subglottic injury plus infection,[309] and subglottic injury plus GER.[247]

Because subglottic stenosis seems to have three different clinical presentations: *1.* massive, soft, obstructing edema, *2.* exuberant granulation, and *3.* firm, mature scar, it is likely that these three types of stenosis may represent different mechanisms or stages of stenosis formation.

Clearly, intubation followed by tracheotomy, with the introduction of pathogenic bacteria in large numbers to denuded areas within the larynx, can result in stenosis, as reported by Sasaki, *et al.*[309] In intubated patients who do not undergo subsequent tracheotomy, infection is still a possible etiologic factor; however, based upon the data of this study, GER seems a more likely cause.

If a prior mucosal injury has occurred, GER will result in further damage to the underlying perichondrium and cartilage. The endotracheal tube itself produces laryngeal injury, and the cuff in the trachea below also creates a basin-like effect in the larynx, so that refluxed material may be held within the damaged area for an extended period of time.

Following injury, the initial reparative process takes the form of exuberant granulation tissue. With time, if the GER improves (decreases), this granulation tissue may undergo maturation to fibrous tissue, and subsequent reepithelialization may occur. (Thus, in patients with firm, stenotic scar tissue, GER may have gone into remission spontaneously, allowing maturation of the lesion.)

Goode and Shinn[394] and Schuller[395] have advocated long-term stenting in subglottic stenosis, presumably to allow epithelialization and cicatrix formation to occur around the stent, leaving an adequate subglottic lumen at the time of stent removal. The beneficial effects of long-term stenting may be related to allowing GER and its accompanying inflammatory response to subside. (This process of resolution apparently may occur spontaneously, since many patients with GERD seem to have chronic intermittent disease associated with remission even without antireflux treatment.[87,89]) Gray, *et al.*[246] have noted that stent placement in laryngotracheal reconstruction in the presence of GER may lead to unremitting exuberant granulation.

When a patient undergoes surgical treatment for subglottic stenosis and granulation tissue persists, the clinician should consider GERD as the etiologic factor in perpetuating the inflammatory process. (Within our series are patients with total obstruction of the larynx by granulation treated with antireflux therapy alone, whose stenosis resolved without surgical treatment.)

Not all patients with stenosis have exuberant granulation tissue. Some patients have extended segments of severe, obstructing soft-tissue edema. This may involve the larynx and/or the trachea. When such edema occurs in the trachea, the "collapse" may mimic tracheomalacia. Such diffuse and persistent collapse due to mucosal and submucosal edema may be due to chronic GER. The lack of granulation and scar tissue may be explained by the fact that the overlying mucosa has remained intact. In such cases, however, surgical intervention, such as endoscopic excision with the carbon dioxide laser or open surgical repair (both of which denude mucosal surface), is likely to result in subsequent granulation tissue formation with worsening of the condition.

Acquired laryngeal webs occur as a result of fusion of the two vocal cords along a portion of their length from the anterior commissure posteriorly. This complication is supposed to occur as a result of injudicious laryngeal surgery when mucosal surfaces on both vocal cords are denuded to the anterior commissure. Clinicians occasionally encounter web formation in a patient in whom great care has been exercised to preserve some of the lining membrane of the anterior larynx (Appendix C, Case 3). It seems likely in these cases that GERD may also have played a role.

In consideration of the clinical data, it is recommended that all patients with glottic, subglottic, and tracheal stenosis be evaluated by 24-hour pH manometry and barium swallow esophagography. When patients are in the proliferation stage of granulation or have widespread and severe mucosal edema, surgical treatment is contraindicated until such time as GER is under control; such control may take months of treatment. Furthermore, it must be emphasized that medical treatment may or may not be adequate since, in this series, the incidence of medical treatment failure in the stenosis group was 55%. Fortunately, fundoplication is effective in abolishing GER; hydrogen ion blockers may also play an important therapeutic role in adult patients.

Tracheotomy should be avoided whenever possible, because it puts the larynx to rest and invariably introduces local wound sepsis. When a tracheotomy is present, however, meticulous tracheotomy care must include the use of topical antibiotic solutions and ointments, frequently applied to the "peristomal" site. If the clinician notes exuberant granulation and inflammation at the skin level (on the outside), he or she can be certain that a comparable inflammatory response is taking place within the larynx and trachea. Therefore, in such cases when granulation is present at the tracheotomy site, cultures, local wound treatment and systemic antibiotic treatment are indicated before surgical correction is initiated. These measures and aggressive antireflux therapy will lead to a much higher success rate in the management of upper airway stenosis. Indeed, in the series reported herein, 25 (81%) of 31 patients have good airways and only 6 (19%) of 31 still have a tracheotomy. Of the six patients who still have tracheotomies in place, all have the potential for decannulation when either reflux is brought under control or surgical procedures are performed to reestablish an adequate airway. (Many of the stenosis cases in this series represented absolutely recalcitrant cases that defied treatment until GERD was controlled.)

The model presented has potential implications for all aerodigestive tract surgery. Randomized studies using hydrogen ion blockers should be used to evaluate the benefit of routine prophylactic antireflux therapy in patients undergoing laryngeal, pharyngeal, or esophageal surgery. In cases in which either raw mucosal surfaces are created or a suture line is present, such treatment may prevent wound breakdown, stenosis, and other complications. Prophylactic antireflux treatment may also be of benefit in patients undergoing microlaryngeal surgery.

Gastroesophageal reflux disease may also be related to a form of acquired esophageal stenosis, namely, esophageal lye burns. Although there is no question, either experimentally or clinically, that transmural esophageal burns result in stricture formation (or perforation), in all likelihood such burns do not constitute the major cause of stenosis.[396,397] If GERD can produce secondary LES function and secondary esophageal dysmotility, then it seems likely that an esophageal lye burn could also adversely affect sphincter competence and esophageal acid clearance. Furthermore, the stress of such injury may lead to gastric hypersecretion. Thus, with mucosal or submucosal lesions within the esophagus, the stage is set for GERD to accelerate, exacerbate, and complicate the injury created by lye ingestion. Future study of GER and its relationship to stricture formation in esophageal lye burns seems warranted, because such injuries may share a great deal with laryngeal and tracheal stenosis.

In summary, the combination of raw mucosal surfaces and either infection or GER may lead to a cycle of injury and attempted repair with secondary stenosis formation in the larynx, tracheobronchial tree, or esophagus. So-called subglottic and tracheal "collapse" (soft, diffuse laryngeal stenosis) may be related to GER in the absence of mucosal breakdown. Routine and aggressive treatment of GERD in stenosis of the aerodigestive tract is recommended.

Group III: Reflux Laryngitis

Overall, 60% of the patients in this group had abnormal pH studies, but only 17% had pharyngeal reflux. Even when only the patients not treated with antireflux therapy are considered, the rate of positivity only rises to 67%. Also notable in this patient group, supine reflux predominated over upright reflux in a ratio of almost 2:1.

The most common laryngeal finding in the reflux laryngitis group was posterior laryngitis (74%). This finding represented a spectrum of interarytenoid mucosal thickening and posterior erythema. Clearly, many of these patients had developed chronic throat clearing, but very few of the patients were otherwise vocal abusers.

Chronic throat clearing probably develops due to the inflammatory condition created by GER. Throat clearing then contributes to a vicious cycle in which inflammation and swelling cause a sensation of a foreign body; throat clearing is then utilized as a remedial tactic, but this further traumatizes the already damaged and/or swollen laryngeal tissues.

Patients in the reflux laryngitis group also were often noted to have significant variation in the laryngeal findings from examination to examination over a period of years. It was not infrequent to have a patient return for examination with red arytenoids and swollen interarytenoid mucosa (an exacerbation of reflux laryngitis) and report "I refluxed last night." Although most of the patients denied heartburn and regurgitation, many patients, after having started treatment, became aware of some symptom that they could associate with reflux.

Nineteen percent (9/48) of the patients in the reflux laryngitis group had vocal process granulomas at the time of presentation, but only 5 of the 9 patients had abnormal pH studies. Three granuloma patients underwent laser excision of the lesions, because the granulomas were symptomatic due to their large size (an example of which is shown in Figure 1-B). All 9 of the patients with granulomas responded to antireflux therapy; however, in some, the granulomas did not disappear for a year.

Solitary granulomas of the vocal cord (not necessarily on the vocal process) were common in the carcinoma-of-the-larynx group following initial treatment (usually endoscopic laser excision). Such patients experienced a considerable delay in healing due to granulation tissue. Case 1 (Appendix C) describes a nondrinking, nonsmoking man who developed three small laryngeal carcinomas over a period of 8 years. One of the clinical clues that he had reflux as an etiologic factor was related to his poor healing with granuloma formation at the surgical site following each local excision. Indeed, when granulation tissue appears in the postoperative period following vocal cord surgery, it may be due to vocal abuse and/or reflux laryngitis. Therefore, when a patient develops postoperative granulation, the clinician should investigate, usually simultaneously, both of these possibilities.

Within the study group were six patients with small areas of reversible leukoplakia on the vocal cords, three of whom were in the reflux laryngitis group. All six were smokers. This patient group is shown in Table XXXVI. Each of these patients had small lesions; each underwent diagnostic testing; and each was willing both to quit smoking and to undergo antireflux therapy. All of the lesions resolved spontaneously without surgical intervention. In one case, a leukoplakic lesion vanished in only 3 weeks.

The laryngeal findings in reflux laryngitis do not follow any one pattern. Diffuse edema, with or without erythema; classic "posterior laryngitis"; granulation tissue, with or without apparent signs of inflammation; leukoplakia; and ulceration all seem to occur with reflux laryngitis. The data from this patient group do not provide an answer to which pattern of GER might be associated with which lesion. It is clear, for example, that there is no obvious relationship between posterior laryngitis and supine nocturnal reflux. In addition, patients with vocal process granulomas frequently do not have associated clinical posterior laryngitis.

TABLE XXXVI.
Patients With Laryngeal Leukoplakia Which Disappeared With Antireflux Therapy and Cessation of Smoking.

Patient*	Group*	Esophagography	pH-Metry
SK (14)	I	Reflux	Normal
GB (64)	III	Esophagitis	Abnormal
JS (96)	III	Ring	Normal
JO (106)	III	Esophagitis	Abnormal
HM (125)	IV	Reflux	Abnormal
WM (135)	IV	Esophagitis	Normal

*Refer to Appendix B (raw data).

Finally, with posterior laryngitis, there is a tremendous variation in the clinical appearance of the larynx, as is true for the appearance of the posterior commissure of normal subjects. Under normal circumstances, the posterior commissure appears rounded and concave. When the posterior interarytenoid mucosa gives the appearance of a straight line across the posterior larynx or even bulges in a convex fashion, then it is reasonable to consider the posterior interarytenoid mucosa to be hypertrophic. When it bulges into the glottic lumen, creating the appearance of a mass, then reflux laryngitis is almost a certainty.

In summary, reflux laryngitis, whether or not associated with ulceration or granuloma formation, is frequently marked by periods of exacerbation and remission. Surgery for pyogenic granulomas should be reserved for patients who develop airway obstruction as the result of their lesions. Medical antireflux treatment often needs to be carried beyond 6 months to achieve resolution of laryngeal granulomas.

Group IV: Globus Pharyngeus

Patients in the globus group complained primarily of the sensation of a lump in the throat without dysphagia. Each patient was carefully examined and some patients underwent thyroid scanning in addition to transnasal fiberoptic laryngoscopy, barium swallow esophagography, and pH manometry. Within the last 2 years, many of the patients have also undergone upper esophageal manometry and pharyngeal pressure analysis. Seventy-nine percent (19/24) of the patients were nonsmokers and none were found to have an "organic" lesion. Abnormal reflux was demonstrated in 14 (58%) of 24 patients. Patients with abnormal studies had supine reflux 86% (12/14) of the time, and upright reflux 78% (11/14) of the time, with pharyngeal reflux occurring 45% (5/11) of the time. This population had the highest incidence of supine reflux. There was considerable variability in the laryngeal findings; however, patients most commonly had normal examinations or posterior laryngitis.

Based upon analysis of the data, three separate mechanisms of globus sensation due to GER are postulated. In Appendix C, these are illustrated by cases 12, 13, and 14. In case 12, the patient had a normal laryngeal examination, abnormal pH manometry, and endoscopic evidence of esophagitis. In case 13, the patient had posterior laryngitis, abnormal esophageal reflux, and no gastrointestinal symptoms. In the third case (14), the patient had supine nocturnal reflux with positive pharyngeal reflux, and a hypertensive UES—177 mm Hg pressure (normal 45 to 107 mm Hg). After 3 months of antireflux treatment, his UES pressure was within normal limits, and his symptoms had disappeared. Thus, as one mechanism, globus pharyngeus may be due to referred discomfort from esophagitis (without pharyngolaryngeal reflux), presumably mediated by the vagus. Second, direct local irritation due to reflux may produce inflammation and swelling of laryngopharyngeal structures. Third, hypertension of the cricopharyngeus in response to esophageal acid exposure may cause the symptom. Of the three mechanisms proposed, patients in the study group seemed to demonstrate one or more of these mechanisms. Occasionally, a patient might have all three (esophagitis, posterior laryngitis, and hypertensive UES).

Globus pharyngeus may also have causes unrelated to GER. Clearly, it is the first obligation of the clinician to rule out a neoplastic or an inflammatory cause; it is unlikely that hysteria is often the cause of globus pharyngeus. The clinical data suggest that GERD may be among the primary group of etiologic factors that should be considered when a patient presents with the sensation of a lump in the throat.

Group V: Dysphagia

Dysphagia occasionally is caused by GERD. Note that the dysphagia group represents the smallest diagnostic subgroup presented: over a 4-year period, only 22 patients were entered into the study. The clinical characteristics that suggest the possibility of a reflux-related cause are the chronic-intermittent nature of the symptoms associated with laryngeal findings that suggest GER. Occasionally, a patient will have nonhealing ulceration in a single area or recurrent aphthous ulcers, and it may be reasonable to consider GER as a possible precipitating factor.

Patients in the dysphagia group had the lowest incidence of pharyngeal probe positivity (10%, 2/20). Indeed, the overall yield for abnormal pH-metry results was only 45% (10/22). Nevertheless, most of the patients responded to antireflux treatment by resolution of their symptoms. Of note, 38% (8/21) of the dysphagia group had lower esophageal rings, and this may have contributed to the dysphagia; however, lower esophageal ring is a lesion that may be associated with GERD.

Group VI: Chronic Cough

The chronic cough group had a relatively low incidence of documented GER (52%, 13/25). Nevertheless, of patients with abnormal studies, 45% had abnormal pharyngeal reflux. It is not clear whether this relatively low yield represents patients with chronic intermittent disease or chronic cough due to other causes. Although the number of abnormal pH studies in this treatment group was relatively small, when GERD was found the patients often responded dramatically to treatment (Appendix C, Case Report 17).

Future Studies and Future Therapy

At its inception 7 years ago, the initial focus of this project was to establish, if possible, a relationship between GERD (particularly with regard to the incidence of occult and intermittent reflux) and the six diagnostic subgroups that have been discussed. GERD may, however, account for other conditions that might be encountered in otolaryngologic practice. Recurrent laryngospasm,[253] Zenker's diverticulum,[61,271] sudden infant death syndrome,[272,274] and torticollis,[282] are some of those conditions (Table XV).

These studies suggest that GERD is multifactorial. Clearly, an infant with severe postcibal reflux and subglottic stenosis requires treatment different from that required by an obese, heavy drinker/smoker who consumes fatty foods late at night. The data of this study suggest that reflux may be intermittent; however, the precise incidence and the patterns of reflux (when intermittent) have not yet been definitively established.

In this study, esophageal motility was investigated by barium examination (12% abnormal motility). Because abnormal esophageal acid clearance and esophageal dysmotility appear to be major factors in the development of GERD, at least in the development of esophagitis, and because esophagitis and heartburn are strongly associated, one might speculate that patients with occult GERD may have a different primary pathogenic mechanism. Otolaryngology patients (such as those in this study) may have relatively good esophageal clearance, accounting for the low incidence of heartburn and esophagitis, or esophageal dysmotility may be associated with the development of some upper aerodigestive tract conditions (*e.g.*, globus) but not others (*e.g.*, carcinoma). Future studies evaluating esophageal motility and acid clearance may relate specific mechanisms to the subgroups in this study.

Multiple-probe pH study appears useful. In this study, pharyngolaryngeal reflux has been demonstrated to be associated with upper aerodigestive tract disease. Additional studies are needed to define the patterns of life-style–related GERD. GERD may depend upon fluctuation in diet, ethanol and tobacco consumption, and other factors. In this study, a significant number of patients presented after having had surgery or having suffered trauma. ICU patients who are intubated need to be studied in a systematic fashion to determine the incidence and risk of developing laryngopharyngeal and pulmonary complications of GERD.

The relationship between GERD and neoplastic conditions of the aerodigestive tract remains primarily speculative; however, the data concerning adenocarcinoma in Barrett's esophagus are convincing. The evidence presented herein with regard to carcinoma of the larynx is convincing as well, but does not clearly establish GERD as the cause of laryngeal carcinoma. A large consecutive series of smokers and nonsmokers should be evaluated, using a full battery of tests for GER, including 24-hour pH manometry. Unquestionably, the relationship between cigarette smoking and GERD needs to be further investigated to determine the degree to which each of these factors may independently contribute to neoplastic conditions of the aerodigestive tract.

Cytoprotective agents such as sucralfate, new prokinetic agents such as cisapride, and hydrogen ion pump blockers such as omeprazole may revolutionize the medical treatment of GERD. In the future, it is possible that these modalities, singularly and in combination, will be used in specific ways. For example, patients who have undergone radiation therapy or have xerostomia for some other reason, but in whom LES pressure and esophageal motility are normal, may benefit from sucralfate alone as a prophylactic and therapeutic agent. Patients with recalcitrant esophagitis or GER-related upper airway disorders may receive either pulsed or long-term therapy with omeprazole, H_2 blockers, sucralfate, and/or cisapride.

Until the clinical introduction of omeprazole, no medical therapy had been documented to be as effective as surgery in severe forms of GERD; however, omeprazole therapy may change the role of antireflux surgery in the future management of GERD.

Just as prophylactic antibiotic treatment substantially reduces the risk of postoperative wound breakdown and fistula formation in head and neck surgery, through further study, prophylactic suppression of gastric secretion may be shown to provide a similar benefit.

LABORATORY INVESTIGATION

BACKGROUND

Anatomically, the subglottic region represents the smallest fixed cross-sectional area in the upper airway, and extends from just below the vocal cords to the lower border of the cricoid cartilage, where the cricoid joins the trachea. Thus, the subglottic region is coterminous with the intracricoid region. Because of its anatomic configuration, mucosal injury of the intracricoid subglottic region is almost universally observed in patients intubated for more than 48 hours, and ulceration of the perichondrium and cartilage is frequently observed at autopsy in patients intubated more than 72 hours.[300,301]

This laboratory investigation was designed to investigate the role of acid and pepsin in producing subglottic injury in a canine model. Unlike most previous animal studies that employed perfusion techniques to produce injury to structures covered by intact mucosa, these experiments were specifically designed to mimic the effects of intermittent reflux on the larynx following mucosal injury.

MATERIALS AND METHODS

Experimental Design

On the first day of study, each animal had a mucosal subglottic lesion created, which was then painted with a control substance, acid, or acid with pepsin 3 days a week for 2 weeks. Each animal was killed 4 days after the final painting, and the larynx was harvested. Histologic findings of the subglottic region were graded in a standard fashion by a pathologist not knowing which substance had been used.

Twenty adult beagles weighing 9 to 12 kg were used in this study. Thiopental sodium (International Medication Systems, Ltd.) supplied in Min-i-Mix™ packets was used as the anesthetic. During each procedure, each dog was administered 250 to 500 mg of thiopental intravenously.

Following induction, each animal was placed supine on the operating table and an adult Jako laryngoscope was inserted. Subglottic measurements (anteroposterior and transverse) were made using an adapted alligator forceps. Each measurement was made to the nearest 0.5 mm and was repeated three times, and the results were averaged. Measurements were made at the beginning of each procedure before any manipulation of the subglottic region.

At the initial procedure, a standard subglottic lesion was created using a Hall-Air drill with a 10-inch diamond burr. The intracricoid mucosa was removed, with care being taken to remove only the mucosa. The lesion was made circumferentially; the perichondrium was exposed, but not removed. Following the mucosal removal, the subglottis was painted with one of the tests solutions (Table XXXVII). Only one test substance was employed in each dog. With each microlaryngeal procedure, subsequent to the initial lesioning procedure, the duration of anesthesia was brief. Following each microlaryngeal procedure, the dogs were returned to a postsurgical recovery area.

The painting of the subglottic region was accomplished by placing a saturated cotton ball on a microsurgical sponge carrier and then inserting it through the laryngoscope into the subglottis. The cotton ball was large enough to contact all the posterior laryngeal mucosa as it was pushed into the subglottic lumen. Care was taken not to saturate the cotton

TABLE XXXVII.
Experimental Schema.

I. Control Groups		
A. *Saline* (pH 5.4–5.8)		Animals 1 & 2
B. *Pepsin only* (pH 5.9–6.5)		Animals 3 & 4
C. *"Neutralized" acid* (pH 7.0) (HCl & NaOH)		Animals 5 & 6
D. *"Neutralized" acid and pepsin* (pH 7.0) (HCl and NaOH and pepsin 0.3 mg/ml)		Animals 7 & 8
II. Experimental Groups		
Acid* Only	*pH*	Acid* and Pepsin†
A. Animals 9 & 10	1.5	Animals 11 & 12
B. Animals 13 & 14	2.5	Animals 15 & 16
C. Animals 17 & 18	4.0	Animals 19 & 20

*0.1 N HCl, buffered to desired pH using 0.1 N NaOH.
†Porcine pepsin 0.3 mg/ml.

TABLE XXXVIII.
Schedule of Procedures (20 Animals).

	M	T	W	T	F
Animal No.	Day 1 1–5 M		Day 3 1–5		Day 5 1–5
Animal No.	Day 8 1–5		Day 10 1–5		Day 12 1–5
Animal No.	Day 15 6–10 M	Day 16 1–5 K	Day 17 6–10		Day 19 6–10
Animal No.	Day 22 6–10		Day 24 6–10		Day 26 6–10
Animal No.	Day 29 11–15 M	Day 30 6–10 K	Day 31 11–15		Day 33 11–15
Animal No.	Day 36 11–15		Day 38 11–15		Day 40 11–15
Animal No.	Day 43 16–20 M	Day 44 11–15 K	Day 45 16–20		Day 47 16–20
Animal No.	Day 50 16–20		Day 52 16–20		Day 54 16–20
Animal No.		Day 56 16–20 K			

M = mucosal lesions created; K = killed.

ball so fully that the test solution ran down the trachea into the tracheobronchial tree. Care also was taken not to further abrade any of the laryngeal mucosa.

Each animal was painted with one test solution six times over a 2-week period (Monday, Wednesday, Friday, Monday, Wednesday, Friday). In other words, all initial lesions were created on a Monday, followed by painting on each of the scheduled days (Table XXXVIII). On the Tuesday of the third week, dogs were killed with a lethal intravenous injection of T61 and each dog's larynx was removed, labeled with an identification number, and sent for histologic evaluation.

Controls

Four control groups consisting of two dogs each were employed. The first group was painted with normal saline only (0.9% NaCl, pH 5.4 to 5.8). In the second group, pepsin alone, in a concentration of 0.3 mg/ml in water, was applied (pH 5.9 to 6.5). In the third group, 0.1 N acid that had been neutralized with sodium hydroxide to pH of 7.0 (this constitutes a weak saline solution) was applied. In the final (fourth) group, acid with pepsin 0.3 mg/ml neutralized to a pH of 7.0 with sodium hydroxide was applied.

Experimental Groups

There were two experimental groups, each consisting of three pairs of dogs. In the first group, the animals, in pairs, were painted with 0.1 N acid titrated with 0.1 N sodium hydroxide to pH levels of 1.5, 2.5, and 4.0. Two dogs were painted with each of the three different pH solutions. Dogs were assigned randomly to each pH group.

The second experimental group likewise consisted of three pairs of animals. In this case, the test solution consisted of acid with pepsin 0.3 mg/ml at the same pH levels 1.5, 2.5, and 4.0. The protocol otherwise remained the same.

End-Point Measurement and Histologic Grading

Following the sacrifice of each animal and removal of the larynx, each larynx was decalcified and sectioned. A pathologist, with no knowledge of whether or not a specimen belonged to the experimental or control groups, studied the histologic specimens and recorded a histologic inflammation score for each. The lowest possible score was 0 and the highest possible score was 17. The scoring system included a grading of intraepithelial inflammation, squamous metaplasia, epithelial attenuation, erosion or superficial ulceration, and deep ulceration. Subepithelial changes included stromal inflammation, periglandular inflammation, granulation, and fibrosis. The scoring system is shown in Table XXXIX.

Procedures for Preparing Acid, Pepsin, and Control Solutions

All instruments were calibrated and all solutions were prepared daily. Before the use of each solution, the pH was checked and recorded by a second investigator to ensure that the solution was within 0.1 pH unit of the desired pH.

Instruments used to prepare the various solutions include the Mettler Analytical balance (Mettler Instrument Company, Heightstown, NJ); the Fisher Scientific Accumet pH meter model 600, and the Fisher Scientific Thermix stirrer model 220T (Fisher Scientific, Fairlawn, NJ). Acid and base were also obtained from Fisher Scientific. The acid was supplied as certified 0.1000 ± 0.0005 N HCl. The base was certified NaOH, assayed as 98.4% pure. The pepsin employed was chromatographically purified pepsin crystalline from porcine stomach mucosa. It was listed as 3700 U/mg solid and 3900 U/mg protein. It was obtained from Sigma Chemical Company, St. Louis, Mo., and assayed at this institution. The solid was stored at less than 0°C, and asbestified until mixing and use.

The Mettler analytical balance allows measurements to the nearest 0.0001 g and was serviced by Rightway, Inc. (Duluth, Ga.) just before the beginning of the experiments. The pH meter from Fisher Scientific allows pH readings to the nearest 0.1 U. It was standardized before each use with certified buffer solutions, pH 4.00 ± 0.01 and 7.00 ± 0.01 at 25°C (standard solutions also from Fisher Scientific). Sodium hydroxide solution was prepared to 0.100 N by dissolving 1.016 g of NaOH in 250.0 ml of water. The control solutions were prepared as follows: (A) The saline-only solution consisted of 0.9 NaCl (Abbott Laboratories). (B) The pepsin-only solution was prepared daily by a Mettler balance: 0.0300 ± 0.0001 g pepsin added to 100.0 ± 0.1 ml distilled water measured in a 100 ml pyrex graduated cylinder. It was mixed until dissolved completely. (C) Neutralized acid was prepared by titrating 0.1000 ± 0.0005 N acid stock solution to a pH level of 7.0 with 0.100 ± 0.005 N NaOH. The end point was determined by continuous pH monitoring using the Fisher Accumet pH meter. (D) Pepsin and neutralized acid solution was prepared daily by dissolving 0.0300 ± 0.0001 g pepsin and 100.0 ± 0.1 ml of the solution in (C). This produced 0.300 mg pepsin per milliliter neutralized acid.

The test solutions were produced by titrating 0.1000 ± 0.0005 N acid stock solution to pH 1.5, 2.5, and 4.0 with 0.100 ± 0.005 N NaOH. The end points were determined by continuous pH measurement. These solutions were prepared daily and pH was tested before each use. Also a daily small portion (50.0 ± 0.1 ml) of each of the above acid solutions was added to 0.0150 ± 0.0001 g pepsin to produce three acidic solutions of pH 1.5, 2.5, and 4.0, each with 0.300 mg pepsin per milliliter of solution.

TABLE XXXIX.
Inflammation Scoring System.

I. Epithelial Changes
A. Intraepithelial inflammation
0 = ≥rare PMN
1 = ≥2 PMN/HPF in <5 HPF
2 = ≥2 PMN/HPF in 5–15 HPF
3 = ≥2 PMN/HPF in >15 HPF
B. Squamous metaplasia
0 = Absent
1 = Present
C. Epithelial attenuation, erosion, very superficial ulcer
0 = Absent
1 = Mild to moderate in extent
2 = Marked
D. Deep Ulcer
0 = Absent
2 = Into glandular tissue
4 = Into cartilage
II. Subepithelial Changes
A. Stromal inflammation
0 = Absent
1 = 1–5 PMN/HPF in <10 HPF
2 = Between 1 and 3
3 = >10 PMN/HPF in >10 HPF
B. Periglandular inflammation
0 = Absent
1 = Rare PMN
2 = >3 PMN in ≥glandular units
C. Granulation/fibrosis
0 = Absent/trace
1 = Between 0 and 2
2 = Involves entire linear extent of ≥2 LPF

PMN = polymorphonuclear leukocyte; HPF = high-power field; LPF = low-power field.

RESULTS

All dogs easily tolerated the microlaryngeal procedures. One dog in the acid-only group (pH 1.5; dog 3846) developed a suppurative laryngotracheobronchitis and was started on ampicillin (250 mg orally b.i.d.) 5 days after the initial procedure. He was maintained on that dose of antibiotic until killed.

No injury to the vocal processes of the arytenoids was noted in any animal, even though each vocal process was painted at the time of each procedure. Rather, all macroscopic (and microscopic) abnormalities were confined to the subglottic region.

All control animals had healed subglottic regions macroscopically within 3 to 7 days. With the exception of the infected dog (3846), all acid-treated animals had "healed" by the time they were killed, but none was healed before day 8. Of the acid with pepsin-treated animals, only dog 3839 appeared clinically to have healed. Granulation tissue was present in the subglottic regions of both of the acid-only (pH 1.5) dogs (3846 and 3845), as well as all of the acid-with-pepsin–treated dogs.

In the control animals at the second endoscopic procedure (day 3), there was frequently a friable, gray circumferential band of granulation-like tissue in the subglottis. By the fourth postoperative day (day 5), some animals had complete healing and others had some small localized areas of similar friable granulation tissue; by day 7, all had healed.

In the acid-only animals, the progression was similar in terms of the observed changes, but the progression to apparent healing took roughly twice as long. None of the acid and pepsin-treated animals healed; all had ulcerations and/or granulations.

Microscopic Findings

The mean inflammation score for the control animals was 5.75 ± SD 1.83. The scores ranged from 3 to 9. For the acid-only group, the mean inflammation score was 7.67 ± SD 2.88 (range, 4 to 12). One animal with ulceration in the acid-only group (3846) was the animal that developed postoperative infection and was treated with ampicillin. The animals with pH 1.5 treatment appeared to have higher inflammation scores than the controls, but the scores were not significantly different from those of the controls (P = .0987).

For the acid with pepsin-treated dogs, the mean inflammation score was 11.33 ± SD 1.03. The scores ranged from 10 to 13, and three dogs treated with pH 1.5, 2.5, and 4.0 (acid + pepsin) demonstrated frank ulceration with exposed cricoid cartilage. The P value comparing the acid with pepsin-treated animals with controls was 0.0002 (a high degree of statistical significance). A summary of the results is shown in Table XL.

DISCUSSION

The most striking finding of these experiments was the degree of nonhealing and inflammation in all of the acid-with-pepsin–treated animals and the relatively rapid healing in the control and acid only-treated animals. Furthermore, comparable inflammatory damage occurred in the acid-with-pepsin–treated animals at pH 1.5, 2.5, and 4.0.

Noteworthy also was the lack of breakdown of the overlying mucosa of the vocal processes. (The posterior vocal cords had been intentionally swabbed at the time of inserting the cotton ball into the subglottis.) Thus, intermittent application, such as was used in this study (six "reflux episodes" over a 2-week period), was insufficient to break down the mucosal barrier.

When these results are compared to those of Little, *et al.*,[24] who demonstrated the development of subglottic stenosis within 2 weeks, it may be concluded either that the lesions created by Little, *et al.* were deeper than "mucosal only" or that, in the current study, the reparative process (granulation, fibrosis, epithelialization) had not yet begun at the time the animals were killed.

The results of these experiments have important clinical implications. First, when a preexisting mucosal injury has occurred, such as with laryngeal intubation, intermittent GERD can produce severe laryngeal injury. Second, such injury is primarily dependent upon the presence of pepsin, which appears to be biologically active even at pH 4.0. (This observation is particularly important since many patients treated with antireflux therapy will have an intragastric pH of greater than 4.0 at points of therapeutic nadir.) Third, these findings suggest that patients who fail medical antireflux therapy may do so because they continue to reflux, whereas those who respond to medical therapy may actually reconstitute competent gastroesophageal defenses. Fourth, "peptic laryngitis" may be a more appropriate name than "reflux laryngitis" or "acid laryngitis."

TABLE XL.
Results: The Role of Acid and Pepsin in the Development of Subglottic Laryngeal Damage Using a Canine Model.

Group	Dog No.	Inflammation Score*	*P* Value†
I. Controls			
A. Saline	3797	9	
	3799	6	
B. Pepsin	3796	4	
	3798	3	
C. Neutralized acid	3818	6	
	3824	6	
D. Neutralized acid and pepsin	3823	5	
	3502	7	
II. Acid			
A. pH 1.5	3846‡	12§	
	3845	9	
B. pH 2.5	3840	8	0.28
	3843	4	
C. pH 4.0	3844	5	
	3825	8	
III. Acid and Pepsin			
A. pH 1.5	3892	12§	
	3891	11§	
B. pH 2.5	3890	11	0.0002¶
	3841	10	
C. pH 4.0	3839	11	
	3842	13§	

*Pathologist was blinded to group assignment.

†Comparisons with the control group via Bonferroni-adjusted Student's *t* test.

‡This dog developed suppurative tracheobronchitis, possibly accounting for the high inflammation score.

§Frank ulceration of the cricoid cartilage.

¶Highly significant difference.

Based on the Animal Data: A Model of Intermittent GERD in Otolaryngology Patients with Atypical GERD

Within the context of the clinical study, the results of the experiments described herein allow one to postulate a unified but multifactorial theory of laryngeal injury in GERD. Since the pathophysiology and pattern of GER may vary from subgroup to subgroup (carcinoma, stenosis, globus, etc.), the mechanism of injury may also differ from group to group.

Although one might reasonably postulate that GERD is simply more "severe" in patients in the carcinoma and stenosis groups compared with that in the other subgroups, this postulate is only in part supported by the data. In support is the observation that patients in the carcinoma and stenosis groups had a higher incidence of pharyngeal reflux, and thereby one might assume greater contact time of the refluxate with laryngopharyngeal structures. On the other hand, pH-metry data from individual subjects within the different diagnostic subgroups varied enough so that there was considerable overlap in the degree of abnormality. That is, some patients with carcinoma had only mildly abnormal studies, while some patients in other groups had grossly abnormal pH-metry data (Appendix B, "Raw Data"). "Severity" (*i.e.*, total acid exposure time) may not be the entire answer.

The data on pepsinogen levels in duodenal ulcer patients suggest that there may be a genetic predisposition for pepsinogen hypersecretion.[385] (Pepsinogen is the precursor of pepsin; pepsin is "acid-activated" pepsinogen.) Abnormally high levels of pepsin (pepsinogen) could account for some of the variations in degree and type of tissue damage in GERD. According to this theory, the severity of tissue damage may be a function of the potency of the refluxate with pepsin concentration being the key variable. Although there are no data at present to support or refute this theory, future study of pepsinogen levels in groups of otolaryngology patients with various GERD disorder types may shed light on this potential pathophysiologic mechanism (factor).

A comparison of the carcinoma and globus groups reveals a difference in reflux patterns. Of patients with abnormal studies, 86% of the globus patients and only 54% of the carcinoma patients demonstrated supine reflux. In addition, the incidence of pharyngeal probe positivity in the globus group was only half that of the carcinoma group.

In a series of patients with esophagitis, 91% had abnormal supine reflux and the majority had gastrointestinal symptoms.[8] Thus, prolonged esophageal acid exposure may be associated with esophageal dysmotility and recumbent LES dysfunction, whereas in a carcinoma of the larynx group, upright reflux seems to predominate. Furthermore, since 57% of the patients in the entire study population denied typical gastrointestinal symptoms, it is likely that most of the study patients did not have esophagitis. (Of the carcinoma group, 75% experienced no esophageal or only mild esophageal symptoms.) These observations suggest the possibility that most otolaryngology patients have relatively good esophageal motor function and acid clearance mechanisms, but relatively poor UES function, so that "high" (pharyngeal) reflux commonly occurs.

In consideration of the findings of Ossakow, *et al.*,[251] whose series more closely resembles that of the globus and dysphagia groups, esophageal dysmotility and dysfunction seem more likely in patients with globus and dysphagia. Indeed, the available data suggest that patients in the dysphagia and globus groups have symptom patterns and reflux patterns that more closely resemble those of patients with esophagitis.

Otolaryngology patients also have a high incidence of throat clearing as a secondary symptom, as well as hoarseness and chronic cough. Reflux episodes in otolaryngology patients may therefore be characterized by upright reflux (into the pharynx), followed by throat clearing causing "nebulization" of the refluxate, followed by swallowing and relatively prompt esophageal acid clearance. The available data on esophageal dysmotility in otolaryngology patients with GERD are conflicting, but clearly deserve further investigation.

The response to treatment of otolaryngology patients was superior to that customarily reported in gastroenterology patients with GERD.[58,88,91] In the series presented, 65% of the patients resolved their symptoms at follow-up. This suggests the possibility that if such patients are intermittent refluxers, the pattern may be more episodic and less chronic than that observed in esophagitis patients. This hypothesis is supported by the observation that many of the otolaryngology patients had disease-free intervals of several years but nonetheless had significant recurrent GERD.

Indiscretions of life-style, such as excessive drinking and smoking, coincidentally timed with events that produce mucosal abrasion in the larynx (*e.g.*, viral infection, cough, intubation, etc.), coincident with stressful life events (leading to gastric hypersecretion) such as trauma or surgery, may tip the balance in favor of a clinical situation analogous to these "intermittent reflux" experiments in dogs.

Within the context of a patient population with occult, intermittent GERD and potentially life-threatening complications, systematic study of GERD may yield major clinical breakthroughs in the management of many upper aerodigestive inflammatory and neoplastic conditions. However, GERD has a complex, multifactorial etiology and its different manifestations are, in part, determined by its different causes. One diagnostic test—even pH manometry—cannot possibly provide the answers to the questions raised by this and other studies. The data from these studies suggest that GERD is common in otolaryngologic, especially laryngologic, practice and that the otolaryngologist must develop and use sophisticated diagnostic tools to understand its manifestations.

CONCLUSIONS

1. The 182 consecutive patients studied by ambulatory 24-hour pH monitoring, herein reported, serve as a unique reference point for the future study of gastroesophageal reflux disease (GER, GERD) in otolaryngology—head and neck surgery.
2. From the study of these patients, it can be seen that:
   A. Many otolaryngology patients have a pattern of GERD that is distinctly different from the pattern seen in gastroenterology patients with esophagitis. The most important differences are:
      1. In otolaryngology patients, complications of GER may occur without the symptoms considered typical of GERD; reflux is often occult.
      2. Esophageal dysmotility (poor esophageal clearance), which is a common feature of GERD patients with esophagitis, may be relatively uncommon in otolaryngology patients with GER-related conditions (only 12% had dysmotility on barium study); this may account for the relative lack of esophagitis and its symptoms in otolaryngology patients.
      3. Otolaryngology patients may demonstrate significant day-to-day variation in the GER pattern (intermittency), making diagnosis of GERD occasionally difficult.
   B. The finding of a high association of GERD (71%) with documented pharyngeal reflux (58%) in patients with carcinoma of the larynx strongly suggests a possible etiologic role for GERD in the pathogenesis of laryngeal carcinoma. Further support for this possibility is provided by the observation that of the six nonsmokers studied in this group, all had significant GERD.
   C. The finding of a high association of GERD (78%) with documented pharyngeal reflux (56%) in patients with laryngeal stenosis and tracheal stenosis suggests that GERD is probably of primary importance in the development of these complications.

D. The highest incidence of medical treatment failure requiring fundoplication (55%) was found in the stenosis group. Nevertheless, subsequent to fundoplication, successful decannulation was virtually assured, although, in some cases, irreversible laryngeal damage prevented a full return of laryngeal function.

E. Early recognition and antireflux treatment of patients in the previous two groups may reduce the risk of complications. Due to the high risk of GERD associated with carcinoma and stenosis of the larynx, routine prophylactic antireflux therapy may be indicated.

F. Reflux laryngitis, with or without ulceration or granulation, was associated with GERD in 60% of the cases studied. The degree of reflux and the incidence of pharyngeal-probe positivity was less severe than that in the identified carcinoma and stenosis groups.

G. Globus pharyngeus was associated with pH-documented GERD in 58% of the cases. Three separate mechanisms of globus are postulated:

1. Reflex cricopharyngeal hypertension secondary to distal esophageal acid exposure.
2. Referred globus sensation (presumably mediated via the vagus nerve) secondary to distal esophagitis.
3. Inflammation (swelling and irritation) of laryngopharyngeal structures secondary to direct laryngopharyngeal acid exposure.

H. Patients in the chronic cough and dysphagia groups also frequently demonstrated reflux, but the incidence of positive pH manometry (52% and 45%, respectively) was less than in the other groups.

3. From the experimental studies it can be seen that:

A. In the subglottic larynx, mucosal injury substantially reduces the threshold of tolerance for the development of a GER-related complication.

B. Pepsin is the primary injurious component of the refluxate.

C. Even though pepsin requires acid activation, it is still active enough to cause severe damage at pH 4.0.

D. Intermittent "reflux" (three episodes per week) is sufficient to produce laryngeal damage when a mucosal injury is present.

4. From these two studies it can be concluded that:

A. The relative ratio of abnormal esophageal reflux (62%) to abnormal pharyngeal reflux (30%) suggests that exposure time in the upper aerodigestive tract is much less than in the esophagus; however, the threshold for peptic injury of the upper aerodigestive tract is probably much lower as well.

B. The principal limitations of diagnostic methods for GER are *sampling error* and *the definition of normal*. With the exception of technical probe failure and the above considerations, pH-metry is both 100% sensitive and 100% specific for GER. False-negative and false-positive pH studies can only occur for these reasons.

C. Ambulatory 24-hour pH-metry allows the antireflux treatment of each patient to be tailored to his or her reflux pattern; effective therapy must reflect the etiologic and predisposing variables.

D. Use of a pharyngeal probe is *strongly recommended* in otolaryngology patients and increases the sensitivity of pH-metry.

E. Pharmacologic control of gastric acid secretion does not prevent GER or aspiration, but it is frequently remedial because it positively influences antireflux mechanisms, thereby allowing restoration of damaged defenses. (GER itself may produce secondary esophageal dysmotility and lower esophageal sphincter (LES) dysfunction. Esophageal injury may therefore lead to a vicious cycle in which GER causes secondary LES dysfunction and esophageal motor dysfunction, which lead to further GER). Therefore, successful medical antireflux treatment depends upon correction of the reflux cycle.

5. Xerostomia, which occurs frequently in otolaryngologic patients, is identified as a significant risk factor for GERD.

6. Since treatment with H_2-blockers fails in approximately 30% to 40% of patients, the "therapeutic trial" is a questionably valid diagnostic test. In the future, a therapeutic trial with one of the hydrogen ion blockers may be considered diagnostic.

7. Routine perioperative antireflux treatment may be beneficial in otolaryngology patients with raw mucosal surfaces or suture lines in the larynx, pharynx, or esophagus, thereby reducing the incidence of postoperative complications, such as wound breakdown, infection, fistula, and stenosis.

ACKNOWLEDGMENTS

Many people provided valuable assistance in carrying out these investigations and in the preparation of the manuscript; I would like to recognize and thank them all. Thanks first to Dr. Donald O. Castell, the world-renown gastroenterologist with whom I worked most closely during the years of these studies, for his steady support, good counsel, and willing collaboration. It was in his clinical laboratory that the actual pH studies were carried out by Chris Dalton and Jane Sinclair. Both of these skilled professionals deserve credit and thanks for performing the consistently high quality work that is reported in the clinical study; thanks also for your flexibility in scheduling procedures.

I wish to thank three other fine gastroenterologists for their assistance and support: Drs. Gregory Wiener, Joel Richter, and Wally Wu. Gregory was the G.I. fellow when we first began to investigate otolaryngology patients using pH-manometry; he actively encouraged and participated in the earliest studies. Drs. Richter and Wu also provided friendly advice on a day-to-day basis, as well as help in managing many of the more difficult patients.

In the animal laboratory, Dr. Richard Cooper and Janet Talcott made it all possible. As a senior medical student, Dr. Cooper was an endoscopic whiz and helped in every aspect of the animal studies; Janet Talcott kept the animals healthy and ready. Without these two, it would not have been possible for me to do this project while simultaneously maintaining a busy clinical practice. A special thanks to Dr. Kim Geisinger in the department of pathology who adapted the inflammation score for the dog larynges from his previous work with an esophagitis animal model; it was he who actually examined and scored the larynges.

For assistance in the tasks of data collection and manuscript preparation, many, many thanks to David Koury, Patty Reece, Judith MacMillan, Alma Doub, and Libby Childress. (It was tough to meet the deadline). To my mentors, Dr. Stuart Strong and Dr. Robert Kohut, who read the manuscript and who served as friendly critics, many thanks. Finally, thanks to my family, especially to my wife Marsha, for being patient and understanding during the 2-plus years of my preoccupation with this consuming project, and double thanks for enduring the months of actual writing.

BIBLIOGRAPHY

1. Casselberry, W.E.: American Laryngological Association Twenty-first Annual Congress, Held at Chicago, May 22–24, 1899. *Ann Otol Rhinol Laryngol,* 8:177–185, 1899.
2. Castell, D.O., Wu, W.C. and Ott, D.J. (Eds.): *Gastro-esophageal Reflux Disease. Pathogenesis, Diagnosis, Therapy.* Futura Publishing Company, Inc., Mount Kisco, NY, p. 325, 1985.
3. Benz, L.J., Hootkin, L.A., Margulies, S., *et al.*: A Comparison of Clinical Measurements of Gastroesophageal Reflux. *Gastroenterology,* 62:1–5, 1972.
4. Bianchi Porro, G. and Pace, F.: Comparison of Three Methods of Intraesophageal pH Recordings in the Diagnosis of Gastroesophageal Reflux. *Scand J Gastroenterol,* 23:743–750, 1988.
5. Fuchs, K.H., DeMeester, T.R. and Albertucci, M.: Specificity and Sensitivity of Objective Diagnosis of Gastroesophageal Reflux Disease. *Surgery,* 102:575–580, 1987.
6. Jamieson, G.G. and Duranceau, A. (Eds.): *Gastroesophageal Reflux.* W. B. Saunders Co., Philadelphia, p. 281, 1988.
7. Johnson, L.F.: New Concepts and Methods in the Study and Treatment of Gastroesophageal Reflux Disease. *Med Clin North Am,* 65(6):1195–1222, 1981.
8. Johnson, L.F.: 24-Hour pH Monitoring in the Study of Gastroesophageal Reflux. *J Clin Gastroenterol,* 2:387–399, 1980.
9. Cherry, J. and Margulies, S.I.: Contact Ulcer of the Larynx. LARYNGOSCOPE, 78:1937–1940, 1968.
10. Delahunty, J.E. and Cherry, J.: Experimentally Produced Vocal Cord Granulomas. LARYNGOSCOPE, 78:1941–1947, 1968.
11. Feder, R.J. and Michell, M.J.: Hyperfunctional, Hyperacidic, and Intubation Granulomas. *Arch Otolaryngol,* 110:582–584, 1984.
12. Goldberg, M., Noyek, A.M. and Pritzker, K.P.H.: Laryngeal Granuloma Secondary to Gastro-esophageal Reflux. *J Otolaryngol,* 7:196–202, 1978.
13. Öhman, L., Olofsson, J., Tibbling, L., *et al.*: Esophageal Dysfunction in Patients with Contact Ulcer of the Larynx. *Ann Otol Rhinol Laryngol,* 92:228–230, 1983.
14. Olson, N.R.: Effects of Stomach Acid on the Larynx. *Proc Am Laryngol Assoc,* 104:108–112, 1983.
15. Ward, P.H., Zwitman, D., Hanson, D., *et al.*: Contact Ulcers and Granulomas of the Larynx: New Insights into Their Etiology as a Basis for More Rational Treatment. *Otolaryngol Head Neck Surg,* 88:262–269, 1980.
16. Delahunty, J.E.: Acid Laryngitis. *J Laryngol Otol,* 86:335–342, 1972.
17. Kambic, V. and Radsel, Z.: Acid Posterior Laryngitis. Aetiology, Histology, Diagnosis and Treatment. *J Laryngol Otol,* 98:1237–1240, 1984.
18. Olson, N.R.: The Problem of Gastroesophageal Reflux. *Otolaryngol Clin North Am,* 19:119–133, 1986.
19. Ward, P.H. and Berci, G.: Observations on the Pathogenesis of Chronic Non-Specific Pharyngitis and Laryngitis. LARYNGOSCOPE, 92:1377–1382, 1982.
20. Wilson, J.A., White, A., von Haacke, N.P., *et al.*: Gastroesophageal Reflux and Posterior Laryngitis. *Ann Otol Rhinol Laryngol,* 98:405–410, 1989.
21. Morrison, M.D.: Is Chronic Gastroesophageal Reflux a Causative Factor in Glottic Carcinoma? *Otolaryngol Head Neck Surg,* 99:370–373, 1988.
22. Ward, P.H. and Hanson, D.G.: Reflux as an Etiological Factor of Carcinoma of the Laryngopharynx. LARYNGOSCOPE, 98:1195–1199, 1988.
23. Bain, W.M., Harrington, J.W., Thomas, L.E., *et al.*: Head and Neck Manifestations of Gastroesophageal Reflux. LARYNGOSCOPE, 93:175–179, 1983.
24. Little, F.B., Koufman, J.A., Kohut, R.I., *et al.*: Effect of Gastric Acid on the Pathogenesis of Subglottic Stenosis. *Ann Otol Rhinol Laryngol,* 94:516–519, 1985.
25. Henderson, R.D.: *The Esophagus: Reflux and Primary Motor Disorders.* Williams & Wilkins, Baltimore, p. 279, 1980.
26. Berenberg, W. and Neuhauser, E.B.D.: Cardio-esophageal Relaxation (Chalasia) as a Cause of Vomiting in Infants. *Pediatrics,* 5:414–420, 1950.
27. Winkelstein, A.: Peptic Esophagitis. A New Clinical Entity. *JAMA,* 104:906–909, 1935.
28. Meltzer, S.J.: On the Causes of the Orderly Progress of Peristaltic Movements in the Oesophagus. *Am J Physiol,* 2:266–272, 1899.
29. Tileston, W.: Peptic Ulcer of the Oesophagus. *Am J Med Sci,* 132:240–265, 1906.
30. Mosher, H.P.: The Liver Tunnel and Cardiospasm. *Ann Otol Rhinol Laryngol,* 30:1065–1067, 1921.
31. Jackson, C.: The Diaphragmatic Pinchcock in So-Called "Cardiospasm." LARYNGOSCOPE, 32:139–142, 1922.
32. Allison, P.R.: Reflux Esophagitis, Sliding Hiatal Hernia, and the Anatomy of Repair. *Surg Gynecol Obstet,* 92:419–431, 1951.
33. Fyke, F.E., Jr., Code, C.F. and Schlegel, J.F.: The Gastroesophageal Sphincter in Healthy Human Beings. *Gastroenterologia [Basel],* 86:135–150, 1956.
34. Ingelfinger, F.J.: Esophageal Motility. *Physiol Rev,* 38:533–584, 1958.
35. LoPresti, P., Scherl, N.D., Greene, L., *et al.*: Clinical Experience with a Glass-Fiber Gastroscope. *Am J Dig Dis,* 7:95–101, 1962.
36. LoPresti, P.A. and Hilmi, A.M.: Clinical Experience with a New Foroblique Fiber Optic Esophagoscope. *Am J Dig Dis,* 9:690–697, 1964.
37. Burnett, W.: An Evaluation of the Gastroduodenal Fibrescope. *Gut,* 3:361–365, 1962.
38. Bernstein, L.M. and Baker, L.A.: A Clinical Test for Esophagitis. *Gastroenterology,* 34:760–781, 1958.
39. Miller, F.A., DoVale, J. and Gunther, T.: Utilization of Inlying pH Probe for Evaluation of Acid-Peptic Diathesis. *Arch Surg,* 89:199–203, 1964.
40. Spencer, J.: Prolonged pH Recording in the Study of Gastro-oesophageal Reflux. *Br J Surg,* 56:912–914, 1969.
41. DeMeester, T.R. and Johnson, L.F.: The Evaluation of Objec-

tive Measurements of Gastroesophageal Reflux and Their Contribution to Patient Management. *Surg Clin North Am,* 56(1):39–53, 1976.

42. DeMeester, T.R., Johnson, L.F., Joseph, G.J., *et al.*: Patterns of Gastroesophageal Reflux in Health and Disease. *Ann Surg,* 184:459–470, 1976.
43. Dent, J., Holloway, R.H., Toouli, J., *et al.*: Mechanisms of Lower Oesophageal Sphincter Incompetence in Patients With Symptomatic Gastrooesophageal Reflux. *Gut,* 29:1020–1028, 1988.
44. Dodds, W.J., Dent, J., Hogan, W.J., *et al.*: Mechanisms of Gastroesophageal Reflux in Patients with Reflux Esophagitis. *N Engl J Med,* 307:1547–1552, 1982.
45. Dodds, W.J., Hogan, W.J., Helm, J.F., *et al.*: Pathogenesis of Reflux Esophagitis. *Gastroenterology,* 81:376–394, 1981.
46. Helm, J.F.: Esophageal Acid Clearance. *J Clin Gastroenterol,* 8(Suppl 1):5–11, 1986.
47. Henderson, R.D.: *Esophageal Manometry in Clinical Investigation.* Praeger Publishers, New York, p. 258, 1983.
48. Kirchner, J.A.: The Motor Activity of the Cricopharyngeus Muscle. LARYNGOSCOPE, 68:1119–1159, 1958.
49. Jackson, C.: *The Life of Chevalier Jackson: An Autobiography.* Macmillan Co., New York, p. 229, 1938.
50. Killian, G.: The Mouth of the Esophagus. LARYNGOSCOPE, 17:421–428, 1907.
51. Jackson, C.: Peptic Ulcer of the Esophagus. *JAMA,* 92:369–372, 1929.
52. Barrett, N.R.: Chronic Peptic Ulcer of the Oesophagus and Oesphagitis. *Br J Surg,* 38:175–182, 1950.
53. Ingelfinger, F.J. and Abbott, W.O.: Intubation Studies of Human Small Intestine: Diagnostic Significance of Motor Disturbances. *Am J Dig Dis,* 7:468–474, 1940.
54. Nissen, R.: Gastropexy and "Fundoplication" in Surgical Treatment of Hiatal Hernia. *Am J Dig Dis,* 6:954–961, 1961.
55. Stiegmann, G.V., Pearlman, N.W. and Teter, A.: Upper Aerodigestive Manifestation of Gastroesophageal Reflux. *Gastroenterology,* 92:1654, 1987. Abstract.
56. Deschner, W.K. and Benjamin, S.B.: Extraesophageal Manifestations of Gastroesophageal Reflux Disease. *Am J Gastroenterol,* 84:1–5, 1989.
57. Wiener, G.J., Copper, J.B., Wu, W.C., *et al.*: Is Hoarseness an Atypical Manifestation of Gastroesophageal Reflux (GER)? An Ambulatory 24 Hour pH Study. *Gastroenterology,* 90A:1691, 1986. Abstract.
58. Toohill, R.J., Mushtag, E., Grossman, T.W., *et al.*: Pharyngeal, Laryngeal and Tracheobronchial Manifestations of Gastroesophageal Reflux. *Proceedings of the XXIV World Congress of Otolaryngology—Head and Neck Surgery.* Kugler and Ghedini Publishing, Berkeley, Calif. In press.
59. Malcomson, K.G.: Globus Hystericus vel Pharyngis (A Reconnaissance of Proximal Vagal Modalities). *J Laryngol Otol,* 82:219–230, 1968.
60. Delahunty, J.E. and Ardran, G.: Globus Hystericus—A Manifestation of Reflux Oesophagitis? *J Laryngol Otol,* 84:1049–1054, 1970.
61. Delahunty, J.E., Margulies, S.I., Alonso, W.A., *et al.*: The Relationship of Reflux Esophagitis to Pharyngeal Pouch (Zenker's Diverticulum) Formation. LARYNGOSCOPE, 81:570–577, 1971.
62. Chodosh, P.L.: Gastro-Esophago-Pharyngeal Reflux. LARYNGOSCOPE, 87:1418–1427, 1977.
63. Fearon, B.: Management of Subglottic Stenosis of the Larynx in Infants and Children. *Adv Otorhinolaryngol,* 23:97–103, 1978.
64. Glanz, H. and Kleinsasser, O.: Chronische Laryngitis und Carcinom (with English abstract). *Arch Otorhinolaryngol,* 212:57–75, 1976.
65. Bogdasarian, R.S. and Olson, N.R.: Posterior Glottic Laryngeal Stenosis. *Otolaryngol Head Neck Surg,* 88:765–772, 1980.
66. Logemann, J.A.: *Evaluation and Treatment of Swallowing Disorders.* College-Hill Press, Inc., San Diego, p. 249, 1983.
67. Nelson, J.L. III and Castell, D.O.: Reflux Esophagitis: An Update. *South Med J,* 78:452–457, 1985.
68. Helm, J.F., Dodds, W.J., Hogan, W.J., *et al.*: Acid Neutralizing Capacity of Human Saliva. *Gastroenterology,* 83:69–74, 1982.
69. Zaninotto, G., DeMeester, T.R., Bremner, C.G., *et al.*: Esophageal Function in Patients with Reflux-Induced Strictures and Its Relevance to Surgical Treatment. *Ann Thorac Surg,* 47:362–370, 1989.
70. Nelson, J.B. and Castell, D.O.: Esophageal Motility Disorders. *DM,* 34:299–389, 1988.
71. Castell, D.O.: Physiology and Pathophysiology of the Lower Esophageal Sphincter. *Ann Otol Rhinol Laryngol,* 84:569–575, 1975.
72. Castell, D.O. and Harris, L.D.: Hormonal Control of Gastroesophageal-Sphincter Strength. *N Engl J Med,* 282:886–889, 1970.
73. Gerhardt, D.C., Shuck, T.J., Bordeaux, E.A., *et al.*: Human Upper Esophageal Sphincter. Response to Volume, Osmotic, and Acid Stimuli. *Gastroenterology,* 75:268–274, 1978.
74. Hellemans, J., Pelemans, W. and Vantrappen, G.: Pharyngoesophageal Swallowing Disorders and the Pharyngoesophageal Sphincter. *Med Clin North Am,* 65:1149–1171, 1981.
75. Cohen, S. and Harris, L.D.: Does Hiatus Hernia Affect Competence of the Gastroesophageal Sphincter? *N Engl J Med,* 284:1053–1056, 1971.
76. Siegel, C.I. and Hendrix, T.R.: Esophageal Motor Abnormalities Induced by Acid Perfusion in Patients with Heartburn. *J Clin Invest,* 42:686–695, 1963.
77. Blackwell, J.N. and Castell, D.O.: Motility Disorders of the Lower Esophagus. *Surv Dig Dis,* 1:157–168, 1983.
78. Di Lorenzo, C., Piepsz, A., Ham, H., *et al.*: Gastric Emptying with Gastro-oesophageal Reflux. *Arch Dis Child,* 62:449–453, 1987.
79. Gill, R.C., Kellow, J.E. and Wingate, D.L.: Gastro-oesophageal Reflux and the Migrating Motor Complex. *Gut,* 28:929–934, 1987.
80. Hunt, P.S., Connell, A.M. and Smiley, T.B.: The Cricopharyngeal Sphincter in Gastric Reflux. *Gut,* 11:303–306, 1970.
81. Kahrilas, P.J., Dodds, W.J., Dent, J., *et al.*: Effect of Sleep, Spontaneous Gastroesophageal Reflux, and a Meal on Upper Esophageal Sphincter Pressure in Normal Human Volunteers. *Gastroenterology,* 92:466–471, 1987.
82. Winans, C.S.: The Pharyngoesophageal Closure Mechanism: A Manometric Study. *Gastroenterology,* 63:768–777, 1972.
83. Dent, J., Dodds, W.J., Hogan, W.J., *et al.*: Factors that Influence Induction of Gastroesophageal Reflux in Normal Human Subjects. *Dig Dis Sci,* 33:270–275, 1988.
84. Ferguson, M.K., Ryan, J.W., Little, A.G., *et al.*: Esophageal Emptying and Acid Neutralization in Patients with Symptoms of Esophageal Reflux. *Ann Surg,* 201:728–735, 1985.
85. Mattioli, S., Pilotti, V., Spangaro, M., *et al.*: Reliability of 24-Hour Home Esophageal pH Monitoring in Diagnosis of Gastroesophageal Reflux. *Dig Dis Sci,* 34:71–78, 1989.
86. Orlando, R.C.: Esophageal Epithelial Resistance. *J Clin Gastroenterol,* 8(Suppl 1):12–16, 1986.
87. Flood, C.A. and Hennig, G.C.: Results of Medical Treatment in Hiatus Hernia. *Gastroenterology,* 35:62–73, 1958.
88. Lieberman, D.A.: Medical Therapy for Chronic Reflux Esophagitis. Long-term Follow-up. *Arch Intern Med,* 147:1717–1720, 1987.
89. Palmer, E.D.: The Hiatus Hernia-Esophagitis-Esophageal Stricture Complex. Twenty Year Prospective Study. *Am J Med,* 44:566–579, 1968.
90. Rex, J.C., Andersen, H.A., Bartholomew, L.G., *et al.*: Esophageal Hiatal Hernia—A 10-Year Study of Medically Treated Cases. *JAMA,* 178:271–274, 1961.
91. Behar, J., Sheahan, D.G., Biancani, P., *et al.*: Medical and Surgical Management of Reflux Esophagitis. A 38-Month Report on a Prospective Clinical Trial. *N Engl J Med,* 293:263–268, 1975.
92. Hetzel, D.J., Dent, J., Reed, W.D., *et al.*: Healing and Relapse of Severe Peptic Esophagitis after Treatment with Omepra-

zole. *Gastroenterology,* 95:903–912, 1988.
93. Graham, D.Y., Larkai, E., Opekun, A.R., *et al.*: Sensitivity of the Esophageal Mucosa to pH in Gastroesophageal Reflux. *Gastroenterology,* 92:A1412, 1987. Abstract.
94. Fearon, B. and Brama, I.: Esophageal Hiatal Hernia in Infants and Children. *Ann Otol Rhinol Laryngol,* 90:387–391, 1981.
95. Urschel, H.C., Jr. and Paulson, D.L.: Gastroesophageal Reflux and Hiatal Hernia. Complications and Therapy. *J Thorac Cardiovasc Surg,* 53:21–32, 1967.
96. Ward, P.H., Ippoliti, A.F., Simmons, D.H., *et al.*: Complications of Gastroesophageal Reflux. *West J Med,* 149:58–65, 1988.
97. Helm, J.F., Allendorph, M., Dodds, W.J., *et al.*: Loss of the Salivary Response to Esophageal Acid Perfusion in Patients With Peptic Stricture. *Gastroenterology,* 90:A1456, 1986. Abstract.
98. Helm, J.F., Dodds, W.J. and Hogan, W.J.: Salivary Response to Esophageal Acid in Normal Subjects and Patients With Reflux Esophagitis. *Gastroenterology,* 93:1393–1397, 1987.
99. Helm, J.F., Dodds, W.J., Riedel, D.R., *et al.*: Determinants of Esophageal Acid Clearance in Normal Subjects. *Gastroenterology,* 85:607–612, 1983.
100. Johansson, K.E., Ask, P., Boeryd, B., *et al.*: Oesophagitis, Signs of Reflux, and Gastric Acid Secretion in Patients with Symptoms of Gastro-Oesophageal Reflux Disease. *Scand J Gastroenterol,* 21:837–847, 1986.
101. Feldman, M. and Richardson, C.T.: Role of Thought, Sight, Smell, and Taste of Food in the Cephalic Phase of Gastric Acid Secretion in Humans. *Gastroenterology,* 90:428–433, 1986.
102. McConnel, F.M.S.: Analysis of Pressure Generation and Bolus Transit During Pharyngeal Swallowing. LARYNGOSCOPE, 98:71–78, 1988.
103. Bonanno, P.C.: Swallowing Dysfunction after Tracheostomy. *Ann Surg,* 174:29–33, 1971.
104. Cameron, J.L., Reynolds, J. and Zuidema, G.D.: Aspiration in Patients with Tracheostomies. *Surg Gynecol Obstet,* 136:68–70, 1973.
105. Hanks, J.B., Fisher, S.R., Meyers, W.C., *et al.*: Effect of Total Laryngectomy on Esophageal Motility. *Ann Otol Rhinol Laryngol,* 90:331–334, 1981.
106. Kilman, W.J. and Goyal, R.K.: Disorders of Pharyngeal and Upper Esophageal Sphincter Motor Function. *Arch Intern Med,* 136:592–601, 1976.
107. McConnel, F.M.S., Cerenko, D. and Mendelsohn, M.S.: Dysphagia after Total Laryngectomy. *Otolaryngol Clin North Am,* 21(4):721–726, 1988.
108. McConnel, F.M.S., Cerenko, D. and Mendelsohn, M.S.: Manofluorographic Analysis of Swallowing. *Otolaryngol Clin North Am,* 21:625–635, 1988.
109. McConnel, F.M.S. and Mendelsohn, M.: The Effects of Surgery on Pharyngeal Deglutition. *Dysphagia,* 1:145–151, 1987.
110. Bonavina, L., Evander, A., DeMeester, T.R., *et al.*: Length of the Distal Esophageal Sphincter and Competency of the Cardia. *Am J Surg,* 151:25–34, 1986.
111. Miller, A.J.: Swallowing: Neurophysiologic Control of the Esophageal Phase. *Dysphagia,* 2:72–82, 1987.
112. Moore, J.G. and Wolfe, M.: The Relation of Plasma Gastrin to the Circadian Rhythm of Gastric Acid Secretion in Man. *Digestion,* 9:97–105, 1973.
113. Richter, J.E. and Castell, D.O.: Drugs, Foods, and Other Substances in the Cause and Treatment of Reflux Esophagitis. *Med Clin North Am,* 65(6):1223–1234, 1981.
114. Radmark, T. and Pettersson, G.B.: The Contribution of the Diaphragm and an Intrinsic Sphincter to the Gastroesophageal Antireflux Barrier. An Experimental Study in the Dog. *Scand J Gastroenterol,* 24(1):85–94, 1989.
115. Higgs, R.H., Smyth, R.D. and Castell, D.O.: Gastric Alkalinization: Effect on Lower-Esophageal-Sphincter Pressure and Serum Gastrin. *N Engl J Med,* 291:486–490, 1974.
116. Rosman, A.S., Goldberg, H., Federman, Q., *et al.*: Chronic Xerostomia Alters 23 Hour Esophageal pH and is Associated With Esophageal Inflammation. *Gastroenterology,* 94:A387, 1988. Abstract.
117. Reichert, T.J. and Faw, K.D.: The Cricopharyngeus in the Neonate. *Ann Otol Rhinol Laryngol,* 89:446–449, 1980.
118. Green, W.E.R., Castell, J.A. and Castell, D.O.: Upper Esophageal Sphincter Pressure Recording: Is an Oval Manometry Catheter Necessary? *Dysphagia,* 2:162–165, 1988.
119. Schatzki, R.: Die Beweglichkeit von Oesophagus und Magen Innerhalb des Zwerchschlitzes Beim Alten Menschen. *Fortschr Geb Rontgenstr Nukearmed Erganzungsband,* 45:177–187, 1932.
120. Wolf, B.S., Brahms, S.A. and Khilnani, M.T.: The Incidence of Hiatus Hernia in Routine Barium Meal Examinations. *Mt. Sinai J Med,* 26:598–600, 1959.
121. Dyer, N.H. and Pridie, R.B.: Incidence of Hiatus Hernia in Asymptomatic Subjects. *Gut,* 9:696–699, 1968.
122. Conway-Hughes, J.H.L.: Oesophageal Reflux: An Analysis of 453 Consecutive Barium Meal Examinations. *Br J Radiol,* 29:331–334, 1956.
123. Wright, R.A. and Hurwitz, A.L.: Relationship of Hiatal Hernia to Endoscopically Proved Reflux Esophagitis. *Dig Dis Sci,* 24:311–313, 1979.
124. Becker, D.J., Sinclair, J.W., Wu, W.C., *et al.*: Fatty Foods and Reflux: Evidence of Increased Esophageal Acid Exposure after a High Fat Meal. *Gastroenterology,* 94:A29, 1988. Abstract.
125. Murphy, D.W. and Castell, D.O.: Chocolate and Heartburn: Evidence of Increased Esophageal Acid Exposure After Chocolate Ingestion. *Am J Gastroenterol,* 83:633–636, 1988.
126. Knuff, T.E., Benjamin, S.B., Worsham, G.F., *et al.*: Histologic Evaluation of Chronic Gastroesophageal Reflux. An Evaluation of Biopsy Methods and Diagnostic Criteria. *Dig Dis Sci,* 29:194–201, 1984.
127. Behar, J.: The Role of the Lower Esophageal Sphincter in Reflux Prevention. *J Clin Gastroenterol,* 8(Suppl 1):2–4, 1986.
128. Mittal, R.K. and McCallum, R.W.: Characteristics and Frequency of Transient Relaxations of the Lower Esophageal Sphincter in Patients With Reflux Esophagitis. *Gastroenterology,* 95:593–599, 1988.
129. Eastwood, G.L., Castell, D.O. and Higgs, R.H.: Experimental Esophagitis in Cats Impairs Lower Esophageal Sphincter Pressure. *Gastroenterology,* 69:146–153, 1975.
130. Baldi, F., Ferrarini, F., Longanesi, A., *et al.*: Oesophageal Function Before, During, and After Healing of Erosive Oesophagitis. *Gut,* 29:157–160, 1988.
131. Katz, P.O., Knuff, T.E., Benjamin, S.B., *et al.*: Abnormal Esophageal Pressures in Reflux Esophagitis: Cause or Effect? *Am J Gastroenterol,* 81:744–746, 1986.
132. Gudmundsson, K.; Johnsson, F. and Joelsson, B.: The Time Pattern of Gastroesophageal Reflux. *Scand J Gastroenterol,* 23:75–79, 1988.
133. Arana, J., Tovar, J.A. and Garay, J.: Abnormal Preoperative and Postoperative Esophageal Peristalsis in Gastroesophageal Reflux. *J Pediatr Surg,* 21:711–714, 1986.
134. Kahrilas, P.J., Dodds, W.J. and Hogan, W.J.: Effect of Peristaltic Dysfunction on Esophageal Volume Clearance. *Gastroenterology,* 94:73–80, 1988.
135. Gerhardt, D.C., Castell, D.O., Winship, D.H., *et al.*: Esophageal Dysfunction in Esophagopharyngeal Regurgitation. *Gastroenterology,* 78:893–897, 1980.
136. Gill, R.C., Bowes, K.L., Murphy, P.D., *et al.*: Esophageal Motor Abnormalities in Gastroesophageal Reflux and the Effects of Fundoplication. *Gastroenterology,* 91:364–369, 1986.
137. Moses, F.M.: Reversible Aperistalsis as a Complication of Gastroesophageal Reflux Disease. *Am J Gastroenterol,* 82:272–275, 1987.
138. Eckardt, V.F.: Does Healing of Esophagitis Improve Esophageal Motor Function? *Dig Dis Sci,* 33:161–165, 1988.
139. Scobey, M.W. and Castell, D.O.: Esophageal Motility: Effects of Collagen Vascular Diseases and Aging. *Soc Gastrointest Assist J,* (Spring):16–21, 1986.
140. Stringer, D.A., Sprigg, A., Juodis, E., *et al.*: The Association of Cystic Fibrosis, Gastroesophageal Reflux, and Reduced Pul-

monary Function. *Can Assoc Radiol J,* 39:100–102, 1988.
141. Dab, I. and Malfroot, A.: Gastroesophageal Reflux: A Primary Defect in Cystic Fibrosis? *Scand J Gastroenterol,* 23(Suppl 143):125–131, 1988.
142. Stentoft, P., Hendel, L. and Aggestrup, S.: Esophageal Manometry and pH-Probe Monitoring in the Evaluation of Gastroesophageal Reflux in Patients With Progressive Systemic Sclerosis. *Scand J Gastroenterol,* 22:499–504, 1987.
143. Barish, C.F. and Castell, D.O.: Dysphagia and Weight Loss: A Particular Concern for the Elderly. *J Fam Med,* 3–8, June 1985.
144. Gillen, P., Keeling, P., Byrne, P.J., *et al.*: Experimental Columnar Metaplasia in the Canine Oesophagus. *Br J Surg,* 75:113–115, 1988.
145. Radigan, L.R., Glover, J.L., Shipley, F.E., *et al.*: Barrett Esophagus. *Arch Surg,* 112:486–491, 1977.
146. Dubois, A.: Clinical Relevance of Gastroduodenal Dysfunction in Reflux Esophagitis. *J Clin Gastroenterol,* 8(Suppl 1):17–25, 1986.
147. Sutphen, J.L. and Dillard, V.L.: Effect of Feeding Volume on Early Postcibal Gastroesophageal Reflux in Infants. *J Pediatr Gastroenterol Nutr,* 7:185–188, 1988.
148. Little, A.G., Martinez, E.I., DeMeester, T.R., *et al.*: Duodenogastric Reflux and Reflux Esophagitis. *Surgery,* 96:447–454, 1984.
149. Miller, G., Palmer, K.R., Smith, B., *et al.*: Smoking Delays Gastric Emptying of Solids. *Gut,* 30:50–53, 1989.
150. Vitale, G.C., Cheadle, W.G., Patel, B., *et al.*: The Effect of Alcohol on Nocturnal Gastroesophageal Reflux. *JAMA,* 258:2077–2079, 1987.
151. Dubois, A. and Castell, D.O. (Eds.).: *Esophageal and Gastric Emptying.* CRC Press, Inc., Boca Raton, Fla., p. 159, 1984.
152. Hagen, J., Deitel, M., Khanna, R.K., *et al.*: Gastroesophageal Reflux in the Massively Obese. *Int Surg,* 72:1–3, 1987.
153. Nebel, O.T., Fornes, M.F. and Castell, D.O.: Symptomatic Gastroesophageal Reflux: Incidence and Precipitating Factors. *Am J Dig Dis,* 21:953–956, 1976.
154. Motil, K.J., Ostendorf, J., Bricker, J.T., *et al.*: Exercise-Induced Gastroesophageal Reflux in an Athletic Child. *J Pediatr Gastroenterol Nutr,* 6:989–991, 1987.
155. Wolfe, M.M. and Soll, A.H.: The Physiology of Gastric Acid Secretion. *N Engl J Med,* 319:1707–1715, 1988.
156. Peters, M.N. and Richardson, C.T.: Stressful Life Events, Acid Hypersecretion, and Ulcer Disease. *Gastroenterology,* 84:114–119, 1983.
157. Mittelmann, B. and Wolff, H.G.: Emotions and Gastroduodenal Function: Experimental Studies on Patients with Gastritis, Duodenitis and Peptic Ulcer. *Psychosom Med,* 4:5–61, 1942.
158. Lenz, H.J., Ferrari-Taylor, J. and Isenberg, J.I.: Wine and Five Percent Ethanol are Potent Stimulants of Gastric Acid Secretion in Humans. *Gastroenterology,* 85:1082–1087, 1983.
159. Aylwin, J.A.: The Physiological Basis of Reflux Oesophagitis in Sliding Hiatal Diaphragmatic Hernia. *Thorax,* 8:38–45, 1953.
160. Ott, D.J., Gelfand, D.W. and Wu, W.C.: Reflux Esophagitis: Radiographic and Endoscopic Correlation. *Radiology,* 130:583–588, 1979.
161. Battle, W.S., Nyhus, L.M. and Bombeck, C.T.: Gastroesophageal Reflux: Diagnosis and Treatment. *Ann Surg,* 177:560–565, 1973.
162. Krejs, G.J., Seefeld, U., Brändli, H.H., *et al.*: Gastrooesophageal Reflux Disease: Correlation of Subjective Symptoms with 7 Objective Oesophageal Function Tests. *Acta Hepato Gastroenterol,* 23:130–140, 1976.
163. Sonnenberg, A., Lepsien, G., Müller-Lissner, S.A., *et al.*: When is Esophagitis Healed? Esophageal Endoscopy, Histology and Function Before and After Cimetidine Treatment. *Dig Dis Sci,* 27:297–302, 1982.
164. Benjamin, S.B., Gerhardt, D.C. and Castell, D.O.: High Amplitude, Peristaltic Esophageal Contractions Associated With Chest Pain and/or Dysphagia. *Gastroenterology,* 77:478–483, 1979.
165. Donner, M.W., Silbiger, M.L., Hookman, P., *et al.*: Acid-Barium Swallows in the Radiographic Evaluation of Clinical Esophagitis. *Radiology,* 87:220–225, 1966.
166. Fisher, R.S., Malmud, L.S., Roberts, G.S., *et al.*: Gastroesophageal (GE) Scintiscanning to Detect and Quantitate GE Reflux. *Gastroenterology,* 70:301–308, 1976.
167. Ott, D.J., Cowan, R.J., Gelfand, D.W., *et al.*: The Role of Diagnostic Imaging in Evaluating Gastroesophageal Reflux Disease. *Postgrad Radiol,* 6:3–14, 1986.
168. Kuriloff, D.B., Chodosh, P., Goldfarb, R., *et al.*: Detection of Gastroesophageal Reflux in the Head and Neck: The Role of Scintigraphy. *Ann Otol Rhinol Laryngol,* 98:74–80, 1989.
169. Nussbaum, E., Maggi, J.C., Mathis, R., *et al.*: Association of Lipid-Laden Alveolar Macrophages and Gastroesophageal Reflux in Children. *J Pediatr,* 110:190–194, 1987.
170. Corwin, R.W. and Irwin, R.S.: The Lipid-Laden Alveolar Macrophage as a Marker of Aspiration in Parenchymal Lung Disease. *Am Rev Respir Dis,* 132:576–581, 1985.
171. Skinner, D.B. and Booth, D.J.: Assessment of Distal Esophageal Function in Patients with Hiatal Hernia and/or Gastroesophageal Reflux. *Ann Surg,* 172:627–637, 1970.
172. DeMeester, T.R., Bonavina, L. and Albertucci, M.: Nissen Fundoplication for Gastroesophageal Reflux Disease. Evaluation of Primary Repair in 100 Consecutive Patients. *Ann Surg,* 204:9–20, 1986.
173. Johnson, L.F. and DeMeester, T.R.: Twenty-Four-Hour pH Monitoring of the Distal Esophagus. A Quantitative Measure of Gastroesophageal Reflux. *Am J Gastroenterol,* 62:325–332, 1974.
174. Johnson, L.F., DeMeester, T.R. and Haggitt, R.C.: Esophageal Epithelial Response to Gastroesophageal Reflux. A Quantitative Study. *Dig Dis,* 23:498–509, 1978.
175. Tuttle, S.G., Rufin, F. and Bettarello, A.: The Physiology of Heartburn. *Ann Intern Med,* 55:292–300, 1961.
176. Boesby, S.: Gastro-oesophageal Acid Reflux and Sphincter Pressure in Normal Human Subjects. *Scand J Gastroenterol,* 10:731–736, 1975.
177. Ward, B.W., Wu, W.C., Richter, J.E., *et al.*: Ambulatory 24-Hour Esophageal pH Monitoring. Technology Searching for a Clinical Application. *J Clin Gastroenterol,* 8(Suppl 1):59–67, 1986.
178. Fink, S.M. and McCallum, R.W.: The Role of Prolonged Esophageal pH Monitoring in the Diagnosis of Gastroesophageal Reflux. *JAMA,* 252:1160–1164, 1984.
179. Weisskopf, A.: Reflux Esophagitis: A Cause of Globus. *Otolaryngol Head Neck Surg,* 89:780–782, 1981.
180. Johnsson, F. and Joelsson, B.: Reproducibility of Ambulatory Oesophageal pH Monitoring. *Gut,* 29:886–889, 1988.
181. Pujol, A., Grande, L., Ros, E., *et al.*: Utility of Inpatient 24-Hour Intraesophageal pH Monitoring in Diagnosis of Gastroesophageal Reflux. *Dig Dis Sci,* 33:1134–1140, 1988.
182. Smout, A.J.P.M., Breedijk, M., van der Zouw, C., *et al.*: Physiological Gastroesophageal Reflux and Esophageal Motor Activity Studied with a New System for 24-Hour Recording and Automated Analysis. *Dig Dis Sci,* 34:372–378, 1989.
183. Euler, A.R. and Byrne, W.J.: Twenty-Four-Hour Esophageal Intraluminal pH Probe Testing: A Comparative Analysis. *Gastroenterology,* 80:957–961, 1981.
184. Sondheimer, J.M. and Haase, G.M.: Simultaneous pH Recordings from Multiple Esophageal Sites in Children With and Without Distal Gastroesophageal Reflux. *J Pediatr Gastroenterol Nutr,* 7:46–51, 1988.
185. Vandenplas, Y. and Sacré-Smits, L.: Continuous 24-Hour Esophageal pH Monitoring in 285 Asymptomatic Infants 0–15 Months Old. *J Pediatr Gastroenterol Nutr,* 6:220–224, 1987.
186. Schindlbeck, N.E., Heinrich, C., König, A., *et al.*: Optimal Thresholds, Sensitivity, and Specificity of Long-Term pH-Metry for the Detection of Gastroesophageal Reflux Disease. *Gastroenterology,* 93:85–90, 1987.
187. Murphy, D.W., Yuan, Y. and Castell, D.O.: Does the Intraesophageal pH Probe Accurately Detect Acid Reflux? Simultaneous Recording with Two pH Probes in Humans. *Dig Dis*

Sci, 34:649–656, 1989.
188. Murphy, D.W., Faust, K.B., Chiantella, V.M., *et al.*: Assessment of Accuracy of Intra-Esophageal pH Probe in a Dog Model. *Dig Dis Sci*, 34:1079–1084, 1989.
189. Castell, D.O.: Ambulatory Monitoring in Esophageal Disease. *Viewpoints on Digestive Diseases*, 21:1–4, 1989.
190. Bozymski, E.M.: Gastroesophageal Reflux Disease. *Hosp Med*, 24:73–86, 1988.
191. Berstad, A., Weberg, R., Frøyshov Larsen, I., *et al.*: Relationship of Hiatus Hernia to Reflux Oesophagitis. A Prospective Study of Coincidence, Using Endoscopy. *Scand J Gastroenterol*, 21:55–58, 1986.
192. Brunner, G., Creutzfeldt, W., Harke, U., *et al.*: Therapy with Omeprazole in Patients with Peptic Ulcerations Resistant to Extended High-Dose Ranitidine Treatment. *Digestion*, 39:80–90, 1988.
193. Lieberman, D.A.: 24-Hour Esophageal pH Monitoring Before and After Medical Therapy for Reflux Esophagitis. *Dig Dis Sci*, 33:166–171, 1988.
194. Lieberman, D.A. and Keeffe, E.B.: Treatment of Severe Reflux Esophagitis with Cimetidine and Metoclopramide. *Ann Intern Med*, 104:21–26, 1986.
195. McHardy, G.: Reflux Esophagitis. *Ann Otol Rhinol Laryngol*, 81:761–769, 1972.
196. Clouse, R.E., Eckert, T.C. and Staiano, A.: Hiatus Hernia and Esophageal Contraction Abnormalities. *Am J Med*, 81:447–450, 1986.
197. Cucchiara, S., Staiano, A., Di Lorenzo, C., *et al.*: Pathophysiology of Gastroesophageal Reflux and Distal Esophageal Motility in Children With Gastroesophageal Reflux Disease. *J Pediatr Gastroenterol Nutr*, 7:830–836, 1988.
198. DiPalma, J.A. and Meyer, G.W.: A Rational Clinical Approach to Esophageal Motor Disorders. *Dysphagia*, 2:97–108, 1987.
199. Mahony, M.J., Migliavacca, M., Spitz, L., *et al.*: Motor Disorders of the Oesophagus in Gastro-oesophageal Reflux. *Arch Dis Child*, 63:1333–1338, 1988.
200. Chen, Y.M., Gelfand, D.W., Ott, D.J., *et al.*: Natural Progression of the Lower Esophageal Mucosal Ring. *Gastrointest Radiol*, 12:93–98, 1987.
201. Barrett, N.R.: The Lower Esophagus Lined by Columnar Epithelium. *Surgery*, 41:881–894, 1957.
202. Khoury, G.A. and Bolton, J.: Age: An Important Factor in Barrett's Oesophagus. *Ann R Coll Surg Engl*, 71:50–53, 1989.
203. Lee, F.I. and Isaacs, P.E.T.: Barrett's Ulcer: Response to Standard Dose Ranitidine, High Dose Ranitidine, and Omeprazole. *Am J Gastroenterol*, 83:914–916, 1988.
204. Naef, A.P., Savary, M. and Ozzello, L.: Columnar-Lined Lower Esophagus: An Acquired Lesion with Malignant Predisposition. Report on 140 Cases of Barrett's Esophagus with 12 Adenocarcinomas. *J Thorac Cardiovasc Surg*, 70:826–835, 1975.
205. Reid, B.J., Haggitt, R.C., Rubin, C.E., *et al.*: Barrett's Esophagus. Correlation Between Flow Cytometry and Histology in Detection of Patients at Risk for Adenocarcinoma. *Gastroenterology*, 93:1–11, 1987.
206. Spechler, S.J. and Goyal, R.K.: Barrett's Esophagus. *N Engl J Med*, 315:362–371, 1986.
207. Goodwin, W.J., Jr., Larson, D.L. and Sajjad, S.M.: Adenocarcinoma of the Cervical Esophagus in a Patient With Extensive Columnar Cell-Lined (Barrett's) Esophagus. *Otolaryngol Head Neck Surg*, 91:446–449, 1983.
208. Mannell, A.: Carcinoma of the Esophagus. *Curr Probl Surg*, 19:554–647, 1982.
209. Tuyns, A.J., Péquignot, G. and Abbatucci, J.S.: Oesophageal Cancer and Alcohol Consumption. Importance of Type of Beverage. *Int J Cancer*, 23:443–447, 1979.
210. Berlatzky, Y., Cohen, O.M., Freund, H.R., *et al.*: Surgical Treatment of Gastroesophageal Reflux With Esophageal Stricture in Infancy and Childhood. *Am J Surg*, 143:205–208, 1982.
211. Smart, H.L., Mayberry, J.F. and Atkinson, M.: Achalasia Following Gastro-oesophageal Reflux. *J R Soc Med*, 79:71–73, 1986.
212. Giuffre, R.M., Rubin, S. and Mitchell, I.: Antireflux Surgery in Infants with Bronchopulmonary Dysplasia. *Am J Dis Child*, 141:648–651, 1987.
213. Hrabovsky, E.E. and Mullett, M.D.: Gastroesophageal Reflux and the Premature Infant. *J Pediatr Surg*, 21:583–587, 1986.
214. Baer, M., Maki, M., Nurminen, J., *et al.*: Esophagitis and Findings of Long-Term Esophageal pH Recording in Children With Repeated Lower Respiratory Tract Symptoms. *J Pediatr Gastroenterol Nutr*, 5:187–190, 1986.
215. Barish, C.F., Wu, W.C. and Castell, D.O.: Respiratory Complications of Gastroesophageal Reflux. *Arch Intern Med*, 145:1882–1888, 1985.
216. Belsey, R.: The Pulmonary Complications of Oesophageal Disease. *Br J Dis Chest*, 54:342–348, 1960.
217. Buts, J.P., Barudi, C., Moulin, D., *et al.*: Prevalence and Treatment of Silent Gastro-oesophageal Reflux in Children with Recurrent Respiratory Disorders. *Eur J Pediatr*, 145:396–400, 1986.
218. Kinni, M.E. and Stout, M.M.: Aspiration Pneumonitis: Predisposing Conditions and Prevention. *J Oral Maxillofac Surg*, 44:378–384, 1986.
219. Olsen, A.M.: The Spectrum of Aspiration Pneumonitis. *Ann Otol Rhinol Laryngol*, 79:875–888, 1970.
220. Pellegrini, C.A., DeMeester, T.R., Johnson, L.F., *et al.*: Gastroesophageal Reflux and Pulmonary Aspiration: Incidence, Functional Abnormality, and Results of Surgical Therapy. *Surgery*, 86:110–119, 1979.
221. Rothstein, F.C. and Halpin, T.C.: High Incidence of Pulmonary Symptoms in Infants Evaluated for Esophageal Disease. *Ann Otol Rhinol Laryngol*, 89:450–453, 1980.
222. Zavala, D.C.: The Threat of Aspiration Pneumonia in the Aged. *Geriatrics*, 132:46–51, 1977.
223. Allen, C.J. and Newhouse, M.T.: Gastroesophageal Reflux and Chronic Respiratory Disease. *Am Rev Respir Dis*, 129:645–647, 1984.
224. Crausaz, F.M. and Favez, G.: Aspiration of Solid Food Particles Into Lungs of Patients with Gastroesophageal Reflux and Chronic Bronchial Disease. *Chest*, 93:376–378, 1988.
225. Gonzalez, E.R. and Castell, D.O.: Respiratory Complications of Gastroesophageal Reflux. *Am Fam Physician*, 37:169–172, 1988.
226. Iverson, L.I.G., May, I.A. and Samson, P.C.: Pulmonary Complications in Benign Esophageal Disease. *Am J Surg*, 126:223–228, 1973.
227. Mays, E.E., Dubois, J.J. and Hamilton, G.B.: Pulmonary Fibrosis Associated with Tracheobronchial Aspiration. A Study of the Frequency of Hiatal Hernia and Gastroesophageal Reflux in Interstitial Pulmonary Fibrosis of Obscure Etiology. *Chest*, 69:512–515, 1976.
228. McArthur, M.S.: Pulmonary Complications of Benign Esophageal Disease. *Am J Surg*, 151:296–299, 1986.
229. Pearson, J.E.G. and Wilson, R.S.E.: Diffuse Pulmonary Fibrosis and Hiatus Hernia. *Thorax*, 26:300–305, 1971.
230. Benjamin, S.B.: Extra-Esophageal Complications of Gastroesophageal Reflux. *J Clin Gastroenterol* 8(Suppl 1):68–71, 1986.
231. Fitzgerald, J.M., Allen, C.J., Craven, M.A., *et al.*: Chronic Cough and Gastroesophageal Reflux. *Can Med Assoc J*, 140:520–524, 1989.
232. Irwin, R.S., Corrao, W.M. and Pratter, M.R.: Chronic Persistent Cough in the Adult: The Spectrum and Frequency of Causes and Successful Outcome of Specific Therapy. *Am Rev Respir Dis*, 123:413–417, 1981.
233. Andersen, L.I., Schmidt, A. and Bundgaard, A.: Pulmonary Function and Acid Application in the Esophagus. *Chest*, 90:358–363, 1986.
234. Babb, R.R., Notarangelo, J. and Smith, V.M.: Wheezing: A Clue to Gastroesophageal Reflux. *Am J Gastroenterol*, 53:230–233, 1970.
235. Boyle, J.T., Tuchman, D.N., Altschuler, S.M., *et al.*: Mechanisms for the Association of Gastroesophageal Reflux and Bronchospasm. *Am Rev Respir Dis (Suppl)*, 131:S16–S20,

1985.
236. Ekström, T., Lindgren, B.R. and Tibbling, L.: Effects of Ranitidine Treatment on Patients With Asthma and a History of Gastro-oesophageal Reflux: A Double Blind Crossover Study. *Thorax,* 44:19–23, 1989. Abstract.
237. Evander, A., Little, A.G., Riddell, R.H., *et al.*: Composition of the Refluxed Material Determines the Degree of Reflux Esophagitis in the Dog. *Gastroenterology,* 93:280–286, 1987.
238. Goodall, R.J.R., Earis, J.E., Cooper, D.N., *et al.*: Relationship Between Asthma and Gastro-oesophageal Reflux. *Thorax,* 36:116–121, 1981.
239. Harper, P.C., Bergner, A. and Kaye, M.D.: Antireflux Treatment for Asthma. Improvement in Patients with Associated Gastroesophageal Reflux. *Arch Intern Med,* 147:56–60, 1987.
240. Hughes, D.M., Spier, S., Rivlin, J., *et al.*: Gastroesophageal Reflux During Sleep in Asthmatic Patients. *J Pediatr,* 102:666–672, 1983.
241. Mansfield, L.E. and Stein, M.R.: Gastroesophageal Reflux and Asthma: A Possible Reflex Mechanism. *Ann Allergy,* 41:224–226, 1978.
242. Martin, M.E., Grunstein, M.M. and Larsen, G.L.: The Relationship of Gastroesophageal Reflux to Nocturnal Wheezing in Children With Asthma. *Ann Allergy,* 49:318–322, 1982.
243. Mitsuhashi, M., Tomomasa, T., Tokuyama, K., *et al.*: The Evaluation of Gastroesophageal Reflux Symptoms in Patients with Bronchial Asthma. *Ann Allergy,* 54:317–320, 1985.
244. Sontag, S., O'Connell, S., Greenlee, H., *et al.*: Is Gastroesophageal Reflux a Factor in Some Asthmatics? *Am J Gastroenterol,* 82:119–126, 1987.
245. Holinger, P.H., Kutnick, S.L., Schild, J.A., *et al.*: Subglottic Stenosis in Infants and Children. *Ann Otol Rhinol Laryngol,* 85:591–599, 1976.
246. Gray, S., Miller, R., Myer, C.M. III, *et al.*: Adjunctive Measures for Successful Laryngotracheal Reconstruction. *Ann Otol Rhinol Laryngol,* 96:509–513, 1987.
247. Gaynor, E.B.: Gastroesophageal Reflux as an Etiologic Factor in Laryngeal Complications of Intubation. LARYNGOSCOPE, 98:972–979, 1988.
248. Hallewell, J.D. and Cole, T.B.: Isolated Head and Neck Symptoms Due to Hiatus Hernia. *Arch Otolaryngol,* 92:499–501, 1970.
249. Wiener, G.J., Koufman, J.A., Wu, W.C., *et al.*: The Pharyngoesophageal Dual Ambulatory pH Probe for Evaluation of Atypical Manifestations of Gastroesophageal Reflux (GER). *Gastroenterology,* 92:A1694, 1987. Abstract.
250. Katz, P.O., Bishop, S.G. and Lumpkin, S.M.M.: Chronic Dysphonia Secondary to Gastroesophageal Reflux (GER). Diagnosis With Continuous Simultaneous Dual Ambulatory pH Monitoring. (CDApHM). *Gastroenterology,* 94:A219, 1988. Abstract.
251. Ossakow, S.J., Elta, G., Colturi, T., *et al.*: Esophageal Reflux and Dysmotility as the Basis for Persistent Cervical Symptoms. *Ann Otol Rhinol Laryngol,* 96:387–392, 1987.
252. Belmont, J.R. and Grundfast, K.: Congenital Laryngeal Stridor (Laryngomalacia): Etiologic Factors and Associated Disorders. *Ann Otol Rhinol Laryngol,* 93:430–437, 1984.
253. Bortolotti, M.: Laryngospasm and Reflex Central Apnoea Caused by Aspiration of Refluxed Gastric Content in Adults. *Gut,* 30:233–238, 1989.
254. Curtis, D.J. and Crain, M.: Aerosol Regurgitation as a Laryngeal Sensitizing Event Explaining Acute Laryngospasm. *Dysphagia,* 2:93–96, 1987.
255. Orenstein, S.R., Kocoshis, S.A., Orenstein, D.M., *et al.*: Stridor and Gastroesophageal Reflux: Diagnostic Use of Intraluminal Esophageal Acid Perfusion (Bernstein Test). *Pediatr Pulmonol,* 3:420–424, 1987.
256. Bradley, P.J. and Narula, A.: Clinical Aspects of Pseudodysphagia. *J Laryngol Otol,* 101:689–694, 1987.
257. Gage-White, L.: Incidence of Zenker's Diverticulum With Hiatus Hernia. LARYNGOSCOPE, 98:527–530, 1988.
258. Henderson, R.D., Woolf, C. and Marryatt, G.: Pharyngoesophageal Dysphagia and Gastroesophageal Reflux. LARYNGOSCOPE, 86:1531–1539, 1976.
259. Hurwitz, A.L., Nelson, J.A. and Haddad, J.K.: Oropharyngeal Dysphagia. Manometric and Cine Esophagographic Findings. *Am J Dig Dis,* 20:313–324, 1975.
260. Batch, A.J.G.: Globus Pharyngeus (Part I). *J Laryngol Otol,* 102:152–158, 1988.
261. Batch, A.J.G.: Globus Pharyngeus (Part II). Discussion. *J Laryngol Otol,* 102:227–230, 1988.
262. Caldarelli, D.D., Andrews, A.H., Jr. and Derbyshire, A.J.: Esophageal Motility Studies in Globus Sensation. *Ann Otol Rhinol Laryngol,* 79:1098–1100, 1970.
263. Flores, T.C., Cross, F.S. and Jones, R.D.: Abnormal Esophageal Manometry in Globus Hystericus. *Ann Otol Rhinol Laryngol,* 90:383–386, 1981.
264. Freeland, A.P., Ardran, G.M. and Emrys-Roberts, E.: Globus Hystericus and Reflux Oesophagitis. *J Laryngol Otol,* 88:1025–1031, 1974.
265. Linsell, J.C. and Owen, W.J.: The Globus Sensation (Editorial). *Clin Otolaryngol,* 11:303–305, 1986.
266. Mair, I.W.S., Schroder, K.E., Modalsli, B., *et al.*: Aetiological Aspects of the Globus Symptom. *J Laryngol Otol,* 88:1033–1040, 1974.
267. Moloy, P.J. and Charter, R.: The Globus Symptom. Incidence, Therapeutic Response, and Age and Sex Relationships. *Arch Otolaryngol,* 108:740–744, 1982.
268. Richter, J.E., Bradley, L.A. and Castell, D.O.: Esophageal Chest Pain: Current Controversies in Pathogenesis, Diagnosis, and Therapy. *Ann Intern Med,* 110:66–78, 1989.
269. Watson, W.C. and Sullivan, S.N.: Hypertonicity of the Cricopharyngeal Sphincter: A Cause of Globus Sensation. *Lancet,* 2:1417–1419, 1974.
270. Wilson, J.A., Heading, R.C., Maran, A.G.D., *et al.*: Globus Sensation Is Not Due to Gastro-oesophageal Reflux. *Clin Otolaryngol,* 12:271–275, 1987.
271. Smiley, T.B., Caves, P.K. and Porter, D.C.: Relationship Between Posterior Pharyngeal Pouch and Hiatus Hernia. *Thorax,* 25:725–731, 1970.
272. Baccino, E., Le Goff, D., Lancien, G., *et al.*: Exploration of Acid Gastroesophageal Reflux by 24-h pH Metry in Infants at Risk of Sudden Infant Death Syndrome: A Study of 50 Cases. *Forensic Sci Int,* 36:255–260, 1988.
273. Herbst, J.J., Minton, S.D. and Book, L.S.: Gastroesophageal Reflux Causing Respiratory Distress and Apnea in Newborn Infants. *J Pediatr,* 95:763–768, 1979.
274. Paton, J.Y., MacFadyen, U.M. and Simpson, H.: Sleep Phase and Gastro-oesophageal Reflux in Infants at Possible Risk of SIDS. *Arch Dis Child,* 64:264–269, 1989.
275. Castell, D.O.: Diagnosis of Noncardiac Chest Pain in Older Patients. *Geriatrics,* 40:61–86, 1985.
276. Castell, D.O.: Gastroesophageal Reflux—The Great Imitator (Editorial). *West J Med,* 149:81–82, 1988.
277. Castell, D.O. and Richter, J.E.: Editorial: Esophageal Symptoms and the "Irritable Esophagus." *Dysphagia,* 2:109–111, 1987.
278. Davies, H.A., Jones, D.B. and Rhodes, J.: "Esophageal Angina" as the Cause of Chest Pain. *JAMA,* 248:2274–2278, 1982.
279. Greenblatt, D.J. and Shader, R.I.: Drug Therapy. Anticholinergics. *N Engl J Med,* 288:1215–1219, 1973.
280. Katz, P.O. and Castell, D.O.: Chest Pain: Is It of Esophageal Origin? *Med Grand Rounds,* 3:335–343, 1984.
281. Peters, L., Maas, L., Petty, D., *et al.*: Spontaneous Noncardiac Chest Pain. Evaluation by 24-Hour Ambulatory Esophageal Motility and pH Monitoring. *Gastroenterology,* 94:878–886, 1988.
282. Bray, P.F., Herbst, J.J., Johnson, D.G., *et al.*: Childhood Gastroesophageal Reflux. Neurologic and Psychiatric Syndromes Mimicked. *JAMA,* 237:1342–1345, 1977.
283. Järvinen, V., Meurman, J.H., Hyvärinen, H., *et al.*: Dental Erosion and Upper Gastrointestinal Disorders. *Oral Surg,* 65:298–303, 1988.
284. Maxton, D.G., Ainley, C.C., Grainger, S.L., *et al.*: Teeth and Benign Oesophageal Stricture. *Gut,* 28:61–63, 1987.
285. Axelrod, F.B., Maayan, C., Hazzi, C., *et al.*: Bradycardia Asso-

ciated with Hiatal Hernia and Gastroesophageal Reflux Relieved by Surgery. *Am J Gastroenterol,* 82:159–161, 1987.
286. Chakraborty, T.K., Ogilvie, A.L., Heading, R.C., *et al.*: Abnormal Cardiovascular Reflexes in Patients With Gastro-oesophageal Reflux. *Gut,* 30:46–49, 1989.
287. Wright, R.A.: Bronchial and Cardiac Responses to Intraesophageal Acid and Saline Infusion. *Gastroenterology,* 94:A503, 1988. Abstract.
288. Henderson, R.D. and Pearson, F.G.: Surgical Management of Esophageal Scleroderma. *J Thorac Cardiovasc Surg,* 66:686, 1973.
289. Belsey, R.: Functional Disease of the Esophagus. *J Thorac Cardiovasc Surg,* 52:164–188, 1966.
290. Smith, J.L., Opekun, A.R., Larkai, E., *et al.*: Sensitivity of the Esophageal Mucosa to pH in Gastroesophageal Reflux Disease. *Gastroenterology,* 96:683–689, 1989.
291. Richter, J.E. and Castell, D.O.: Gastroesophageal Reflux. Pathogenesis, Diagnosis, and Therapy. *Ann Intern Med,* 97:93–103, 1982.
292. Cann, C.I., Fried, M.P. and Rothman, K.J.: Epidemiology of Squamous Cell Cancer of the Head and Neck. *Otolaryngol Clin North Am,* 18:367–388, 1985.
293. Wynder, E.L. and Stellman, S.D.: Comparative Epidemiology of Tobacco-Related Cancers. *Cancer Res,* 37:4608–4622, 1977.
294. McGuirt, W.F., Matthews, B. and Koufman, J.A.: Multiple Simultaneous Tumors in Patients with Head and Neck Cancer. A Prospective, Sequential Panendoscopic Study. *Cancer,* 50:1195–1199, 1982.
295. Shapshay, S.M., Hong, W.K., Fried, M.P., *et al.*: Simultaneous Carcinomas of the Esophagus and Upper Aerodigestive Tract. *Otolaryngol Head Neck Surg,* 88:373–377, 1980.
296. Stanciu, C. and Bennett, J.R.: Smoking and Gastro-oesophageal Reflux. *Br Med J,* 3:793–795, 1972.
297. Dennish, G.W. and Castell, D.O.: Inhibitory Effect of Smoking on the Lower Esophageal Sphincter. *N Engl Med J,* 284:1136–1137, 1971.
298. Gabriel, C.E. and Jones, D.G.: The Importance of Chronic Laryngitis. *J Laryngol Otol,* 74:349–357, 1960.
299. Burns, H.P., Dayal, V.S., Scott, A., *et al.*: Laryngotracheal Trauma: Observations on Its Pathogenesis and Its Prevention Following Prolonged Orotracheal Intubation in the Adult. LARYNGOSCOPE, 89:1316–1325, 1979.
300. Healy, G.B.: An Experimental Model for the Endoscopic Correction of Subglottic Stenosis With Clinical Applications. LARYNGOSCOPE, 92:1103–1115, 1982.
301. Papsidero, M.J. and Pashley, N.R.T.: Acquired Stenosis of the Upper Airway in Neonates. An Increasing Problem. *Ann Otol Rhinol Laryngol,* 89:512–514, 1980.
302. Gates, G.A. and Fernandez, A.T.: Laryngotracheoplasty for Acquired Subglottic Stenosis in Infants and Children: Experience With Six Cases. LARYNGOSCOPE, 88:1468–1476, 1978.
303. Hawkins, D.B.: Glottic and Subglottic Stenosis From Endotracheal Intubation. LARYNGOSCOPE, 87:339–346, 1977.
304. Acquired Subglottic Stenosis in Infants. Proceedings of Round Table Meeting, Royal Society, London, October, 1987. *J Laryngol Otol (Suppl),* 17:1–48, 1988.
305. Bergström, J., Moberg, A. and Orell, S.R.: On the Pathogenesis of Laryngeal Injuries Following Prolonged Intubation. *Acta Otolaryngol,* 55:342–346, 1962.
306. Hedden, M., Ersoz, C.J., Donnelly, W.H., *et al.*: Laryngotracheal Damage After Prolonged Use of Orotracheal Tubes in Adults. *JAMA,* 207:703–708, 1969.
307. Hilding, A.C.: Laryngotracheal Damage During Intratracheal Anesthesia. Demonstration by Staining the Unfixed Specimen with Methylene Blue. *Ann Otol Rhinol Laryngol,* 80:565–581, 1971.
308. McGovern, F.H., Fitz-Hugh, G.S. and Edgemon, L.J.: The Hazards of Endotracheal Intubation. *Ann Otol Rhinol Laryngol,* 80:556–564, 1971.
309. Fan, L.L., Flynn, J.W. and Pathak, D.R.: Risk Factors Predicting Laryngeal Injury in Intubated Neonates. *Crit Care Med,* 11:431–433, 1983.
310. Koufman, J.A., Fortson, J.K. and Strong, M.S.: Predictive Factors of Cricoid Ring Size in Adults in Relation to Acquired Subglottic Stenosis. *Otolaryngol Head Neck Surg,* 91:177–182, 1983.
311. Donnelly, W.H.: Histopathology of Endotracheal Intubation. An Autopsy Study of 99 Cases. *Arch Pathol,* 88:511–520, 1969.
312. Strome, M. and Ferguson, C.F.: Multiple Postintubation Complications. *Ann Otol Rhinol Laryngol,* 83:432–438, 1974.
313. Whited, R.E.: A Prospective Study of Laryngotracheal Sequelae in Long-Term Intubation. LARYNGOSCOPE, 94:367–377, 1984.
314. Sasaki, C.T., Horiuchi, M. and Koss, N.: Tracheostomy-Related Subglottic Stenosis: Bacteriologic Pathogenesis. LARYNGOSCOPE, 89:857–865, 876–877, 1979.
315. Gray, S., Miller, R., Myer, C.M. III, *et al.*: Adjunctive Measures for Successful Laryngotracheal Reconstruction. *Ann Otol Rhinol Laryngol,* 96:509–513, 1987.
316. Koufman, J.A., Thompson, J.N. and Kohut, R.I.: Endoscopic Management of Subglottic Stenosis with the CO_2 Surgical Laser. *Otolaryngol Head Neck Surg,* 89:215–220, 1981.
317. Strong, M.S., Healy, G.B., Vaughan, C.W., *et al.*: Endoscopic Management of Laryngeal Stenosis. *Otolaryngol Clin North Am,* 12(4):797–805, 1979.
318. Cotton, R.T. and Seid, A.B.: Management of the Extubation Problem in the Premature Child. Anterior Cricoid Split as an Alternative to Tracheotomy. *Ann Otol Rhinol Laryngol,* 89:508–511, 1980.
319. Cotton, R.T. and Evans, J.N.G.: Laryngotracheal Reconstruction in Children. Five-Year Follow-Up. *Ann Otol Rhinol Laryngol,* 90:516–520, 1981.
320. Finnegan, D.A., Wong, M.L. and Kashima, H.K.: Hyoid Autograft Repair of Chronic Subglottic Stenosis. *Ann Otol Rhinol Laryngol,* 84:643–649, 1975.
321. Borowiecki, B. and Croft, C.B.: Experimental Animal Model of Subglottic Stenosis. *Ann Otol Rhinol Laryngol,* 86:835–840, 1977.
322. Klainer, A.S., Turndorf, H., Wu, W.H., *et al.*: Surface Alterations Due to Endotracheal Intubation. *Am J Med,* 58:674–683, 1975.
323. Wynne, J.W., Ramphal, R. and Hood, C.I.: Tracheal Mucosal Damage after Aspiration. A Scanning Electron Microscope Study. *Am Rev Respir Dis,* 124:728–732, 1981.
324. Kuriloff, D.B.: Laryngeal Complications of Intubation: GER. LARYNGOSCOPE, 99:227–228, 1989. Letter to Editor.
325. Brodnitz, F.S.: Contact Ulcer of the Larynx. *Arch Otolaryngol,* 74:70–80, 1961.
326. Coffin, L.A.: Response to: The Relations of the Upper Air Passages to Diseases of the Gastrointestinal Tract. *Ann Otol Rhinol Laryngol,* 12:521–526, 1903.
327. Jackson, C.: Contact Ulcer of the Larynx. *Ann Otol Rhinol Laryngol,* 37:227–230, 1928.
328. Baker, D.C., Jr.: Contact Ulcers of the Larynx. LARYNGOSCOPE, 64:73–78, 1954.
329. Bloch, C.S. and Gould, W.J.: Vocal Therapy in Lieu of Surgery for Contact Granuloma: A Case Report. *J Speech Hear Disord,* 39:478–485, 1974.
330. Peacher, G. and Holinger, P.: Contact Ulcer of the Larynx. II. The Role of Vocal Reeducation. *Arch Otolaryngol,* 46:617–623, 1947.
331. Hill, F.T.: Granuloma of Larynx Following Endotracheal Anesthesia. *Ann Otol Rhinol Laryngol,* 57:910–913, 1948.
332. Pratt, L.W., Tobin, W.H. and Gallagher, R.A.: Globus Hystericus—Office Evaluation by Psychological Testing With the MMPI. LARYNGOSCOPE, 86:1540–1551, 1976.
333. Cherry, J., Siegel, C.I., Margulies, S.I., *et al.*: Pharyngeal Localization of Symptoms of Gastroesophageal Reflux. *Ann Otol Rhinol Laryngol,* 79:912–915, 1970.
334. Wallin, L., Boesby, S. and Madsen, T.: The Effect of HCl Infusion in the Lower Part of the Oesophagus on the Pharyngo-oesophageal Sphincter Pressure in Normal Subjects. *Scand J Gastroenterol,* 13:821–826, 1978.
335. Labrousse, J.-M. and Poliquin, J.F.: Paresthésies Pharyngées

et Reflux Gastro-oesophagien. *J Otolaryngol,* 12:261–262, 1983.
336. Ellis, F.H., Jr. and Crozier, R.E.: Cervical Esophageal Dysphagia. Indications for and Results of Cricopharyngeal Myotomy. *Ann Surg,* 194:279–289, 1981.
337. Henderson, R.D. and Marryatt, G.: Cricopharyngeal Myotomy as a Method of Treating Cricopharyngeal Dysphagia Secondary to Gastroesophageal Reflux. *J Thorac Cardiovasc Surg,* 74:721–725, 1977.
338. Sutherland, H.D.: Cricopharyngeal Achalasia. *J Thorac Cardiovasc Surg,* 43:114–126, 1962.
339. Falor, W.H., Miller, J., Kraus, J., *et al.*: Twenty-Four-Hour Monitoring of Esophagopharyngeal pH in Outpatients. Use of Four-Channel pH Probe and Computerized System. *J Thorac Cardiovasc Surg,* 91:716–722, 1986.
340. Kennedy, J.H.: "Silent" Gastroesophageal Reflux: An Important but Little Known Cause of Pulmonary Complications. *Dis Chest,* 42:42–45, 1962.
341. Ducolone, A., Vandevenne, A., Jouin, H., *et al.*: Gastroesophageal Reflux in Patients With Asthma and Chronic Bronchitis. *Am Rev Respir Dis,* 135:327–332, 1987.
342. Kelly, K., Latimer, J. and Johnson, L.: Dual pH Probes for the Evaluation of Gastroesophageal Reflux in Pediatric Patients with Chronic Pulmonary Symptoms. *Gastroenterology,* 90:1489, 1986. Abstract.
343. Mays, E.E.: Intrinsic Asthma in Adults. Association With Gastroesophageal Reflux. *JAMA,* 236:2626–2628, 1976.
344. Mansfield, L.E.: Gastroesophageal Reflux and Respiratory Disorders: A Review. *Ann Allergy,* 62:158–163, 1989.
345. Ekström, T. and Tibbling, L.: Influence of Theophylline on Gastro-oesophageal Reflux and Asthma. *Eur J Clin Pharmacol,* 35:353–356, 1988.
346. Hubert, D., Gaudric, M., Guerre, J., *et al.*: Effect of Theophylline on Gastroesophageal Reflux in Patients With Asthma. *J Allergy Clin Immunol,* 81:1168–1174, 1988.
347. Fordtran, J.S. and Collyns, J.A.H.: Antacid Pharmacology in Duodenal Ulcer. Effect of Antacids on Postcibal Gastric Acidity and Peptic Activity. *N Engl J Med,* 274:921–927, 1966.
348. McHardy, G.: A Multicentric, Randomized Clinical Trial of Gaviscon in Reflux Esophagitis. *South Med J,* 71(Suppl 1):16–21, 1978.
349. Graham, D.Y., Lanza, F. and Dorsch, E.R.: Symptomatic Reflux Esophagitis: A Double-Blind Controlled Comparison of Antacids and Alginate. *Curr Ther Res,* 22:653–658, 1977.
350. Johnson, L.F. and DeMeester, T.R.: Evaluation of Elevation of the Head of the Bed, Bethanechol, and Antacid Foam Tablets on Gastroesophageal Reflux. *Dig Dis Sci,* 26:673–680, 1981.
351. Richter, J.E.: A Critical Review of Current Medical Therapy for Gastroesophageal Reflux Disease. *J Clin Gastroenterol,* 8(Suppl 1):72–80, 1986.
352. Castell, D.O.: Long-Term Therapy for Chronic Gastroesophageal Reflux (Editorial). *Arch Intern Med,* 147:1701–1702, 1987.
353. Feldman, M., Richardson, C.T., Peterson, W.L., *et al.*: Effect of Low-Dose Propantheline on Food-Stimulated Gastric Acid Secretion. Comparison with an "Optimal Effective Dose" and an Interaction with Cimetidine. *N Engl J Med,* 297:1427–1430, 1977.
354. Koelz, H.R., Birchler, R., Bretholz, A., *et al.*: Healing and Relapse of Reflux Esophagitis during Treatment with Ranitidine. *Gastroenterology,* 91:1198–1205, 1986.
355. Johansson, K.-E., Boeryd, B., Johansson, K., *et al.*: Double-Blind Crossover Study of Ranitidine and Placebo in Gastro-oesophageal Reflux Disease. *Scand J Gastroenterol,* 21:769–778, 1986.
356. Sontag, S., Robinson, M., McCallum, R.W., *et al.*: Ranitidine Therapy for Gastroesophageal Reflux Disease. Results of a Large Double-Blind Trial. *Arch Intern Med,* 147:1485–1491, 1987.
357. Stalnikowicz-Darvasi, R.: H_2 Antagonists in the Treatment of Reflux Esophagitis: A Critical Analysis. *Am J Gastroenterol,* 84:245–248, 1989.
358. Johansson, K.-E. and Tibbling, L.: Maintenance Treatment with Ranitidine Compared with Fundoplication in Gastro-oesophageal Reflux Disease. *Scand J Gastroenterol,* 21:779–788, 1986.
359. Sandmark, S., Carlsson, R., Fausa, O., *et al.*: Omeprazole or Ranitidine in the Treatment of Reflux Esophagitis. Results of a Double-Blind, Randomized, Scandinavian Multicenter Study. *Scand J Gastroenterol,* 23:625–632, 1988.
360. Vantrappen, G., Rutgeerts, L., Schurmans, P., *et al.*: Omeprazole (40 mg) is Superior to Ranitidine in Short-Term Treatment of Ulcerative Reflux Esophagitis. *Dig Dis Sci,* 33:523–529, 1988.
361. Richards, D.A.: Comparative Pharmacodynamics and Pharmacokinetics of Cimetidine and Ranitidine. *J Clin Gastroenterol,* 5(Suppl 1):81–93, 1983.
362. Baldi, F., Bianchi Porro, G., Dobrilla, G., *et al.*: Cisapride Versus Placebo in Reflux Esophagitis. A Multicenter Double-Blind Trial. *J Clin Gastroenterol,* 10(6):614–618, 1988.
363. Klinkenberg-Knol, E.C., Jansen, J.M.B.J., Festen, H.P.M., *et al.*: Double-Blind Multicentre Comparison of Omeprazole and Ranitidine in the Treatment of Reflux Oesophagitis. *Lancet,* 1:349–351, 1987.
364. Scarpignato, C.: Pharmacological Bases of the Medical Treatment of Gastroesophageal Reflux Disease. *Dig Dis,* 6:117–148, 1988.
365. Walan, A.: Clinical Perspectives of Drugs Inhibiting Acid Secretion—H^+K^+-ATPase Inhibitors. *Scand J Gastroenterol (Suppl 125),* 21:50–53, 1986.
366. Castell, D.O.: Future Medical Therapy of Reflux Esophagitis. *J Clin Gastroenterol,* 8(Suppl 1):81–85, 1986.
367. Schweitzer, E.J., Bass, B.L., Johnson, L.F., *et al.*: Sucralfate Prevents Experimental Peptic Esophagitis in Rabbits. *Gastroenterology,* 88:611–619, 1985.
368. Tytgat, G.N.J.: Clinical Efficacy of Sucralfate in Reflux Oesophagitis. *Scand J Gastroenterol (Suppl 140),* 22:29–31, 1987.
369. Katz, P.O., Geisinger, K.R., Hassan, M., *et al.*: Acid-Induced Esophagitis in Cats is Prevented by Sucralfate but not Synthetic Prostaglandin E. *Dig Dis Sci,* 33:217–224, 1988.
370. Little, A.G., Ferguson, M.K. and Skinner, D.B.: Reoperation for Failed Antireflux Operations. *J Thorac Cardiovasc Surg,* 91:511–517, 1986.
371. Low, D.E., Mercer, C.D., James, E.C., *et al.*: Post Nissen Syndrome. *Surg Gynecol Obstet,* 167:1–5, 1988.
372. St. Cyr, J.A., Ferrara, T.B., Thompson, T.R., *et al.*: Nissen Fundoplication for Gastroesophageal Reflux in Infants. *J Thorac Cardiovasc Surg,* 92:661–666, 1986.
373. Stirling, M.C. and Orringer, M.B.: Continued Assessment of the Combined Collis-Nissen Operation. *Ann Thorac Surg,* 47:224–230, 1989.
374. Stuart, R.C., Dawson, K., Keeling, P., *et al.*: A Prospective Randomized Trial of Angelchik Prosthesis Versus Nissen Fundoplication. *Br J Surg,* 76:86–89, 1989.
375. Turnage, R.H., Oldham, K.T., Coran, A.G., *et al.*: Late Results of Fundoplication for Gastroesophageal Reflux in Infants and Children. *Surgery,* 105:457–464, 1989.
376. Waters, P.F. and DeMeester, T.R.: Foregut Motor Disorders and Their Surgical Management. *Med Clin North Am,* 65(6):1235–1268, 1981.
377. Csendes, A., Braghetto, I., Korn, O., *et al.*: Late Subjective and Objective Evaluations of Antireflux Surgery in Patients With Reflux Esophagitis: Analysis of 215 Patients. *Surgery,* 105:374–382, 1989.
378. Johnsson, F., Joelsson, B., Gudmundsson, K., *et al.*: Effects of Fundoplication on the Antireflux Mechanism. *Br J Surg,* 74:1111–1114, 1987.
379. Benjamin, S.B., Kerr, R., Cohen, D., *et al.*: Complications of the Angelchik Antireflux Prosthesis. *Ann Intern Med,* 100:570–575, 1984.
380. Benjamin, S.B., Knuff, T.K., Fink, M., *et al.*: The Angelchik Antireflux Prosthesis. Effects on the Lower Esophageal Sphincter of Primates. *Ann Surg,* 197:63–67, 1983.
381. Henderson, R.D., Marryatt, G. and Henderson, R.F.: Review of

the Surgical Management of Recurrent Hiatal Hernia: 5-Year Follow-Up. *Can J Surg,* 31:341–345, 1988.
382. Rokkas, T. and Sladen, G.E.: Ambulatory Esophageal pH Recording in Gastroesophageal Reflux: Relevance to the Development of Esophagitis. *Am J Gastroenterol,* 83:629–632, 1988.
383. Smith, V.M.: Gastroesophageal Reflux, *JAMA,* 245:406, 1981.
384. Stirling, M.C. and Orringer, M.B.: Surgical Treatment after the Failed Antireflux Operation. *J Thorac Cardiovasc Surg,* 92:667–672, 1986.
385. Samloff, I.M. and Taggart, R.T.: Pepsinogens, Pepsins, and Peptic Ulcer. *Clin Invest Med,* 10:215–221, 1987.
386. Lillemoe, K.D., Johnson, L.F. and Harmon, J.W.: Role of the Components of the Gastroduodenal Contents in Experimental Acid Esophagitis. *Surgery,* 92:276–284, 1982.
387. Johnson, L.F. and Harmon, J.W.: Experimental Esophagitis in a Rabbit Model. Clinical Relevance. *J Clin Gastroenterol,* 8(Suppl 1):26–44, 1986.
388. Penagini, R., Yuen, H., Misiewicz, J.J., *et al.*: Alkaline Intraoesophageal pH and Gastro-oesophageal Reflux in Patients with Peptic Oesophagitis. *Scand J Gastroenterol,* 23:675–680, 1988.
389. Goldberg, H.I., Dodds, W.J., Gee, S., *et al.*: Role of Acid and Pepsin in Acute Experimental Esophagitis. *Gastroenterology,* 56:223–230, 1969.
390. Piper, D.W. and Fenton, B.H.: pH Stability and Activity Curves of Pepsin with Special Reference to Their Clinical Importance. *Gut,* 6:506–508, 1965.
391. Wiener, G.J., Morgan, T.M., Copper, J.B., *et al.*: Ambulatory 24-Hour Esophageal pH Monitoring. Reproducibility and Variability of pH Parameters. *Dig Dis Sci,* 33:1127–1133, 1988.
392. Haase, G.M., Ross, M.N., Gance-Cleveland, B., *et al.*: Extended Four-Channel Esophageal pH Monitoring: The Importance of Acid Reflux Patterns at the Middle and Proximal Levels. *J Pediatr Surg,* 23:32–37, 1988.
393. Baldi, F., Ferrarini, F., Longanesi, A., *et al.*: Extension of Acid Gastroesophageal Reflux and Its Relation With Symptoms: An Assessment with Double Esophageal pH Recording. *Gastroenterology,* 94:A19, 1988. Abstract.
394. Goode, R.L. and Shinn, J.B.: Long-Term Stenting in the Treatment of Subglottic Stenosis. *Ann Otol Rhinol Laryngol,* 86:795–798, 1977.
395. Schuller, D.E.: Long-Term Stenting for Laryngotracheal Stenosis. *Ann Otol Rhinol Laryngol,* 89:515–520, 1980.
396. Thompson, J.N.: Corrosive Esophageal Injuries. I. A Study of Nine Cases of Concurrent Accidental Caustic Ingestion. LARYNGOSCOPE, 97:1060–1068, 1987.
397. Thompson, J.N.: Corrosive Esophageal Injuries. II. An Investigation of Treatment Methods and Histochemical Analysis of Esophageal Strictures in a New Animal Model. LARYNGOSCOPE, 97:1191–1202, 1987.

APPENDICES

APPENDIX A: DATA FLOW SHEET: AMBULATORY 24-HOUR pH MONITORING

(1) Series #: ____________
Patient Name: ____________ Unit Number: ____________
Telephone Number: (H) ____________, (W) ____________ Date: ____________
(2) Presumptive Dx(s): ____________
(3) Age: ______ (4) Sex: /1/ Male /2/ Female
(5) Race: /1/ Caucasian /2/ Black /3/ Oriental /4/ Other: ____________

(6) pH probe:
/1/ Single Probe
/2/ Double Probe
/3/ Other: ____________

(7) /1/ Diagnostic
/2/ On Treatment
/3/ Call-Back
/4/ Other: ____________

(8) Cohort
/1/ Carcinoma
/2/ Stenosis
/3/ Laryngitis
/4/ Globus
/5/ Dysphagia
/6/ Chr. Cough
/7/ Other: ____________

(9) Study Number: /1/ First /2/ Second /3/ Third

HISTORY

(10) Never Used Tobacco

Tobacco Consumption

(11) Cigarettes	(12) PPD: ______	(13) Pack years: ______
(14) Ex-Smoker	(15) Pack years: ______	(16) Years ago quit: ______
(17) Smokeless	(18) Hours/day: ______	(19) Years: ______
(20) Cigar	(21) Cigars/day: ______	(22) Years: ______
(23) Pipe	(24) Bowls/day: ______	(25) Years: ______

Alcohol Consumption

(26) None
(27) Social
(28) Social binger
(29) Moderate
(30) Heavy

(31) Medication History
/1/ Med's associated with GI symptoms
/2/ Med's not associated with GI symptoms
/3/ Other: ____________

Past Medical Hx

(32) Ulcer hx: /1/ no /2/ yes (year: ______)
(33) Previous UGI tract surgery: /1/ no /2/ yes
(34) Diabetes: ____________
(35) ASCVD: ____________
(36) Other: ____________

Dietary Hx

(37) Coffee:	/1/ None	/2/ 1–3 cups/day	/3/ ≥4 cups/day
(38) Tea:	/1/ None	/2/ 1–3 cups/day	/3/ ≥4 cups/day
(39) Soda:	/1/ None	/2/ 1–3 cans/day	/3/ ≥4 cans/day
(40) Chocolate:	/1/ None	/2/ ≥4 × /wk	/3/ daily
(41) Mints:	/1/ None	/2/ ≥4 × /wk	/3/ daily
(42) Fried Food:	/1/ None	/2/ ≥4 × /wk	/3/ daily

(43) Dietary Score (Total of items 37–42): ______

SYMPTOMS

(44) **Heartburn or Regurgitation**
/1/ None
/2/ 0–1 episodes per week
/3/ 2–4 episodes per week
/4/ Frequently (daily)
/5/ Most of the time

OTHER SYMPTOMS

(45) Intermittent hoarseness
(46) Chronic hoarseness
(47) Globus
(48) Dysphagia
(49) Throat clearing
(50) Chronic cough

(51) Use Tums, Rolaids, or other antacids: /1/ no /2/ yes

FINDINGS

(52) Height (in.): ____________ (53) Weight (lbs.): ____________

(54) **Laryngeal Examination:** /1/ not done /2/ normal /3/ abnormal

(55) Mild edema	(58) Posterior erythema	(61) Granulation	(64) Carcinoma
(56) Moderate edema	(59) Diffuse erythema	(62) Leukoplakia	(65) Other: ____
(57) Severe edema	(60) Ulceration	(63) Stenosis	______

(66) **Barium Swallow:** /1/ Not done /2/ Normal /3/ Abnormal

(67) Hiatal hernia	(72) Dysmotility
(68) Stricture	(73) Achalasia
(69) Radiological reflux	(74) Ring
(70) Esophagitis	(75) Other: ____________
(71) Esophagitis w/erosions	

(76) **Endoscopy:** /1/ Not done /2/ Normal /3/ Abnormal

(77) Erythema/mild esophagitis
(78) Esophagitis w/Erosions
(79) Barrett's esophagitis
(80) Stricture
(81) Cancer
(82) Other: ____________

(83) **Manometry:** /1/ Not done /2/ Normal /3/ Abnormal

(84) Achalasia
(85) "Nutcracker" esophagus
(86) Diffuse spasm (DES)
(87) Nonspecific motility disorder
(88) Other: ____________

pH MONITORING RESULTS

	Esoph	Normal	Pharynx
% Time pH ≤4, upright ______	(89) ______	≤5.85	(92) ______
% Time pH ≤4, supine ______	(90) ______	≤1.81	(93) ______
% Time pH ≤4, total ______	(91) ______	≤4.39	(94) ______

(95) **pH Probe Interpretation**
/1/ Normal
/2/ Abnormal esophagus
/3/ Abnormal pharynx
/4/ Both abnormal
/5/ Pseudo pharynx reflux
/6/ Other: ____________

(96) **Medical Treatment**
/1/ None
/2/ ART
/3/ ART & H_2: ____________
/4/ Other: ____________

(97) Duration of Rx (months): ______
(98) Follow Up (months): ____________

(99) **Outcome:** /1/ Resolved
/2/ Relapses
/3/ Persistent Sx
/4/ Dead
/5/ Lost to Follow Up
/6/ Other: ____________

(100) Fundoplication: ____________

COMMENTS ____________

KEY TO APPENDIX B

Group:
A—pH manometry performed before initiation of antireflux therapy, "Clean Diagnostic Tests"
B—Diagnostic pH manometry performed 3 weeks to 3 months after initiation of antireflux therapy, "Already on ART"

Barium Swallow Esophagogram: (Ba Sw)
nl = Normal
b = Barrett's esophagus
c = Cricopharyngeal abnormality
d = Dysmotility
e = Esophagitis
h = Hiatal hernia
r = Free reflux
rl = Lower esophageal ring
s = Stricture

Esophageal pH Manometry Results: [ ] indicate abnormal values

Pharyngeal Probe Results:
Phx Probe = Pharyngeal Probe
N = normal
A = abnormal
– = not done

Other Data:
F = Fundoplication
D = Died
L = Leukoplakia
T = Tracheotomy in place
G = Granuloma or granulation
NS = lifetime nonsmoker (group I only)
UESP = Upper esophageal sphincter pressure
X—Patient underwent pH-metry on two occasions (the first study was normal, the second was abnormal)
Y—pH-metry normal, but barium esophagogram (BA SW) demonstrated free reflux and/or esophagitis
Z—Pharyngeal probe positive for reflux with a normal esophageal study

APPENDIX B: RAW DATA GROUP I: CARCINOMA.

				Ambulatory 24-Hour pH Manometry				
				Esophageal Probe*				
Patient	Group	Age/ Sex	BA SW	Upright	Supine	Total	Phx Probe	Other Data
1. MB	A	56F	nl	[11.6]	1.6	[8.0]	A	F
2. JB	A	75M	h,e,ri	3.4	[2.5]	2.9	–	NS,G,F
3. MB	A	57F	–	[18.0]	[3.0]	[13.0]	A	G,F
4. RB	A	46M	h	3.0	0.0	2.2	N	G
5. HB	A	63M	h	[6.2]	0.0	4.1	A	
6. SC	A	37F	–	[6.9]	0.0	[4.7]	–	NS
7. HC	A	53M	h	[17.0]	[12.7]	[15.4]	A	
8. ED	A	70M	h,r,d	[23.0]	0.1	[11.4]	A	
9. FG	A	42M	h,e,ri	1.0	[15.0]	[8.0]	A	NS,G,X
10. HH	A	66M	–	[22.1]	[32.1]	[42.0]	A	NS
11. WH	A	67M	d	[8.0]	[9.7]	[8.8]	A	NS,G,F
12. HH	A	76M	–	[6.6]	[3.5]	[5.3]	A	
13. FJ	A	58F	nl	[30.0]	[42.0]	[35.0]	A	
14. SK	A	45M	h,r	1.0	1.0	1.0	N	L Y
15. FM	A	51M	h	[7.5]	[19.3]	[12.9]	–	F,D
16. TM	A	68M	–	2.0	0.0	1.0	A	Z
17. MS	A	57F	–	[7.0]	0.0	[4.5]	A	
18. BS	A	56M	–	1.0	0.0	1.0	A	G Z
19. JS	A	56M	–	0.6	0.0	0.4	A	Z
20. MT	A	72M	h,d,ri	[16.1]	[5.2]	[11.5]	N	
21. MT	A	56M	h	[6.0]	[2.0]	0.0	–	D
22. HD	A	48M	h	[10.1]	[7.8]	[9.2]	–	
23. RH	A	53M	h,s	2.1	0.1	1.5	N	
24. RP	A	54M	h,d	[9.8]	0.0	[5.8]	N	
25. JL	A	72M	h	2.4	0.0	1.7	N	
26. RB	B	53F	–	0.3	0.0	0.1	N	G
27. SB	B	67M	h,e	2.0	0.0	1.0	N	D Y
28. AD	B	34F	h	2.0	1.0	2.0	N	
29. RO	B	66M	h,r,d	0.0	0.0	0.0	N	NS,D,Y
30. AS	B	74M	h	2.4	1.8	2.2	N	
31. HS	B	55F	–	[6.8]	0.0	[4.8]	A	G

*[ ] indicate abnormal values.

Group Key

A = "clean" diagnostic tests; B = already on antireflux therapy; NS = lifetime nonsmoker.

APPENDIX B: RAW DATA GROUP II: SUBGLOTTIC STENOSIS.

				Ambulatory 24-Hour pH Manometry				
				Esophageal Probe*				
Patient	Group	Age/ Sex	BA SW	Upright	Supine	Total	Phx Probe	Other Data
32. HH	A	.5F	r	[10.4]	[3.9]	[5.0]	A	F,T
33. BR	A	2M	–	[9.4]	[33.3]	[26.7]	–	F
34. SW	A	2M	–	[13.5]	[16.6]	[15.4]	–	
35. ML	A	2M	–	0.7	[2.2]	1.3	–	X
36. CL	A	3M	–	[21.0]	[3.0]	[13.0]	–	
37. JT	A	5M	nl	[23.9]	0.0	[11.7]	–	
38. CC	A	6M	–	[18.5]	[5.7]	[12.7]	–.	
39. JW	A	6F	–	2.0	1.0	3.0	–	
40. KC	A	12M	–	[29.0]	[13.4]	[23.4]	A	F X
41. JD	A	37M	nl	[15.5]	[3.2]	[10.9]	–	
42. LS	A	48M	h	5.0	[18.0]	[10.0]	–	F
43. CZ	A	21M	h	1.8	0.0	1.0	A	F X,Z
44. WA	A	47M	–	[39.7]	[32.8]	[38.0]	–	
45. RH	A	21M	–	[8.4]		[8.4]	A	F,T
46. RP	A	42F	h	1.0	0.0	1.0	N	
47. CS	A	30F	h,r	1.0	[11.0]	[6.8]	A	F
48. EH	A	56F	h,r	[23.7]	[6.7]	[15.9]	N	
49. JH	A	24F	–	3.0	[3.0]	3.0	N	
50. KD	A	29F	–	2.6	0.0	1.6	A	Z
51. BE	A	53F	–	[23.0]	1.5	[13.5]	A	
52. MK	A	69F	h	[20.0]	[3.4]	[16.3]	A	
53. VP	A	62F	h	[32.3]	0.0	[9.8]	A	T X
54. DL	A	73F	h	[8.0]	1.0	4.0	–	F
55. LF	A	65F	nl	[10.1]	1.4	[8.1]	N	T
56. PM	A	63F	–	0.2	0.0	0.2	A	Z
57. SR	B	.3M	–	0.0	0.5	1.0	–	
58. JC	B	7M	nl	0.0	0.2	0.1	–	T
59. CS	B	51M	–	0.3	0.0	0.2	N	
60. TH	B	19M	–	2.0	0.0	1.0	N	
61. BC	B	44F	–	[9.0]	0.0	[5.9]	–	T
62. FA	B	53M	nl	[8.1]	[10.6]	[9.0]	N	
63. RB	B	39F	h,r	3.3	0.0	1.8	N	F,T,Y

*[ ] Indicate abnormal values.

Group Key

A = "clean" diagnostic tests; b = already on antireflux therapy.

APPENDIX B: RAW DATA GROUP III: REFLUX LARYNGITIS.

				Ambulatory 24-Hour pH Manometry					
				Esophageal Probe*					
Patient	Group	Age/ Sex	BA SW	Upright	Supine	Total	Phx Probe	Other Data	
64. GB	A	49F	h,e	2.0	[8.0]	4.0	N	L	
65. PB	A	45F	–	3.6	[10.9]	[6.2]	N		
66. FB	A	66M	–	[5.8]	0.0	3.9	A		
67. JC	A	56M	–	[17.5]	0.0	[10.0]	N		
68. MC	A	20M	–	1.0	[2.0]	1.0	N	G	
69. RC	A	63M	h	1.0	0.0	1.0	N		
70. BC	A	34F	–	[7.0]	[4.0]	[6.0]	N		
71. WC	A	63M	h,e,s	[22.7]	[30.7]	[26.0]	–		
72. FC	A	61M	nl	1.0	0.0	1.0	N		
73. MC	A	42M	nl	3.1	[5.4]	3.8	–	F	
74. MD	A	62F	nl	1.2	[7.6]	4.0	–	G	
75. ED	A	37M	–	1.0	0.0	1.0	N		
76. EF	A	42M	nl	1.0	[3.0]	1.0	–		
77. DG	A	36M	e	1.0	0.0	1.0	N		Y
78. PH	A	70F	h,r,d	[28.1]	[2.3]	[19.3]	N		
79. KH	A	30F	h	[12.6]	[2.6]	[8.9]	A		
80. CH	A	30F	nl	[13.6]	0.0	[6.9]	N		
81. LL	A	50F	–	[12.8]	[5.5]	[10.1]	N		
82. WL	A	36M	h	1.0	1.0	1.0	N		
83. CM	A	36M	h	4.6	0.2	2.9	N		
84. VM	A	55F	h	[5.9]	[7.2]	[6.5]	N	F	
85. OM	A	68F	h,d	1.3	[3.3]	2.2	A		
86. WN	A	56M	–	2.0	0.0	1.0	N	G	
87. SN	A	30F	nl	1.0	1.0	1.0	N		
88. EP	A	63F	h,e	1.0	0.0	1.0	N		Y
89. RR	A	51M	–	5.6	[8.0]	[9.3]	N	G	
90. GR	A	31M	h	3.0	[3.0]	3.0	A		
91. JR	A	50M	h,rl,b	5.2	1.0	3.6	A		Z
92. RS	A	45M	–	1.0	[9.0]	[5.0]	N		
93. VS	A	67F	–	3.9	0.0	2.3	N		
94. GS	A	56M	h	[16.2]	0.7	3.1	N	G	X
95. ES	A	73M	h,e,d	[11.7]	1.0	[7.0]	N		
96. JS	A	50M	h,rl	2.3	0.1	1.2	N	L	
97. JW	A	59M	h,d,r	[7.0]	[27.0]	[12.0]	A		
98. MW	A	55F	d	[14.6]	[3.3]	[9.0]	–	G	
99. JW	A	38M	h,e	4.7	0.7	3.3	N	G	Y
100. MB	B	36M	h	2.0	1.0	1.0	N		
101. SB	B	55M	h,rl	4.0	1.0	3.0	N		
102. BB	B	41F	nl	0.0	1.0	1.0	N		
103. EC	B	73M	h	0.0	0.0	0.0	N	G	
104. JE	B	60M	h	1.0	1.0	0.0	N	G	
105. BM	B	55F	–	0.9	0.0	0.4	N		
106. JO	B	47M	h,e,rl	[9.0]	1.0	[5.0]	N	L	
107. MP	B	52F	h	3.0	[4.0]	3.0	–		
108. DR	B	37M	nl	4.0	[7.0]	4.0	N		
109. JS	B	38F	nl	0.6	0.0	0.9	N		
110. SS	B	31F	nl	3.9	0.3	2.4	A	Z	
111. MW	B	59F	h	4.9	[13.0]	[6.5]	N		

*[ ] indicate abnormal values.

Group Key

A = "clean" diagnostic tests; B = already on antireflux therapy.

APPENDIX B: RAW DATA GROUP IV: GLOBUS.

Patient	Group	Age/ Sex	BA SW	Ambulatory 24-Hour pH Manometry: Esophageal Probe* Upright	Supine	Total	Phx Probe	Other Data
112. WA	A	24M	–	0.8	1.6	1.3	N	
113. FB	A	42F	nl	3.0	0.0	3.0	–	
114. RB	A	67F	h,c	[6.9]	[9.0]	[8.0]	A	
115. EC	A	53F	nl	1.0	0.0	0.0	–	
116. RD	A	53M	–	3.3	[8.8]	[5.7]	A	UESP 177
117. RF	A	73M	h,r,s,e,b	[56.0]	[17.0]	[61.0]	–	F
118. PG	A	68M	h,ri	[7.0]	[18.0]	[11.0]	N	
119. WH	A	38F	nl	3.9	0.2	3.0	A	Z
120. SH	A	38M	h	[7.3]	[12.0]	[9.7]	–	
121. BK	A	67F	h	1.3	0.4	1.0	N	
122. TK	A	30M	h,e	3.0	1.0	2.0	N	Y
123. JL	A	45M	h	[9.5]	[2.6]	[7.4]	N	
124. DM	A	58M	nl	[16.0]	0.0	[11.0]	–	
125. HM	A	60M	h,r,b	3.2	[5.7]	[4.9]	A	L
126. MM	A	66F	h	[19.7]	[7.4]	[12.7]	N	
127. RN	A	26M	h,e	[19.7]	[7.4]	[12.7]	N	
128. JN	A	60M	–	[8.8]	[5.9]	[7.5]	N	
129. RR	A	31M	e	[20.0]	[24.0]	[25.0]	N	
130. MS	A	25F	d	0.0	0.0	0.0	N	
131. SV	A	39F	nl	1.0	0.0	1.0	N	
132. JW	A	59M	–	[7.0]	[27.0]	[12.0]	A	
133. CW	A	57M	h,d	1.0	0.0	1.0	–	
134. CM	B	54M	h,e,ri	1.0	0.0	1.0	N	G Y
135. WM	B	44M	h,d,e	0.0	0.0	1.7	N	L Y

*[ ] indicate abnormal values.

Group Key

A = "clean" diagnostic tests; B = already on antireflux therapy.

APPENDIX B: RAW DATA GROUP V: SORE THROAT/DYSPHAGIA.

Patient	Group	Age/Sex	BA SW	Ambulatory 24-Hour pH Manometry: Esophageal Probe* Upright	Supine	Total	Phx Probe	Other Data
136. GB	A	62F	h,ri,s	3.4	[8.7]	[5.3]	N	
137. BB	A	34F	nl	2.5	0.0	1.6	N	
138. LB	A	87F	h,d,ri	1.0	1.0	1.0	N	
139. EB	A	45M	ri	5.0	[3.0]	4.0	A	
140. GD	A	44F	h	[6.1]	0.0	3.5	–	
141. CG	A	73F	h,e,ri	1.0	0.0	1.0	N	Y
142. MH	A	27M	h,d	1.0	[22.0]	[14.0]	N	
143. RH	A	44M	nl	2.0	0.0	1.0	N	
144. SJ	A	45F	h,r	[6.2]	[4.6]	[5.7]	N	
145. AL	A	41M	h,e	1.0	1.0	1.0	N	Y
146. PL	A	46M	h,e,ri	5.0	[3.0]	4.0	N	
147. CM	A	45M	h	0.0	0.0	0.0	N	
148. MM	A	61F	–	[31.9]	0.1	[25.0]	–	
149. FP	A	54F	h	2.5	0.4	1.8	N	
150. OR	A	65F	h	0.0	0.0	0.0	N	
151. LR	A	35M	h,d	1.0	0.0	1.0	N	
152. CT	A	30F	h,e	0.0	0.0	0.0	N	Y
153. ET	A	80F	h,ri	[14.0]	0.0	[10.0]	N	
154. SW	A	19F	h,ri	3.0	1.0	2.0	N	
155. CW	A	24M	nl	1.0	0.0	1.0	N	
156. FC	B	51F	h,ri	[8.8]	[9.7]	[9.2]	N	
157. DM	B	22F	h	[15.3]	[5.7]	[10.6]	A	

*[ ] indicate abnormal values.

Group Key

A = "clean" diagnostic tests; B = already on antireflux therapy.

APPENDIX B: RAW DATA GROUP VI: CHRONIC COUGH.

Patient	Group	Age/ Sex	BA SW	Ambulatory 24-Hour pH Manometry: Esophageal Probe*				Other Data
				Upright	Supine	Total	Phx Probe	
158. WB	A	48F	h,d	0.0	0.0	0.0	N	
159. WB	A	43M	h,r,e,d	1.0	0.0	1.0	A	Z
160. EC	A	56F	nl	1.0	0.0	1.0	N	
161. JC	A	62M	—	[7.0]	1.0	3.0	N	
162. HH	A	39F	h,d	1.0	0.0	1.0	N	
163. RH	A	50M	—	1.0	0.0	1.0	N	
164. CH	A	73M	h,e	1.0	0.0	1.0	N	F Y
165. WH	A	28M	nl	[6.0]	0.0	4.0	N	
166. HK	A	56F	—	[8.0]	1.0	[7.0]	N	
167. EL	A	63F	nl	1.0	0.0	1.0	N	
168. WL	A	72M	—	[10.0]	[10.0]	[10.0]	A	
169. CM	A	1M	—	[6.8]	[27.3]	[17.4]	–	
170. SR	A	37F	h	2.0	1.0	1.0	N	
171. SR	A	35M	e	[9.8]	[13.5]	[11.4]	–	
172. SS	A	37F	—	1.0	0.0	1.0	N	
173. CS	A	61F	—	0.5	[6.3]	3.0	N	
174. JS	A	70M	—	3.0	1.0	2.0	A	Z
175. ET	A	59F	h,rl	[14.0]	0.0	[10.0]	N	
176. DT	A	37M	nl	1.0	1.0	1.0	N	
177. MW	A	59F	h	4.9	[13.0]	[6.5]	N	
178. MB	B	30F	h	1.3	[8.3]	4.3	A	F
179. PD	B	52F	h	1.0	1.0	1.0	N	
180. EE	B	49F	nl	1.0	0.0	1.0	N	
181. DW	B	54F	—	1.0	0.0	1.0	N	
182. LW	B	65F	—	0.0	0.8	0.3	A	Z

*[ ] indicate abnormal values.
Group Key
A = "clean" diagnostic tests; B = already on antireflux therapy.

APPENDIX B: RAW DATA GROUP VII: MISCELLANEOUS.

Patient	Group	Age/ Sex	BA SW	Ambulatory 24-Hour pH Manometry: Esophageal Probe*				Other Data
				Upright	Supine	Total	Phx Probe	
183. MB	A	39F	nl	0.1	0.0	0.8	N	
184. PB	A	42F	—	0.0	1.0	1.0	A	
185. CB	A	79M	—	0.7	0.0	0.5	N	
186. BC	A	53F	—	1.0	1.0	1.0	N	
187. WC	A	58M	—	1.0	0.0	1.0	N	
188. AC	A	65F	d	1.0	0.0	1.0	N	
189. JD	A	45F	—	2.0	0.0	1.0	–	
190. BH	A	63F	h,r	[22.6]	[9.9]	[15.2]	–	
191. FL	A	40F	—	0.0	0.0	0.0	–	
192. JN	A	46F	—	1.5	0.0	1.0	N	
193. GR	A	73M	h,e,d	1.0	1.0	1.0	N	Y
194. JW	A	70M	—	1.0	1.0	1.0	N	
195. OS	B	62M	h	2.0	0.0	1.0	N	F
196. JS	B	53M	nl	0.0	0.0	3.0	N	
197. JW	B	37F	—	1.0	0.0	1.0	N	

*[ ] indicate abnormal values.
Group Key
A = "clean" diagnostic tests; B = already on antireflux therapy.

APPENDIX C: REPRESENTATIVE CASE REPORTS

Case 1: Recurrent Mucosal Carcinoma of the Larynx in a Nonsmoker (Patient 9)

In March of 1980, a 42-year-old, nondrinking, nonsmoking, real estate broker presented with a 1-month history of hoarseness. For the previous 5 years, he had had a history of intermittent hoarseness. His medical history was noncontributory and he specifically denied heartburn, regurgitation, dysphagia, odynophagia, or cough.

Examination revealed a red, 3-ml dome-shaped lesion on the free edge of the midleft vocal cord. In April of 1980, he underwent suspension microlaryngoscopy and laser excision of the lesion. The histopathology was reported as microinvasive carcinoma. Postoperatively, granulation tissue appeared at the operative site, which had a gray, shaggy, gelatinous appearance with little surrounding erythema. After 3 months without change, the granuloma was excised and the histopathology was benign. The second biopsy site did not heal for 2 months.

The patient was followed closely, and in March of 1983 the superior surface of the left true cord at the anterior commissure appeared to have an area of erythroplakia. One month later, the area of erythroplakia had grown in size; 1 month after that, the lesion involved the anterior third of the vocal cord. In March of 1983, the patient underwent microlaryngeal excision of the vocal cord lesion, which proved histologically to be carcinoma *in situ*. Postoperatively, granulation tissue persisted for 2 months.

The patient did well until September of 1986, when he was found to have a left vocal process granuloma. Twenty-four-hour pH manometry was obtained. The esophageal probe demonstrated time pH was less than 4 to be 1.6% upright, 0% supine, and 1.07% total; there were no episodes of pharyngeal reflux (pH manometry was within normal limits). The "granulation tissue" persisted and was removed 2 months later. The excised lesion again was reported as carcinoma *in situ*. Repeat pH-metry was obtained, as well as a barium swallow. Barium esophagography revealed a hiatal hernia with mild esophagitis and a lower esophageal ring. This time the pH results demonstrated 1% upright reflux, 15% supine, and 8% total. During the supine period, there were five documented episodes of pharyngeal acid exposure.

The patient was placed on antireflux therapy, consisting of dietary modification, elevation of the head of the bed, antacids, and cimetidine (300 mg q.i.d.). Seven months after initiation of antireflux treatment, he again developed hoarseness and laryngeal erythema; he was referred for fundoplication. Since that time (now 3 years postfundoplication), the patient has maintained a normal laryngeal examination.

Comment: This patient developed three small mucosal carcinomas over a 6-year period and, when the lesions were removed endoscopically, on each occasion he developed exuberant granulation at the excisional biopsy site. He had no gastrointestinal symptoms and his hoarseness was intermittent. Indeed, his first pH study was within normal limits, whereas the second was grossly abnormal. This patient typifies a pattern of GERD that is both occult (silent) and intermittent.

Case 2: Carcinoma of the Larynx in the Nonsmoker Complicated by Postradiation Glottic Stenosis (Patient 2)

On March 8, 1988, a 75-year-old man presented with chronic cough, dyspnea, and aphonia. The dyspnea had been progressive over a 6-month period. His medical history was significant in that he had had a chronic cough for 3 years, dating back to October 1985. In addition, he had asthma-like symptoms and was under treatment by a pulmonologist. Also in 1985, a right vocal cord lesion had been found. He was treated with Cobalt 60 radiation in 30 fractions, receiving a total of 6000 rad, completed in December 1986. His medical history was otherwise noncontributory.

Examination of the larynx revealed marked edema with crusting and impaired mobility of the vocal cords bilaterally. There was an anterior glottic web and a posterior stenosis and the glottic chink was elliptical, measuring approximately 2 × 6 mm. (The intensity of the crusting was unusual. It had been assumed by his physicians that the crusting and stenosis were complications of radiation therapy.)

The patient underwent 24-hour pH manometry and barium swallow esophagography. The percentage of time pH was less than 4 in the supine position was abnormal (2.5%); the pharyngeal probe malfunctioned. Barium esophagography revealed hiatal hernia, lower esophageal ring, and moderate esophagitis.

The patient was started on an antireflux program, including antacids, dietary modification, elevation of the head of the bed, and ranitidine (150 mg b.i.d.). Six weeks later, there was no significant improvement and the patient continued to complain bitterly of his cough. The dose of ranitidine was increased to 300 mg b.i.d. After 6 months, there was marked improvement in the appearance of the larynx. Much of the crusting had subsided. An endoscopic laser procedure was carried out to open the glottic stenosis. The patient's postoperative course was uncomplicated, and epithelialization occurred rapidly, with improvement in the airway and moderate improvement of the voice.

Two months later, stenosis had redeveloped. A repeat pH study with the patient on antireflux therapy revealed abnormal upright and supine reflux, with one episode of pharyngeal positivity. The patient underwent fundoplication in January of 1989. At that time, the recurrent stenosis was opened. One month later, the larynx appeared pink, minimally edematous, and well-healed; the postfundoplication appearance of the larynx was dramatically improved.

Comment: This case was included because it illustrates that radiation therapy and other forms of treatment are often blamed for complications that may be the result of GERD.

Case 3: Carcinoma of the Larynx and Web Formation in the Nonsmoker (Patient 6)

A 37-year-old nonsmoking woman insurance adjuster presented with a vocal polyp in March of 1985. There was a small lesion on the opposite cord. Both were removed endoscopically with the carbon dioxide laser, leaving a substantial island of tissue at the anterior commissure on the left. Postoperatively, the patient developed a 70% glottic web and was referred to the author.

The patient underwent 24-hour pH manometry, which revealed abnormal upright reflux (6.9%). She was treated with an antireflux regimen and remained on medical antireflux treatment for 1 year. Three years later, she returned with recurrent (relative) glottic stenosis; repeat pH manometry was abnormal. She again was started on antireflux therapy. (This recurrence was recent and, therefore, the outcome of therapy remains to be seen.)

Comment: The postoperative complication (web formation) in this case was in all likelihood due to GERD, as was, perhaps, the development of her carcinoma as well. The recurrence of GERD after several "disease-free" years is evidence of the chronic intermittent nature of GERD in many otolaryngology patients. The relatively long duration of this patient's remission is not unusual.

Case 4: Carcinoma of the Larynx in a Nonsmoker; Uncontrolled GER Postoperatively (Patient 11)

A 67-year-old nondrinking, nonsmoking retired man presented with a 6-month history of hoarseness and a sensation of a lump in the throat. His medical history was noncontributory. Examination revealed an infiltrating lesion of the right true vocal cord with normal mobility of the arytenoid but impaired mobility of the vocal fold itself. The tongue base and hypopharynx appeared to have a purulent exudate and diffuse erythema.

Twenty-four-hour pH manometry revealed abnormal upright pH (8.0%), abnormal supine pH (9.7%), abnormal total pH (8.8%), and pharyngeal reflux. The patient was started on an antireflux program, including ranitidine (150 mg b.i.d.). One week later, he underwent a right vertical hemilaryngectomy and all the margins were free. The initial postoperative course was uneventful, although the patient did complain of some aspiration. He was discharged on the 12th postoperative day with his tracheotomy plugged.

Two weeks later, he was decannulated by his referring otolaryngologist. Four weeks after that, he presented to the emergency room in respiratory distress with inspiratory stridor, and complaining of increasing heartburn and regurgitation. The tracheotomy was replaced; however, even with the tracheotomy cuff inflated, he continued to aspirate gastric contents. Indeed, as the antireflux medications were increased, so were the symptoms. After 3 weeks of hospitalization, fundoplication was performed. The larynx appeared immobile and, even with the cuff inflated, aspiration of secretions still occurred. Six weeks later, a total laryngectomy was carried out. There was no evidence of carcinoma in the specimen. The patient is alive and well without any evidence of new or recurrent disease at 9 months' follow-up.

Comment: In this case, reflux was apparent, but this patient had a severe medical treatment failure and the stress of his surgery seemed to exacerbate his GERD to the point that his larynx became functionless (but acted as a funnel). Of the various options that were proposed to the patient, he elected total laryngectomy as the most expeditious. (In the future, cases of this type will probably be managed from the beginning with a hydrogen ion blocker, such as omeprazole.)

Case 5: Carcinoma of the Larynx in a Nonsmoker (Patient 29)

This 66-year-old nonsmoker presented to an otolaryngologist in February 1987, complaining of hoarseness. He underwent suspension microlaryngoscopy and removal of a right midcord lesion, which was diagnosed as a benign nodule. Postoperatively, he remained hoarse, the operated cord became ulcerated, and the ulcerative lesion began to enlarge. During this period, he complainted of severe reflux symptoms of heartburn and regurgitation. He was treated with cimetidine without benefit. A second microlaryngeal procedure was performed in June 1987. The histologic diagnosis was well-differentiated squamous cell carcinoma. He then underwent radiation therapy with Cobalt 60, receiving 6400 rad to the laryngeal port, which was completed in August 1987. Subsequently, because of persistent hoarseness and ulceration, a third microlaryngeal procedure was carried out. Again, the diagnosis was moderately well-differentiated squamous cell carcinoma, involving both cords.

The medical history was significant. He had undergone ulcer surgery in 1962, but the type of surgery was unknown. At time of presentation, he was on a regimen of ranitidine (300 mg b.i.d.), dietary modification, and elevation of the head of his bed. pH manometry was performed and revealed no episodes of reflux (pH less than 4.0). Barium swallow esophagogram demonstrated a hiatal hernia with esophageal dysmotility and free reflux with a patulous gastroesophageal junction.

An attempt was made to perform an endoscopic laryngeal resection, but the tumor was found to involve the deep margins and to abut the anterior portion of the thyroid cartilage bilaterally. A total laryngectomy was performed. The patient's postoperative course was complicated by severe reflux. Dehiscence of his neck wound occurred and a large fistula developed. Enteral hyperalimentation was instituted through a feeding jejunostomy. A celestine tube was placed to divert salivary flow from the stoma. Six weeks after laryngectomy, a pectoralis myocutaneous flap was brought up to close the anterior neck wound dehiscence and fistula. Two weeks later, an area of breakdown was noted inferiorly and biopsy revealed recurrent squamous cell carcinoma. One week later, the patient was discharged. He died at home 3 months later.

Comment: This man's ulcer surgery in 1962 probably contributed to his demise. This is the only case of alkaline reflux in the series presented. pH manometry did not reveal the extent of his problem because of the alkaline reflux. (In general, alkaline reflux is not a problem except in patients, such as this one, who have had previous gastric surgery.)

Case 6: Squamous Cell Carcinoma of the Larynx in a Nonsmoker (Patient 10)

This 66-year-old man presented in February of 1987 with a 3-year history of intermittent hoarseness. His medical history was noncontributory, except that he did have daily and frequent heartburn. Examination revealed a diffusely red larynx with a granular lesion of the right true vocal cord with normal mobility. Twenty-four-hour pH manometry was abnormal: upright (22.1%), supine (32.1%), and total (42%). The pharyngeal probe was positive 9.5% in the supine position, and 2.9% in the upright position.

This patient underwent laser excision of the vocal cord lesion and was placed on an antireflux regimen, including the use of ranitidine (150 mg b.i.d.). At this time, 30 months after laser excision, he has no evidence of new or recurrent disease. He has been maintained on long-term antireflux therapy. His laryngeal examination is within normal limits.

Comment: This patient's pH manometry was highly abnormal. For almost 90 minutes, the pharyngeal probe was positive, indicating acid in the hypopharynx for at least that long. He has done well on antireflux treatment.

Case 7: An 18-Year-Old Man With Laryngeal Stenosis Following Maxillofacial Trauma (Patient 43)

On November 26, 1986, an 18-year-old man was involved in a motorcycle accident and suffered a midface fracture with craniofacial separation (LeFort III), an intracranial injury, and orthopedic injuries. There was no history of laryngeal trauma. A tracheotomy was performed and, at that time, he was described as having immobile vocal cords bilaterally with subglottic and tracheal stenosis. The tracheotomy tube was then removed and a Montgomery T-tube placed. At this point, the patient was transferred to the author for treatment.

On initial examination, the patient had exuberant granulation tissue arising from the larynx, no glottic aperture, and no mobility of either vocal cord. Twenty-four-hour double-probe pH ambulatory manometry was performed and found to be normal. Nevertheless, the patient was started on an antireflux program, consisting of life-style and dietary modification, as well as ranitidine (300 mg b.i.d.). The T-tube was removed in October 1987, and the carbon dioxide laser was used to remove granulation tissue from the larynx and trachea. A small tracheotomy tube was placed. The patient continued on antireflux therapy, and the granulation tissue ceased. An endoscopic procedure was performed to open the posterior commissure, and this resulted in a modest improvement of the posterior glottic fixation with approximately a 4- to 5-mm posterior glottic chink and some mobility, and a reasonably good airway and voice. The tracheotomy was removed in March 1987. At that time, pulmonary function tests showed a normal inspiratory/expiratory flow-volume loop with a forced expiratory volume in 1 second (FEV_1) of 4.67 liters (108% of that predicted) and a forced vital capacity (FVC) of 5.22 liters (102% of that predicted).

The patient did well for 7 months and then redeveloped laryngeal stenosis. Repeat pH manometry with the patient on an antireflux regimen revealed positive pharyngeal reflux in the supine position. The patient then underwent fundoplication. Subsequently, a second endoscopic procedure was carried out. At 7 months' follow-up, the larynx appeared healthy, pink, and uninflamed. The posterior glottis was open, the airway was excellent, and the voice was good.

Comment: This patient demonstrates that GERD may fluctuate in severity; furthermore, the complication of restenosis occurred while he was under medical surveillance. Fundoplication was the next treatment for this patient, who wanted to smoke cigarettes and drink alcohol.

Case 8: Subglottic Stenosis in a 52-Year-Old Woman (Patient 56)

This 52-year-old, previously healthy woman was involved in an automobile accident and sustained injuries to her left shoulder, clavicle, ribs, and liver, and developed bilateral pneumothoraces. She was in intensive care for 41 days and in the hospital for 50 days. After 10 days of intubation, a tracheotomy was performed; however, it was removed before she was discharged.

Within a few weeks of discharge, the patient developed progressive airway difficulties. In February 1988, she underwent 24-hour pH manometry, which revealed normal esophageal values but three episodes of pharyngeal reflux. On the following day, she underwent laser resection of obstructing granulation tissue in the posterior subglottis and on the anterior tracheal wall. Her airway was reestablished without replacing her tracheotomy, and antireflux treatment was started. One month later, transnasal fiberoptic laryngoscopy was performed and the airway appeared entirely normal. She has remained asymptomatic without any evidence of reflux laryngitis.

Comment: Many patients with acquired laryngeal stenosis present at the time of failed extubation. This case, in which the development of stenosis was delayed, is, nevertheless, not unusual.

Case 9: A 69-Year-Old Woman With Subglottic Stenosis and No History of Endotracheal Intubation or Trauma (Patient 52)

In March 1987, a previously healthy, 69-year-old woman presented with cough, dyspnea, and stridor, and a presumptive diagnosis of reflux laryngitis. She had no previous history of trauma, intubation, diphtheria, or any disorder of the upper aerodigestive tract. She had mild symptoms of heartburn and throat clearing. She was a nonsmoker.

Examination revealed severe inflammation of the larynx with edema, erythema, and decreased vocal cord mobility; there was an approximately 2- to 3-mm glottic gap posteriorly. Barium esophagogram revealed only hiatal hernia. The patient underwent 24-hour pH manometry with a double probe. The esophageal tracing was abnormal (upright: 7%); the rest of the study was unremarkable. The patient was started on antireflux treatment.

The posterior commissure appeared to have a submucous mass, and the patient was taken to the operating room for examination and biopsy. The arytenoids were found to be relatively immobile. The biopsy results revealed acute and chronic inflammation of a nonspecific type. Postoperatively, she was continued on antireflux therapy and continued to have findings consistent with posterior laryngitis. One month later, the appearance of the larynx was much improved. The return of vocal cord mobility provided her with a 6- to 7-mm posterior glottic aperture; the edema subsided.

The patient continued to do well until December 1988, at which time the larynx appeared similar to its initial condition at presentation. The patient underwent repeat pH manometry while on antireflux treatment. This time the results were more abnormal: upright (20%), supine (3.4%), and total (16.3%), and there were four episodes of pharyngeal reflux. Fundoplication was recommended but the patient refused. The dose of ranitidine was increased from 150 mg b.i.d. to 300 mg b.i.d. By August of 1989, the laryngeal examination was again normal.

Comment: This case illustrates glottic hypomobility—"posterior glottic stenosis"—developing as a consequence of GERD. In years past, this patient might have been misdiagnosed as having ankylosis of the cricoarytenoid joint due to some form of "rheumatism." The fact that this woman responded well to therapy and then had a recrudescence despite therapy is not unusual. She perhaps should undergo fundoplication, but she still does not want to have the surgery performed.

Case 10: Reflux Laryngitis in a Healthy 20-Year-Old Singer (Patient 68)

A 20-year-old college music student presented with a 3-week history of hoarseness. His medical history was entirely unremarkable. Examination revealed massive edema and erythema of the posterior glottis. The intra-arytenoid mucosa was so swollen that it overhung the posterior half of the glottic aperture. Twenty-four hour-pH manometry showed only slight abnormality in the supine position (2.0%). The patient was started on antireflux therapy, including ranitidine (150 mg b.i.d.). Two months after initial treatment, the appearance of the larynx had improved but the posterior arytenoids still appeared erythematous. By 5 months of therapy, the larynx appeared normal. The patient was maintained on treatment for another month, at which point he discontinued treatment and was lost to follow-up for 16 months. Recently, he returned with a mild recrudescence, and antireflux therapy was reinstituted.

Comment: This patient illustrates the variability in severity seen in chronic, intermittent GERD.

Case 11: A 56-Year-Old Man With a Left Vocal Process Granuloma (Patient 94)

This 56-year-old choir director presented with a 3-month history of hoarseness. He had no history of infection, trauma, intubation, or gastroesophageal reflux. He specifically denied heartburn, regurgitation, dysphagia, or cough. He was a nonsmoker and was vocally well-trained. Other than chronic throat clearing, he did not abuse his voice.

Six weeks before presentation, a vocal cord granuloma had been removed, but had recurred immediately. Histologic examination showed acute and chronic inflammation without evidence of malignancy. Twenty-four-hour pH manometry was obtained and revealed abnormal supine reflux (8.10%).

The patient was started on antireflux therapy, including ranitidine (150 mg b.i.d.). After 1 month of treatment, the lesion had grown somewhat and was causing the patient to have a foreign body sensation. The lesion was removed endoscopically, but recurred. The antireflux treatment was intensified (ranitidine 300 mg t.i.d.). After 5 months, the lesion appeared unchanged. The patient was referred to a gastroenterologist and a surgeon for consideration of fundoplication. The patient declined to have a fundoplication. Navertheness, the lesion healed spontaneously within 2 months. At 1-year follow-up, the patient remains well without any evidence of recurrent granulation.

Comment: This patient's granuloma took 8 months to heal despite antireflux therapy and good patient compliance.

Case 12: Globus Pharyngeus in a 58-Year-Old Man (Patient 128)

A 58-year-old man presented with a 1-year history of a sensation of a lump in the throat. He denied dysphagia, odynophagia, hoarseness, or chronic throat clearing. He did have a chronic dry cough. He was a nondrinker and nonsmoker, and the remainder of his medical history was noncontributory.

Examination revealed normal transnasal fiberoptic laryngoscopy and pharyngoscopy. The patient underwent 24-hour pH-manometry with a double probe. The results were abnormal: upright (9.8%), supine (5.9%), total (7.5%), without any episodes of documented pharyngeal reflux. Upper esophageal sphincter studies were carried out. Pharyngeal propulsion and coordination were normal, but the UES resting pressure was 38 mm Hg (normal, 45 to 107 mm Hg). At the time of manometry, endoscopy was carried out and revealed esophagitis. The patient was placed on an antireflux treatment program, including ranitidine (150 mg b.i.d.). Within 2 months, his symptoms had abated and by 5 months, he was well.

Comment: In this case, the patient demonstrated none of the signs and symptoms of reflux laryngitis, and yet still had a sensation of a lump in the throat. Consequently, one might propose that the globus sensation in this patient was due to symptoms of reflux esophagitis referred via the vagus nerve (referred "pain") from the distal esophagus.

Case 13: Globus Pharyngeus in a 65-Year-Old Man with Chronic Throat Clearing (Patient 118)

A 65-year-old man presented with a 2-year history of a sensation of a lump in the throat, intermittently associated with chronic throat clearing. His medical history was unremarkable and he neither drank alcohol nor smoked. Examination revealed intense erythema and edema of the arytenoids with piling up the interarytenoid mucosa.

Barium swallow esophagogram revealed a hiatal hernia with lower esophageal ring. Twenty-four-hour pH manometry revealed abnormal supine and upright reflux but no evidence of pharyngeal reflux (upright (7.0%), supine (18.0%), total (11.0%)). The patient began a regimen of antireflux therapy, including ranitidine, 150 mg in the morning and 300 mg at night. Within 2 months, his symptoms had improved and, by 4 months, he was completely well; repeat examination was normal.

After 6 months of treatment, he elected to discontinue his antireflux treatment. Within 3 months, signs and symptoms of reflux laryngitis and globus had redeveloped. He was again placed on an antireflux regimen, and within 3 months he was again asymptomatic.

Comment: In this case, the presumed mechanism of globus was actual laryngopharyngeal acid exposure with considerable local inflammation.

Case 14: Globus Pharyngeus and a Hypertensive UES in a 53-Year-Old Man (Patient 116)

A 53-year-old man presented with a 3-year history of chronic cough and a sensation of a lump in the throat. He was a nonsmoker and drank wine socially. His medical history was noncontributory. Examination revealed mild posterior laryngitis.

Twenty-four-hour pH manometry was abnormal: 8.8% supine and 5.7% total, and there were several episodes of pharyngeal reflux. Upper esophageal sphincter (UES) studies were performed and the resting pressure of the UES was 177 mm Hg (normal 45 to 107 mm Hg).

The patient was started on antireflux therapy, including famotidine (40 mg b.i.d.). Two months later, his examination was normal and repeat UES manometry revealed a return to normal UES pressure (101 mm Hg). He was asymptomatic at that time.

Comment: This is the first case in the medical literature that documents a hypertensive UES associated with globus and GERD, with a response to medical treatment. (The hypertensive UES returned to normal resting pressure following treatment of the GERD.)

Case 15: Chronic Intermittent Throat Pain and Hoarseness in a 46-Year-Old Man (Patient 146)

A 46-year-old man presented with a 6-month history of recurrent throat pain, dysphagia, and hoarseness. He complained of heartburn and had a history of a duodenal ulcer, which had been treated with cimetidine. Examination revealed posterior laryngitis. Barium esophagography revealed a hiatal hernia with esophagitis and a lower esophageal ring. Twenty-four-hour pH manometry was abnormal: 3.0% supine; there was no pharyngeal reflux demonstrated. Treatment was initiated, including the use of ranitidine (150 mg b.i.d.), and within 3 months, the patient was asymptomatic.

Comment: The mechanism of intermittent throat pain in this case was related to intermittent laryngopharyngeal GER.

Case 16: Sore Throat and Persistent Pharyngeal Ulceration in a 45-Year-Old Man (Patient 139)

A 45-year-old school administrator presented with a 6-week history of ulceration of the lateral pharyngeal wall just below the tonsil. He was known to have a hiatal hernia and reflux and had been treated with ranitidine. Examination revealed diffuse pharyngitis with a shallow ulceration below the left tonsil and extending for approximately 1 cm inferiorly. The larynx revealed mild erythema and edema.

Barium esophagography demonstrated a lower esophageal ring and pH manometry demonstrated supine reflux (3%) and six episodes of documented pharyngeal reflux. Treatment was initiated, including ranitidine (150 mg b.i.d.), and the patient was healed in 3 weeks.

Comment: The relationship between GERD and aphthous or herpetic ulcers is not known. However, it is possible that chronic irritation from GERD may both trigger and complicate the natural evolution of such ulcerative diatheses.

Case 17: Chronic Cough in a 35-Year-Old Insurance Salesman (Patient 171)

A 35-year-old insurance salesman had a 1-year history of severe chronic cough. When bouts of coughing started, he would sometimes cough until he vomited. This problem complicated his occupation as an insurance agent, because when he would go to interview a client, he would begin coughing and have to leave the interview in embarrassment. He noted that his symptoms were worse on weekdays as opposed to weekends.

Over a course of 10 months, he had sought the advice of 17 physicians without benefit, had undergone bronchoscopy twice, and had been treated with courses of antibiotics 14 times. At the time of presentation to the author, he was under allergy and psychiatric treatment. The remainder of his medical history was noncontributory. The patient was a nonsmoker and his weight was 260 pounds. Otolaryngologic examination was unremarkable.

Barium esophagography revealed esophagitis, and 24-hour pH manometry was abnormal: 9.8% supine, 13.5% upright; a pharyngeal probe was not used. The patient underwent endoscopy with biopsy (diagnostic of esophagitis) and was started on antireflux treatment, including ranitidine (150 mg b.i.d.). Within 2 months, he had become asymptomatic. One year later, he discontinued his antireflux therapy and again became symptomatic. (He continues to be followed by another physician and has reportedly done well on long-term antireflux treatment.)

Comment: This patient's history is not atypical of patients with chronic cough due to GERD. Many such patients have seen many doctors and have undergone a variety of treatments before having the correct diagnosis made. In this particular patient, the response to treatment was dramatic, and so was his relapse when treatment was discontinued.

Commentary

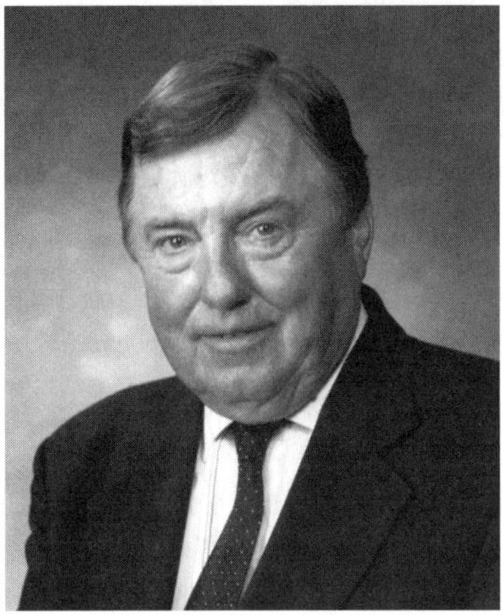

Robert J. Toohill, MD, FACS

In the mid-1970s, a patient presented with severe attacks of paroxysmal laryngospasm. The workup of this patient was extensive but no obvious etiology was found. These episodes were frightening to the patient and led to several emergency visits. For more than a year, these episodes continued to the discouragement of the patient, his internist and myself. His internist in response to mild symptoms of gastroesophageal reflux disease (GERD) prescribed Cimetidine. This resulted in a complete cessation of his laryngospasm attacks. This case was of great interest to me and I began a search of literature and consultations with other colleagues. A realization that many of my patients with voice and laryngeal problems were undiagnosed despite thorough evaluations and treatments. There was frustration from the lack of results with speech and vocal hygiene therapy. These factors inspired me to look deeper at the possibilities that gastroesophageal reflux (GER) was present in many patients with laryngologic disorders. In the early 1980s, several studies had accumulated suggesting a relationship and possible etiology of some vocal and laryngeal problems. Relying on the only test available at that time, I would order a barium esophagram and in at least two-thirds of the patients an esophageal abnormality suggestive of GER was found. In these studies I was greatly aided by several intellectually curious G.I. radiologists. When the above findings were present, I would place the patients on acid suppression mostly using H_2 receptor antagonists with good resolution of their laryngeal symptoms.

In 1988, realizing that my approach was nonscientific concerning the etiology and treatment of LPR, I did a 10 year review of my patients whom I suspected had laryngeal or pharyngeal problems with GER. Two hundred seven out of a total of 5421 new patients seen over the 10-year period were suspected of having extraesophageal reflux (EER). The diagnosis, treatment and follow-up constituted this retrospective review and was presented at the XIV World Congress of Otorhinolaryngology in Madrid, Spain (Proceedings of the XIV World Congress, 1989:3000-3005). This review gave further credence in my mind that LPR was a true entity that had great impact on voice and laryngology problems. There was a realization, however, that much investigation and study were necessary to delineate the importance of GER and its relationship with the larynx.

In the 1990s, the development of ambulatory 24-hour pH monitoring utilizing simultaneous pharyngeal and lower esophageal pH testing was a giant step in the diagnosis of LPR. With coinvestigators from gastroenterology, we performed controlled studies of the vocal nodule, reflux laryngitis and laryngotracheal stenosis patients. These studies offered very significant information as to relationship and etiology in patients with LPR. We felt from our studies that the etiology of "idiopathic" subglottic stenosis was likely due to LPR. Treatment of these patients with acid suppression greatly improved the surgical and nonsurgical management. In this period, in addition to LPR, there were very important investigations to support GER as etiologic in pulmonary disorders such as chronic cough, asthma, and chronic bronchitis. There were also studies that indicated that chronic rhinosinusitis combined with LPR was associated in both disorders. The development of sophisticated autonomic nervous system testing laboratories clearly defined the etiology of vasomotor rhinitis. It was found that this disorder was frequently associated with LPR and indicated that chronic nasal and sinus disease in some cases was the result of regurgitations of refluxate to nasopharynx. It should be noted that pepsin in middle ear effusions in children has led to new and greater insights into pediatric GER. The future will see further analyses of the contents of GER in the lungs, pharynx, nasopharynx, and the nose and sinuses.

The 2000s produced investigations that duodenogastroesophageal reflux (DGER) containing not only acid but pepsin, bile, and pancreatic enzymes are very much involved in causing LPR-related damage or disease. The advent of impedance testing, bile detection by Bilitec, and investigational nasopharyngeal pH-probe testing (Restech) is adding greatly to our diagnostic methods for DGER. There are now immunohistologic and immunoblot tests that will detect pepsin in laryngeal tissue from biopsies taken in patients with LPR. In the near future, it is likely there will be fairly simple analyses of sputum samples for pepsins in patients with EER. The advent of noninvasive studies of pharyngeal secretions not only for pepsin but also for bile will be of great benefit in the diagnosis of LPR. These methods will be a great supplement to present methods of reflux testing by pH probe and impedance.

History and Physical

Several comments and opinions based on my experience have influenced the diagnostic and treatment methods for LPR. From a historical prospective, the adult presenting with the chief complaint of hoarseness must be questioned in detail about other relevant problems that might cause this symptom. These would include trauma or surgery in the head and neck region, recent severe throat infection, and severe situations requiring excessive use of the voice. A strong history of smoking must be noted. If one does not get positive information to the above questioning, the diagnosis of LPR might be entertained. In addition to the hoarseness, throat clearing, excess throat mucus or postnasal drip, swallowing difficulty, cough, breathing difficulty, choking, sensations of sticking, or a lump in the throat are symptoms associated with LPR. Symptoms of GERD include heartburn, chest pain, indigestion, or a regurgitation of acid are important, but it should be noted that 80% of patients with LPR do not have symptoms of GERD. Inquiry into the timing of symptoms is important. The above complaints of LPR will be noted more during the upright daytime hours and less so when supine. The exact opposite is true when a patient mainly has symptoms of GERD. The recently developed reflux symptom index (RSI) is helpful in categorizing the severity of the LPR.

The findings of erythema and hyperemia especially of the arytenoid and aryepiglottic fold area, ventricular obliteration, subcordal edema, vocal cord edema, diffuse laryngeal edema, and posterior commissure changes are findings associated with LPR. Vocal fold nodules, polyps, and granuloma may also be part of the findings. The nature of endolaryngeal mucous if it is thick and tenacious will point to LPR. Any or all of these findings can occur. A recently developed reflux finding score (RFS) is quite useful in categorizing the severity of the LPR.

Diagnostic Evaluation

Diagnostic methods have improved but the use of the classical barium esophagram has been underestimated and underutilized. This procedure is mostly noninvasive, requires no more than 30 minutes to perform, and is available in most clinical facilities and is inexpensive. The dynamic fluoroscopic aspect of the study performed by the radiologist will give many clues that might lead the clinician to a better understanding of the individuals future evaluation and treatment. The observant radiologist can document motility and peristalsis problems, tumors, diverticula, stricture,, esophagitis, spontaneous reflux, and lower esophageal sphincter (LES) dysfunction. All of these findings can add to gastroesophageal reflux (GER) and impact LPR. The sensitivity of the esophagram is the range of 60 to 70%. The fact that 30 to 40% of patients with suspected LPR have negative esophagrams does not rule our GER as the cause. It also can be stated that on occasions a positive study will not be indicative of LPR.

The technical aspects of pH-probe testing have become consistent. The equipment is now readily available and the ease or probe placement via endoscopic technique has eliminated the need for cumbersome manometric study. The upper probe is placed in a consistent zone from the upper esophageal sphincter (UES) to 2 cm above it. This allows the lower control probe to be placed in a zone approximately 5 cm above the LES. The LPR patient is positive when pH drops to 4 or below at the upper probe with a simultaneous drop to 4 or below at the lower probe. When the acid exposure time (AET) at the upper probe is more than 0.01% of the time (more than 7–8 sec) this is considered a positive study and many times this will be during one reflux event in the 24-hour period. As with barium esophagram, 20 to 30% of patients with LPR have negative pH study, but this also does not rule out GER as the causative factor. Likewise, a positive probe study may be present in the absence of symptoms or findings of LPR. The major disadvantages of probe testing are the invasiveness and expense of the procedure. This methodology will conclusively find whether the acid reflux events are upright or supine. Upright reflux events are very characteristic for LPR.

Impedance testing has become another effective method of identifying GER and LPR. It will measure the entire elements of gastric refluxate but only the acid component of such can be delineated. For the most part, use of pH-probe testing or impedance gives the same information. The indication for using both tests is very rare and one must decide which method is to be used for these patients. An exception is that combined impedance pH monitoring will detect nonacid reflux that is not detected using pH monitoring alone. It should be noted that pepsin and bile are injurious at weakly and nonacidic pH. Both methods are similarly invasive and expensive. I feel that, when pharyngeal acid is present, we can assume that the other elements of gastric reflux (ie, pepsin, bile, and pancreatic enzymes) have also reached the pharynx. When LPR is associated with symptoms of GERD, transnasal esophagoscopy is indicated to identify distal esophageal problems.

Management

Treatment of LPR formerly seemed fairly simple. However we have found that acid suppression alone is not sufficient in some cases. The use of proton pump inhibitors (PPI) has become widespread despite their expense and the need for long-term therapy. We have overlooked the use of H_2 blockers, which are less expensive and may be safer when used on a long-term basis. The long-term use of acid suppressive drugs has not been investigated in detail. The recent suspicions of osteoporosis and cardiac complications should be in the minds of those treating LPR in the long term.

At present, the most logical and successful treatment of DGER is surgery and the advent of laparoscopic Nissen fundoplication made this technique the best that can be offered to the refractory patient.

There is a promising medical therapy in the form of liquid alginate that may lead to more conservative management. Alginate is harvested off the coast of northern Norway from the stem of the seaweed, *laminaria hyperborea*. When taken orally, it forms a strong, coherent, voluminous, and buoyant alginate gel raft over the gastric mucosa, thus preventing refluxate from leaving the stomach. Alginate is not available in the United States. but has widespread utilization in Europe. Hopefully, we will see this available in our country. Further investigations of conservative treatments such as this will greatly simplify the management of DGER to the extraesophageal structures for the clinician.

Conclusion

One could speculate as to the recent findings of LPR in voice and laryngologic patients. Is this a modern day problem of lifestyles in our population? Have problems with LPR been present in past generations but undiagnosed? The clinically curious laryngologist who has long been puzzled by the elusive problems in the larynx would indicate that this has been a problem for many past years. The concept of a "unified aerodigestive tract" in which disorders of the extraesophageal structures will influence the stomach and duodenum. Evidence indicates that this occurs vice-versa. The presence of the vagus nerve and autonomic nervous system in the aerodigestive tract is immense and abnormalities of this neural input likely play an important role in many cases of GER.

The lead role that otolaryngologist-head and neck surgeons have taken in the appreciation of LPR makes one proud of our specialty. Basic and clinical science from our colleagues has introduced a remarkable new part of our specialty. Opportunities from this clinical problem will promote further studies and answers to important questions for the years ahead. I am very grateful to have been involved in the appreciation of LPR and its profound effects on the larynx and voice.

Role of Refluxed Acid in Pathogenesis of Laryngeal Disorders

Robert J. Toohill, MD, FACS, Joan C. Kuhn, MS, CCC-Sp, *Milwaukee, Wisconsin*

The neuroanatomic proximity of the larynx to the hypopharynx and proximal esophagus make it particularly vulnerable to diseases that occur in those 2 areas. This is particularly true of gastroesophageal reflux disease (GERD). There is increasing awareness of this relationship, and dysphonias from gastroesophageal reflux (GER) are far more common than previously realized. The symptoms and findings of reflux laryngitis, vocal nodules, Reinke's edema, contact ulcer and granuloma, laryngeal stenosis, and paroxysmal laryngospasm are presented, and diagnostic protocols for each disorder are suggested. The treatment varies with the severity of each problem. Conservative lifestyles and dietary control are helpful, but long-term medical therapy with H_2, H_1, and prokinetic drugs are usually needed. Surgical therapy may be indicated for such life-threatening problems as laryngeal stenosis and paroxysmal laryngospasm. The need for physician and patient awareness, research, and improved and less expensive therapy are discussed. ***Am J Med.*** **1997;103(5A):100S–106S. © 1997 by Excerpta Medica, Inc.**

From the Department of Otolaryngology and Human Communication, The Medical College of Wisconsin, Milwaukee, Wisconsin.
Requests for reprints should be addressed to Robert J. Toohill, MD, FACS, the Department of Otolaryngology and Human Communication, The Medical College of Wisconsin, 9200 W. Wisconsin Avenue, Milwaukee, Wisconsin 53226.

The suggestions that gastroesophageal reflux (GER) has an impact on laryngeal and pharyngeal disorders have arisen in the last 30 years. Studies that actually relate causality have been more recent but are unfortunately few in number. During the last several years, a substantial number of reports have been published relating chronic pharyngeal and laryngeal symptoms to GER. Unfortunately, there remains a significant portion of the medical establishment that is unaware of the very significant problems that GER causes in the pharynx and larynx, and this includes otolaryngologists (ORL).[1] To date, most investigators describe disorders of the larynx as being caused by or cofactored with GER or GER disease (GERD). It has been recently suggested that a better term for this association would be laryngo-pharyngeal reflux (LPR). The major factors that have led clinicians to associate GER and chronic laryngeal disorders are 2-fold. The first factor is the frequent lack of an etiology for chronic laryngeal symptoms or findings. Second, many inquisitive and thoughtful investigators employed antireflux therapy and found that the laryngeal problem disappeared. This latter factor is thus far the best diagnostic indicator and the best proof that GER is pertinent, although the parallel is scientifically inadequate.[2] A recent retrospective review of 205 dysphonic patients in our institutions showed that 191 (93%) responded to antireflux therapy.[3]

INCIDENCE

Koufman has estimated that 10% of patients presenting to an ORL practice will have symptoms and/or findings related to GER.[4] A recent report from our institution placed the incidence at 4%.[5] In a general practice of primary care medicine, the incidence would likely be in the range of 1%. Koufman estimates that almost two-thirds of ORL patients with laryngeal and voice disorders have GERD as the primary cause, or as a significant etiological cofactor.[6]

SYMPTOMS

The symptoms are listed in **Table I**. Patients with laryngeal disorders due to GER will not consistently complain of the typical distal symptoms of reflux, such as heartburn or indigestion. Our review found only 20% of patients with upper aerodigestive problems had distal symptoms.[5] Dysphonia manifested by hoarseness is the most significant and common laryngeal complaint. The hoarseness may be intermittent and may occur later in the day as a result of vocal fatigue. Professional voice users will frequently note a breaking of their voice sometimes to the point of aphonia. Chronic throat clearing, excessive throat mucous, and postnasal drip are invariably present. Patients will describe the mucous that is expectorated as clear, white, yellow, or green. The coloration of the mucous represents gastric content in many cases. Most of these patients will tell you or have been told by their physician that this mucous is from the nose and sinuses as postnasal drip, even though the vast majority of these patients have no nasal or sinus disease whatsoever. It is clear that the mucociliary transportation of secretion to the throat that is then swallowed is a neutral nonirritating and nonsymptom-producing phenomena. The words "postnasal drip" are invariably a misnomer, and physicians should not use this term. When patients use this term, it is a likely clue that they are refluxing. Many patients with a laryngeal disorder from GER will have symptoms of chronic cough, sore throat, and dysphagia in the 3 nearby structures of the tracheo-bronchial tree, pharynx, and esophagus.

TABLE I

Laryngeal Symptoms Associated with Gastroesophageal Reflux

- Lack of typical reflux symptoms
- Chronic or intermittent hoarseness
- Voice fatigue and/or breaks
- Chronic throat clearing
- Excessive throat mucus
- Postnasal drip
- Chronic cough
- Sore throat
- Dysphagia

TABLE II

Laryngeal Findings Associated with Gastroesophageal Reflux

- Reflux laryngitis
- Vocal nodules
- Polypoid degeneration (Reinke's edema)
- Contact ulcers and granulomas
- Laryngeal stenosis
- Paroxysmal laryngospasm

LARYNGEAL FINDINGS

The benign conditions of the larynx as the result of GER are listed in **Table II** and will be described in the order of decreasing incidence.

1. Reflux laryngitis is most common and in many instances can be identified by routine mirror indirect laryngoscopy. The predominant symptoms will be hoarseness, voice fatigue, and breaking of the voice. A functional voice disorder (FVD) is nearly always present, and the frequent question arises as to which is most prevalent: (1) the vocal abuse, misuse, or overuse, or (2) GERD. In most cases, it is likely that the GER precipitated the FVD. The laryngitis is most predominate in the posterior larynx, with erythema involving the arytenoids and posterior commissure. In advanced cases the posterior commissure will have edematous, hyperkeratotic epithelium that will tend to crust and desquamate (pachydermia laryngis). The erythema will frequently extend to the true and false vocal cords, subglottic mucosa, and to the pharyngeal mucosa. The finding of laryngitis is quite subtle on occasion. The advent of videoendoscopy has allowed for identification of small areas of erythema in the interarytenoid area or on the vocal cords. Increased mucous in the larynx is probably the result of a local tissue inflammation from GER, and in many instances this can only be visualized by video technique. Treatment of reflux laryngitis is almost always medical, and results are quite good with modern antireflux medications along with voice therapy.

2. Vocal nodules are likely a unique result of subtle reflux laryngitis in the adult population. Although GER may play a role in some cases of childhood vocal nodules, the majority of children develop such from FVD that are psychosomatic in origin.[7] Vocal nodules most often occur in adults who are professional voice users, i.e., singers, actors, public speakers, and teachers. The nodules are seen at the junction of the anterior and middle thirds of the phonating surface of the true vocal cords (TVC), are bilateral, and are usually associated with minimal laryngeal erythema and increased mucous production (**Figure 1**) Though most remain as small nodules, those that are untreated may progress to a polyp; the polypoid nodule may require phonosurgical removal. Nearly all patients have FVD and require voice therapy with antireflux management.

3. Polypoid degeneration or Reinke's edema is likely the end result of untreated vocal nodules. The patient population has a predominance of elderly females who do not rely on voice for their profession. Many have a long history of smoking. A progressive increase in the fluid and edema in Reinke's space traverses the entire length of the TVC. This space is between the mucosa of the TVC and the vocal ligament, which covers the vocalis muscle. Various degrees of erythema are present in the larynx, and on occasion there is leukoplakia of the TVC (**Figure 2**) Antireflux therapy, smoke cessation, and voice therapy will aid in reducing this edema, but phonosurgical removal is usually necessary. It is important to continue the above-mentioned conservative mea-

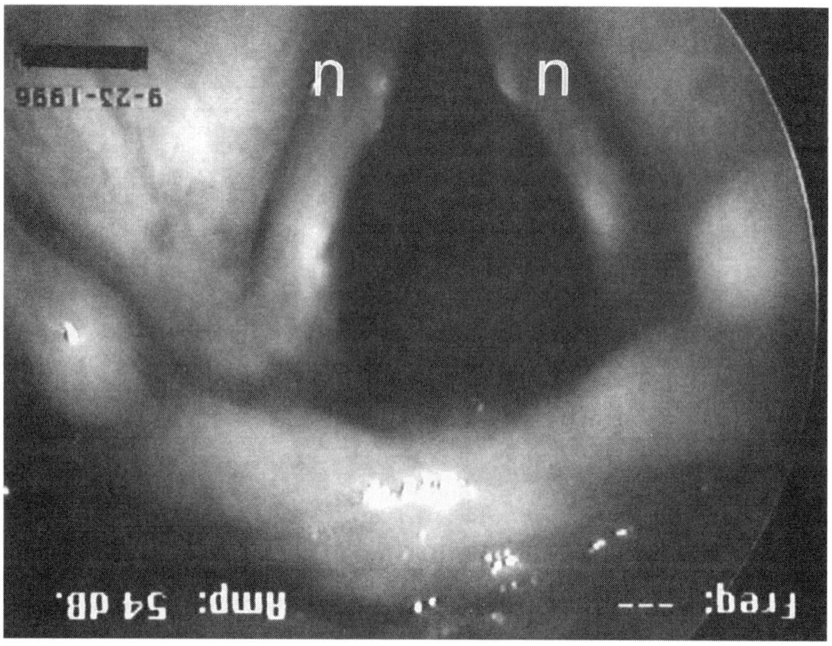

Figure 1. Videoendoscopic view of larynx with bilateral true vocal cord (TVC) nodules (n).

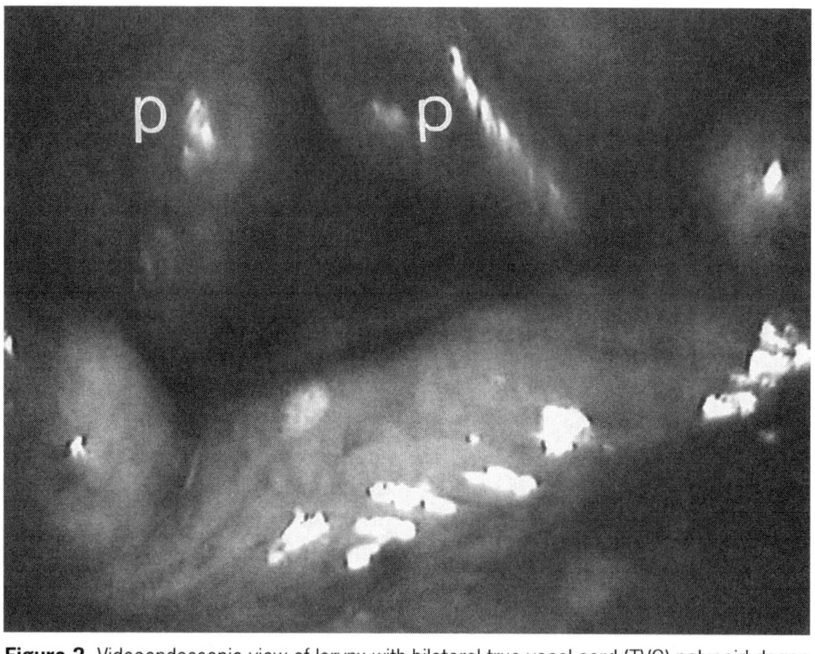

Figure 2. Videoendoscopic view of larynx with bilateral true vocal cord (TVC) polypoid degeneration (p).

sures for a prolonged period postoperatively to insure a better rehabilitation of voice.[6]

4. Contact ulcers and granulomas occur at the vocal process of the arytenoid cartilage, which attaches to the posterior end of the vocalis muscle. The vocal process is the key in regards to vocal dysfunction and GER. All adduction and abduction movements of the TVC are hinged on the vocal process and therefore are subjected to vocal abuse and hard glottal attack. Because of their posterior position, they are influenced by posterior laryngitis from GER. Constant throat clearing is characteristic of these patients. Eventually ulceration over the thin mucosa of the vocal process occurs followed by perichondritis, which subsequently causes the granuloma. Although vocal abuse and GER cause the majority of contact ulcers and granulomas, intubation, particularly on a prolonged basis, with GER will cause the same problem (**Figure 3**). Vigorous antireflux therapy over a prolonged period along with voice therapy to reduce vocal hyperfunction is successful in ridding most patients of granuloma. On occasions, surgical removal

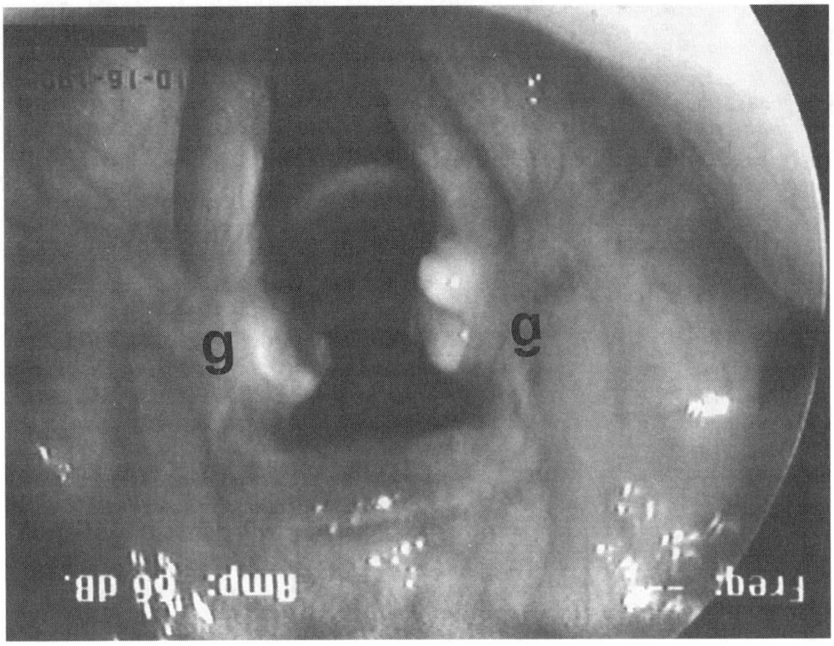

Figure 3. Videoendoscopic view of larynx with bilateral true vocal cord (TVC) contact granulomas (g).

is indicated when the granuloma persists after prolonged conservative treatment, when it becomes large and obstructing, or when there is suspicion of carcinoma and a biopsy is indicated[6,8,9] Injection of 5–10 mg of triamcinolone into the vocal process after surgical removal is helpful. There are rare occasions where neither conservative nor surgical therapy will clear the granuloma. Nasri et al[10] have utilized botulinum toxin injections of 10–15 units into the TVC to paralyze the larynx partially and reduce vocal hyperfunction. They have been highly successful in clearing the refractory granuloma, and our initial use of this technique has supported their results.

5. Laryngeal stenosis (LS) is a severe sequella of GER and in some cases may be life threatening. LS is the result of ongoing reflux laryngitis. Those patients who have a traumatized larynx, most often from trauma or intubation, with associated GER are good candidates for LS. If there is no GER present, the traumatized larynx will heal and not develop significant stenosis.[11] The most common areas of LS are the posterior commissure and subglottic area (**Figure 4**). The scars of these patients are frequently immature, soft, erythematous, and usually not mature because of the ongoing influence of GER. When GER is managed, the scar matures and becomes effectively managed by surgery. Koufman[12] studied 32 patients in 1991 with laryngeal and tracheal stenosis and demonstrated significant reflux in 75% of his patients. Both Koufman and our group manage patients with LS at first contact and continue vigorous antireflux measures until patients are fully rehabilitated.[6,11] Idiopathic subglottic stenosis, occurring predominantly in women, has been an enigma, because it was difficult to rehabilitate. It is now thought that GER is the etiology of these stenoses. With associated management of reflux, this group of patients has been much easier to manage, and once rehabilitated the stenoses do not recur.[13]

6. Paroxysmal laryngospasm is likewise a life-threatening form of GER, but fortunately it is rare. Patients who experience laryngospasm are very concerned by this event, which usually occurs without warning. It occurs mostly at night by frightfully awakening the patient with severe stridor and dyspnea. The patient can detail the event with the bitter taste of refluxate in the mouth. Studies will invariably show severe GER. The attacks will recur unless GER is vigorously managed. Strong consideration for fundal plication should be given to this group of patients to prevent the attacks of potentially fatal laryngospasms.[6]

DIAGNOSIS

Diagnosis of larngeal disorders associated with GER is summarized in **Table III**.

1. Detailing a patient's complaints plus a thorough review of history will often lead to a nonobvious cause of laryngeal complaints. The importance of voice, the nagging pharyngeal complaints, chronic cough, dysphagia, and airway obstruction without a history of obvious pharyngeal or laryngeal disease will lead to a suspicion of GER. Diagnosis will be accomplished by an organized approach.

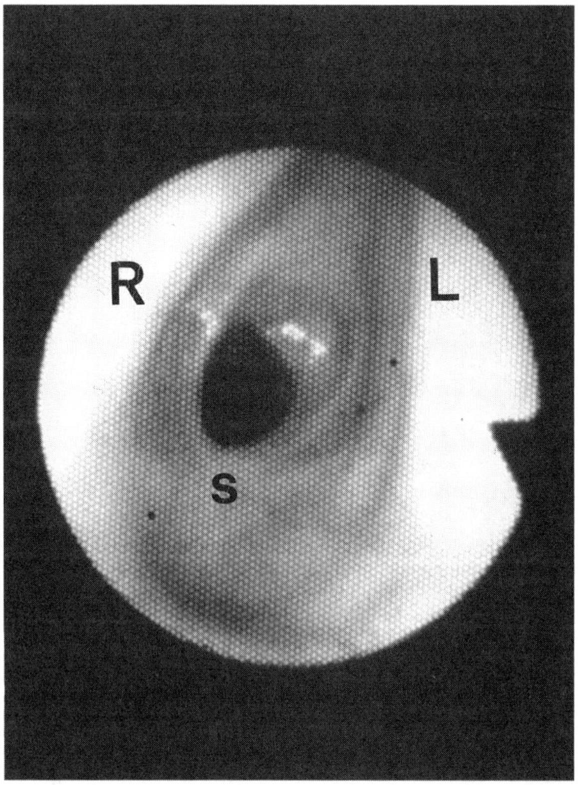

Figure 4. Flexible fiberoptic laryngoscopic view of larynx showing right (R) and left (L) true vocal cords (TVC) and subglottic stenosis (s).

2. Laryngoscopy by the head mirror–laryngeal mirror indirect technique is an invaluable, inexpensive, time-honored method of evaluating the hypopharynx and larynx. This should be routine on every patient with laryngeal symptoms, will give clues as to the diagnosis, and will give rationale to the patient for further recommended studies.

3. Fiberoptic laryngoscopy is relatively simple to perform via either the nasal or oral cavities under topical anesthesia. The visual field is small, but near normal neuromuscular functions can be assessed, such as vocal cord movement and swallowing function. Videostroboscopy can be performed, but there is a limited visual field. The cost of equipment is moderate.

4. Rigid angulated laryngoscopy has been an excellent addition to the clinician's ability to evaluate the hypopharynx and larynx. These periscopic instruments angulate and magnify the view of the involved areas at 70–90 degrees; 70 degrees appears to be more optimal. These scopes are moderately priced and are likely needed in the average modern otolaryngology practice. These are the preferred instruments when performing videostroboscopy, although the technique does involve extrusions of the tongue to move the anterior pharynx forward, which some feel distorts the muscular functions of the larynx. This distortion is actually minimal, and standards of the stroboscopic evaluation include this factor. This methodology is patient comfortable, frequently does not require any topical anesthesia, and gives excellent visualization and documentation of laryngeal disease.

5. Videostroboscopy has greatly enhanced our ability to evaluate pathology and function of the larynx. The personnel and equipment to perform videostroboscopy is expensive, and this technology is mostly limited to modern voice laboratories. In many instances, the clinician will not need the services of a voice lab or videostroboscopy, but it is fortunate that these facilities are available in the United States with good access to most patients. When there are diagnostic problems, the video exam will document laryngeal problems, such as erythema, mucous production, small lesions, adynamic vocal cord segments, paralysis, small scars, and lesions that might escape other visual examining techniques. The cost to the patient for a videostroboscopy is not excessive, and the value of such study is very cost effective.

6. Microlaryngoscopy must be performed under general anesthesia in most instances. The visualization is superb, and the ability to obtain biopsy material is at times essential. The expense of this procedure is moderate.

7. The barium esophagram is essential for all patients who are suspected of having GER as a cause or cofactor for laryngeal disease. This radiologic study is convenient, inexpensive, noninvasive, and highly informative. The inquisitive and concerned radiologist will identify motility and peristaltic abnormalities; esophageal lesions, such as tumors; diverticula; strictures; esophagitis; spontaneous reflux; hiatal hernia; and disorders of the lower esophageal sphincter (**Table IV**). All of these factors have been associated with GER and have implications for the laryngeal disease. This information will be of value to the patient and clinician for future needs. We have recently performed esophagram on 286 dysphonia patients for various laryngeal disorders. Abnormalities listed above were found in 79.9% of the patients. This finding further suggests the strong relationship of GER and laryngeal disease. This fact, plus the suspicion that a normal barium esophagram does not always identify a GER problem, projects an overwhelming relation.[3]

8. Ambulatory pH monitoring has had great impact on the understanding of GER.[6] The results of this study for laryngeal disease have been inconclusive.[14] The study is invasive and uncomfortable to patients, it is expensive, and there are many factors during the study that lead to false-positive and false-negative results. At present, this study is not routinely used for reflux laryngitis, vocal nodules, and

polypoid degeneration. We recommend pH monitoring for contact ulcers and granulomas, laryngeal stenosis, and paroxysmal laryngospasm. At present, we are conducting prospective studies of ambulatory pH monitoring on all laryngeal disorders plus laryngeal, hypopharyngeal and pharyngeal cancer, pharyngitis, and sphenoid sinusitis.

TREATMENT

The larynx, pharynx, and tracheo-bronchial tree are more susceptible to the ravages of GER as compared to the esophagus. The treatment for these areas, therefore, must be vigorous, persistent, and for longer periods of time as compared to gastroesophageal problems.[6] The therapeutic approaches are largely dictated by the laryngeal findings and barium esophagram study (**Table V**).

1. Reflux laryngitis is treated with cimetidine or ranitidine. The local tissue effects of these H_2 blockers are helpful in addition to the good acid reduction.[15] If the esophagram demonstrates motility, peristaltic, or lower esophageal sphincter dysfunction cisapride will be added to the therapy. Treatment must be 3–6 months. In the upper midwest, treatment is more often needed in spring and fall, very much like the treatment for duodenal ulcer. H_1 blockers or surgical therapy are rarely indicated.

2. Vocal nodules are mostly a manifestation of spontaneous GER, as identified on barium esophagram. H_1 blockers for pure acid reduction, such as omeprazole or lansoprazole, are highly effective. H_2 blockers are less expensive and effective, but there is less need for the anti-inflammatory properties of these drugs. If propulsion defects are demonstrated, cisapride can be added. Phonosurgical removal is rarely indicated.

3. Polypoid degeneration or Reinke's edema is managed in the same fashion as vocal nodules, with the exception that phonosurgical removal is almost always indicated.

4. Contact ulcers and granulomas respond to the acid reduction and anti-inflammatory properties of H_2 blockers on a prolonged basis—at least 6 months. Cisapride should be used if the esophagram is suggestive, as mentioned above. Surgical removal, intralesional steroid injection, and botulinum toxin injection may be necessary.

5. Laryngeal stenosis requires maximum, continued acid reduction over long periods of time. Combinations of H_1 blockers and cisapride will be needed. Surgical fundal plication should be strongly considered, especially if the patient is young and has a long life expectancy. Surgical therapy for the stenosis is almost always needed, but preoperative antireflux therapy and prolonged postoperative maintenance are essential.

TABLE III

Diagnosis of Laryngeal Disorders Associated with Gastroesophageal Reflux

- History
- Indirect laryngoscopy
- Fiberoptic laryngoscopy
- Rigid angulated laryngoscopy
- Videostroboscopy
- Microlaryngoscopy
- Barium esophagram
- Ambulatory pH monitoring

TABLE IV

Barium Esophagram and Its Role in Gastroesophageal Reflux and Laryngeal Disorders

- Motility and peristalsis problems
- Tumors and diverticula
- Strictures
- Esophagitis
- Spontaneous reflux
- Hiatal hernia
- Lower esophageal sphincter integrity

TABLE V

Treatment of Laryngeal Disorders Associated with Gastroesophageal Reflux

- Reflux laryngitis
  - Acid suppressive therapy
  - Seasonal therapy
- Vocal nodules
- Polypoid degeneration (Reinke's edema)
  - Acid suppressive therapy
- Contact ulcers and granulomas
  - Acid suppressive therapy
  - Surgical removal and steroid injection
  - Botulinum toxin injection
- Laryngeal stenosis
- Paroxysmal laryngospasm
  - Acid auppressive therapy
  - Fundoplication
  - Surgical repair of stenosis

6. Paroxysmal laryngospasm is life threatening and should be treated vigorously, as mentioned with laryngeal stenosis above.

OUTCOME

Limited data reveal a remarkably good therapeutic outcome in most patients who have laryngeal disorders as the result of GER. The data concerning results of antireflux therapy for these disorders are outstanding, real, but only known to those who have knowledge and conviction to treat the problem. A recent quote summarizes the difficulties that we in otolaryngology and gastroenterology must face: "The extraesophageal manifestations of GERD can be difficult to manage. Although otolaryngological complications are increasingly recognized, and these have been shown responsive to medical or surgical GERD therapy, the poor parallel between the esophageal and otolaryngological manifestation of GERD make it difficult to prove causality."[2] The major concerns are (1) to increase physician and patient awareness of the relationships, (2) to develop better methods to prove the causality of GER-related laryngeal disease, and (3) to develop less expensive and effective methods of medical and surgical therapy for these often chronic and morbid disorders.

REFERENCES

1. Koufman J, Sataloff FT, Toohill R. Laryngopharyngeal reflux: consensus conference report. *J Voice.* 1996;10:215–216.
2. Kahrilas PJ. Gastroesophageal reflux disease. *JAMA.* 1996;276:983–988.
3. Kuhn JC, Massick D, Toohill RJ, et al. Role of the esophagram in management of dysphonia. Presented at the Middle Section Meeting of the Triological Society, Kansas City, Missouri, January 24–26, 1997.
4. Koufman JA, Wiener GJ, Wallace CW, et al. Reflux laryngitisis and its sequela: the diagnostic role of ambulatory 24-hour monitoring. *J Voice.* 1988;2:78–79.
5. Toohill RJ, Mushtag E, Lehman RH. Otolaryngologic manifestations of gastroesophageal reflux. In: *Proceedings of XIV World Congress of Otolaryngology, Head and Neck Surgery.* Sacristan T, Alvarez–Vincent JJ, Bartual J, Antolf-Candela F, et al. Amsterdam, Berkeley, Milano: Kugler & Ghedini Publications, 1990:3005–3009.
6. Koufman JA. Gastroesophageal Reflux and Voice Disorders. In: Rubin JS et al, eds. *Diagnosis and Treatment of Voice Disorders.* New York: Igaku-Shoin, 1995:161–175.
7. Toohill RJ. The psychosmatic aspects of children with vocal nodules. *Arch Otolaryngol.* 1975;101:591–595.
8. Cherry J, Margulies SI. Contact ulcer of the larynx. *Laryngoscope.* 1968:78:1937–1940.
9. Ohman L, Olfsson J, Tibbling L, et al. Esophageal dysfunction in patients with contact ulcer of the larynx. *Ann Otol Rhinol Laryngol.* 1983;92:228–230.
10. Nasri S, Sercarz JA, McAlpin T, et al. Treatment of vocal fold granuloma using botulinum toxin type A. *Laryngoscope.* 1995;105:585–588.
11. Toohill RJ. Gastroesophageal reflux and laryngotracheal stenosis. Presented at the Second International Symposium on Laryngeal and Tracheal reconstruction, Monte Carlo, Monaco, May 23, 1996.
12. Koufman JA. The otolaryngologic manifestations of gastroesophageal reflux disease (GERD): a clinical investigation of 225 patients using ambulatory 24-hour pH monitoring and an experimental investigation of the role of acid and pepsin in the development of laryngeal injury. *Laryngoscope.* 1991;101:1.
13. Jindal JR, Milbrath MM, Shaker R, et al. Gastroesophageal reflux disease as a likely cause of "idiopathic" subglottic stenosis. *Ann Otol Rhinol Laryngol.* 1994;186–191.
14. Wilson JA, White A, Von Haacke NP, et al. Gastroesophageal reflux and posterior laryngitis. *Ann Otol Rhinol Laryngol.* 1989;98:405–410.
15. Richtsmeier WJ, Styczynski P, Johns ME. Selective, histamine-mediated immuno-suppression in laryngeal cancer. *Ann Otol Rhinol Laryngol.* 1987: 96:569–572.

Laryngopharyngeal reflux: Position statement of the Committee on Speech, Voice, and Swallowing Disorders of the American Academy of Otolaryngology–Head and Neck Surgery

JAMES A. KOUFMAN, MD, JONATHAN E. AVIV, MD, ROY R. CASIANO, MD, and **GARY Y. SHAW, MD,** Winston-Salem, North Carolina, New York, New York, Miami, Florida, and Kansas City, Missouri

The term *reflux* (derived from the Latin words *re* ["back"] and *fluere* ["to flow"]) literally means *backflow*. The term *gastroesophageal reflux* (GER) refers to the backflow of stomach contents into the esophagus. GER may be physiologic, and indeed up to 50 GER episodes a day, occurring mostly after meals, is accepted as being within the normal range.[1-3] *Gastroesophageal reflux disease* (GERD) is a clinical term that refers to GER that is excessive and that causes tissue damage (eg, esophagitis) and/or clinical symptoms (eg, heartburn).[1]

Laryngopharyngeal reflux (LPR) refers to the backflow of stomach contents into the throat, that is, into the laryngopharynx. There are numerous synonyms for LPR in the medical literature; the most accepted of these terms is *extraesophageal reflux* (Table 1). Most commonly, patients presenting to gastroenterologists have GERD, but most otolaryngologic patients have LPR. LPR differs in many ways from classic GERD.[1,4-9]

LPR DIFFERS FROM CLASSIC GERD

Patients with LPR appear to have different pathophysiologic mechanisms and patterns of reflux, as well as different symptoms, manifestations, and responses to treatment compared with patients with GERD.[1,4-14] The most significant difference between LPR and GERD is that the majority of patients with LPR do not have esophagitis or its primary symptom, heartburn.[1,4,6,9] Indeed, in a number of studies, the incidence of heartburn in patients with LPR is <40%, and the incidence of esophagitis is approximately 25%.[1,4-6] Thus, the vast majority of patients with LPR do not have esophagitis, the diagnostic sine qua non of GERD.[1,6,9]

It appears that the mechanisms of LPR are different from those of GERD.[4-9] Patients with LPR are predominantly upright (daytime) refluxers, whereas GERD patients are predominantly supine (nocturnal) refluxers.[1-6] There are prolonged periods of acid exposure in GERD but not in LPR.[1,2] In addition, patients with GERD have dysmotility and prolonged esophageal acid clearance, whereas those with LPR do not.[1,7] It is believed that the primary defect in GERD is lower esophageal dysfunction, whereas the primary defect in LPR is upper esophageal sphincter dysfunction. It is likely that these differences in mechanisms and patterns account for the differences in symptoms and manifestations of LPR and GERD. It is important to note that although most patients with LPR do not have GERD, some patients do indeed have both LPR and GERD.

SYMPTOMS OF LPR

The symptoms of LPR are protean; however, the most common are hoarseness, globus pharyngeus, dysphagia, cough, chronic throat clearing, and sore throat (Table 2). These symptoms are often intermittent or "chronic-intermittent."

CLINICAL MANIFESTATIONS

The most common manifestation of LPR is reflux laryngitis with or without granulation or gran-

From the Center for Voice Disorders of Wake Forest University, Winston-Salem, NC (Dr Koufman), Department of Otolaryngology–Head and Neck Surgery, New York Presbyterian Hospital, College of Physicians and Surgeons, Columbia University, New York, NY (Dr Aviv), Department of Otolaryngology, University of Miami Medical Center, Miami, FL (Dr Casiano), and Kansas City, MO (Dr Shaw).

Reprint requests: James A. Koufman, MD, FACS, Center for Voice Disorders of Wake Forest University, Medical Center Boulevard, Winston-Salem, NC 27157-1034; e-mail, jkoufman@wfubmc.edu.

Otolaryngol Head Neck Surg 2002;127:32-35

0194-5998/2002/$35.00 + 0 **23/1/125760**

doi:10.1067/mhn.2002.125760

Table 1. Synonyms for laryngopharyngeal reflus

Reflux laryngitis
Laryngeal reflux
Gastropharyngeal reflux
Pharyngoesophageal reflux
Supraesophageal reflux
Extraesophageal reflux
Atypical reflux

uloma formation.[11-17] In addition, reflux has been reported to be associated with subglottic stenosis, laryngeal carcinoma, polypoid degeneration, laryngospasm, paradoxical vocal fold movement, and vocal nodules[1,4,6,10-24] (Table 2). Other manifestations in the head and neck that have been reported include asthma, sinusitis, and otitis media.[25-30] In addition, pediatric LPR is now receiving considerable attention.[29-34]

It has been estimated that up to half of patients with laryngeal and voice disorders have reflux.[35] The prevalence of LPR in other disorders of the head and neck remains unknown.

Table 2. Symptoms and clinical manifestations reported to be related to laryngopharyngeal reflux

Symptoms	Conditions
Chronic dysphonia	Reflux laryngitis
Intermittent dysphonia	Subglottic stenosis
Vocal fatigue	Carcinoma of the larynx
Voice breaks	Endotracheal intubation injury
Chronic throat clearing	Contact ulcers and granulomas
Excessive throat mucus	Posterior glottic stenosis
"Postnasal drip"	Arytenoid fixation
Chronic cough	Paroxysmal laryngospasm
Dysphagia	Paradoxical vocal fold movement
Globus	Globus pharyngeus
Intermittent airway obstruction	Vocal nodules
Chronic airway obstruction	Polypoid degeneration
Wheezing	Laryngomalacia
	Pachydermia laryngis
	Recurrent leukoplakia
	Sudden infant death syndrome
	Sinusitis
	Otitis media
	Sleep apnea
	Exacerbation of asthma

DIAGNOSIS

The diagnosis of LPR can be made on the basis of the symptoms and laryngeal findings,[1,4,36] but ambulatory 24-hour double-probe (simultaneous esophageal and pharyngeal) pH monitoring remains the gold standard for the diagnosis of LPR when the diagnosis is in question.[1-3,37-39] In addition, double-probe pH testing is often used to evaluate drug efficacy. Other diagnostic tests, such as barium esophagraphy or esophagoscopy, are far less sensitive for LPR.[1,40] Even though barium studies and esophagoscopy are not usually used to diagnose LPR, it may be advisable to screen the esophagus for related pathology with one of these methods.[1,9]

TREATMENT

H_2-antagonists and proton pump inhibitors (PPIs) have been used to treat both GERD and LPR.[41-53] In general, treatment for LPR needs to be more aggressive and prolonged than that for GERD.[1,4,14-17,50-55] It has been shown that as few as 3 experimental LPR episodes a week can result in severe laryngeal damage.[1,20] The larynx is more susceptible to reflux injury than the esophagus, because it lacks both the extrinsic and intrinsic epithelial defenses of the esophagus.[1,20,56]

The type of treatment is dependent on the symptoms and severity of LPR and on the patient response to treatment. Patients with mild and/or intermittent symptoms can be treated with dietary and lifestyle modifications as well as with H_2-antagonists such as ranitidine.[1,4,14,17] The majority of patients with LPR, however, require at least twice-daily dosing with PPIs.[4,36,50-53,57] The reason for the twice-daily dosing is that none of the PPIs exert acid suppression (intragastric pH >4) for >16.8 hours.[51,52] In some patients, it is necessary to treat with both a PPI and an H_2-antagonist.[50]

Within 2 to 3 months of treatment, most patients report significant symptomatic improvement; however, it takes 6 months or longer for the laryngeal findings of LPR to resolve.[57,58] Thus, twice-daily dose PPI treatment is recommended for a minimum initial treatment for a period of 6 months in many patients with LPR. Some patients may require prolonged tapering and/or chronic treatment. As an alternative to medical treatment, fundoplication has been shown to be an effective therapy for LPR.[59,60]

CONCLUSIONS

Patients with LPR have upper aerodigestive manifestations of reflux disease rather than classic GERD (ie, esophagitis and its sequelae). The manifestations and symptoms of LPR are different because the mechanisms and patterns of reflux are different than those of GERD. For most patients with LPR, twice-daily dosing with a PPI is recommended for an initial treatment for a period of no less than 6 months, and lifetime treatment may be required.

REFERENCES

1. Koufman JA. The otolaryngologic manifestations of gastroesophageal reflux disease (GERD): a clinical investigation of 225 patients using ambulatory 24-hour pH monitoring and an experimental investigation of the role of acid and pepsin in the development of laryngeal injury. Laryngoscope 1991;101(Suppl 53):1-78.
2. Richter JE, editor. Ambulatory esophageal pH monitoring: practical approach and clinical applications. New York: Igaku-Shoin; 1991.
3. Postma GN. Ambulatory pH monitoring methodology. Ann Otol Rhinol Laryngol 2000;109(suppl 184):10-4.
4. Koufman J, Sataloff RT, Toohill R. Laryngopharyngeal Reflux: Consensus Report. J Voice 1996;10:215-6.
5. Ossakow SJ, Elta G, Colturi T, et al. Esophageal reflux and dysmotility as the basis for persistent cervical symptoms. Ann Otol Rhinol Laryngol 1987;96:387-92.
6. Wiener GJ, Koufman JA, Wu WC, et al. Chronic hoarseness secondary to gastroesophageal reflux disease: documentation with 24-h ambulatory pH monitoring. Am J Gastroenterol 1989;84:1503-8.
7. Postma GN, Tomek MS, Belafsky PC, et al. Esophageal motor function in laryngopharyngeal reflux is superior to that of classic gastroesophageal reflux disease. Ann Otol Rhinol Laryngol 2001;110:1114-6.
8. Aviv JE, Takoudes TG, Ma G, et al. Office-based esophagoscopy: a preliminary report. Otolaryngol Head Neck Surg 2001;125:170-5.
9. Belafsky PC, Postma GN, Koufman JA. Transnasal esophagoscopy (TNE). Otolaryngol Head Neck Surg 2001;125:588-9.
10. Bain WM, Harrington JW, Thomas LE, et al. Head and neck manifestations of gastroesophageal reflux. Laryngoscope 1983;93:175-9.
11. Al Sabbagh G, Wo JM. Supraesophageal manifestations of gastroesophageal reflux disease. Semin Gastrointest Dis 1999;10:113-9.
12. Toohill RJ, Kuhn JC. Role of refluxed acid in pathogenesis of laryngeal disorders. Am J Med 1997;103:100S-6S.
13. Koufman JA, Wiener GJ, Wu WC, et al. Reflux laryngitis and its sequelae: The diagnostic role of ambulatory 24-hour pH monitoring: J Voice 1988;2:78-89.
14. Ulualp SO, Toohill RJ. Laryngopharyngeal reflux: state of the art diagnosis and treatment. Otolaryngol Clin North Am 2000;33:785-01.
15. Koufman JA. Contact ulcer and granuloma of the larynx. In Gates G, editor. Current Therapy in Otolaryngology–Head and Neck Surgery. 5th ed. St Louis: Mosby Publishers; 1993. p. 456-9.
16. Havas TE, Priestley J, Lowinger DS. A management strategy for vocal process granulomas. Laryngoscope 1999;109:301-6.
17. Hanson DG, Jiang JJ. Diagnosis and management of chronic laryngitis associated with reflux. Am J Med 2000;108:112S-9S.
18. Kuhn J, Toohill RJ, Ulualp SO, et al. Pharyngeal acid reflux events in patients with vocal cord nodules. Laryngoscope 1998;108:1146-9.
19. Ross JA, Noordzji JP, Woo P. Voice disorders in patients with suspected laryngo-pharyngeal reflux disease. J Voice 1998;12:84-8.
20. Little FB, Koufman JA, Kohut RI, et al. Effect of gastric acid on the pathogenesis of subglottic stenosis. Ann Otol Rhinol Laryngol 1985;94:516-9.
21. Ward PH, Hanson DG. Reflux as an etiological factor of carcinoma of the laryngopharynx. Laryngoscope 1988; 98:1195-9.
22. Koufman JA, Burke AJ. The etiology and pathogenesis of laryngeal carcinoma. Otolaryngol Clin North Am 1997;30:1-19.
23. Loughlin CJ, Koufman JA. Paroxysmal laryngospasm secondary to gastroesophageal reflux. Laryngoscope 1996;106:1502-5.
24. Loughlin CJ, Koufman JA, Averill DB, et al. Acid-induced laryngospasm in a canine model. Laryngoscope 1996;1506-9.
25. Bowrey DJ, Peters JH, DeMeester TR. Gastroesophageal reflux disease in asthma: effects of medical and surgical antireflux therapy on asthma control. Ann Surg 2000; 231:161-72.
26. Harding SM, Richter JE, Guzzo MR, et al. Asthma and gastroesophageal reflux: acid suppressive therapy improves asthma outcome. Am J Med 1996;100:395-405.
27. Harding SM, Richter JE. The role of gastroesophageal reflux in chronic cough and asthma. Chest 1997;111: 1389-402.
28. Bothwell MR, Parsons DS, Talbot A, et al. Outcome of reflux therapy on pediatric chronic sinusitis. Otolaryngol Head Neck Surg 1999;121:255-62.
29. Rozmanic VM, Bonifacic M. Gastroesophageal reflux, allergy and chronic tubotympanal disorders in children. Int J Pediatr Otorhinolaryngol 2000;55:187-90.
30. Tasker A, Dettmar PW, Panetti M, et al. Reflux of gastric juice and glue ear in children. Lancet 2002;359:493.
31. Halstead LA. Role of gastroesophageal reflux in pediatric upper airway disorders. Otolaryngol Head Neck Surg 1999;120:208-14.
32. Little JP, Matthews BL, Glock MS, et al. Extraesophageal pediatric reflux: 24-hour double-probe pH monitoring of 222 children. Ann Otol Rhinol Laryngol 1997; suppl 169:1-16.
33. Wetmore RF. Effects of acid on the larynx of the maturing rabbit and their possible significance to the sudden infant death syndrome. Laryngoscope 1993;103:1242-54.

34. Duke SG, Postma GN, McGuirt WF Jr, et al. Laryngospasm and diaphragmatic arrest in the immature canine after laryngeal acid exposure: a possible model for sudden infant death syndrome (SIDS). Ann Otol Rhinol Laryngol 2001;110:729-33.
35. Koufman JA, Amin MR, Panetti M. Prevalence of reflux in 113 consecutive patients with laryngeal and voice disorders. Otolaryngol Head Neck Surg 2000;123:385-8.
36. Belafsky PC, Postma GN, Koufman JA. The validity and reliability of the reflux finding score (RFS). Laryngoscope 2001;111:1313-7.
37. Grontved AM, West F. pH monitoring in patients with benign voice disorders. Acta Otolaryngol Suppl 2000; 543:229-31.
38. Johnson PE, Amin MA, Postma GN, et al. pH monitoring in patients with laryngopharyngeal reflux (LPR): why the pharyngeal probe is essential. Otolaryngol Head Neck Surg (in press)
39. Johnson PE, Koufman JA, Nowak LJ, et al. Ambulatory 24-hour double-probe pH monitoring: the importance of manometry. Laryngoscope 2001;111:1970-5.
40. Ott DJ. Gastroesophageal reflux disease. Radiol Clin North Am 1994;32:1147-66.
41. Klinkenberg-Knol EC, Meuwissen SG. Treatment of reflux oesophagitis resistant to H2-receptor antagonists. Digestion 1989;suppl 1:47-53.
42. Vigneri S, Termini R, Leandro G, et al. A comparison of five maintenance therapies for reflux esophagitis. N Engl J Med 1995;333:1106-10.
43. Maton PN, Orlando R, Joelsson B. Efficacy of omeprazole versus ranitidine for symptomatic treatment of poorly responsive acid reflux disease: a prospective, controlled trial. Aliment Pharmacol Ther 1999;13:819-26.
44. Jansen JB, Van Oene JC. Standard-dose lansoprazole is more effective than high-dose ranitidine in achieving endoscopic healing and symptom relief in patients with moderately severe reflux oesophagitis. The Dutch Lansoprazole Study Group. Aliment Pharmacol Ther 1999; 13:1611-20.
45. Scott M, Gelhot AR. Gastroesophageal reflux disease: diagnosis and management. Am Fam Physician 1999;59: 1161-99.
46. Smith JT, Gavey C, Nwokolo CU, et al. Tolerance during 8 days of high-dose H2-blockade: placebo-controlled studies of 24-hour acidity and gastrin. Aliment Pharmacol Ther 1990;suppl 1:47-63.
47. Skoutakis VA, Joe RH, Hara DS. Comparative role of omeprazole in the treatment of gastroesophageal reflux disease. Ann Pharmacother 1995;29:1252-62.
48. Leite LP, Johnston BT, Just RJ, et al. Persistent acid secretion during omeprazole therapy: a study of gastric acid profiles in patients demonstrating failure of omeprazole therapy. Am J Gastroenterol 1996;91:1527-31.
49. Peghini PL, Katz PO, Bracy NA, et al. Nocturnal recovery of gastric acid secretion with twice-daily dosing of proton pump inhibitors. Am J Gastroenterol 1998;93: 763-7.
50. Bough ID Jr, Sataloff RT, Castell DO, et al. Gastroesophageal reflux laryngitis resistant to omeprazole therapy. J Voice 1995;9:205-11.
51. Chiverton SG, Howden CW, Burget DW, et al. Omeprazole (20 mg) daily given in the morning or evening: a comparison of effects on gastric acidity, and plasma gastrin and omeprazole concentration. Aliment Pharmacol Ther 1992;6:103-11.
52. Kahrilas PJ, Falk GW, Johnson DA, et al. Esomeprazole improves healing and symptom resolution as compared with omeprazole in reflux oesophagitis patients: a randomized controlled trial. Aliment Pharmacol Ther 2000; 14:1249-58.
53. Shaw GY, Searl JP. Laryngeal manifestations of gastroesophageal reflux before and after treatment with omeprazole. South Med J 1997;90:1115-22.
54. Wong RK, Hanson DG, Waring PJ, et al. ENT manifestations of gastroesophageal reflux. Am J Gastroenterol 2000;95(suppl 8):515-20.
55. Harding SM, Richter JE, Guzzo MR, et al. Asthma and gastroesophageal reflux: acid suppressive therapy improves asthma outcome. Am J Med 1995;100:395-05.
56. Axford SE, Sharp N, Ross PE, et al. Cell biology of laryngeal epithelial defenses in health and disease: preliminary studies. Ann Otol Rhinol Laryngol 2001;1099-08.
57. Belafsky PC, Postma GN, Koufman KA. Laryngopharyngeal reflux symptoms improve before changes in physical findings. Laryngoscope 2001;111:979-81.
58. Aviv JE, Liu H, Parides M, et al. Laryngopharyngeal sensory deficits in patients with laryngopharyngeal reflux and dysphagia. Ann Otol Rhinol Laryngol 2000;109: 1000-6.
59. Hunter J. Laparoscopic fundoplication. Ann Surg 1996; 223:673-87.
60. Dallemagne B, Weerts JM, Jeahes C, et al. Results of laparoscopic Nissen fundoplication. Hepatogastroenterology 1998;45:1338-43.

6

Endoscopic Laryngeal Surgery

Introduction

It is mystifying that the mainstay procedure in laryngologic surgery, laryngoscopy, is so sparsely represented in this collection of classic articles. The transition from surgery with the naked eye to microscopic surgery occurred at least partially within the timeframe covered, articulated as a complete system of surgery in Kleinsasser's 1968 monograph *Microlaryngoscopy and Endolaryngeal Microsurgery*.[1] The change was so dramatic that one surgeon remarked that the individual using standard endoscopic instruments under the microscope "feels as if he is working with crowbars."[2] Yet, of all the subsequent refinements, only the introduction of the CO_2 laser meets the classic criteria. It would appear that much of the technical and instrument innovations took place off of the stage of peer-reviewed literature, perhaps in panels, courses, discussions, or instrument catalogs. Were the benefits so self-evident that they did not need validation or debate in the journals? Nonetheless, it is striking that so much clinical evolution took place with so little apparent ado.

Microlaryngeal surgery was certainly no sterile advance, and has evolved into an increasingly sophisticated repertoire of techniques; mastery of these is one of the elements that has justified the establishment of fellowship training programs in the field. The introduction of the CO_2 laser was indeed a large and—as Dr. Strong's recollection clearly conveys—a brave step forward, with obvious advantages for hemostasis and, at the time, for minimizing tissue injury. The laser-tissue interaction, which seemed exemplary at the time of its introduction, is regarded with rather more reservation today, especially at the vibratory margin of the vocal fold; this reveals not only how far microlaryngopscopic technique and expectations have evolved, but also the challenging environment in which Dr. Strong and his colleagues were innovating.

The CO_2 laser has not yet reached its full potential, even now more than three decades after its introduction, and in fact continues to expand into endoscopic cancer surgery, even as it is replaced at the membranous vocal fold by its angiolytic cousins. As for microlaryngoscopy, it will probably continue to hold pride of place in the laryngeal surgeon's repertoire. There will likely be no medical or molecular cure for the bulk of its targets, lesions which are the products of trauma, any more than there will be a nonsurgical cure for fractures and lacerations. Surgical finesse and precision are not likely to become obsolete.

References

1. Kleinsasser O. *Microlaryngolscopy and Endolaryngeal Microsurgery.* Philadelphia, Pa: Saunders; 1968.
2. Scalco AN, Shipman WF, Tabb HG. Microscopic suspension laryngoscopy. *Ann Otol.* 1960;69:1134–1138.

Classic Articles

• Reprint of article included in this chapter.
♦ Commentary on this article.

•♦ Strong MS, Jako GJ. Laser surgery in the larynx. Early clinical experience with continuous CO_2 laser. *Ann Otol Rhinol Laryngol.* 1972;81(6):791–798.

Commentary

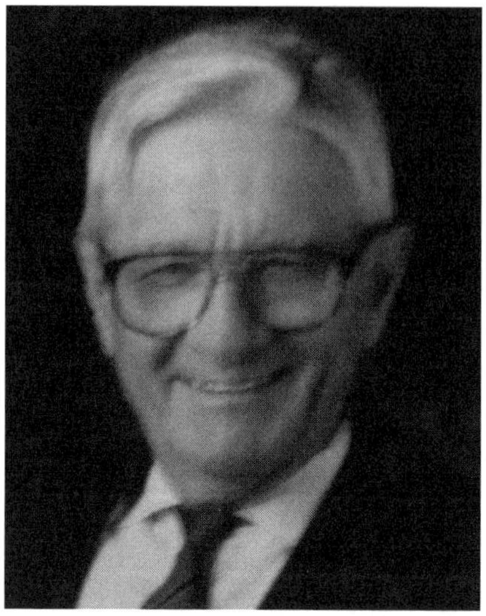

M. Stuart Strong, MD

When Geza Jako first mentioned to me that he thought we might have access to a surgical laser in 1969, I thought it was a flight of fancy; I could see no prospect of it being useful in Otolaryngology. He did press me (knowing that I was a bit of a gadgeteer) and eventually I did consent to go and see the new laser in the American Optical Gas Laser Research lab in Southborough Massachusetts; the instrument had been developed by Dr. Thomas Polanyi and his team of engineers. The machine was very crude and unwieldy and I thought there was little hope of it being useful in our field. I did notice, however, that the lesions we created on the dog's vocal folds did not bleed and were followed by no immediate postoperative swelling.

Geza persevered with encouragement from Dr. Polanyi's team to develop an attachment to a Zeiss surgical microscope. Six months later when I saw the micromanipulator with the laser attached to it, I finally became interested that just maybe a surgical laser had possibilities in laryngology—in endoscopic surgery. One doubt in my mind was, "could it made safe to use clinically?" and secondly, "would it prove to be a dependable and useful instrument?" Geza and I spent almost 2 years in the dog lab attempting to establish the exact nature of the soft tissue-laser interaction and what precautions needed to be taken to avoid unwanted tissue injury or fire in an oxygen- enriched atmosphere. The first part was easy but making the system fireproof was more difficult—identifying an endotracheal tube that would not combust when impacted with the laser in an oxygen enriched atmosphere. We were keenly aware that if we had one single clinical dangerous accident, the project would be dead. The use of a red rubber endotracheal tube wrapped with reflective tape was as good as we could come up with.

We knew it was not perfect but we were very anxious to see if we could duplicate the favorable features of the laser-tissue interaction in the human larynx. We were attracted especially by the bloodless field, the lack of postoperative swelling, the prompt healing with minimal scarring, and the accuracy of the removal of a specimen by a surgeon with average dexterity. We knew that sometimes a price would have to be paid in vocal fold function by the loss of some vocal fold cover.

We were cautiously optimistic so that we proceeded to obtain the sanction of the Hospital Human Studies' Committee and the concurrence of the anesthesiologists. The clinical trial started on April 1, 1971 in the Boston Veterans Administration Hospital after which we found, as expected, that the effects on human tissue were exactly the same as on the animal tissue. We were off and running and the outcome was the manuscript of 1972. It was quite soon that our activity was noticed by the one laryngologist on the East Coast who had the trust of many of the New York singing elite, Dr James Gould of Lennox Hill Hospital. Dr Gould did more to bring about the inclusion of voice into the repertoire of the laryngology than anybody else. He came up to Boston to see how we were dealing with tiny lesions of the larynx and was sufficiently impressed that he asked us to take care of a few special singers whose careers were likely to come to an end unless we could remove the offending lesion without causing too much damage to the vocal fold cover. It was a great privilege for us to take care of these world class artists, perhaps the most gratifying part of my career. Soon we felt confident that we could remove tiny lesions or coagulate offending bleeding vessels predictably so that they could get them back to performing on stage.

Another very important source of satisfaction was the knowledge that the use of a CO_2 laser in this fashion was transferable to others—that others with average dexterity could duplicate the outcomes in their patients —provided that they observed the constraints of caution and caring and only consented to try and help when there was no other option. It was an immense advance over what we had been able to do with conventional microsurgical cold instrument techniques. Others (eg, Dr Steve Zeitels, who was one of our trainees) have since shown that, in exceptional hands, cold instrument technique can be brought to the next level of sheer excellence. I just know that he could not have trained me to copy him. He is gifted with an extraordinary level of manual skill.

It wasn't long before we wanted to try more extensive dissections within and around the larynx; this part of the project was lead by my colleague of over 45 years, Dr. Charles W. Vaughan. He found that it was possible to carry out a subtotal laryngectomy with laser and without a tracheotomy, all because of the special attributes of the laser-soft tissue interaction. Soon our pulmonary colleagues were wondering if we could clear the tracheal and bronchial airways of obstructing masses—benign tumors, malignant tumors (for temporary relief, prior to further treatment) and so forth. Following on with the principle that "if you can see it, you can impact with a laser," it wasn't long before the Research Group came up with a bronchoscopic attachment—a laser bronchoscope! The instrument had an aiming light that could be manipulated within the confines of the scope; it was tedious work but we showed that it could be done safely—endoscopic surgery.

With refinements being made in the equipment, others who came after us were able to advance the use of the laser in areas that we had not imagined and also identified areas where its use had no particular advantage over conventional techniques. This was all very gratifying to those of us who had "made a beginning." There were some who wanted to exploit the laser, making it an end in itself for financial reasons; that made us very uncomfortable and we regretted that we could not do anything to control such misuse.

Overall, however, some 30 years later, the introduction of a surgical laser into laryngology has proven to be of benefit to countless patients and because of that I feel the project was worthwhile.

LASER SURGERY IN THE LARYNX

EARLY CLINICAL EXPERIENCE WITH CONTINUOUS CO_2 LASER

M. STUART STRONG, M.D.

GEZA J. JAKO, M.D.

BOSTON, MASSACHUSETTS

Although lasers have been available for ten years or more, physicians in general have had a nebulous idea of their properties and have been skeptical regarding their use in medicine. Probably this attitude has been fostered by their publicity in popular cartoons and movie thrillers!

Initial experience with pulsed lasers in the ablation of experimental tumors demonstrated an explosive effect and the scattering of viable tumor cells; this effect of pulsed lasers has frequently discouraged potential investigators from pursuing the possibilities of laser application in surgery.

Certain lasers, depending on their wave length, have properties making them specifically applicable to a particular problem; the energy of an argon laser, for example, will pass through the cornea and be selectively absorbed by the pigmented retina. In contrast a continuous CO_2 laser is almost completely absorbed by biologic tissues and can be used to achieve controlled destruction of preselected areas of tissue.

Development and Application of CO_2 Laser. The continuous CO_2 laser was discovered in 1965 and shortly thereafter the gas laser research group of the American Optical Laser Research Laboratories developed methods of producing, transmitting and focusing this energy; it rapidly became apparent that this form of nonionizing electromagnetic radiation had potential as a surgical tool. After the development of the basic surgical laser with the handpieces containing lenses of various focal lengths,[1] the development of the laser endoscope and the stereomicroscope laser attachment quickly followed.[2]

The coupling of the CO_2 surgical laser to the Zeiss surgical microscope made it possible to study the effect of laser impacts on the canine larynx. It was found that the new type of energy could be controlled and applied to preselected areas of the vocal cords with microscopic precision; a lesion no deeper than the epithelium could be created or the entire vocal cord could be systematically destroyed.

Properties of the Continuous CO_2 Laser. As a surgical tool the continuous CO_2 laser presented certain distinct advantages over other types of lasers. The safety precautions needed in the use of a CO_2 laser are much less than with many other lasers; the operating room personnel need only wear ordinary eye glasses to protect their corneas from injury[3] if the laser beam should be accidentally reflected from a metal surface. If an area of tissue close to the target area needs to be protected, it can be adequately shielded by covering it with moist gauze, since water dissipates the energy effectively.

From the Department of Otolaryngology, Boston University School of Medicine, University Hospital and Boston Veterans Administration Hospital, Boston, Mass.

Presented at the meeting of the American Broncho-Esophagological Association, Palm Beach, Florida, April 24-25, 1972.

While many lasers are absorbed in proportion to the degree or type of pigmentation of the target area, the CO_2 laser has the great advantage of being absorbed by all biological tissues. Mucosa, skin, fat, muscle, cartilage, bone, etc., can all be vaporized in a controlled fashion using the appropriate amounts of laser energy. Since the CO_2 laser operates at a wave length of 10.6 μ in the infrared region of high tissue absorption, the injury is entirely a thermal process.

The early high power pulsed lasers had the disadvantage of exerting considerable pressure on the target area so that soft tissue such as tumor would tend to "explode" and scatter. The continuous CO_2 laser, whether it is used intermittently or as a continuous beam, has little or no "pulsive effect."

Experience with Soft Tissue Destruction in Dogs. In addition to the first series of experiments done on the canine larynx,[2] further experiments were carried out to explore the horizons of the stereomicroscope laser attachment and to gain expertise in its use. Small areas of the canine vocal cords were impacted creating very superficial lesions or deep lesions; in others the entire vocal cord was excised and in some the arytenoid cartilage was vaporized. The instrument was used to excise 2.0 cm "wedges" of the canine soft palate and tongue. In half of these experiments the animals were sacrificed immediately and the impacted areas studied histologically; in the other half the animals were sacrificed at four weeks so that the healed laser wounds could be examined by light microscopy.

Features of Laser Surgery. After this animal surgery it became apparent that laser surgery of the vocal cords using a continuous CO_2 laser had some very important attributes. In laser surgery of the larynx *the target area which has an approximate diameter of 2 mms is continuously under binocular vision* so that the progress of tissue destruction can be carefully monitored; this is in contrast to the use of a diathermy probe or a cryoprobe, where the view of the area being destroyed is often obscured. Vaporization of soft tissues by laser causes steam, and with low energy levels, smoke which would obscure the field, if they are not removed through a strategically placed suction tip.

Microsurgery is only practical so long as the field can be kept free of blood. Laser radiation has an extraordinary *hemostatic effect* when tissue is destroyed,[4] so that maximum visibility is maintained. Segmental resections of the canine tongue and soft palate could be carried out with no bleeding, unless a vessel greater than 0.5 mm was sectioned, and even these vessels could be secondarily coagulated by the laser. Conventional forms of tissue destruction such as diathermy and cryosurgery are often accompanied by marked postoperative edema in the tissues adjacent to the wound; in laser surgery, *postoperative edema is conspicuous by its absence.* This suggests that the laser injury is sharply demarcated from the surrounding nonirradiated tissue and that there is not an area of gradually decreasing tissue injury surrounding the impacted area.

Histological examination of fresh laser wounds reveals a very *clean line of tissue destruction*; surrounding the wound there is a thin layer (5 to 10 cells in thickness) of heat coagulation and beyond that, the tissue architecture is undisturbed. In this latter zone, capillaries maintain their circulation and there is no evidence of increased interstitial fluid. A laser wound appears as if it had been created by a searing scalpel! *Healing, after laser surgery is very rapid.* In some experiments, extensive lesions were re-epithelialized in 10 to 12 days. Probably rapid healing ensues because of the minimal disturbance that is found in the tissues immediately adjacent to the impacted area. *Laser surgery causes minimal postoperative scarring*; after extensive resections of the tongue, palate and vocal cords of the dog, excellent mobility was maintained. This appears to be due to the localized nature of the laser injury.

Clinical Trial. The laboratory experience suggested that laser surgery might

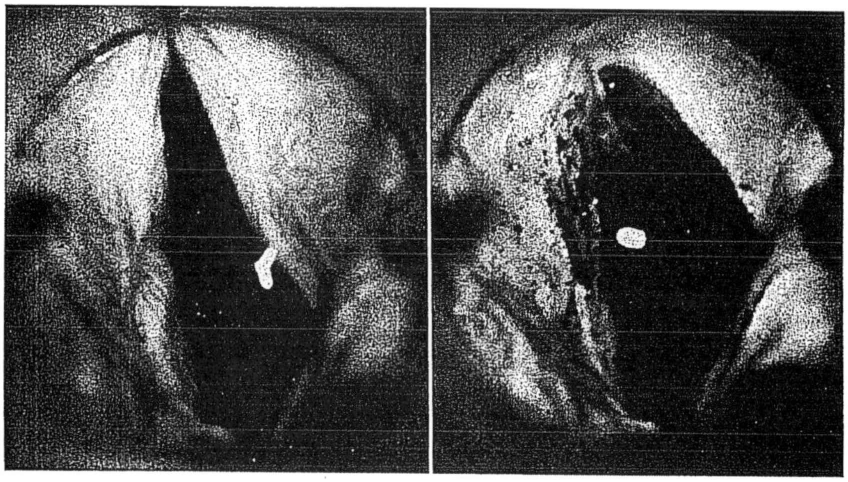

Fig. 1. Focussing light on the larynx about to be excised for carcinoma of the pyriform sinus.

Fig. 2. A superficial lesion has been created on the left cord and a deep lesion on the right cord of larynx in Fig. 1.

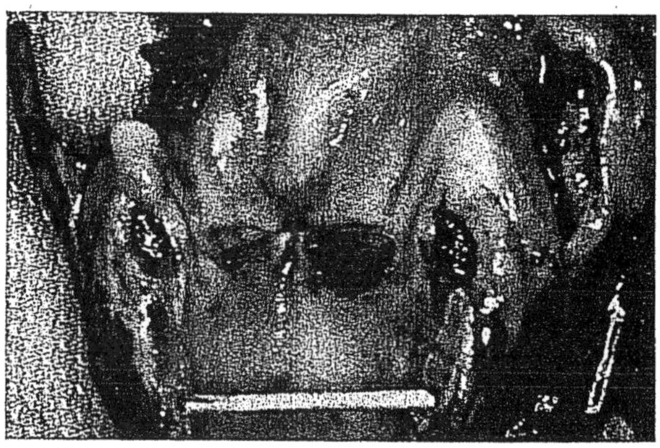

Fig. 3. The laryngectomy specimen of Fig. 1 showing superficial lesion on left cord and deep lesion on right cord.

be ideal for the management of certain localized problems where preservation of function is important. Prior to applying the CO_2 laser therapeutically, it was decided to "treat" the vocal cord area of patients about to have laryngectomy for advanced carcinoma; in this way any discrepancy between the effect of the laser on the canine larynx and human larynx would be detected. This was carried out in four patients.

After carrying out a tracheotomy and inducing general anesthesia, the larynx was exposed with the Jako-Pilling Laryngoscope. The laryngoscope was placed on the suspension apparatus and the microscope with the laser attachment brought into position. A wide variety of lesions were created on the normal cord and tumor bearing area using various combinations of power (in watts) and time settings (in fractions of a second).

It was found that the lesions created were entirely predictable, as they had been in the canine experiments. Using low power (5 watts) and short duration of exposure (1/20 sec) a very superficial lesion could be produced, merely vaporizing the epithelium and exposing Reinke's space (Figs. 1, 2 and 3); by

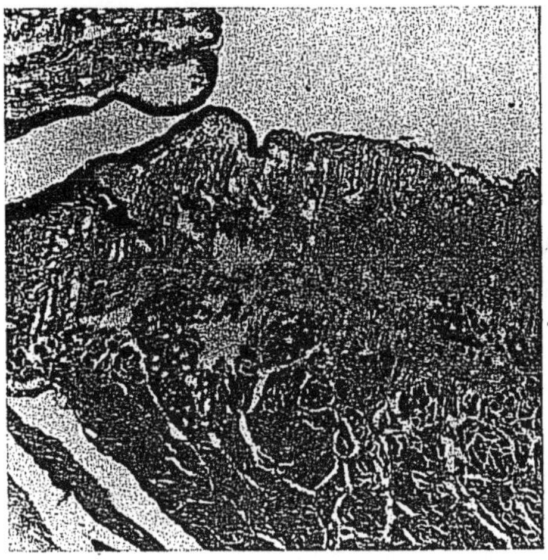

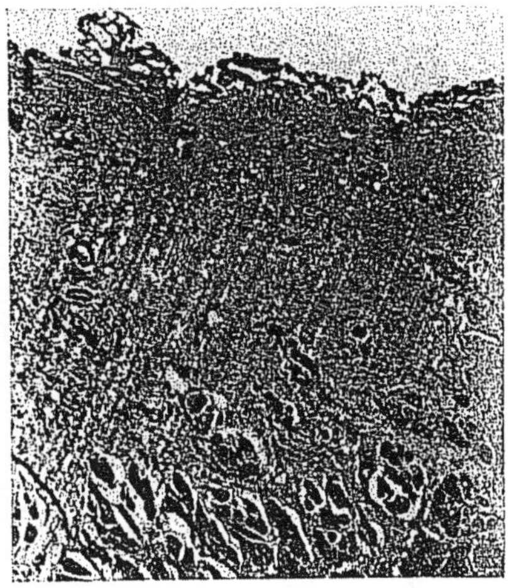

Fig. 4. Low power view (40x) of upper surface of left vocal cord at inlet of ventricle; the epithelium has been vaporized by laser.

Fig. 5. Medium power view (100x) of cord in Fig. 4 showing flecks of carbon on the surface with a thin layer of heat coagulum.

focusing the beam on an adjacent area after each impact this superficial lesion could be extended indefinitely on the vocal cord (Figs. 4 and 5). With higher power (20 watts) and longer duration (1/5 sec), a deeper lesion could be created; if several impacts of the beam were made on the same target area, the vocalis muscle (Figs. 6 and 7) or elastic fibers of the cord could be rapidly exposed and the entire cord vaporized. The ease with which the depth of tissue destruction could be controlled was very striking.

It was felt that the beam could be confidently controlled at all times with perfect precision so that there was no danger to the patient or the operating room personnel. Consequently cases were selected for therapeutic trial in which soft tissue was to be destroyed and where preservation of function was paramount.

Technique. The surgical microscope is fitted with a 400 mm front lens and the CO_2 laser attachment (Figs. 8 and 9). The laser attachment to the microscope is checked for accuracy on an inert target area (e.g., an asbestos block). The patient is then prepared for microscopic laryngoscopy under general anesthesia in the usual manner;[5] with a No. 26 French (6 mm) cuffed endotracheal tube in position, the Jako-Pilling Laryngoscope is used to expose the vocal cords and the instrument placed on the suspension apparatus (Fig. 10).

The microscope, with the laser attachment in place, is swung into position and the larynx exposed with 10X magnification. The aiming light for the laser beam is manipulated into position with the joy stick control on the laser attachment (Fig. 11) and the laser is activated. A 2 mm self-retaining suction tip is clipped onto the inner wall of the laryngoscope so that steam and smoke can be immediately removed from the target area. Depending on the volume of tissue that is to be vaporized, power and time settings for the laser are selected. Using a footswitch to control each timed impact and the joy stick to change the target area, the lesion is progressively destroyed. The suction tip within the laryngoscope tube keeps the target area from being obscured by steam, etc. When necessary, a straight or curved probe may be used to bring the lesions into better view; the cord may need to be retracted to expose a lesion in the subglottic area.

If the histologic nature of the lesion is not known, a fragment is held under

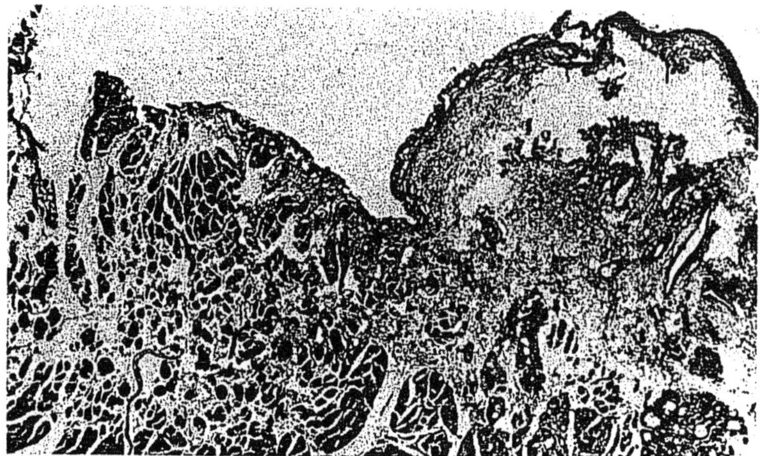

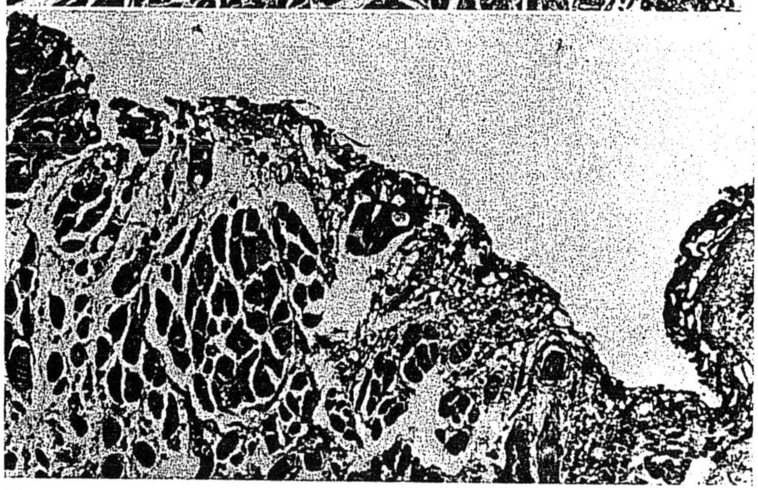

Fig. 6. Medium power view (100x) of right cord in Fig. 2 adjacent to ventricle in which the vocalis muscle has been exposed by laser.

Fig. 7. High power view (200x) of cord in Fig. 6 showing carbon particles and layer of heat coagulum in exposed muscle bundles.

tension with a cup forceps and then cleanly detached with several laser impacts. The biopsy specimen is sent for histologic study and the remainder of the lesion is destroyed. Laser excision of a biopsy specimen causes minimal distortion of the tissue, which appears to be even less than that seen after avulsion of a specimen by a cup forceps. Any residual bleeding provoked by a mechanical manipulation with the suction tip or probes can be controlled with the laser. The microscope is removed from the operative field, the laryngoscope is withdrawn and the procedure concluded in the usual fashion.

Clinical Experience. A variety of pathologic entities have been treated with laser surgery (Table I). If the lesion had not been biopsied previously, a biopsy was taken. Plaque-like lesions such as keratoses and carcinoma *in situ* were vaporized by multiple superficial impacts until all of the involved area had been eradicated (Figs. 12 and 13). Small sessile lesions, such as vocal cord nodules, were treated in a similar fashion leaving the free edge of the cord perfectly smooth. Pedunculated lesions such as polyps and cysts were usually put on the stretch with a cup forceps and then excised through the base with the laser.

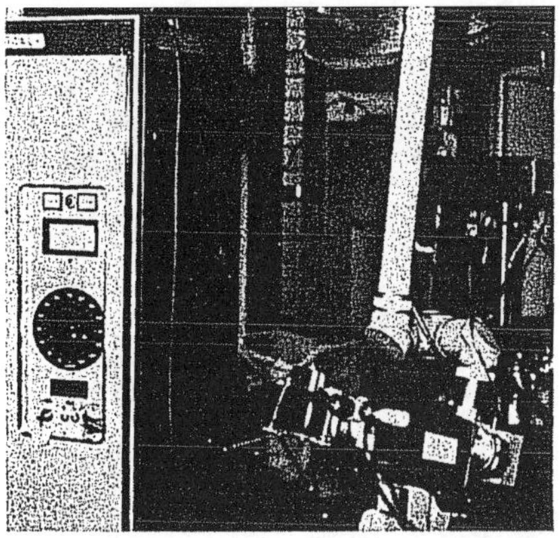

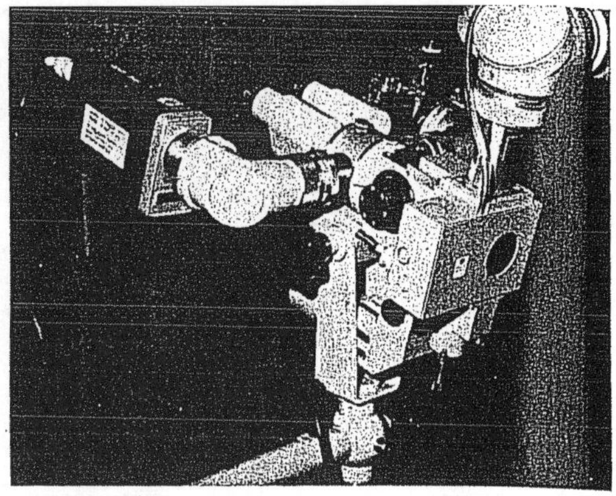

Fig. 8. Control panel of American Optical Corporation CO_2 surgical laser.
Fig. 9. CO_2 laser attachment fitted over the front lens of the microscope. Still and TV cameras are fitted to the beam splitter.

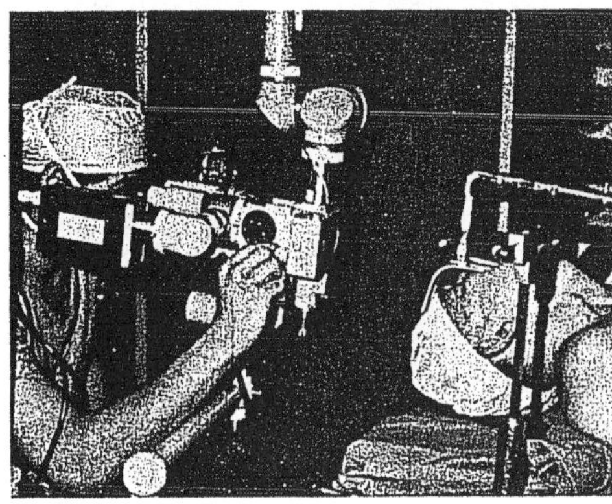

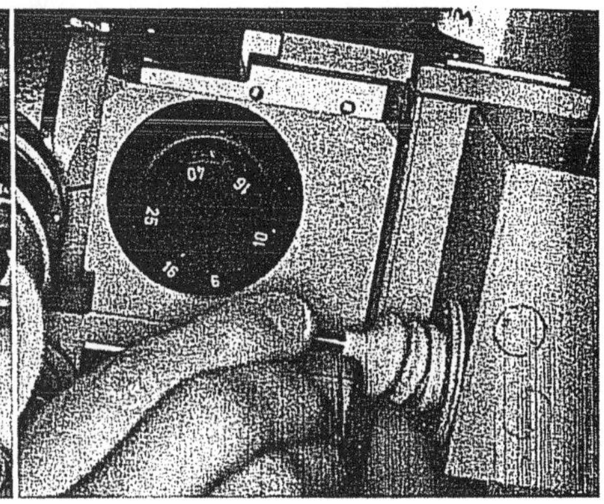

Fig. 10. The laryngoscope is on the suspension gallows and the laser attachment is in the operating position.
Fig. 11. The joy stick control of the laser attachment.

TABLE I

LESIONS TREATED BY LASER SURGERY

Nodules	2	
Polyps	4	
Cysts	1	
Keratosis	4	
Carcinoma in situ	1	(x2)
Papilloma	3	(1x3)
Total	15	

Papillomas were treated by progressive destruction without manipulation in order to avoid bleeding and perhaps further seeding. The lack of bleeding during this method of excision was particularly striking (Figs. 14 and 15).

All cases were returned to the ward on awakening, allowed to talk softly and were discharged the day following operation. The treated areas of the larynx were seen to be covered with a white fibrinous exudate and no edema was noted around the treated area. There was no postoperative discomfort other than associated with the use of the laryngoscope or muscle relaxants. Patients were seen at weekly intervals for one month so that the rate of healing could be observed. At the end of one week most cases were healed and epithelization was complete in all cases after three weeks; residual disease was absent in all cases except in one case of extensive papilloma which required three treatments to clear the larynx and a case

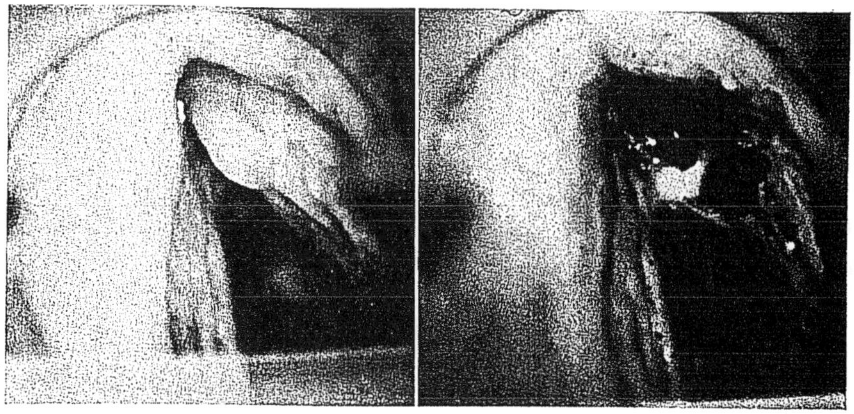

Fig. 12. Polyp with keratosis on the right vocal cord which has been previously biopsied.

Fig. 13. The polyp and keratosis of Fig. 12 have been destroyed. Aiming light still in position.

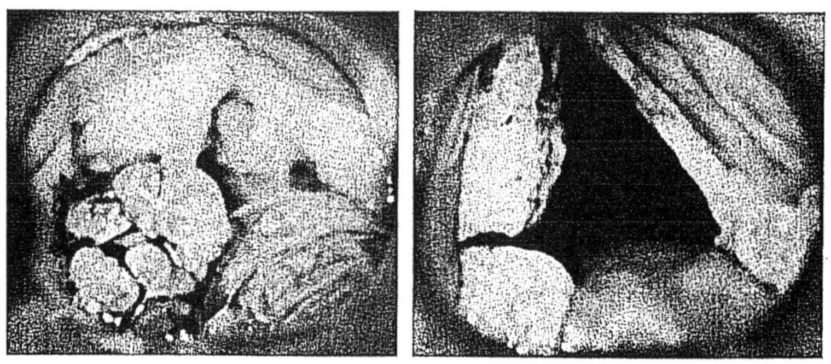

Fig. 14. Multiple papillomas of 14-year-old male following 28 conventional endoscopic procedures.

Fig. 15. One month after a single laser excision of papillomas seen in Fig. 14; larynx was cleared of all visible papilloma remnants after two further laser excisions.

of carcinoma in situ in which each cord was treated separately. Prolonged follow-up will be necessary to determine if the disease has been arrested.

Precautions and Potential Complications. Although it is only remotely possible that the CO_2 laser beam could strike a metal object (such as the end of the laryngoscope) and be reflected as a focussed beam, personnel in the operating room should wear ordinary glasses; in this way protection of their corneas is assured. Care must be taken to avoid injury of the balloon of the endotracheal tube in the trachea; if it cannot be safely advanced down the trachea out of sight, it should be protected with a strip of moist selvage gauze.

The endotracheal tube should be kept out of the target area, although it is not possible to penetrate the rubber wall of the tube with twenty-five 0.5 second impacts of the energy values that have been used above. Using maximum power (40 watts) and exposing the tube experimentally to a continuous beam, it is possible to penetrate the wall of the tube. With a high oxygen flow rate, the tube can be made to burn.

The subglottic area and anterior tracheal wall will sometimes receive an impact as a lesion is removed from the edge of the cord; because the beam is defocussed at this level, the energy density is lower and the resulting injury trivial. Initially the mucosa blanches without charring, and at the end of the procedure an area of slight erythema persists. The redness may or may not be visible on examination on the following day.

It was found during the dog experiments that symmetrical lesions on the anterior third of the cords healed with web formation; consequently lesions involving the anterior commissure should be treated one side at a time. Postoperative swelling of mucosa adjacent to the target area was not seen either experimentally or in the treated patients. No doubt the finding is related to the absence of thermal injury beyond 5 to 10 cells from the edge of the crater.

The Future. From our experience in the laboratory and in the operating room it appears that the CO_2 surgical laser is full of potential as a method of tissue destruction and incision. The only limiting factor is that the target area must be continuously visible, preferably with binocular vision. The precision with which laser surgery can be carried out suggests that it will be most useful in the management of small lesions within the larynx; where delicate surgery with preservation of function is important, laser surgery promises to be most beneficial. Acoustic and stroboscopic methods of voice analysis are now available and these will be used to make pre- and postoperative comparison of vocal dynamics using laser surgery and other modalities in phonosurgery. The best method of managing specific problems will then become apparent.

SUMMARY.

1. The CO_2 surgical laser is a practical instrument for incision or excision of tissue.

2. The microsurgical laser attachment to the operating microscope allows laser surgery of the vocal cords to be carried out with exquisite precision.

3. Laser surgery has been used successfully in the treatment of vocal cord keratosis, carcinoma *in situ*, nodules, polyps and papillomas.

4. Following laser surgery, healing is prompt and associated with a minimum of postoperative swelling and scarring.

5. Further applications of laser surgery in Otolaryngology will be forthcoming as experience and expertise accumulates.

750 Harrison Ave., Boston, Mass. 02118

Acknowledgment—The authors wish to express their appreciation to Dr. T. G. Polanyi, Mr. H. D. Bredemeier and Mr. T. W. Davis, Jr., members of the Surgical Laser Research Group of the American Optical Corporation, who provided the laser equipment and technical expertise which made these studies possible.

Request for reprints should be sent to M. Stuart Strong, M.D., University Hospital, 750 Harrison Ave., Boston, Mass. 02118.

REFERENCES

1. Leibowitz HM, Peacock GR: Corneal injury produced by carbon dioxide laser radiaion. Arch Ophthal 81:713-721, 1969

2. Gonzalez R, Edlich RF, Bredemeier HC et al: Rapid control of massive hepatic hemorrhage by laser irradiation. Surg Gynec Obst 121:198-200, 1970

3. Polanyi TG, Bredemeier HC, Davis TW, Jr: A CO_2 laser for surgical research. Med Biol Engng 8:541-548, 1970

4. Strong MS: Microscopic laryngoscopy. A review and appraisal. Laryngoscope 80: 1540-1552, 1970

5. Jako GJ: Laser surgery of the vocal cords. Laryngoscope (In press)

7

Benign Laryngeal Lesions

Introduction

Among the many articles on benign processes of the vocal folds, only two articles qualify as classics providing the entire foundation for our limited understanding of the processes involved in the development of benign pathology of the vocal folds, issues of standardized nomenclature, diagnostic accuracy, and therapeutic decision-making. This is not completely surprising. Dr. DeSanto is truly a pioneer in this regard, providing a fundamental description of laryngeal cysts. Confirming its place as a classic, this classification schema has withstood 4 decades, and is the only publication providing such thorough information regarding any benign laryngeal lesion.

Although many clinicians and scientists have made significant contributions to the establishment of laryngology and vocology as a true subspecialty within otolaryngology and the speech sciences, few contributed as much as Dr. Steven Gray. Dr. Gray was a professor in the Department of Otolaryngology, Head and Neck Surgery at the University of Utah. In addition to his robust clinical practice, Dr. Gray is considered the father of "voice biology," Dr. Gray's scientific contributions are vast including the biologic composition of the vocal folds, the effects of aging on the vocal fold tissue, and tissue engineering in the larynx. In 2002, Dr. Gray passed away.

His legacy lives on, however, through the many he trained. Dr. Susan Thibeault, in her commentary, provides unique insight into the scientific accomplishments of Dr. Gray, the evolution of his research program, and most importantly, the personal side of Dr. Gray, a truly great man. Dr. Gray is missed every day.

Classic Articles

● Reprint of article included in this chapter.
♦ Commentary on this article.

● DeSanto LW, Devine KD, Weiland LH. Cysts of the larynx—classification. *Laryngoscope.* 1970;80(1):145–176.

●♦ Gray SD, Hammond E, Hanson DF. Benign pathologic responses of the larynx. *Ann Otol Rhinol Laryngol.* 1995;104(1):13–18.

CYSTS OF THE LARYNX — CLASSIFICATION.*

LAWRENCE W. DESANTO, M.D.,
KENNETH D. DEVINE, M.D.,
and
LOUIS H. WEILAND, M.D.,
Rochester, Minn.

True cysts of the larynx are a group of benign lesions that usually are easily recognized and simply managed. Among them are several cysts distinctive enough to be considered clinical or pathologic entities, but a comprehensive classification is not available to assist the laryngologist in separating distinct entities from the heterogenous group of cysts.

With the objective of formulating a working classification, a study was made of a large amount of previously unreported material from the case files and tissue registry of the Mayo Clinic.

HISTORICAL REVIEW OF CLASSIFICATIONS.

The early classifications of laryngeal cysts were based on location of the lesion within the larynx;[1,2,3,4,5] thus, they were designated (in order of frequency) as cysts of the epiglottis, the true cords, ventricle, false cords, aryepiglottic fold, etc.

In 1881, Abercrombie reported a cyst of the newborn which he called a "congenital cyst."[6] For many years this kind of lesion was considered to occur only in the newborn infant, but now the designation is used as a descriptive diagnosis for a particular type of cyst found in patients of any age. The mucous or retention cyst appears regularly in various classifications. This is the lesion that is thought to develop from dilation of a mucous gland after obstruction of its duct.[7,8]

Other categories that have been suggested are "implanta-

*From the Mayo Clinic and Mayo Foundation.

Editor's Note: This manuscript received in THE LARYNGOSCOPE Office and accepted for publication September 3, 1968.

Request for reprints should be sent to Section of Publications, Mayo Clinic, Rochester, Minn. 55901.

tion" or acquired cysts, which were thought to be due to accidental or surgical implantation of surface epithelium below the laryngeal mucosa,[9] lymph cysts,[10] blood cysts,[10] and branchiogenic cysts.[11]

A glandular cyst or "cystadenoma" was described by Howarth and Chamings[12] in 1934. Much of the literature pertaining to it is quite separate from that written about other cysts.

In 1955, Pereira[13] of Brazil, after a thorough review of the subject and a report of three new cases, proposed an elaborate classification of true cysts:

- Neoplastic
  - Disembryoplastic
    - Congenital
    - Acquired
  - Traumatic
    - Accidental
    - Surgical
  - Cystic lymphangioma
  - Cystic hemangioma
- Non-neoplastic (retention)
  - Glandular
  - Amygdaloid
  - Lymphatic

The congenital and acquired disembryoplastic cysts are clinical lesions. The former is said to develop *in utero* and appear at birth, and the latter occurs later in life. These are the same growths that are called "congenital cysts" in other classifications. Traumatic cysts are identical to the implantation type suggested by Dean and Gregg[9] and are considered very rare. Retention cysts are thought to be due to retained secretions in glands, lymph crypts (amygdaloid), or lymphatics. Other classifications combine various items listed separately here.

Congenital Cyst. A good deal of confusion surrounds discussions of the so-called congenital cyst, which is poorly defined

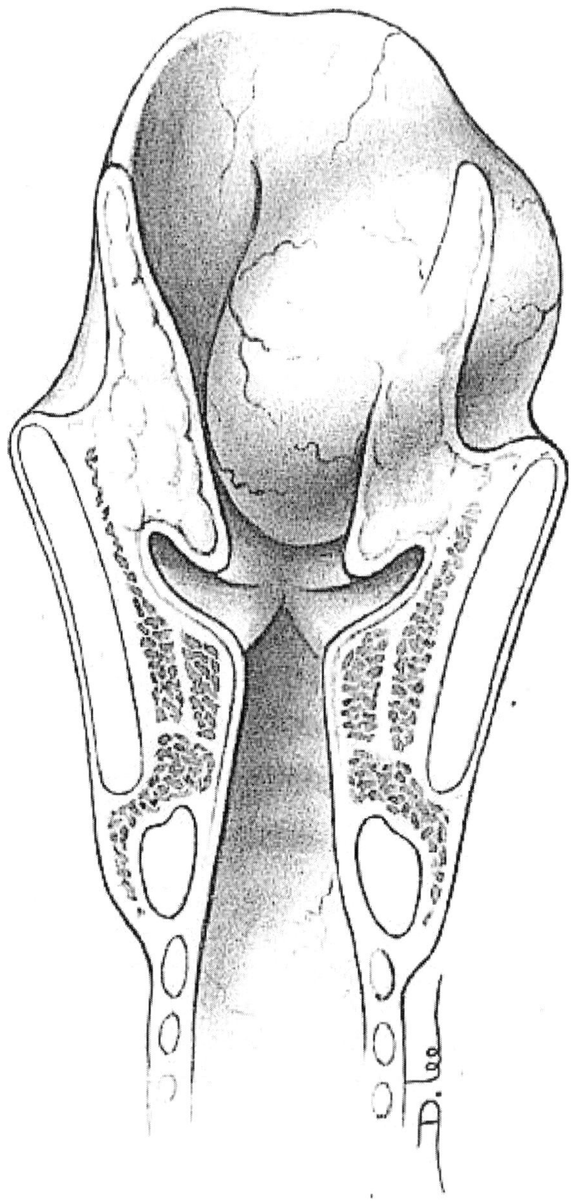

Fig. 1-A. Typical congenital cyst — the lateral saccular cyst in proposed classification. As exposed by section of larynx.

both clinically and pathologically. A wealth of hypotheses exists to explain its pathogenesis. Lesions that are essentially identical have been called embryonic,[14] dysontogenic,[15] cysts of the newborn,[16] distention cyst of the saccule,[17] ventricular-area cyst,[18,19] laryngeal dermoid,[20] epithelial laryngeal cyst,[21] inborn cyst of the larynx,[22] and disembryoplastic cyst.[13]

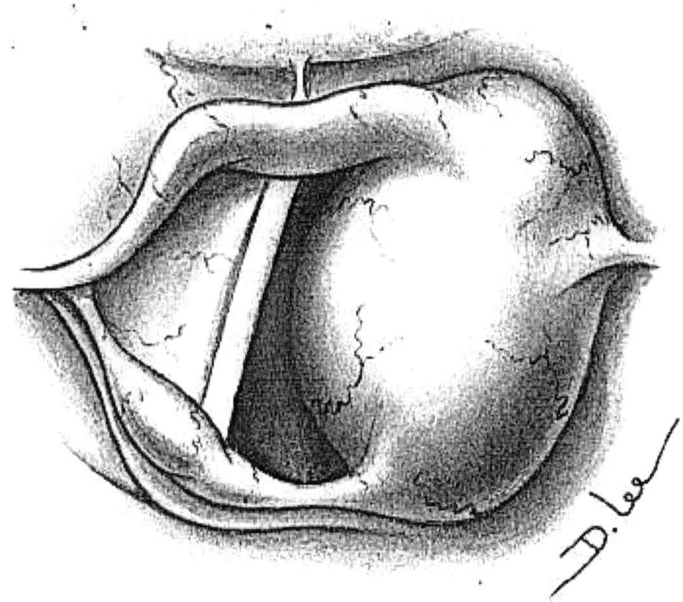

Fig. 1-B. As seen at laryngoscopy.

The feature common to each diagnosis is location. All of the sites are lateral supraglottic and distinctly beneath the normal laryngeal mucosa. Depending on its size, this cyst can distort the aryepiglottic fold, the false cord, or the ventricle — alone or in combinations. These structures are displaced and distorted as they are pushed into the laryngeal lumen. Larger cysts can also bulge laterally into the pyriform sinus, and superiorly to elevate the floor of the vallecula. They often overhang the true cords and at least partially obscure the glottis (Fig. 1 A and B).

Extralaryngeal extension of this cyst has been well documented.[18,19,21,23,24] It enters the neck through the foramen of the superior laryngeal bundle in the thyrohyoid membrane and reaches into the upper portion of the anterior cervical triangle. A review of the literature disclosed about 50 reports sufficiently detailed for identification of the so-called congenital cyst. Edis,[25] Abercrombie,[6] Greene,[26] and Chamberlin[4] reported cysts with such characteristics in newborn or very young infants. Lorie and Lux[27] commented on the rarity of such cysts in infants and the fact that they seldom are found prior to death. They suggested that cysts or other laryngeal lesions frequently are responsible for asphyxia of the newborn, rather than the often-blamed thymus gland; and they appealed for laryngoscopic examination of infants with dyspnea, obstructed respiration, or absent or distorted cry.

A clinical syndrome in infants with a congenital cyst was proposed by Jacobi and Rascoff[28] on the basis of the 11 case reports available to them in 1935: onset of symptoms shortly after birth; labored respiration; increase of respiratory difficulty during feeding; change in respirations for either better or worse with change in head position; a cry that is hoarse, feeble, or absent; and a cystic mass in the neck. For many years the diagnosis "congenital cyst" was reserved for lesions found in infants. Reported under different diagnoses,[11,20,29,30,31] however, were lesions in adults that would now be considered congenital cysts.

New and Erich[8] provided a link between the similar cysts of infants and adults when they reported lesions with the characteristic location and appearance in girls 14 and 17 years old. Both patients had had symptoms from birth, and their lesions were diagnosed as congenital cysts. After introduction of the idea that such cysts were not peculiar to the very young, reports were published of a number of similar lesions — all considered congenital — in individuals varying in age from newly born to 71 years.[18,19,21,22,23,24,32,33,34,35,36,37,38] Communication between a cystic mass in the neck and a supraglottic lesion was documented in six of these cases.[18,19,21,23,24,38]

Symptoms vary with age, cyst size, and the presence or absence of extension into the neck. In adults the symptoms are those common to any space-occupying lesion of the larynx, such as a tumor, laryngocele, or other cyst. Hoarseness or weakness of the voice is usual. The voice abnormality may have been present from the beginning of speech. Intermittent hoarseness, in one case reported by Cody,[30] was attributed to filling of the cyst with mucus, rupture, and then refilling.

Dyspnea and difficult respiration are variable symptoms. These are the primary problems in newborns and infants because of their small larynges. Fox and Dinolt,[39] however, treated an adult for two episodes of acute respiratory distress from large obstructing cysts. El Mofty's[24] patient experienced dyspnea only when pressure was applied to an extralaryngeal extension of the cyst. Death from asphyxia has occurred in at least two instances in adults.[29,40]

Dysphagia has been an occasional symptom.

The combination of a swelling in the neck and an internal cyst can be an aid to diagnosis. This combination has long been associated with laryngocele.

The size of reported congenital cysts has varied from that of a "hemp seed" (in an infant) to as large as 7.5 by 5 cm. No sex predilection has been noted. These cysts have been observed in all decades of life from the first to the seventh; though the sixth decade provided the largest number of cases (nine).

Some investigators have considered the histologic character of the wall of the cyst important in deciding which cysts truly merit the designation "congenital." Crynes and Yinger[33] restricted the diagnosis to those having a stratified squamous lining with underlying lymphocytes in the subepithelial tissue. Myerson[7] believed the essential feature to be a combination of ectodermally derived cells at the surface, with subepithelial mesodermal structures, but he did not elaborate. A comparison of all cases cited as congenital (or one of the synonyms) showed a considerable variation in histology. More than half of the cysts were said to be lined with typical respiratory epithelium. Others had a stratified squamous epithelial lining. Still others were lined with unciliated columnar cells or with cuboidal cells, or partially or totally with fibrous tissue. A few combinations of these patterns have been observed.[24,37,41] Some authors[19,37] suggested that the histologic appearance of a given cyst was not sufficiently characteristic to support a precise diagnosis. The importance of diffuse or follicular subepithelial lymphocytes to the congenital cyst has been emphasized;[8,33] but the cases with and without lymphocytes beneath the cyst lining were about equal in number. Holinger and Steinmann[37] discounted the importance of these ubiquitous cells by noting that they are not especially characteristic of any particular tissue or lesion but can be found almost anywhere in the body near recent or chronic inflammation.

A number of hypotheses have been proposed to explain the pathogenesis of the congenital cyst:

1. The cysts are visceral-pouch anomalies — that is, branchial-cleft cysts within the larynx.[11,30,38,41] This idea is opposed to the accepted understanding of embryologic development, which locates the visceral pouches lateral to the embryonic larynx.

2. The cysts are related in some way to isolation of the embryonic saccule or sequestration of embryonic cells from this laryngeal appendage.[14,15,39] The appearance of the cysts during adult life is explained by either of two mechanisms: a very slow growth of the isolated saccular elements in the adult, allowing the cysts to become apparent only after many years, whereas saccular isolation and cyst growth occur very rapidly in infants; or dormancy of embryonic cells isolated off the saccule until some stimulus occurs to trigger growth. (This latter is known as the Blastomeric Theory of Wilms.[42])

3. The cysts are isolated laryngoceles.[17,19,35,36,40] This idea would be identical to the preceding if "laryngocele" were defined merely as a distended saccula laryngis. There seems to be a distinction between the two, however, as the laryngocele is an air sac and the cyst contains mucus.

4. The cysts result from obstruction of ducts of mucous glands.[43] Considering the number of mucous glands within the larynx, the consistent location of this cyst is hard to reconcile with this concept.

5. Other theories mentioned are that the cysts result from fusion failure of the epiglottis,[44] that they are thyroglossal-duct anomalies,[3] and that they develop from displaced embryonal thyroid tissue.[45]

Cystadenoma. The so-called cystadenoma of the larynx is another cystic lesion that merits separate consideration. The diagnosis "cystadenoma" implies cystic spaces in a benign adenoma. That this is not completely applicable was demonstrated by Kuhn,[46] who also summarized four hypotheses of the pathogenesis of this rare lesion: *1.* cystic changes in a solid adenoma; *2.* inflammation, with obstruction of the ducts of mucous glands followed by epithelial hyperplasia of the ducts; *3.* tumor resulting from neoplastic proliferation of gland-duct epithelium; and *4.* a unique process, different from that of adenoma. A fifth explanation, advanced by Stewart,[47] is that the cystadenoma in a case he reported had developed from bronchial-adenoma cells implanted traumatically by a bronchoscope.

Of the various growths of the larynx, a true adenoma is perhaps the most rare. Some laryngologists doubt that there is such an entity. This rarity is surprising when one considers the number of submucosal glands throughout the larynx, yet Moore,[48] searching the literature up to 1920, was able to collect reports of only 13 cases of adenoma; and he noted that in a number of these the diagnosis was open to question. Although the first case appears to have been reported by Koschier in 1897,[49] Howarth and Chamings introduced the diagnosis of cystic adenoma or cystadenoma in 1934.[12] They described bilateral cystic swellings in both ventricles of their patient. After excision, histologic examination showed cystic spaces lined with columnar epithelial cells having finely granular eosinophilic cytoplasm; and the authors considered the lesion to be derived from dilation of salivary acini. Including their report, a total of at least 29 laryngeal lesions removed from 22 patients have been classified as cystic adenoma, cystadenoma, or papillary cystadenoma,[12,46,47,49,50,51,52,53,54] or under synonyms such as some type of oncocytoma,[55,56] oncocytic cystadenoma,[57] eosinophilic granular-cell cyst,[58] and eosinophilic granular-cell cystadenoma.[59]

Figi and associates[50] believed the cystadenoma to be a true glandular neoplasm and attributed its cystic character to cystic degeneration of solid adenoma. Of the five lesions in their four cases, two were on the false cords, one within the ventricle, and two on the true vocal cords.

Nohteri[51] described a cystic lesion called cystadenoma from within the substance of the right aryepiglottic fold of a 66-year-old man. He was particularly impressed with the staining properties of the lining cells, which were large and brightly eosinophilic with a fine granular cytoplasm — the type of cell that was made familiar as the "onkocyte" by Hamperl.[60] Later this oncocyte or oxyphilic granular cell was to be considered a necessary feature for the diagnosis of cystadenoma of the larynx; but it remains an enigma today — a large epithelial cell derived from other cells of the organ in which it is found. Its outstanding feature is a finely granular eosinophilic cytoplasm which renders it easily identifiable. Similar cells have been identified in the normal tissue of the tongue, pharynx, nasal mucosa, uvula, trachea, bronchi, larynx, esophagus, liver, gallbladder, pancreas, testes, uterus, fallopian tube, lacrimal sac and gland, and major and minor salivary glands.

Two studies indicate that the number of oncocytes in normal tissue of the upper airway increases with age.[60,61] Mollica and Rossi,[61] investigating the normal histology of the larynx, were impressed with the absence of oncocytes before puberty and their increasing frequency after adolescence. Among the very old, oncocytes were seen in large numbers in the glands and ducts of the larynx. The investigators believed that the oncocytic change was an "early physiopathologic manifestation of senility of the tissues." In four of the 29 reported cystadenomas, the oncocytic cells were found in combination with typical respiratory epithelial cells within the lining of the cyst.[57,59] One of these instances was noteworthy in that after removal of one cyst a second developed at the same site on the false cord but with different histologic makeup. The initial cyst was lined with typical respiratory epithelium. The second cyst, removed 15 months later, was totally lined with oncocytic cells. In three cases ciliated oncocytic epithelium was found in the lining of the cyst.

These observations of combination patterns and an apparent change from respiratory to oncocytic lining suggest that the oncocytic or oxyphilic granular cystadenoma is in part a respiratory epithelial cyst that for some reason undergoes the oncocytic change. Kroe and associates[54] have recently reviewed 12 cases of papillary cystadenoma of the larynx reported in the literature and presented two cases of their own. They considered that the tumors probably arise from oncocytic transformation of submucosal glands and possibly from oncocytic transformation of respiratory epithelium.

Of the 22 reported patients with cystadenomas or related lesions, at least 19 were more than 50 years old. The locations of the lesions varied: nine within the ventricles, eight on the false cords, six subglottic, two at the anterior commissure, and one each on the true cord and the aryepiglottic fold.

The similarity between cystadenoma of the larynx and Warthin's tumor of the parotid gland has been considered by several authors. Pinkerton and Beck[58] dismissed the idea that they were in some way related. They noted the lack of an intimate relationship between oncocytic epithelium and lymphoid tissue and the absence of two-layered epithelium, both features usually seen in the parotid tumor. The lesion in Kuhn's[46] case, however, matched the histopathology of the parotid lesion in respect to the double-layered epithelium but lacked the submucosal lymphoid tissue. Kuhn considered the laryngeal cystadenoma different from its parotid counterpart only in that it did not grow within lymphoid tissue. Both, he thought, were neoplasms of the mucous-gland ducts.

Electron microscopic examination of the cytoplasm of oncocytes reveals that they are packed with mitochondria, although the basis for oncocytic transformation and its functional status has not been established.[54]

Others. The majority of cysts fall into neither the congenital nor the cystadenoma category. These lesions have been called acquired, retention, epidermoid, or simply "other" laryngeal cysts. Being more ordinary, they have not stimulated such interest as the cystadenomas and congenital cysts; and most reports of them have been made incidentally to complete studies of the more unusual lesions. Often these other laryngeal cysts were categorized only by location.

Epiglottic cysts are considered the most common.[7,14,62,63] Only Holinger and Johnston's[23] large series of benign tumors is an exception to this consensus. Of the 73 cysts in their material, 38 (52 percent) were from the true cords and 27 (37 percent) were from the epiglottis. The rest were found on the aryepiglottic fold, arytenoids, and false cords.

Obstruction of mucous-gland ducts, with consequent retention of mucus and dilation of the glands, is thought generally to be the origin of these cysts. Chronic inflammation is cited as the usual cause of the duct obstruction.

Many epiglottic or vallecular cysts are asymptomatic. Among symptoms, the most common is the sensation of having a foreign body in the throat. Vallecular cysts are often multiple. Size varies, and those reported in the literature range from 2 mm to 3.0 cm in their greatest diameter. Epiglottic cysts are most often found in adults, but a few have been observed in children.[28,64] Simple excision through the laryngoscope usually is adequate treatment for symptomatic epiglottic cysts. Many require no treatment, as their benign nature is quite obvious on mirror examination.

The vocal-cord cysts cause hoarseness early when they are quite small. Most of them are less than 5 mm in size when treated, but lesions up to 1 cm have been reported. Transoral removal with the laryngoscope usually suffices.

The cellular lining of the epiglottic, vocal-cord, and other so-called acquired or retention cysts is usually described as stratified squamous epithelium. Cuboidal, columnar, and ciliated pseudostratified columnar epithelial linings have been reported infrequently.[65]

MATERIALS AND METHODS.

Review was made of all cases of laryngeal cyst seen by the laryngology service of the Mayo Clinic in the 20 years from 1945 through 1964. Instances of cystic myxomatous polyp and cystic change in solid tumors were excluded, leaving for study the clinical records of 238 patients. Among these, 48 patients had been examined but not treated; preserved gross specimens and paraffin-blocked tissue were available from the remaining 190. All gross specimens were inspected, and multiple sections were prepared with hematoxylin and eosin for examination with the light microscope. Follow-up data were obtained from the clinical records, from reexamination of patients on return visits, or from follow-up letters in selected cases. To trace

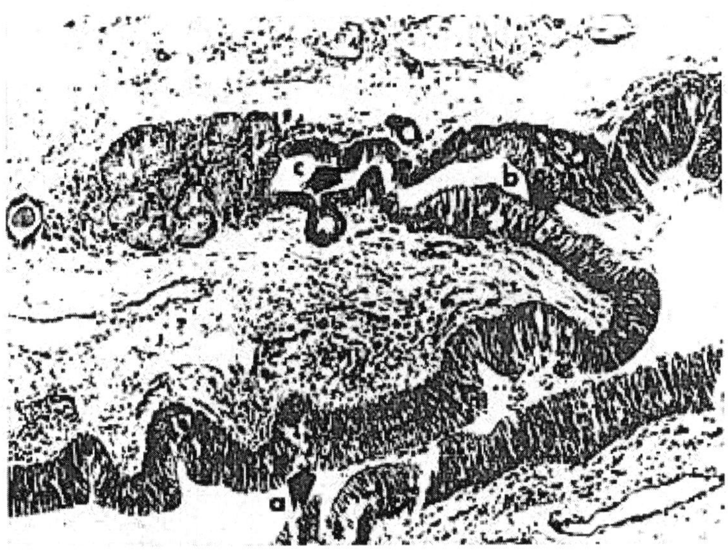

Fig. 2. Laryngeal duct system. Sections taken from the false cord. Note ciliated pseudostratified columnar collecting ducts (A), and goblet cells (B), and cuboidal epithelium (C) lining intralobular duct. (Hematoxylin and eosin; x90.)

every patient was not attempted, but the desired information was obtained in more than two-thirds of the cases studied.

Secondary Study of Normal Histology. For a proper understanding of the origin of the cysts it was thought necessary to determine the normal histology of the laryngeal gland system. Material for this was obtained from 10 larynges that had been removed for carcinoma of that organ or of the hypopharynx. Representative blocks were taken from where the surface epithelium was grossly and microscopically normal, as far as possible from the neoplasms. The sites sampled were the vallecula, base of the epiglottis, lingual surface of the epiglottis, false cords, ventricle, true cords, and subglottic region. Six sections were taken from each block at right angles to the mucous membrane, and each was prepared and stained with hematoxylin and eosin. A total of 1,480 sections were examined to establish a concept of the normal gland-duct system of the larynx. The study of these sections of mucous membrane from the various sites throughout the larynx enabled us to divide

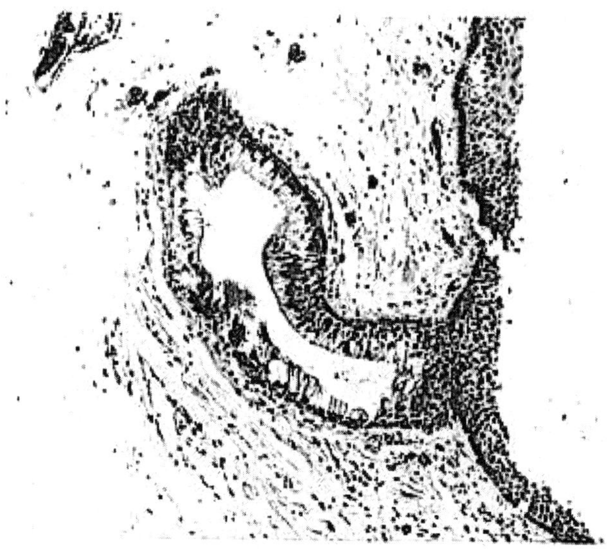

Fig. 3. Ciliated, pseudostratified, columnar-epithelial collecting duct arising from stratified squamous epithelial surface of vallecula. (Hematoxylin and eosin; x90.)

the gland ducts into three types: collecting, interlobular, and intralobular (Fig. 2).

The collecting ducts are the large proximal ducts that open onto the lumen of the larynx. They are lined by one of two types of epithelium, depending upon location. Consistently, the ducts of the false cords, ventricle, base of the epiglottis, and subglottic region are lined with respiratory epithelium; and some collecting ducts of the anterior epiglottis, vallecula, and true cords also exhibit this histologic pattern. The respiratory epithelium, interestingly, is seen to join the stratified squamous surface of the false cord and epiglottis as shown in Figure 3. Other collecting ducts of the epiglottis, vallecula, and true cords have a stratified squamous epithelial lining. Occasionally oxyphilic granular (oncocytic) cells, alone or in small clumps, are seen in the collecting ducts (Fig. 4).

The interlobular ducts lie between acinar groups in the gland and are quite short. Their lining cells consistently are

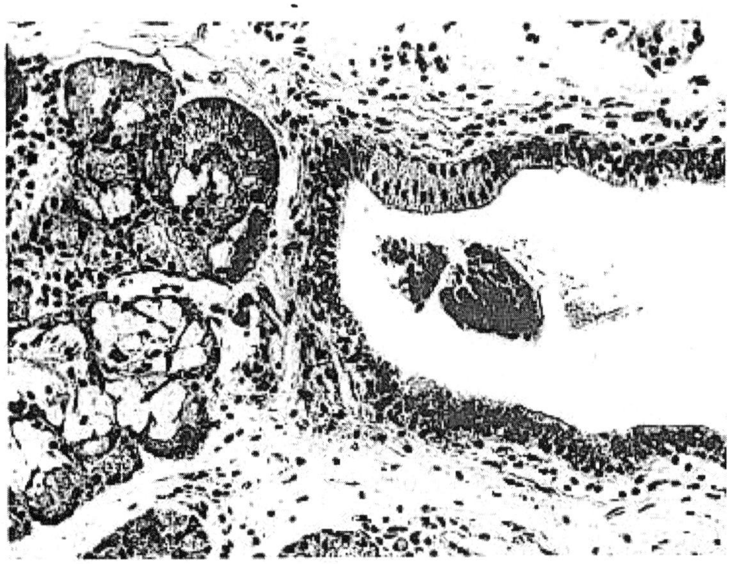

Fig. 4. Group of oxyphilic granular (oncocytic) cells in collecting duct. (Hematoxylin and eosin; x250.)

globlet cells. Some of these, too, stain with an oxyphilic character and have granular cytoplasm. Interlobular ducts were found in all sites studied.

The intralobular ducts lie within the acinar groups. They are lined with unciliated cuboidal epithelium and are found throughout the larynx.

PROPOSED CLASSIFICATION.

The review of our gross, microscopic, and clinical material led to the following classification of laryngeal cysts.

Saccular cysts (with or without oxyphilia).
Ductal cyst (with or without oxyphilia).
Thyroid-cartilage foraminal cyst.

Saccular cysts are those supraglottic lesions located in the anatomic plane of the saccule which appear to result from cystic distention of that laryngeal appendage. Under this interpretation, a laryngocele differs from a saccular cyst only in that it contains air, whereas the cyst contains mucus. A laryngopyocele is an infected air cyst.

Ductal cysts are those found at any site within the larynx that result from retention of mucus in the collecting ducts of the submucosal glands.

The third group, the thyroid-cartilage foraminal cyst, is a very rare but quite distinct entity. No record of a similar cyst has been found in the literature. An instance is reported in detail below, and a theory of pathogenesis suggested.

For classifying a laryngeal cyst the following clinical features are considered pertinent: *1.* its site in the larynx; *2.* its size and content; and *3.* its relation to the laryngeal mucosa. As will be noted, the histologic character of the cyst lining is not particularly helpful in classification.

To be sure, a given cyst cannot always be categorized by these criteria. For example, there is no reason to assume that the multiple submucosal gland ducts within the wall of the saccule are not subject to obstruction and cystic distortion that would produce a ductal cyst there; but this should be rare, and in most instances a clinical distinction can be made by the criteria detailed here.

Saccular Cysts. Site. Saccular cysts are supraglottic lesions. They may develop at any site in the plane of the saccule, and thus can distort the aryepiglottic fold, the false cord, the ventricle, or the vallecula — either singly or in various combinations. Two subcategories of saccular cysts appear appropriate for more precise clinical differentiation: the anterior and the lateral.

The anterior saccular cysts are those located near the saccular orifice at the anterior ventricle. These are the lesions that bulge from deep within the ventricle and usually overhang the anterior glottis. Some are large enough to fill the entire ventricle (Fig. 5). These are the lesions that others have called "ventricular-area cysts," but in our material there were enough having the more specific characteristics to merit this separate designation. Many instances of what has been called

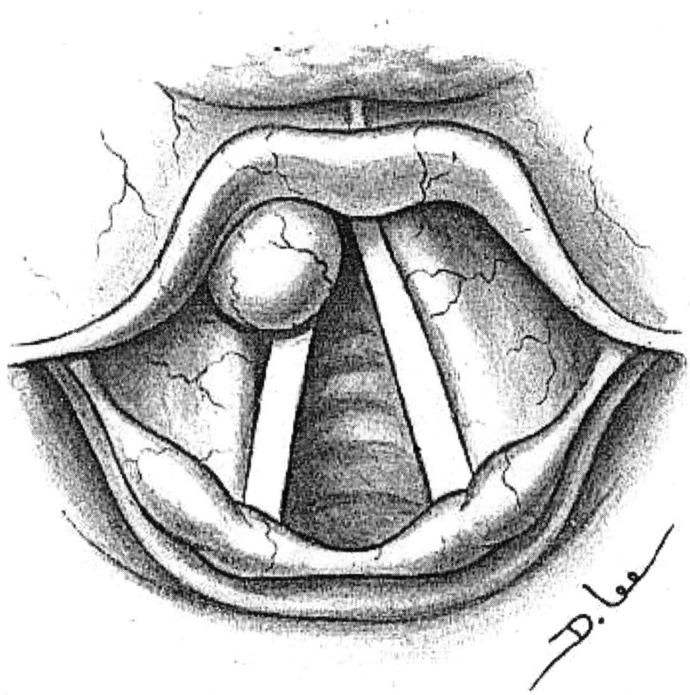

Fig. 5. Anterior saccular cyst as seen at laryngoscopy.

"eversion of the saccule" may have been in actuality this form of the saccular cyst.

The lateral saccular cyst in our classification is the same lesion that is usually termed the "congenital" cyst of the larynx. That is the very large lesion that bulges the false cord, aryepiglottic fold, or ventricle, or the entire supraglottic larynx (Fig. 1 A and B). Some extend to or even through the thyrohyoid membrane into the neck (Fig. 6).

Size. Saccular cysts as a group are the largest cysts of the larynx. They rarely are less than 1 cm in diameter in the adult and often are much larger.

Relation to Mucosa. Saccular cysts are distinctly submucosal lesions and are covered with normal mucous membrane.

Ductal Cysts. Site. Ductal cysts can form at any site within the laryngopharynx where there are mucosal glands. This excludes only the gland-free area on the free edge of the true cords.

Size. Generally, ductal cysts are the smaller lesions. Most

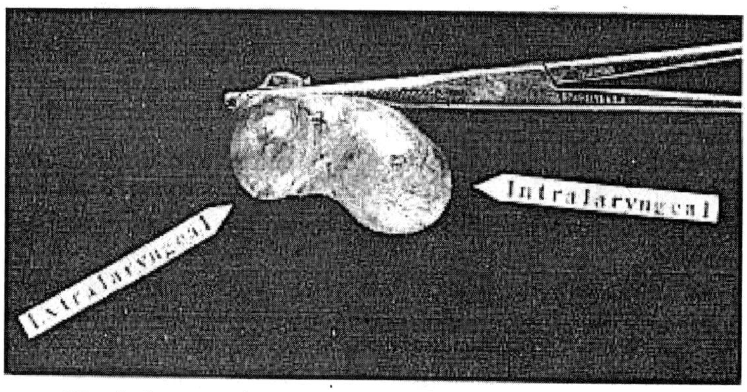

Fig. 6. Gross specimen of lateral saccular cyst, 4.5 by 2.5 cm.

are less than 1 cm in diameter. Exceptions exist, but the larger ductal cysts usually can be classified precisely by location and depth.

Relation to Mucosa. In contrast to the saccular type, ductal cysts appear quite superficial, being located within the mucous membrane.

Thyroid-Cartilage Foraminal Cyst. This category is included in our classification on the basis of a single lesion found in our material. It does not satisfy the criteria for the other types and seems to merit a separate designation because of its uniqueness.

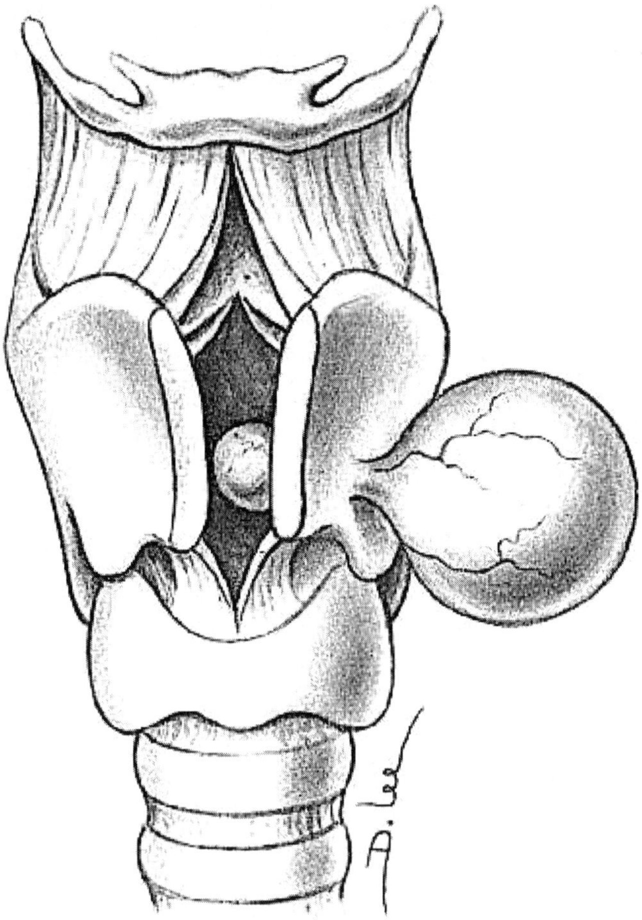

Fig. 7. Thyroid-cartilage foraminal cyst.

CASE REPORT.

The patient, a 17-year-old girl, was first seen at this clinic because of her complaint of a mass in the left side of the neck. She had been born with a marble-sized swelling there which had varied, usually increasing during an upper respiratory infection. During the six months preceding admission she had been hoarse.

Examination verified the presence of a cystic swelling, 3 by 2 cm, adjacent to the left lower thyroid-cartilage ala. Mirror examination of the larynx revealed a 1 cm dark-blue mass below the left true cord.

At suspension laryngoscopy, the internal swelling was incised and a dark-blue liquid evacuated. An incision was then made over the neck swelling, which had deflated partially after the incision and drainage of the internal mass. A partially filled cyst was identified directly lateral to the lower thyroid cartilage. With blunt dissection it was found to narrow down and continue through a small defect in the thyroid ala. This neck joined the internal and external components (Fig. 7). It was possible to remove both extremities of the dumbbell-shaped cyst without entering the larynx. Grossly it was obvious that the lesion was a cyst, and histologic examination showed it to be lined with ciliated pseudostratified columnar epithelium.

Follow-up revealed no subsequent difficulty.

TABLE I.

Anatomic Distribution of Saccular and Ductal Cysts.

Site	Saccular		Ductal		Total	
	No.	Percent	No.	Percent	No.	Percent
Vocal cords	0	0	72	40	72	30
Epiglottis	0	0	67	37	67	28
Ventricle	33	58	10	6	43	18
Aryepiglottic fold	8	14	9	5	17	7
False cord	0	0	13	7	13	5
Lateral larynx "congenital"	7	12	0	0	7	3
Arytenoid	0	0	6	3	6	3
False cord and aryepiglottic fold	5	9	0	0	5	2
False cord and ventricle	4	7	0	0	4	2
Anterior commissure	0	0	1	<1	1	<1
Pyriform sinus	0	0	1	<1	1	<1
Subglottic region	0	0	1	<1	1	<1
Total	57	100	180	100	238*	100

*Includes one thyroid-cartilage foraminal cyst.

No report of a similar lesion was found in the literature. A hypothesis that seems appropriate is that the cyst was formed by a projection of the mucosa lining the larynx, likely as a herniation, through a foramen that sometimes remains at this particular site in the larynx. The foramen is attributed to persistent fetal vessels that penetrate the mesenchyma at this point and persist after condensation and chondrification of this mesenchyma.[66] With isolation of the herniated mucosa and continued secretion of mucus, the cyst develops.

APPLICATION OF SCHEME WITHIN SERIES.

Table I relates the types and sites of the cysts in our series.

Saccular Cysts. Of the 238 cysts, 57 (24 percent) were classified as saccular derivatives by the criteria stated. Among these 57 lesions, 33 were so consistent in presenting as a dome-shaped bulge from the anterior ventricle that they merited specific classification as the anterior subtype; and the remaining 24 were considered lateral. All but four were available for gross and microscopic examination. Two of the four not available were large lateral cysts of infants who were treated by aspiration and injection of a sclerosing solution.

TABLE II.

Histology of Lining Membrane of Saccular Cysts.

Location of cyst	Type of Lining: Respiratory	Squamous	Oxyphilic (Columnar)	Fibrous	Combination	Not Removed
Lateral (congenital)	4	0	0	0	1*	2
False cord and ventricle	4	0	0	0	0	0
False cord and aryepiglottic fold	2	1	2	0	0	0
Aryepiglottic fold	3	3	0	0	2†	
Anterior (ventricular)	15	0	13	1	3‡	1

*Respiratory and squamous.
†One respiratory and squamous; one respiratory and oxyphilic granular.
‡Respiratory and oxyphilic granular.

Another patient was not treated because of other medical difficulties that contraindicated removal of the obviously benign lesion.

Table II shows the variety in the histologic character of the saccular cysts. Respiratory epithelium lined more than half of them (28 of 54). Fifteen cysts were lined exclusively with oxyphilic columnar (oncocytic) epithelial cells (Fig. 8) usually at least two layers in thickness (Fig. 8) or focally pseudostratified with variable papillary infoldings. Cilia were rarely seen on oxyphilic linings. Four cysts were lined partly with oxyphilic columnar epithelium and the remainder by respiratory epithelium. This suggests to us that the oxyphilic cells are modified respiratory epithelial or ductal cells and not an entirely distinct type nor a specific tissue. No reason for the oxyphilic change is apparent from our study. Nearly all (98 percent) of the patients with an oxyphilic cyst were more than 50 years old, so age may well be a variable as suggested in other studies;[60,61] however, 77 percent of all the patients were in the sixth or later decades of life, so a significant overlap

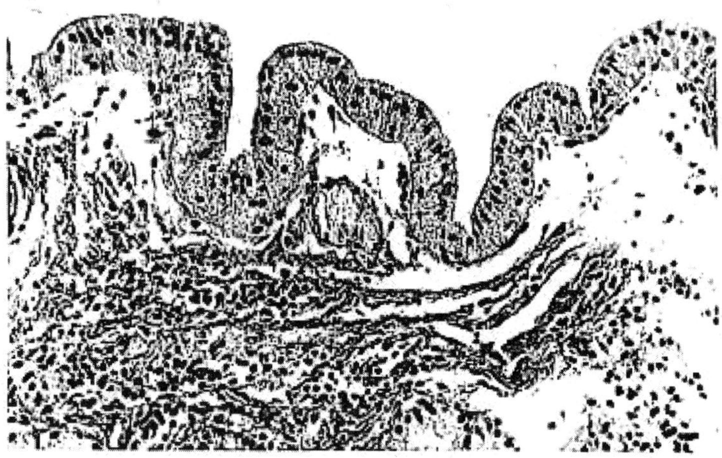

Fig. 8. Typical oxyphilic granular epithelial lining from portion of wall of anterior saccular cyst.

exists in the comparison of age and histology. One other cyst was lined with a combination of oxyphilic columnar cells and stratified squamous epithelium. One saccular cyst had a fibrous lining.

The saccular cysts as a group were the largest cysts of the larynx. None was less than 1 cm in diameter, even in the infants. The largest measured 7.5 cm in its greatest dimension. This particular lesion extended into the neck through the thyrohyoid membrane (Fig. 6). Three others had similar neck extensions.

Hoarseness or other voice change was the nearly universal

complaint among patients with cysts that were classified as saccular. The two infants having cysts of this kind were unable to cry at birth. Both had labored respiration, did not tolerate feedings, and were intermittently cyanotic. Tracheotomy was performed within the first hour of life in both cases. The cysts so distorted the larynx that the glottis was nearly obliterated and the anatomy of the supraglottic region unrecognizable.

In adults the voice changes had been present from one month to eight years prior to examination at this clinic. Most patients, however, sought treatment within the first year of symptoms.

Four patients complained of acute or recurring throat pain that was thought to be due to infected cyst, as the pain terminated with antibiotic therapy. Four other patients had a cystic neck mass along with alteration of voice. Each had a large cyst that extended through the thyrohyoid membrane and expanded in the neck:

The surgical procedure for removing these cysts varied. The anterior saccular cysts, which generally are smaller, were usually managed by means of suspension laryngoscopy and transoral excision. In most instances the cyst was grasped with large cup forceps, the overlying ventricular mucosa was slit with a laryngeal knife, and the cyst was evulsed. In all but a few cases the cyst ruptured in the course of excision. Among the 29 cases in which anterior cysts were removed by this method, recurrence required further treatment in only one. Laryngofissure was used then to excise the lesion totally.

Laryngofissure was employed initially for one anterior saccular cyst. This was a large left-sided lesion (3.5 by 3 cm) that was seen one year after laryngofissure and excision of a low-grade squamous-cell carcinoma of the left true cord. At operation it was perceived that the cyst was actually the distended saccule on the left side of the larynx.

In two other instances anterior saccular cysts were associated with carcinoma of the larynx. A 0.9 cm cyst deep in the right ventricle was noted incidentally in a larynx that had been removed because of a right supraglottic squamous-cell carcinoma; and careful dissection of the specimen led us to conclude that this lesion — like the one described above — was a cyst of the distended saccule. In the second instance, a cyst was seen in the same region at laryngoscopy two years after extensive electrocautery and intralaryngeal skin grafting to the site of a squamous-cell carcinoma of both true cords and the anterior commissure.

Laryngofissure was the preferred approach to the large lateral saccular cysts, and 14 patients were so treated — preliminary tracheotomy, with local anesthesia, having been performed in five of the cases. Eight patients underwent lateral thyrotomy, a procedure that permits submucosal excision of the cyst. The conventional midline thyrotomy was performed on the remaining patients. Each of the procedures appears satisfactory, as all cysts were removed completely and did not recur, and every patient was found to have a satisfactory voice afterward. Seven smaller cysts of the aryepiglottic-fold or the aryepiglottic-fold and false-cord region were excised perorally after exposure of the larynx with the suspension laryngoscope, and none of these recurred. Currently the large lateral saccular cysts are approached through a transverse incision between hyoid and thyroid cartilage without splitting the thyroid cartilage.

One lateral saccular cyst was discovered in a laryngectomy specimen that had been removed as the initial treatment for a squamous-cell carcinoma, Grade 2, involving the base of the epiglottis and the right false cord. The cyst measured 2 by 3 cm, and extended from the right ventricle to the thyrohyoid membrane but did not communicate directly with the ventricle. Careful dissection of the specimen did not demonstrate the sacculus, and the opposite ventricular appendix was quite normal. The cyst itself, therefore, seemed to be the distended sacculus, isolated from the ventricle. The tumor did not close off the saccular orifice grossly or microscopically. This cyst was lined with typical respiratory epithelium.

Ductal Cysts. A varied group of cysts considered ductal in origin were the most common type in our series, totaling 180 (75 percent) of the 238 lesions studied. Table I shows their anatomic distribution.

Since glands and ducts are present in the mucous lining of all the larynx except the free edge of the true cords, ductal cysts could be anticipated in almost any site with that one exception; and this was verified in our study.

The most common site of ductal cysts was the *true vocal cords*, 72 (40 percent) of the 180 having that location. More than half (54 percent) of these cordal cysts were lined with squamous epithelium, and 31 percent were lined with respiratory epithelium. These facts are consistent with the observation of both squamous epithelial and pseudostratified columnar epithelial collecting ducts on the superior and inferior surfaces of the true cords with only a few millimeters of the free edge devoid of glandular elements. The others had cuboidal, nonciliated columnar, or fibrous surfaces, and one was lined with the oxyphilic columnar epithelial cells. Vocal-cord cysts as a group were much smaller than ductal cysts from elsewhere in the larynx: 90 percent measured only 1 to 5 mm in greatest diameter, and none was larger than 1 cm.

Hoarseness or weakness of the voice affected 69 of the 72 patients having vocal-cord cysts. In each of the other three, a tiny cyst was found near the posterior extremity of the cord. All 72 vocal-cord cysts were removed with use of the suspension laryngoscope, and none recurred.

Ductal cysts about the *epiglottis* were seen in 67 patients, 48 (72 percent) of these lesions being within the vallecula or on the lingual surface of the epiglottis. Sixteen (24 percent) were on the free edge and three (5 percent) on the laryngeal surface. Nearly two-thirds of the patients were asymptomatic, and most of the cysts were found in the course of an otolaryngologic examination for another reason. Several were discovered by the patient's dentist or by the patient himself.

Only 38 of the 67 epiglottic cysts were removed. The others were left without treatment because the patients were asymptomatic, and the innocent nature of the lesions was obvious on indirect examination. Of the cysts removed, 85 percent were lined with stratified squamous epithelium. Respiratory epithelium, cuboidal cells, and fibrous tissue lined two cysts each.

A total of 41 ductal cysts were removed from *other loca-*

tions: the false cord (13), ventricles (10), aryepiglottic folds (9), arytenoid cartilage (6), anterior commissure (1), pyriform sinus (1), and subglottic larynx (1). Six patients of this group had had other laryngeal surgery prior to removal of the cyst: cautery excision of superficial cordal carcinoma in four, multiple excision and cautery treatments for papilloma in one, and transoral excision and cautery for contact ulcer with granuloma in one. A single arytenoid cyst was observed in a laryngectomy specimen. The histologic lining of these cysts was essentially the same as those observed in the cordal and epiglottic cysts; that is, the majority were a mixture of respiratory and stratified squamous epithelium. Three cysts from the false cords and three from the ventricle had the oxyphilic epithelium with variable papillary development, the so-called cystadenoma pattern.

COMMENT.

Normal Structure of Ducts. Four observations seem pertinent from the study of the laryngeal duct system: *1.* the division of the gland ducts into what we have termed collecting, interlobular, and intralobular is applicable consistently throughout the larynx; *2.* two histologic patterns can be found in the collecting ducts: either stratified squamous epithelium or ciliated pseudostratified columnar epithelium; *3.* respiratory epithelial collecting ducts can be seen to penetrate the stratified squamous surfaces, whereas stratified squamous epithelial collecting ducts are seen to blend into such surfaces; and *4.* oxyphilic granular cells (oncocytes) are seen at any level of the ductal system.

Hopp[67] noted that all laryngeal surface epithelium is derived from a single embryonal cell type. The ducts, as surface derivatives, undoubtedly share the same parent cell type. At birth, the entire laryngeal lumen except the free margins of the true cords and the interarytenoid region have a ciliated, pseudostratified surface. These exceptions are unciliated and remain so throughout life, but other regions undergo adaptation to their functions. To illustrate, the edges of the false cords and vallecula at three months of age have a ciliated respiratory epithelial surface but by age six months are covered with stratified squamous epithelium and remain so covered throughout life. This change is termed "physiologic metaplasia," as an adaptation to the wear and tear of phonation, swallowing, and the other functions of the laryngeal sphincter.

The stratified squamous epithelial ducts of the epiglottis, vallecula, and true cords undoubtedly undergo this same kind of metaplasia, as they are exposed to these same stresses. Other collecting ducts, less exposed, retain their ciliated respiratory type of lining; and this provides an explanation of why the collecting ducts that underlie the stratified squamous surface have respiratory epithelial lining in some laryngeal regions and stratified squamous lining in others.

Saccular Cysts. The cysts classified as saccular are so considered for the following reasons.

1. They all appear in the anatomic plane of the ventricular appendage.

2. The anatomic structure of the saccule, with its narrow ventricular opening, would lend itself easily to obstruction and subsequent cystic dilation. Similarly, at one time during embryonic development the saccule is physically obliterated by the pressure of the surrounding mesenchyma, but normally it recanalizes. A failure to recanalize would provide a setting for a cyst of the newborn or very young.

3. There is a remarkable clinical similarity between these cysts and the various forms of laryngocele, an accepted saccular derivative.

4. In both of the two larynges available for dissection that contained cysts fulfilling the criteria of the saccular type, the ipsilateral saccule was not identified on sectioning, whereas the opposite member was quite easily demonstrated. It seems that these cysts were truly distended saccules.

The normal anatomic variations between various appendages of the saccule, considered along with what is known of its embryologic development, reasonably explain how saccular obstruction can be responsible for the various clinical lesions. To illustrate, obstruction of a small appendage (5 to 10 mm) at the ventricular extremity would result in an anterior (ventricular) cyst. A cyst developed from a longer saccule (10 to 15 mm) would extend beyond the ventricle and beneath the false cord and aryepiglottic fold. If the obstruction occurred a few millimeters up from the ventricle, the ventricular component would be smaller or absent and the clinical appearance would be that of a cyst beneath the false cord or aryepiglottic fold. The precise location would depend upon how far distal from the ventricle the obstruction developed and how large the normal saccule was before obstruction.

Any etiologic discussion of this category of cysts can only be speculative. The lateral cyst or so-called congenital cyst that appears at birth can be explained as a product of developmental arrest. It has been observed[62] that in the course of embryonic growth the sacculo-ventricular outgrowth as well as the laryngeal lumen is pressed together by expanding fourth and fifth arch mesenchyma. With failure of separation of adherent endoderm, the saccule can be isolated from the ventricle at any point along its length, permitting a saccular cyst of any type to evolve. It seems unnecessary to speculate about isolated embryonic cells or activated blastomeres to explain these cysts.

For cysts acquired after birth, another mechanism of saccular isolation must be sought. Association with carcinoma, cautery trauma, and intralaryngeal skin grafts affords rather obvious explanations; and tumor growths, inflammation, and fibrosis also can easily close off the millimeter-sized orifice.

Ductal Cysts. The literature consistently refers to duct obstruction as the genesis of many cysts. The question of what becomes distended — the duct or the glands — seems to be resolved by comparing cyst histology with gland-system histology. Except the few with fibrous linings, all cysts in our study were lined with cells of a ductal cell type rather than with acinar cells; so it seems that the cysts are dilated ducts and not distended glands. The length of the collecting ducts would accommodate distention to the size of the cysts found in our study. The tiny size of the cysts of the true cords corresponds with the shortness of ducts in this location; and larger cysts are found in places where the collecting ducts are correspondingly longer, such as the false cord and epiglottis.

Finally, the interesting observation that a number of cysts are lined with respiratory epithelium beneath stratified squamous laryngeal surfaces supports the thought that many of the cysts originate from obstructed collecting ducts. A similar situation is seen in the nasopharynx, where it has been nicely demonstrated that cysts found there follow obstruction of collecting ducts.[68]

The actual causes of duct obstruction and cyst formation remain to be proven. Instances associated with carcinoma, leukoplakia, and particularly cautery trauma provide a clue to other mechanisms. Whether the granular oxyphilic transformation precedes or develops in the wall of a preformed cyst is uncertain, although it is not considered indicative of neoplasia. Oxyphilia is often seen in some neighboring submucosal ducts outside of the cyst wall. Epithelial hypertrophy due to the increased amount of oxyphilic cytoplasm in addition to hyperplasia may account for the infolding and development of a papillary lining in some of these cysts.

The thyroid-cartilage foraminal cyst appears to be a distinct and extremely rare lesion, but an embryologic explanation for it is available (that is, a projection of the subglottic laryngeal mucosa as a herniation through the persistent foramina occasionally seen in the anterior lateral thyroid ala).

SUMMARY.

The need for a satisfactory clinicopathologic classification of the cysts of the larynx was recognized after surveying the number and diversity of those available in the literature. The entire experience of the Mayo Clinic with laryngeal cysts over the 20-year period 1945 through 1964 was reviewed to gather sufficient data to formulate a working classification that could be useful to the laryngologist.

This review provided 238 clinical records and 190 pathologic specimens of laryngeal cysts. A secondary study was made of the histology of submucosal glands and ducts in 10 larynges from cases outside the series to provide a basis for comparison with the abnormal histology.

A classification was formulated which is based on anatomic location and probably pathogenesis, and includes the air cyst or laryngocele and relates it to the other cysts. The series was divided into three basic categories: saccular cysts (24 percent), ductal cysts (75 percent), and thyroid-cartilage foraminal cyst (one case).

Saccular cysts are the large cysts found along the plane of the sacculus deep to the false cords, aryepiglottic fold, and anterior ventricle. They are thought to result from cystic distention of the sacculus laryngis. The so-called congenital cyst represents the extreme in size of the saccular cyst. In our classification this is termed "lateral saccular cyst," and use of the diagnosis "congenital cyst" is discouraged. The cyst of the anterior ventricle is a clinical entity, considered a variant of the saccular cyst, and designated "anterior saccular cyst." The laryngocele is a cyst of the lateral saccular type, but is distinguished from the others by containing air rather than mucus. The laryngopyocele is an infected air cyst.

Ductal cysts, formed by distention of obstructed collecting ducts, are the most common type of laryngeal cyst. The cyst of the true cords was the most numerous of this group, but the epiglottic cyst was seen almost as frequently. Granular oxyphilic (oncocytic) columnar-lined cysts, or so-called cystadenomas of the larynx, were found in 35 percent of the saccular and 4 percent of the ductal groups. Their location and behavior were similar to those of the non-oxyphilic cysts. The oxyphilic cyst is considered a histologic variant without known special clinical significance, although its pathogenesis remains undetermined.

Histologic patterns alone are not specific enough for classifying laryngeal cysts; clinically, their location, depth, and size are more useful.

The single case of a cyst ballooning through a foramen of the thyroid ala is reported. This lesion is designated "thyroid-cartilage foraminal cyst." Its apparent basis is a subglottic epithelial projection through a congenital defect in the cartilage at the site of vessel penetration.

BIBLIOGRAPHY.

1. Casselberry, W. E.: Cystoma of the Arytenoid Region of the Larynx, With the Report of a Case. *Jour. A.M.A.*, 16:338-341, March, 1891.

2. Horne, J.: Cyst of Epiglottis. *Jour. Laryngol.*, 13:65, Feb., 1898.

3. Beck, J. C.: Cyst of Epiglottis. The Laryngoscope, 19:704, Sept., 1909.

4. Chamberlin, W. B.: Report of a Case of Cyst of the Larynx. The Laryngoscope, 27:622-624, Aug., 1917.

5. Oppikofer, A. Cited by M. Jacobi and H. Rascoff.[28]

6. Abercrombie, J.: Congenital Cyst in Larynx. *Trans. Path. Soc. London*, 32:33-34, 1881.

7. Myerson, M. C.: Cysts of the Larynx. *Arch. Otolaryngol.*, 18:281-290, Sept., 1933.

8. New, G. B., and Erich, J. B.: Congenital Cysts of the Larynx: Report of a Case. *Arch. Otolaryngol.*, 30:943-949, Dec., 1939.

9. Dean, L. W., and Gregg, J. B.: An Implantation Cyst of the Larynx. The Laryngoscope, 28:74-77, Jan., 1918.

10. Chiari.: Über Larynxcysten. Cited by W. Salomon. *Z. Ohrenheilk.*, 62:49-68, 1910.

11. Imperatori, C. J.: Branchiogenetic Cyst of Larynx Removed by Thyrotomy. The Laryngoscope, 39:679-683, Oct., 1929.

12. Howarth, W., and Chamings, A. J.: Cystic Adenomata of the Ventricles of Morgagni. *Jour. Laryngol.*, 49:324-325, May, 1934.

13. Pereira, C.: Quistos do laringe. *Revista brasileira de oto-rino-laringologia*, 23:159-200, Sept.-Dec., 1955.

14. Woodruff, G. H.: Cyst of the Epiglottis and Other Laryngeal Cysts. *Ill. Med. Jour.*, 66:569-572, Dec., 1934.

15. Schneider, P.: Zur Genese der kongenitalen Larynxcysten. *Z Ohrenheilk.*, 64:358-374, 1912.

16. Kleinfeld, L.: Laryngeal Cysts in the New-Born. *Arch. Otolaryngol.*, 19:590-593, May, 1934.

17. Thomas, R.: Operation (Thyrotomy) for Distention Cysts of Laryngeal Saccule. *Jour. Laryngol.*, 62:537-539, Aug., 1948.

18. Black, J. I. M.: A Cyst of the Laryngeal Ventricle. *Jour. Laryngol.*, 65:735, Oct., 1951.

19. Laff, H. I.: Cysts in the Ventricular Area of the Larynx. The Laryngoscope, 63:227-240, March, 1953.

20. Adams, W. S.: A Laryngeal Dermoid Cyst. *Jour. Laryngol.*, 45:266-269, 1930.

21. Portmann, G., and Guillen, D.: Présentation d'un cas de kyste épithélial laryngé. *Rev Laryng (Bordeaux)*, 81:119-121, Jan.-Feb., 1960.

22. Di Blasi, A.: Sulle cisti congenite della laringe. *Otorinolaring Ital*, 21:399-406, 1952.

23. Holinger, P. H., and Johnston, K. C.: Benign Tumors of the Larynx. *Ann. Otol.*, 60:496-509, June, 1951.

24. El Mofty, A.: A Huge Trilobed Laryngeal Cyst. *Jour. Laryngol.*, 73:768-771, Nov., 1959.

25. EDIS, A. W.: Specimen of Cyst in the Larynx Removed Post Mortem from An Infant. Report of An Exhibit. *Jour. Trans. Obstet. Soc. London*, 18:2, 1876.

26. GREENE, D. C., JR.: An Unusual Cyst of the Larynx. THE LARYNGOSCOPE, 17:800-804, Oct., 1907.

27. LORIE, A. J., and LUX, P.: Congenital Cyst of the Larynx. THE LARYNGOSCOPE, 42:957-960, Dec., 1932.

28. JACOBI, M., and RASCOFF, H.: Cysts of the Larynx in Infancy. *Amer. Jour. Dis. Child*, 49:448-459, Feb., 1935.

29. DAVIS, E. D. D.: Cysts of the Larynx. *Jour. Laryngol.*, 38:473-476, 1923.

30. CODY, C. C., JR.: Cysts of the Larynx. *Tex. Jour. Med.*, 33:581-583, Dec., 1937.

31. NEVILLE, W. S. T.: Cyst with Displacement of the Sacculus. *Jour. Laryngol.*, 53:127-128, Feb., 1938.

32. SNAITH, L.: Congenital Cyst of the Larynx Causing Fatal Asphyxia Neonatorum. *Arch. Dis. Child*, 15:274-276, 1940.

33. CRYNES, S. F., and YINGER, S. C.: Congenital Cyst of the Larynx. *Arch. Otolaryngol.*, 34:170-173, July, 1941.

34. NEW, G. B.: The Treatment of Cysts of the Larynx. *Trans. Pacific Coast Oto-Ophthal. Soc.*, 27:17-18, 1942.

35. DAVIDSON, J. I.: Congenital Cyst of the Larynx. *Lancet*, 2:508-509, Oct., 1943.

36. AHLÉN, G., and RANSTRÖM, S.: Congenital Laryngeal Cysts in Early Infancy. *Acta Otolaryngol.*, (Stockholm), 32:483-495, 1944.

37. HOLINGER, P. H., and STEINMANN, E. P.: Congenital Cysts of the Larynx. *Prac. Oto-Rhino-Laryngol.*, (Basel), 9:129-137, 1947.

38. TAYLOR, J. N. S.: Laryngeal Cysts of Developmental Origin. *Jour. Laryngol.*, 79:15-18, Jan., 1965.

39. FOX, N., and DINOLT, R.: Cysts of the Larynx. *Arch. Otolaryngol.*, 37:552-557, April, 1943.

40. BEAUTYMAN, W.; HAIDAK, G. L., and TAYLOR, M.: Laryngopyocele: Report of a Fatal Case. *New Eng. Jour. Med.*, 260:1025-1027, May, 1959.

41. EL-HAKEEM, A.: A Large Trilobed Congenital Laryngeal Cyst. *Jour. Laryngol.*, 65:41-43, Jan., 1951.

42. WILMS. Cited by A. Di Blasi.[22]

43. ROSENBERGER, H. C.: Cyst of the Larynx and Lobus Azygos of Lung: A Case Report. THE LARYNGOSCOPE, 37:360-366, May, 1927.

44. KAHLER, O. Cited by P. Schneider.[15]

45. WASSLER, H.: Histopathology of the Ear, Nose and Throat. Cited by A. A. Eggston and D. Wolff. Williams & Wilkins Company, Baltimore, Md., pp. 944-945, 1947.

46. KUHN, A. J.: Cystadenoma of the Parotid Gland and Larynx. *Arch Otolaryngol.*, 73:404-406, April, 1961.

47. STEWART, E. F.: Cystadenoma of Larynx. *Jour. Laryngol.*, 74:325-330, May, 1960.

48. MOORE, I.: Adenomata (Glandular Tumors) of the Larynx. *Jour. Laryngol.*, 35:65-75, March, 1920.

49. KOSCHIER, H.: Ueber Prolapsus sinus Morgagni. *Wien Klin Wschr*, 10:815-820, 1897.

50. FIGI, F. A.; ROWLAND, W. D., and NEW, G. B.: Cystadenoma of the Larynx: Report of Four Cases. *Arch. Otolaryngol.*, 40:445-450, Dec., 1944.

51. NOHTERI, H.: A Case of Laryngeal Cyst Composed of Oncocytes and the Appearance of Oncocytes in the Mucous Membrane of the Nose and the Larynx. *Acta Path. Microbiol. Scand.*, 23:473-483, 1946.

52. RANGER, D., and THACKRAY, A. C.: Papillary Cystadenoma of the Larynx. *Jour. Laryngol.*, 67:609-614, Sept., 1953.

53. ASH, J. E., and RAUM, M.: An Atlas of Otolaryngic Pathology. American Registry of Pathology, Washington, D. C., p. 355, 1956.

54. KROE, D. J.; PITCOCK, J. A., and COCKE, E. W.: Oncocytic Papillary Cystadenoma of the Larynx: Presentation of Two Cases. *Arch. Path.*, 84: 429-432, Oct., 1967.

55. MØLLER, J., and ØRNTOFT, I.: Laryngeal Oncocytoma. *Acta Otolaryngol*, (Stockholm), 60:239-242, 1965.

56. CAPO, O. A.: Oxyphilic Adenoma (Oncocytoma) of the Larynx. *Arch. Otolaryngol.*, 82:42-44, July, 1965.

57. SOM, M. L., and PEIMER, R.: Oncocytic Cystadenoma of the Larynx. *Ann. Otol.*, 58:234-242, March, 1949.

58. PINKERTON, P. H., and BECK, J. S.: Eosinophilic Granular-Cell (Oncocytic) Cysts of the Larynx. *Jour. Path. Bact.*, 81:532-534, April, 1961.

59. HEATH, D.: Eosinophilic Granular-Cell Cystadenoma of the Larynx. *Jour. Laryngol.*, 75:679-684, July, 1961.

60. HAMPERL, H.: Onkocytes and the So-Called Hürthle Cell Tumor. *Arch. Path.*, 49:563-567, May, 1950.

61. MOLLICA, V., and ROSSI, G.: Il problema degli oncociti e loro significato nella mucosa laringea in condizioni normali. *Riv Anat Pat Oncol*, 4:1179-1200, 1951.

62. NEW, G. B., and ERICH, J. B.: Benign Tumors of the Larynx: A Study of Seven Hundred Twenty-Two Cases. *Arch. Otolaryngol.*, 28:841-910, Dec., 1938.

63. SCHILLING, H. H.: Über Retentionsynsten and Stimmbandknötchen. *Der Hals, Nasen, und Ohrenarzt*, 28:195-206, May, 1937.

64. PARK, J. H., JR., and ISRAEL, S.: Epiglottic Cysts in Infancy. *South. Med. Jour.*, 18:128-131, Feb., 1925.

65. ERICH, J. B.: Cysts of the Larynx: Report of Case. *Proc. Staff Meet., Mayo Clin.*, 15:44-47, Jan, 1940.

66. FRAZER, J. E.: A Manuel of Embryology: The Development of the Human Body. Edition 1, William Wood and Company, New York, N. Y., pp. 223-253, 1932.

67. HOPP, E. S.: The Development of the Epithelium of the Larynx. THE LARYNGOSCOPE, 65:475-499, July, 1955.

68. ALI, M. Y.: Pathogenesis of Cysts and Crypts in the Nasopharynx. *Jour. Laryngol.*, 79:391-402, May, 1965.

Commentary

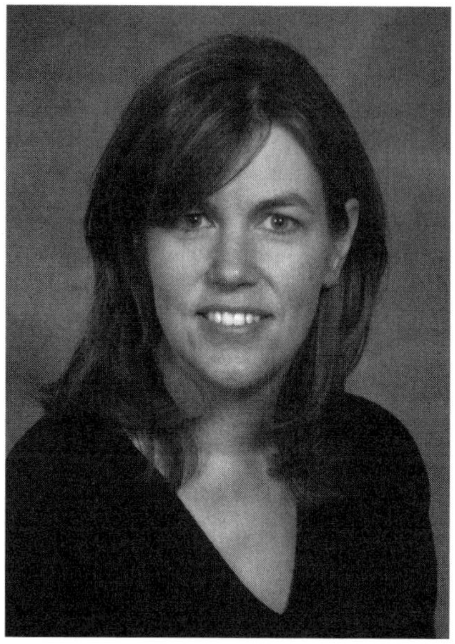

Susan L. Thibeault, PhD

Hirano[1,2] was one of the first to identify the importance of the microstructure of the vocal fold. According to Hirano, five histological layers of increasing density break down into two biomechanical layers (the body and the cover). The body is composed primarily of muscle whereas the cover has been described as being composed primarily of collagen and elastin. For over 50 years, it has been recognized that the shape and tension of the vocal fold determined the vibratory characteristics and subsequent vocal quality. More recently, it has been recognized that the cover, the vibratory source, is passive tissue acted upon by muscle contractions of the body and other intrinsic laryngeal muscles, serving as the primary source of vocal quality. Until recently, the primary foci of cover descriptions were the shape and thickness of the structure and the presence or absence of collagen and elastin. Scientists began to suspect this was not the whole picture that the normal lamina propria structure is constructed of a great deal more than collagen and elastin, after Gray, Hammond, and Hansen published their 1995 work. Gray, Hammond, and Hanson's paper describing "filler" proteins in benign lesions—nodules, Reinke's edema, and polyp—is the first of his work to characterize the extracellular matrix (ECM) of the vocal folds beyond collagen and elastin. The work is noteworthy because of the description of the basement membrane zone and lamina propria with speculation about correlation to function in disease states. This work laid the foundation for Gray's later triological thesis, which investigated levels of various glycoaminoglycans and proteoglycans (fillers) of the ECM and relative contribution to mucosal wave function in normal and disease states.[3,4] The notion that all of the constituents of the lamina propria and their subsequent organization contributes to its biomechanical properties was revolutionary in that it meant there might be other ways to treat laryngeal pathologies than those that existed at the time.

Steve Gray worked with Elizabeth Hammond, a pathologist who was the first to explain to him, while reading a set of vocal fold slides with Steve, that other stains and/or immunohistochemistry could be utilized to look at things that may not necessarily show up on trichome or H&E slides. Steve described the sense of excitement that he had, that there was more to the vocal fold structure than simply collagen and elastin—that there were other things that may be responsible for its structure and function. He said that these things needed to be investigated, things that researchers in the field of voice had no idea about, concepts that would change the field of laryngology. Steve had the insight to recognize that vocal fold biology needed to use more than histology that it was necessary to incorporate biochemistry, bioengineering, mechanics, genetics, and molecular biology for future development and growth in this area. He embraced scientists from other fields and enticed them into studying vocal fold biology while he simultaneously convinced young scientists interested in voice to study outside conventional coursework. Considering the prolific publication and grant funding history of Gray, his seminal work that has incorporated the aforementioned methodologies, including polymerase chain reaction, microarray, and genetics, are those that will no doubt become future "citation classics" in the field of voice and laryngology. Gray was the first to use the now prevalent vernacular—gene expression, proteome, tissue engineering, tissue regeneration, and bioreactors—in our field.

It should be evident that we're discussing two classics: the often cited article; subsequent work and its impact on the field; and the visionary man, Steve Gray. Steve loved what he did; he was a bright star, a most gentle soul, and remarkable mentor. Steve helped provide the foundation to what is now a diverse and ever expanding field of vocal fold biology. However, to think of Steve simply in terms of his vast scientific accomplishments would be to minimize the impact he had on the field and the people around him. Steve established a career as a surgeon and researcher that has become a template for others and that has been unparalleled. He brought the concept of molecular biology and genetics into laryngology and has been its heart and soul from the beginning. He set a standard so high it has been virtually impossible to replicate. He is deeply missed.

References

1. Hirano M. Morphological structure of the vocal cord as a vibrator and its variations. *Folia Phoniatr.* 1974; 26:89–94.
2. Hirano M, Kakita Y. Cover-body theory of vocal fold vibration. In: Daniloff RG, ed. *Speech Science.* San Diego, Calif: College-Hill Press; 1985:1–34.
3. Gray SD, Alipour F, Titze IR, Hammond TH. Biomechanical and histological observations of vocal fold fibrous proteins. *Ann Otol Rhinol Laryngol.* 2000;109: 77–85.
4. Gray SD, Titze IR, Chan R, Hammond TH. Vocal fold proteoglycans and their influence on biomechanics. *Laryngoscope.* 1999;109(6):845–854.

BENIGN PATHOLOGIC RESPONSES OF THE LARYNX

STEVEN D. GRAY, MD

ELIZABETH HAMMOND, MD DARRIN F. HANSON, MD

SALT LAKE CITY, UTAH

Benign laryngeal lesions were examined for patterns of injury indicated by deposition of fibronectin and collagen type IV. An immunoperoxidase technique was used to compare 33 fresh or paraffin-embedded tissues with regard to their staining of monoclonal antibodies directed against fibronectin and collagen type IV. Two types of patterns were recognized. One pattern showed intense fibronectin deposition in the superficial layer of the lamina propria, often coupled with basement membrane zone injury, indicated by thick collagen type IV bands. The other pattern showed rare basement membrane zone injury and very little fibronectin deposition. The first pattern correlated more with nodules, the second pattern more with Reinke's edema and some polyps. A better understanding of the effects of excessive deposition of structural glycoproteins such as fibronectin and of abnormal proteoglycan deposition may lead to a better characterization of vocal fold disease and its causation and, ultimately, better treatment.

KEY WORDS — collagen type IV, fibronectin, larynx, nodules, pathology.

INTRODUCTION

Pathologic responses to benign laryngeal injury have traditionally been described by means of hematoxylin and eosin (H & E) staining. However, electron and light microscopic identification techniques have revealed that the laryngeal responses to injury are varied and cannot be adequately characterized by using only H & E staining. This paper discusses laryngeal injury in terms of immunohistochemical techniques for protein identification in the lamina propria.

The vocal fold lamina propria consists of two important tissue components: cellular and extracellular. Only the extracellular tissue is likely to have a determining biomechanical role, since the cellular tissue in the lamina propria is sparse.[1]

The extracellular tissue, called a matrix, embodies two families of macromolecules: those molecules that provide a fibrous scaffolding of the lamina propria, which are the collagens and elastins, and those molecules that provide the "filling" around the fibrous scaffolding.[2] This latter family contains two macromolecular groups: the proteoglycans and the structural glycoproteins.

Traditionally, attention has been given to those molecules of the fibrous network as being a key influencing factor in determining tissue vibration. Hirano[3] has observed the elastin and collagen fibers histologically. Elastin and sparse collagen fibers are present in the superficial aspect of the lamina propria. The elastin fibers are prominent in the intermediate layer and then decrease in the deep layer. Collagen fibers are more numerous in the intermediate and deep layers.[3]

The anatomic distribution of the fibrous scaffolding, correlated with vibratory observations of the vocal folds, led to the cover-body theory of vibration.[4] Vocal fold disease was correlated with a disturbed fibrous network.[2,5] The fibrous proteins became the focus in studying normal and impaired vibration. As a result, the "filler" proteins of the extracellular matrix have been forgotten.

This paper describes one of the filler proteins of the extracellular matrix, fibronectin, which is a critical structural glycoprotein found in the lamina propria, and its relationship to basement membrane zone injury. We have chosen fibronectin because of its deposition as a result of tissue injury, and collagen type IV because of its location only in the basement membrane zone,[6] which makes it a good indicator of basement membrane zone thickness and location.[7]

METHODS

Polyps, nodules, and Reinke's edema specimens were obtained from the University of Iowa from 1984 to 1989 and from the LDS Hospital in Salt Lake City from 1980 to 1993. Specimens were analyzed only if the epithelium, basement membrane zone, and recognizable components of the superficial layer of the lamina propria were present. Because of the limited surgical excision involved with this type of surgery,

From the Division of Otolaryngology, University of Utah (Gray, Hanson), and the Department of Pathology, LDS Hospital (Hammond), Salt Lake City, Utah. This work was supported by Public Health Service Grant 5 K08 DC00036-06.

Presented at the meeting of the American Broncho-Esophagological Association, Palm Beach, Florida, May 9-11, 1994. Winner of the Broyles-Maloney Award.

REPRINTS — Steven D. Gray, MD, Division of Otolaryngology, University of Utah Medical Center, 3C 120, Salt Lake City, UT 84132.

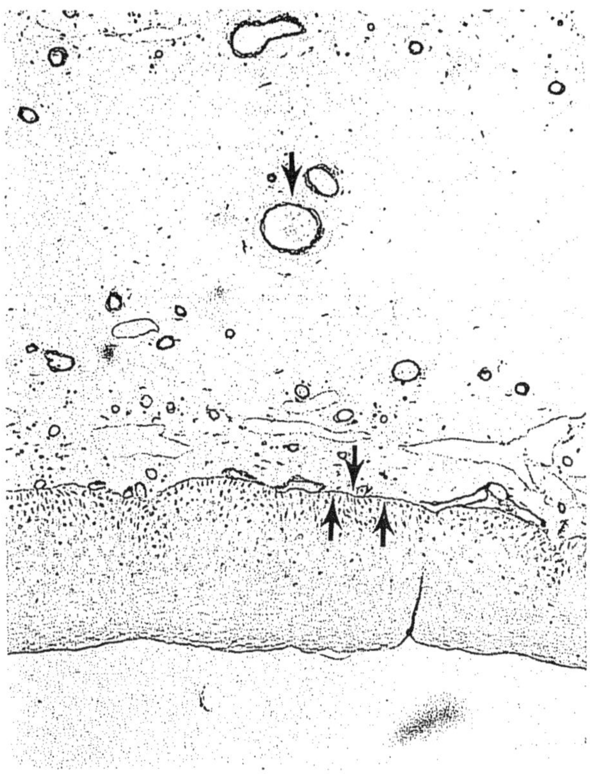

Fig 1. Normal human vocal fold (original ×25) stained for collagen type IV (arrows). Note thin black staining of basement membrane around arteriole and capillary structures, which serves as control to verify accuracy of staining technique. Basement membrane zone of epidermis is represented as very thin black line. Lamina propria appears amorphous and nondescript.

specimens were often excluded because of insufficient tissue. Thirty-three specimens were acceptable.

Initially our goal was to correlate the tissue diagnosis and clinical diagnosis with our findings, but we realized that often the H & E stains of nodules and polyps look alike. Consequently, pathologists called the specimen a nodule or a polyp if the surgeon clinically indicated it as one or the other. Furthermore, occasionally the lesions were not labeled consistently by the surgeon, and hence we had little clinical information to use in interpretation. Therefore, although the pathologic processes are described in this paper, the clinical correlation is performed cautiously and should be considered preliminary. The specific effect of fibronectin and collagen type IV on vibratory behavior has not yet been quantified.

For the immunocytochemical studies, fresh and paraffin-embedded tissues were compared with regard to their staining of monoclonal antibodies directed against fibronectin and collagen type IV; an immunoperoxidase (peroxidase-antiperoxidase, using diaminobenzidine as a substrate) technique was used. Antibodies were obtained from Dako Corp, Carpinteria, Calif. This procedure assured us that we could identify the components of fibronectin and collagen type IV protein that survived the fixation process. Controls of kidney and skin (fixed and unfixed with known staining distributions) were used with each staining process.

RESULTS

We found that normal adult vocal fold lamina propria has fairly moderate fibronectin deposition. This fibronectin deposition is intense through the superficial layer, and it remains fairly intense through the intermediate layer. In the deep layer, where the collagen fiber predominates, fibronectin staining becomes less intense. Although we are currently working on a technique to quantify the amount of fibronectin in vocal folds, so far we can only report our observations in degrees of intensity.

It is curious that normal, noninjured vocal folds should have much fibronectin deposition, since fibronectin is a prominent extracellular protein only in scar or densely cellular tissue (such as kidney).[8] We presume normal folds are not scarred, and the lamina propria is generally sparsely cellular; therefore, little fibronectin should be present. However, in the normal superficial layer of the lamina propria, one of the major filler proteins is fibronectin. In view of the sparse fibrous components in the superficial layer, the filler components may be the predominant determinant of tissue deformability.

In normal human vocal folds, the basement membrane zone is similar to human skin in construction and thickness (Fig 1). This normally consists of a thin, highly organized structure securing the epithelium to the lamina propria. No increase in basement membrane zone thickness is seen. Collagen type IV staining can be seen around arterioles and just below the basal cells as a thin black line. Filler proteins of the lamina propria found in these normal specimens are fibronectin, hyaluronic acid, and other, as yet unidentified mucopolysaccharides.[9]

We identified two general types of pathologic responses in the vocal fold lesions examined. One response, characterized by intense fibronectin deposition (more than normal) in the superficial layer of the lamina propria (Fig 2), is often associated with basement membrane zone injury (Fig 3B[10]). The second type of response is noted for its lack of fibronectin (less than normal) in the superficial layer (Fig 4). Staining for fibronectin shows minimal or no fibronectin. This second type of pathologic injury usually shows no basement membrane zone injury, and the disorder may be confined to the lamina propria. Some specimens occasionally showed variations of these findings.

Fig 2. Human vocal fold lesion described as nodule showing fibronectin deposition. A) Hematoxylin and eosin stain (original ×25). Note lack of lamina propria detail. B) Fibronectin stain (original ×10). Notice intense brown stain throughout lamina propria. Arrows show region of intense fibronectin; compare with Figs 3 and 4. Note no fibronectin basement membrane involvement in this lesion. C) Collagen type IV stain (arrows; original ×10). Normal basement membrane zone confirmed.

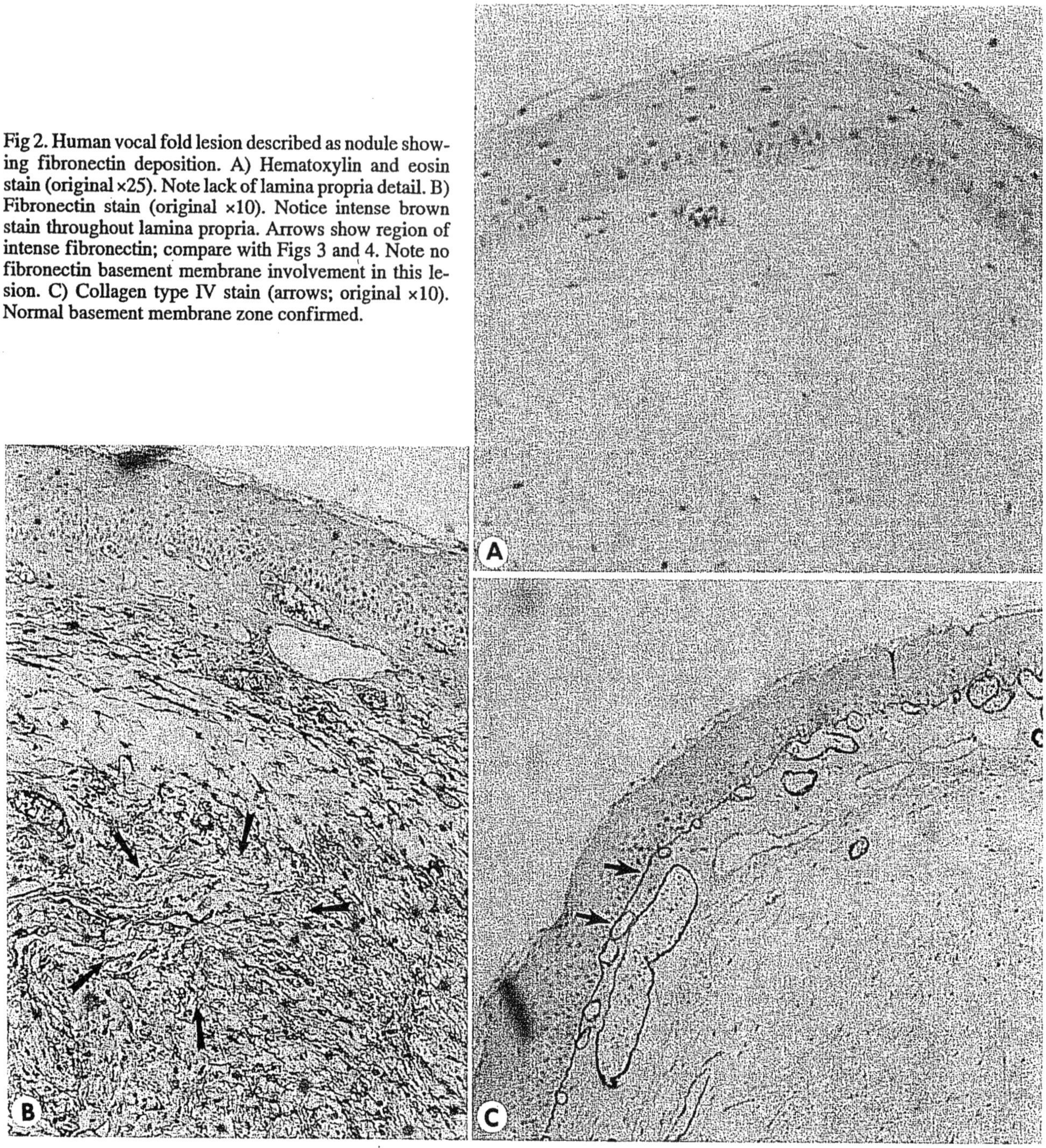

DISCUSSION

The cause of vocal fold injury and the pathologic response to that injury have been debated for years. Vocal fold polyps have been attributed to vocal abuse that has resulted in a hemorrhagic event or increased vascular permeability.[11] Nodules have also been attributed to vocal abuse that has caused a thickening of the epithelium or lamina propria.

The results of this work indicate that one type of injury is due to lamina propria disruption, usually associated with severe basement membrane zone injury. This injury leads to an aggravated healing response marked by fibronectin deposition in amounts exceeding that found in normal vocal folds. Since the basement membrane zone shows thickening and disorganization, this injury involves more than the lamina propria. The thickness of the collagen type IV band confirms the extent and aggravation of basement membrane zone injury sustained.

Normal basement membrane zones heal within days or weeks following injury. Basement membrane zone thickening and disruption to the degree seen in

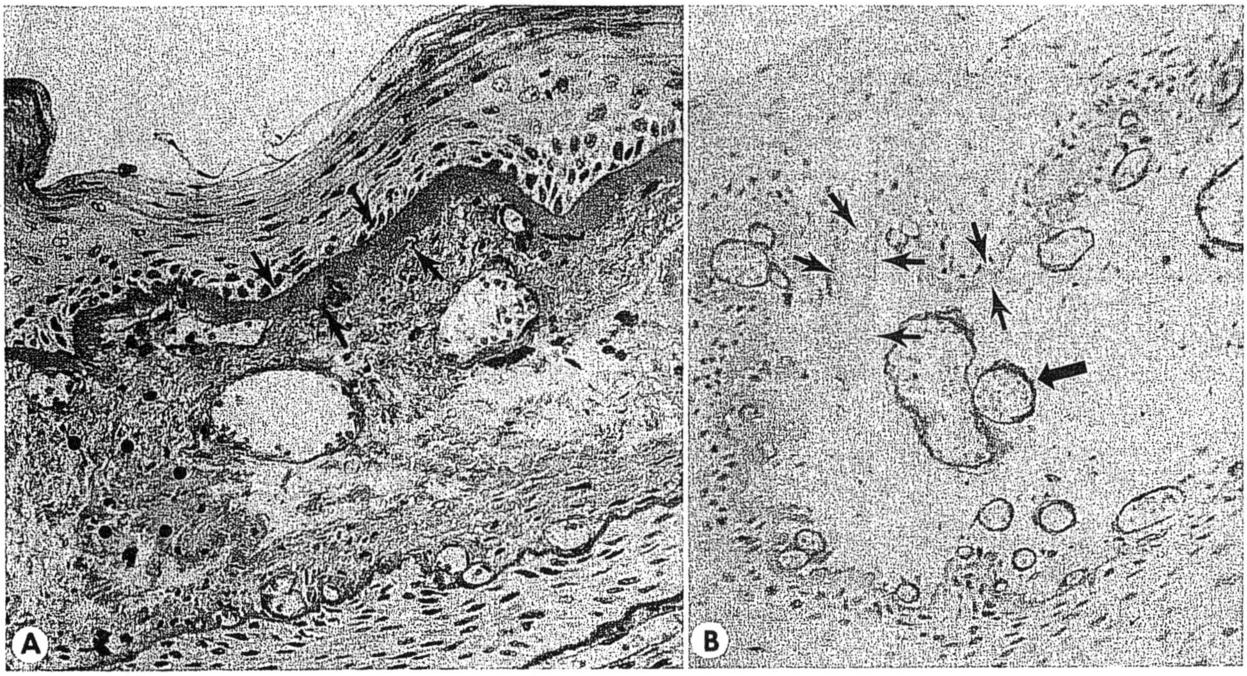

Fig 3. Another vocal fold lesion described as nodule, showing both fibronectin and collagen type IV deposition (original ×25). A) Fibronectin stain. Basement membrane zone (arrows) is abundant with fibronectin. Lamina propria, although partially surgically crushed, displays much fibronectin (dots) throughout. Compare with polyp in Fig 4. B) Collagen type IV stain. This stain is interesting in two regards. Basement membrane zone (small arrows) stains broadly, but weakly. Weak staining probably indicates incomplete assembly of protein. Broad band indicates extensive basement membrane zone disorganization and injury.[10] Large arrow indicates normal basement membrane zone around arteriole.

this vocal injury pattern are rarely seen anywhere else in the body. This pattern is likely due to the repetitive and chronic nature of reinjury that the vocal folds frequently sustain. This inability to let the vocal folds rest enough to heal probably leads to the aberrant healing responses seen in these specimens.

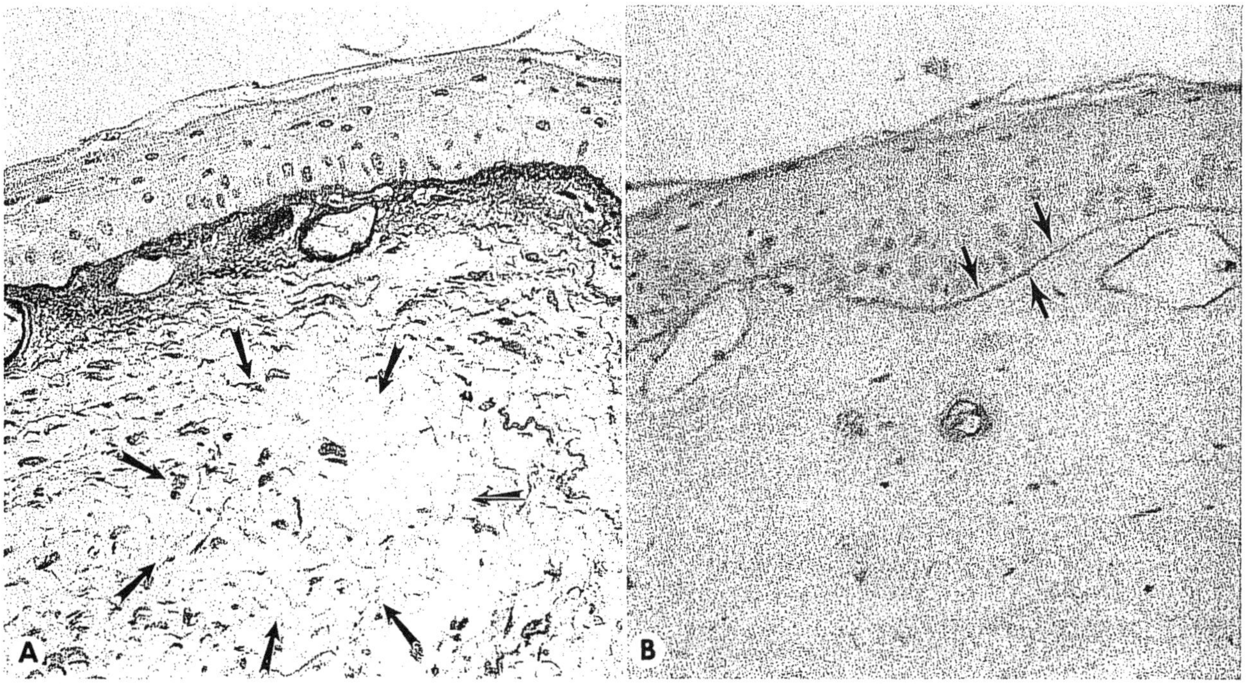

Fig 4. Human vocal fold lesion described as polyp (original ×25). A) Fibronectin stain shows very little fibronectin in lamina propria. Arrows surround region of sparse fibronectin. Compare to Figs 2 and 3. Fibronectin is deposited normally in basement membrane zone, however. B) Collagen type IV stain shows normal basement membrane zone, with no increased thickness. Arrows indicate collagen type IV band.

Fibronectin is a structural glycoprotein deposited by fibroblasts in response to interstitial injury. Structural glycoproteins permeate the areas between and around the fibrous structures. Fibronectin is a large macromolecule with a structure that promotes binding to several other macromolecules. Fibronectin and vitronectin (another structural protein found in extracellular matrix) bind to the collagens, other structural proteins, and proteoglycans.[12] Fibronectin is one of the early macromolecules deposited in wound healing and is a prominent protein in wound repair.[13]

Fibronectin is a precursor for collagen deposition and scar formation. However, in vocal fold benign laryngeal lesions, increased collagen or scar is not often seen. The increased fibronectin found in these lesions indicates that enough interstitial injury has occurred to cause a cellular fibroblastic response to repair the extracellular matrix. This response seems to be aborted before the phase of collagen type I (scar) deposition is achieved.

These findings lead to formation of the following picture of causation and pathologic response in vocal fold lesions severe enough to require excision. The vocal folds sustain enough injury to lead to basement membrane zone disruption and injury to the superficial layer of the lamina propria. The injury, if repetitive, leads to aberrant healing and a fibroblastic response involving increased fibronectin deposition. The clinical implications are that in the acute phase, treatment must allow healing to occur without repetitive injury, as fibronectin deposition is usually a permanent event.[6,13] Because of the biologic characteristics of this macromolecule, which are molecular binding, adhesion, and strength, its presence (in excess) probably does not contribute to efficient tissue vibration.[2,12]

This type of injury was seen in nodules and, occasionally, in polyps. The deposition of fibronectin may explain why some nodules do not respond to voice therapy, even though voice habits to reduce abuse are strictly followed by the patient. Clinically, a patient with vocal nodules may show vastly improved phonatory habits while stroboscopy examination continues to show nodules or areas of stiffness. Fibronectin deposition would likely lead to either or both clinical findings. The disordered basement membrane and lamina propria may also predispose the patient to recurrence of the lesion, since the pathologic state is less likely to be as resilient to voice abuse as the original, uninjured state. In cases of chronic injury, because these proteins are permanent, surgical excision may be required for improved voice.

The second type of pathologic finding shows few structural proteins such as collagen or elastin, and little or no fibronectin.[10] Clinically, this absence of the structural glycoproteins and fibrous proteins would lead to a vocal fold with excessive propensity for deformability (like a bag of jelly). The effect is then opposite to that of the first type of disorder described.

The pathogenesis of this second type of injury is not clear. The injury often seems to be confined to the lamina propria only and apparently does not consist of a fibroblastic response of tissue repair. This second type of pathologic response is seen more often in Reinke's edema, polypoid corditis, and some polyps.

CONCLUSION

The extracellular matrix of the vocal fold consists of many structural and filler proteins. The above descriptions represent only a few of them. Diseases such as some polyps, polypoid corditis, or Reinke's edema may be disorders of increased abnormal proteoglycan deposition. Diseases leading to dampening of the mucosal wave or decreased tissue vibration may be due to increases in collagen fibers (scar), but also may be due to excessive deposition of structural glycoproteins such as fibronectin, as shown in this research. Further studies of normal and abnormal vocal folds will lead to a better characterization of fold disorders and their causes and, hence, better treatment.

REFERENCES

1. Gray SD, Titze I, Lusk RP. Electron microscopy of hyperphonated vocal cords. J Voice 1987;1:109-15.

2. Labat-Robert J, Bihari-Varga M, Robert L. Extracellular matrix. FEBS Lett 1990;268:386-93.

3. Hirano M. Structure of the vocal fold in normal and disease states. Anatomical and physical study. ASHA Rep 1981; 11:11-30.

4. Hirano M, Kakita Y. Cover-body theory of vocal fold vibration. In: Daniloff RG, ed. Speech science. San Diego, Calif: College-Hill Press, 1985:1-46.

5. Hirano M, Kurita S, Sakaguchi S. Aging of the vibratory tissue of human vocal folds. Acta Otolaryngol (Stockh) 1989;107: 428-33.

6. Grinnell F. Fibronectin and wound healing. J Cell Biochem 1984;26:107-16.

7. Lauri WG, Leblong CP, Martin GR. Localization of type 4 collagen, laminin, heparin sulfate proteoglycan, and fibronectin to the basal lamina of basement membranes. J Cell Biol 1982;95: 340-4.

8. D'Ardenne AJ, Burns J, Sykes BC, Kirkpatrick P. Comparative distribution of fibronectin and type III collagen in normal human tissues. J Pathol 1983;141:55-69.

9. Matsuo D, Watanabe S, Hirano M, Kamimura M, Tanaka Y, Takazono I. Acid mucopolysaccharide and glycoprotein in the

vocal fold. Alterations with aging. Pract Otol (Kyoto) 1984;77: 817-22.

10. Mossallam I, Kotby MN, Ghaly AF, Nassar AM, Barakah MA. Histopathological aspects of benign vocal fold lesions associated with dysphonia. In: Kirchner JA, ed. Vocal fold histopathology. San Diego, Calif: College-Hill Press, 1986:65-80.

11. Frenzel H. Fine structural and immunohistochemical studies on polyps of human vocal folds. In: Kirchner JA, ed. Vocal fold histopathology. San Diego, Calif: College-Hill Press, 1986:39-50.

12. Ruoslahti E. Fibronectin and its receptors. Annu Rev Biochem 1988;57:375-413.

13. Nagata H, Ueki H, Moriguchi T. Fibronectin. Arch Dermatol 1985;121:995-9.

≈

FIRST WORLD CONFERENCE ON THE PREVENTION AND TREATMENT OF CAUSTIC ESOPHAGEAL BURNS IN CHILDREN

The First World Conference on the Prevention and Treatment of Caustic Esophageal Burns in Children will be held April 3-5, 1996, in Izmir, Turkey. For information, contact Prof Oktay Mutaf, Dept of Pediatric Surgery, Ege University Faculty of Medicine, TR-35100 Izmir, Turkey; fax +90(232) 375 1288 and 342 2142; e-mail mutafp@cakabey.ege.edu.tr.

≈

FOURTH INTERNATIONAL CONFERENCE ON HEAD AND NECK CANCER

The American Society for Head and Neck Surgery and the Society of Head and Neck Surgeons will sponsor the Fourth International Conference on Head and Neck Cancer, to be held from July 28 to August 2, 1996, in Toronto, Canada. For further information, contact We Plan Meetings, Inc, Ruth C. Enquist, President, 1503 15th St NE, Rochester, MN 55906; telephone (507) 285-1523; fax (507) 281-8328.

8

Laryngeal Scarring and Stenosis

Introduction

Scarring—both in the sense of circumferential airway narrowing and changes in the tissues of the membranous vocal fold—represents an important remaining hurdle in laryngology. Despite quantum leaps in the delicacy of instruments and technique under surgical magnification, unpredictable and harmful tissue response remains troublesome. The vocal folds themselves punish casual or ham-handed tissue handling with a loss of pliability of the mucosal cover. Even small alterations in the tissues of the membranous vocal fold will have consequences for voice quality. The lumen of the airway also seems to never forget an injury, following many efforts at repair with repeat contracture and narrowing.

Dr. Shapshay speaks from a vast experience dealing with airway stenosis, spanning the introduction of a number of new materials and technologies. He describes in detail efforts to prevent restenosis by altering post-instrumentation tissue proliferation using mitomycin-C. Dr. Benninger recalls the genesis and evolution of a landmark review paper on vocal fold scar, and highlights the fact that there remains no good replacement for native superficial lamina propria. That the best advice seems to be to prevent scarring in the first place highlights underlines our relative helplessness in dealing with scar, and outlines the challenge for the future.

Classic Articles

●Reprint of article included in this chapter.
♦Commentary on this article.

●♦Benninger MS, Alessi D, Archer S, Bastian R, et al. Vocal fold scarring: current concepts and management. *Otolaryngol Head Neck Surg.* 1996;115(5):474–482.

Eliashar R, Eliachar I, Esclamado R, Gramlich T, Strome M. Can topical mitomycin prevent laryngotracheal stenosis? *Laryngoscope.* 1999;109(10):1594–1600.

●♦Rahbar R, Shapshay SM, Healy GB. Mitomycin: effects on laryngeal and tracheal stenosis, benefits, and complications. *Ann Otol Rhinol Laryngol.* 2001;110(1):1–6.

Commentary

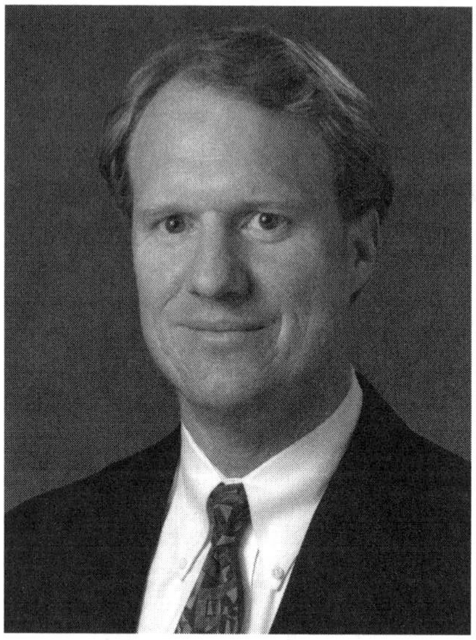

Michael S. Benninger, MD

For laryngologists who frequently deal with complex voice and laryngology disorders, one of the most frustrating treatment dilemmas is the management of the patient with vocal fold scarring. To further complicate the problem, vocal fold scarring is often iatrogenic secondary to overaggressive treatment or the improper use of instruments or technology. Another problem with scarring is that there are no reliable treatments that work in a majority, or even a good subset, of patients. Although the literature has numerous articles regarding various aspects of vocal fold scarring, the clinical studies are all low level evidence. There are no randomized, controlled trials nor is there enough level A and B evidence to prompt an evidence-based review of the literature. Nonetheless, scarring is common and laryngologists have long been looking for a guide that will help them manage these difficult and distressed patients.

In 1994, the Committee on Speech, Voice and Swallowing of the American Academy of Otolaryngology created a miniseminar for the annual meeting of that organization to try to address what was the state of the art about the pathogenesis and treatment of vocal fold scarring. Although the Committee felt that this would be an esoteric topic that would be of interest to a select group of laryngologists, the auditorium was overflowing with otolaryngologists, many of whom were general ENTs, and it seemed that every speech-language pathologist who attended the meeting was there. The discussion continued long after the presentations concluded and extended into the early parts of the Neurolaryngology Study Group later that meeting.

The interest in the topic was so overwhelming that the presenters decided that we should pull together as much as was known regarding scarring and present it as a review article. "Vocal Fold Scarring; Current Concepts and Management" was published in *Otolaryngology-Head and Neck Surgery* in 1996. The presenters were all recognized laryngologists and it was felt that together we could come up with some concrete recommendations regarding the causes, prevention, and subsequent treatment of vocal fold scarring. The paper was organized into sections that allowed even the relatively unknowledgeable reader to understand the intricate anatomy and physiology of the vocal folds and the impact of scarring on subsequent vocal fold function. It began with a definition of scar, "the fibrous tissue replacement of normal tissue destroyed by injury and disease." A long list of potential causes of scarring was presented, although much of the focus of the paper was on the preventable, mostly iatrogenic, causes.

We decided that it was an excellent place to describe the histology of the vocal folds and to identify changes that occurred with injury, and how these changes affected normal vocal fold function. This was one of the first articles in the general, nonbasic science English literature that described the multiple different fibers that make up the normal architecture of the vocal fold and how disruption of this architecture could result in alteration in vibratory function and voice. The therapeutic options that were discussed included voice therapy, revision surgery, collagen or adipose injections, and vocal fold medialization. All of these techniques are still being used over a decade later. In fact, although there are some newer options for treatment, including more specific replacements such as hyaluronic acid, there has really not been a major, reliable improvement in therapy for this difficult problem.

What was unique about this article was the remarkable group of authors who were well recognized for their basic science, clinical research, and practice experience in assessment and management of vocal fold scarring. Although most of the presentations were the cutting edge at the time, the fundamental approaches have stood the test of time and continue to be the standard of therapy to this date. This article did help to reinforce the critical principles of safe primary voice surgery to prevent scarring, including careful dissection of vocal fold lesions, an admonition against vocal fold stripping (which was still being performed at that time), and the cautious, appropriate use of technology such as lasers. Vocal fold scarring remains one of the major dilemmas of treatment for the laryngologist and the search continues for better approaches to these patients. Our summary in 1996 has become a sentinel description of this complex entity and the information presented there has remained a valuable resource until this day.

REVIEW ARTICLE

Vocal fold scarring: Current concepts and management

MICHAEL S. BENNINGER, MD, DAVID ALESSI, MD, SANFORD ARCHER, MD, ROBERT BASTIAN, MD, CHARLES FORD, MD, JAMES KOUFMAN, MD, ROBERT T. SATALOFF, MD, JOSEPH R. SPIEGEL, MD, and PEAK WOO, MD, Detroit, Michigan, Los Angeles, California, Lexington, Kentucky, Chicago, Illinois, Madison, Wisconsin, Winston-Salem, North Carolina, Philadelphia, Pennsylvania, and Boston, Massachusetts

Scarring of the vocal folds can occur as the result of blunt laryngeal trauma or, more commonly, as the result of surgical, iatrogenic injury after excision or removal of vocal fold lesions. The scarring results in replacement of healthy tissue by fibrous tissue and can irrevocably alter vocal fold function and lead to a decreased or absent vocal fold mucosal wave. The assessment and treatment of persistent dysphonia in patients with vocal fold scarring presents both diagnostic and therapeutic challenges to the voice treatment team. The common causes of vocal fold scarring are described, and prevention of vocal fold injury during removal of vocal fold lesions is stressed. The anatomic and histologic basis for the subsequent alterations in voice production and contemporary modalities for clinical and objective assessment will be discussed. Treatment options will be reviewed, including nonsurgical treatment and voice therapy, collagen injection, fat augmentation, endoscopic laryngoplasty, and Silastic medialization. (Otolaryngol Head Neck Surg 1996;115:474-82.)

Vocal fold scarring can occur after blunt or penetrating neck trauma, as a result of prolonged or traumatic intubation, after caustic or thermal burns, and after radiation therapy for small glottic carcinomas. Scarring is the single greatest cause of poor voice after vocal fold surgery.[1] It is also poorly recognized after surgery because there may be little evidence of a mass lesion or a visible abnormality. Although the following discussion will address the prevention, evaluation, and treatment of these causes of vocal fold scarring, postsurgical scarring will be emphasized.

From the Department of Otolaryngology–Head and Neck Surgery, Henry Ford Hospital (Dr. Benninger); and the Departments of Otolaryngology at the University of California–Los Angeles (Dr. Alessi), the University of Kentucky–Lexington (Dr. Archer), Loyola University Medical Center (Dr. Bastian), the University of Wisconsin–Madison (Dr. Ford), Bowman-Gray School of Medicine (Dr. Koufman), Thomas Jefferson University (Drs. Sataloff and Spiegel), and Tufts University School of Medicine (Dr. Woo).

Presented at the Annual Meeting of the American Academy of Otolaryngology–Head and Neck Surgery, San Diego, Calif., Sept. 18-21, 1994.

Received for publication Sept. 13, 1995; accepted Nov. 7, 1995.

Reprint requests: Michael S. Benninger, MD, Chairman, Department of Otolaryngology–Head and Neck Surgery, Henry Ford Hospital, 2799 West Grand Blvd., Detroit, MI 48202.

0194-5998/96/$5.00 + 0 **23/76/70639**

CAUSE AND PREVENTION OF VOCAL FOLD SCARRING

Stedman's Medical Dictionary defines scar as "the fibrous tissue replacement of normal tissue destroyed by injury or disease."[2] A scar is therefore a natural late sequelae of injury and repair. In the larynx, and more specifically on the vocal folds, scarring produces a functional deficit because of the loss of mucosal pliability and inability to modulate airflow to produce the glottal sound source. Scar tissue in the membranous vocal fold disrupts normal vibratory function by changing the physical properties of the tissue destroying the body-cover interface. Increased effort to overcome the localized mucosal stiffness caused by the scar results in a poor voice, often with glottal insufficiency. The voice quality may be strained, harsh, diplophonic, or hoarse. Pathophysiologically, anatomic alterations caused by the disease or surgical injury result in loss of the normal layered structure of the vocal fold. This results in poor mucosal pliability, poor airflow modulation, altered voice source production, and hoarse voice.

Vocal fold scar may occur through either disease or injury. The most common causes are listed in Table 1. After surgical excision of the vocal fold epithelium, the superficial ulceration and fibrin deposition is filled by acute and chronic inflammatory cells, macrophages, and plasma cells. Fibroblasts and collagen deposition occur below the epithelial layer, and healing by secondary intention and wound contracture occurs if the deficit is too large to permit primary wound healing.

With vocal fold surgery, the creation of larger defects requires secondary healing. Poorer results are expected more often after large defect creation than after smaller defect creation. Repeated surgery, especially when vocal fold epithelium is removed for dysplasia, leukoplakia, or papilloma, also contributes to progressive scarring. Anatomic sites of involvement, such as the anterior commissure and vocal ligament, and the presence of bilateral vocal fold pathology contribute to the risk of vocal fold scar development.

Careful preoperative, operative, and postoperative management can reduce the risk of scar and poor voice. Patients with untreated chronic inflammation of the larynx who undergo laryngeal surgery often have prolonged or significant postoperative inflammation. The patients most at risk are those with untreated gastroesophageal reflux, those with chronic tracheobronchitis, and those who are heavy smokers. In the preoperative assessment, it is important to identify these risk factors and reverse the causes of chronic inflammation before surgery. The local milieu is optimized with hydration and mucolytic agents, treatment of reflux laryngitis, mucosal hygiene instructions, and preoperative consultation by a speech-language pathologist before surgery to reduce inflammation and decrease voice abuse. Reduction of environmental irritants, allergens, and smoking is advised before surgery.

Operative technical advancements allow the phonosurgeon better tools than those available even a few years ago. These include more precise microsurgical instruments, dissectors and knives, and microspot CO_2 lasers with superpulse modes. Operative techniques should include the principles of careful dissection, sparing of normal tissue, and avoidance of injury to the vocal ligament. By limiting the dissection to the layer of vocal fold involvement, the epithelium can often be spared while vocal fold cysts are removed. When epithelial resection is necessary, preservation of the superficial and deep layers of the lamina propria should prevent scarring. When deeper dissection is needed, attempts to preserve the deep layer of the lamina propria are critical.

Table 1. Causes of vocal fold scarring

Traumatic
Blunt trauma (with or without fracture)
Penetrating injury (e.g., knife, bullet, dog bite)
Neoplastic
Carcinoma of the vocal cord
Prior radiation therapy
Prior surgical treatment
Iatrogenic
Prior polytef (Teflon) injection
Injudicious vocal cord surgery (e.g., polpectomy)
Prolonged endotracheal intubation
Prolonged nasogastric intubation
Tracheotomy
Inflammatory
Gastroesophageal (laryngopharyngeal) reflux disease
Acute (thermal) inhalation injury
Rheumatoid arthritis
Relapsing polychondritis
Bacterial laryngotracheitis
Other acute necrotizing infections
Chronic granulomatous disorders
Miscellaneous
Sulcus vocalis
Congenital webs
Radiation injury (e.g., fibrosis)
Intracordal cysts

Microsutures of 6-0 absorbable gut may be used to close the vocal fold defect, thereby reducing epithelial healing by secondary intention.

During the postoperative period, the patient is examined frequently to monitor wound healing. Mucolytics and antireflux dietary regimens and medications are routinely used. Systemic steroids and antibiotics are also occasionally used to reduce inflammation and treat infection. Voice rest may be valuable for a short time after surgery. Adjunctive measures such as the use of a multidisciplinary evaluation, formation of a contract with the patient to change his or her lifestyle, and careful documentation of results as feedback to the phonosurgeon are useful to refine surgical results. Voice therapy should be a vital part of postoperative rehabilitation, and caution should be used to ensure that the patient does not resume full voice use until recovery has occurred.

ANATOMY OF THE VOCAL FOLDS AND PHYSIOLOGY OF PHONATION

Voice is produced as a result of the interaction of three basic anatomic units. The infraglottic respiratory tract, consisting of the lungs, supporting thoracic muscles, back muscles, and diaphragm, with the support of the abdominal musculature, creates the power source. The larynx serves as the oscillator. Parts of the supraglottic vocal tract, including the supraglottic larynx, pharynx, oral cavity, nasal cavity, and paranasal sinuses, serve as

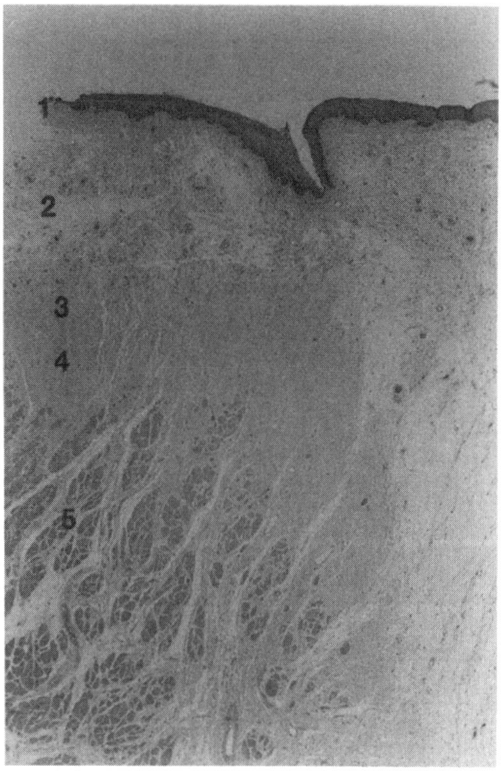

Fig. 1. Hematoxylin and eosin-stained coronal section of vocal fold showing normal vocal fold mucosa. Numbers *1*, *2*, *3*, *4*, and *5* refer to the stratified squamous epithelium, superficial layer of the lamina propria (Reinke's space), intermediate layer of the lamina propria, deep layer of the lamina propria, and vocalis muscle, respectively.

resonators, although the infraglottic vocal tract may also have resonating functions.

The larynx is composed of four basic units: mucosa, intrinsic muscles, extrinsic muscles, and skeleton. The thyroarytenoid muscle originates anteriorly from the inner surface of the thyroid cartilage and inserts into the lateral base of the arytenoid cartilage from the vocal process to a portion of the muscular process. The medial portion of this muscle is known as the vocalis muscle. It adducts, lowers, shortens, and thickens the vocal fold, rounding the vocal fold edge. The posterior cricoarytenoid muscle abducts, elevates, elongates, and thins the vocal fold. The lateral cricoarytenoid muscle adducts, lowers, elongates, and thins the vocal fold with stiffening of the vocal fold edge, allowing a more angular and sharp contour. The interarytenoid muscles adduct the cartilaginous portion of the vocal folds but have relatively little effect on the stiffness of the membranous portion. The cricothyroid muscle rotates the cricoid cartilage in relationship to the thyroid cartilage, resulting in elongation, thinning, and lowering of the vocal fold. This longitudinal tension is important in the control of pitch and loudness.

At the beginning of each phonatory cycle, the vocal folds are approximated, and the glottis is obliterated. This permits infraglottic pressure to increase, typically to a level of about 7 cm of water for conversational speech. The subglottic air pressure pushes the vocal folds progressively further apart from the bottom up until a gap develops and air begins to flow. Bernoulli forces created by the air passing between the vocal folds and the tension and mechanical properties of the vocal folds begin to close the lower portion of the glottis even while the upper edges are still separating. The upper portions of the vocal folds have strong elastic properties that tend to make the vocal folds snap back to the midline. This force becomes more dominant as the upper edges are stretched further apart and the force of the airstream diminishes. Thus the upper portion of the vocal folds returns to the midline, completing the glottic cycle. Subglottal air pressure then begins to build again until this overcomes the glottal pressures, and the cycle is repeated.

The frequency of vibration (number of cycles of openings and closings per second), measured in hertz, is dependent on the air pressure, the mass of the vocal folds, and the mechanical properties of the vocal folds such as length and tension. Frequency corresponds closely with the perception of pitch, although the sound from the larynx is a complex tone containing the fundamental frequency and many overtones or higher harmonic partials. The resonators attenuate some frequencies and enhance others. Sundberg[3] has shown that the vocal tract has four or five important resonant frequencies called *formants*. Formant frequencies are established by vocal tract shape, which can be altered by laryngeal, pharyngeal, and oral cavity musculature. Control mechanisms for two vocal characteristics are particularly important: fundamental frequency and intensity. Fundamental frequency can be altered by changing either the air pressure or the mechanical properties of the vocal folds, with the latter being more efficient under most conditions.

Vocal fold scarring primarily inhibits the production of the mucosal wave across the vibratory margin. The patient will often try to compensate for this deficit by altering the mechanical properties of the vocal folds with the intrinsic laryngeal muscles, changing the shape and position of the larynx with the extrinsic muscles, increasing the infraglottic air pressure, or changing the shape of the supraglottic resonators. It is often just as important to treat these compensatory mechanisms as it is to diagnose and treat the primary vocal fold pathology.

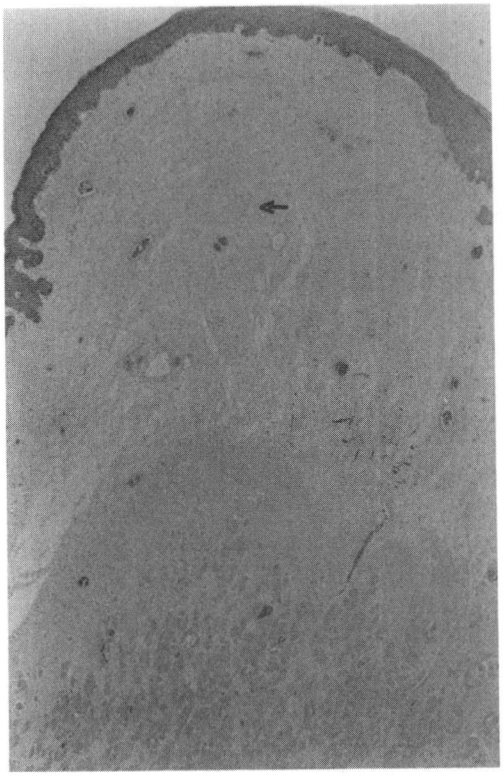

Fig. 2. Elastin van Gieson's stain shows relatively fewer elastic fibers in the superficial layer of the lamina propria *(arrow)* and much more in the intermediate and deep layers of the lamina propria.

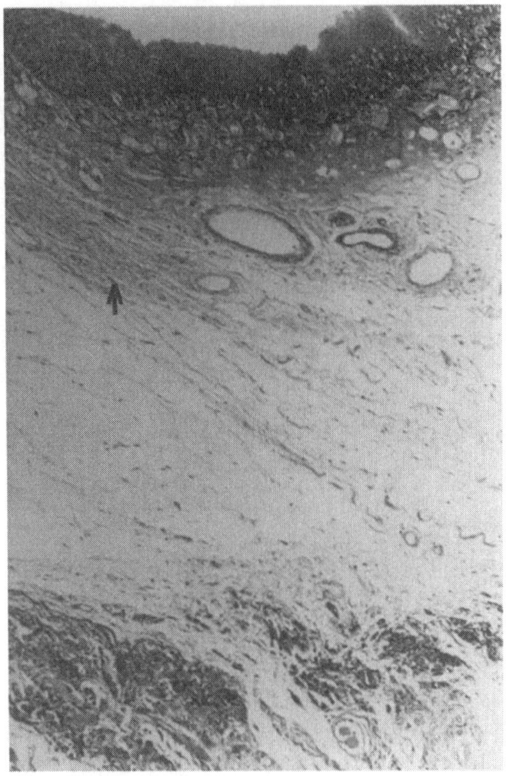

Fig. 3. Reticulin stain of section of vocal fold. Reticulin stain is sensitive for reticular fibers, which are primarily loose, nonorganized type III collagen fibers saturated with proteoglycans. Staining is heavy in the superficial layer of the lamia propria *(arrow)*.

SURGICAL HISTOLOGY OF THE VOCAL FOLD

On the basis of the knowledge of vocal fold anatomy, techniques have been developed to operate in areas of the vocal fold that have the least propensity for scar formation and subsequent hindrance of mucosal waveform. One of the most important concepts advocates that dissection be kept as superficial as possible. This is done by operating within the superficial layer of the lamina propria (Reinke's space). This concept is based on the fact that the paucicellular Reinke's space contains few fibroblast cells, which are responsible for production of most extracellular matrix and can contribute to scar formation. This section describes the microarchitecture of the vocal folds.

The histology review was based on evaluation of six specimens from the Department of Pathology at Cedars-Sinai Medical Center, which were resected for squamous cell carcinoma and had one fold grossly and microscopically free of disease and therefore were suitable for study. The hematoxylin and eosin–stained sections allowed review of the normal histology of the vocal fold (Fig. 1). The most superficial layer of the vocal fold consisted of pseudostratified ciliated columnar epithelium (respiratory epithelium). However, the adducting edge of the vocal fold was lined predominantly with stratified squamous epithelium. Seromucinous glands are found throughout the mucosa, except along the adducting surface. The epithelium rested on a continuous basement membrane.

The lamina propria was identified beneath the basement membrane of the epithelium. This could be divided anatomically into three layers. The superficial or Reinke's space contained a sparse number of fibroblasts with a relatively high content of reticulum fibers and a few elastic (Fig. 2) or collagen fibers (Fig. 3). The intermediate layer had slightly more extracellular matrix and collagen fibers, as identified by trichrome stain (Fig. 4), with moderate numbers of elastic fibers. Fibroblasts were also moderate in number. The intermediate layer merged into the deep layer, and in most areas it was not possible to completely distinguish them. However, the deep layer appeared to consist of a dense accumulation of extracellular matrix material as high-

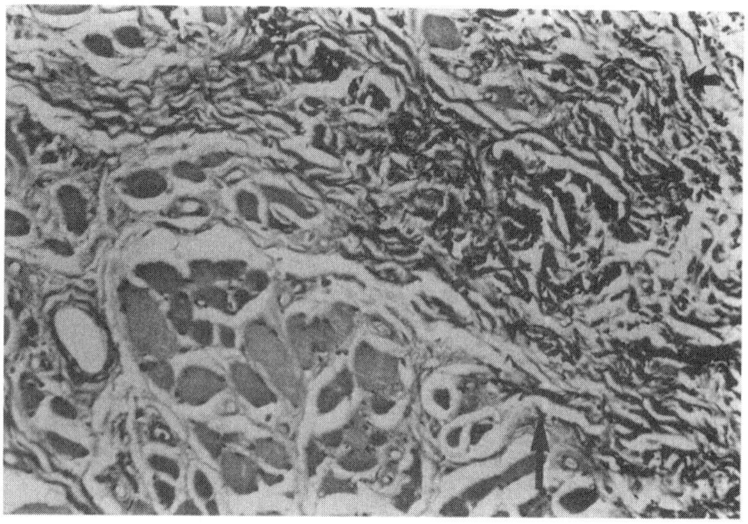

Fig. 4. Trichrome stain shows collagen bundles in large numbers in the deep layer of the lamina propria *(small arrow)*. The superficial layer (not shown) had relatively little staining for collagen with trichrome stain. These bundles appear to be contiguous with the collagen surrounding the muscle fibers in the vocalis muscle *(large arrow)*.

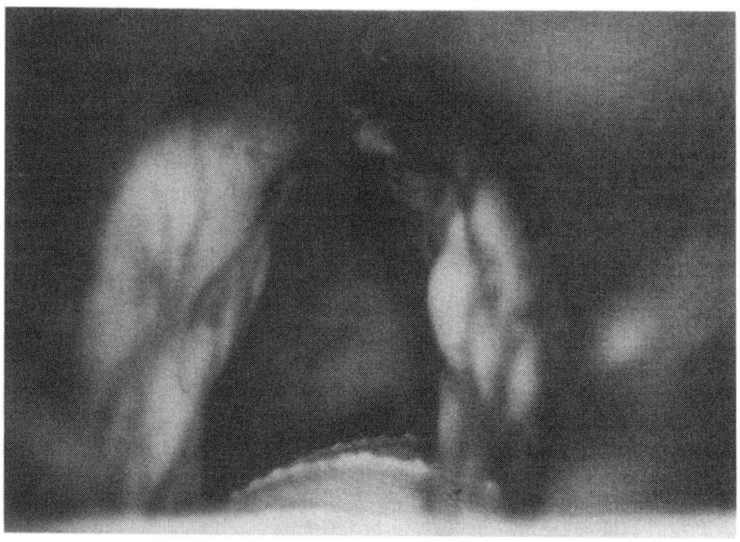

Fig. 5. Laryngeal examination of an aphonic patient with prior vocal fold stripping for dysplasia. Note irregularly thickened vocal folds with areas of mucosal hypertrophy and atrophy.

lighted with the trichrome stain (Fig. 4), with many elastic and collagen fibers and an intermediate number of fibroblasts.

Studies with the elastin van Gieson's stain confirmed that the elastic fibers were sparse, moderate, and frequent in number within the superficial, intermediate, and deep layers, respectively, of the lamina propria (Fig. 2). Reticulin fiber stain showed numerous fibers in the superficial layer, forming an extensive, fine fibular network that often courses to join larger bundles of extracellular matrix (probable collagen) in the intermediate and deep layers (Fig. 3). As indicated from the hematoxylin and eosin and trichrome stain sections (Figs. 1 and 4), dense accumulation of extracellular matrix material, which most likely contains a high content of collagen, is identified mainly in the deep layers. This matrix is in continuity with that found in close association with the vocalis muscle bundles.

The avidin-biotin peroxidase method was used for immunohistochemical studies because micrometer sections were deep paraffinized and stained with commercially available antibodies to human type 4 collagen and laminin.[4] Laminin type 4 collagen was found to be distributed within the basement membrane throughout the entire vocal fold mucosa, as well as along the basement membrane of blood vessels and mucosal glands.

Tissues with higher levels of collagen and fibroblasts have a greater potential for adverse scarring. Because of this, penetration of the vocal ligament during mucosal surgery confers a relatively high risk of causing the vocal fold mucosa adhesion to the vocal ligament. Some have theorized that surgery in Reinke's space can be done without any chance of scar formation because this layer has no scar tissue–forming capabilities. We now know that to be false. However, minimal disruption of the mucosa and superficial layer of the lamina propria will result in a minimal chance of scar formation.[5,6] On the basis of the aforementioned concepts, certain rules should be followed when operating on benign mucosal lesions. First, stripping of the vocal fold mucosa must be avoided (Fig. 5). The more mucosa is excised, the more the scar-forming activity of the lamina propria is stimulated.[7] Second, mucosal excision needs to be limited to precisely what is diseased or absolutely required. Third, because fibroblast collagen is highest in the deeper layers of the lamina propria, the dissection must be kept superficial. With the thickness of the vocal fold epithelium in the lamina propria being approximately 1.1 mm, accurate surgery of the layers within this 1.1-mm area necessitates relatively high magnification. Laser should be used cautiously for benign laryngeal lesions. To prevent thermal stimulation of fibroblast activity, lasers should generally be avoided. However, the microspot CO_2 laser has a much smaller chance of thermal damage and may be safe for the treatment of mucosal lesions.[8]

EVALUATION OF A PATIENT WITH VOCAL SCARRING

In addition to a good history and meticulous physical examination, reliable and valid objective voice assessment is essential in diagnosing vocal fold scarring. Familiarity with the measures currently available and in clinical use is extremely helpful.[9,10] A fully equipped voice laboratory measures the phonatory ability, aerodynamic function, acoustic output, vibration, and electromyographic signals, and often includes psychoacoustic evaluation. Many laboratory measures are helpful in assessing and treating patients with vocal scar and in evaluating the successive treatment. Measures of aerodynamic function, phonatory ability, and acoustic analysis, such as pitch and perturbation, are particularly important. However, accurate assessment of vibration is critical, and strobovideolaryngoscopy is virtually indispensable to proper diagnosis and management of vocal fold scar.[11]

Integrity of the vibratory margin of the vocal fold is essential for the complex motion required to produce good voice quality. Under continuous light, the vocal folds vibrate approximately 250 times per second while phonating at middle C. Naturally, the human eye cannot discern necessary details during such rapid motion. Assessment of the vibratory margin may be performed through high-speed photography, strobovideolaryngoscopy, electroglottography, or photoglottography. Only stroboscopy provides the necessary clinical information in a practical fashion.

Stroboscopy is the single most important technologic advance in diagnostic laryngology, with the possible exception of fiberoptic laryngoscopy. Stroboscopic light allows routine, slow-motion evaluation of the mucosal cover layer of the leading edge of the vocal fold. This improved physical examination permits detection of vibratory asymmetries, structural abnormalities, small masses, submucosal scars, and other conditions that are invisible under normal light.[11] For example, in a patient with a poor voice after laryngeal surgery and a "normal-looking larynx," stroboscopic light may reveal adynamic segments (scar) that explain the problem even to an untrained observer such as the patient. With more significant scarring, a white, stiffened area of the vocal fold that fails to vibrate when viewed videostroboscopically is often seen. Okamura et al.[12] have studied canine vocal fold wound healing after vocal fold surgery and have shown reduced amplitude of vibration after secondary healing of vocal fold defects. In the patients with suspected scarring as a cause of persistent hoarseness, stroboscopy can be used to identify localized or diffuse stiffness of the vocal fold. Stroboscopic features of stiffness and a scar include (1) asymmetric amplitude of vibration, with the scarred side having reduced or absent amplitude of vibration with loss of mucosal wave, (2) incomplete closure because of the high pressure needed to sustain phonation, and (3) a nonvibrating segment that prevents mucosal wave propagation. Many patients with such a stiff vocal fold develop compensatory hyperfunctional vocal gestures, such as ventricular phonation, squeezed supraglottal attack, and abnormal pitching. These laryngeal compensatory behaviors after previous surgery should be suspected and evaluated before a diagnosis of muscular hyperfunction.

MANAGEMENT OF VOCAL FOLD SCARRING

Although there is no ideal method to resolve significant vocal scarring, there are several treatment approaches that have proved useful. Behavioral management with voice therapy and antireflux measurers can be effective over time. Medical treatment with steroids and antibiotics occasionally plays a role in prophylaxis and early management of scarring. Aspects of the problem can be addressed with a variety of surgical techniques, from scar lysis to tissue replacement with flaps and grafts. Injection of aloplastics can be used in some instances to augment deficient vocal fold tissue, but the resultant fibrosis might aggravate the problem. Bioimplants such as fat and collagen are more suitable fillers for the scar vocal fold, and soluble bovine collagen has been demonstrated to soften scar tissue.

VOICE THERAPY AS AN INITIAL APPROACH TO VOCAL FOLD SCARRING

The loss of frequency range, strength, control, and quality associated with the scarred, impaired larynx can often be reversed to some degree through voice therapy and conditioning. Under the circumstances of significant scarring, voice therapy alone will usually not restore a normal voice, but it may improve the voice considerably beyond its condition when the pathology was first diagnosed, including when the patient is past the point of scar maturation, which is generally about 6 months from the injury. The involvement of a voice therapist early in the rehabilitation of a patient with voice scarring will allow for the development of appropriate voice behaviors and prevention of hyperfunctional compensatory behaviors that may result in further deterioration of the voice. The speech pathologist should initiate a voice therapy program, taking into consideration the patient's degree of scarring, vocal fold incompetence and air wastage, stiffness of the mucosa and loss of normal mechanical decoupling of the vocal fold body and cover, and irregular matching of the two vocal folds, leading to turbulence in the transglottic airstream. Furthermore, the patient's needs and desires for improved voice should be taken into consideration. Significant improvement in voice can occur in some patients with vocal fold scarring with voice therapy alone.[13] If surgical therapy is indicated, a voice-language pathologist can work with the patient in the immediate postoperative period to develop a program for strengthening the voice and returning to normal voice behaviors.

COLLAGEN INJECTIONS

Encouraged by studies showing softening of facial scars with repeated injections of Zyderm collagen implant (Collagen Corp., Palo Alto, Calif.),[14,15] Ford et al.[16,17] performed a series of experiments injecting canine larynges with bovine collagen preparations. These implants promoted minimal inflammatory response, seemed to be rapidly invaded by host fibroblasts, and were partially replaced by new host collagen within 6 to 12 months. It was postulated that metabolically active invading fibroblasts produced sufficient collagenase to affect the equilibrium between scar production and breakdown to amino acids. A series of 119 patients with glottic insufficiency, nearly half of whom had scarred larynges, were subsequently treated with bovine collagen injections.[18] The voice results of collagen injection in patients with glottic insufficiency caused by scarring were less dramatic than in groups without scarring; nevertheless, these patients showed objective and subjective voice improvement without serious complications. These findings were perhaps more significant because of the selected patient population, in whom other treatment options were limited, and collagen injection addressed both the glottic insufficiency and the physical properties of the damaged vocal fold tissues. In a limited study of scarred larynges, three groups of patients were treated with collagen injection: (1) patients who had undergone cordectomy for cancer, (2) patients in whom Teflon injection failed, with fibrosis status after removal of Teflon granulomas, and (3) patients who had iatrogenic injury caused by aggressive vocal fold stripping procedures.[19] The functional voice results were proportional to the amount of residual normal tissue; patients with stripped vocal folds did the best, and those who had extensive tissue loss with only a residual scar tissue band after cordectomy did the worst. Multiple injections were used in several patients. Good results were also associated with preservation of at least one intact vocal fold. It appeared that voice therapy played an important adjunctive role and improved results, but other metabolic and functional factors may have occurred naturally over time that might have favorably affected outcome.

Ford and Bless[19] conclude that injectable collagen plays a role in the management of dysphonia caused by vocal fold scarring. Although there are other options for filler substances to displace the vocal fold and correct the glottic insufficiency, collagen injection appears to promote softening of existing scar tissue and should be considered as a primary or adjunctive measure in the management of scarred vocal folds. Bovine cross-linked collagens (Phonagel or Zyplast; Collagen Corp.) remain restricted because of Food and Drug Administration concerns about possible immune reactions, but there is currently investigation to assess the use of autologous collagen as a safe substitute injectable implant. It is important to recognize components of the pathology in every case of scarred larynx and to design treatments accordingly. Major musculoskeletal strictures that might require open surgical procedures and framework surgery can play a role in cases of severe glottic insufficiency. That component of the dysphonia caused by stiffness of the vocal fold proper can be addressed by vocal fold collagen injection.

AUTOLOGOUS FAT AUGMENTATION

Dedo[20] first introduced the concept of free fat grafting under a local mucosal advancement flap for construction of a neocord after vertical hemilaryngectomy. He reported "phonatory voices with minimal hoarseness or breathiness" in all of his cases.[20] All of his observations were subjective, and no follow-up or patient numbers were cited. Human autologous fat injection was first reported by Mikaelian et al.,[21] who made autologous lipoinjections lateral to the vibratory margin in the location where Teflon was traditionally placed. Recent studies by Wexler et al.[22] have demonstrated that fat autographs performed through a laryngofissure into injured canine vocal folds had lower threshold pressures for phonation, greater vocal intensity, and more efficient acoustic output than injured vocal folds without the fat grafting. This technique appears also to restore the stability (periodicity) of the acoustic output. It has been shown by Wetmore[23] that augmentation can be obtained by autograph fat injections for improving body contour. Up to 40% of fat cells survive for at least 52 weeks, but the degree of resorption was not predictable. Microscopic studies of this behavior have led to controversy as to whether the graft ultimately was made of surviving graft adipocytes or host adipocytes. In a host replacement-type fashion, further investigations provided evidence for the dynamic nature of the adipose tissue strongly supporting the cell survival theory, giving explanations for the unpredictable behavior of free fat autographs. In a similar fashion, Sataloff et al.[24] have recently reported implantation of autologous fat into a pocket elevated along the vibratory margin of scarred vocal folds. Preliminary results have been most encouraging, with marked voice improvement and return of mucosal wave in previously adynamic vocal folds.

Using the canine model, Archer and Banks (Personal communication, 1994) have studied autologous fat injected into mucosally damaged vocal folds. At 1 year, all augmented vocal folds had evidence of increased bulk compared with the nonaugmented group. Histologic evaluation showed evidence of residual fat in all the augmented animals. Statistical analysis demonstrated a significant difference in vocal fold thickness in the augmented group compared with the mucosally damaged group. Several authors have reported the use of fat for augmentation of the paralyzed vocal fold, and the method of harvesting the fat for lipoinjection may play a role in the degree of graft survival.[25]

Autogenous fat has been demonstrated to be a safe, minimally reactive substance that is universally available, is easy to harvest, and will remain viable and stable for more than 1 year. Adipose tissue may be the only bioinjectable material presently available that can be implanted submucosally to improve the viscoelastic properties of the vocal fold without an open surgical procedure. A mild chronic inflammatory process noted histologically may be related to the fat-harvesting technique. Further clinical studies are necessary to examine long-term results objectively in larger groups of patients. The optimal fat-harvesting technique also needs to be established to ensure consistent results. It is clear that, for fat to remain clinically viable, overinjection is necessary. The success that has been had with the use of autologous fat injections will likely lead to greater use as further data become available.

MEDIALIZATION LARYNGOPLASTY IN PATIENTS WITH SCARRED VOCAL FOLDS

Medialization laryngoplasty for unilateral paralysis has been shown to be an effective surgical treatment; however, whether this approach is as beneficial in patients with vocal fold scarring is less certain. For the last decade, Koufman and Isaacson[26] have performed laryngoplastic procedures on approximately 20 patients with vocal fold/laryngeal scarring. After laryngeal fracture with scarring, when one side of the larynx is fixed (including the arytenoid), a medialization procedure or a medialization laryngoplasty combined with arytenoid adduction may fail to adequately reposition the affected vocal fold because of pericapsular cricoarytenoid joint fibrosis and soft tissue inelasticity. In these cases, the posterior commissure seems to hold the most important key to success because, if the posterior commissure is not open, medialization laryngoplasty may be relatively effective in achieving glottic closure. At times, failure to adequately reposition the arytenoid by arytenoid adduction seems to be the primary obstacle to achieving adequate closure. As an alternative, when external arytenoid adduction fails, an endoscopic arytenoid repositioning may be successful in medializing a fixed arytenoid.

The most effective use of medialization laryngoplasty for vocal fold scarring is for cases in which there is relatively normal arytenoid mobility, but a fibrotic, adynamic vocal fold with incomplete glottic closure. The best results are seen in patients whose soft tissue deficiency is anterior (near the anterior commissure).

Medialization laryngoplasty is recommended for patients with glottal gaps of 1.5 mm or greater. In these cases, medialization may help the patient achieve closure, and if necessary, submucosal lipoinjection or collagen injection may be used as a secondary procedure to help reestablish mucosal vibrations. For defects smaller than 1.5 mm and for isolated adynamic segments, lipoinjection or collagen injection alone, and not medialization laryngoplasty, is recommended.

In performing medialization laryngoplasty for cordal fibrosis, the surgeon must be careful not to introduce an implant with a posterior phalange that impinges on the vocal process, thereby interfering with arytenoid mobility. In addition, the size and location of the laryngoplasty window should be customized so that it is coterminous with the glottal gap to be narrowed. A goal of treatment with medialization for the scarred vocal fold should be vocal improvement (closure) and not normal voice; however, sometimes the results are surprisingly excellent.

CONCLUSION

The scarred vocal fold is a challenge to the phonosurgeon. The best management is prevention of scarring with appropriate microsurgical techniques and careful use of the laser for laryngeal surgery. Should scarring occur, appropriate assessment of the patient's needs and adequate voice therapy are beneficial in improving voice quality and for presurgical and postsurgical planning. At present, there are multiple surgical techniques available to treat individual cases of vocal fold scarring, although none is optimal for all circumstances. Currently, autologous fat, collagen, and medialization laryngoplasties are being used alone or in combination to improve glottic closure, decrease glottic insufficiency, and improve mucosal waveform.

REFERENCES

1. Woo P, Casper J, Colton R, Brewer D. Diagnosis and treatment of persistent dysphonia after laryngeal surgery: a retrospective analysis of 62 patients. Laryngoscope 1994:104:1084-91.
2. Spraycar M. Stedman's medical dictionary. 26th ed. Baltimore: Williams and Wilkins, 1995.
3. Sundberg J. The science of the singing voice. Northern Illinois University Press, 1987.
4. Nicolai P, Cappiello J, Peretti G, et al. Distribution of laminin, type IV collagen and fibronectin in normal, dysolastic and neoplastic laryngeal tissue. Acta Otorhinol Italica. 1990;10:139-49.
5. Bastian R. Treatment of benign mucosal disorders of the larynx. Ear Nose Throat J June 1988;67:408-10.
6. Hirano M, Hirade Y, Yoshida T, Sanada T. Improved surgical technique for epidermoid cysts of the vocal fold. Ann Otol Rhinol Laryngol 1989;98:791-5.
7. Ford C, Bless D. Phonosurgery: assessment and surgical management of voice disorders. New York: Raven Press, 1991.
8. Shapshay S, Rebeiz E, Bohigian R, Hybels R. Benign lesions of the larynx: should laser be used? Laryngoscope 1990;100:953-60.
9. Jacobson BH. Objective voice analysis: the clinical voice laboratory. In: Benninger MS, Jacobson BH, Johnson AF, eds. Vocal arts medicine: the care and prevention of professional voice disorders. New York: Thieme Medical Publishers, Inc., 1994: 135-52.
10. Baken RJ. Clinical measurement of speech and voice. Boston: College Hill Press, Little, Brown, 1987.
11. Sataloff RT, Spiegel JR, Hawkshaw MJ. Strobovideolaryngoscopy. Results and clinical value. Ann Otol Rhinol Laryngol 1991;100:725-57.
12. Okamura H, Yumoto E, Okamoto K. Wound healing of canine vocal folds after phonosurgery. Ann Otol Rhinol Laryngol 1987; 96:425-8.
13. Casper JK, Cotton RH, Woo P, Brewer DW. Efficacy of treatment for the post-surgically dysphonic patient. Presented at the Voice Foundation, Care of the Professional Voice, Philadelphia, June 15-20, 1992.
14. Knapp TR, Kaplan EN, Danies JR. Injectable collagen for soft tissue augmentation. Plast Reconstr Surg 1977;60:398-405.
15. Stedman SJ, Tromovitch TA. Implantation of collagen for depressed scars. J Dermatol Surg Oncol 1980;6:450-3.
16. Ford CN, Martin DW, Warner TF. Injectable collagen in laryngeal rehabilitation. Laryngoscope 1984;94:513-8.
17. Ford CN. Histologic study of injectable collagen in the canine larynx. Laryngoscope 1986;96:1248-57.
18. Ford CN, Bless DM, Loftus JM. Role of injectable collagen in the treatment of glottic insufficiency: a study of 199 patients. Ann Otol Rhinol Laryngol 1992;101:237-47.
19. Ford CN, Bless DM. Collagen injection in the scarred vocal fold. J Voice 1987;1:116-8.
20. Dedo H. A technique for vertical hemilaryngectomy to prevent stenosis and aspiration. Laryngoscope 1995;85:978-84.
21. Mikaelian D, Lorry LD, Sataloff RT. Lipoinjection for unilateral vocal cord paralysis. Laryngoscope 1991;101:465-8.
22. Wexler D, Gray S, Jiang J, et al. Phonosurgical studies: fat-graft reconstruction of injured canine vocal cords. Ann Otol Rhinol Laryngol 1989;98:668-73.
23. Wetmore S. Injection of fat for soft tissue augmentation. Laryngoscope 1989;99:50-7.
24. Sataloff RT, Spiegel JR, Hawkshaw MJ, Rosen DC, Heuer RJ. Autologous fat implantation for vocal fold scar: a preliminary report. J Voice (in press).
25. Mikus JL, Koufman JA, Kilpatrick SE. Fate of liposuctioned and purified autologous fat injections in the canine vocal fold. Laryngoscope 1995;105:17-22.
26. Koufman JA, Isaacson. Laryngoplastic phonosurgery. Otolaryngol Clin North Am 1991;24:1151-71.

Commentary

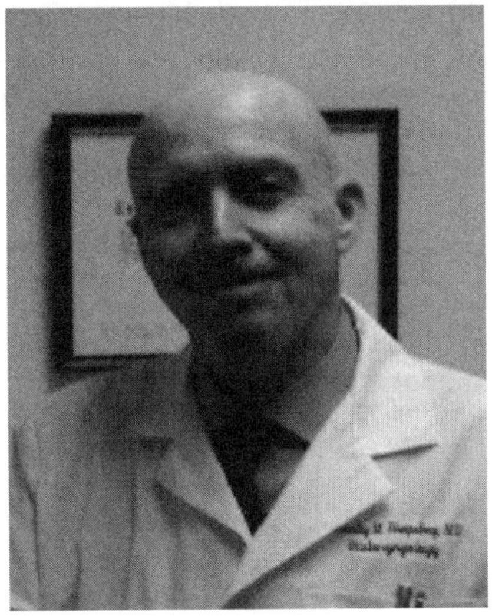

Stanley M. Shapshay, MD, FACS

The first two sentences of this paper written in 2001 are still unfortunately an accurate statement to the present day, "Treatment of laryngeal and tracheal stenosis remains one of the most difficult and perplexing problems in the area of head and neck surgery. Scar formation and restenosis remains the main cause of failure in the surgical management of airway stenosis." This report, as noted in the paper, was the first to describe the use of mitomycin-C as an adjuvant treatment in the endoscopic management of laryngeal and tracheal stenosis in both the pediatric (6 patients) and adult populations (9 patients). This small prospective clinical trial from two academic teaching centers (Tufts-New England Medical Center and The Childrens Hospital in Boston) was done to test the safety and efficacy of mitomycin-C used as an adjuvant to endoscopic laser surgery. Fourteen patients (93%) showed an improvement in the degree of airway stenosis and resolution of their preoperative symptoms. The use of mitomycin-C proved to be safe without any soft tissue breakdown or other complications. This small clinical study supported the excellent experimental data presented by Eliashar et al in 1999 from the Cleveland Clinic showing the effectiveness of mitomycin-C in preventing laryngotracheal stenosis in a canine model.[1] A very impressive reduction in the severity of stenosis was noted in the mitomycin group as compared to the control group without any complications.

Endoscopic laser applications in the airway has been a career-long interest of mine since my Otolaryngology residency at the Boston University School of Medicine (1972–1975) where the CO_2 laser was first applied by Drs. Strong, Vaughan, and Jako to treat conditions affecting the laryngotracheal airway. The CO_2 laser was quite crude back in those days when compared to the present day refinements in laser beam quality and beam spot impact. The CO_2 laser beam profile in 1972 was uneven with a "cold spot" in the middle, the beam impact or "spot size" was 2 mm using a 400-mm lens on the operating microscope. In comparison, the present day microspot micromanipulator delivery system has a spot size of 0.25 mm, an enormous increase in power density allowing for much lower power applications with less collateral tissue damage. To apply the CO_2 laser in the mid to distal trachea, a somewhat awkward bronchoscopic coupling system was devised as there are no readily available quartz fibers to transmit the CO_2 wavelength. This laser coupler had only minimal proximal magnification and a difficult to align aiming light. In addition, the laser coupler for the bronchoscope had to be a closed system making simultaneous suctioning of secretions and blood very difficult. Only within the past

2 years have we had efficient, flexible waveguide delivery systems for tracheobronchial application of the CO_2 laser wavelength.[2] Endoscopic CO_2 laser treatment of glottic, subglottic, and tracheal stenosis was certainly possible; however, the long-term results were not impressive. It became obvious to me that resecting the stenosis in its entirety despite dilation and steroid injection was prone to failure in most cases. More complex endoscopic techniques such as creating microtrapdoor mucosal flaps and excision of underlying scar were described but, due to their complexity, widespread adoption of this technique did not occur. Endoscopic approach to limited areas of airway stenosis remained appealing; however, new techniques and adjuvant therapy to alter the predictive reformation of stenosis and scar contracture was needed.

During my residency, particularly during rotation at the Boston Veterans Hospital, laryngectomy stoma stenosis was a common problem probably as a result of technical error in stoma construction. Rather than embarking on a complex stoma reconstruction with tissue flaps, a simple and very effective approach was to make radial incisions through the stenotic scarred tissue with a needle-tip cautery and place a large laryngectomy tube. The tube was kept in place for up to 6 months and invariably the stoma was large and well healed. This simplicity appealed to me, and after thinking about why this worked so well, it occurred to me that preservation of normal skin and gentle incision/dilation of scar tissue was the key to success. This approach was applied to patients with limited scarring in the subglottis and upper trachea using radial incisions and dilating with increasing sized rigid ventilating bronchoscopes. Early results of this method was published in 1987 and this method has been used by me ever since.[3] Poor prognostic features for success with endoscopic laser radial incision and dilation were pointed out by Simpson et al,[4] namely, circumferential scarring, vertical length greater than 1 cm, posterior commissure scarring with arytenoid fixation, and loss of cartilage support. It was also noted that certain medical conditions such as prior tracheotomy with infection, Wegener's granulomatosis, or other vasculitis conditions, or medical conditions prone to poor wound healing such as hypothyroidism, diabetes, and chronic steroid use would lead to poor outcome in treatment. When patients were carefully selected, endoscopic laser treatment was the first option; failures were usually treated by open cricotracheal resection and reanastomosis. All of the endoscopic procedures were done under general anesthesia using intravenous technique and Venturi jet ventilation. The exposure was obtained using a standard anterior commisure laryngosocope inserted between the vocal cords exposing the subglottic scarring. The Venturi jet needle injector was placed on the proximal lip of the laryngoscope. The operating microscope is used at magnification of 16× with the attached microspot CO_2 laser micromanipulator. It is to be emphasized that the laser was used judiciously in the suprapulsed mode to cut precisely with power just above the threshold of vaporization. Short pulses were used to allow for the thermal relaxation of tissue and the smoke of vaporization was removed at the site of impact to minimize collateral tissue thermal damage. Gentle dilation in a corkscrew-type fashion starting with a 6.5-mm rigid ventilating bronchoscope (Karl Storz Co, Culver City, Calif) using venturi jet ventilation and gradually increasing to a 8.5-mm rigid bronchoscope would allow the dilation to occur along the lines of laser incisions through the scar tissue. After satisfactory dilation up to 10 mm, the laryngoscope exposure is again used on a suspension system and any loose fibrous scar is removed with the laser. Unfortunately, despite this very atraumatic technique, the long-term results were disappointing with a high (60%) recurrence rate. Should there be an attempt to stent the wounds? Could we use an adjuvant to alter wound healing in a beneficial fashion? Endoscopic stents were not appealing particularly in the subglottic area—tolerance of a foreign body close to the vocal cords, migration and plugging of the stent were of great concern. An adjuvant therapy to modify wound healing was appealing prompting a need to search the literature!

Prior to the advent of computer search engines such as Medline and Google there was a very common source of information known as the medical library. It was my habit at least on a monthly schedule to go to the library and scan the medical journals of other allied specialties such as *Chest, Annals of Thoracic Surgery, Archives of Ophthalmology, Cancer, Lancet, Nature,* and the *New England Journal of Medicine*, to name a few. It was of some interest to see what research was taking place on basic themes such as wound healing and scar contracture as well as the treatment of airway stenosis and to my surprise an adjuvant therapy was being used in Ophthalmology for many years with great success! Mitomycin-C, an antineoplastic antibiotic that acts as an alkylating agent by inhibiting DNA and protein synthesis, was being used to alter scarring in a number of eye procedures and conditions with great success. The safety record was good with a small single topical application (0.2 to 0.4 mg/mL). After a review of 13 papers on the subject, I decided to test this on a subglottic stenosis model in the laboratory. Because we had a ready supply of 5-fluorouracil a study was designed to treat subglottic stenosis in a rabbit model using an antimetabolite with a very well known toxicity. There was a very significant modulation of wound healing in this model prompting a clinical study. Because mitomycin-C had a long track record in Ophthalmology and the Cleveland Clinic Study showed a beneficial effect in the canine model, it was decided to use mitomycin-C with the same dose and method of topical application as used in the Ophthalmology series of cases (0.4 mg/mL for 4 minutes). A prospective clinical study was designed with Dr. Rahbar at The Childrens Hospital in Boston to include both children and adults with glottic and subglottic stenosis using laser incision, dilation, and mitomycin-C as an adjuvant therapy. Mitomycin-C was applied on a 4-mm neurosurgical cottonoid pattie and carefully placed on each laser incision for 4 minutes and then washed off with 30 cc of saline.

Scarring in the larynx as pointed out by an excellent review article, "Vocal Cord Scarring: Current Concepts and Management" by Benninger et al[5] is best prevented as treatment options are limited. Operative techniques such as careful dissection, sparing of normal tissue, and avoiding injury to fibroblast-rich areas such as the vocal ligament are key to the prevention of scar development. Operative trauma to the deeper layers of the lamina propria or removal of the mucosal cover with subsequent development of a nonvibrating segment of the vocal fold are the most common causes of laryngeal scarring. Unfortunately, scar contracture in the larynx can be devastating for vocal function. Scar contracture in a circular tube, however, such as the subglottis and trachea can be relentless and slowly progressive causing airway distress. A combination of glottic and subglottic scarring with narrowing of both airways may present the ultimate challenge for the clinician and, in fact, may not be "fixable"—permanent tracheotomy perhaps the only solution. In the natural course of events, ulceration proceeds on to granulation tissue and then fibroblast ingrowth and scar formation. Prevention of scarring, as pointed out in the above review study, is to be stressed as we still do not have the solution to the problem of treating scar contracture. Mitomycin-C application during the granulation tissue phase of wound healing may prove to be beneficial. Careful surgery in the proper surgical planes, meticulous handling of soft tissue, minimal and careful use of thermal devices such as lasers for dissection, and preservation of the mucosal lining are all important principles in surgery of the larynx and trachea.

Over the past 32 years of clinical practice, I have been fascinated by the uncommon condition of idiopathic subglottic stenosis which has served as an interesting model of altered wound healing. I have treated over 40 patients, all female ages 30 to 55 with this condition and remain puzzled by the etiology and progression of this disease. The female preponderance would suggest some hormonal contribution to abnormal wound healing. All of these patients have been worked up for the usual causes of subglottic stenosis such as history of trauma most commonly endotracheal intubation, vasculitis, inflammatory conditions, and acid reflux and most have had a biopsy of their stenosis showing nonspecific chronic inflammatory tissue fibrosis. My suspicion based on careful history taking is that many of these patients had a prior severe tracheobronchitis with severe cough. A sloughing of the subglottic mucosa may have taken place with subsequent granulation tissue and circumferential scarring. Because most of the scar tissue is in the posterior larynx/subglottis, perhaps reflux plays a role in the altered wound-healing process. The effect of hormonal status on wound healing in this female population remains an interesting area for further research investigation. Mitomycin-C has improved the results of laser radial incision and dilation but there still is a 30% failure rate in my hands dictating further treatment usually a cricotracheal resection and reconstruction. Most of these open surgical procedures, albeit sometimes very technically demanding, are successful. Once the damaged subglottis and tracheal scar is removed, healing proceeds normally with normal ciliary flow and clearance of secretions.

How often should mitomycin-C be applied? What is the optimum dose of mitomycin-C? Is topical mitomycin the best delivery method? Is there a better adjuvant than mitomycin-C to disrupt fibroblast ingrowth and scar formation/contracture? Would fibroblast "targeting" by antibody tagging techniques be a better approach to this problem? Further research studies are needed to address these questions. Presently, I am suggesting an empiric three endoscopic laser incisions and dilations followed by 0.4 mg/mL topical application of mitomycin-C for 4 minutes (washed off with 30 cc of saline). The procedures are timed every 3 to 4 months to coincide with the beginning of wound contracture in an attempt to "stay ahead of the curve" of scar formation. My impression thus far with 10 patients is that sequential treatment is more effective than the wait and watch approach. Long-term follow-up of at least 18 months will be necessary to determine any beneficial effect of this new approach which has the disadvantage of three general anesthesias.

Laryngeal, subglottic, and tracheal stenosis remain challenging problems for the head and neck surgeon. Great progress has been made over the past 30 years with better technology and certainly a better understanding of the pathophysiology of this condition. I am grateful to the editors of *Classics in Voice and Laryngology* to be asked to submit a commentary on my research paper. I would also wish to acknowledge the outstanding contributions of my coauthors, Dr. Reza Rahbar and Dr. Gerald B. Healy.

References

1. Eliashar R, Eliashar I, Esclamado R, Gramlich T, Strome M. Can topical mitomycin prevent laryngotracheal stenosis? *Laryngoscope.* 1999;1594–1600.
2. Devaiah AK, Shapshay SM, Desai U, et al. Surgical utility of a new carbon dioxide laser fiber: functional and histological study. *Laryngoscope.* 2005;115:1463–1468.
3. Shapshay SM, Beamis JF Jr, Hybels RL, Bohigian RK. Endoscopic treatment of subglottic and tracheal stenosis by radial laser incision and dilation. *Ann Otol Rhinol Laryngol.* 1987;96:661–664.
4. Simpson GT, Strong MS, Healy GB, Shapshay SM, Vaughan CW. Predictive factors of success or failure in the endoscopic management of laryngeal and tracheal stenosis. *Ann Otol Rhinol Laryngol.* 1982;91:384–348.
5. Benninger MS, Alessi D, Archer S, et al. Vocal fold scarring: current concepts and management. *Otolaryngol Head Neck Surg.* 1996;115:474–482.

MITOMYCIN: EFFECTS ON LARYNGEAL AND TRACHEAL STENOSIS, BENEFITS, AND COMPLICATIONS

REZA RAHBAR, DMD, MD

STANLEY M. SHAPSHAY, MD GERALD B. HEALY, MD

BOSTON, MASSACHUSETTS

The management of laryngeal and tracheal stenosis continues to challenge us, despite advances in surgical techniques and better understanding of the wound healing process. Injury to the airway mucosa is the inciting event, regardless of the cause of the stenosis. Mitomycin-C is an antineoplastic antibiotic that acts as an alkylating agent by inhibiting DNA and protein synthesis. It can inhibit cell division, protein synthesis, and fibroblast proliferation. Topical application of mitomycin-C (0.4 mg/mL) was used as an adjuvant treatment in the endoscopic laser management of laryngeal and tracheal stenosis in 15 patients. Fourteen patients (93%) have shown improvement of their airway and resolution of their preoperative symptoms. After a mean follow-up of 18 months, no complication was noted with regard to the application of mitomycin-C. This study gives promising findings on the efficacy and safety of mitomycin-C as an adjuvant treatment in the management of selected cases of laryngeal and tracheal stenosis.

KEY WORDS — endoscopic surgery, laryngeal stenosis, laser surgery, mitomycin-C, subglottic stenosis, tracheal stenosis.

INTRODUCTION

Treatment of laryngeal and tracheal stenosis remains one of the most difficult and perplexing problems in the area of head and neck surgery. Scar formation and restenosis remains the main cause of failure in the surgical management of airway stenosis. Modulation of the wound healing process to prevent excessive scar formation can play a major role in improving the success rate and decreasing the need for further surgery.

Mitomycin-C is an antiproliferative agent that can inhibit fibroblast proliferation and activity. It has been successfully used as an adjuvant treatment in a number of ophthalmologic procedures to decrease scar formation and restenosis.

A multicenter prospective clinical trial was undertaken in an effort to evaluate the efficacy and safety of the topical application of mitomycin-C in the prevention and treatment of airway stenosis. Mitomycin-C was used as an adjuvant treatment in the endoscopic laser management of laryngeal or tracheal stenosis in 15 patients. The preliminary results of some of these patients have been reported.[1]

MATERIALS AND METHODS

Fifteen patients underwent endoscopic laser management of laryngeal or tracheal stenosis and the topical application of mitomycin-C at New England Medical Center and The Children's Hospital, Boston, between January 1998 and December 1999. There were 8 male patients and 7 female patients. The patients' ages ranged from 2 to 78 years (mean, 32 years). The patients presented with preoperative symptoms of dyspnea interfering with routine daily activity, poor voice quality and vocal fatigue, and/or the inability to cap their tracheotomy tube. Included were 3 cases of glottic stenosis, 10 cases of subglottic stenosis, and 2 cases of tracheal stenosis (see Table).

Glottic Stenosis. One patient (No. 1) presented with a congenital anterior glottic web. Two patients (Nos. 2 and 3) were referred with posterior glottic stenosis and arytenoid fixation: 1 patient had undergone a tracheotomy and laryngofissure for repair of a blunt laryngeal trauma, and the other had undergone a tracheotomy and partial arytenoidectomy for bilateral vocal cord paralysis caused by a brain stem infarct. Only patient 3 was tracheotomy-dependent at the time of our evaluation, with an inability to cap the tracheotomy tube and poor voice quality.

Subglottic Stenosis. Three patients (Nos. 5, 11, and 13) presented with subglottic stenosis due to prolonged intubation because of cardiac surgery, pneumonia, and thalamic infarct, respectively. One patient (No. 4) presented with restenosis after a laryngotracheal reconstruction for a congenital subglottic stenosis (grade IV). No cause could be identified in

From the Department of Otolaryngology and Communication Disorders, The Children's Hospital (Rahbar, Healy), the Department of Otology and Laryngology, Harvard Medical School (Rahbar, Healy), the Department of Otolaryngology–Head and Neck Surgery, New England Medical Center (Shapshay), and Tufts University School of Medicine (Shapshay), Boston, Massachusetts.

Presented at the meeting of the American Laryngological Association, Orlando, Florida, May 13-14, 2000.

CORRESPONDENCE — Reza Rahbar, DMD, MD, Dept of Otolaryngology and Communication Disorders, The Children's Hospital, 300 Longwood Ave, Boston, MA 02115.

PATIENT DATA

Pt No.	*Sex*	*Age (y)*	*Location of Stenosis*	*Etiology*	*Tracheo-tomy-Dependent*	*No. of Procedures*	*Initial Airway Stenosis*	*Thick-ness (mm)*	*Current Airway Stenosis*	*Initial Symptoms*	*Current Status*	*Follow-up (mo)*
1	F	5	Glottic	Congenital web	No	2	60%	4	20%	B	F	12
2	M	14	Glottic	Laryngeal trauma	No	1	4-mm opening		7-mm opening	A, B	F	23
3	M	78	Glottic	Bilateral vocal cord paralysis	Yes	3	2-mm opening		5-mm opening	B, C	D, E	25
4	M	14	Subglottic*	Congenital	Yes	1	80%	4	20%	B, C	D, E	6
5	M	17	Subglottic	Prolonged intubation	No	1	80%	5	30%	A, B	F	13
6	F	33	Subglottic*	Idiopathic subglottic stenosis	No	1	80%	15	20%	A, B	F	25
7	F	38	Subglottic	Idiopathic subglottic stenosis	No	1	50%	12	20%	A, B	F	27
8	F	40	Subglottic*	Idiopathic subglottic stenosis	No	1	80%	4	20%	A, B	F	15
9	F	42	Subglottic*	Idiopathic subglottic stenosis	No	1	50%	7	10%	A, B	F	15
10	F	45	Subglottic*	Idiopathic subglottic stenosis	No	2	70%	10	10%	A, B	F	20
11	M	48	Subglottic	Prolonged intubation	Yes	2	95%	4	40%	A, B, C	D, E	19
12	M	53	Subglottic	Wegener's granuloma-tosis	No	1	50%	5	10%	A	F	15
13	M	56	Subglottic	Prolonged intubation	No	2	70%	5	30%	A, B	F	29
14	M	2	Tracheal	Prolonged intubation	No	1	70%	5	60%	Prolonged intubation	Tracheot-omy	15
15	F	5	Tracheal	Congenital stenosis	No	2	70%	3	10%	A, B	F	13

A — dyspnea on routine daily activity; B — poor voice quality and vocal fatigue; C — inability to cap tracheotomy tube; D — improved voice quality; E — ability to cap tracheotomy tube during day; F — resolution of preoperative symptoms.

*Circumferential scarring.

5 cases (patients 6 through 10), which were classified as idiopathic subglottic stenosis. Wegener's granulomatosis was the cause of subglottic stenosis in 1 patient (No. 12). Only 2 patients from this group (Nos. 4 and 11) were tracheotomy-dependent, with an inability to cap the tracheotomy tube and poor voice quality.

Tracheal Stenosis. One patient (No. 14), with a history of trisomy 21, presented with tracheal stenosis after prolonged intubation because of cardiac and pulmonary status. A second patient (No. 15) presented with tracheal stenosis after laryngotracheal reconstruction for a congenital subglottic and tracheal stenosis.

All patients underwent endoscopic examination and treatment under inhalational general anesthesia provided via a tracheotomy tube, when present, or intravenous anesthesia and Venturi jet ventilation. The airway size and length of stenosis were measured with an open tube ventilating bronchoscope or an endotracheal tube through a laryngoscope. Surgical exposure was obtained by placing the tip of a laryngoscope (Dedo, Healy-Jako, or anterior commissure scope) through the vocal cords for subglottic and tracheal stenosis. The laryngoscope was suspended from a Boston University suspension apparatus, and an operating microscope was used at 16× magnification for all cases. The CO_2 laser at a power setting of 4 to 6 W (time, 0.1 to 0.3 second), in a

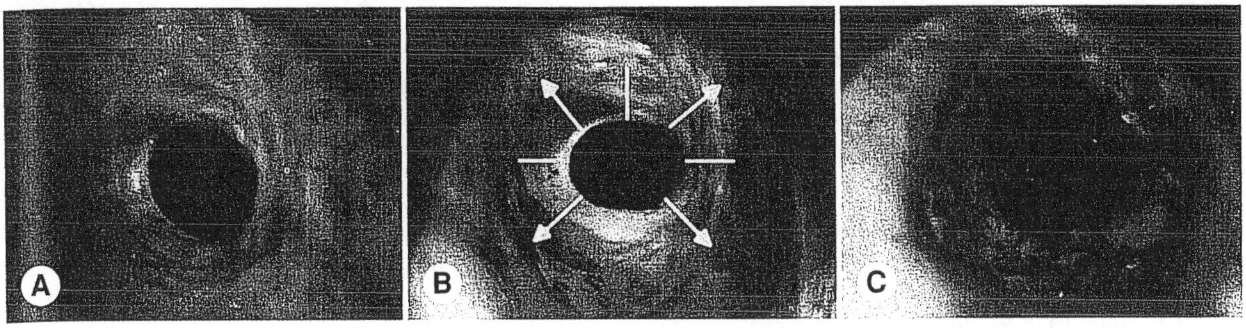

Fig 1. Subglottic stenosis. A) Preoperative. B) Radial laser incision. C) Postoperative.

superpulsed mode (0.25- to 0.3-mm spot size) was used to make radial incisions through the subglottic or tracheal stenosis (Fig 1). Ventilating open tube bronchoscopes were then used for dilation of the stenotic segment. The radial incisions in subglottic or tracheal stenotic areas served to guide the dilating forces in a controlled manner to preserve viable epithelium within the incision.[2] A similar laser setting was used for excision of glottic stenosis (Fig 2). Thereafter, a 10-mm cottonoid sponge was soaked with mitomycin-C 0.4 mg/mL and topically applied to the surgical site for 4 minutes. Then the area was irrigated with 20 to 30 mL of normal saline solution. All patients were observed for a minimum of 24 hours after the procedure. Success was defined as an improvement in the size of the airway and elimination of the preoperative symptoms.

RESULTS

A total of 22 procedures were performed in 15 patients (average, 1.5 procedures): 9 patients had 1 procedure each, 5 patients had 2 procedures each, and 1 patient had 3 procedures. The follow-up ranged from 6 to 29 months, with an average of 18 months. Open tube bronchoscopes and/or endotracheal tubes were used for the measurement of the postoperative length and degree of stenosis under general anesthesia, or the measurements were made with fiberoptic laryngoscopy and still photographs taken by means of a 70° rigid telescope under topical anesthesia. Fourteen patients (93%) showed an improvement in the degree of airway stenosis and resolution of their preoperative symptoms (see Table). The postoperative length of the subglottic or tracheal stenosis could only be measured in patients who underwent general anesthesia because of the need for further surgery. There was no significant improvement noted in the length of the stenosis.

Glottic Stenosis. A total of 6 procedures were performed in 3 patients. Before operation, 1 patient demonstrated a 60% stenosis, and 2 patients had posterior airway openings of 4 and 2 mm, respectively, compared to a postoperative stenosis of 20% and airway openings of 7 and 5 mm, respectively. Two patients are completely asymptomatic with regard to their preoperative symptoms. One patient was tracheotomy-dependent, was unable to cap the tracheotomy tube, and had poor voice quality. Currently, the tracheotomy tube is capped during the day without dyspnea on exertion, and the patient has good voice quality.

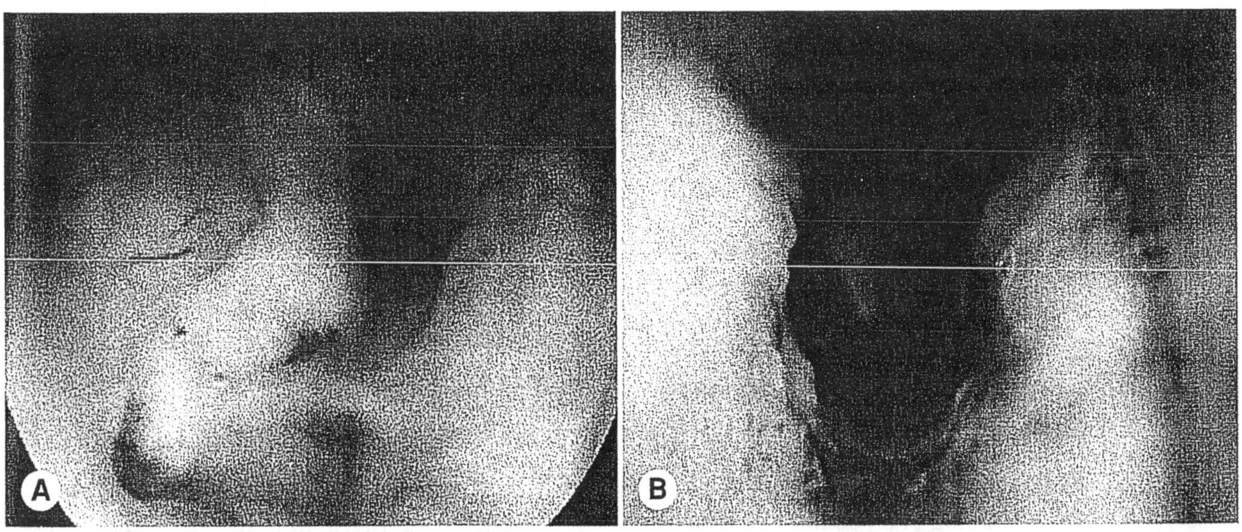

Fig 2. Posterior glottic stenosis. A) Preoperative. B) Postoperative.

The patient has not been decannulated because of his general medical condition following a brain stem infarct.

Subglottic Stenosis. A total of 13 procedures were performed in 10 patients. The preoperative stenosis ranged from 50% to 95% (mean, 71%), and the postoperative stenosis ranged from 10% to 40% (mean, 21%). The length of the stenosis ranged from 4 to 15 mm (average, 7 mm). Three patients had a length of stenosis equal to or greater than 1 cm. Before operation, 9 patients had moderate dyspnea with routine daily activity; currently, they are all free of symptoms. Two patients were tracheotomy-dependent before the procedure, with an inability to cap the tracheotomy tube and poor voice quality. Currently, both patients tolerate capping the tracheotomy tubes during the day and have improved voice quality. One patient (No. 11) has not been decannulated because of his general medical condition (diabetes and recurrent pneumonia); the second patient (No. 4) is scheduled for decannulation in the near future.

Tracheal Stenosis. A total of 3 procedures were performed in 2 patients. The preoperative degree of stenosis was 70% in both patients; the stenoses were 3 and 5 mm long, respectively. One patient (No. 15) is asymptomatic with 10% airway obstruction. The second patient (No. 14), whose history is significant for trisomy 21, tetralogy of Fallot, and pulmonary arteriovenous malformation, presented with restenosis and underwent tracheotomy because of worsening of his pulmonary and cardiac status.

DISCUSSION

The management of laryngeal and tracheal stenosis remains difficult, requiring accurate diagnosis and a proper treatment plan. The goal of any treatment is the restoration of an adequate airway, the provision of a competent larynx for protection against aspiration, and the achievement of a satisfactory voice. The first decision is whether an open surgical technique is necessary, or whether an endoscopic approach is adequate. Factors such as 1) age, 2) general medical condition, 3) cause, location, degree, length, and consistency of stenosis, and 4) previous treatment should be considered. There is still controversy with regard to the optimum approach in the treatment of laryngeal and tracheal stenosis.

Endoscopic management of laryngeal and tracheal lesions has undergone tremendous advancement in the past 2 decades. The development of microlaryngoscopy and adaptation of the binocular operating microscope, the introduction of endolaryngeal CO_2 laser surgery, the coupling of an endoscopic adapter to a ventilating bronchoscope, and the development of the microspot manipulator allow microprecision and hemostatic ability, which were lacking with the standard instrumentation of conventional endoscopic techniques.[3-6]

Multiple endoscopic techniques have been described: microcauterization, dilation with local and systemic steroids, and cryosurgery have all had some success.[7,8] Strong and Jako[6] first published their experience with endoscopic CO_2 laser management of laryngeal stenosis in 1972. The CO_2 laser appears to be the most effective means for treating mild to moderate stenosis of the larynx and trachea endoscopically.[9-12]

With the advancements in endoscopic surgical technique and a better understanding of the wound healing process, and even with the introduction of mucosa-preserving laser surgery such as the microtrapdoor flap technique (Dedo and Sooy[13]) and radial incision and dilation (Shapshay et al[2]), there is still a high degree of scar formation and restenosis. A review of the literature reveals a wide range of success for endoscopic management of laryngeal and tracheal stenosis: Strong et al,[14] 50% success; Andrews and Horowitz,[15] 66% success; Simpson et al,[16] 44% success; Carruth,[17] 50% success; Shapshay and Simpson,[5] 40% success; and Ossoff et al,[18] 57% success. Although there are fundamental differences between these studies (definition of success; location, severity, and type of stenosis; length of follow-up), restenosis and scar formation remains the primary cause of failure.

Regardless of the surgical techniques, there is further injury to the airway mucosa that leads to fibroblast proliferation and collagen formation, which are the key to scar formation. Modulation of the wound healing response to prevent excessive scar formation can play a major role in increasing the success of surgical treatment and reducing the need for further surgery. In the past decade, the role of growth factors and fibrogenic peptides in the regulation and modulation of wound healing leading to fibrosis and scar formation has been reported.[19-21] Pharmacological agents such as 5-fluorouracil and β-aminopropionitrile (βAPN) have been shown to inhibit the development of collagen cross-linking, thus minimizing scar formation.[22,23]

Kunitomo and Mori[24] presented the first clinical use of mitomycin-C in the prevention and treatment of scar formation in pterygium surgery. Later, Chen,[25] Palmer,[26] and Bergstrom et al[27] reported its use for prevention of restenosis in glaucoma surgery.

Mitomycin-C is an antibiotic produced by *Streptomyces caespitosus*. It is referred to as mitomycin-C to differentiate it from mitomycins A and B. It has both antineoplastic and antiproliferative properties. Its antineoplastic activity is similar to that of the alkylating agents, causing cross-linking of DNA and inhibiting RNA and protein synthesis. Mitomycin-C also acts as an antiproliferative agent that can inhibit fibroblast activity and suppress fibrosis and scar formation.

The exact mechanism by which mitomycin-C exerts an antifibroblast activity is unknown. There is evidence to suggest that the reduction of fibroblast activity may be mediated by apoptosis, which is a gene-directed process causing cell death. Apoptotic cells display a characteristic morphology that includes condensation of the nucleus and cytoplasm, nuclear fragmentation, and cytoplasmic blebbing with an intact cell membrane.[28] Lee et al[29] showed that mitomycin has antifibroblastic properties in vivo. Khaw et al[30] showed that in vitro, a single application of mitomycin could inhibit fibroblast proliferation. Mitomycin has been successfully used for prevention of stenosis in glaucoma surgery, dacryocystorhinostomy, optic nerve sheath fenestration, and pterygium recurrence.[31-35] The fibroblast population and collagen formation are substantially increased during the wound healing response that follows a mucosal insult such as a surgical procedure. The rationale of the use of mitomycin-C is to inhibit fibroblast proliferation during the postoperative phase without damaging the mucosal and epithelial growth.[36]

Historically, endoscopic management of patients with circumferential scarring, a vertical scar greater than 1 cm, posterior scarring with arytenoid fixation, and loss of cartilaginous support had a high failure rate.[16] We have presented 15 patients with laryngeal and tracheal stenosis. A group of these patients have characteristics of airway stenosis that falls into the category of high failure rate based on historical experience: 5 patients with circumferential stenosis of the subglottic area; 2 patients with posterior glottic stenosis and arytenoid fixation; and 3 patients with length of subglottic stenosis greater or equal to 1 cm. The endoscopic management of airway stenosis has produced a success rate of 40% to 68%, as reported by experienced investigators, with most results being closer to 50%. We have defined success as clinical improvement of the degree of stenosis and the resolution of preoperative symptoms. We have shown improvement of the size of the airway and resolution of preoperative symptoms in 14 patients (93% success rate), without any complications, with a mean follow-up of 18 months. Three of our patients were tracheotomy-dependent at the time of our evaluation. They have shown improvement of their airway, allowing capping of their tracheotomy tube during the day, and improvement of their voice quality. Two of these patients have not been decannulated because of their general medical condition, and 1 is scheduled for decannulation in the near future.

Our results demonstrate that the topical application of mitomycin-C can be beneficial in the modulation of wound healing and in decreasing scar formation in the treatment of airway stenosis. Our study is the first to describe the use of mitomycin-C as an adjuvant treatment in the endoscopic management of laryngeal and tracheal stenosis in both pediatric and adult populations. Further research and randomized prospective clinical trials are needed to determine the most effective concentration and time of exposure of mitomycin-C, and the difference in efficacy and safety between single and multiple applications.

CONCLUSION

Treatment of laryngeal and tracheal stenosis remains a therapeutic challenge. Different surgical techniques have been proposed, and no single approach has proven satisfactory for all cases. With the advances in the surgical techniques and the recognition of the importance of mucosal preservation, the potential for endoscopic surgical techniques has expanded. Restenosis and scar formation remains the main cause of failure in these cases. This study reveals promising results in terms of the efficacy and safety of mitomycin-C as an adjuvant method for the management of laryngeal and tracheal stenosis.

REFERENCES

1. Rahbar R, Valdez TA, Shapshay SM. Preliminary results of intraoperative mitomycin C in the treatment and prevention of glottic and subglottic stenosis. J Voice 2000;14:282-6.

2. Shapshay SM, Beamis JF Jr, Hybels RL, Bohigian RK. Endoscopic treatment of subglottic and tracheal stenosis by radial laser incision and dilation. Ann Otol Rhinol Laryngol 1987; 96:661-4.

3. Kleinsasser O. Microlaryngoscopy and endolaryngeal microscopy. Philadelphia, Pa: WB Saunders, 1968.

4. Polanyi TG, Bredemeier HC, Davis TW. A CO_2 laser for surgical research. Med Biol Eng Comput 1970;8:541-8.

5. Shapshay SM, Simpson GT. Lasers in bronchology. Otolaryngol Clin North Am 1983;16:879-86.

6. Strong MS, Jako GJ. Laser surgery in the larynx. Early clinical experience with continuous CO_2 laser. Ann Otol Rhinol Laryngol 1972;81:791-8.

7. Strome M. Cryosurgery: the effect on the canine endolaryngeal structures. Laryngoscope 1971;81:1057-65.

8. Friedman EM, Healy GB, McGill TJ. Carbon dioxide laser management of subglottic and tracheal stenosis. Otolar-

yngol Clin North Am 1983;16:871-7.

9. Strong MS, Healy GB, Vaughan CW, Fried MP, Shapshay SM. Endoscopic management of laryngeal stenosis. Otolaryngol Clin North Am 1979;12:797-805.

10. Healy GB. An experimental model for the endoscopic correction of subglottic stenosis with clinical applications. Laryngoscope 1982;92:1103-15.

11. Shapshay SM, Beamis JF Jr, Dumon J-F. Total cervical tracheal stenosis: treatment by laser, dilation, and stenting. Ann Otol Rhinol Laryngol 1989;98:890-5.

12. Strong MS, Jako GJ, Polanyi TG, Wallace RA. Laser surgery in the aerodigestive tract. Am J Surg 1973;126:529-33.

13. Dedo HH, Sooy CD. Endoscopic laser repair of posterior glottic, subglottic, and tracheal stenosis by division or micro-trapdoor flap. Laryngoscope 1984;94:445-50.

14. Strong MS, Vaughan CW, Polanyi G, Wallace R. Bronchoscopic carbon dioxide laser surgery. Ann Otol Rhinol Laryngol 1974;83:769-76.

15. Andrews AA, Horowitz SL. Bronchoscopic CO_2 laser surgery. Lasers Surg Med 1980;1:35-9.

16. Simpson GT, Strong MS, Healy GB, Shapshay SM, Vaughan CW. Predictive factors of success or failure in the endoscopic management of laryngeal and tracheal stenosis. Ann Otol Rhinol Laryngol 1982;91:384-8.

17 Carruth AS. The role of lasers in otolaryngology. World J Surg 1983;7:719-22.

18. Ossoff RH, Tucker GF, Duncavage JA, Toohill RJ. Efficacy of bronchoscopic carbon dioxide laser surgery for benign strictures of the trachea. Laryngoscope 1985;95:1220-3.

19. Sera VR, Hall K, Low H, eds. Growth factors: from genes to clinical application. New York, NY: Raven Press, 1990.

20. Border WA, Ruoslahti E. Transforming growth factor–β in disease: the dark side of tissue repair. J Clin Invest 1992;90: 1-7.

21. Crouch E. Pathobiology of pulmonary fibrosis. Am J Physiol 1990;259:159-84.

22. Doolin EJ, Strande LF, Tsuno K, Santos MC. Pharmacologic inhibition of collagen in an experimental model of subglottic stenosis. Ann Otol Rhinol Laryngol 1998;107:275-9.

23. Ingrams DR, Ashton P, Dhingra J, Shah R, Shapshay SM. Slow-release 5-fluorouracil and triamcinolone reduces subglottic stenosis in a rabbit model. Ann Otol Rhinol Laryngol 2000; 109:422-4.

24. Kunitomo N, Mori S. Studies on the pterygium. Part IV. A treatment of the pterygium by mitomycin-C instillation. Acta Soc Ophthalmol Jpn 1963;67:601-7.

25. Chen C. Enhanced intraocular pressure controlling effectiveness of trabeculectomy by local application of mitomycin-C. Trans Asia-Pacific Acad Ophthalmol 1983;9:172-7.

26. Palmer S. Mitomycin as adjunct chemotherapy with trabeculectomy. Ophthalmology 1991;98:317-21.

27. Bergstrom TJ, Wilkinson WS, Skuta GL, Watnick RL, Elner VM. The effects of subconjunctival mitomycin-C on glaucoma filtration surgery in rabbits. Arch Ophthalmol 1991;109: 1725-30.

28. Desmouliere A, Redard M, Darby I, Gabbiani G. Apoptosis mediates the decrease in cellularity during the transition between granulation tissue and scar. Am J Pathol 1995;146:56-66.

29. Lee DA, Lee TC, Cortes AE, Kitada S. Effects of mithramycin, mitomycin, daunorubicin, and bleomycin on human subconjunctival fibroblast attachment and proliferation. Invest Ophthalmol Vis Sci 1990;31:2136-44.

30 Khaw PT, Doyle JW, Sherwood MB, Grierson I, Schultz GS, McGorray S. Prolonged localized tissue effects from 5-minute exposures to fluorouracil and mitomycin C. Arch Ophthalmol 1993;111:263-7.

31. Palmer SS. Mitomycin as adjunct chemotherapy with trabeculectomy. Ophthalmology 1991;98:317-21.

32. Urban RC Jr, Kaufman LM. Mitomycin in the treatment of hypertrophic conjunctival scars after strabismus surgery. J Pediatr Ophthalmol Strabismus 1994;31:96-8.

33. Kao SCS, Liao CL, Tseng JHS, Chen MS, Hou PK. Dacryocystorhinostomy with intraoperative mitomycin. Ophthalmology 1997;104:86-91.

34. Rubinfeld RS, Stein RM. Topical mitomycin-C for pterygia: is single application appropriate? Ophthalmic Surg Lasers 1997;28:662-9.

35. Schipper I, Suppelt C, Gebbers J. Mitomycin-C reduces scar formation after excimer laser (193) photorefractive keratectomy in rabbits. Eye 1997;11:649-55.

36. Lee DA. Antifibrosis agent in glaucoma surgery. Invest Ophthalmol Vis Sci 1994,35:3789-91.

9

Recurrent Respiratory Papillomatosis

Introduction

It has been said that a robust papilloma practice is the sign of a mature laryngology practice. That is an indirect way of acknowledging the huge frustration of treating patients with papilloma—and the frustration of those patients themselves. Despite our best clinical efforts, they occupy a greater proportion of office and operating room schedules every successive year in practice, simply because we fail to effect a cure. The infection itself is subtle, present in many—possibly most—adults without a sign. Most factors which lead to gross disease remain elusive, as are the aspects that differentiate aggressive, multiply recurrent lesions from those instances of disease that burn out quickly. And the consequences of surgical treatment, particularly when repeated half a dozen times or more, are discouraging and demoralizing. Finally, the virus has resisted successive waves of treatment tools, seeming sometimes to respond just enough to raise our hopes.

Yet, even a modest historical perspective reveals good reason for hope. Dr. Steinberg's recapitulation of the advances of the last quarter-century plainly reveals how much information has been uncovered about papillomatosis and the changes in its treatment. This is recapitulated in the classic papers in this section: Viral etiology, asymptomatic infection, CO_2 laser, interferon, phototherapy, and, most recently, cidofovir. Dr. Derkay also notes the advent of the HPV vaccine, developed for nonlaryngeal disease, which may put an end to the adage that opened this introduction. A mere 7 years after his state of the art review article in *Laryngoscope,* Dr. Derkay recently published an update. That is both telling and encouraging.

Classic Articles

● Reprint of article included in this chapter.
♦ Commentary on this article.

Strong MS, Vaughan CW, Cooperband SR, Healy GB, Clemente MA. Recurrent respiratory papillomatosis. Management with the CO2 laser. *Ann Otol Rhinol Laryngol.* 1976;85(4 pt 1):508–516.

Haglund S, Lundquist PG, Cantell K, Strander H. Interferon therapy in juvenile laryngeal papillomatosis. *Arch Otolaryngol.* 1981;107(6):327–332.

Mounts P, Shah KV, Kashima H. Viral etiology of juvenile- and adult-onset squamous papilloma of the larynx. *Proc Nat Acad Sci USA.* 1982;79(17):5425–5429.

●♦Steinberg BM, Topp WC, Schneider PS, Bramson AL. Laryngeal papillomavirus infection during clinical remission. *N Engl J Med.* 1983;308(21):1261–1264.

Abramson AL, Steinberg BM, Winkler B. Laryngeal papillomatosis: clinical, histopathologic and molecular studies. *Laryngoscope.* 1987;97(6):678–685.

Leventhal BG, Kashima HK, Mounts P, et al. Long-term response of recurrent respiratory papillomatosis to treatment with lymphoblastoid interferon alfa-n1. *N Eng J Med.* 1991;325(9):613–617.

Kashima HK, Shah F, Lyles A, Glackin R, et al. A comparison of risk factors in juvenile-onset and adult-onset recurrent respiratory papillomatosis. *Laryngoscope.* 1992;102(1);9–13.

Snoeck R, Wellens W, Desloovere C, et al. Treatment of severe laryngeal papillomatosis with intralesional injections of cidofovir [(S)-1-(3-hydrox-2-phosphoylmethoxypropyl) cystine]. *J Med Vir.* 1998;54(3):219–225.

Shikowitz MJ, Abramson AL, Freeman K, Steinberg BM, Nouri M. Efficacy of DHE photodynamic therapy for respiratory papillomatosis: immediate and long-term results. *Laryngoscope.* 1998;108(7):962–967.

Armstrong LR, Derkay CS, Reeves WC. Initial results from the National Registry for Juvenile-Onset Recurrent Respiratory Papillomatosis. *Arch Otolaryngol.* 1999;125(7):743–748.

•Pransky SM, Magit AE, Kearns DB, Kang D, Duncan NO. Intralesional cidofovir for recurrent respiratory papillomatosis in children. *Arch Otolaryngol.* 1999;125(10):1143–1148.

Pransky SM, Brewster DF, Magit AE, Kearns DB. Clinical update on 10 children treated with intralesional cidofovir injections for severe recurrent respiratory papillomatosis. *Arch Otolaryngol.* 2000;126(10):1239–1243.

•♦Derkay CS. Recurrent respiratory papillomatosis. *Laryngoscope.* 2001;111(1);57–69.

Commentary

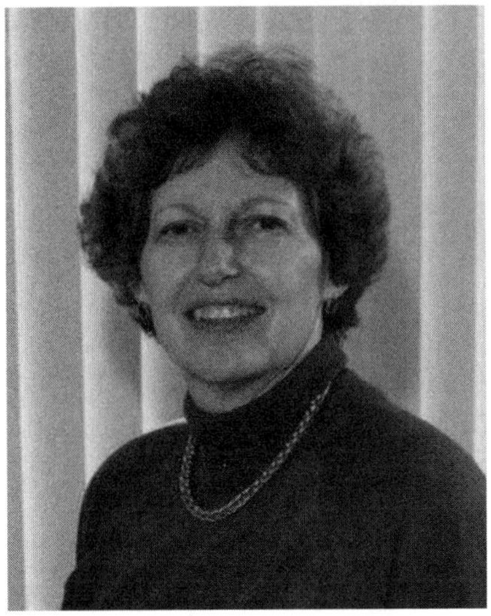

Bettie M. Steinberg, PhD

Understanding the biology of recurrent respiratory papillomatosis (RRP) has been a team effort from the time I started my studies in 1980. I was recruited to LIJ by Dr. Allan Abramson, at that time Chief of the Division of Otolaryngology and Communicative Disorders and subsequently chairman of the independent Department of Otolaryngology and Communicative Disorders, who had developed expertise using the CO_2 laser and was treating many patients with RRP. He held the deep belief that a major commitment to research would be necessary to address all the unanswered questions and find better ways to treat the disease based on those discoveries. Moreover, he felt that partnering with a scientist who had research experience in virology and tumor biology was the right way to begin. Joining Allan was the beginning of a long-standing, fruitful collaboration. It has taken us from our early descriptions of the biology and etiology of RRP to our present state, where a therapeutic clinical trial of celecoxib therapy is in progress, based on our understanding of the molecular basis of papilloma formation.

Like all science, our studies were built on a strong foundation established by others. The first papillomavirus had been described in the 1930s, the Shope rabbit virus (now named the cottontail rabbit papillomavirus), with subsequent initial studies focusing on morphology based on electron microscopy and chemical properties of the coat proteins after isolation and purification of virus from large warts on the skin of wild rabbits.[1] By the early 1950s, investigators were exploring the biology of the Shope virus, and its abilities to contribute to malignancy.[2] Subsequent studies described the presence of similar papillomaviruses in human warts and in genital condyloma,[3,4] and Crawford described the structure of human papillomavirus (HPV) DNA in 1965.[5] Investigators subsequently learned that there was more than one HPV, and that the different types were associated with lesions in different parts of the body.[6] Meanwhile, others were postulating that papilloma viruses caused RRP, based on electron microscopy visualization of viral particles in the papilloma tissues.[7,8] Together, these reports set the stage for the discovery of specific HPVs that cause genital condyloma in[9] and laryngeal papillomas.[10,11] These data, although still preliminary and unpublished, were discussed at a conference on human papillomaviruses held at Cold Spring Harbor in 1980, just as I was starting my research on RRP.

The research started simply, with the goal of devising a way to grow papilloma cells in culture, derived from biopsies of the papilloma tissues, in order to have material that we could manipulate to dissect the biology of the disease. We accomplished this initial goal, and published the study in 1982,[12] the same year that Gissmann et al[10] published the DNA sequence of HPV 11 cloned from a laryngeal papilloma. Dr. Gissmann and his colleagues were extremely generous in sharing the HPV DNAs they had cloned with others in the scientific community. Thus, we had a critical tool for our future studies, and their openness and willingness to share meant that future studies from multiple laboratories could be compared as we all used the same viral probes.

Studying short-term cultured cells, and comparing the results to analysis of biopsy samples when possible, became the standard approach to our research on RRP. We made an early commitment to study cells and biopsy material derived from patients, rather than tissue culture systems using that established genital tumor lines containing HPVs that are used by most investigators studying HPVs. We were studying RRP, not just the virus. In retrospect, a wise choice, but one that restricted the pace of research and introduced the problem of variability from one patient to another.

Nonscientists often think, based on cartoons, that significant scientific discoveries occur in a "Eureka moment," based on years of study in isolation in the laboratory. Most of our discoveries were based on conversations over coffee that started with the word "why." Why did patients have recurrent disease when all visible papilloma were removed? Why was the disease pattern so variable from one patient to another? Why was the disease so rare, when genital tract HPV infections were so common, and mounting data suggested that subclinical or latent HPV infection was relatively common in the airway of people with no history of RRP? Why did all of the myriad therapies that had been described seem to help a subset of the patients but not most, and if we understood the molecular pathology of the disease could we find a treatment that might be better? Those were among the questions that led the direction of our research, resulting in the publication of more than 80 papers on RRP, and continue to drive it today.

One of our biggest breakthroughs occurred early in our studies: the discovery of widespread latent HPV infection in the clinically normal airway epithelium of patients with RRP,[13] including those in remission who were free of disease. Now, we understood why patients had recurrent disease. It was not possible to remove all the infection surgically. We also now knew that recurrence was not iatrogenic spreading of virus during surgery, and that when patients had extension of disease into the trachea was not due to "seeding," because the virus already infected the trachea. With this knowledge, like all of science, came new questions. What activates the latent infection? Why does the immune system not prevent recurrent activation? Can any therapy be considered "curative" if latent infection remains? Those questions are still being studied.

We, as a large scientific community of biologists and clinicians, have come a long way since 1980. We know the cause of RRP, and know a great deal more about the molecular biology of HPVs and the diseases they cause (although with answers to many questions still pending). We understand better the risk factors that contribute to development of RRP and possibly to severity. These include demographic factors, mechanism of transmission of HPV, relationship of HPV type to disease severity, genetic susceptibility, and the relationship between genetic variation and the ability of the immune response to control recurrent disease in patients with RRP. We have tested a number of promising therapies, including interferon, photodynamic therapy, and intralesional cidofovir. Many patients have benefited, although it is clear that there is no "magic bullet" that will cure or even prevent recurrence in all patients. Examples of this increased knowledge are included in the classic papers selected for this volume. These studies are continuing, and hopefully before too long we will have even better therapies or better ways to optimize current therapies. Meanwhile, development of a preventive HPV vaccine holds the promise that RRP eventually will become a historical curiosity and patients will no longer suffer with this disease.

References

1. Scherp HW, Syverton JT. A chemical investigation of keratin and carcinomas deriving from rabbit papillomas (Shope). *Cancer Res.* 1949;9(1):12–16.
2. Rogers S, Rous P. Joint action of a chemical carcinogen and a neoplastic virus to induce cancer in rabbits; results of exposing epidermal cells to a carcinogenic hydrocarbon at time of infection with the Shope papilloma virus. *J Exp Med.* 1951;93(5):459–488.
3. Bunting H. Close-packed array of virus-like particles within cells of a human skin papilloma. *Proc Soc Exp Biol Med.* 1953;84(2):327–332.
4. Melnick JL, Bunting H, Banfield WG, Strauss MJ, Gaylort WH. Electron microscopy of viruses of human

papilloma, molluscum contagiosum, and vaccinia, including observations on the formation of virus within the cell. *Ann N Y Acad Sci.* 1952;54(6):1214–1225.
5. Crawford LV. A study of human papilloma virus DNA. *J Mol Biol.* 1965;13(2):362–372.
6. Orth G, Favre M, Croissant O. Characterization of a new type of human papillomavirus that causes skin warts. *J Virol.* 1977;24(1):108–120.
7. Bartual R. [Laryngeal papilloma (current status of the problem)]. *Acta Otorinolaryngol Iber Am.* 1966;17(4): 374–384.
8. Bouchet JM. [Viral etiology of laryngeal papillomatosis]. *Ann Otolaryngol Chir Cervicofac.* 1967;84(9):695–696.
9. Gissmann L, deVilliers EM, zur Hausen H. Analysis of human genital warts (condylomata acuminata) and other genital tumors for human papillomavirus type 6 DNA. *Int J Cancer.* 1982;29(2):143–146.
10. Mounts P, Shah KV, Kashima H. Viral etiology of juvenile- and adult-onset squamous papilloma of the larynx. *Proc Nat Acad Sci USA.* 1982;79(17):5425–5429.
11. Gissmann L, Diehl V, Schultz-Coulon HJ, zur Hausen H. Molecular cloning and characterization of human papilloma virus DNA derived from a laryngeal papilloma. *J Virol.* 1982;44(1):393–400.
12. Steinberg BM, Abramson AL, Meade RP. Culture of human laryngeal papilloma cells in vitro. *Otolaryngol Head Neck Surg.* 1982;90(6):728–735.
13. Steinberg BM, Topp WC, Schneider PS, Abramson AL. Laryngeal papillomavirus infection during clinical remission. *N Engl J Med.* 1983;308(21):1261–1264.

LARYNGEAL PAPILLOMAVIRUS INFECTION DURING CLINICAL REMISSION

Bettie M. Steinberg, Ph.D., William C. Topp, Ph.D., Patricia S. Schneider, Ph.D., and Allan L. Abramson, M.D.

Abstract Biopsy samples from 20 patients with a history of laryngeal papillomas were analyzed by Southern blot hybridization for the presence of human papillomavirus DNA. All papillomas examined contained papillomavirus DNA sequences. Four samples from uninvolved sites in two patients with active disease and eight samples from patients in remission also contained viral DNA. No human papillomavirus DNA was detected in a third patient seen during remission. These results explain the clinical pattern of frequent recurrences even after long-term remission in laryngeal papillomatosis. (N Engl J Med 1983; 308: 1261-4.)

LARYNGEAL papillomas are rapidly growing, non-invasive tumors that are located primarily on the vocal cords and epiglottis, but that can also involve the oral cavity, trachea, and lungs. They consist of connective-tissue stalks covered by well-differentiated stratified squamous epithelium, and are similar to common cutaneous and genital warts. At present, there is no system of subclassifications for laryngeal papillomas. Presenting symptoms include hoarseness, stridor, and if severe, dyspnea and acute respiratory obstruction. The age at initial onset of symptoms is equally distributed between children and adults and ranges from 3 months to 70 or more years. The clinical course of the disease is characterized by multiple recurrences after surgical removal, with surgery necessary as frequently as every four weeks, interspersed with periods of remission lasting for months or years. The success of treatment with various hormones and drugs, autogenous vaccines, cautery, and cryosurgery has been reported to be mixed and limited.[1] The results of preliminary studies in which interferon has been used to control this disease appear promising,[2,3] and carefully controlled studies are currently in progress.

From the Department of Otolaryngology and Communicative Disorders, Long Island Jewish–Hillside Medical Center, New Hyde Park, N.Y., and the Cold Spring Harbor Laboratory, Cold Spring Harbor, N.Y. Address reprint requests to Dr. Steinberg at the Department of Otolaryngology, Long Island Jewish–Hillside Medical Center, New Hyde Park, NY 11042.

Supported in part by grants from the New York State Health Research Council (13-031), the Morris S. and Florence H. Bender Foundation, the Voice Foundation (042), the National Institutes of Health (CA 28638), and the Otolaryngology Fund.

Laryngeal papillomas are caused by one or more of the human papillomaviruses. Viral capsid antigen has been shown to be present in superficial cells of the papillomas,[4-6] and human papillomavirus DNA has been reported in papilloma tissues.[7-9] However, the presence of the virus in the papilloma itself has not explained the clinical pattern of regrowth of the tumors after surgical removal, termination of interferon therapy, or a period of spontaneous remission. We have investigated the possibility that human papillomavirus DNA is present not only in the tumors but also in tissues that appear normal during visual endoscopic examination. This latent infection may thus serve as a source of new lesions. Biopsy samples from 20 patients have shown that the virus is present not only in the overt papilloma but in apparently normal tissues taken both from patients with active disease and from patients in spontaneous remission.

Methods

Biopsies

Biopsy samples were removed before microlaryngeal laser surgery[10] and were immediately frozen in liquid nitrogen or transferred to tissue culture, as previously described.[11] The ages of the patients ranged from 1.5 to 78 years, and the duration of disease from 1 to 24 years. The diagnosis of papillomatosis was based on both clinical findings and histopathological evaluation.

DNA Isolation and Hybridization

Tissues were thawed and digested with proteinase K; deproteinized with phenol, phenol–chloroform (1:1), and chloroform; precipitated with two volumes of 100 per cent ethanol at −70°C; resuspended and treated with ribonuclease A; re-extracted with phenol and chloroform; and reprecipitated with alcohol, as previously described.[12] Cells grown in culture were scraped from the cell-culture dish into the same solution used to extract DNA from the biopsy samples and were processed in the same way.

DNA was digested with restriction endonucleases (Bethesda Research Laboratories) under the conditions specified by the vendor. Whenever possible, 6 to 8 μg of DNA was used, but in some cases, only 1 to 2 μg was available. The DNA fragments were separated in 0.9 per cent agarose gel and transferred to nitrocellulose filters (Schleicher and Schuell) by the procedure of Southern.[13] Hybridization was done as previously described,[12] except that either 30 or 50 per cent formamide was included and incubation was at 41°C. The probe was human papillomavirus 6b. It was isolated from a vaginal papilloma, cloned into the *Escherichia coli* plasmid pBR 322,[14] and labeled in vitro with alpha [^{32}P]deoxynucleotide triphosphates (Amersham) by the method of Rigby et al.[15] Filters were washed extensively with 0.03 M sodium chloride and 0.03 M sodium citrate (for 30 per cent formamide filters) or 0.015 M sodium chloride and 0.015 sodium citrate (for 50 per cent formamide filters) at 50°C. To prepare the filters for reuse we incubated them for two hours at 68°C in 50 per cent formamide to remove all probe bound to the DNA.

Results

Using the method of Southern,[13] we separated DNA fragments by size, with smaller fragments near the bottom of the gel, and hybridized them to the radioactive probe. Only viral fragments that were homologous to the viral probe formed stable hybrids, which appeared as thickened black bands on the x-ray film. Cellular DNA fragments from papillomavirus-infected cells were not detected by the human papillomavirus-specific probe. Under nonstringent conditions (30 per cent formamide) all of the human papillomaviruses (over 15) will cross-hybridize, permitting detection of any human papillomavirus, whether it is the same as or different from the probe. If stringent conditions are used (50 per cent formamide) only human papillomaviruses with a high degree of homology will be detected.

Figure 1 shows the results of hybridizing the human papillomavirus-6b probe to DNA from 12 different biopsy samples, as well as to DNA from in vitro cultured papilloma cells. Under nonstringent conditions (30 per cent formamide), all the laryngeal papillomas (Lanes 5, 7, 8, 9, 11, 12, and 14) were found to contain human papillomavirus sequences. Lanes 3, 4, 5, and 7 (Fig. 2a) and Lane 2 (Fig. 2b) showed viral sequences detected in five additional papillomas.

Three vocal-cord biopsy samples from patients in remission still contained human papillomavirus DNA. This is especially clear in Lane 10 of Figure 1. The patient, an eight-year-old girl, had a history of rapidly recurring papilloma but had been free of all papillomas for 19 months. No papilloma was visualized at the time of biopsy during surgery for a laryngeal web. The samples shown in Lanes 2 and 3 of Figure 1 were taken from children who had been free of papilloma for more than two years. The faintness of the bands probably reflects the very small amounts of DNA available from unusually small biopsy samples rather than reduced amounts of viral DNA per cell. The human papillomavirus sequences in Lane 2 were more easily visualized under stringent conditions (50 per cent formamide), as was a new band in Lane 3. Three additional patients in remission (two girls and a boy) were also found to have human papillomavirus sequences in their vocal cords at subsequent biopsies (Fig. 2a, Lanes 1, 6, and 10 through 12, respectively).

The biopsy sample used in Lane 13 of Figure 1 was also from a patient in remission, a six-year-old boy who at the time of the study had been free of disease for almost one year. This patient may have no longer had human papillomavirus DNA in his laryngeal tissues, since none could be detected. However, less than 1 μg of tissue DNA was available for assay. The level of human papillomavirus may simply have been below detectable limits.

Heterogeneity in the viruses became apparent when we compared hybridization under stringent and nonstringent conditions. Papillomavirus sequences were readily visualized in samples from two girls with active papillomas (Fig. 1, Lanes 9 and 14) when 30 per cent

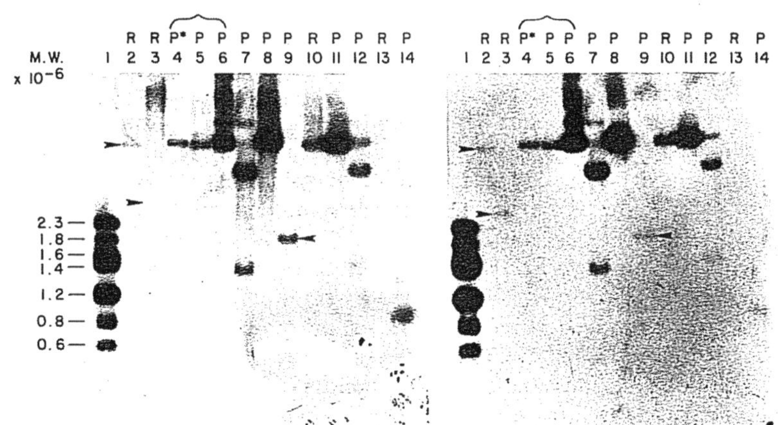

Figure 1. Southern Blot Hybridization to Human Papillomavirus-6b Probe under Nonstringent and Stringent Conditions.

DNA was extracted from tissues or cells, digested with *Hinc*II, and analyzed for human papillomavirus sequences, as described in Methods.

In Lane 1 human papillomavirus-6 probe, cut with *Eco*RI, *Bam*I, and *Ava*I, was used as the molecular-weight standard.

Lanes 2 through 14 show tissue and cell DNA. R denotes patient in remission, and P papilloma tissue. Asterisks denote cells grown in culture, and brackets group samples obtained from one patient during a single surgical procedure. Arrows indicate locations of hybridized fragments that are either faint or show differences between nonstringent (30 per cent formamide) and stringent (50 per cent formamide) conditions (see description in Results).

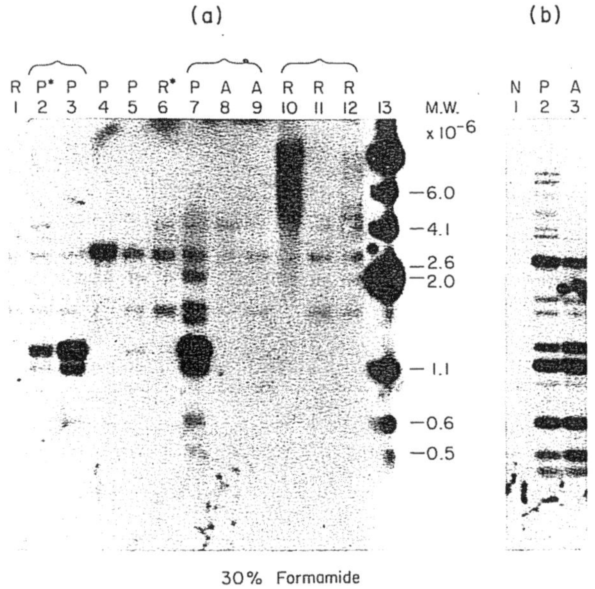

Figure 2. Southern Blot Hybridization to Human Papillomavirus-6b Probe under Nonstringent Conditions.

DNA from tissues or cells was digested with a mixture of *Eco*RI, *Bam*I, and *Pst*I, as described in Methods.

In Panel a, Lanes 1 through 12 show experimental DNA. Lane 13 shows human papillomavirus-6b DNA on same gel as Lanes 1 through 12. In Panel b, Lanes 1 through 3 show experimental DNA on second gel. R denotes patient in remission, P papilloma, A "normal" tissue from patient with papilloma, and N normal tissue from patient with carcinoma but no history of papilloma. Asterisks denote cells grown in culture, and brackets group samples obtained from one patient during a single surgical procedure.

formamide was used. With 50 per cent formamide Lane 9 was barely detectable, and Lane 14 did not hybridize at all. These two patients had a type of human papillomavirus that was different from the type found in the other patients and was much less closely related to the condyloma virus used as the probe, although their diseases were not atypical. On the other hand, although not all identical in restriction pattern, the samples from papillomas in an adult woman, a boy, a girl, and an adult man (Fig. 1, Lanes 4 through 6, 7 and 12, 8, and 11) were closely related to the condyloma virus, since they showed similar intensities of hybridization under different conditions of stringency.

Multiple biopsy samples from the same patient did not appear to be heterogeneous. Lanes 4, 5, and 6 (Fig. 1) contained, respectively, DNA from a vocal-cord papilloma grown in tissue culture for two months, the original vocal-cord papilloma before cell culture, and a uvula papilloma from the same patient (a 24-year-old woman). Both papillomas were removed during the same surgical procedure. All three samples contained human papillomavirus, which was cut once with *Hinc*II, generating linear molecules from the circular viral DNA. The uvula papilloma also contained human papillomavirus DNA with higher molecular weights, which were possibly concatenate. The papilloma tissues in Lanes 7 and 12 were also from the same patient, a young boy, but were removed in two separate procedures four months apart. Again, the *Hinc*II restriction patterns were the same for this patient.

Since we had found human papillomavirus sequences in "normal" tissues removed from patients in remission, we screened several samples obtained from biopsies of other apparently uninvolved laryngeal sites, as well as "normal" tissue from patients with carcinoma. The results of these experiments are shown in Figure 2. For this assay, the DNA was cut with a mixture of three enzymes to generate a more complex pattern of fragments.

Biopsy samples from a young boy (Fig. 2a, Lane 10) were taken from two additional sites in the larynx: the epiglottis (Lane 11) and the false cord (Lane 12). Both sites were positive in this asymptomatic patient, as they were in an adult with active papilloma of the true cord (Fig. 2a, Lanes 7 through 9). Biopsies of papilloma and opposite normal cord (Fig. 2b, Lanes 2 and 3) from a patient with adult-onset disease also support these findings.

DNA from normal vocal cord in a patient with a base-of-tongue carcinoma did not hybridize to the probe (Fig. 2b, Lane 1). DNA from two additional patients with carcinoma of the larynx and from two with vocal-cord polyps who had no history of papillomatosis was also negative for human papillomavirus (data not shown).

There may have been less viral DNA in the tissues that appeared to be normal at the time of surgery, but this may reflect the small amount of DNA usually available from normal tissues. Clearly, sequences related to human papillomavirus can be detected in morphologically normal laryngeal tissues from patients with active papillomatosis and from patients in remission.

Discussion

The presence of a latent infection in the "normal" tissues of patients with papilloma and patients in remission explains the clinical pattern of laryngeal papillomatosis. Removal of all papilloma tissue during surgery does not eliminate infected tissue, and therefore new papillomas can grow. In addition, these findings explain the observation that patients in remission for long periods can suddenly have a recurrence of active disease. Although we have no biochemical evidence that latent virus persists for longer than two years, recurrence has been documented after as many as 20 years without symptoms.

We are unable to state with certainty that the human papillomavirus sequences we have seen in "normal" tissues represent functional or infectious viral DNA. Clearly, the clinical implications of our results will vary according to the characteristics of the sequences in nonpapilloma tissue. At present, there is no way to grow papillomaviruses in vitro, and since human papillomavirus will not infect animals, the viability of the DNA cannot be tested in this way either.

Although defective variants can be detected in some human papillomavirus-1-induced skin lesions, where they may account for up to 25 per cent of the viral DNA molecules,[16] this is not necessarily common, and DNA/DNA homoduplex analysis of DNA extracted from a number of cutaneous warts gives no indication of the presence of a large number of defective variants (Chow L: personal communication).

Laryngeal papillomatosis is a relatively rare disease as compared with vaginal condyloma, although the two are epidemiologically related.[7] It is estimated that as many as 2 to 10 per cent of the women of child-bearing age in the United States currently have vaginal human papillomavirus infections.[17] If the route of infection in infants is through aspiration of infected material during birth, many more children could be infected than actually contract the disease. The condyloma virus may be only slightly infectious, or perhaps only a subset of the condyloma viruses is responsible for laryngeal papillomatosis. A third possibility is that most infections are "silent" and are never expressed as papillomas. Our results suggest that silent or latent infections do occur in laryngeal tissues, so it is possible that a large number of infants have been infected.

Two important conclusions may be tentatively drawn from our findings. First of all, the actual involved tissue extends far beyond the morphologically apparent laryngeal papilloma. The generality of this conclusion will need to be extended to papillomatosis of other body sites. We do not know whether similar latent infections are associated with cutaneous warts or genital condyloma. Secondly, the presence of papillomavirus sequences is not itself sufficient to ensure the appearance of a tumor. Other influences must be present, and those influences trigger only some of the infected tissue to proliferate. Frequent regression of papillomas in both boys and girls at puberty and occasional clinical changes during pregnancy[1] suggest that steroid hormones may somehow play a part in this process. The mechanism of hormonal action is completely unknown. Delineation of the hormonal and environmental factors that regulate the expression of the human papillomavirus may eventually allow us either to prevent these infections or to prevent the activation of a latent infection.

References

1. Holinger PH, Schild JA, Maurizi DG. Laryngeal papilloma: review of etiology and therapy. Laryngoscope 1968; 78:1462-74.
2. Haglund S, Lundquist P-G, Cantell K, Strander H. Interferon therapy in juvenile laryngeal papillomatosis. Arch Otolaryngol 1981; 107:327-32.
3. Goepfert H, Sessions RB, Gutterman JU, Cangir A, Dichtel WJ, Sulek M. Leukocyte interferon in patients with juvenile laryngeal papillomatosis. Ann Otol Rhinol Laryngol 1982; 91:431-6.
4. Braun L, Kashima H, Eggleston J, Shah K. Demonstration of papillomavirus antigen in paraffin sections of laryngeal papillomas. Laryngoscope 1982; 92:640-3.
5. Costa J, Howley PW, Bowling MC, Howard R, Bauer WC. Presence of human papilloma viral antigens in juvenile multiple laryngeal papilloma. Am J Clin Pathol 1981; 75:194-7.
6. Lack EE, Jenson AB, Smith HG, Healy GB, Pass F, Vawter GF. Immunoperoxidase localization of human papillomavirus in laryngeal papillomas. Intervirology 1980; 14:148-54.
7. Quick CA, Watts SL, Krzyzek RA, Faras AJ. Relationship between condylomata and laryngeal papillomata: clinical and molecular virological evidence. Ann Otol Rhinol Laryngol 1980; 89:467-71.
8. Mounts P, Shaw KV, Kashima H. Viral etiology of juvenile-onset and adult-onset squamous papilloma of the larynx. Proc Natl Acad Sci USA 1982; 79:5425-9.
9. Gissmann L, Diehl V, Schultz-Coulon H-J, zur Hausen H. Molecular cloning and characterization of human papilloma virus DNA derived from a laryngeal papilloma. J Virol 1982; 44:393-400.
10. Stern LS, Abramson AL, Grimes GW. Qualitative and morphometric evaluation of vocal cord lesions produced by the carbon dioxide laser. Laryngoscope 1980; 90:792-808.
11. Steinberg BM, Abramson AL, Meade RP. Culture of human laryngeal papilloma cells in vitro. Otolaryngol Head Neck Surg 1982; 90:728-35.
12. Botchan M, Topp W, Sambrook J. The arrangement of Simian virus 40 sequences in the DNA of transformed cells. Cell 1976; 9:269-87.
13. Southern EM. Detection of specific sequences among DNA fragments separated by gel electrophoresis. J Mol Biol 1975; 98:503-17.
14. de Villiers E-M, Gissmann L, zur Hausen H. Molecular cloning of viral DNA from human genital warts. J Virol 1981; 40:932-5.
15. Rigby PWJ, Dieckmann M, Rhodes C, Berg P. Labeling deoxyribonucleic acid to high specific activity in vitro by nick translation with DNA polymerase I. J Mol Biol 1977; 113:237-51.
16. Yoshiike K, Defendi V. Presence of deletion molecules in human wart virus DNA. J Virol 1977; 21:415-8.
17. Reid R, Stanhope CR, Herschman BR, Booth E, Phibbs GD, Smith JP. Genital warts and cervical cancer. I. Evidence of an association between subclinical papillomavirus infection and cervical malignancy. Cancer 1982; 50:377-87.

CLINICAL NOTE

Intralesional Cidofovir for Recurrent Respiratory Papillomatosis in Children

Seth M. Pransky, MD; Anthony E. Magit, MD; Donald B. Kearns, MD; D. Richard Kang, MD; Newton O. Duncan, MD

Objective: To assess the potential benefit of intralesional administration of cidofovir, an acyclic nucleoside phosphonate with activity against several DNA viruses, for treating severe respiratory papillomas in pediatric patients.

Design: Prospective case series.

Setting: Tertiary care children's hospitals.

Patients: Five pediatric patients with severe recurrent respiratory papillomatosis requiring laryngoscopy with carbon dioxide laser therapy more frequently than once a month to maintain airway patency. Each patient underwent between 12 and 33 laryngoscopies with laser treatment prior to being injected with cidofovir.

Intervention: Microsuspension laryngoscopy with intralesional injection of cidofovir (Vistide) in conjunction with mechanical debulking and carbon dioxide laser of papillomas.

Main Outcome Measure: Papilloma stage at time of serial laryngoscopies.

Results: One patient was disease free and 3 patients demonstrated a dramatic response to adjuvant therapy with cidofovir at the 9-month follow-up visit after the last injection of cidofovir. One patient showed an improvement in papilloma stage that was possibly related to concurrent therapy with interferon.

Conclusions: Intralesional injection of cidofovir seems to be of benefit in the treatment of severe respiratory papillomatosis in pediatric patients. Larger prospective studies with longer follow-up will be required before cidofovir can be considered an accepted means of managing this difficult disease.

Arch Otolaryngol Head Neck Surg. 1999;125:1143-1148

From Pediatric Otolaryngology, Children's Hospital and Health Center, San Diego, Calif (Drs Pransky, Magit, and Kearns); the Division of Otolaryngology, University of California, San Diego, School of Medicine (Dr Magit); the San Diego Naval Medical Center (Dr Kang); and Texas Ear, Nose & Throat Consultants, Houston (Dr Duncan).

RECURRENT respiratory papillomatosis (RRP) is the most common benign neoplasm of the larynx in children. It is caused by human papillomavirus (HPV), a DNA virus that results in benign epithelial proliferation. There are multiple types of HPV; HPV-6 and HPV-11 are the viral subtypes that are most commonly found in juvenile RRP. Although benign, this process can be life-threatening, and even when remission has occurred, there can often be chronic changes to the airway, resulting in voice problems and chronic airway difficulties.[1,2]

It is estimated that there are between 2000 and 2500 new cases of pediatric RRP per year, with an estimated 6000 active cases in any one year. Because of the difficulty in obtaining accurate data, we thought that it was possible that all these estimates were below the true incidence of cases of pediatric RRP.[3]

Multiple modes of treatment have been used in an attempt to control RRP, the most common of which is repetitive surgical ablation of the lesions with microsuspension laryngoscopies, usually using a carbon dioxide laser.[1,2] Tracheotomy, with its own inherent problems and risks, creates the potential for seeding and spread of the papillomas to the more distal aspect of the airway.[4] Photodynamic therapy with dihematoporphyrin ether has been successfully used, although latent infection has been noted to persist after photodynamic therapy, and photosensitivity can persist for weeks after the therapy has been discontinued.[5]

The mainstay of medical management of RRP to date has been therapy with interferon alfa-2a. This treatment, which consists of subcutaneous injections administered every other day, has resulted in successful eradication of the disease 30% to 50% of the time. Problems with interferon therapy include elevation of hepatic enzyme levels and decreased renal function, both of which require constant monitoring, as well as a significant rebound phenomenon after cessation of interferon therapy. There have also been recent reports that raise concern about central nervous system impairment with the development of spastic diplegia in association with the use of interferon.[1,2,6-9] Anecdotal reports of success include the use of indole-3 carbinol,[10] acyclovir,[11] ribavirin,[12] mumps vaccine,[10] and isotretinoin.[2,8]

Cidofovir (1-[(*S*)-3-hydroxy-2-(phosphonylmethoxy)-propyl]cytosine) is a cytosine nucleotide analog that has been shown to have potent antiviral activity against a broad spectrum of herpes viruses (eg, cytomegalovirus, herpes simplex types 1 and 2, varicella zoster, Epstein-Barr virus, and human herpesvirus types 6 and 8, as well as adenovirus and HPV).[13,14] Its mechanism of action is through the active intracellular metabolite cidofovir dihydrate, which inhibits cytomegalovirus DNA polymerase. It does not require intracellular activation by virally encoded enzymes, and the diphosphonate has an intracellular half-life between 17 and 65 hours, which permits it to continue antiviral efficacy with infrequent dosing.[15] Cidofovir is currently approved by the Food and Drug Administration to treat cytomegalovirus retinitis in patients with acquired immunodeficiency virus.

Van Cutsem et al[16] and Snoeck et al[17] reported the initial successful use of cidofovir for laryngeal papillomatosis, mostly in adult patients. Snoeck et al[17] reported on 11 patients, aged 11 to 54 years, who received between 2 and 13 injections, with excellent results in at least 8 of these patients. These 11 patients were then included in a recent publication[18] that reported on 17 patients with severe RRP, with excellent responses in 14 of these patients. Ten of the 14 responded completely after a mean of 6.6 injections (range, 2-15 injections) and have remained disease free during a follow-up period of 13.3 months (range, 2-27 months).

In several of our patients with RRP, papilloma growth progressed despite our best attempts at control using a carbon dioxide laser as well as adjuvant medical therapies. Encouraged by the successful reports on cidofovir therapy, we prospectively evaluated direct intralesional cidofovir (Vistide) injection as a means to reduce the severity of the disease.

Papillomatosis Staging Sheet

Surgery Date:
Adjuvant Therapy:
Last Procedure:

Severity Rating
1 = Minimal
2 = Moderate
3 = Severe

Larynx

- Epiglottis: Lingual ____ Laryngeal ____
- Aryepiglottic Folds: Right ____ Left ____
- False Vocal Cords: Right ____ Left ____
- True Vocal Cords: Right ____ Left ____
- Anterior Commissure ____
- Posterior Glottis ____

Trachea

- Upper Third: Anterior ____ Posterior ____
- Middle Third: Anterior ____ Posterior ____
- Lower Third: Anterior ____ Posterior ____
- Bronchi: Right ____ Left ____
- Tracheostoma ____

Other

Nose ____ Palate ____ Pharynx ____ Esophagus ____ Lungs ____

Total ____

Figure 1. *Papillomatosis staging sheet.*

Table 1. Patient Data*

Patient No./Sex	Race	Age at Diagnosis/ Date of Diagnosis	HPV Type	Before Cidofovir Therapy		
				No. of Procedures	Routine Laser Interval for 6 mo,† d	Adjuvant Therapy
1/M	White	3 y 2 mo/ 7/13/94	6/11	33	14	Interferon alfa-2a (3/17/95-4/12/96): no significant impact Acyclovir (7/3/95-8/17/95): no improvement, possible exacerbation Indole-3-carbinol (1/24/96-6/7/96): slight improvement initially, then no effect Isoretinoin (6/20/96-8/12/96): no effect
2/F	Hispanic	23 mo/ 8/28/95	6/11	18	7-21	Indole-3-carbinol (7/23/96-8/16/96): no effect Interferon alfa-2a (9/27/96-11/7/96): initial improvement, then significant worsening; discontinued owing to elevation in LFT results
3/M	Black	18 mo/ 1/26/96	11	12	14-28	Interferon alfa-2a (4/2/96-9/6/96): good response initially, then significant worsening
4/M	White	8 mo/ 3/30/94	11	20	28	Indole-3-carbinol (2/15/96-11/22/96): no effect
5/M	White	3 y 10 mo/ 3/17/95	6	12	28-42‡	Interferon alfa-2a (3/21/96-3/24/97): initial improvement, then significant worsening

**HPV indicates human papillomavirus; LFT, liver function test.*
†Interval between procedures needed to maintain airway.
‡Patient came from Philippines to San Diego, Calif, for treatment.

Table 2. Cidofovir Injection Data

Patient No.	No. of Cidofovir Injections	Period of Injections, mo	Follow-up Time From Last Injection, mo	Current Status
1	13	8	8	Minimal papilloma along undersurface mid portion of right true vocal cord; severity score, 1
2	15	8	8	No papilloma; severity score, 0
3	13	7½	9	Moderate papilloma at 2 sites: anterior commissure and laryngeal surface of epiglottis; severity score, 4
4	18	13½	2	Very minimal papilloma at 3 sites: anterior commissure, subglottis, mid trachea; severity score, 3
5	8	3¾	8½	Papilloma at 2 sites: right true vocal cord and anterior half of left true vocal cord; severity score, 3

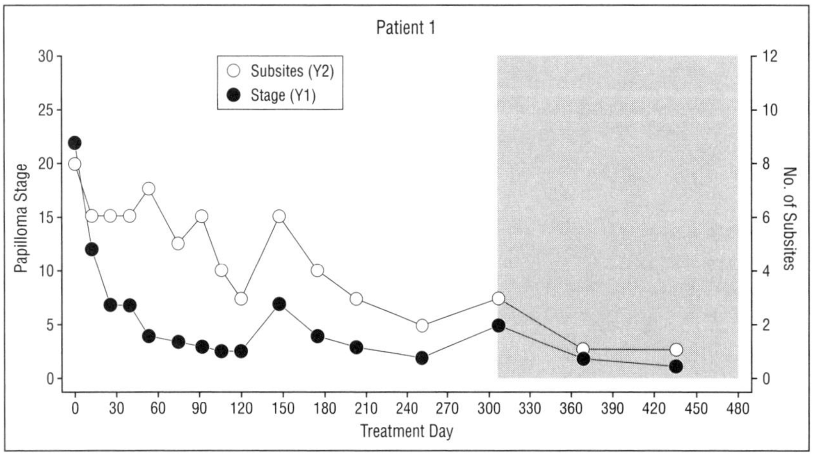

Figure 2. *Treatment response in patient 1.*

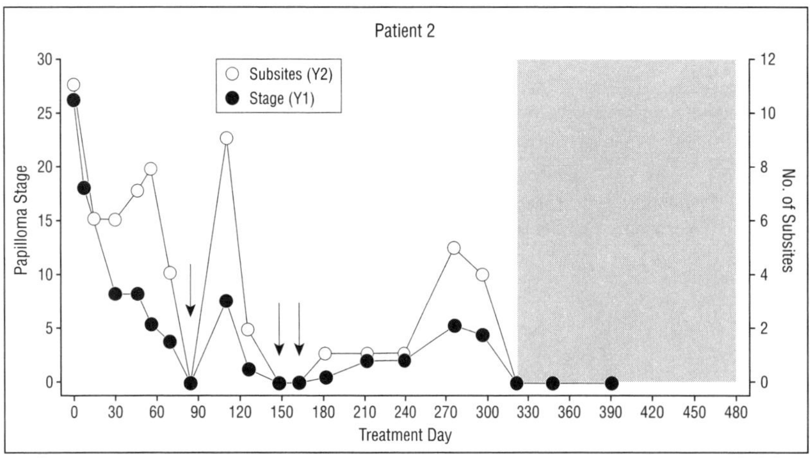

Figure 3. *Treatment response in patient 2.*

PATIENTS AND METHODS

This pilot study included 5 patients with aggressive RRP. These patients were chosen because they required laser therapy more frequently than once a month to maintain airway patency and because other adjuvant medical therapy had not been successful for them. They ranged in age from 2 to 5 years and had no other medical problems, specifically renal or hepatic disease. Informed consent was obtained from their parents according to the policies of Children's Hospital and Health Center, San Diego, Calif, and Texas Children's Hospital, Houston.

Papilloma stage was determined using a uniform grading format developed at the University of Alabama at Birmingham (Brian J. Wiatrak, MD, oral communication, July 20, 1996) (**Figure 1**). This system is designed to quantify the extent of RRP based on involved sites (larynx, trachea, and others) and subsites with severity based on a 4-point rating scale (0, none; 1, minimal involvement; 2, moderate involvement; and 3, severe involvement). A complete blood cell count and a blood chemistry profile were obtained at baseline before the first injection and then again each month.

The cidofovir injection was performed with the patient under general anesthesia using spontaneous ventilation and the Benjamin or Lindholm microsuspension laryngoscope (Karl Storz Endoscopy-America Inc, Culver City, Calif). No patient required endotracheal intubation, either before or after the injection of cidofovir. Debulking of the papillomas was done through a combination of cup forceps and carbon dioxide laser.

The cidofovir injection was administrated at a maximum dose of 1 mg/kg. It was formulated initially at 2.5 mg/mL and injected in the areas most involved with the papillomas using a laryngeal needle (Luerlock Injection Needle, Straight No. 8598B; Karl Storz Endoscopy-America Inc. The injection was performed so as not to generate airway obstruction. As we began to see a response to the medication, and because of the limitation of the injectable volume in these small children, the concentration was changed to 5 mg/mL. The volume of injection was between 1 and 2 mL, with the total dose between 2.5 and 10 mg. The specific dose for each session is not available because of leakage at the injection site. The amount injected was not related to the clinical disease present at the time of injection. All 5 children were discharged to home on the day of surgery. None routinely received treatment with systemic steroids, antibiotics, or probenecid. Based on the original data from Van Cutsem et al[16] and on the clinical course of our patients, cidofovir was injected every 2 to 3 weeks.

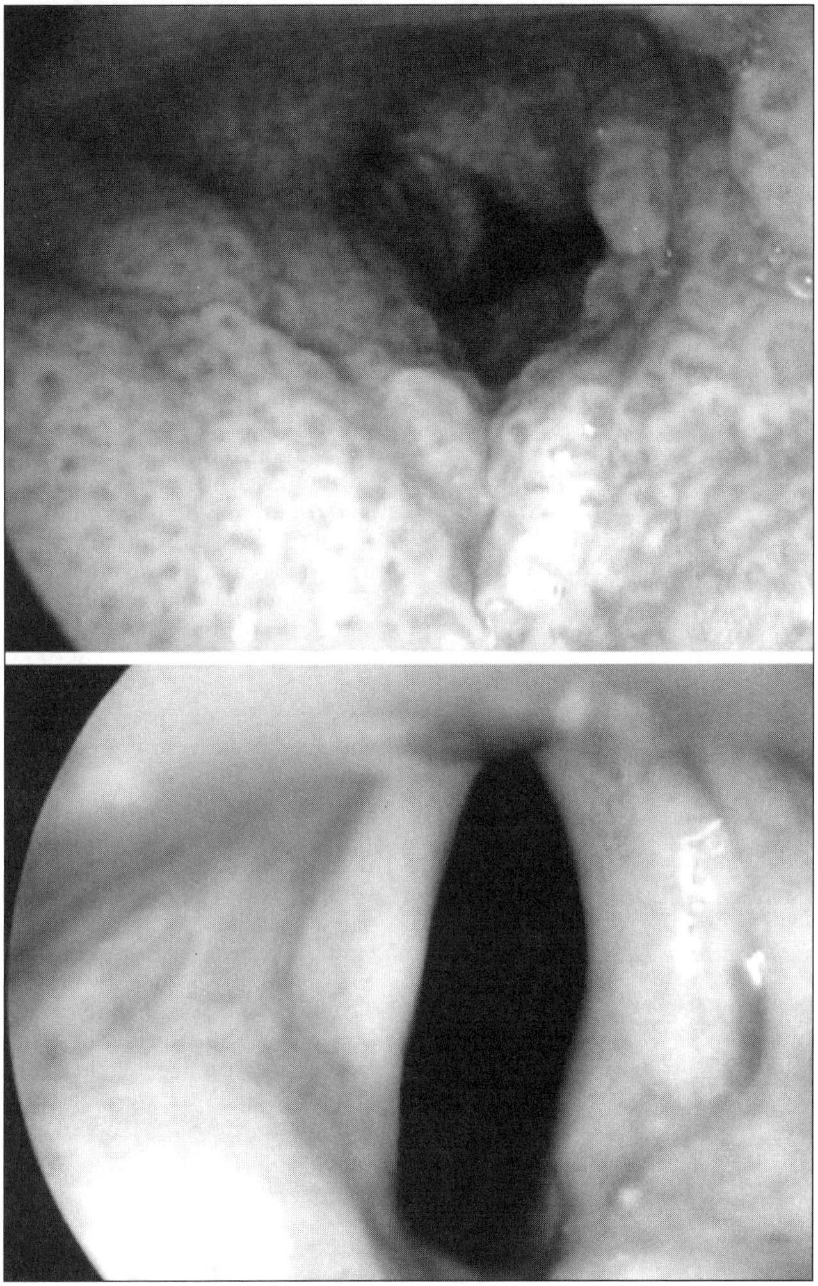

Figure 4. *Endoscopic photograph of patient 2 before cidofovir treatment (top) and 9 months after last injection (bottom).*

RESULTS

Table 1 reviews patient data in regard to age at diagnosis, HPV type, number of procedures undergone prior to initiation of cidofovir therapy, intervals between laser treatments needed to maintain control of the airway for 6 months prior to initiation of cidofovir therapy, and adjuvant therapy and response to it. Four of 5 patients underwent laser ablation at intervals of every 4 weeks or less. Patient 5, whose interval of treatment was every 4 to 6 weeks, was treated slightly differently because his family had to commute from the Philippines to San Diego for each treatment.

Table 2 reviews the cidofovir injection data and patient response. Of the 5 patients injected, 4 (Nos. 1, 2, 3, and 5) showed a marked reduction in their papilloma severity score and significant improvement of the status of their airway. Operative intervention, which had been necessary on the average of every 2 weeks (range, 7-28 days), has decreased to an average of every 3 months (range, 2-6 months), with longer intervals planned as office surveillance identifies minimal regrowth or disease-free states. Patient 4 had a transient improvement in his papilloma severity score and less fulminant regrowth in involved areas. His course was variable and his improvement was not sustained until interferon was added to his regimen.

Patient 1 was the first patient to be offered cidofovir injections. The results of his therapy are outlined in **Figure 2**. He received a total of 13 injections over a 9-month period and had only minimal residual papilloma along the undersurface of the right true vocal cord 9 months after the last injection. Although there is still one small area of papilloma that remains, his last operative procedure as of this writing was 3 months ago and recent office flexible laryngoscopy showed no significant regrowth. His voice is excellent.

Patient 2 is the only patient in whom cidofovir therapy completely cleared her RRP. She started with diffuse disease, and her clinical course progressed dramatically, with the intervals between laser treatments decreasing to 2 to 3 weeks. Her response to cidofovir injections was quite dramatic (**Figure 3**), to the point where she was clear of macroscopic papillomas after the seventh injection. She had a recurrence 1 month later; however, by the 15th injection, her larynx was essentially clear. Her last injection was 9 months ago, and her most recent endoscopy showed no evidence of macroscopic papilloma (**Figure 4**). Her voice is excellent.

Patient 3, one of twins born prematurely and intubated for 2 months, had his RRP identified initially at 18 months of age. He underwent a total of 13 cidofovir injections over a 7.5-month period, and although he did show marked improvement (**Figure 5**), he still had mild disease involving 2 subsites (anterior commissure and laryngeal surface of the epiglottis) 9 months after the cidofovir therapy was discontinued. His current interval of treatment has decreased to 10 weeks, and he still has a somewhat raspy voice.

Patient 4 underwent his first 7 endoscopic laser procedures in Houston and then moved to San Diego. He underwent 11 injections in San Diego

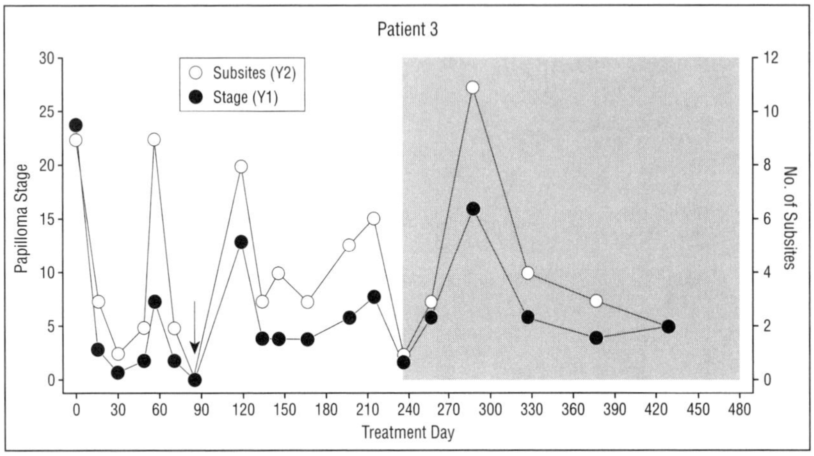

Figure 5. *Treatment response in patient 3.*

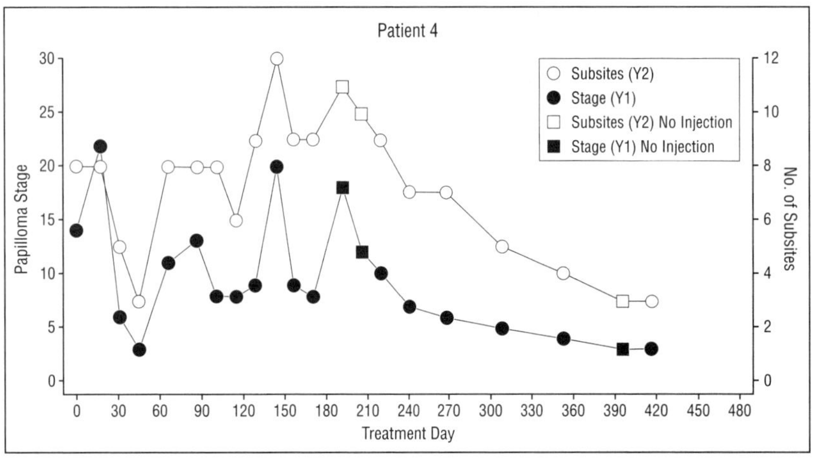

Figure 6. *Treatment response in patient 4.*

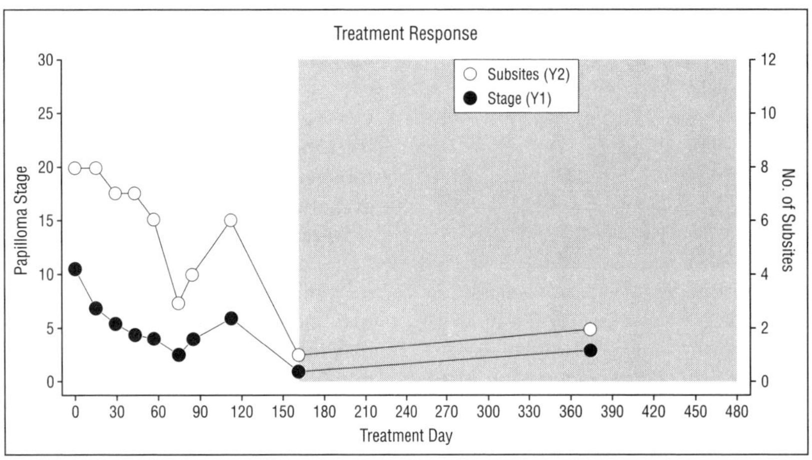

Figure 7. *Treatment response in patient 5.*

over a 5-month period and then subsequently moved back to Houston. His response to cidofovir therapy was the least noteworthy of all of the patients' responses (**Figure 6**). On his return to Houston, the cidofovir therapy was not initially restarted, and his disease became more severe. Cidofovir therapy was restarted, but this time interferon alfa-2a was added to the regimen, and the response was dramatic. The cidofovir and interferon therapy was discontinued after 5 months, and at the last follow-up visit, the patient had minimal disease involving 3 sites: the anterior commissure, the subglottis, and the midtrachea. His voice is excellent.

Patient 5 was the one patient whose routine laser interval was more than 4 weeks. When he did undergo microsuspension laryngoscopy, his disease was growing increasingly diffuse and severe. A mitigating factor in his starting cidofovir therapy was the fact that he lived in the Philippines and needed to fly to San Diego for treatment. His response to the injections was excellent (**Figure 7**). He received 8 injections over 3.5 months, and since his last injection, 10 months ago, he has required only 2 procedures and has minimal residual disease involving the true vocal cords bilaterally.

Although the target dose of cidofovir was to be 1 mg/kg injected at a concentration of 2.5 mg/mL, the small size of the pediatric airway limited the volume that could be injected and effectively reduced the amount of drug delivered. As we began to see significant clinical response, we changed the concentration of the cidofovir to 5 mg/mL, which allowed us to more closely achieve the target dose.

One patient had complete response to the medication; 3 patients have had a significant response, with only mild residual papilloma; and 1 patient has had an erratic response. There has also been less concern regarding airway obstruction; voice quality is markedly better; and the intervals between treatments are longer. No local nor systemic sequelae have been identified, and there were no significant changes in blood chemistry profiles during cidofovir therapy.

COMMENT

To our knowledge, this is the first report on the use of cidofovir for pediatric patients with severe RRP. The results of this preliminary report are quite promising and offer hope to those who are most severely affected with RRP. Although our findings do not confirm the complete eradication of the disease in most of the patients, in contrast to the report of Snoeck et al,[18] the marked improvement in the airways (as well as the improvement in voice) and the significant reduction in the need for repetitive operative intervention suggest that this form of therapy has tremendous value in pediatric patients with severe RRP.

The significant improvement noted in our patients after the initiation of cidofovir therapy does not appear to be coincident with the anticipated spontaneous improvement of this disease that generally comes about after years of therapy and at adolescence. All our patients had increasing disease, demanding more frequent and aggressive operative intervention simply to maintain airway patency. The cidofovir injections brought about an impressive response quite rapidly and seem to have permitted a sustained response in 4 of the 5 patients.

There are several issues relating to the dosage and technique of the injections. Initially, we started with a concentration of 2.5 mg/mL, as had been used in Belgium.[18] When confronted with overwhelming involvement of the larynx during the initial injections, it was difficult to get an adequate amount of volume injected and not generate airway obstruction. Once a response was obtained and the amount of papilloma decreased, it became easier to inject regions that could not be visualized previously (such as the subglottis), and a more effective and larger injection could be achieved.

Cidofovir can be toxic. Animal studies have identified nephrotoxicity, which appears to be related to dosage and schedule, as the major adverse event. Neutropenia has also been reported. In one study,[18] patients who received intralesional injection of cidofovir did not have any of these problems, but in another study[15] approximately 10% of the patients with human immunodeficiency virus who received intravenous cidofovir therapy had some adverse reactions, mainly asymptomatic proteinuria or neutropenia. None of our patients experienced any of these problems.

Of greater concern is the possible development of carcinoma. The Food and Drug Administration had approved a phase 1/2 study that was to be performed by the National Institute of Allergy and Infectious Diseases Collaborative Antiviral Study Group to establish the safety of cidofovir directly injected into HPV lesions of the larynx, but expressed some reluctance at the time of approval owing to reports of the development of adenocarcinoma in an animal model of Sprague-Dawley rats (which are predisposed to developing mammary tumors). Recently, a disturbing anecdotal report of the development of carcinoma at the injection site in 2 (and possibly 3) of 34 patients in Belgium resulted in the Food and Drug Administration–approved study being placed on hold. This is currently being investigated, with initial information revealing that the 2 confirmed cases involve adult patients who smoked and apparently had laryngeal biopsy specimens showing atypical cells that may have actually been verrucous carcinoma rather than RRP.

Several distinctions need to be made between our report and that of Snoeck and colleagues.[18] First, the age range in our 5 children was between 2 years 8 months and 5 years 10 months, in contrast to the primarily adult population in the study of Snoeck and coworkers. Second, all our patients had HPV typing of either HPV-11 or HPV-6, in contrast to Snoeck and colleagues' study, in which biopsy specimens were obtained but HPV typing was only performed in 2 patients and 2 patients had lesions that were microscopically compatible with verrucous carcinoma.

There are multiple questions that remain to be answered. Once the basic safety profile of the medication has been established, areas of investigation include (1) the appropriate dosage level, (2) the appropriate interval between injections, (3) the appropriate number of injections, and (4) which patients should receive the drug (should the medication be reserved for those patients who are most severely affected, or can it be used in small concentrations in those with only 1 or 2 papillomatous lesions?).

We intend to continue long-term follow-up of our patients to look for the recurrence of disease and to obtain laryngeal biopsy specimens to evaluate histopathologic changes. We suggest that if cidofovir is to be used, it should be as part of a multicenter trial with a uniform staging system, injection technique, dosing schedule, and follow-up.

Accepted for publication June 18, 1999.

Reprints: Anthony E. Magit, MD, Pediatric Otolaryngology, Children's Hospital and Health Center, 3030 Children's Way, Suite 402, San Diego, CA 92123.

REFERENCES

1. Pransky SM, Kang DR. Tumors of the larynx, trachea, and bronchi. In: Bluestone CD, Stool SE, Kenna MA, eds. *Pediatric Otolaryngology.* Vol 2. Philadelphia, Pa: WB Saunders Co; 1996:1402-1414.
2. Bauman NM, Smith RS. Recurrent respiratory papillomatosis. *Pediatr Clin North Am.* 1996;43:1385-1401.
3. Derkay CS. Task force on recurrent respiratory papillomatosis: a preliminary report. *Arch Otolaryngol Head Neck Surg.* 1995;121:1386-1391.
4. Kashima H, Leventhal B, Mounts P, Hruban RH. Sites of predilection in recurrent respiratory papillomatosis. *Ann Otol Rhinol Laryngol.* 1993;102:580-583.
5. Abramson A, Shikowitz M, Rullooly V, Steinberg B, Amella C, Rothstein H. Clinical effects of photodynamic therapy on recurrent laryngeal papillomas. *Arch Otolaryngol Head Neck Surg.* 1992;118:25-29.
6. Healy GB, Gelber RD, Trowbridge AL, et al. Treatment of recurrent respiratory papillomatosis with human leukocyte interferon: results of a mulitcenter randomized clinical trial. *N Engl J Med.* 1988;319:401-407.
7. Leventhal B, Kashima H, Mounts P, et al. Long-term response of recurrent respiratory papillomatosis to treatment with lymphoblastoid interferon alfa-N1. *N Engl J Med.* 1991;325:613-617.
8. Avidano M, Singleton G. Adjuvant drug strategies in the treatment of recurrent respiratory papillomatosis. *Otolaryngol Head Neck Surg.* 1995;112:197-202.
9. Barlow CF, Priebe CJ, Mulliken JB, et al. Spastic diplegia as a complication of interferon alfa-2A treatment of hemangionas of infancy. *J Pediatr.* 1998;132:527-530.
10. *Recurrent Respiratory Papillomatosis Newsletter.* Lawrenceville, NJ: RRP Foundation; Spring 1998.
11. Endres D, Bauman N, Burke D, Smith R. Acyclovir in the treatment of recurrent respiratory papillomatosis: a pilot study. *Ann Otol Rhinol Laryngol.* 1994;103:301-305.
12. McGlennen R, Adams G, Lewis C, Faras A, Ostrow R. Pilot trial of ribavirin for the treatment of laryngeal papillomatosis. *Head Neck.* 1993;15:504-513.
13. De Clercq E. Therapeutic potential of cidofovir (HPMPC, Vistide) for the treatment of DNA virus (i.e. herpes-, papova-, pox- and adenovirus) infections. *Verh K Acad Geneesk Belg.* 1996;58:19-47.
14. Ho H, Woods K, Bronson J, DeBoeck H, Martin J, Hitchcock M. Intracellular metabolism of the antiherpes agent (*S*)-1-[3-hydroxy-2-(phosphonylmethoxy)propyl]cytosine. *Mol Pharmacol.* 1991;41:197-202.
15. Lalezari J, Stagg R, Kuppermann B, et al. Intravenous cidofovir for peripheral cytomegalovirus retinitis in patients with AIDS. *Ann Intern Med.* 1997;126:257-263.
16. Van Cutsem E, Snoeck R, Van Ranst M, et al. Successful treatment of a squamous papilloma of the hypopharynx-esophagus by local injections of (*S*)-1-(3-hydroxy-2-phosphonylmethoxypropyl) cytosine. *J Med Virol.* 1995;45:230-235.
17. Snoeck R, Wellens W, Desloovere C, Van Ranst M, De Clercq E, Feenstra L. Treatment of severe recurrent laryngeal papillomatosis by local injections of (*S*)-1-(3-hydroxy-2-phosphonylmethoxypropyl) cytosine (cidofovir). In: Programs and Abstracts of the Ninth International Conference on Antiviral Research; May 19-24, 1996; Fukushima, Japan.
18. Snoeck R, Wleens W, Desloovere C, et al. Treatment of severe laryngeal papillomatosis with intralesional injections of cidofovir [(*S*)-1-(3-hydroxy-2-phosphonylmethoxypropyl) cytosine]. *J Virol.* 1998;54:219-225.

Commentary

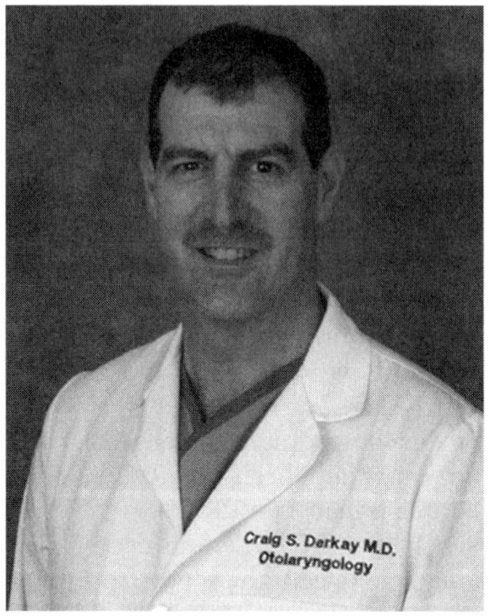

Craig S. Derkay, MD

It is a pleasure to reflect back on this work for *Classics in Voice and Laryngology*. Since the publication of this "state of the art" clinical review, many exciting developments have occurred in the pursuit of a "cure" for recurrent respiratory papillomatosis (RRP).

We have seen the recent introduction of the quadrivalent HPV vaccine (Gardasil), which could conceivably do for future RRP patients what the HiB vaccine has done for children previously affected by acute epiglotitis. Ongoing collaboration with the vaccine's manufacturer in the United States and worldwide with the RRP Task Force aims to measure the impact of the vaccine on future generations. Through a proposed serology study looking at the level of anti-HPV 6 and 11 antibodies in existing RRP patients, we also hope to identify a therapeutic role for this vaccine.

Recent years have also seen advancements in the development of pulse- dye lasers capable of treating patients with RRP in the office setting as well as improved optics for our rigid and flexible endoscopes enhancing our diagnostic skills and providing less invasive treatment options in the ambulatory setting.

The search for an effective adjuvant medical therapy for RRP patients continues. Cidofovir has shown some promise but is not universally effective, is not FDA-approved for treatment of RRP, and has adverse effects that may make it an unacceptable option in patients. Hsp-E7 is a biologic modifier with activity against HPV and RRP demonstrated in a phase II trial but is not commercially available. Other potential RRP therapies such as cox-2 inhibitors are currently under investigation.

A commercially available HPV subtyping assay is on the horizon and, based upon recent research regarding the more aggressive nature of HPV 11, this may help us to better educate our families regarding the prognosis for further surgical and medical care.

As a follow-up to the article included in this volume, a new "state of the art" clinical review for *Laryngoscope* was published with Brian Wiatrak, MD as coauthor.

CLINICAL STATE OF THE ART REVIEW

Recurrent Respiratory Papillomatosis

Craig S. Derkay, MD

Recurrent respiratory papillomatosis (RRP) is the most common benign neoplasm of the larynx in children. Despite its benign histology, RRP has potentially morbid consequences and is often difficult to treat because of its tendency to recur and spread throughout the respiratory tract. Long neglected from an epidemiological standpoint, recent initiatives to better understand this disease process have been launched through coordination between the Centers for Disease Control and Prevention and the American Society of Pediatric Otolaryngology. In this clinical review, I discuss what we currently know regarding the etiology, epidemiology, and transmission of this disease. Clinical features including pertinent aspects of the history, physical examination, airway endoscopy, and other considerations are highlighted. A detailed description of the surgical and anesthetic management of these challenging cases is presented. Adjuvant modalities of surgical and nonsurgical treatment and their indications are discussed. Ongoing research initiatives and the Practice Guidelines of the Recurrent Respiratory Papillomatosis Task Force are also included. *Key Words:* Recurrent respiratory papillomas, laser, microdebrider, cidofovir, interferon.

***Laryngoscope*, 111:57–69, 2001**

INTRODUCTION

Recurrent respiratory papillomatosis (RRP) is a disease of viral origin that is caused by human papillomavirus types 6 and 11 (HPV 6 and HPV 11) and is associated with exophytic lesions of the airway. Although it is a benign disease, RRP has potentially morbid consequences because of its involvement of the airway and the risk of malignant conversion.

Recurrent respiratory papillomatosis is both the most common benign neoplasm of the larynx among children and the second most frequent cause of childhood hoarseness.[1] The disease is often difficult to treat because of its tendency to recur and spread throughout the respiratory tract. Although it most often involves the larynx, RRP may involve the entire aerodigestive tract. The course of the disease is variable; some patients have spontaneous remission and others have aggressive papillomatous growth, requiring multiple surgical procedures over many years.

In most pediatric series, RRP is diagnosed between 2 and 4 years of age with a delay in diagnosis from the time of onset of symptoms averaging about 1 year.[2] Seventy-five percent of the children have been diagnosed before their fifth birthday.[3] It is estimated that between 1500 and 2500 new cases of childhood-onset RRP occur in the United States each year. The incidence among children in the United States is estimated at 4.3 per 100,000 children, translating into more than 15,000 surgical procedures at a total cost of more than $100 million per year.[4] Anecdotal observations suggest that most patients are firstborn; have young, primigravid mothers; and come from families of low socioeconomic status.[4–6] The clinical course is unpredictable, with malignant transformation possible in chronic invasive papillomatosis.

Recurrent respiratory papillomatosis may have its clinical onset during either childhood or adulthood. Two distinct forms are generally recognized: a juvenile or aggressive form and an adult or less aggressive form. The aggressive form, although most prevalent in children, can also occur in adults. Children whose RRP was diagnosed at younger ages (<3 y) have been found to be 3.6 times more likely to have more than four surgeries per year and almost 2 times more likely to have two or more anatomical sites affected than children whose RRP was diagnosed at later ages (>3 y).[7]

DISCUSSION

Etiology

Human papillomavirus. Human papillomavirus (HPV) is a small, DNA-containing, nonenveloped icosahedral (20-sided) capsid virus with a double-stranded circular DNA that is 7900 base pairs (bp) long. The present understanding is that HPV establishes itself in the basal layer, where viral DNA enters the cell and elaborates RNA to produce viral proteins. Until the 1990s, HPV had been suspected but not confirmed as the causative agent in RRP. This uncertainty developed from an inability to culture the virus in vitro and from the failure to demonstrate viral particles consistently in papilloma lesions

From the Department of Otolaryngology and Pediatrics, Eastern Virginia Medical School, Norfolk, Virginia.

Editor's Note: This Manuscript was accepted for publication October 5, 2000.

Send Correspondence to Craig S. Derkay, MD, Department of Otolaryngology and Pediatrics, Eastern Virginia Medical School, Norfolk, VA 23507, U.S.A.

using electron microscopy or HPV antibodies. Today, with the use of viral probes, HPV DNA has been identified in virtually every papilloma lesion studied. The most common types identified in the airway are HPV 6 and HPV 11, the same types that are responsible for genital warts. Specific viral subtypes may be correlated with disease severity and clinical course. Children infected with HPV 11 appear to have a more obstructive airway course early in the disease and a greater need for tracheotomy.[8] At least 90 different types of HPV have been identified and are designated by numbers (e.g., HPV 6). The closer the numbers are, the more similar the viral subtypes are in their clinical manifestations.

An association between cervical HPV infection in the mother and the incidence of RRP has been well established. Viral DNA has been detected in areas of "normal-appearing mucosa" adjacent to papilloma lesions, suggesting a possible explanation for the recurrence of the disease following thorough surgical removal.[9] Adult-onset respiratory papillomas could reflect either activation of virus present since birth or an infection acquired in adolescence or adult life.

The universality of HPV in the lower genital tract rivals that of any other sexually transmitted disease in humans. It is estimated that at least 1 million cases of genital papillomas occur per year in the United States.[10] These most often manifest as condylomata acuminata involving the cervix, vulva, or other anogenital sites in women or the penis of male sexual partners of affected women. HPV has been noted to be present in the genital tract of as many as 25% of all women of child-bearing age worldwide. The incidence of HPV infections in sexually active young college women is high with a cumulative incidence of 43% over a 36-month period in a recent study.[11] Clinically apparent HPV infection has been noted in 1.5% to 5% of pregnant women in the United States.[12] As in RRP, HPV 6 and HPV 11 are the most common subtypes identified in cervical condylomata.

Histology

Histologically, RRP appears as pedunculated masses with fingerlike projections of nonkeratinized stratified squamous epithelium supported by a core of highly vascularized connective tissue stroma (Fig. 1). The basal layer may be either normal or hyperplastic, and mitotic figures are generally limited to this layer. Cellular differentiation appears to be abnormal, with altered expression and production of keratins. The degree of atypia may be a sign of premalignant tendency. RRP lesions occur most often at anatomical sites in which ciliated and squamous epithelium are juxtaposed.[13] The most common sites for RRP are the limen vestibuli, the nasopharyngeal surface of the soft palate, the midline of the laryngeal surface of the epiglottis, the upper and lower margins of the ventricle, the undersurface of the vocal folds, the carina, and at bronchial spurs.[5] In tracheotomized patients, RRP lesions are often encountered at the stoma and in the midthoracic trachea, areas that might be considered iatrogenic squamociliary junctions. Papilloma lesions may be sessile or pedunculated and often occur in irregular exophytic clusters (Fig. 2). Typically, the lesions are pinkish to white. Iatrogenic implantation of papilloma may be preventable by avoiding injury to nondiseased squamous or ciliated epithelium adjacent to areas of frank papilloma. Ciliated epithelium undergoes squamous metaplasia when exposed to repeated trauma and is replaced with nonciliated epithelium that creates an iatrogenic squamociliary junction. This may also explain the observation that RRP flourishes in the presence of uncontrolled gastroesophageal reflux.[14]

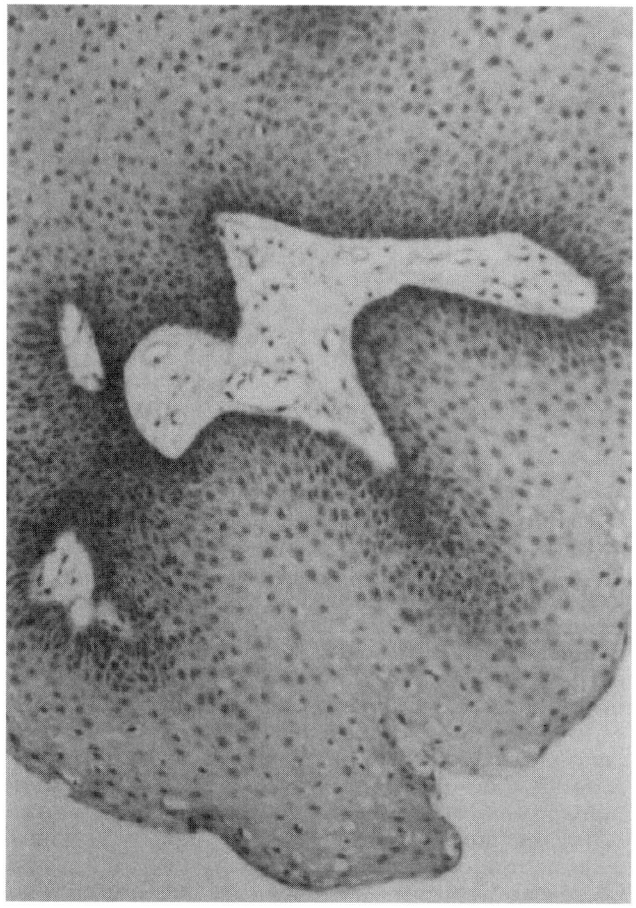

Fig. 1. Histological section of papilloma, demonstrating finger-like projection of nonkeratinized stratified squamous epithelium and vascularized connective tissue stroma.

Epidemiology

Recurrent respiratory papillomatosis may affect people of any age, with the youngest patient identified at 1 day of age and the oldest at 84 years.[4] Childhood-onset RRP (arbitrarily defined as patients diagnosed at less than 12 y of age) is most often diagnosed between 2 and 4 years of age. Adult RRP peaks between the ages of 20 and 40 and has a slight male predilection; distribution among boys and girls is approximately equal and there are no apparent differences in surgical frequencies by gender or ethnicity.[7] Childhood-onset RRP is more common and is more aggressive than its adult counterpart. The National Registry of children with RRP, comprising the clinical practices at 22 pediatric otolaryngology sites, calculates a mean number of procedures at 19.7 per child with an average of 4.4 procedures per year.[7] Children diagnosed at younger than 3 years of age were found to be 3.6 times more likely to require more than four surgical procedures per year and 2.1 times more likely to have two or more anatomical sites involved than those diagnosed after their fourth birthday.[7] In a survey of practicing otolaryngologists in the United States, half of the adults with RRP had required fewer than five procedures over their lifetime compared with less than 25% of the children. Approximately equal percentages of children and adults (17% children vs. 19% adults) had aggressive RRP (defined as requiring more than 40 lifetime operations), although adults had more years to accumulate these operations.[4] True incidence and prevalence of RRP are uncertain. In a Danish subpopulation incorporating 50% of the population of that country, the incidence of laryngeal papillomatosis was 3.84 cases per 100,000.[15] The rate among children was 3.62 per 100,000, whereas adult-onset cases occurred at a rate of 3.94 per 100,000. These data are comparable with those found in a recent U.S. survey, which estimated an incidence in the pediatric population of 4.3 per 100,000 children and 1.8 per 100,000 adults. This translates into approximately 2300 new pediatric cases per year in the United States.[4]

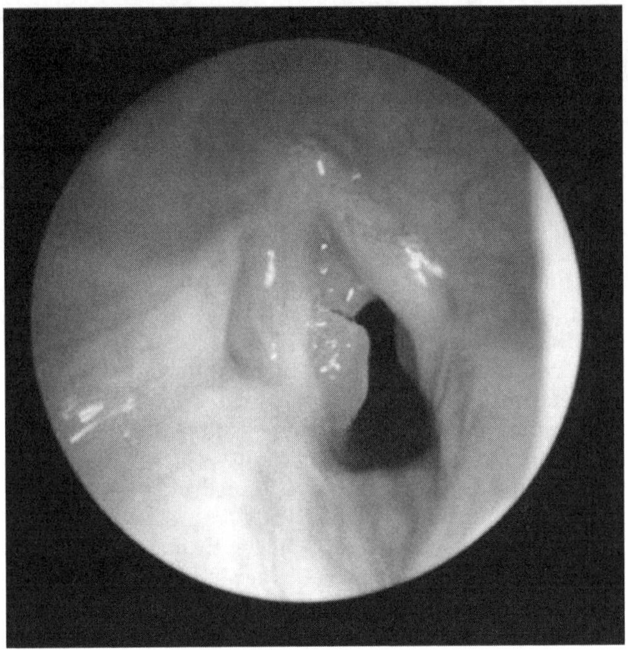

Fig. 2. Sessile papilloma lesions involving the true vocal folds.

Transmission

The precise mode of HPV transmission remains unclear. Several studies have convincingly linked childhood-onset RRP to mothers with genital HPV infections, whereas circumstantial evidence suggests that adult disease may be associated with oral-genital contact. Retrospective and recent prospective studies have confirmed that HPV may be passed by vertical transmission from mother to child.[16–18] In addition, Kashima et al.[5] found that patients with childhood-onset RRP were more likely to be firstborn and vaginally delivered than were control patients of similar age. The authors hypothesized that primigravid mothers are more likely to have a long second stage of labor and that the prolonged exposure to the virus leads to a higher risk of infection in the firstborn child. The authors also suggested that newly acquired genital HPV lesions are more likely to shed virus than long-standing lesions, thus explaining the higher incidence of papilloma disease observed among the offspring of young mothers of low socioeconomic status, the same group that is most likely to acquire sexually transmitted diseases such as HPV. Despite the apparent close association between maternal condylomata and the development of RRP, few children exposed to genital warts at birth develop clinical symptoms.[19,20] Why RRP develops in so few children whose mothers have condylomata is not well understood. The most likely method of maternal-fetal HPV transmission is through direct contact in the birth canal. This would explain the clinical observation that most children in whom RRP lesions develop are delivered vaginally to mothers with a history of genital condylomatas.[19] Although HPV could be recovered from the nasopharyngeal secretions of 30% of infants exposed to HPV in the birth canal,[20] the number of infants expected to manifest evidence of RRP is only a small fraction of this percentage. Clearly, other factors (patient immunity, timing, length and volume of virus exposure, and local trauma) must be important determinants of development of RRP. Even though cesarean section would seem to reduce the risk of transmission of the disease, this procedure is associated with a higher morbidity and mortality for the mother and a much higher economic cost than elective vaginal delivery. Shah et al.[19] estimated that the risk of a child contracting the disease from a mother who has an active condylomatous lesion and delivers vaginally is only about 1 in 400. The characteristics that differentiate this one child from the other 399 are elusive. In light of the uncertainty surrounding intrapartum exposure, there is presently insufficient evidence to support delivery by cesarean section in all pregnant women with condylomata.[21] Reports of neonatal papillomatosis suggest that, in at least some cases, development of the disease may occur in utero. Since cesarean section still does not prevent the development of papilloma disease in all cases, a better understanding of the risk factors associated with RRP is needed before the efficacy of cesarean delivery in preventing papilloma disease can be fully assessed.

Clinical Features

Because the most common symptoms of RRP are related to airway obstruction, it is not uncommon for children to be misdiagnosed initially as having asthma, croup, or chronic bronchitis. The hallmark of RRP in children is the triad of relentlessly progressive hoarseness, stridor, and respiratory distress. Although hoarseness in children tends to be overlooked or, at least, accepted until it reaches a certain level of severity, any infant or young child with symptoms of voice change, along with obstructive airway symptoms or recurrent croup, warrants laryngoscopy to rule out neoplasia, with RRP being the most likely lesion.

Children with RRP most often present with some degree of dysphonia. However, particularly in young children, changes in voice may go unnoticed. Stridor is often the second clinical symptom to develop, beginning as an inspiratory noise and becoming biphasic with progression of the disease. Less commonly, chronic cough, recurrent pneumonia, failure to thrive, dyspnea, dysphagia, and acute life-threatening events may be the presenting symptoms. The duration of symptoms before diagnosis varies. Not uncommonly, a mistaken diagnosis of asthma, croup, allergies, vocal nodules, or bronchitis is entertained before a definitive diagnosis is made.

Because of the rarity of RRP and the slowly progressive nature of the disease, some cases may go unrecognized until respiratory distress results from papillomas obstructing the airway. The result is a relatively high need for tracheotomy to be performed in these children. Shapiro et al.[22] noted that RRP tracheotomy patients presented at a younger age and with more widespread disease, often involving the distal airway, before tracheotomy. In the authors' experience with 13 patients, they did not think that the tracheotomy itself led to spread of disease outside the larynx. In the Centers for Disease Control and Prevention (CDC) registry, children with tracheotomy were initially diagnosed with RRP at a younger age (2.7 y) than those without a tracheotomy (3.9 y).[7] Other authors have suggested that tracheotomy may activate or spread disease lower in the respiratory tract. Cole et al.[23] reported that tracheal papillomas developed in half of their tracheotomy patients and that, despite attempts to avoid this procedure, 21% of their patients required a long-term tracheotomy. Prolonged tracheotomy and the presence of subglottic papilloma at the time of tracheotomy have been associated with an increased risk of distal tracheal spread. Most authors have agreed that tracheotomy is a procedure to be avoided unless absolutely necessary. When a tracheotomy is unavoidable, decannulation should be considered as soon as the disease is managed effectively with endoscopic techniques. Children with bronchopulmonary dysplasia who require prolonged endotracheal intubation may also be at increased risk for development of RRP. Through interruption of the continuous respiratory mucosal surface, an endotracheal tube may have the same role in the mechanical dissemination or implantation of RRP as tracheotomy. Gastroesophageal reflux disease has also been identified as a potential risk factor for disease persistence, although additional research is necessary to verify this anecdotal observation.

Extralaryngeal spread of respiratory papillomas has been identified in approximately 30% of children and in 16% of adults with RRP. The most frequent sites of extralaryngeal spread were, in order of frequency, the oral cavity, trachea, and bronchi.[4] A possible link between RRP and immunodeficiency states has also been observed. Both children and adults with AIDS or congenital immunodeficiencies or those on a regimen of immunosuppression after organ transplantation have been identified with RRP.[4] Malignant transformation of RRP into squamous cell carcinoma has been documented in several case reports. A total of 26 patients was identified as having progressed to squamous cell carcinoma in the Recurrent Respiratory Papillomatosis Task Force survey.[4] When death occurs, it is usually associated with a complication of frequent surgical procedures or caused by respiratory failure attributable to distal disease progression. RRP presenting in the neonatal period is thought to be a negative prognostic factor with a greater likelihood for mortality and need for tracheotomy.

Patient Assessment

History. Persistent or progressive stridor and dysphonia, with the possible development of respiratory distress, are the most consistent signs and symptoms of RRP in children. In the absence of severe respiratory distress, a careful history should be obtained. Information regarding the time of onset of symptoms, possible airway trauma including a history of previous intubation, and characteristics of the cry are, obviously, important. Hoarseness, although a common and often benign clinical complaint in young children, always indicates some abnormality of structure or function. Because of the precision of laryngeal mechanics, hoarseness may result from a remarkably small lesion and thus be an early sign in the course of a disease process. On the other hand, if the lesion's origin is remote from the vocal cords, hoarseness may present as a late sign. Although histologically the same lesion, a papilloma that produces hoarseness in one patient may produce stridor and obstruction in another, depending on the size and location of the lesion. The quality of the voice change may give only limited clues to its etiology, while other characteristics such as age of onset, rate of progression, associated infection, history of trauma or surgery, and the presence of respiratory or cardiac distress may be of much greater significance. A low-pitched, coarse, fluttering voice suggests a subglottic lesion, whereas a high-pitched, cracking voice; aphonia; or a breathy voice suggests a glottic lesion. Associated high-pitched stridor also suggests a glottic or subglottic lesion. Although stridor that has been present since birth is more often associated with laryngomalacia, subglottic stenosis, vocal cord paralysis, or a vascular ring, it should be realized that neonates can also present with papillomatosis. Associated symptoms such as feeding difficulties, allergic symptoms, vocal abuse, and the presence of hereditary congenital anomalies may help distinguish RRP from alternative diagnoses, including vocal fold nodules, vocal fold paralysis, subglottic cysts, subglottic hemangioma, and subglottic stenosis. In the absence of any history suggesting these lesions, review of the perinatal period may reveal a history of maternal or paternal condylomata. If the onset of stridor and dysphonia is gradual and progressive over weeks or months, neoplastic growth compromising the airway must be considered and investigated.

Certainly, not every child with a hoarse voice or cry merits investigation beyond an assessment of the symptom. However, in the presence of hoarseness with respiratory distress, tachypnea, decreased air entry, tachycardia, cyanosis dysphagia, chronic cough, failure to thrive, recurrent pneumonia, or dysphagia, the larynx must be visualized, and a firm diagnosis of the cause of hoarseness must be made. Any child with slowly progressive hoarseness merits investigation, and the clinician should not wait until total aphonia or airway problems occur.

Physical examination. Children presenting with symptoms consistent with RRP must undergo a thorough and organized physical examination. The child's respiratory rate and degree of distress must be assessed first. The physician should observe the child for tachypnea or the onset of fatigue that may indicate impending respiratory collapse. The child should be observed for flaring of the nasal ala and the use of accessory neck or chest muscles. Increasing cyanosis and air hunger may cause the child to sit with the neck hyperextended in an attempt to improve airflow. If a child is gravely ill, additional examination should not be undertaken outside the operating room (OR), the emergency room, or the intensive care unit, where resuscitation equipment for intubation of the airway, endoscopic evaluation, and possible tracheotomy are readily available. In the stable, well-oxygenated child additional examination can proceed. The most important part of the examination is auscultation with the aid of a stethoscope. The physician should listen over the nose, open mouth, neck, and chest to help localize the probable site of the respiratory obstruction. The authors prefer to pull the bell off the stethoscope and listen over these areas with the open tube. The respiratory cycle, which is normally composed of a shorter inspiratory phase and a longer expiratory phase, should be observed. Stridor of a laryngeal origin is most often musical and may begin as inspiratory, but progresses to biphasic with worsening airway narrowing. Infants with stridor should be placed in various positions to elicit any changes in the stridor. A child with RRP would not be expected to demonstrate much change in the stridor with position change, in contrast to infants with laryngomalacia, a vascular ring, or a mediastinal mass. Pulse oximetry can add an accurate quantitative analysis of the child's respiratory state. In the stable patient in whom asthma is a likely diagnosis, pulmonary function testing combined with arterial blood gas evaluation may also be helpful.

Airway endoscopy. The preoperative diagnosis of RRP is best made with a flexible fiberoptic nasopharyngoscope. Careful, sequential inspection of the pharynx, hypopharynx, larynx, and subglottis provides the critical information necessary to make the diagnosis of RRP and allows estimation of lumen size, vocal cord mobility, and the urgency of operative intervention. Advances in instrumentation of flexible nasopharyngoscopes have resulted in instruments as small as 1.9 mm in diameter that allow passage in even the smallest newborns. Even the smallest-diameter scopes provide images that can be seen on a video monitor and recorded for later review. Topical decongestion and local anesthesia can be applied by spray, dropper, or pledget. Oxymetazoline is the decongestant of choice because of its lack of cardiac side effects. Either topical tetracaine or lidocaine may be used to enhance patient cooperation, but the dosage must be critically monitored in the young infant to avoid cardiotoxicity.

Most clinicians find that visualization with the flexible nasopharyngoscope is far superior to that obtained with indirect mirror laryngoscopy in young children. However, patient cooperation is required even with good topical anesthesia. In infants, this is not a large issue because they can easily be restrained in a sitting-up position in the parent's or nurse's lap for evaluation. Likewise, most children older than 6 or 7 years of age can be "talked into" cooperating for the examination. It is patients in the intermediate age group, between 1 and 6 years of age, who may be the most difficult to examine, taxing the patience and skill of even the most experienced clinicians. Although dynamic evaluation is be appreciated when children are spontaneously breathing, endoscopy in the OR under anesthesia is warranted in any child suspected to have RRP who cannot be fully examined in the outpatient setting.

Other considerations. Children who are newly diagnosed with RRP warrant a substantial time commitment on the part of the otolaryngologist to engage the family in a frank and open discussion of the disease and its management. Support groups such as the Recurrent Respiratory Papilloma Foundation (telephone: 609-530-1443; website: www.RRPF.org) can be a vital resource for information and support. Patients with RRP require frequent office visits and endoscopic procedures at the outset to establish the aggressiveness of their disease. They are encouraged to return to the office or call as often as necessary while family members and the health care team become familiar with the child's symptoms and level of distress. While infant home intercom-type monitors are often recommended, apnea/bradycardia monitors and pulse oximetry are generally not necessary. Repeat flexible fiberoptic laryngoscopy may be used in the office setting, as well as speech and language therapy if offered early in the course of the disease. Control of other medical factors such as reflux and asthma is also aggressively pursued.

Surgical Management

Classic management. No single modality has consistently been shown to be effective in eradication of RRP. The current standard of care is surgical therapy with a goal of complete removal of papillomas and preservation of normal structures. In patients in whom anterior or posterior commissure disease or highly aggressive papillomas are present, the goal my be subtotal removal with clearing of the airway. It is advisable to "debulk" as much disease as possible while preserving normal morphological appearance and anatomy and preventing the complications of subglottic and glottic stenosis, web formation, and a diminished airway.

The CO_2 laser has been favored over cold instruments in the treatment of RRP involving the larynx, pharynx, upper trachea, and nasal and oral cavities.[4] When coupled to an operating microscope, the laser vaporizes the lesions with precision, causing minimal bleeding. When used with a no-touch technique, it minimizes damage to the vocal cords and limits scarring. The CO_2 laser has an emission wave length of 10,600 nm and converts light to thermal energy. It provides a controlled destruction of tissues with vaporization of water. It also cauterizes tissue surfaces. The smoke plume contains water vapor and destroyed tissue material. Although the CO_2 laser allows for precision of surgery and excellent hemostasis, multiple procedures are often necessary. Frequent-interval laser laryngoscopies are recommended in an attempt to avoid tracheotomy and permit the child to develop good phonation with preservation of normal vocal cord anatomy. The newest generation of laser microspot micromanipulator enables the surgeon to use spot sizes of 250 mm at 400-mm focal length and 160 mm at 250-mm focal length. The 710 AccuSpot Sharplan laser (ESC Sharplan, Yokneam, Israel) is our current choice in management of RRP of the larynx. This unit allows direct visualization of the surgical target with elimination of the parallax problem inherent in earlier models. The AccuSpot is used in the defocused mode to debulk papilloma initially and then focus the 250 mm spot size to excise papillomas from potentially tricky areas such as near the anterior or posterior commissure and along the true vocal cords. Although the CO_2 laser is the most commonly used laser for RRP in the larynx, the KTP, as well as the Argon laser, could also be used. Papillomas that have extended down the tracheobronchial tree often require use of the KTP laser coupled to a ventilating bronchoscope for removal. Occasionally, the ventilating resectoscope can also be used in these circumstances.

Emerging technologies. The use of the CO_2 laser on the true vocal folds must be judicious, because of the potential for significant postoperative scar tissue formation from unrecognized heat transfer. To minimize the risk of scar formation in the true vocal folds, cold steel excision can be used successfully using the principles of phonomicrosurgery, submucosal infusion, and microinstrumentation. This approach may have treatment advantages over CO_2 laser surgery, especially in the adult RRP patient.[24,25] In their initial series, Zeitels and Sataloff[25] reported recurrence of papilloma in none of six adults who underwent resection for primary disease at 2 years' follow-up. Of those who presented with recurrent papillomatosis, 6 of 16 (38%) continued to have recurrence after their microflap procedure.

Recent publications have highlighted the potential benefits of newer surgical technologies in managing RRP. Bower et al.[26] evaluated the feasibility and safety of the flash pump dye laser in nine children and found good early results. McMillan et al.[27] have published preliminary results regarding their positive experience with the 585-nm pulsed dye laser in three patients. Bergler et al.[28] reported on the successful use of argon plasma coagulation to treat a 3-year-old with recalcitrant RRP.

Currently, a number of investigators are complementing and, in some cases, replacing their use of the CO_2 laser with the endoscopic microdebrider as means of quickly debulking laryngeal disease.[29] Although this technique is relatively new, with the development of smaller (<2 mm) shaver blades, it may offer the patient benefits in terms of reduced laryngeal scarring in relation to the CO_2 laser.

Surgery

Preoperative planning. Before the child enters the operating suite, the surgeon, anesthesiologist, and OR team must select the proper sizes of endotracheal tubes, laryngoscopes, and bronchoscopes and ascertain that all ancillary equipment, including telescopes, light cords, suction tips, and forceps, are available and properly functioning. The surgeon, along with the OR team, should check that all equipment used for the procedure, including the surgical microscope with appropriate size lens, the laser unit, the micromanipulator, and filtered suction and smoke evacuation units, are all properly functioning. At Children's Hospital of the King's Daughter's, the surgeon personally checks the laser for beam alignment by test-firing it before the child enters the room. Laser safety is carefully monitored in our institution by the Laser Safety Committee, which includes a laser safety officer, a physician for each specialty that uses the laser, nurses from the OR, a hospital administrator, and a biomedical engineer. All OR personnel are required to wear eye protection whenever working around the laser. It is required that specially designed laser masks be worn by OR personnel during the surgery to prevent the inhalation of viral particles liberated during the laser procedure.

Before the institution of any anesthesia, the surgeon should discuss the disease with the anesthesiologist. In addition, the staff within the OR should also be informed of the surgeon's concerns so that appropriate instrumentation is ready. Intraoperative teamwork is enhanced with the availability of video monitors during the operation because this allows the entire OR staff to follow the operation as it progresses. Dialogue between the surgeon and the anesthesiologist continues throughout the procedure regarding the current status of ventilation, the amount of bleeding encountered, the motion of the vocal cords, the timing of laser use in conjunction with respiration, and the concentration of oxygen in the anesthesia mix. The ultimate decision about the technique of anesthesia should be shared between the anesthesiologist and the surgeon when an endotracheal tube is being used. The smallest possible laser-safe endotracheal tube should be used that allows for adequate ventilation. If a cuffed tube is necessary, the cuff should be filled with saline so that, if it is inadvertently struck by the laser beam, the saline acts as a heat sink and fire extinguisher. Some surgeons prefer to use methylene blue–colorized saline to provide an additional warning in case the cuff is penetrated. The laser-ignited airway explosion is a shocking emergency. Prompt, appropriate management is facilitated if the OR team has previously "rehearsed" and discussed this potential disaster.

Operative technique. After informed consent has been obtained from the appropriate family members, including a discussion regarding potential laser complications, the child is brought back into an OR that has been prepared and inspected by the surgeon and the laser team. When performing surgery for RRP, it is advisable to have an experienced team of OR nurses who are familiar with the sequence in which equipment is used and instructed in the proper use of the laser. In our facility we also have a laser safety team and provide yearly updates for the OR staff to ensure everyone's familiarity with the equipment and its potential complications. All of our pediatric anesthesiologists are familiar and comfortable with microlaryngoscopy laser surgery in children. However, in a non-pediatric hospital or nonacademic setting, if there are only one or two anesthesiologists who are experienced with these techniques, they should be exclusively used whenever possible. This type of surgery is not well suited to the novice surgeon, anesthesiologist, or OR nurse. It is our practice to insist that the attending anesthesiologist be present and involved "hands-on" with all critical portions of the surgical procedure, including induction, securing of the endotracheal tube, positioning of the patient, changing of anesthesia techniques from a laser-safe tube to apnea technique, and extubation.

In our facility the laser team consists of a scrub nurse, a circulating nurse, and a laser nurse. The laser is the responsibility of the laser nurse, allowing the circulator and scrub nurses to concentrate on their duties. All OR personnel are equipped with micropore laser filtration masks and approved goggles. The room is set up in advance with a suspension microlaryngoscope (Lindholm, Karl Storz Endoscopy-America, Culver City, CA), a full set of Parson's laryngoscopes (Karl Storz Endoscopy-America), two appropriately sized ventilating bronchoscopes, and 7200A and 8700A Hopkins Rod telescopes (Karl Storz Endoscopy-America). A microscope with a 400-mm lens is fitted with the AccuSpot 710 micromanipulator. An assortment of suctions, alligator forceps, cup forceps, and light cords, as well as a pack of "neuro-patties" and topical Neo-Synephrine, is also standard. An endoscopy video cart equipped with color TV monitor, video cassette recorder, three-chip camera, and Xenon light source are also used. Still photography through the endoscope is also available as needed. In addition, a pediatric tracheotomy set is brought into the room, although the pack is not opened.

The surgical sequence begins with the mask induction using halothane and the establishment of intravenous (IV) access. Dexamethasone 0.5 mg/kg and cefazolin 20 mg/kg are routinely administered preoperatively. The larynx is exposed using the Parson's laryngoscope attached to 6 L/min of oxygen flow through its insufflation port, and the vocal folds are sprayed with 2% lidocaine using a syringe attached to a Cass needle. A diagnostic laryngoscopy is performed using the 7200A telescope under video control to assess the degree of papilloma disease and its encroachment on the laryngeal airway. Depending on the extent of disease, the child's history and the interval since the previous endoscopy, a full tracheoscopy and bronchoscopy may also be performed. Again, depending on the child's level of preoperative and operative distress, the surgeon may choose to perform this maneuver with either the 7200A telescope (if there is a low likelihood of discovering distal disease) or with an appropriately sized ventilating bronchoscope (if there is high likelihood of discovering distal disease). Still photography with the 8700A telescope is performed at this stage, if desirable. If no distal disease is present, the trachea may be intubated by the surgeon with a laser-safe tube (metal Xomed-Treace, Medtronics, Minneapolis, MN) of the smallest caliber that will allow the anesthesiologist to provide adequate ventilation. Once the airway has been secured with the endotracheal tube, the anesthesiologist is given the option to administer muscle relaxants. As an alternative, the child may be maintained on a regimen of propofol. It should be emphasized that no muscle relaxants are administered until the surgeon has assessed the degree of laryngeal obstruction and ascertained that the airway has been secured. This precaution serves to prevent the situation in which the child has lost his or her respiratory drive and airway obstruction results from the presence of papilloma, blood, or mucus, precipitating hypoxia and a possible laryngospasm. Once the airway has been secured, the endotracheal tube is taped in place with a single piece of tape (allowing the surgeon easy access for removal of the endotracheal tube in the case of an airway fire) and the child suspended for microlaryngoscopy with the Lindholm microlaryngoscope. I prefer to suspend the Lindholm to a Mayo stand attached to the OR table. This device allows the microsuspension system to be moved along with the patient and allows angulation of the laryngoscope over a 120° range. The child's eyes are protected against any stray laser beam exposure with moist, saline-soaked gauze eye pads. Lubricant is placed in the eyes, and the operative field is draped with moistened towels. OR personnel all are equipped with ocular protection including side shields, and a sign is posted outside the OR warning that a laser procedure is occurring. A spare set of safety glasses is left outside the door for OR personnel who wish to come inside the room while the laser is in operation. Special laser masks with extremely small pores are worn to minimize exposure to the laser plume. A high-volume smoke evacuator is attached to one port of the Lindholm device to collect the laser plume. A second suction attached to the smoke evacuator is used by the surgeon. At this time, the fractional concentration of oxygen in inspired gas (FIO_2) that is delivered to the patient should be as close to a room-air mixture as possible. Ideally, the laser is not used until the oxygen in the mixture is between 26% and 30%. In selected circumstances, it may be warranted to proceed with an FIO_2 at or below 40%. These precautions are taken to minimize the possibility of a laser-induced endotracheal tube fire.

As an initial procedure, a microcup forceps is used for obtaining a biopsy specimen from the bulkiest portion of papilloma. I use the AccuSpot laser at initial settings of 4-W power, 0.1-s intervals, and repeat mode. Bulky papilloma is handled by defocusing the laser. Moistened neuro-patties are placed in the subglottis to decrease the air leak and to provide a back-stop for errant laser shots. These must be kept moist because they too can act as a source of combustion. With the laser refocused, lesions are gradually vaporized to the level of the mucosa, avoiding entry into Reinke's space and the deeper vocalis muscle. I prefer using low-power settings to limit thermal injury to the surrounding tissue, although this does result in longer operating time. A small-caliber suction device is kept close to the laser impact site to remove the hot steam of vaporization and to remove eschar. Neuro-patties soaked in Neo-Synephrine are also used for removal of eschar and debris, as well as hemostasis. The blunt tip of the suction device can also be used as a probe and retractor of the false cord, or to roll the true cord for exposure of the subglottic region. Care is taken to avoid injuring the anterior commissure, and at least 1 mm of untreated mucosa should be left in this region so that a web does not develop during the healing period. Similar considerations are taken for the posterior commissure. I normally begin the procedure with removal of papillomas in the supraglottic larynx followed by the anterior half of both true vocal cords. If disease has been noted in the posterior half of the glottis or in the subglottic region, I find that the endotracheal tube obstructs exposure to these areas of the operative field and I seek an alternative means of anesthesia. I prefer an apneic technique whereby the endotracheal tube is removed intermittently and work is performed while the patient's oxygen saturation is monitored. Another alternative would be spontaneous ventilation, although I find increased circulation of anesthesia gases into the OR with this technique to be an undesirable side effect. Many centers prefer the use of jet ventilation and sevoflurane. I have found all of these techniques to be workable. Once a decision is made to "go apneic," the anesthesiologist increases the FIO_2 to 100%. The trachea is extubated, although the child is not removed from suspension from the microlaryngoscope, and the smoke evacuation port of the Lindholm is disconnected and oxygen tubing connected to this port to flow 6 L/min of O_2. While using an apneic technique, the laser is used for 90- to 120-s intervals initially and the trachea is reintubated with a polyvinyl chloride endotracheal tube directly through the microlaryngoscope, using a stylet to stiffen the tube and improve the angulation. The CO_2 and O_2 levels are closely monitored, and the duration of "laser-on" time is adjusted appropriately. Typically, the lungs are reoxygenated for the same period of time that they were apneic before proceeding with the next cycle.

Since there is currently no therapeutic regimen that reliably eradicates the HPV, when there is a question about whether papilloma in an area must be removed, it is prudent to accept some residual papilloma rather than risking damage to normal tissue and producing excessive scarring. Even with the removal of all clinically evident papilloma, latent virus may remain in adjacent tissue, which may explain the recurrent nature of RRP.[13] Therefore, the aim of therapy in extensive disease should be to reduce the tumor burden, decrease the spread of disease, create a safe and patent airway, improve voice quality, and increase the time interval between surgical procedures. Staged papilloma removal for disease in the anterior commissure is appropriate to prevent the apposition of two raw mucosal surfaces. The surgeon who is not aware of injury to deeper tissue layers with injudicious laser usage may encounter unacceptable scarring and subsequent abnormal vocal fold function. Inappropriate and aggressive use of the laser may also cause injury to unaffected tissues and create an environment suitable for implantation of viral particles. Use of CO_2 laser can also result in delayed local tissue damage, which may be related to the total number of laser surgeries and the severity of RRP disease.

At the end of the procedure, the trachea is reintubated with a standard endotracheal tube using a Selinger technique to avoid any difficulty in re-establishing the airway on removal of the Lindholm microlaryngoscope. The trachea is then extubated only when the child is fully awake. High humidity and, occasionally, racemic epinephrine are administered postoperatively in the recovery room. The patient is closely monitored for several hours before discharge, and often an overnight stay in a monitored bed unit is necessary. As a general rule, the more extensive the papilloma disease and the more compromised the airway, the more important it is for the child to be monitored postoperatively in an intensive care or step-down unit. Additional doses of steroids can be administered at 6-hour intervals if needed while continuous pulse oximetry is mandatory.

Another anesthetic alternative is the use of jet ventilation for microsurgery of the larynx. Jet ventilation eliminates the potential fire hazard of the endotracheal tube and allows good visualization of the vocal cords. A limitation of this technique is the possibility of transmission of HPV particles into the distal airway. The jet cannula can be placed either above or below the vocal cords; each has its own particular benefit. I prefer placement of the cannula proximal to the end of the laryngoscope to decrease the risk of possible pneumothorax or pneumomediastinum. With large laryngeal lesions, narrowed airways, and ball-valve lesions, there may develop a high degree of outflow obstruction, which could lead to increased intrathoracic pressure and a subsequent pneumothorax. This may also result if there is inadequate muscle relaxation. Jet ventilation also requires constant communication between the operating surgeon and the anesthesiologist. Excessive mucosal drying and damage can occur, as can insufflation of air into the stomach with gastric distention. As mentioned, there is also the potential risk of disseminating papilloma or blood into the tracheobronchial tree.

Postoperative care. Children with stable papilloma disease requiring fewer than four laser procedures per year and whose parents reliably bring them in before they show signs of respiratory distress can be monitored at home with commercially available infant home intercom-type monitors. Those with rapidly reforming papillomas and those whose parents wait until the child is in distress before seeking medical attention may warrant home pulse oximetry with frequent home health care visits. Children with RRP are encouraged to return to the office or call as often as necessary. I give their parents "carte blanche" within my practice and explain to them that their children have a special problem which allows them access to speak with the doctors and nurses and show up unexpectedly at the office whenever they believe their child is in need. I have yet to experience a family that has abused this privilege; on the contrary, it has enhanced their trust in the health care team and has averted urgent and emergent laser procedures.

Staging

It is helpful, when tracking the progression of a child's disease, communicating with other surgeons, and treating patients in a protocol format, to have a surgical scoring system to assess severity and clinical course of RRP disease. Although several scoring and staging systems have been proposed, clinicians and researchers have not yet adopted a uniformly acceptable nomenclature for describing RRP lesions that is simple, yet comprehensive.

This has created confusion in the RRP literature and in physician-to-physician communications regarding patients' response to therapies. In addition, the absence of a universally accepted staging system has hampered our abilities to accurately report the results of adjuvant therapies or document the natural course of the disease. We have proposed a new severity and staging system for RRP (Fig. 3) in a format that incorporates the best qualities of the existing systems by numerically grading the extent of papillomatosis at defined aerodigestive sub-sites, assesses functional parameters, diagrammatically catalogues subsite involvement, and assigns a final numerical score to the patient's current extent of disease.[30] Using software designed at the University of Washington (Seattle, WA) and licensed to the American Society of Pediatric Otolaryngology, this staging system is currently computerized and available to pediatric otolaryngologists and bronchoesophagologists to allow them to objectively and subjectively measure an individual patient's clinical course and response to therapy over time. Encryption technology with this software offers promise to allow clinicians from around the world to anonymously share patient data to enhance our knowledge of this disease and promote multi-institutional investigations.

Adjuvant Treatment Modalities

Although surgical management remains the mainstay therapy for RRP, ultimately, as many a 10% of patients with the disease require some form of adjuvant therapy. The most widely adopted criteria for initiating adjuvant therapy are a surgery requirement of more than four procedures per year, distal multisite spread of disease, and/or rapid regrowth of papilloma disease with airway compromise. The most commonly recommended adjuvant therapy is α-interferon.[4] The exact mechanism by which interferon elicits its response is unknown. It appears to modulate host immune response by increasing production of a protein kinase and endonuclease that in-

PATIENT INITIALS:_____ DATE OF SURGERY________ SURGEON__________________

PATIENT ID#_____________________ INSTITUTION_____________________________

1. How long since the last papilloma surgery? _______days _______weeks _______months _______years _______don't know _______this is the child's first surgery

2. Counting today's surgery, how many papilloma surgeries in the past 12 months? ____________
3. Describe the patient's voice today:
normal______(0) abnormal_____(1) aphonic_____(2)
4. Describe the patient's stridor today:
absent______(0) present with activity______(1) present at rest____(2)
5. Describe the urgency of today's intervention:
scheduled___(0) elective___(1) urgent___(2) emergent_____(3)
6. Describe today's level of respiratory distress:
none_____(0) mild_____(1) Mod___(2) severe____(3) extreme____(4)
Total score of questions 3-6 = ___________

FOR EACH SITE, SCORE AS: 0 = None, 1 = surface lesion, 2 = raised lesion, 3 = bulky lesion

LARYNX
Epiglottis
Lingual surface_______ Laryngeal surface_______
Aryepiglottic folds: Right_____ Left____
False vocal cords: Right_____ Left____
True vocal cords: Right_____ Left____
Arytenoids: Right_____ Left____
Anterior commissure_________ Posterior commissure_________
Subglottis ________

TRACHEA:
Upper one-third ___________
Middle one-third ___________
Lower one-third ___________
Bronchi: Right_______ Left_______
Tracheotomy stoma ___________

OTHER:
Nose ______
Palate ______
Pharynx ______
Esophagus _____
Lungs ______
Other ______

TOTAL SCORE ALL SITES: __________ TOTAL CLINICAL SCORE: ____________

Fig. 3. Coltrera/Derkay staging and severity scheme.

hibits viral protein synthesis. Interferons are a class of proteins manufactured by cells in response to a variety of stimuli, including viral infection. The enzymes that are produced block the viral replication of RNA and DNA and alter cell membranes to make them less susceptible to viral penetration.

Common interferon side effects fall into two categories: acute reactions (fever and generalized flulike symptoms, chills, headache, myalgias, and nausea that seem to decrease with prolonged therapy) and chronic reactions (decrease in the growth rate of the child, elevation of liver transaminase levels, leukopenia spastic diplegia, and febrile seizures). Thrombocytopenia has been reported, as have rashes, dry skin, alopecia, generalized pruritus, and fatigue. Acetaminophen has been found to effectively relieve the fevers, and interferon injections are best tolerated at bedtime. Interferon produced by recombinant DNA techniques appears to have fewer side effects and better efficacy than blood bank–harvested interferon. Therapy is initiated at 5 million units/m^2 body surface area administered by subcutaneous injection on a daily basis for 28 days, then 3 days per week for at least a 6-month trial. After 6 months in children with excellent responses, and if side effects are severe, the dosage can be decreased to 3 million units/m^2 administered 3 days per week with further slow weaning as tolerated.

Photodynamic therapy (PDT) in the treatment of RRP has been studied extensively at Long Island Jewish Hospital (New York, NY) by Shikowtiz et al.[31] PDT is based on the transfer of energy to a photograph-sensitive drug. The original drug used was dihematoporphyrin ether (DHE), which has a tendency to concentrate within papillomas to a greater degree than in surrounding normal tissue. Patients are typically treated intravenously with 4.25 mg/kg DHE before photoactivation with argon pump dye laser. A small but statistically significant decrease in RRP growth, especially in patients with the most severe disease, was seen with the use of PDT and DHE. The drawback of this therapy is that patients become markedly photograph sensitive for periods lasting 2 to 8 weeks. A new drug, m-tetra (hydroxyphenyl) chlorine (Foscan®), has shown efficacy in HPV-induced tumors in rabbits with minimal tissue damage and less photograph sensitivity. A clinical trial using this drug at a dose of 0.15 mg/kg is currently under way. The preliminary results in adults are encouraging, and children have been added to the protocol.

Recent interest has focused on chemically pure indole-3-carbinol (I3C), a non–U.S. Food and Drug Administration (FDA)–approved dietary supplement, which has been shown to inhibit papilloma formation in mice.[32] This compound is found in high concentration in cruciferous vegetables such as cabbage, broccoli, and cauliflower. A small dietary study at Long Island Jewish Hospital showed promise, although there were concerns regarding how much active drug the patients were actually receiving. The supplement I3C is currently available in pure chemical form, and a current trial is ongoing at the University of Pittsburgh (Pittsburgh, PA). There are concerns regarding whether the pure I3C will maintain its effectiveness when taken with antacids or histamine type 2 (H_2) blockers. A new product, Indoplex, available in capsule form or as flavored sprinkles, is purported to overcome this limitation. Preliminary data suggest a linear relationship between the ratio of estrogen metabolism pathways (2-hydroxylation:16 α-hydroxylation) and the severity of RRP disease. Ratios of less than 1 are associated with severe disease, and those of greater than 3 are associated with mild disease. Rosen et al.[33] reported preliminary results in 18 children who were treated with pure I3C, demonstrating safety and efficacy, with 6 patients sharing a complete response, 6 a partial response, and 6 no response.

Ribavirin is an antiviral drug, which is used to treat respiratory syncytial virus pneumonia in infants, that has also shown promise in the treatment of aggressive laryngeal papillomatosis. McGlennen et al.[34] at the University of Minnesota (Minneapolis) have recently completed a small trial in eight patients using ribavirin in an oral form at 23 mg/kg per day divided four times daily after an initial IV loading dose, showing an increase in surgical interval in those who were treated.

An antiviral treatment that has been advocated in the treatment of RRP is acyclovir. Although the activity of acyclovir depends on the presence of virally encoded thymidine kinase, an enzyme that is not known to be encoded by papillomavirus, conflicting clinical results have been obtained in several small series. Theoretically, it would not be expected to have a positive effect. However, it has been postulated that perhaps acyclovir is most effective when there are co-disease factors such as a simultaneous infection with herpes simplex virus. Such viral co-infections with herpes simplex virus type 1, cytomegalovirus, and Epstein-Barr virus have been demonstrated in both adult[35] and pediatric[36] RRP patients. Adult patients with viral co-infections appear to have a more aggressive clinical course.

Two recent reports have stimulated interest in the intralesional injection of cidofovir (Vistide®) (s)-1-(3-hydroxy-2-phosphonylmethoxypropyl)cytosine [HPMPC]), a drug currently FDA approved for use for patients with human immunodeficiency virus (HIV) who have cytomegalovirus-retinitis. Snoeck et al.[37] reported that 14 patients in a series of 17 patients with severe RRP who were treated with cidofovir at 2.5 mg/mL injected directly into the papilloma bed after laser surgery experienced a complete response. Pranksy et al.[38,39] have used this therapy in 10 children with severe RRP with short-term follow-up showing a response in 10 of 10. Neither of these studies used a control group. Two open-label multisite protocols have been initiated to further study the safety and efficacy of this promising drug.

Optimal control of extraesophageal reflux disease has been advocated as a means of improving patient outcomes, along with surgical therapy. Koufman and McGuirt (personal communication, May 2000) have reported anecdotal improvements in both children and adults with RRP who are aggressively treated with H_2 blockers, proton pump inhibitors, and Nissen fundoplication. A prospective clinical evaluation is currently underway at Bowman Gray (Winston-Salem, NC) to validate this finding.

TABLE I.

RRP Task Force Practice Guidelines for Management of Children With RRP

Diagnosis and work-up

History: Persistent or progressive stridor and dysphonia, with the possible development of respiratory distress characterizes the child with newly diagnosed RRP. A maternal or paternal history of genital papilloma or abnormal pap should be sought. Associated symptoms such as feeding difficulties, allergic symptoms, vocal abuse, and a history of choking or aspiration of foreign bodies may help to distinguish RRP from other diagnoses.

Physical exam: Findings are dependent on site and size of papilloma. Note the quality of voice, presence of stridor, level of respiratory distress, use of accessory muscles of respiration, and the resting oxygen saturation. The presence of congenital anomalies such as cutaneous hemangiomas may help to distinguish RRP from other diagnoses.

Imaging: Airway fluoroscopy with barium may be helpful to rule out other diagnoses such as FB, GERD, laryngomalacia, vascular ring. No role for CT or MRI in initial diagnosis but may be helpful to follow for pulmonary extension of disease.

Endoscopy: Flexible fiberoptic laryngoscopy (FFL), (or indirect laryngoscopy in older child), is essential to make the diagnosis outside of the OR. If not technically feasible or child is in such distress that you fear that instrumenting the airway outside of the OR would be hazardous, then operative endoscopy with a rigid telescope/ventilating bronchoscope or FFL in the OR would be the alternative. Making the diagnosis (or strongly suspecting the diagnosis) before the operative procedure is desirable for facilitating the education and expectations of the family and the preparation of the anesthesiologist, surgeon, and/or nursing personnel.

Other considerations: Children newly diagnosed with RRP warrant a substantial time commitment on the part of the otolaryngologist to engage the family in a frank and open discussion of the disease and its management. Support groups such as the Recurrent Respiratory Papilloma Foundation (609-530-1443) can be a vital resource for information and support. While infant home intercom-type monitors are often recommended, apnea/bradycardia monitors and pulse oximetry are generally not necessary. Speech and language therapy is offered early in the course of the disease. Control of other medical factors such as reflux and asthma is also aggressively pursued.

Surgical management

Preparation: Room should be set up in advance and the equipment checked by the surgical team to ensure that appropriate-sized bronchoscopes and telescopes are available, suctions are of proper length to fit through bronchoscopes, video equipment functioning (desirable for education of families and to allow anesthesia and OR team to follow the progress of the surgery), microlaryngoscopes, light cables, and light sources all available. Procedure should not be performed in a facility that does not have the necessary complement of equipment to safely instrument a child's airway. CO_2 laser (when used) should be tested before the child enters the room to make sure it is functioning properly. Informed consent from the family should include discussion of possible scarring, airway edema, and airway fire with the use of the laser (at least on first visit to the OR).

Anesthesia technique: A number of acceptable techniques ranging from ventilation through a laser-safe tube with an FiO_2 of $<30\%$, to insufflation techniques using Propafol with intermittent intubation if needed, to jet-ventilation (either supraglottic or subglottic). Key is good communication between surgeon and anesthesiologist before and during the procedure so that approach is coordinated. Additional key is to use experienced anesthesiologist comfortable with managing obstructed pediatric airways. If no such individual is available, then should consider delaying the procedure or transferring the child to a facility where one is available.

Surgical technique: A number of acceptable techniques are available to the surgeon including use of the CO_2 laser, KTP/ND:Yag laser, microlaryngoscopy forceps, and powerized laryngeal shavers. New technologies that are just coming available with limited long-term follow-ups that may ultimately prove superior to standard techniques include use of the microdebriders, flash pump dye and 585-mm pulse dye lasers, argon plasma coagulation, and phonomicrosurgical resection techniques.

When there is a question about whether papilloma in an area needs to be removed, it is prudent to accept some residual papilloma rather than risk damage to normal tissue and producing excessive scarring. Even with the removal of all clinically evident papilloma, latent virus may remain in adjacent tissue, which may explain the recurrent nature RRP. Therefore, the aim of therapy in extensive disease should be to reduce the tumor burden, decrease the spread of disease, create a safe and patent airway, improve voice quality, and increase the time interval between surgical procedures. Staged papilloma removal for disease in the anterior commissure is appropriate to prevent the apposition of two raw mucosal surfaces. The surgeon who is not aware of injury to deeper tissue layers with injudicious laser use may encounter unacceptable scarring and subsequent abnormal vocal fold function. Inappropriate and aggressive use of the laser may also cause injury to nonaffected tissues and create an environment suitable for implantation of viral particles.

Biopsy: There is controversy among clinicians regarding the need to send a tissue biopsy with each papilloma surgery. It is our recommendation that a biopsy specimen be sent at the time of the initial diagnosis of RRP. HPV-typing may be performed at that time though its value in terms of predicting prognosis is currently limited. Subsequent surgeries should have specimens sent for monitoring of progression to atypia and malignant transformation to SCCA. Additional HPV-typing would only seem to be needed if there is a significant clinical change (surgical interval shortens substantially, new onset of spread to an extra-laryngeal site). In children who require frequent surgeries, it would certainly seem reasonable to send specimens with every other or every third surgery. An additional benefit that may be derived from serial biopsies is the opportunity to study the archival tissue in the future for clues to prognosis using techniques or markers not currently available.

Documentation: It is highly desirable to have a consistent staging and severity scale to follow progression of RRP disease. A computerized tracking system developed by Coltrera and soon to be available in CD-ROM format through an ASPO grant should simplify this problem by standardizing the nomenclature for describing RRP. This system is ideally suited for tracking results of clinical trials of adjuvant therapies and for physician-to-physician communications.

Follow-up: Individualized follow-up needs to be arranged between the families and their doctors. Circumstances that would influence the timing and location of this follow-up would include the travel distance to the medical center, the reliability of the family and the reliability of their transportation, the rapidity at which the papillomas recur, and the degree of airway compromise caused by the papillomas. An acceptable regimen might include monthly follow-up in the office in the first year of disease diagnosis with FFL performed every-other-month and whenever the clinical situation warrants with follow-up extended to every 2–4 months in subsequent years in a local child with stable disease with reliable transportation and guardians. Surgical intervention would then be planned according to clinical needs. In contrast, a family that lives quite a distance from the hospital might be scheduled for interval operating room exams once a pattern of recurrence has been established with use of e-mail or phone contact between the surgeon and the family to monitor the clinical situation between surgeries.

Adjuvant therapy: The decision to embark on adjuvant therapy should also be individualized and based on the frequency of surgical interventions, the morbidity of frequent surgeries, and the recurrence pattern of the papillomas. A basic rule of thumb to follow would suggest the need for adjuvant therapies if surgery is being required more frequently than four times a year for 2 years or if the papillomas begin spreading outside of the endolarynx. Additionally, children who present with disease in their trachea should have early consideration for adjuvant therapy.

Choice of therapy depends on informed consent and evidence-based research. Ideally, patients should be enrolled in clinical studies whenever possible.

Adjuvant therapies currently recommended would include:

Recombinant Interferon alpha-N2 administered initially at 5 million units per meter squared body surface area by subcutaneous injection daily for 30 days and then three times weekly for at least a 6-month trial. The dose can be reduced to 3 million units/m^2 three times a week if side effects are severe. Weaning should be slow to prevent a rebound effect. Reinstitution of therapy after discontinuation has been shown to be effective. Children under the age of a year should be monitored for the possibility of spastic diplegia and should have a baseline neurologic exam. Children on chronic interferon therapy need to have their liver enzymes and leukocytes monitored on at least a quarterly basis.

Indole-3-carbinol, a derivative of cruciferous vegetables, has been shown to alter the growth of papilloma in mice by altering estrogen metabolism. The National Toxicology Program at the National Institute of Environmental Health Sciences has recently embarked on a toxicology testing program to certify its safety. A large scale, multi-institutional trial based at University of Pittsburgh is still enrolling new patients using chemically pure I3C.

Photodynamic therapy is currently being investigated at LIJ in a study headed by Abramson and Shikowitz. Preliminary studies using DHE showed promise in reducing surgical intervals but photosensitivity limited its usefulness. The present study using Foscan has shown early promise with minimal tissue damage and less photosensitivity.

Cidofovir (Vistide) has demonstrated promise in clinical series from San Diego and Belgium in adults and children with aggressive RRP disease. This drug, which is approved for use in HIV patients with CMV retinitis, is designed to be injected into the papilloma bed after debulking surgery. This has prompted interest in pursuing a multi-institutional open trial. The protocol for the open trial is being formulated currently and will likely include an arm for children with severe disease as well as a randomized, placebo-controlled arm for children with newly diagnosed papilloma. An ASPO grant and support from the Gilead Pharmaceutical company are being sought to administer the study. A multi-institutional safety study is also in the process of development.

Reflux: Preliminary data from Bowman Gray (Cummins and Koufman) and Great Britain (Harcourt et al) suggests that achieving optimal control of gastro-esophageal reflux disease may have significant benefits in children with laryngeal papillomas. It would seem prudent to investigate and control reflux in RRP patients while this relationship is studied further.

RRP = recurrent respiratory papillomatosis; FB = foreign body; GERD = gastroesophageal reflux disease; CT = computed tomography; MRI = magnetic resonance imaging; HPV = human papilloma virus; SCCA = squamous cell carcinoma; ASPO = American Society of Pediatric Otolaryngology; LIJ = Long Island Jewish; DHE = dihematoporphyrin ether; CMV = cytomegalovirus.

Recurrent Respiratory Papillomatosis Registry and Task Force Initiatives

It should be emphasized that participation in national and regional protocols of adjuvant treatment modalities is essential for the scientific community to learn more about RRP. A national registry of patients with RRP has been formed through the cooperation of the American Society of Pediatric Otolaryngology and the CDC.[7] The registry currently tracks nearly 600 children at 22 sites with data on more than 11,000 surgical procedures. It is hoped that the national registry will aid in the identification of patients who are suitable for enrollment in multi-institutional studies of adjuvant therapies and will better define the risk factors for transmission of HPV and the cofactors that may determine the aggressiveness of RRP. The Recurrent Respiratory Papilloma Task Force has been formed, which is made up of the principal investigators at each of the registry sites, to facilitate research initiatives. The Task Force has recently completed a set of Practice Guidelines (Table I) to help guide the clinician in the diagnosis and management of children with RRP. The Task Force is currently working on establishing an RRP Tissue Bank, coordinating a multicenter cidofovir clinical trial, facilitating an interleukin investigation, and distributing the RRP staging software through the American Society of Pediatric Otolaryngology.

CONCLUSION

1. Recurrent respiratory papillomatosis is a frustrating, capricious disease with the potential for morbid consequences because of its involvement of the airway and the risk of malignant degeneration.
2. The goals of surgical therapy are to maintain a safe airway with a serviceable voice while avoiding excessive scarring.
3. No single modality of therapy has been consistently shown to be effective in eradicating RRP. When children are requiring laser therapy more frequently than 6 times in 12 months or have evidence of distal spread of RRP outside the larynx, adjuvant medical therapy should be considered.
4. Many adjuvant therapies have been investigated to supplement surgical therapy. These range from dietary supplements and control of extraesophageal reflux disease to potent antiviral and chemotherapeutic agents and photograph-dynamic therapies. Although several of these modalities have shown promise, no adjuvant therapy to date has "cured" RRP.
5. Strides are being made in learning more about the natural history of the disease. A registry of RRP patients at the CDC has been established, and software to help clinicians share information on and accurately follow their patients with RRP has been developed.
6. Future research is needed regarding prevention of transmission of HPV from mother to child. Specifically, the roles of cesarean section and gynecological surgery during pregnancy must be elucidated. Development of an HPV vaccine and refinements in surgical techniques to minimize laryngeal scarring also must be studied.
7. Surgical therapy for RRP requires a skilled team consisting of otolaryngologists, anesthesia providers, and OR personnel working together in a facility properly equipped to manage difficult pediatric airways. Whenever possible, use the most experienced pediatric-trained anesthesiologist and OR staff available.
8. Check your laser and bronchoscopic equipment before the operation. Make certain that your OR staff understands and practices laser precautions for the patient as well as themselves.
9. Because of the recurrent nature of papilloma disease and the potential for airway obstruction, parental support and education can be invaluable to the safety of the child with RRP.

BIBLIOGRAPHY

1. Morgan AH, Zitsch RP. Recurrent respiratory papillomatosis in children: a retrospective study of management and complications. *Ear Nose Throat J* 1986;65:19–28.
2. Mounts P, Shah KV, Kashima H. Viral etiology of juvenile and adult onset squamous papilloma of the larynx. *Proc Natl Acad Sci U S A* 1982;79:5425–5429.
3. Cohn AM, Kos JT, Taber LH, Adam E. Recurring laryngeal papilloma. *Am J Otolaryngol* 1981;2:129–5429.
4. Derkay CS. Task force on recurrent respiratory papillomas. *Arch Otolaryngol Head Neck Surg* 1995;121:1386–1391.
5. Kashima H, Shah F, Lyles A, et al. Factors in juvenile-onset and adult onset recurrent respiratory papillomas. *Laryngoscope* 1992;102:9–13.
6. Shah KV, Stern WF, Shaf PK, Bishai D, Kashima H. Risk factors for juvenile-onset recurrent respiratory papillomatosis. *Pediatr Infect Dis J* 1998;17:372–376.
7. Armstrong LR, Derkay CS, Reeves WC. Initial results from the National Registry for juvenile-onset recurrent respiratory papillomatosis. *Arch Otolaryngol Head Neck Surg,* 1999;125:743–748.
8. Rimell FL, Shoemaker DL, Pou AM, Jordan JA, Post CJ, Ehrlich GD. Pediatric respiratory papillomatosis: prognostic role of viral subtyping and cofactors. *Laryngoscope* 1997;107:915–918.
9. Rihkaren H, Aaltonen LM, Syranen SM. Human papillomavirus in laryngeal papillomas and in adjacent normal epithelium. *Clin Otolaryngol* 1993;18:470–474.
10. Koutsky LA, Wolner-Hanssen P. Genital papillomavirus infection: current knowledge and future prospects. *Obstet Gynecol Clin North Am* 1989;16:541–561.
11. Ho, GYF, Bierman R, Beardsley L, Chang CJ, Burk RD. Natural history of cervicovaginal papillomavirus infection in young women. *N Engl J Med* 1998;338:423–428.
12. Bennett RS, Powell KR. Human papillomavirus: association between laryngeal papillomas and genital warts. *Pediatr Infect Dis J* 1987;6:229–232.
13. Kashima H, Mounts P, Leventhal B, Hruban RH. Sites of predilection in recurrent respiratory papillomatosis. *Ann Otol Rhinol Laryngol* 1993;102:580–583.
14. Cummins MM, Koufman JA. Reflux and recurrent laryngeal papillomas. 2000 (submitted).15. Lindeberg H, Elbrond O. Laryngeal papillomas: the epidemiology in a Danish subpopulation: 1965–1984. *Clin Otolaryngol* 1991;15:125–131.
16. Puranen M, Yliskoski M, Saarikoski S, Syrjanen K, Syrjanen S. Vertical transmission of human papillomavirus from infected mothers to their newborn babies and persistence of the virus in childhood. *Am J Obstet Gynecol* 1996;174: 694–699.
17. Smith EM, Johnson SR, Pignaari S, Cripe TP, Turek L.

Perinatal vertical transmission of human papilloma virus and subsequent development of respiratory tract papillomatosis. *Ann Otol Rhinol Laryngol* 1991;100:479–483.

18. Tseng C, Liang C, Soong Y, Pao C. Perinatal transmission of human papillomavirus in infants: relationship between rate and mode of delivery. *Obstet Gynecol* 1998;91:92–96.
19. Shah K, Kashima H, Polk BF, Shah F, Asbbey H, Abramson A. Rarity of caesarean delivery in cases of juvenile-onset respiratory papillomatosis. *Obstet Gynecol* 1986;68: 795–799.
20. Tenti P, Zappatore R, Migliora P, Spinillo A, Belloni C, Carnevalli L. Perinatal transmission of human papillomavirus from gravidas with latest infections. *Obstet Gynecol* 1999;93:475–479.
21. Kosko J, Derkay CS. Role of caesarean section in the prevention of recurrent respiratory papillomas: is there one? *Int J Pediatr Otolaryngol* 1996;1:31–38.
22. Shapiro AM, Rimmel FL, Shoemaker D, Pou A, Stool S. Tracheotomy in children with juvenile-onset recurrent respiratory papillomatosis: the Children's Hospital of Pittsburgh experience. *Am Otol Rhinol Laryngol* 1996;105:1–5.
23. Cole RR, Myer CM, Cotton RT. Tracheotomy in children with recurrent respiratory papillomatosis. *Head Neck* 1989;11: 226–230.
24. Dean C, Sataloff RT, Hawkshaw M. Recurrent vocal fold papilloma: resection using cold instruments. *Ear Nose Throat J* 1998;77:882–884.
25. Zeitels SM, Sataloff RT. Phono-microsurgical resection of glottal papillomatosis. *J Voice* 1999;13:123–127.
26. Bower CM, Wanes M, Flock S, Schaeffer R. Flash pump bye laser treatment of laryngeal papillomas. *Ann Otol Rhinol Laryngeal* 1998;107:1001–1005.
27. McMillan K, Shapshay SM, McGilligan JA, Wang Z, Rebeiz E. A 585 nm meter pulsed dye laser treatment of laryngeal papillomas: preliminary report. *Laryngoscope* 1998;108:968–22.
28. Bergler W, Honig M, Gotte K, Petroianu G, Hormann K. Treatment of recurrent respiratory papillomatosis with argon plasma coagulation. *J Laryngol Otol* 1997;111: 381–384.
29. Myer CM, Wiliging P, Cotton R. Use of a laryngeal microresector system. *Laryngoscope* 1999;109:1165–1166.
30. Derkay CS, Malis DJ, Zalzal G, Wiatrak BJ, Kashima H, Coltrera M. A staging system for assessing severity of disease and response to therapy in recurrent respiratory papillomatosis. *Laryngoscope* 1998;108:935–937.
31. Shikowitz MJ, Abramson AL, Freeman K, Steinberg BM, Nouri M. Efficacy of DHE photodynamic therapy for respiratory papillomatosis: immediate and long-term results. *Laryngoscope* 1998;108:962–967.
32. Newfield L, Goldsmith A, Bradlow HL, Auborn K. Estrogen metabolism and human papillomavirus-induced tumors of the larynx: chemo-prophylaxis with indole-3-carbinol. *Anticancer Res* 1993;13:337–341.
33. Rosen CA, Woodson GE, Thompson JW, Hengesteg AP, Bradlow HL. Preliminary results of the use of indole-3-carbinol for recurrent respiratory papillomatosis. *Otolaryngol Head Neck Surg* 1998;118:810–815.
34. McGlennen RC, Adams GL, Lewis CM, Faras AJ, Ostrow RS. Pilot trial of ribavirin for the treatment of laryngeal papillomatosis. *Head Neck* 1993;15:504–512.
35. Pou AM, Rimell FL, Jordan JA, et al. Adult respiratory papillomatosis: human papillomavirus type and viral confections as predictors of prognosis. *Am Otol Rhinol Laryngol* 1195;104:758–762.
36. Stanley JJ, Robinson RA, Post JC, Ehrlich GD, Smith RJH. Viral confections in pediatric respiratory papillomatosis. *Arch Oto-HNS* 2001 (*in press*).
37. Snoeck R, Wellens W, Desloovere C, et al. Treatment of severe laryngeal papillomatosis wit intralesional injections of Cidofovir. *J Med Virol* 1998;54:219–225.
38. Pranksy SM, Magit AE, Kearns DB, Kang DR, Duncan NO. Intralesional Cidofovir for recurrent respiratory papillomatosis in children. *Arch Otolaryngol Head Neck Surg* 1999;125:1143–1148.
39. Pransky SM, Brewster DF, Magit AE, Kearns DB. Clinical update on 10 children treated with intralesional cidofovir injections for severe recurrent respiratory papillomatosis. *Arch Otolaryngol Head Neck Surg* 2000;126:1239–1243.

10

Laryngeal Malignancy and Vocal Outcomes

Introduction

Cancer can only be discussed in a volume devoted to vocal issues because of aspects specific to the laryngeal —or at least the vocal fold—manifestation of the disease. First, squamous cell carcinoma is, for a malignancy, relatively disciplined. That is to say, both its cellular progression, from mild atypia to carcinoma in situ, and its anatomic progression following invasion, from the epithelium of the vocal fold to deeper laryngeal tissues, is generally orderly and contiguous, if occasionally hard to assess. Furthermore, the anatomic barriers of the larynx, so elegantly described by Kirchner and others, create barriers, speed bumps and predictable avenues of spread for malignancy. Finally, glottic carcinoma has a built-in early warning system—hoarseness—that permits high cure rates simply because the disease usually reveals itself early, provided the patient and the physician are alert. Together, these three factors allow laryngeal surgeons the luxury of concern about factors beyond simple survival. Voice quality is principal among these.

Dr. McGuirt recounts the evolution of otolaryngologists' concern regarding voice outcomes after cancer surgery, as the consequences of degrees and configurations of tumor resection began to be examined. This thinking took place at the intersection of the fields of tumor biology and laryngeal anatomy and function. Dr. Zeitels follows with a broad historical perspective on the evolution of laryngologic approaches to vocal fold carcinoma, and includes a view of evolving tools and approaches likely to be useful in the future. Both of these author's classic articles and commentaries are landmarks in the evolution of an explicitly physiologic—yet oncologically sound —treatment of vocal fold cancer, and are landmark instances in laryngology of intellectual synthesis and of the integration of basic science into clinical practice.

Classic Articles

● Reprint of article included in this chapter.
♦ Commentary on this article.

McNeil BJ, Weichselbaum R, Pauker SG. Speech and survival. Tradeoffs between quality and quantity of life in laryngeal cancer. *N Eng J Med.* 1981;305(17):982–987.

Steiner W. Results of curative laser microsurgery of laryngeal carcinomas. *Am J Otolaryngol.* 1993;14(2): 116–121.

Cragle SP, Brandenburg JH. Laser cordectomy or radiotherapy: cure rates, communication, and cost. *Otolaryngol Head Neck Surg.* 1993;108(6):648–654.

●♦ McGuirt WF, Blalock D, Koufman JA, et al. Comparative voice results after laser resection or irradiation of T1 vocal cord carcinoma. *Arch Otolaryngol Head Neck Surg.* 1994;120(9):951–955.

●♦Zeitels SM. Premalignant epithelium and microinvasive cancer of the vocal fold: the evolution of phonomicrosurgical management. *Laryngoscope.* 1995;105 (3 pt 2):1–51.

Rydell R, Schalen L, Fex S, Elner A. Voice evaluation before and after laser excision vs. radiotherapy of T1A glottic carcinoma. *Acta Otolaryngol.* 1995;115(4): 560–565.

Commentary

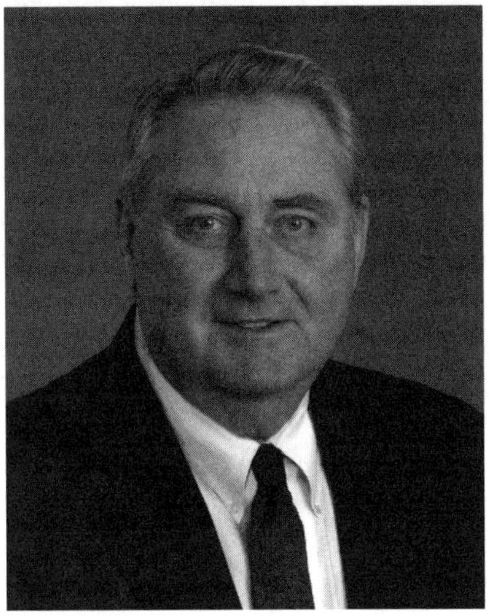

W. Frederick McGuirt, Sr, MD

In the mid to late 1970s, the standard of care for early laryngeal cancer was either radiation or hemilaryngectomy popularized by Dr. Joseph Ogura and his trainees from St. Louis. The surgical option, despite its equally good cure rate when compared to radiation, resulted in poor voice quality due to the degree of tissue sacrificed by the technique. Therefore, it became the opinion of many that radiation therapy for early laryngeal cancer was preferable due to the impaired voice result of surgical external resection. This use of irradiation resulted in total laryngectomy for recurrence or later second primary cancer development in the larynx. In the early 1970s, utilization of the operating microscope and CO_2 laser advocated by Drs. Strong and Jako in Boston began to be accepted management for benign laryngeal lesions such as papillomas. This teaching, technology, and their trainees spread outward from Boston as did its potential application for limited neoplastic conditions of the larynx. Through my contacts with friend and former resident mate, Dr. Arnie Katz, a junior faculty member under Dr. Strong, we at Wake Forest University, were able to recruit Dr. Jamie Koufman, a Boston trainee, to join our faculty. With Dr. Koufman's background knowledge of laryngeal laser surgery techniques, a CO_2 laser was obtained for laryngeal disease management. Living in the tobacco belt where tobacco was grown, manufactured, transported, and, most importantly, used in recreational and social settings by an inordinately high percentage of the population, a large number of laryngeal cancer patients presented to us for management. A significant portion of these cancers presented early in their development due to voice changes from involvement of the vibratory surface of the vocal fold. Extrapolating from ablation of benign growths with good voice preservation, I postulated that similar voice results could occur from limited resection of the vocal cord using the microscope and CO_2 laser. In addition, this technique would allow us to perform the resection at the time of the diagnostic biopsy and additionally save patients distant travel and lost time from employment. During the time of implementation of treating T1A laryngeal cancers by this method, Dr. Koufman, working with Mr. David Blalock of our Hearing and Speech Department, established a Voice Center Clinic with full vocal acoustic measurement capability. I proposed to them that we study the voice outcome of early stage endoscopically laser resected laryngeal cancer patients who were 3 years free of disease and considered cured by this therapeutic modality. Together we developed a three-level investigation of voice outcome that included perceptual subjective ratings of recorded standard voice passages by three independent panels of patients, otolaryngologists, and speech therapists, each group blinded according to patient identification. Additionally, objective measurement of voice quality parameters of the study patients were compared by the speech therapists to normative values of nonlaryngeal patients. This was published in February of 1992 in the *Annals of Otology, Rhinology and Laryngology* as the first evaluation of voice findings in patients treated solely by endoscopic laser resection. The subjective grading of voice function was found to be inversely related to the raters' level of training in voice pathology. Voice function rated normal to near normal by patients was rated nearly normal to mildly abnormal by both otolaryngologists and speech pathologists. Objective recordings compared to historical norms indicated a slightly higher fundamental frequency, decreases in intensity and phonatory duration, and markedly higher airway resistance. Chart review by senior resident, Dr. Bob Feehs, and me revealed that greater degrees of vocalis resection resulted in higher or worse scores by spectrographic analysis and greater attenuation of mucosal waves by videostroboscopy as evaluated by Dr. Koufman and Mr. Blalock. The degree of muscle resection though in these early staged cases resulted in only minimal differences in objective acoustic measurements and subjective voice ratings. The videostroboscopic findings had little correlation with voice function scores but did indicate significant muscle tension dysfunction as a compensatory mechanism to control airflow in the laser resected patients.

The above study findings served as the background for this currently published article, which was a study with our radiation therapy colleagues at Wake Forest published in 1994 in the *Archives of Otolaryngology*. It was performed to compare and to attempt to answer the question of whether radiation therapy resulted in a better voice result than endoscopic laser resection for comparable early neoplastic lesions of the vocal fold. The same protocol for evaluation was used as in the prior study. Only T1A lesions were included. All patients were greater than 6 months out from their clinical treatments. It had been my perceived experience that, if greater than 50% of the vocalis muscle depth measured medial to lateral from the free margin of the vocal fold to the thyroid ala was resected, then a significantly greater functional muscle volume was lost and compensatory closure on phonation did not occur and resulted in a breathy dysphonic voice. If intraoperative microscopic observation and palpation indicated a greater depth of involvement than described above, these patients were predicted to have poor voice outcomes and were radiated rather than resected. Our T1A laser resected patients studied were compared to radiated T1A patients directly referred to radiation therapy from outside our institution but judged by clinical nonoperative exams to be comparably staged lesions.

The study results showed no significant differences between the two study groups, laser resection versus radiation. On a scale of 1 to 5 with 1.5 to 2.5 noting nearly normal voices, patients and physicians rated the radiated group as 1.5 to 2.0 and the laser group as 2.0 to 2.4, both nearly normal. Speech pathologists rated the two groups as indistinguishable at 2.75 and 2.73 or mildly abnormal. Parenthetically included, the YAG laser resected group were a judge, a teacher, and an accountant all of whom returned to their jobs with no functional communication difficulties. With resection of less than one half of the depth of the vocalis muscle, two thirds of the muscle mass remains to activate the resulting scar band formed medially. There is often mild incomplete glottic closure though, which results in decreased phonatory duration and increased muscle tension contraction and increased airway resistance. This was noted in the initial study and the result is seen as well in irradiated patients as referenced by Lehman et al in our report. European authors subsequently classified and staged resection levels as mucosal, ligamentous, and varied muscular levels.

This comparative objective and subjective study indicated that selected patients with early glottic carcinoma could be treated as outpatients in a single operative experience and achieve equally good results to a prolonged radiation protocol therapy course. Preservation of future treatment options and reduced cost of care were other important considerations, as well as obviating the dry throat sensation of irradiated patients.

Extended endoscopic laser resection has evolved as therapy for more advanced laryngeal cancer but little has been studied as to voice outcome in these extended procedures and such information is needed to determine the quality of voice results in these patients so treated. In limited numbers of our patients with more extended intraoperative directed resection, poorer voice outcome has been subjectively noted and some patients have undergone endoscopic augmentation and/or external displacement procedures to improve vocal results but these patients are too few and of too varied methodologies of augmentation to study as a separate group to date. It remains for individuals of the current generation of laryngological oncologists and voice specialists to report the objective results of the pre- and post-therapy results in this group of patients to answer the question of how aggressive can the vocal resection with secondary augmentation be and still result in a subsequent voice comparable to lesser resections or irradiated patients.

I am honored to have our work recognized in this text and wish to thank my colleagues, especially Dr. Jamie Koufman and Mr. David Blalock, for their collaboration for having made this work possible.

ORIGINAL ARTICLE

Comparative Voice Results After Laser Resection or Irradiation of T1 Vocal Cord Carcinoma

W. Frederick McGuirt, MD; David Blalock, MA; James A. Koufman, MD; Robert S. Feehs, MD; Anita J. Hilliard, MD; Kathy Greven, MD; Mark Randall, MD

Objective: To compare voice results following laser resection or radiation therapy for T1a glottic carcinomas.

Design: Objective recordings of acoustical data that were analyzed and calculated by an acoustic analyzer and subjective scores by patients, speech therapists, surgeons, and radiation therapists are compared.

Setting: Academic medical center speech laboratory at an institution where patients had been treated. Archival files were searched and patients were solicited by letter to participate in this analysis.

Patients: Men treated at least 6 months previously and who were without active laryngeal disease. Criteria were unilateral vocal cord carcinomatous involvement with no subglottic, anterior commissure, or arytenoid extension and tumor invasion clinically judged to be less than half of the cordal depth.

Interventions: Thirteen patients had received approximately 63 Gy in 28 fractions, five fractions a week, with laterally opposed fields using a linear accelerator. Eleven patients had had resection of less than half of the cordal depth by using a carbon dioxide laser with a 300-μm spot size working at a 400-mm distance; 13- to 15-W power intensity with a one tenth of a second burn in a noncontinuous mode.

Results: No statistically significant differences between the two study groups were found. Patients and physicians subjectively rated (1 indicates normal; 5, aphonic) the quality of voices of patients in the irradiation group (1.5 and 2.0) as slightly better than the quality of voices of patients in the laser group (2.0 and 2.4). Speech pathologists rated the voices of patients in the laser and irradiation group as indistinguishable and mildly abnormal (2.75 and 2.73).

Conclusion: Voice quality in highly selected patients with vocal cord carcinoma treated by laser resection can be as good as that in patients whose cancer was similarly staged after radiation therapy.

(Arch Otolaryngol Head Neck Surg. 1994;120:951-955)

From the Departments of Otolaryngology (Drs McGuirt, Koufman, and Feehs), Hearing and Speech (Mr Blalock), and Radiation Therapy (Drs Greven and Randall), The Bowman Gray School of Medicine of Wake Forest University, Winston-Salem, NC.

ENDOSCOPIC laser resection of early laryngeal carcinoma has received increasing attention since its introduction by Strong and Jako[1] in 1972. It has become an excellent alternative to irradiation for early vocal cord lesions and allows simultaneous biopsy, staging, and definitive treatment as an outpatient procedure. Although comparable cure rates have been documented with irradiation or laser surgery,[2] to our knowledge comparison of voice quality has not been documented previously. In 1985, Hirano et al[3] reported little subjective difference in conversational voice results between patients who underwent laser resection and patients who underwent radiation therapy. Their study was not a pure comparison in that 50% of patients who underwent laser resection also had received radiation therapy. In 1989, Koufman[4] also reported subjectively good voice quality in many patients undergoing laser resection of their lesions. The patients with inferior voice quality were those with tumors involving the anterior commissure, those treated previously with radiation therapy, or those undergoing removal of more than

See Patients and Methods on next page

PATIENTS AND METHODS

STUDY GROUP

To eliminate the variability of vocal parameters between sexes, only male patients were studied. Additional selection criteria included a previously untreated, unilateral, clinically staged T1 vocal cord invasive squamous cell carcinoma not having extended to the anterior commissure, periarytenoid, or subglottic areas. In the laser group, all lesions required removal of less than 50% of the vocal cord width. The bulk of disease in the irradiated group could not be quantitated definitively, but by clinical observation the disease was comparable with that of the laser-treated group. The irradiated group was identified through the tumor registry files of the Bowman Gray School of Medicine Section on Radiation Therapy. Of the patients who had received radiation therapy and who agreed to be studied, 13 fit the selection criteria. These patients had received a tumor dose of 63 Gy in 28 fractions, five fractions given each week, with laterally opposed fields using a linear accelerator.

Of the patients who had had endoscopic laser resection of T1 invasive vocal cord carcinomas and who agreed to be studied, 11 fit the staging and resection criteria. Their lesions had been resected using a carbon dioxide laser with a 300-μm spot size at a 400-mm working distance. Generally, the lesions had been placed on stretch with cup forceps and were resected at 13- to 15-W power intensity with a one tenth of a second burn in the noncontinuous mode. Postresection microcup deep-tissue biopsies were performed to verify adequate margins.

Therapy in all patients had been completed at least 6 months before the voice analyses were made, and none of the patients had active laryngeal disease. None of the patients were professional voice users.

VOICE ANALYSES SPEECH SAMPLE

The speech samples obtained for evaluation consisted of two vowels, /a/ and /i/, and a reading of the Rainbow Passage.[6,7] The vowel /a/ was chosen because it is considered to be the most sensitive indicator of differences in voice production.[8] The vowel /i/ was chosen on the basis of the work of Yanagihara,[9] which indicated that this vowel, along with /a/, is among those vowels providing essential information when qualitatively classifying hoarseness. The Rainbow Passage is a phonetically balanced prose passage[10]; the second sentence of the first paragraph was chosen for the analysis of connected speech (*c* speech sample).

EVALUATION PARAMETERS

Evaluation was based on the following parameters: (1) acoustical data for each patient were analyzed and calculated by an acoustic analyzer (Visi-Pitch, model 6095/6097, Kay Elemetrics Corp, Pinebrook, NJ) (fundamental frequency, percentage of perturbation or jitter,[11] average intensity, and percentage of voicing); (2) laryngeal airway resistance was calculated by using Perci-PC Version 1.5 (Microtronics Corp, Chapel Hill, NC) and by following the protocol suggested by Smitheran and Hixon[11]; (3) narrow-band spectrographic recordings of the vowels /a/ and /i/ were evaluated according to spectrographic categories described by Yanagihara[9] (**Table 1**) and were scored by the speech pathologist; (4) voice quality was judged and scored by the patients, by us, and by a panel of speech pathologists "blinded" to the diagnosis and treatment groups (scores were based on the rating scale shown in **Table 2**); and (5) videostroboscopy was used to evaluate glottic closure, mucosal waves, and amplitude; mucosal waves were rated as normal, reduced, or absent; muscle tension dysfunction (primarily supraglottic contraction) was recorded as present or absent, and if present, was rated on a numerical scale.

Instrumentation, recording procedure, and analysis technique for all five parameters studied are detailed in **Table 3** to allow reproducibility and standardization for future comparative studies.

half of the vocal cord mass. These reports stimulated our recent, more in-depth evaluation of the voice quality of patients with laser-resected vocal cord carcinoma.[5]

In this report, we compare the voice results of patients with T1 vocal cord invasive squamous cell carcinoma treated with either laser resection or definitive irradiation. All tumors were unilateral and did not extend to the anterior commissure. To our knowledge, our results represent the first objective comparison of the voices of patients whose cancers were comparably staged and who were treated only by one or the other of these two modalities.

RESULTS

Fundamental frequency was slightly increased for the laser-resected group (157 Hz) compared with the irradiated group (136 Hz) and the historical norm (122 Hz) (**Table 4**). This difference between the laser and irradiation groups was more pronounced for the *c* speech sample.

Intensity measurements (Table 4) revealed a nearly identical decrease for the *c* speech sample for both the irradiation (43.8 dB) and the laser-resected (43.5 dB) groups from the historical norm (70 dB).

Phonatory duration (Table 4) was reduced in the laser-resected group (15.81 seconds) compared with the irradiation group (19.26 seconds) and the historical norm (20 seconds).

For the laser-resected group, the percentage perturbation scores were within the 0.5% to 1.0% normal range for all three speech samples studied (Table 4), whereas the irradiated group had a mean value outside the norm for the *c* speech sample.

Percentage voicing measurements (Table 4) revealed slightly lower values in the irradiated group for the *a* and *i* speech samples. The laser-resected group had more abnormal scores for the *c* speech sample, whereas the irradiated group was indistinguishable from the norm.

The greatest variance from normal for all patients was seen in the measurements of laryngeal airway resistance. The laser-resected group had values three times the norm (118.05 vs 36 to 40 cm H_2O/L per second), and the irradiated group had resistances 4.5 times the norm (177.21 cm H_2O/L per second). Yanagihara scores revealed no differences between the two study groups, with the mean scores of both being 2.8. Statistical analysis indicated no significant differences between the two groups for any of the aforementioned objective parameters tested.

The subjective voice rating scores were directly proportional to the level of voice training of the raters. The greatest differences in scores occurred between the patients and the speech pathologists, with the physician scores being intermediate between the two. The patients and physicians rated the voices of the patients in the irradiation

Table 1. Yanagihara Score*

Type I: The regular harmonic components are mixed with the noise component chiefly in the formant region of the vowels.
Type II: The noise components in the second formant of /a/ and /i/ dominate over the harmonic components, and slight additional noise components appear in the high-frequency region above 3000 Hz in the vowels /a/ and /i/.
Type III: The second formants of /a/ and /i/ are totally replaced by noise components, and the additional noise components above 3000 Hz further intensify their energy and expand their range.
Type IV: The second formants of /a/ and /i/ are replaced by noise components, and even the first formants of all vowels often lose periodic components, which are [supplanted] by noise components. In addition, more intensified high-frequency additional noise components are seen.

**Modified from Yanagihara.[9]*

Table 2. Subjective Rating Scale*

1. Normal (<1.5)
2. Mild dysphonia—nearly normal—only trained listener would detect (1.5-2.5)
3. Moderate dysphonia—mildly abnormal—patient has to explain voice to others (2.5-3.5)
4. Severe dysphonia—moderately abnormal—sounds like severe laryngitis all the time (3.5-4.5)
5. Aphonic—nonserviceable voice (>4.5)

**Arbitrary rating scale of 1 to 5.*

Table 3. Instrumentation, Recording Procedure, and Analysis Technique

Instrumentation and Procedure: All voices were recorded with a microphone positioned approximately 15 cm from the mouth and slightly below the chin to reduce effects of airflow. Signal was recorded on a cassette tape deck. The voice data were also directly stored on 5.25-in floppy disks Visi-Pitch model 6095/6097 (Kay Elemetrics, Pinebrook, NJ), interfaced with a PC/AT compatible computer. Perci-II (palatal efficiency rating computed instantaneously) was used to record data for calculations of laryngeal airway resistance. Perci-II/PC (MicroTronics, Carrboro, NC) is a PC-based system that provides for the collection and interactive analysis of pressure-flow data using the noninvasive measurement method of Smitheran and Hixon.[11] McSpeech Lab program (G. W. Instruments, Cambridge, Mass) with standard Macintosh 512 computer interface was used to produce narrow-band spectrograms of the vowel samples. Testing of normal subjects by these techniques yielded values comparable with previously published normal values, and those values were used in this study for comparison.

Each subject was instructed to take a comfortable but full breath and sustain vowel /a/ at the most comfortable loudness level for as long as possible. The same procedure was used while producing vowel /i/. Subjects were next instructed to read the first paragraph of the Rainbow Passage while being recorded directly onto Visi-Pitch. The second sentence of the passage was extracted and stored for analysis. Subjects were then instructed to sustain vowels /a/ and /i/ for 3 seconds. The approximate middle 2.1 seconds of the vowel was stored for analysis. Following the protocol of Smitheran and Hixon,[11] subjects were required to repeat the syllable /Pi/ in three separate trains of seven productions each. For each train, subjects were instructed to take a breath approximately twice normal depth and to produce the seven productions on a single, continuous expiration at normal loudness, pitch, and quality, with equal stress on each syllable, at a rate of 1.5 syllables per second.

Analysis Techniques: The analysis techniques for five parameters studied were as follows:

Acoustic Measurements: Acoustic data comparisons with those of normal patients for vowels /a/ and /i/ and for connected speech (second sentence of the Rainbow Passage) for each patient were analyzed and calculated by Visi-Pitch for (1) fundamental frequency; (2) percent perturbation; (3) average intensity (decibels); and (4) percent voicing.

Aerodynamic Measurements: Laryngeal airway resistance (LAR) equation used is LAR = (subglottic pressure minus laryngeal pressure) divided by glottic airflow. It is calculated by dividing glottal airflow into the pressure drop across the glottal opening. The middle three pressure-flow measurements of the seven-syllable series are used to calculate LAR. The subglottal pressures needed to calculate LAR are inferred from oral pressures on the peak of the /p/. The computer program then connects a line from the third to the fourth to the fifth pressure peak. This line represents the subglottal pressures occurring on the vowel /i/. The program then drops the cursor onto the flow signal for voicing on each of the three /i/ vowels. This value is the flow value that is used in the resistance equation. The average of the three resistances is the LAR for the trial. Resistance values were expressed in centimeters of water per liters per second and were compared with known normative data from the literature.

Spectrographic Analysis: Narrow-band spectrograms were produced over a range of 0-5 kHz for the vowels /a/ and /i/ using the McSpeech Lab program. Spectrograms were evaluated according to spectrographic categories described by Yanagihara.[9] Judgment of classification was carried out by the senior speech pathologist in a "blinded" fashion.

Videostroboscopic Evaluation: Videostroboscopic segments were evaluated for glottic closure, mucosal waves, and amplitude. Average visual perceptive scores by a panel of the authors were used. Mucosal waves were rated as normal, reduced, or absent. Glottic closure was rated as complete or incomplete. A rating of observed muscle tension dysphonia was recorded as to its presence or absence and was noted to be isometric, false vocal cord voice, partial A-P contraction, or sphincteric closure.

Perceptual Voice Ratings: Judgment ratings of vocal quality were performed by patients, authors, and a panel of speech pathologists (American Speech Language Hearing Association certified and experienced with voice disorders) who were blinded as to the patients' diagnoses and treatment groups. Average scores by the patients, speech pathologists, and authors were based on a rating scale.

Table 4. Acoustical Data

	Laser	Radiation	Normal*
Fundamental frequency, Hz			
/a/	144	127	125±25
/i/	190	174	128±18
/c/	137	106	113±14
Average	157	136	122
Intensity, dB			
/a/	49.7	50.25	. . .
/i/	48.8	51.35	. . .
/c/	43.3	43.5	70
Phonatory duration, s	15.81	19.26	20
Perturbation, %			
/a/	0.54	0.48	0.5-1.0
/i/	0.79	0.70	. . .
/c/	0.88	1.33	. . .
Voicing, %			
/a/	98.93	92.77	100
/i/	96.63	91.65	100
/c/	76.05	65.38	65

Unless otherwise stated, values are presented as mean± SD.

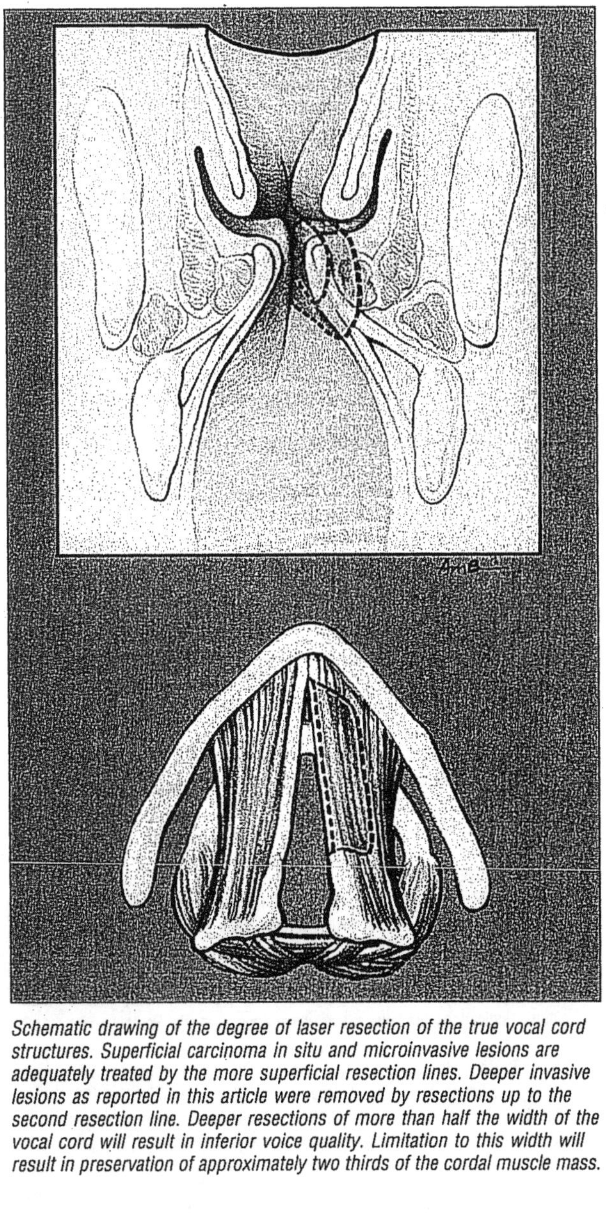

Schematic drawing of the degree of laser resection of the true vocal cord structures. Superficial carcinoma in situ and microinvasive lesions are adequately treated by the more superficial resection lines. Deeper invasive lesions as reported in this article were removed by resections up to the second resection line. Deeper resections of more than half the width of the vocal cord will result in inferior voice quality. Limitation to this width will result in preservation of approximately two thirds of the cordal muscle mass.

group as 1.5 and 2, respectively, which is slightly better than the ratings of 2 and 2.43, respectively, for the voices of patients in the laser group (ie, both the irradiation and laser groups were rated as having nearly normal voices by both panels). The speech therapists rated the laser and irradiated group voices as 2.75 and 2.73, respectively, ie, essentially indistinguishable and mildly abnormal.

Videostroboscopic examination was performed in only five patients in the irradiated group, which allowed for only subjective observations. Glottic closure was seen in all of the irradiated subjects studied and in 80% of the laser-resected subjects. Mucosal waves were abnormal in about two thirds of the patients studied in both groups, but only for the vocal cord operated on in the laser-resected subjects, whereas approximately half of the irradiated subjects had abnormal waves in both vocal cords. Muscle tension dysphonia, evidenced by predominantly false vocal cord voice and partial anteroposterior contractions, was frequently seen in both groups.

COMMENT

Treatment of early laryngeal carcinoma by endoscopic laser resection at the time of laryngoscopic diagnosis and staging is more expedient and cost-effective than treatment by irradiation. Previously published results[2,12,13] have shown that the cure rates in highly selected patients who have had laser resection equal those in similar patients receiving radiation therapy. This study also confirms that when strict criteria are met, the voice resulting from this surgical therapeutic approach is, by objective and subjective measurements, equal to the voice resulting from irradiation of patients with comparable tumors.

When excisional depth is limited to less than half of the vocal cord width, two thirds of the actual working muscle wall remains (**Figure**). With an intact arytenoid and anterior commissure, a functional vocal cord results, with the defect being bridged by scar tissue. Despite the scar-band formation, laser resection does result in some cordal deficiency on the side that underwent operation. This deficiency was manifested by decreases in phonatory duration and in some patients by incomplete glottic closure as well. Often the result is compensatory muscle tension contraction, which was seen by transnasal fiberoptic laryngoscopy.

Increased laryngeal airway resistance was the most abnormal finding in both the laser and irradiation groups. Our values are comparable with those of a postirradiated population described by Lehman et al[8] in which increases in subglottic airway pressure measurements were of a three-times magnitude. We believe this increased airway resistance or subglottic pressure is primarily a glottic and supraglottic muscular functional phenomenon. Although fibrosis and scarring from the treatments are present, the resulting increased resistance is more likely related to a subconscious, persistent compensatory mechanism resulting from the primary disease or the effects of the treatment on laryngeal muscular function. An analogy to other compensatory muscle dysfunction syndromes can be made.

Speech counseling and therapy from the onset of diagnosis may alter the outcome with regard to these parameters and is an area for future prospective study. Such a need for vocal rehabilitation was suggested by Murry et al[14] in their assessment of the postirradiation voice, although they did not suggest any time schedule for therapy.

The patients' and physicians' qualitative voice analyses and ratings were comparable for both the laser-treated and the radiation-treated groups and were in the nearly normal range (1.5 to 2.5). This finding is compatible with the reports of near-normal subjective patient assessment of the postirradiation voice by Schuller et al[15] and Lehman et al.[8] The voices of the irradiated group were rated better than the voices of the laser-treated group by both the patients and the physicians. Although the physicians' ratings of the two groups were comparable with the patients' ratings, they were slightly more abnormal. The patients and the physicians viewed the voice quality resulting from both treatments to be satisfactory, ie, sufficient to allow daily social and employment communication. The opinions of the patients and physicians were most likely related to interpretation of voice intensity, which was not different for the two groups, and interpretation of the fundamental frequency, which was minimally increased compared with normal values.

THE SPEECH pathologists, who have the highest levels of training in detecting speech abnormalities, gave the most critical subjective analysis scores. They rated voice quality of the irradiated group (2.73) to be no different than that of the laser-treated group (2.75), both being rated mildly abnormal. In addition to considering the minimal increase in fundamental frequency and the comparable reductions in intensity, they better appreciated comparable increases in the signal-to-noise ratios above 3000 Hz (as shown by the Yanagihara scores) and were better able to differentiate the percentages of perturbation and voicing differences from the norm.

These voice results indicate that a highly selected group of patients with early glottic carcinoma can be treated in a single outpatient laser-surgery session and can achieve functional results equivalent to those of patients treated with a 6-week course of radiation therapy. The advantages of this treatment may be a lower cost to the patient and the ability to reserve irradiation for possible future needs.

We emphasize that the patients chosen for laser resection are those with highly selected, early lesions, and we do not advocate laser resection for all patients with T1 lesions when vocal quality is the determining factor in choice of treatment modality. Subjective poor speech quality has been reported previously after laser treatment of larger lesions that involve the anterior commissure or arytenoid, as well as deeper T1 lesions that require extensive cordal resections (more than half of the cordal depth).[4] We also recognize that the irradiated group was not an identically matched study group but was studied as a comparable group of patients (T1 unilateral vocal cord carcinoma without anterior commissure involvement) and was matched as closely as possible in a clinically nonsequential, nonrandomized study. In conclusion, if appropriate criteria are met, voice quality in highly selected patients treated surgically by laser resection can be as good as that in similar patients treated with radiation therapy.

Accepted for publication May 18, 1993.

Presented at the Scientific Session of the American Society for Head and Neck Surgery, Waikoloa, Hawaii, May 9, 1991.

We appreciate the statistical evaluations done by Evan Sands of the Department of Prevention and Biometry, as well as the editorial service and manuscript preparation provided by Judith MacMillan and Alma Doub.

Reprint requests to Department of Otolaryngology, Bowman Gray School of Medicine, Medical Center Boulevard, Winston-Salem, NC 27157-1034 (Dr McGuirt).

REFERENCES

1. Strong MS, Jako GJ. Laser surgery in the larynx: early clinical experience with continuous CO_2 laser. *Ann Otol Rhinol Laryngol.* 1972;81:791-798.
2. McGuirt WF, Koufman JA. Endoscopic laser surgery: an alternative in laryngeal cancer treatment. *Arch Otolaryngol Head Neck Surg.* 1987;113:501-505.
3. Hirano M, Hirade Y, Kawasaki H. Vocal function following carbon dioxide laser surgery for glottic carcinoma. *Ann Otol Rhinol Laryngol.* 1985;94:232-235.
4. Koufman JA. The endoscopic management of early squamous carcinoma of the vocal cord with the carbon dioxide surgical laser: clinical experience and a proposed subclassification. *Otolaryngol Head Neck Surg.* 1986;95:531-537.
5. McGuirt WF, Blalock D, Koufman JA, Feehs RS. Voice analysis of patients with endoscopically treated early laryngeal carcinoma. *Ann Otol Rhinol Laryngol.* 1992; 101:142-146.
6. Fairbanks G. *Voice and Articulation Drillbook.* New York, NY: Harper Brothers; 1960.
7. Horii Y. Jitter and shimmer difference among sustained vowel phonations. *J Speech Hear Res.* 1980;25:12-14.
8. Lehman JJ, Bless DM, Brandenburg JH. An objective assessment of voice production after radiation therapy for stage I squamous cell carcinoma of the glottis. *Otolaryngol Head Neck Surg.* 1988;98:121-129.
9. Yanagihara N. Significance of harmonic changes and noise components in hoarseness. *J Speech Hear Res.* 1967;10:531-541.
10. Fitch JL. Consistency of fundamental frequency and perturbation in repeated phonations of sustained vowels, reading, and connected speech. *J Speech Hear Disord.* 1990;55:360-363.
11. Smitheran JR, Hixon TJ. A clinical method for estimating laryngeal airway resistance during vowel production. *J Speech Hear Disord.* 1981;46:138-146.
12. Ossoff RH, Sisson GA, Shapshay SM. Endoscopic management of selected early vocal cord carcinoma. *Ann Otol Rhinol Laryngol.* 1985;94:560-564.
13. Shapshay SM, Hybels RL, Bohigian RK. Laser excision of early vocal cord carcinoma: indications, limitations, and precautions. *Ann Otol Rhinol Laryngol.* 1990; 99:46-50.
14. Murry T, Bone RC, Von Essen C. Changes in voice production during radiotherapy for laryngeal cancer. *J Speech Hear Disord.* 1974;39:194-201.
15. Schuller DE, Trudeau M, Bistline J, LaFace K. Evaluation of voice by patients and close relatives following different laryngeal cancer treatments. *J Surg Oncol.* 1990; 44:10-14.

Commentary

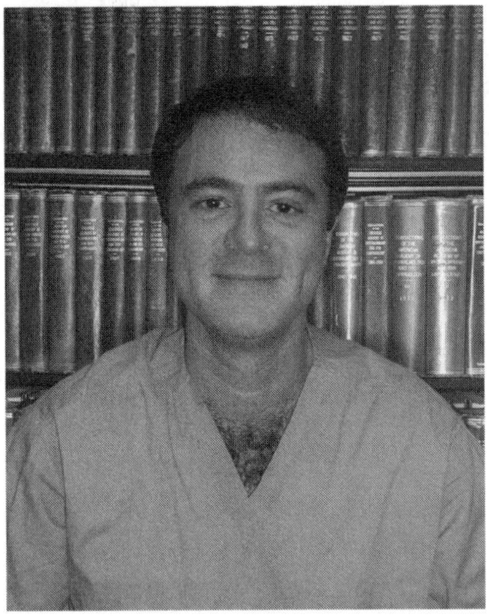

Steven M. Zeitels, MD

The surgical treatment of vocal-fold neoplasms during the last 2 centuries comprises a rich history chronicling the development of minimally invasive endoscopic laryngeal surgery along with our enhanced understanding of phonatory physiology in a normal and a diseased state. Independent and interdependent advances have led to current philosophies in which curative treatment is routine, while optimal vocal outcome remains a pursuit.

Because any adequate treatment for early glottic cancer (endoscopic excision, transcervical excision, radiation therapy) results in a cure rate of ~90 to 95%, the primary metric by which the clinician should judge the success of the treatment is the resulting quality of the voice. *Phonomicrosurgery*[1] can be understood as the convergence of mucosal-wave body-cover theory instituted by Hirano[2] in the 1970s with microlaryngoscopic surgical-technique theory. I believe that the first use of the term "phonomicrosurgery" in the literature was in this manuscript in 1995. I had noted that there was often confusion at meeting when the term phonosurgery (created by von Leden decades earlier) was used as it was unclear whether individuals were referring to open laryngeal framework surgery or endoscopic surgery on the glottal mucosa.

This approach was based on what I had learned about the physiologic principles of laryngeal-sound production from Dr. Hirano and my unique training in laryngeal oncology from Drs. Strong, Vaughan, and Jako. Taken together, detailed elements of glottal sound production were incorporated into the design of cancer procedures of the vocal folds. The goal of phonomicrosurgical treatment of early vocal-fold cancer is to maximally preserve the normal mucosal layered-microstructure, while not compromising oncologic principles. In my Triological thesis,[1] it was established that ultra-narrow margins[3] requiring dissection in the superficial lamina propria were best done with cold instruments[4] for lesions that were not invading the vocal ligament. With the assistance of my scientific partner Robert Hillman, we established that using this surgical approach, near-normal conversational-level voice results could be achieved consistently.

I created the superficial lamina propria infusion technique based on a comment by Charles Vaughan when I was a resident (1987). He had explained to me that the best voice results when endoscopically treating glottic cancer were in those patients who had underlying Reinke's edema. I then decided to create Reinke's edema in all of the dysplasia and early glottic cancer patients and used the mediastinal lymph-node aspiration needle designed by John Tucker.[5] The infusion of saline and epinephrine into the superficial lamina propria substantially enhanced my ability to preserve this anatomic structure critical for human voice. Over time, I modified that needle to optimize its use for phonomicrosurgery in both benign and malignant lesions.[6,7] The subepithelial infusion technique[6,8] allowed for ultra-narrow-margin resections that were oncologically sound.[1,3,9]

It was clear that endoscopic treatment of early glottic cancer provided a number of advantages over open surgical management and radiation therapy included a very low complication rate, which consists mainly of minor postoperative bleeding, and granuloma formation. Endoscopic excision also preserved all treatment modalities including further transoral resections. Unlike radiotherapy, endoscopic resection treated only the areas of concern without distorting the remaining normal anatomy. Postradiotherapy videostroboscopic exams suggested that both normal and cancerous tissues reflect fibrotic changes.[10] We investigated the implications of diminished phonatory mucosal pliability in glottic cancer patients and established that the greatest value of stroboscopy was to identify viable pliable mucosa, which would be the key soft tissue to preserve as it would be the primary sound source; stroboscopy was unreliable in determining the depth of cancer invasion.[11]

Apart from the potential detrimental affect on post-treatment voice quality, the use of radiotherapy for early glottic malignancies precluded this valuable single-use cancer treatment from being employed for tumor recurrence or new primaries in the larynx or in the region. There is even a limited risk in younger patients that radiotherapy may induce carcinogenesis. The cost of endoscopic excision was significantly less than open laryngeal surgery or radiation as either of these procedures is typically preceded by a staging endoscopy.[12,13]

Apart from enhancing voice results associated with phonomicrosurgical treatment of glottic cancer, the other mission in the late 20th century was to extend the indications for what was an acceptable lesion with regards to larger size and more advanced staging. Steiner visited the Boston University group (Strong, Vaughan, Jako) in the 1970s and subsequently championed more extensive endoscopic laryngeal cancer treatment.[14,15] This included lesions deeply invading the thyroarytenoid muscle and anterior-commissure tendon. Other Europeans followed[16,17] substantiating that larger glottal cancers, even in the anterior commissure[18] can be successfully treated endoscopically.

To address the limitations in visualizing the perimeter of many glottic cancers, I introduced the Universal Modular (UM) glottiscope, which provided superior glottal exposure. Although it was conceived in the 1980s, it was not produced until years later.[19,20] The UM glottiscope retains a lancet-arch-shaped speculum that was designed to accommodate to the inner contours of the thyroid laminae thereby providing optimal exposure of the anterior commissure and deep paraglottic space. This had not been previously achieved[21] and now allowed for a majority of glottal cancers to be resected en bloc.[22]

In patients who had paraglottic space tissue loss as a result of cancer treatment, it became clear that improving aerodynamic incompetency would significantly enhance the voice result. To manage this, I employed Ishhiki's techniques for laryngeal framework reconstruction in 1994 to restore glottal competence in patients in whom substantial amount of paraglottic musculature required resection. By medializing the excavated neocord, there would be substantially better entrainment of the noncancerous phonatory mucosa. The techniques were transferred from paraglottic-space augmentation procedures designed to treat vocal-fold paralysis introduced by Brunings,[23] Payr,[24] and Isshiki.[25] This was comprised of stereoscopic lipoinjection[9,26,27] and transcervical medialization laryngoplasty.[9,27–29] Gore-Tex was deemed to be the best synthetic implant because of the malleability of shaping it to complex cancer defects. Adjustments in volume and position of the Gore-Tex are done simultaneously while talking to the patient. If there is minimal or no paraglottic tissue left, it is wiser to collapse the thyroid ala similar to Payr's approach.

Apart from the tissue deficits in the paraglottic region, reconstructing the anterior commissure was initially difficult when part or all of Broyle's ligament was resected. When patients had a substantial keyhole aperture anteriorly, the voice outcome was often poor due to the aerodynamic incompetence. This problem was solved when the author introduced the thyroid-lamina subluxation procedure, which was done under local anesthesia with sedation.[27] This procedure has been adopted more in Europe due to the longer history of extensive endolaryngeal glottic cancer resections.

Our 2002 manuscript[9] was a key report and the culmination of 15 years of phonosurgical development and innovation. We demonstrated that a majority of patients with early glottic cancer could achieve a near-normal conversational-level voice, regardless of depth of invasion. We described several straightforward surgical maneuvers in the work that substantially enhanced voice outcomes, which have not been done in any other report.

Photoangiolysis and Incremental Treatment: The Future

Incremental treatment of laryngeal cancer is routine during the administration of ionizing radiation and chemotherapy to diminish host morbidity. Tumor surgery has developed over hundreds of years and principles developed during the past century mandate that the cancer resection separate the patient from the neoplasm directly to diminish the time of intercurrent disease. Intercurrent disease predisposes patients to regional and distant metastasis. Notwithstanding, incremental radiation was instituted for laryngeal cancer in the beginning of the 20th century based on the premise that the cancer surgery was more morbid than the disease itself, which was a key issue of controversy of Crown Prince Frederick of Germany.[1]

Considering the fact that radiation is employed as the treatment for early glottic cancer in a majority of patients, incremental treatment over a period of 6 weeks is the standard of care in most institutions. Moreover, XRT typically begins approximately 1 month after the microlaryngoscopic biopsy establishes the diagnosis. Pulsed-KTP laser photangiolysis of glottic cancer was instituted to preserve radiation as a valuable single-use cancer treatment and to diminish the treatment time. More importantly, the noncancerous glottal phonatory membranes and the saccular glands that provide lubrication to the glottal valve are spared from the ionizing radiation so that subsequent to photoangiolysis treatment, glottal vibration and voice quality are enhanced.[30]

We have been involuting the microcirculation[31] to treat early glottic cancer[30] for over 6 years and more than 50 patients have been managed successfully with outstanding vocal outcomes. One patient developed a limited recurrence at 18 months, was retreated by pulsed-KTP laser photoangiolysis and is without disease 26 months. No patient currently has cancer, none have been resected at the site of the photoangiolysis, and one has undergone radiotherapy to treat the disease. There is more than 2-year follow-up in a majority of patients. The phonatory outcome revealed that we are now able to achieve voice results in patients with bilateral glottic cancer, comparable to those with one normal vocal fold (unilateral disease),[30] which was not previously done.

Remarkably, the elements of photoangiolysis of glottic cancer were identified almost 40 years ago. Whereas Kleinsasser described the aberrant microcirculation associated with microinvasive vocal fold carcinoma, Jako had already commenced investigations into the utilization of laser technology. "Experiments using laser beams for destruction of discrete areas of vocal folds are presently being conducted"[32]

Staging the surgical treatment of these microinvasive glottic cancers with pulsed-laser photoangiolysis potentially portends another revision of the typical surgical oncologic principle. Surgical treatment usually implies effective management as a solitary intervention. This is in contradistinction to radiotherapy and chemotherapy, which are incremental. For the promise of enhanced function, these nonsurgical cancer treatments have achieved acceptability despite the fact that patients are left with intercurrent disease during months of treatment. Laser photoangiolytic treatment by surgeons using non-ionizing radiation retains elements of current surgery and radiotherapy models synthesizing key assets of both. It is likely to be philosophically acceptable to most otolaryngologists because it is well recognized that early glottic cancer rarely metastasizes. Therefore, selecting smaller lesions initially poses little risk to the patient and preserves all treatment options, while allowing for a better voice result. Accordingly, the surgeon develops his or her comfort-level and learning-curve in a gradual fashion.

If this is deemed acceptable, it is not difficult to envision that laser photoangiolytic treatment may be a single modality or it might serve as a cytoreduction an adjuvant treatment. Induction light treatment could be applied at the time of staging endoscopy. Given our office experience with the pulsed photoangiolytic laser treatment of glottal dysplasia with topical anesthesia,[32-34] it conceivable that further induction treatment could be continued in the clinic prior to full-course radiotherapy. Given the migration of many surgical interventions to be minimally invasive and/or office procedures, these prospects are not inconceivable.

Summary

Endoscopic treatment of early glottic cancer has been demonstrated to have a variety of advantages over other treatment modalities. The procedures are relatively easy and highly successful in properly selected cases. In recent years, transoral treatment of early glottic cancer has received increased attention because there have been innovations in laryngoscopic instrumentation, laser technology, and phonomicrosurgical techniques, as well as improvements in our understanding of laryngeal sound-production and associated reconstruction. This has led to a convergence of microlaryngoscopic surgical-technique theory with body-cover mucosal-wave theory. Taken together, the vocal outcome from these procedures has improved while maintaining >90% cure rates. It is likely that we will be able to achieve near normal voice results in the foreseeable future given research initiatives worldwide to design biomaterials and cellular construct grafts to replace the pliable layered microstructure of the vocal fold replaced by cancer.[35]

Bibliography

1. Zeitels SM. Premalignant epithelium and microinvasive cancer of the vocal fold: the evolution of phonomicrosurgical management. *Laryngoscope.* 1995;105(suppl 67): 1–51.
2. Hirano M. Phonosurgery: basic and clinical investigations. *Otologia (Fukuoka).* 1975;21:239–442.
3. Zeitels SM. Phonomicrosurgical treatment of early glottic cancer and carcinoma in situ. *Am J Surg.* 1996; 172:704–709.
4. Zeitels SM. Laser versus cold instruments for microlaryngoscopic surgery. *Laryngoscope.* 1996;106:545–552.
5. Tucker JA. Mediastinoscopy: 300 cases reported and literature reviewed. *Laryngoscope.* 1972;82(12):2226–2248.
6. Zeitels SM, Vaughan CW. A submucosal vocal fold infusion needle. *Otolaryngol Head Neck Surg.* 1991;105: 478–479.
7. Kass ES, Hillman RE, Zeitels SM. The submucosal infusion technique in phonomicrosurgery. *Ann Otol Rhinol Laryngol.* 1996;105:341–347.
8. Zeitels SM. Microflap excisional biopsy for atypia and microinvasive glottic cancer. *Op Techn Otolaryngol Head Neck Surg. (Phonosurgery ed.).* 1993;4:218–222.
9. Zeitels SM, Hillman RE, Franco RA, Bunting G. Voice and treatment outcome from phonosurgical management of early glottic cancer. *Ann Otol Rhinol Laryngol.* 2002;111(suppl 190):1–20.
10. Lehman JJ, Bless DM, Brandenburg JH. An objective assessment of voice production after radiation therapy for stage I squamous cell carcinoma of the glottis. *Otolaryngol Head Neck Surg.* 1988;98:121–129.
11. Colden D, Zeitels SM, Hillman RE, Jarboe J, Bunting G, Spanou N. Stroboscopic assessment of vocal-fold atypia and early cancer. *Ann Otol Rhinol Laryngol.* 2001; 110:293–298.
12. Cragle SP, Brandenburg JH. Laser cordectomy or radiotherapy: cure rates, communication, and cost. *Otolaryngol Head Neck Surg.* 1993;108:648–653.
13. Myers EN, Wagner R, Johnson JT. Microlaryngoscopic surgery for T1 glottic lesion: a cost-effective option. *Ann Otol Rhinol Laryngol.* 1994;103:28–30.
14. Steiner W. Experience in endoscopic laser surgery of malignant tumours of the upper aerodigestive tract. *Advances Otorhinolaryngol.* 1988;39:135–144.
15. Steiner W. Results of curative laser microsurgery of laryngeal carcinomas. *Am J Otolaryngol.* 1993;14:116–121.
16. Thumfart WF, Eckel HE. [Endolaryngeal laser surgery in the treatment of laryngeal cancers. The current Cologne concept]. *HNO.* 1990;38(5):174–178.
17. Eckel H, Thumfart WF. Laser surgery for the treatment of larynx carcinomas: indications, techniques, and preliminary results. *Ann Otol Rhinol Laryngol.* 1992; 101:113–118.
18. Desloge RB, Zeitels SM. Endolaryngeal microsurgery at the anterior glottal commissure: controversies and observations. *Ann Otol Rhinol Laryngol.* 2000;109: 385–392.
19. Zeitels SM. A universal modular glottiscope system: the evolution of a century of design and technique for direct laryngoscopy. *Ann Otol Rhinol Laryngol.* 1999; 108(suppl 179):1–24.
20. Zeitels SM. *Universal modular laryngoscope/glottiscope system.* United States Patent #5,893,830, 1999.
21. Davis RK, Jako GJ, Hyams VJ, & Shapshay SM. The anatomic limitations of CO_2 laser cordectomy. *Laryngoscope.* 1982;92:980–984.
22. Zeitels SM, Dailey SH, Burns JA. Technique of en block laser endoscopic frontolateral laryngectomy for glottic cancer. *Laryngoscope.* 2004;114(1):175–180.
23. Brunings W. Eine neue Behandlungsmethode der Rekurrenslahmungen. *Verhandl Deutsch Vereins Deutscher Laryngologen.* 1911;18:93–151.
24. Payr E. Plastik am schildknorpel zur Behebung der Folgen einseitiger Stimmbandlahmung. *Dtsch Med Wochensch.* 1915;43:1265–1270.
25. Isshiki N, Morita H, Okamura H, Hiramoto M. Thyroplasty as a new phonosurgical technique. *Acta Otolaryngol (Stockh).* 1974;78:451–457.
26. Burns JA, Kobler JB, Zeitels SM. Microstereolaryngoscopic lipoinjection: practical considerations. *Laryngoscope.* 2004;114(10):1864–1867.
27. Zeitels SM, Jarboe J, Franco RA. Phonosurgical reconstruction of early glottic cancer. *Laryngoscope.* 2001;111: 1862–1865.
28. Zeitels SM, Mauri M, Dailey SH. Medialization laryngoplasty with Gore-Tex for voice restoration secondary to glottal incompetence: indications and observations. *Ann Otol Rhinol Laryngol.* 2003;112:180–184.
29. Zeitels SM. Optimizing voice after endoscopic partial laryngectomy. *Otolaryngol Clin North Am.* 2004;37(3): 627–636.

30. Zeitels SM, Burns JA, Hillman RH, Anderson RR. Photoangiolytic laser treatment of early glottic cancer: a new management strategy. *Ann Otol Rhinol Laryngol Suppl.* 2008;199:3–24.
31. Zeitels SM. Vocal fold atypia/dysplasia and carcinoma. In: Zeitels SM, ed. *Atlas of Phonomicrosurgery and Other Endolaryngeal Procedures for Benign and Malignant Disease.* San Diego, Calif: Singular; 2001;177–218.
32. Jako GJ, Kleinsasser O. *Endolaryngeal micro-diagnosis and microsurgery.* Reprint from the Annual Meeting of the American Medical Association; 1966.
33. Zeitels SM, Franco RA Jr, Dailey SH, Burns JA, Hillman RE, Anderson RR. Office-based treatment of glottal dysplasia and papillomatosis with the 585-nm pulsed dye laser and local anesthesia. *Ann Otol Rhinol Laryngol.* 2004;113(4):265–276.
34. Zeitels SM, Anderson RR, Burns JA, Hillman RE. Office based 532nm pulsed-KTP laser treatment of glottal papillomatosis and dysplasia [Letter to the Editor]. *Ann Otol Rhinol Laryngol.* 2007;116:317–318.
35. Zeitels SM, Blitzer A, Hillman RE, Anderson RR. Foresight in laryngology and laryngeal surgery: a 2020 vision. *Ann Otol Rhinol Laryngol.* 2007;116(suppl 198): 1–16.

Premalignant Epithelium and Microinvasive Cancer of the Vocal Fold: The Evolution of Phonomicrosurgical Management

Steven M. Zeitels, MD, FACS

"Our knowledge has been built up, we have seen, not by the mushroom activity of any one period, or of any school of medicine, or by the premature birth of an idea or theory, but by the patient, painstaking, laborious exertions of many generations of earnest men."

—Jonathan Wright, MD
A History of Laryngology and Rhinology, 1914[1]

Phonomicrosurgical treatment of premalignant vocal fold epithelium and microinvasive cancer combines principles of surgical oncology with advanced laryngoscopic microsurgical-techniques. This treatment is guided by mucosal-wave theory of voice production and strives not only to cure the disease but also to achieve optimal vocal function.

Surgical techniques developed during the past two centuries have improved methods for vocal fold visualization, tissue retrieval, and tissue evaluation. Examination of the evolution of these surgical techniques reveals the incomplete convergence of laryngoscopic surgical theory with both the concept of premalignancy and the anatomical-physiological principles of voice production. This historical review, which helps to explain the lack of consensus about current treatment options, led to a series of four investigations. They were conducted with the aim of developing a laryngoscopic (phonomicrosurgical) management approach for improving the treatment of premalignant and microinvasive vocal fold epithelium.

In the first of four investigations, 42 patients (each of whom had a significant smoking history) underwent microlaryngoscopic biopsy of 52 vocal fold lesions. These lesions, which were suspicious for atypia or malignancy and were confined to the musculomembranous vocal fold, were mapped according to surface involvement and depth of penetration. Review of the maps revealed that 27 of the 52 lesions involved only the superior/ventricular surface. For these patients, the entire layered vocal fold structure could potentially be preserved on the medial/vocalizing surface. Twenty-five of the 52 lesions involved both the superior/ventricular surface and the medial/vocalizing surface. No lesion involved only the medial surface.

These data suggest that (in smokers) geographic localization of keratotic and erythroplastic lesions on the superior/ventricular surface of the musculomembranous vocal fold are likely to contain atypia. This characteristic facilitates the appropriate selection of patients for biopsy and may spare individuals, who have lesions resulting from hyperfunctional dysphonia and/or gastroesophageal reflux, from unnecessary biopsy. These two disorders typically result in pathology on the medial and/or posterior glottal surfaces.

In order to determine whether a directed biopsy or an excisional biopsy approach is preferable for obtaining an accurate diagnosis, all specimens underwent whole-mount sectioning for three-dimensional histopathological analysis. Keratosis was noted: without atypia in 14; with atypia in 27; and with carcinoma in 11. The severity of the atypia usually varied throughout each specimen. The surface appearance of the lesion was not a reliable prognosticator of the severity of dysplasia either between patients or in different areas of the same lesion; therefore, excisional biopsy and whole-mount, multiple-section histopathological analysis were necessary for obtaining an accurate diagnosis.

In the second study, submucosal vocal fold dye infusions were performed to identify where the glottal mucosa was supported by the superficial lamina propria (SLP). The histological sections of these vocal folds demonstrated that the caudal limitation of the SLP was in close proximity to the epithelial surface change from ciliated to nonciliated epithelium (inferior arcuate line). It is generally thought that the inferior arcuate line denotes the proximal subcordal vibratory epithelium. The infusions also demonstrated that dye-induced hydrostatic distension of the SLP would provide more room for surgical dissection in the SLP and would reduce instrumental trauma to the layered vocal-

Presented as a Candidate's Thesis to the American Laryngological, Rhinological and Otological Society, Inc. Recipient of an Honorable Mention. Submitted: September 1993.

From the Department of Otology and Laryngology, Harvard Medical School, Boston, Mass.

Send Reprint Requests to Steven M. Zeitels, MD, Department of Otology and Laryngology, Harvard Medical School, Massachusetts Eye and Ear Infirmary, 243 Charles St., Boston, MA 02114.

fold microstructure. These features assisted in the design of a procedure that, by simulating Reinke's edema, would help to preserve the vocal fold's layered anatomy.

The third investigation employed the anatomical SLP-infusion studies in a clinical trial. A submucosal infusion of saline and epinephrine in conjunction with microflap excisional biopsy was performed on 43 vocal folds. Complete excisional biopsy was accomplished in all. The infusion produced hydrostatic distension of the SLP and the overlying epithelium. This improved the visualization of the lesion's perimeter and resulted in precise placement of incisions around the lesion. The increased depth of the SLP and the hydrodissection of the epithelium from the vocal ligament facilitated both the development of a precise microflap and the maximal preservation of the vocal fold's layered microstructure. The infusion effectively demonstrated invasion through the SLP into the vocal ligament by causing distension of the epithelium and of the SLP not involved with cancer, while leaving a relative depression where the SLP was replaced by cancer.

In the fourth study, a pilot group of 17 patients was assessed to determine which postoperative objective vocal-measurement criteria would be valuable, and to begin to establish expected postsurgical outcome data. The results generally suggested that as the epithelial resection extended from the superior surface to include the medial surface as well, the measures used began to reflect deteriorating vocal function. Specifically, the acoustic data revealed that the most likely aberrations postoperatively were increased jitter (cycle-to-cycle irregularity of pitch) and reduced maximal ranges for both loudness (intensity) and pitch (frequency). These changes appeared to be related to higher levels of stiffness and/or tension in the vocal mechanism. With these changes, there was often an increase in subglottic aerodynamic support (pressure), which could be a compensatory adjustment or the manifestation of persistent (presurgical) hyperfunctional behaviors. While patients did not describe discomfort in conjunction with voice production, the stroboscopic evaluations visually confirmed the presence of increased stiffness/restriction in the glottal valve. The most common abnormal sequela seen with stroboscopy was a decrease in the magnitude of the mucosal wave on the superior/ventricular vocal-fold surface. If a medial/vocalizing surface resection was done, the amplitude of vocal fold vibration (excursion) was also likely to be diminished. The perceptual vocal assessment parameters were typically normal or revealed mild dysphonia.

Phonomicrosurgical treatment of premalignant and microinvasive vocal fold epithelium integrates principles of surgical oncology with those of voice production. The use of submucosal infusion with microflap excisional biopsy *a.* provides a tissue specimen suitable for multiple-section histopathological analysis; *b.* establishes an unequivocal diagnosis; *c.* treats the lesion; *d.* reserves all cancer treatment options; *e.* is simple, repeatable, and cost-effective; *f.* preserves the layered vocal-fold anatomy, and *g.* avoids the medial aspect of the vocal fold (vocalizing surface) as much as is oncologically possible for optimal postoperative voice. The pilot voice evaluations that were done suggest that while patients treated by this approach did not typically achieve "normal" vocal function (according to measures of underlying physiology), most did manage to produce voices that were, acoustically and perceptually, within normal limits during conversational-level speech.

INTRODUCTION

Ideal management of premalignant epithelium and microinvasive cancer of the vocal fold should provide an accurate diagnosis, eliminate the disease, and result in normal voice. But, because of technical biases, philosophical differences, and the unknown results of various interventions on voice, there is no consensus about how to achieve this ideal. Excision of keratotic vocal fold lesions has been accomplished with stripping, controlled microdissection of the vocal fold cover, and cordectomy (the latter, approached transorally or transcervically). Alternatively, these lesions have been destroyed by heat, cold, and ionizing radiation.

Evaluation of laryngological history demonstrates the gradual but incomplete convergence of laryngoscopic surgical theory with the concept of premalignancy and the anatomical-physiological principles of voice production. This history also provides explanations for the variations in management approaches. There are, however, questions that remain unresolved. Among them: *1.* What tissue must be removed for accurate diagnosis and for treatment? *2.* How does the microanatomy of the vocal fold influence management? *3.* What is the best therapeutic technique in light of the answers to questions 1 and 2? and *4.* What are the objective voice results of that technique? Answers to these questions were sought in a series of four studies.

HYPOTHESIS

Management of premalignant epithelium and microinvasive cancer of the vocal fold by phonomicrosurgical excisional biopsy not only integrates mucosal-wave theory of voice production with sound surgical oncology but also preserves "normal" voice.

OBJECTIVES

1. To delineate the historical evolution of laryngoscopy, laryngology, the concept of vocal fold premalignancy, and the theories of voice production as they each relate to *a.* the foundations of transoral management of vocal fold atypia and microinvasive cancer and *b.* the choices of equipment and technique that ultimately determine phonomicrosurgical capabilities.

2. To develop patient-selection criteria for phonomicrosurgical excision of atypical and microinva-

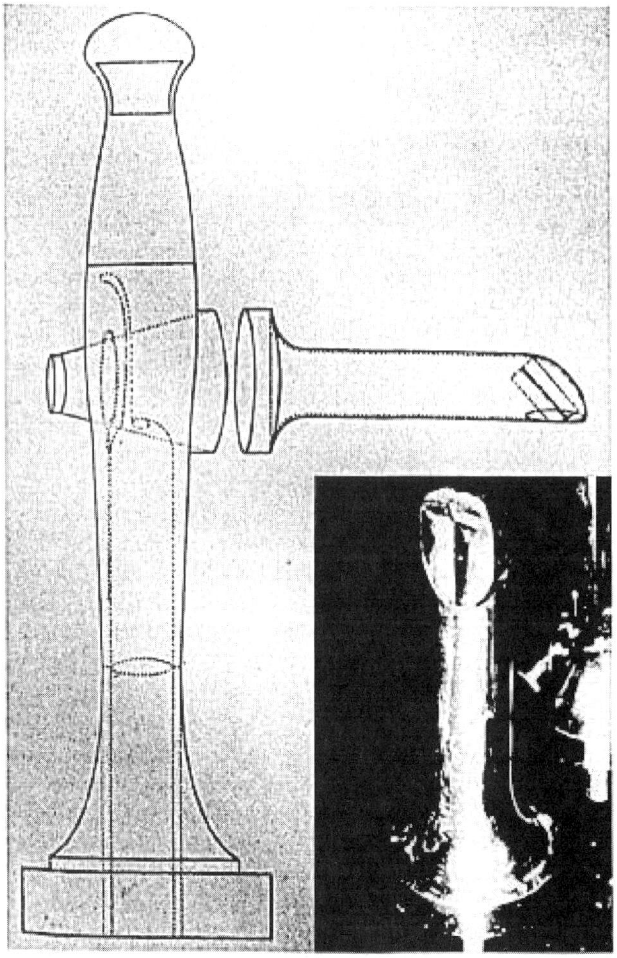

Fig. 1. Philipp Bozzini's (1773-1809) Lichtleiter (1807). (Courtesy of the American College of Surgeons).

sive epithelium by determining the geographic areas of the vocal fold most likely to become involved by this disease.

3. To determine whether the surface appearance of the vocal fold is an accurate prognosticator of underlying cellular morphology; and, thereby, to determine whether directed biopsy or excisional biopsy approaches are necessary for accurate diagnosis and treatment.

4. To design an oncologically sound, phonomicrosurgical, excisional biopsy technique for atypical and microinvasive epithelium *a.* by determining where the vocal fold epithelium is supported by a superficial lamina propria (and, therefore, the vibratory mucosa) and *b.* by incorporating the information in *4a* to help preserve the layered vocal-fold anatomy.

5. To assess the vocal results of this technique by *a.* determining which objective acoustic, aerodynamic, and visual measurement parameters optimally assess postsurgical results of vocal-fold epithelial resections, and *b.* beginning to establish expected outcome data for those parameters.

HISTORY

The evolution of surgical management of premalignant and early malignant lesions of the vocal fold developed from the ability to observe the larynx, to biopsy suspicious tissue precisely, to assess accurately its biological aggressiveness, and ultimately, to excise that tissue without significant vocal or airway impairment. A continuum of instrument and technique development throughout the past 185 years has facilitated progress in managing premalignant vocal-fold epithelium and microinvasive cancer. A comprehensive, detailed review of this evolution provides explanations for current surgical preferences. This history is presented in a topic-oriented fashion for ease of understanding, despite some overlapping events and concepts.

Mirror Laryngoscopy and the Origin of Laryngology

The ability to visualize the larynx during phonation and respiration in both healthy and diseased states was one of the great medical advancements of the 19th century; from this, the field of laryngology was born.

Classical historical teaching indicates that indirect mirror laryngoscopy preceded direct endoscopic examination by approximately 85 years. In 1807, Bozzini[2] published a pamphlet describing a double cannula with an internal mirror (Fig. 1) that was used to observe various internal organs in the body, such as the larynx. He designed a universal handle in which a candle with a reflector provided illumination. A variety of cannulae could be attached to the handle depending on the site in the body to be examined. Bozzini developed the revolutionary concept that an extracorporeal light source should be employed to view inside of the body; this is the guiding premise of present-day minimally-invasive surgery. The device, however, was not perfected and received little attention. Reports of other marginally successful attempts at mirror laryngoscopy were reported by Cagniard de la Tour (1825)[3] and Senn (1827).[4] In 1829, Babington[5] presented his glottiscope to the Hunterian Society. The instrument consisted of an oblong mirror set in silver wire on a long handle (Fig. 2). The mirror was held against the palate while the tongue was depressed by a spatula. Selligue (1832),[6] an ingenious mechanic who suffered from laryngeal phthisis, designed a speculum to visualize his larynx. Liston (1837),[7] in his well-known surgical textbook, described observing laryngeal edema with a dentist's mirror dipped in hot water. Baumes (1838)[8] exhibited a laryngeal mirror at the Medical Society of Lyon. To accompany his headlight, Avery (1844) designed a single cannula speculum (Fig. 3) similar to Bozzini's instrument, which employed a perforated concave mirror. These isolated reports were minimally acknowledged or appreciated be-

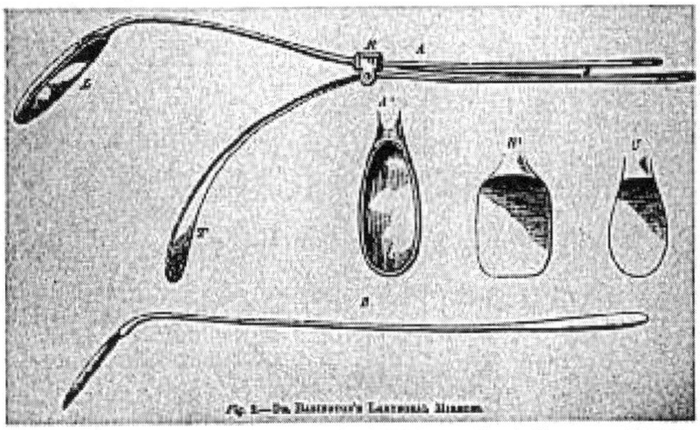

Fig. 2. Benjamin Guy Babington's (1794-1866) glottiscope (1829). (From Mackenzie: "The Use of the Laryngoscope in Diseases of the Throat With an Appendix on Rhinoscopy.")

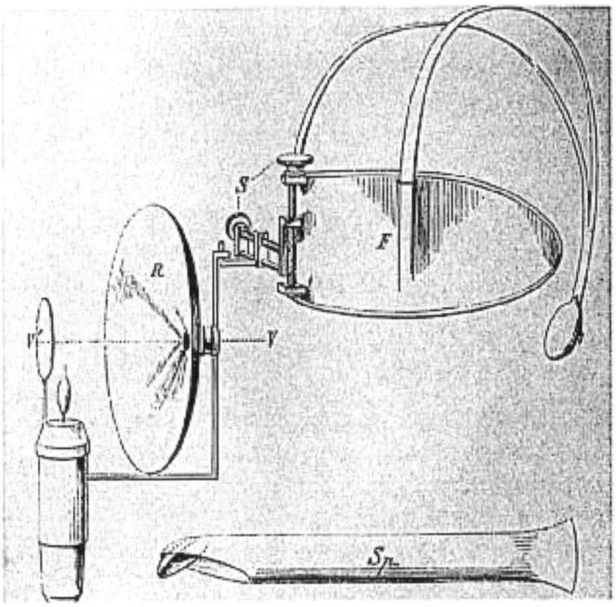

Fig. 3. John Avery's (1807-1855) laryngoscope (1844). (From Mackenzie: "The Use of the Laryngoscope in Diseases of the Throat With an Appendix on Rhinoscopy.")

cause of instrument and/or technique difficulties.

In 1855, Manuel Garcia (Fig. 4) described autolaryngoscopy, which he carried out using two mirrors and reflected sunlight. He presented this technique to the Royal Society of London in his paper entitled "Observations on the Human Voice."[10] Since Garcia was a classical vocal pedagogist, attempting to understand musical phonation, historians believe that he was unaware of the previous reports of laryngoscopy.[11] His ability to observe and describe his own larynx stimulated widespread interest in the technique from which the new specialty of laryngology was born. This won him recognition as the "Father of Laryngoscopy." Garcia lived to be 101 and, on his centennial birthday (1905), Sir Felix Semon organized a celebration to honor him. Laryngologists gathered from around the world for that celebration and commissioned John Singer Sargent to

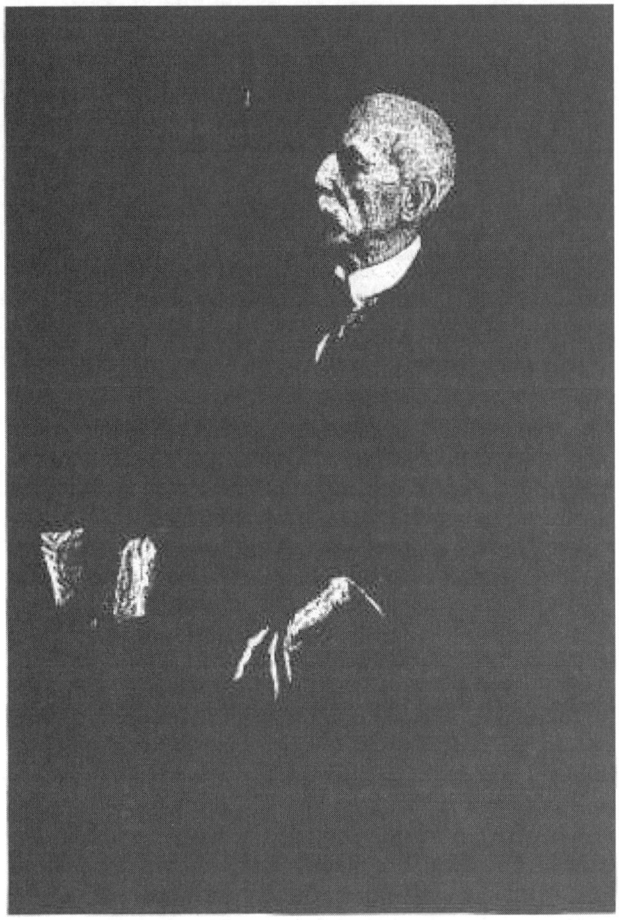

Fig. 4. Manuel Garcia (1805-1906) at 100 years of age in 1905. (Courtesy of the Rhode Island School of Design.)

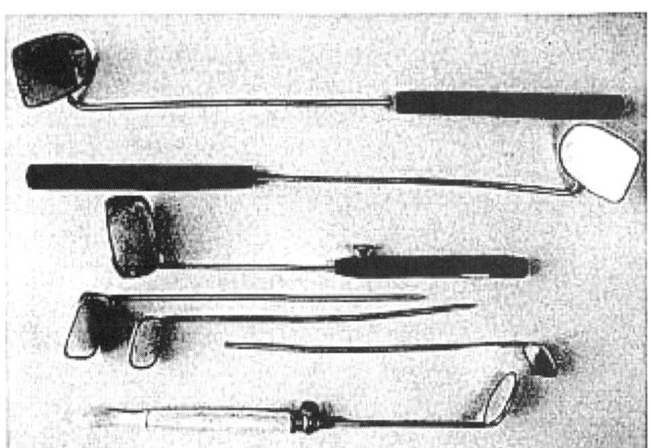

Fig. 5. Various 19th-century laryngoscope mirrors; Johann Czermak used square mirrors similar to those seen here. (Courtesy of the Massachusetts Eye and Ear Infirmary.)

paint Garcia's portrait (Fig. 4).

In 1857, Turck[12] explored, but then abandoned, the clinical application of mirror laryngoscopy. Several months later, his colleague, Czermak,[13,14] borrowed Turck's mirrors (Fig. 5) and commenced similar clinical investigations; he concluded that the

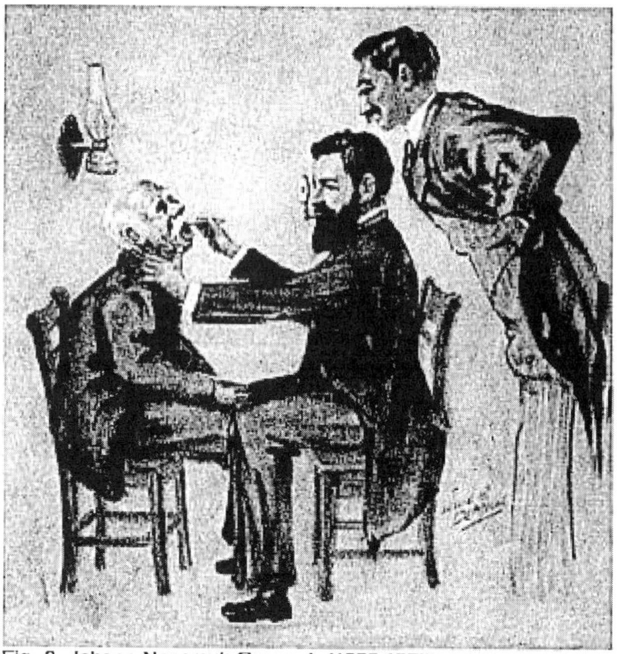

Fig. 6. Johann Nepomuk Czermak (1828-1873) performing indirect laryngoscopy around 1860. Note the head and neck position. (Courtesy of the American Laryngological Association.)

technique was valuable for the understanding and management of laryngeal disorders. Czermak introduced the artificial light source and reintroduced the fenestrated concave mirror; he initially placed the mirror in a frame between his teeth (Fig. 6) before settling on the head mirror. Subsequent to Czermak's success, Turck resumed his investigations and eventually made excellent contributions to descriptive laryngeal pathology.[15] The two quarreled bitterly for many years about academic recognition for the development of indirect mirror laryngoscopy. Czermak is generally considered to be the individual most influential in disseminating the technique and in establishing the value of mirror laryngoscopy throughout the Western world. Without his innovations, the head mirror and the use of artificial light, mirror laryngoscopy would again probably have been a stillborn child.

The feud between Czermak and Turck fueled interest in laryngoscopy, and there was an outpouring of literature describing laryngeal pathology.[15-17] Stoerk (1859)[18] (Figs. 7, 8) reported the first laryngoscopically-controlled manipulation that involved the topical application of silver nitrate to the larynx. Laryngoscopic technique quickly spread throughout the major cities of the Western world.

In 1859, at the age of 21, Sir Morell Mackenzie (Fig. 9) visited Czermak and quickly mastered laryngoscopic technique. In 1863, Mackenzie won the Jackson Prize of the Royal College of Surgeons for his essay, "The Pathology and Treatment of Laryngeal Disease." Mackenzie designed many instruments (Fig. 8) and broadened the appeal of laryngoscopic techniques by perfecting and teaching transoral surgical methods.[19,20] His 1865 textbook, *The Use of the Laryngoscope in Diseases of the Throat*[19] was important for enhancing laryngoscopic training.

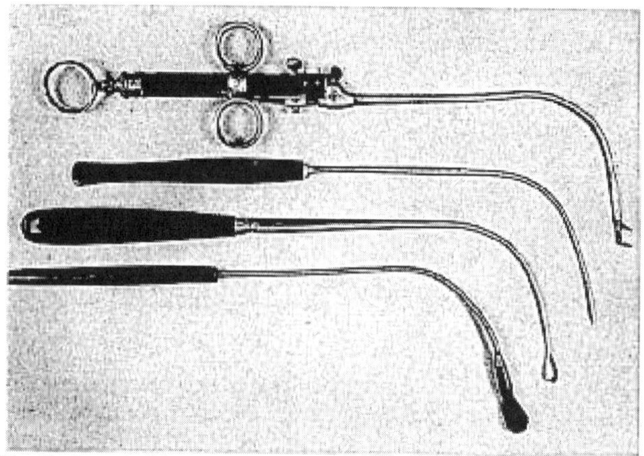

Fig. 7. Assorted transoral instruments; the forceps at the top was designed by Stoerk. (Courtesy of the Massachusetts Eye and Ear Infirmary.)

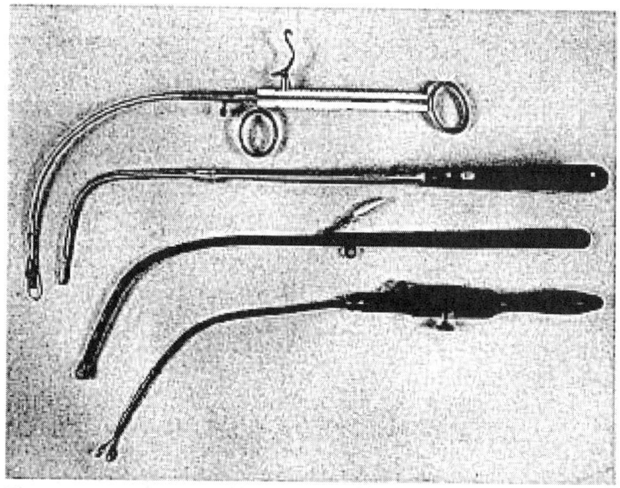

Fig. 8. Assorted transoral instruments; Mackenzie designed the bottom two. (Courtesy of the Massachusetts Eye and Ear Infirmary.)

Ernst Krackowizer, a native of Vienna, was the first to perform laryngoscopy in the United States (1858)[21-23]; however, it was Louis Elsberg (Fig. 10)[24,25] of New York and Jacob Solis-Cohen (Fig. 11)[26] of Philadelphia who were the primary figures in 19th century American laryngology. Elsberg's gold medal, prize-winning presentation[25] to the American Medical Association in 1865 was entitled "Laryngoscopal Surgery, Illustrated in the Treatment of Morbid Growths Within the Larynx." Elsberg[27] and Solis-Cohen,[28] were the major forces in the spreading of laryngoscopic technique in America. In 1879, Elsberg became the first president of the American Laryngological Association (ALA);[22] and after moderating the meeting for the first 2 years, he was succeeded by Solis-Cohen.[29] In 1880, they began the *American Archives of Laryngology*,

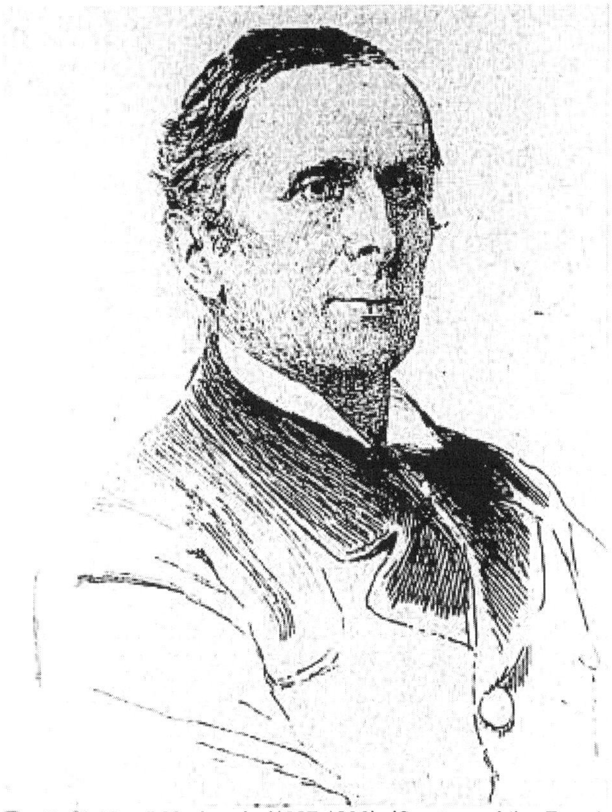

Fig. 9. Sir Morell Mackenzie (1837-1892). (Courtesy of the Francis A. Countway Medical Library.)

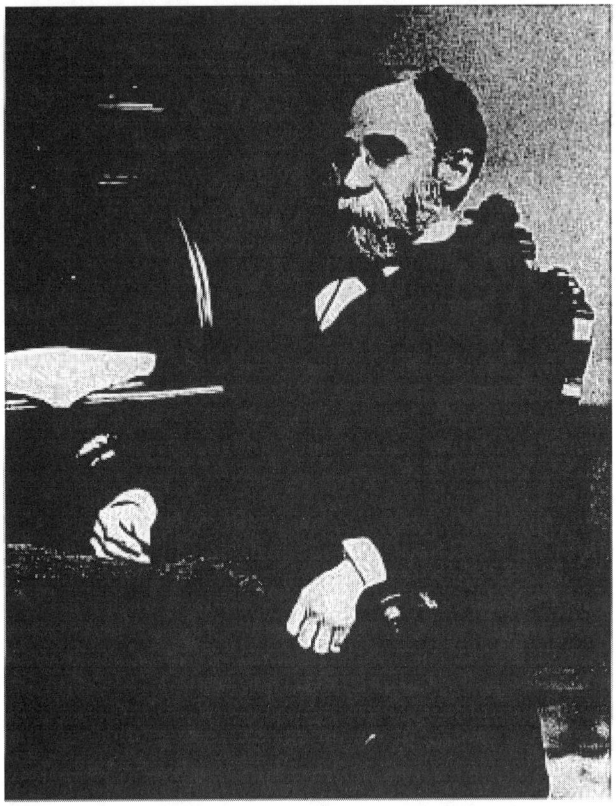

Fig. 11. Jacob de Silva Solis-Cohen (1838-1927). (Courtesy of the Mutter Museum.)

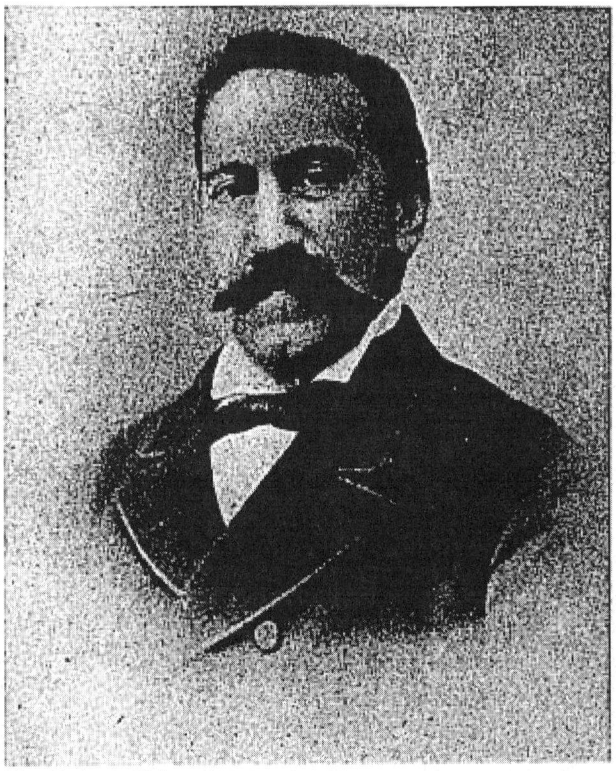

Fig. 10. Louis Elsberg (1837-1885): The first president of the American Laryngological Association. (Courtesy of the *Annals of Otology, Rhinology and Laryngology.*)

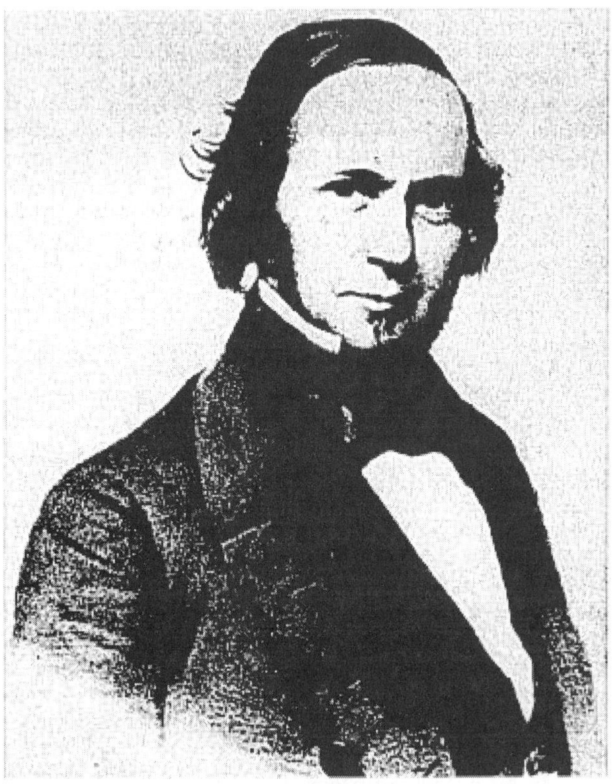

Fig. 12. Horace Green (1802-1866): "The Father of American Laryngology." (Courtesy of the American Laryngological Association.)

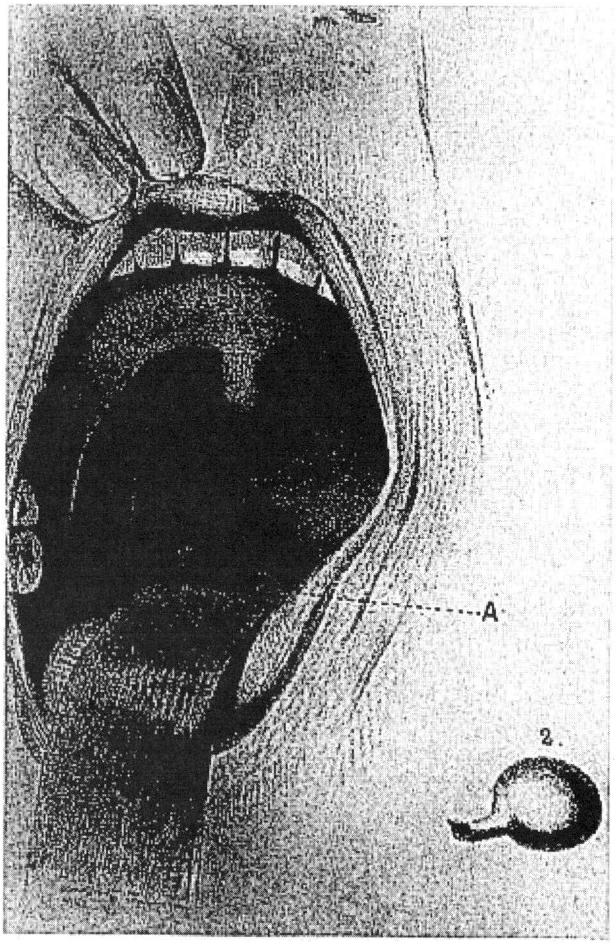

Fig. 13. Laryngeal polyp excised under direct vision by Green. (From Green: "On the Surgical Treatment of Polypi of the Larynx, and Oedema of the Glottis.")

which was published until 1884. This journal was followed in 1896 by The LARYNGOSCOPE.

ENDOLARYNGEAL SURGERY

Before Laryngoscopy

There were several descriptions of excision of intralaryngeal tumors in the prelaryngoscopic era. According to Wright,[30] it was in 1770 that Koederik (in Brussels) reported the first intralaryngeal removal of a neoplasm. To do this, he used some type of malleable instrument to ligate a laryngeal polyp.

In 1852, Horace Green (Fig. 12) of New York reported on the transoral removal of a large laryngeal polyp from an 11-year-old child.[31] He exposed the polyp by forcible tongue depression (Fig. 13), grasped it with a curved hook, and cut it off with a knife. This event is included in the prelaryngoscopy era because it has been recorded as such in all historical documents. It can be argued that this was, in fact, the first example of direct laryngoscopy, predating (by 40 years) Kirstein (1895),[32] who is generally recognized as the first individual to perform

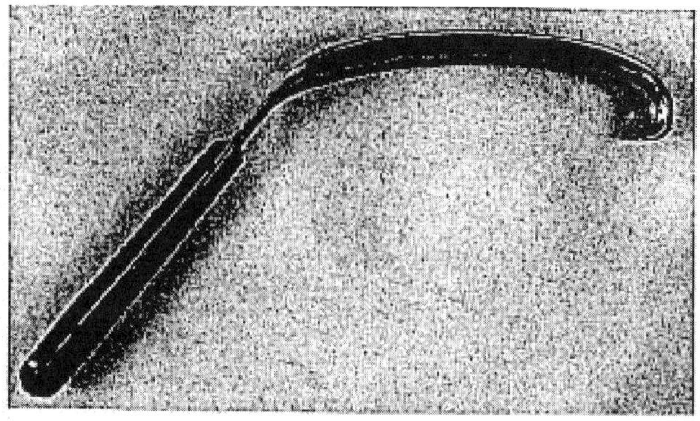

Fig. 14. Nineteenth-century tongue spatula similar to that used by Green. It bears great resemblance to a standard anesthesia-type spatula laryngoscope but without self-contained illumination. (Courtesy of the Massachusetts Eye and Ear Infirmary.)

direct laryngoscopy. Although Green may not have seen the true vocal cords well, his description of that procedure bears similarity to Kirstein's report of direct laryngoscopy with an open spatula blade, which is similar to instrumentation used by anesthesiologists today.

As reported by Elsberg,[22] Green was the first physician to devote his career to the study of the throat and respiratory diseases. This was courageous and bold work during the prelaryngoscopic era, when infectious diseases such as diphtheria, tuberculosis, and syphilis often resulted in lethal membranous laryngeal airway obstruction.[33,34]

Unknowingly, in his comprehensive textbook on rigid endoscopy, Brunings (1912)[35] supported the contention that Green had performed the first direct laryngoscopy. His chapter describing direct laryngoscopic technique begins with a description of having the examiner place a bent spatula on the tongue base to determine the patient's ability to undergo tubular laryngoscopy. "It may even happen, in particularly favorable circumstances, that by introducing the spatula a long way and exercising a strong pressure, a direct view of the arytenoid region may be obtained." Green's description offers the reader the opportunity to decide about the true priority for the first direct laryngoscopy:

> I proceeded to examine this organ [the larynx], with a bent tongue spatula [Fig. 14]. I drew forward and depressed the tongue, so as to enable me to see the condition of the epiglottis. By this procedure, nearly the whole of this cartilage was brought into view, but no deviation from its usual normal aspect was observed. Whilst making this examination and at the very moment when the tongue was depressed, and the epiglottis in full view, the patient gave sudden and rather violent cough, when a round, white, fibrous looking polypus appeared, momentarily at the opening of the glottis, and then seemed as quickly to be drawn into the larynx. Again and again, was this operation repeated; and whenever the patient coughed, at the moment when the

> tongue was depressed, a portion of the polypus could be seen, not over the top of the epiglottis, but at the lateral border of this cartilage. The mobility of the tumor was quite manifest. It appeared to be attached by its pedicle to the left ventricle or the left vocal ligament; for on coughing, the current of air would force the body out of the glottis, sufficient to allow a portion of the tumor to be seen, on the side of the opening, just above the tip of the left arytenoid cartilage.[31]

Green[31] explained that because there was no precedent for performing a laryngotomy to remove such a tumor:

> I determined to make an attempt to remove the polypus through the opening of the glottis.... She was seated in a good light, before an open window, with her head thrown well back, and held firmly, by an assistant, in that position. With the flat handle of my knife, I depressed the tongue, and when the epiglottis was in view, I glided the double hook over the top of this cartilage and a little on its laryngeal face.... I succeeded in catching the hooks into the top of the tumour, and turning quickly the blade of the knife downwards, passed it over the left border of the glottis, I cut from behind forwards, and happily, dividing the pedicle near its attachment, brought the tumour out of the larynx.

The artist who generated the accompanying drawing (Fig. 13) did so from personal visualization. Green's description indicates that he saw significantly more of the laryngeal introitus than is seen in the artist's depiction in Figure 13. His success was due both to his skill and to his wisdom in selecting a child; for the elevated laryngeal position of the child allowed him to achieve direct laryngeal visualization despite as yet undeveloped instrumentation (the laryngoscope) and poor lighting.

Green also described transoral application of caustics to the larynx to treat infectious inflammatory disorders of the laryngeal membranes.[34] He was, however, maligned by his contemporaries, who did not believe that his transoral interventions were possible.[22,36,37] Later, Green resolved this by placing a whalebone probang transorally through the glottis of a patient with a tracheotomy until the probang could be visualized at the tracheotomy site. Transoral laryngeal manipulation via mirror laryngoscopy also helped reinstate Green's reputation before his death in 1866. At the first meeting of the ALA, in recognition of Green's contributions in the prelaryngoscopic era, Elsberg credited Green as the "Father of American Laryngology."

Indirect Laryngoscopy: Benign Tumors and Origin of the Cancer Biopsy

Lewin (1860)[38] was the first to report laryngoscopically guided management of laryngeal tumors. In his series of 50 neoplasms, he excised 3 and applied caustics to 4. During the subsequent decade, there were numerous reports of transoral removal of benign laryngeal tumors. At the time of the Civil War in America, it appears that H.B. Sands (1865)[39] was the first to report performing transoral biopsy of a laryngeal cancer with subsequent transcervical excision of the lesion. Sands has not been given due credit for reporting what is now a standard approach to head and neck cancer: endoscopic biopsy followed by open resection. In 1871, Mackenzie published his treatise on *Growths in the Larynx*.[17] Mackenzie popularized transoral vocal cord biopsy techniques and his skills gained him international fame. He opened the first hospital for diseases of the throat and is considered to be the "Father of British Laryngology."

Mackenzie's fame resulted in a tumultuous period in his professional and personal life. In May 1887, Crown Prince Frederick of Germany, to whom Queen Victoria's eldest daughter was married, developed hoarseness; Mackenzie[40] was sent to examine him. On mirror examination, Mackenzie noted an irregular lesion, which he thought should be biopsied for microscopic diagnosis. He retrieved abnormal vocal cord tissue three times during four attempts in 5 weeks. Despite the repeated biopsies, Rudolf Virchow could not establish the presence of cancer in the specimens, and the laryngectomy that was urged by the prince's surgeon, Van Bergman, was not performed. Because laryngectomy was frequently a lethal procedure, Mackenzie was not in favor of the surgery without a clear diagnosis of cancer. Ultimately, the clinically suspected and pathologically undiagnosed subglottic cancer progressed to create airway obstruction requiring a tracheotomy. The prince died of laryngeal cancer within the year, shortly after becoming emperor of Germany.

By Mackenzie's account,[40] the prince's private physicians were displeased about Mackenzie's involvement and management decisions. The unfortunate outcome fueled simmering intrigue and gossip. Mackenzie was so disturbed by the course of events subsequent to the prince's death that in response to a derogatory report emanating from the prince's private physicians, he felt compelled to record a detailed account of the entire affair. In that book, entitled *The Fatal Illness of Frederick the Nobel*,[40] Mackenzie sought to clear his name; but, many colleagues considered this approach unprofessional and unethical. For this conduct, he was censured by both the Royal College of Surgeons and the British Medical Society and resigned from the Royal College of Physicians.[40,41]

It is ironic that the delay in diagnosis probably prolonged the prince's life (the average survival of Van Bergman's seven previously laryngectomized patients was only 4 months[42,43]). Had Mackenzie's biopsies established the diagnosis of cancer, the prince would probably not have become emperor (kaiser). There are some who suggest that Virchow was aware of this and had purposefully misdiagnosed the biopsy to prevent the prince from undergoing the perilous procedure of laryngectomy.

A review of Virchow's own descriptions of the histology of the biopsies suggests, however, that he simply erred in the diagnosis.[44] Eventually, the German physicians lost confidence in Virchow, and Waldeyer was consulted. Waldeyer had little trouble establishing the diagnosis of cancer. It was Waldeyer who had formulated the epithelial theory of carcinoma that is the foundation for modern theory of mucosal carcinogenesis.[44] Although Virchow was the creator of cellular pathology, he believed that cancer arose from connective tissue and grew to the surface.[44] This fundamental misunderstanding probably caused Virchow's error in diagnosis.

The delayed cancer diagnosis also resulted in a thesis among many respected physicians that Mackenzie had induced the cancer with the biopsy. Earlier in the 1880s, Solis-Cohen in America[45] and Lennox Browne in Britian[46] had already suggested that benign laryngeal neoplasms could undergo malignant degeneration from repeated manipulation. With the death of Frederick, the general concept of tissue biopsy for microscopic diagnosis was discredited.

Semon[47,48] recognized the crippling effect that his notion would have upon the fledgling field of laryngology. In 1889, he gathered data from throughout the world and reported on 10,747 mirror-observed cases of laryngeal lesions. Of that group, 8216 underwent endoscopic removal or biopsy with resultant benign histology, and 2531 were observed. Cancer was ultimately diagnosed in 33 (0.40%) of the 8216 in the operated group and in 12 (0.47%) of the 2531 in the observed patient group. This exhaustive investigation refuted the theory that laryngoscopic biopsy induced malignant degeneration and helped to clear Mackenzie's reputation. The eminent surgeon Henry Butlin,[49] as well as Fraenkel[50] and Chiari,[51] also strongly advised that cancer should be biopsied and submitted for histopathological analysis. At the ALA meeting in 1900, Solis-Cohen[52] altered his position and supported the concept of laryngeal biopsy followed by microscopic analysis. Despite this, the misconceptions that a transoral biopsy could induce neoplastic degeneration, accelerate local neoplastic growth, or induce metastasis persisted into the early 20th century.

The Cancer Biopsy in the 20th Century

John Mackenzie (1906)[53,54] was a chief opponent of the laryngeal biopsy. "The objections which I would urge against removal of tissue for examination (especially when done through the natural passages) are: (1) It subjects the patient at once to the dangers of autoinfection at the point of incision and to metastasis elsewhere; (2) it stimulates local growth of the cancer, and (3) finally, the method is often inconclusive, misleading, and sometimes impossible." He supported naked-eye mirror diagnosis followed by definitive laryngectomy without a histopathological diagnosis. This position de-emphasized the prevalence of infectious diseases, such as tuberculosis and syphilis, that could mimic the appearance of cancer.[55] In the unusual case he would support exploratory laryngofissure to establish the diagnosis. Mackenzie's sentiments were supported by Moore[56] and Mackenty[57] into the early 1920s. Jackson,[58-61] was a staunch advocate of histopathological tissue analysis, and he worked diligently for years to dispel the myths surrounding the laryngeal biopsy.

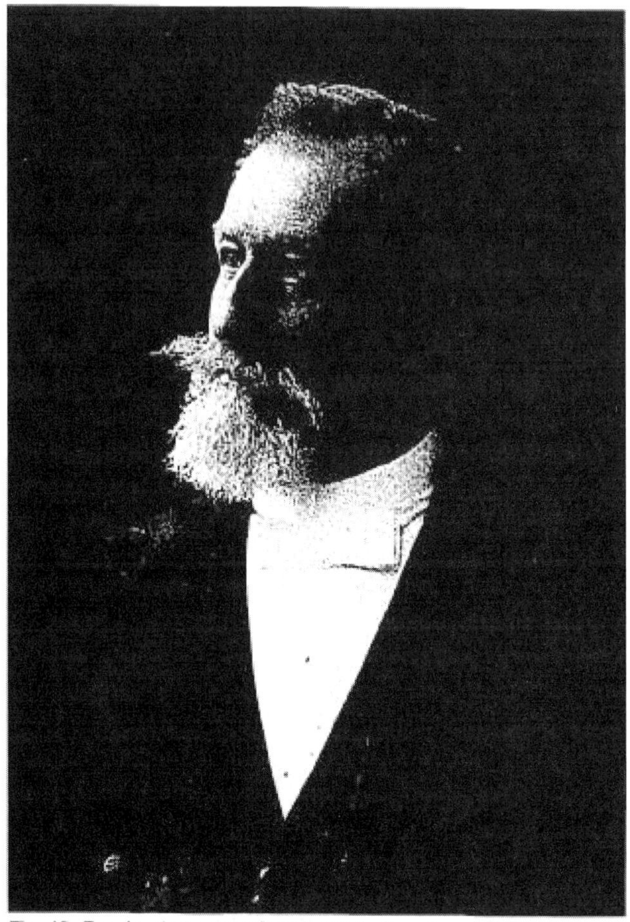

Fig. 15. Bernhard Fraenkel (1836-1911). (Courtesy of the *Annals of Otology, Rhinology and Laryngology.*)

Endolaryngeal Cancer Treatment

Months prior to the prince's illness, Fraenkel (Fig. 15), a renowned German laryngologist of this time, published the first report of transoral excision (1886) as the sole treatment for early glottic cancer.[62]

> The larnyx is a part of the body in which cancer can be recognized very early. Even very small tumors

disturb its function and will be realized by the patient. Laryngoscopy and microscopical examination of the specimen gives reliable diagnosis in a relatively short time.... I would like to report a laryngeal cancer case in which I have succeeded healing through the natural way.... The swelling covered the upper surface of the vocal cord and only the anterior and posterior quarters remained free.... In all cases where technically possible, tissue should be excised endolaryngeally ... using cocaine anesthesia.

After multiple transoral excisions for local recurrences and a modified neck dissection for metachronous regional metastasis, his patient was alive and well more than 5 years after the initial presentation of his disease, which was in 1881.

This report established many of the principles of laryngoscopic management of neoplastic vocal-fold lesions. Fraenkel realized that hoarseness can develop with minimal aberration of the vocal fold cover and that patients will often present with premalignant epithelium or small volume cancers. He noted that the lesion is likely to be situated on the superior surface of the vocal fold, which makes the lesion visible endoscopically. Its location on the musculomembranous fold, without involvement of the arytenoid or anterior commissure, makes it amenable to endoscopic removal.

Despite this report there were only isolated and anecdotal reports of endolaryngeal extirpation of cancer.[63–67] Twenty years after his initial report, Fraenkel would be honored in the *Annals of Otology, Rhinology and Laryngology* for his many contributions to laryngology.[68] It would take further developments in the 20th century, such as the direct laryngoscope, before endoscopic treatment of small volume cancers would become broadly accepted.

In 1915, Lynch[69–71] gradually introduced the concept of direct removal of early vocal fold neoplasia using his modification of the Killian laryngoscope-suspension system. Unlike his predecessors, Lynch resected these lesions en bloc and obtained cancer-free margins with the specimen. He was highly selective and chose lesions that were adequately exposed, of small volume, confined to one vocal fold, and that did not involve the arytenoid or anterior commissure. He emphasized the importance of the surgeon's flexibility in reverting, as necessary, to standard open transcervical techniques.

In 1941, New and Dorton[72] reported curing 9 of 10 patients with carcinoma of the musculomembranous vocal fold by using the Lynch suspension laryngoscope and surgical diathermy. In 1946, as a result of his association with Lynch, LeJeune[73] reported excellent results in 39 patients resected transorally by using the Lynch system. In 1973, Lillie and DeSanto[74] reported a successful series of transorally treated glottic lesions. They used the operating microscope with the Lynch suspension laryngoscope for the treatment of 57 T1 vocal fold carcinomas as well as 41 with carcinoma in situ (CIS). Shortly thereafter, Jako, Strong, and Vaughan[75–78] coupled the carbon dioxide laser (Fig. 16) to the surgical microscope and introduced it to laryngology and surgical oncology. They described a pilot group of patients who had undergone carbon dioxide laser resection of T1 musculomembranous vocal-fold carcinomas. Later, they reported a larger series that included a 3-year follow-up and firmly established the reliability of the technique.[79] This success was later confirmed by others and, today, there is broad acceptance of using the CO_2 laser for transoral excisional biopsy of selected musculomembranous T1 vocal-cord carcinomas.[80–82]

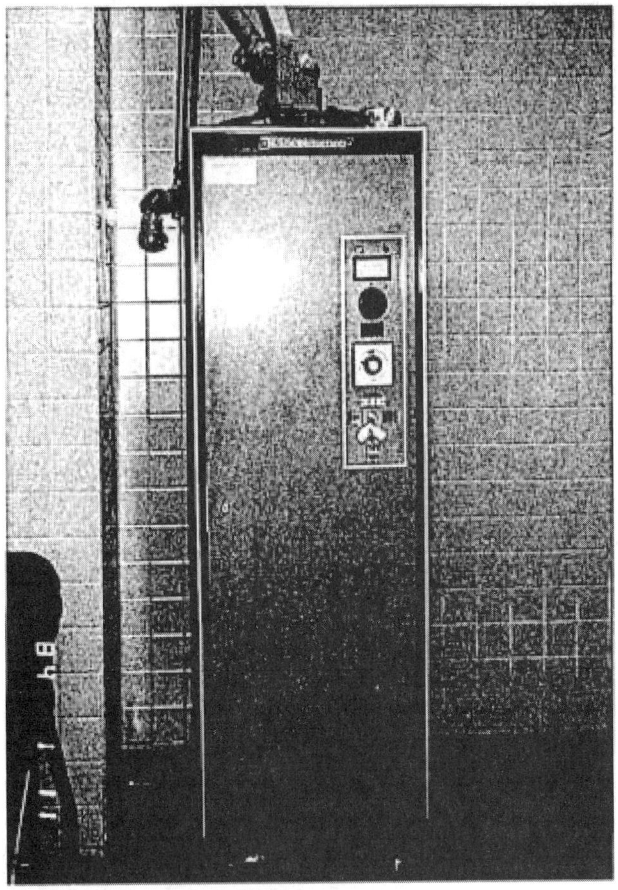

Fig. 16. An early carbon dioxide laser.

Direct Laryngoscopy: The Technique

In 1895, Kirstein[32,83] employed direct laryngoscopy (Fig. 17) in both the sitting and supine positions. He held the laryngoscope with one hand and surgically manipulated the larynx with the other. He believed that the sniffing position (flexion of the neck relative to the chest and extension of the head on the neck[84]) optimized laryngeal visualization during indirect laryngoscopy and was also important for direct laryngoscopic exposure of the anterior commissure in an awake patient. In his text-

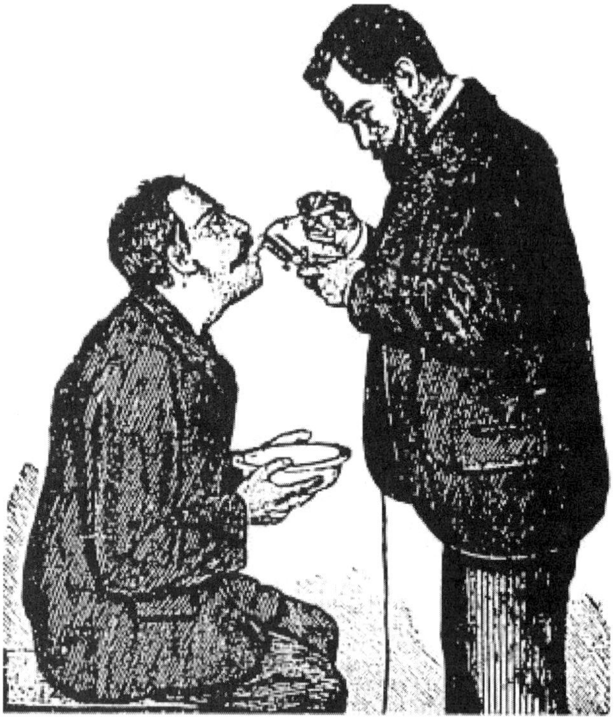

Fig. 17. Alfred Kirstein (1863-1922) performing direct laryngoscopy around 1895. Note the head and neck position.

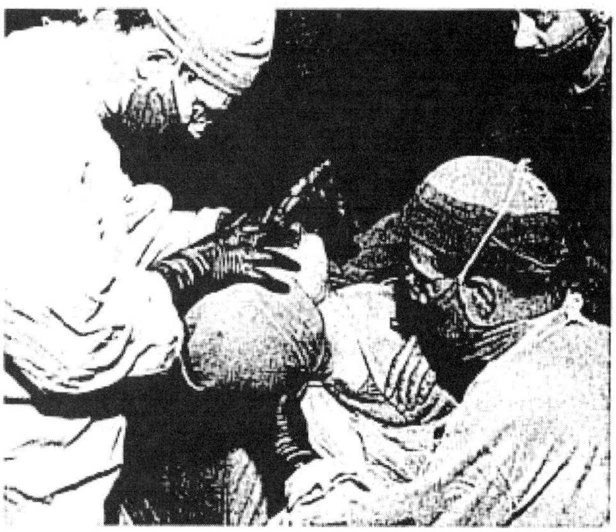

Fig. 18. Boyce-Jackson (1865-1958) head and neck position for supine direct laryngoscopy. (Reprinted with permission from W. B. Saunders Co., Philadelphia.)

book on peroral endoscopy, Jackson explained, "Kirstein position contains the essentials of the best position for direct laryngoscopy.... The extreme anterior displacement of the cervical spine with extension only at the occipito-atloid joint and avoidance of instrumental counter pressure on the upper teeth are fundamental."[59,85]

Around the turn of the century, Jackson concentrated on supine positioning for direct laryngoscopy. Human assistants functioned as head holders

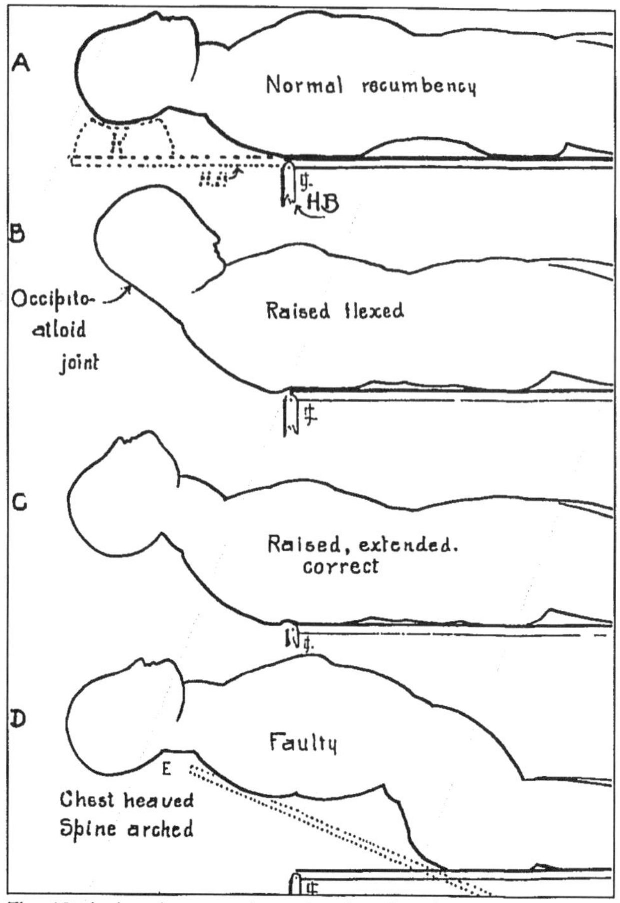

Fig. 19. Jackson's comparison of various head and neck positions for direct laryngoscopy. (From Jackson and Jackson: *Bronchoscopy, Esophagoscopy and Gastroscopy.*)

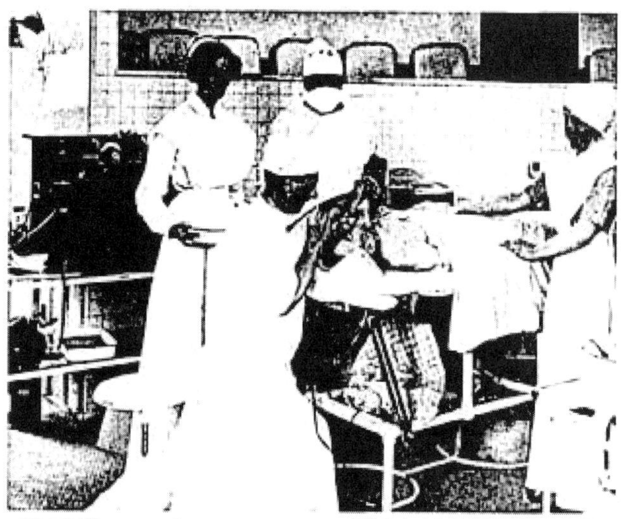

Fig. 20. A demonstration of Jackson's direct laryngoscopy technique without using a holding device to maintain the patient. The patient is in elevated-vector suspension; the examiner's left arm is functioning as the suspension gallows.

to raise the head and neck (Fig. 18). He credits his assistant, Boyce,[86] with adopting the proper head positioning from sitting indirect (Fig. 6) and sitting

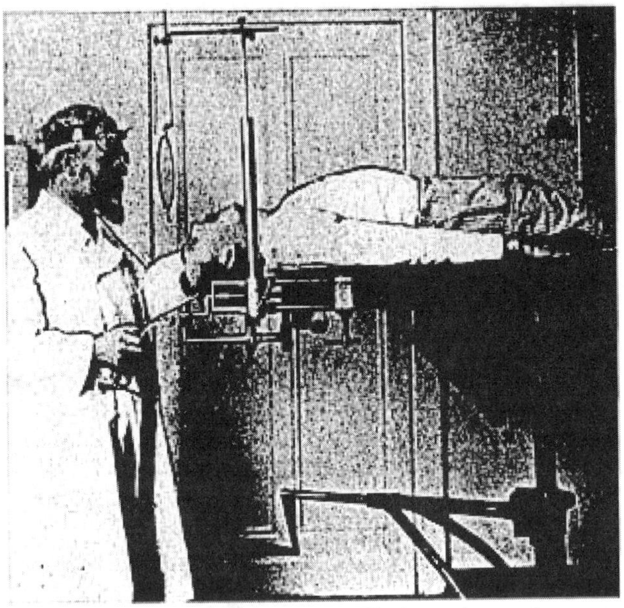

Fig. 21. Gustav Killian (1860-1921) positioning and preparing a patient for suspension laryngoscopy. The circular glass is to provide protection for the surgeon.

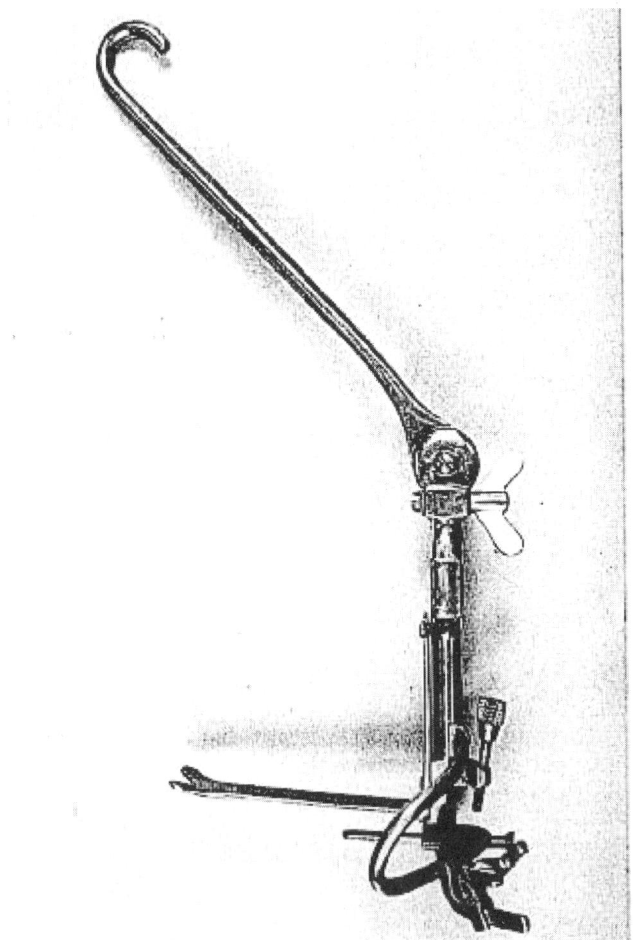

Fig. 22. Killian's spatula laryngoscope. (Courtesy of the Massachusetts Eye and Ear Infirmary.)

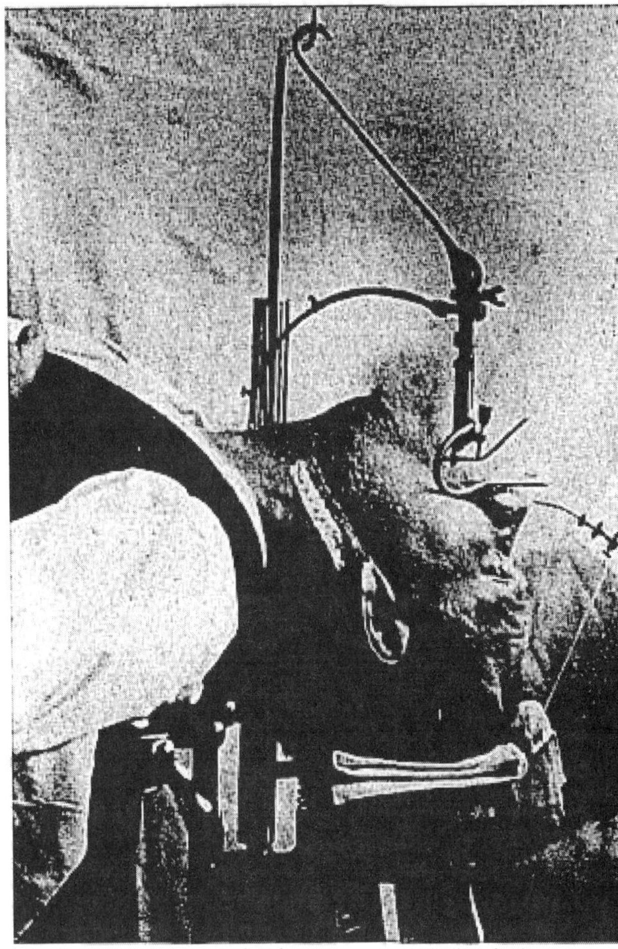

Fig. 23. Killian's suspension laryngoscope with Bruning's counterpressor attachment; note the head position demonstrating extension of the head and neck in relation to the chest.

direct laryngoscopy (Fig. 17) to supine direct laryngoscopy (Fig. 19). The Boyce-Jackson position is understood by rotating Figures 6 and 17 counterclockwise by 90 degrees from a sitting to a supine position.

In Jackson's approach, the surgeon positioned and maintained the laryngoscope with one hand, leaving the other hand free for tissue manipulation. He acknowledged the great skill that was required to perform delicate vocal-fold surgery with one hand, while the other was exerting great force to keep the larynx exposed and the head elevated (Fig. 20). He likened it to playing the piano when the left hand is required to pound out interval chords while the right plays a delicate treble. This technique was suitable for therapeutic laryngoscopy on benign lesions and for diagnostic endoscopy on malignant ones. It was not suitable for therapeutic, surgical, oncological laryngoscopy. The Jacksons[59] did not support the concept of endoscopic excision of vocal-cord cancer (personal communication, J. Tucker). Endoscopy was reserved for obtaining diagnostic tissue.[87] Even the earliest lesions would be treated by

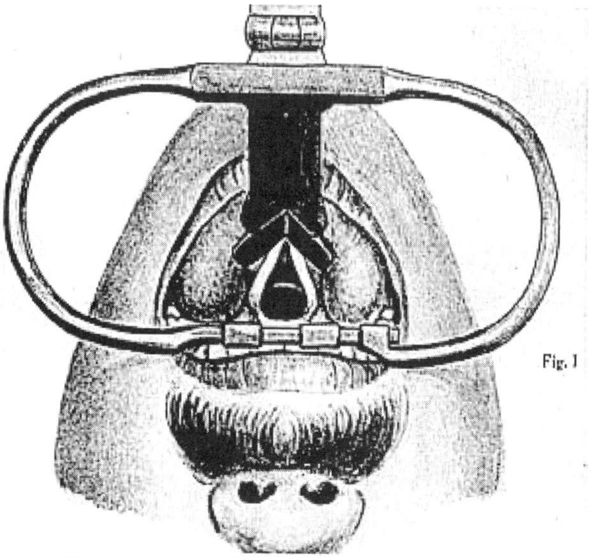

Fig. 24. Killian exposure with an "inverted V" spatula blade. (From Die Schwebelaryngoskopie und ihre praktische Verwertung.)

laryngofissure. In their comprehensive textbook on cancer of the larynx,[88] there is no mention of endoscopic excision of vocal cord cancer, even though there is a short discussion of endoscopic excision of epiglottic carcinoma.

Suspension Laryngoscopy: The Technique

Killian[89-92] designed an elaborate suspension gallows (Fig. 21) to hold his spatula laryngoscope (Fig. 22) in place; this freed the surgeon's hands for surgical manipulation. He reported this innovation, which was an outgrowth of his 1909 cadaver studies, at the Third International Laryngo-Rhinological Congress in 1911. His experiments in laryngeal suspension were initially performed to stabilize the larynx for anatomical illustration. In Jackson's monumental textbook, *Peroral Endoscopy and Laryngeal Surgery*,[91] the only chapter not written by him was "Suspension Laryngoscopy," which was authored by Killian. Observation of Killian working with his suspension gallows reveals that the patient is not in the Boyce-Jackson position but rather in a head-hanging extension position (Figs. 21, 23). There was often inadequate anterior glottal exposure with the extended neck position during suspension laryngoscopy. Although exposure was improved by using Brunings'[93] extrinsic counter-pressor devices to compress the lower larynx (Figs. 23, 24), suspension devices that freed the surgeon's hands did not reliably expose the entire musculomembranous vocal fold.

Jackson must not have been in favor of this technique[87] because there is little recognition or discussion of suspension devices or laryngoscope holders in his later textbooks.[94-96] It is unclear from his writings why Jackson did not build a device that would stabilize the laryngoscope in the head and neck position that he and Boyce utilized. Suspension laryngoscopy done in the extended position often did not provide complete glottal exposure; but without a suspension device and two-handed tissue manipulation, successful excision of vocal fold neoplasms was not possible. Presumably, it was because of this set of conditions that Jackson did not pursue endoscopic excision of vocal fold cancer.

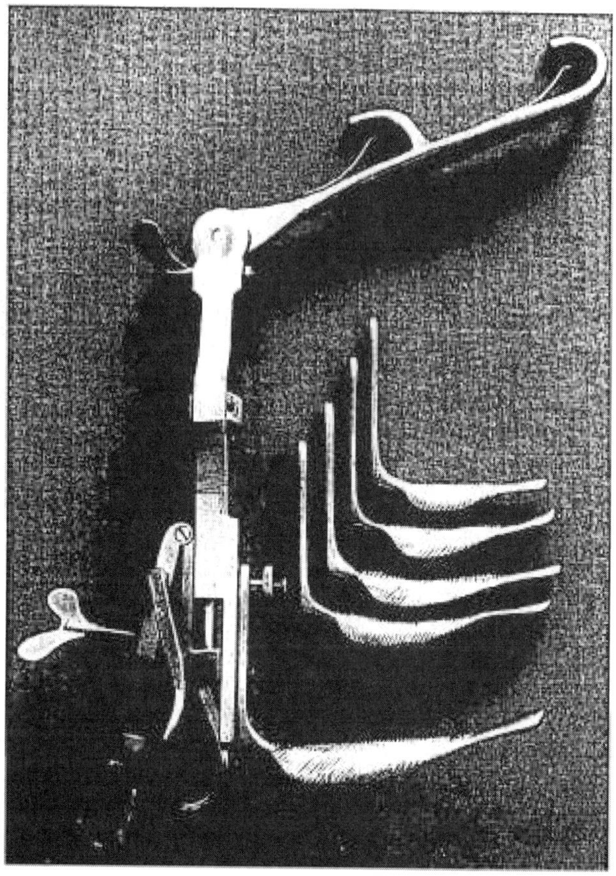

Fig. 25. Richard Clyde Lynch's suspension spatula laryngoscope. (Courtesy of the Massachusetts Eye and Ear Infirmary.)

Although the modifications made by Lynch[69-71] (Fig. 25) to Killian's suspension laryngoscope system made it popular among some surgeons in the United States, there were major disadvantages: a high level of skill was needed by the surgeon and the anesthesiologist, and there was no self-contained light. Scalco, *et al.*,[97] in 1960, described using the Lynch laryngoscope system for microlaryngoscopy. This instrument, however, was ill-suited for endotracheal anesthesia. Without an inferior blade, the endotracheal tube would distract into the region of the musculomembranous vocal fold surgical field. The technical difficulties encountered with suspension laryngoscopy enhanced the popularity of chest support holders, which remain popular today.

Killian and Jackson: De-emphasis of Their Laryngoscopic Teachings

"The difference (between the laryngologist and the pi-

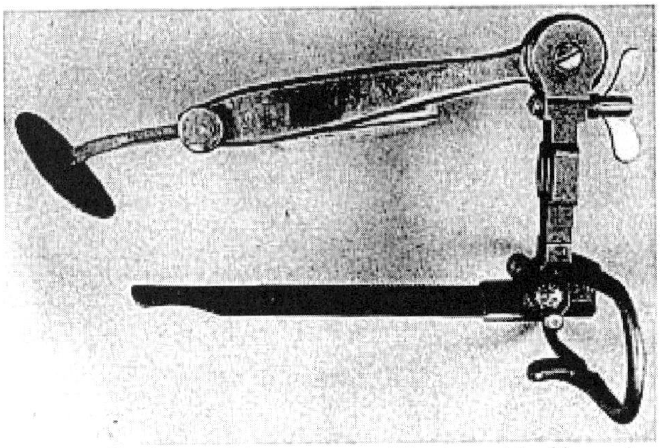

Fig. 26. Seiffert's spatula laryngoscope. (Courtesy of the Massachusetts Eye and Ear Infirmary.)

anist) is that the pianist expects to practice for years to acquire skill, whereas many laryngologists think that long years of laryngology should enable them to do skillful endoscopic work with little practice."

—C. Jackson and C.L. Jackson (1939)[61]

By 1910, Jackson had established the technical principles of glottic exposure using peroral direct laryngoscopy. About that same time, Killian developed the suspension laryngoscope, which freed both of the surgeon's hands for more precise vocal fold surgery. Jackson and Killian collaborated for Jackson's textbook on peroral endoscopy,[91] and there was a commonality to their technical philosophy of exposing the larynx by supporting the lower jaw, tongue, and larynx. Although Jackson did not employ a suspension apparatus, his left arm would function in that capacity (Fig. 20). Killian's laryngoscope applied pressure to the maxilla to maintain an open oral cavity, not to expose the larynx. It would be more than 60 years later that Jackson's concepts of head and neck position would be united with Killian's idea of head and neck suspension to free the surgeon's hands.

Most surgeons use chest-support systems to stabilize the laryngoscope. This approach can not be construed as suspension if one examines the definition of the word and the mechanical forces involved.[84] Contrary to Jackson's and Killian's teachings, these devices depend upon instrumental counter-pressure to the upper jaw to obtain glottal exposure. In the following sections, two fundamental questions will be answered: *1.* Why were the techniques of these masters abandoned? and *2.* Is there adequate reason to return to their teachings today in order to improve our phonomicrosurgical capabilities?

The Origin and Development of the Chest-Support Torsion Laryngoscope Holders

Around 1920, in an effort to overcome the difficulty in performing suspension laryngoscopy, Seiffert, a disciple of Killian, introduced the chest-sup-

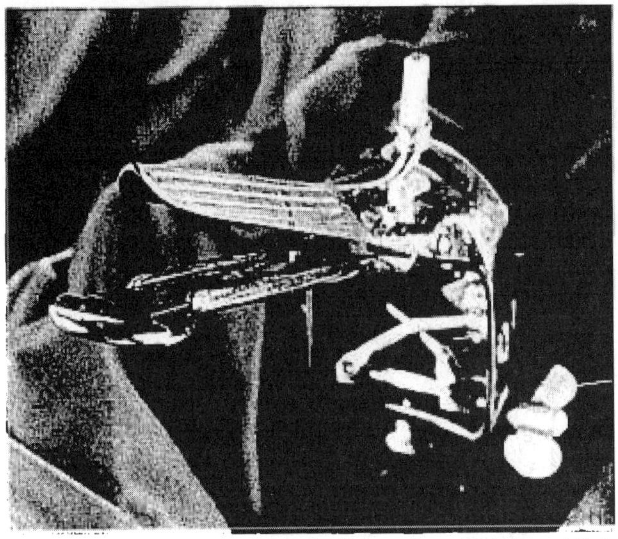

Fig. 27. Haslinger's bivalved spatula directoscope. (Courtesy of Collin S. Karmody, MD.)

port system (Fig. 26). Seiffert altered Killian's spatula suspension-laryngoscope by rotating the distal arm, which initially hung on the gallows, until it was resting on the chest. This modification fundamentally transformed the suspension laryngoscope into a lever laryngoscope-holder that exerted a torsion force on the upper teeth. Roberts[98,99] further modified this instrument and thoughtfully designed special pillows to support the head in the Boyce-Jackson position. (Fig. 27 will be discussed later.)

Jackson did not employ extrinsic devices to maintain his tubed laryngoscopes. King,[100] Sommers,[101] and Lewy,[102] in the 1950s, designed holders (stabilizers) for Jackson-style laryngoscopes. They were constructed to follow the chest-support fulcrum principle. Little attention was given to laryngoscopic head position. These devices employ a stable platform (chest wall or Mayo stand), an extension arm that creates a lever, and a fulcrum in which a torsion force is exerted to the maxilla, which results in undesirable head and neck extension.[84]

Fulcrum laryngoscope-holders can precipitate iatrogenic injury because these devices produce extension forces on the neck. Cervical spine injury may occur in patients in whom degenerative kyphotic cervical fusion has occurred from osteoporosis (Fig. 28).[103] Additionally, the surgeon is less aware of the force being generated and less sensitive to the resistance of a particular position because of the device's gear-power advantage. In the 1950s,[104] further departure from Jacksonian laryngoscopic principles was precipitated by the popularization of general endotracheal anesthesia with paralyzing agents. There was less need for orthodox laryngoscopic technique because of the use of small-lumened monocular laryngoscopes and the anestheti-

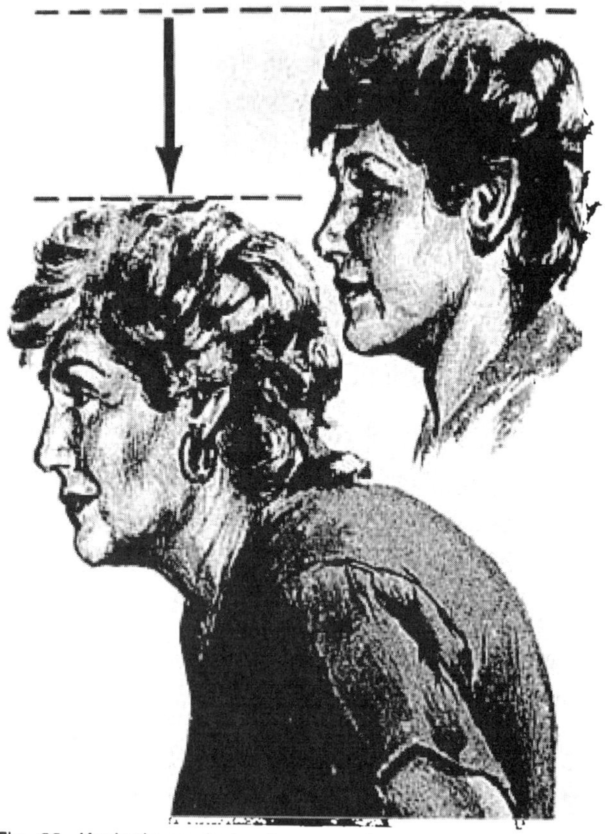

Fig. 28. Kyphotic cervical spine secondary to osteoporosis (Reprinted with permission of Ciba.)

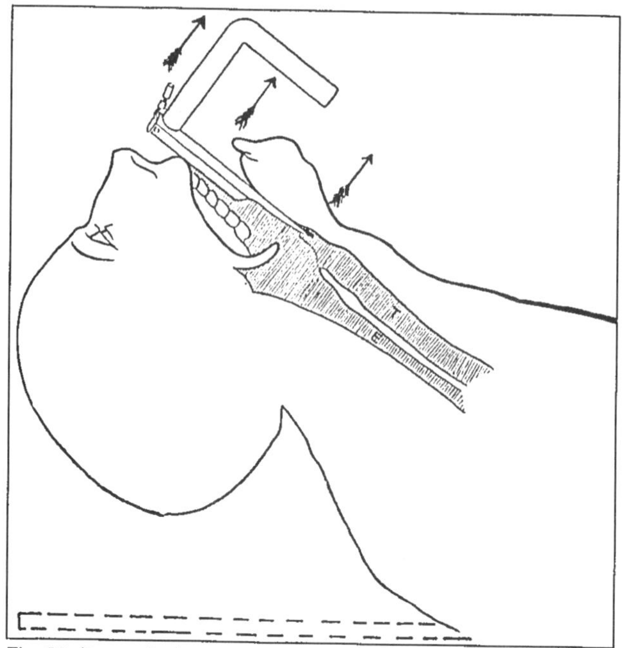

Fig. 29. Boyce-Jackson position demonstrating the vector forces for elevated-vector suspension (Reprinted with permission from W. B. Saunders Co., Philadelphia.)

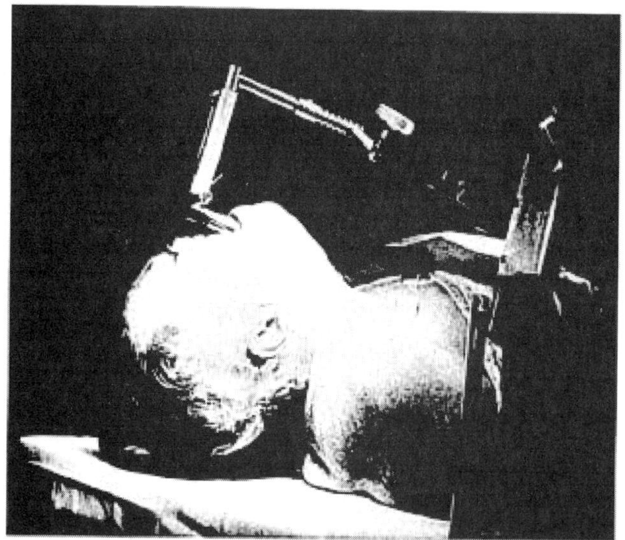

Fig. 30. Patient in elevated-vector suspension with the Boston University suspension apparatus.

cally induced increase in muscular compliance made possible by the neuromuscular paralyzing agents.

Reemergence and Marriage of Jackson's and Killian's Laryngoscopic Philosophies

In 1971, Thomas[105] modified the Lewy laryngoscope holder by attaching it to a telescoping arm and an inverted U-shaped frame. His apparatus allowed for mechanical laryngoscope stabilization in the Boyce-Jackson position. This position, where the head and neck are actually lifted off the table, will be referred to as elevated-vector suspension (Fig. 29) to distinguish it from Killian's head-hanging extension suspension (Figs. 21, 23). In 1978, as a modification of the Killian gallows, Grundfast and the Boston University group[106] developed an apparatus (Pilling Co.) that also provided *elevated-vector suspension* (Fig. 30). The classical tubed laryngoscopes were fitted with extended handles to allow application of a force equal and opposite to that needed to expose the glottis; this eliminated rotation (levers) and worked in varied head and neck positions. The suspension gallows employed a simple window crank for its works.

Direct Laryngoscope Design

Equally important as head positioning in surgical direct laryngoscopy is the shape and contour of the laryngoscope. Kirstein,[32,83] who is generally recognized as the first individual to perform direct laryngoscopy, experimented with both open spatula and tubular designs before settling on the former.[107] All subsequent laryngoscopes are derivatives of one of these designs. Kirstein's autoscope spatula was placed over the middle of the tongue[107] for anterior tongue displacement and direct view of the larynx, a technique reminiscent of Green's description published 40 years earlier. In 1903, Jackson introduced a narrower tubed glottiscope[107] that was placed along the lateral tongue in order to take the path of

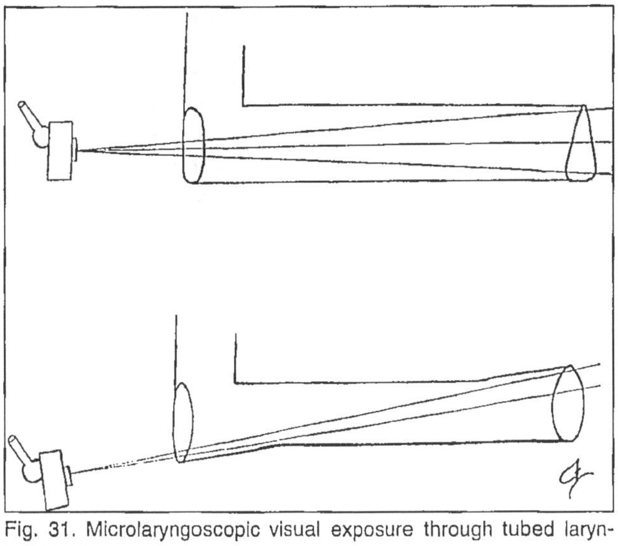

Fig. 31. Microlaryngoscopic visual exposure through tubed laryngoscopes.

least resistance. He also fitted this glottiscope with self-contained distal lighting.

Many of the innovations made with regard to the design, shape, and contour of laryngoscopes helped deal with the problem of inconsistent exposure of the anterior commissure. Just as Kirstein, Killian[89–92] and Lynch[69–71] used single, open-bladed, spatula instruments that were stabilized with their suspension gallows. Killian designed a variety of spatula blades,[91,92,108] including one contoured as an "inverted-V"[108] (Fig. 24), to accommodate the anterior glottal commissure. Both Seiffert (Fig. 26) and Haslinger adopted the "inverted-V" design into their laryngoscopes. Haslinger's[109] design modification (around 1920) provided one of the first adjustable bivalved instruments (Fig. 27). The Haslinger directoscope obtained anterior glottal exposure by internal distension of the laryngopharynx with anterior displacement of the larynx. This approach to the anterior commissure is in contrast to external posterior laryngeal counter-pressure, as suggested by Brunings. Jackson, *et al.*[110] used the "inverted-V" design feature in a tubed glottiscope, which was teardrop-shaped and named the laryngostat.

Apart from these instruments, which were designed to accommodate the anterior commissure and the triangle-shaped glottis, most 20th century glottiscopes were circular or oval. With the introduction of microlaryngoscopy, attention to laryngoscope design was focused on providing wider horizontal dimensions in order to allow for binocular stereoscopic visualization. The "inverted-V" concept for anterior glottal exposure was seemingly lost. Recently, Vaughan[84] designed a wide-lumened, tubed, triangular glottiscope that provides more complete glottal exposure.

Typically, anterior commissure glottiscopes are designed with a distal-vertical flare. The visual surgical field is determined by the narrowest intralumenal diameter of the glottiscope and the position of the surgeon's eye (Fig. 31). Anterior commissure scopes that widen at the distal length of the scope are inefficiently constructed.[84] To use the advantage of the distal-lumenal distension, the proximal lumen is widened creating an hourglass-shaped tube. However, neither the surgeon's distal visual-field nor the carbon dioxide laser can bend along these angulations. To view the anterior commissure, the operating microscope must be inferiorly malpositioned.

Microlaryngoscopy

Microlaryngoscopy arose from the need and desire to perform more precise vocal fold surgery. In the early 1950s, Albrecht[111] used a colposcope for magnified indirect vocal fold examination and for photodocumentation of keratosis. The first report on suspension microlaryngoscopy was made by Scalco, *et al.* in 1960.[97] The microscope provided both a magnified stereoscopic surgical field and improved illumination that fostered a new era in precision vocal fold surgery.

In 1962, Jako (personal communication) performed microlaryngoscopy (using a 200-mm lens) with both a monocular tubed laryngoscope and general endotracheal anesthesia. Later that year, to accompany the requirements of a magnified surgical field, Jako, working with the Stuemer Company (in Germany), developed the first set of microlaryngeal handheld instruments; they were otologic instruments with long handles. In 1963, Jako (personal communication) designed a wide lumened microlaryngoscope (Pilling Co) to enable stereoscopic visualization.[112,113] During the same period, Kleinsasser[114,115] reported stereoscopic microlaryngoscopy. Soon thereafter, the Zeiss Company developed a 400-mm lens for him to facilitate the introduction of hand instrumentation into the proximal lumen of the laryngoscope.[116] After the first decade of microlaryngoscopy, DeSanto and Carney[117] and Strong[118] provided a review and appraisal of the American experience.

Concepts of Phonomicrosurgical Instrumentation

At the turn of the century, when general endotracheal anesthesia was not yet avaialbe, Jackson developed optimal laryngoscopic positioning for small-lumened tubed laryngoscopy. Necessity (the absence of general anesthesia) was the mother of invention (discovering ideal head and neck position). Since the anatomy of the patient cannot be varied and anesthetic techniques have been optimized by general anesthesia with paralysis, the two factors limiting vocal-fold exposure become the surgeon's technique and the choice of equipment.

The trend today is toward the use of laryngoscopes with wider lumens for obtaining greater glottal exposure. Phonomicrosurgery is improved by safely placing the largest well-designed glottiscope that can be admitted from the lips to the vocal folds to provide the widest exposure of the vocal fold surgical field. This should be supported by a device that will maintain the patient in Boyce-Jackson position by employing elevated-vector suspension. The improved exposure of the operative site allows for better exposure of the lesion as well as more room to retract tissue by angulation of the hand instruments. This improved exposure, along with higher magnification and finer hand instruments[119] (such as those designed by Shapshay, Healy (K. Storz Co.), and Ossoff (Pilling Co.), have enhanced the precision of present phonomicrosurgical techniques.

The Concept of Vocal Fold Premalignancy and Atypical Epithelium

The concept of glottal premalignancy developed synchronously with two epidemiological events in the 20th century. First, infectious diseases of the larynx, such as tuberculosis and syphilis, began to recede. Second, mass production of cigarettes was introduced,[120,121] after which irregular vocal fold membrane changes were likely to be smoking-induced metaplasia and/or neoplasia. The popularity of cigarettes was coincident with the decline in popularity of smokeless tobacco use. This change in mores was accompanied by antispitting laws and social unacceptability of smokeless tobacco.

Jackson was developing the concept of precancerous conditions of the larynx by 1915.[122] Pierce (1920)[123] reported two cases of keratosis of the superior surface of the musculomembranous vocal fold, although he did not discuss the concept of premalignancy. Despite the suspicion of malignancy, one patient did not undergo a procedure and was lost to follow-up. The second patient was followed for 3 years and was eventually biopsied because of worsening symptoms and signs. Cancer was observed histologically and treated by laryngofissure and resection. Shortly thereafter, Jackson[124] formally discussed the concept of premalignancy of the glottis at the 1922 ALA meeting; his presentation was entitled, "Cancer of the Larynx: Is It Preceded by a Recognizable Precancerous Condition?" In it, he emphasized the importance of early identification and treatment of keratotic lesions for preventing malignant degeneration. His suggestion in the presentation that there was a window of opportunity to prevent otherwise inevitable larynx cancer was remarkable because it was made before premalignant epithelium was an accepted concept in medicine.

After that presentation, the renowned pathologist James Ewing commented on one of Jackson's cases: "[T]his is the stage in which to treat cancer, not after it gets well advanced." Ewing considered the premalignant stage as a form of cancer. Jackson stated: "... it encourages me in making a plea before this Association for the clinical recognition of a precancerous condition....it will be a step toward the ultimate attainment of such an ideal if we begin by recognizing the fact that there exists a group of cases already cancerous in which the malignant possibilities are so great as to justify wide removal of normal tissue surrounding the lesion."[124]

Throughout the next decade, both laryngologists and pathologists struggled to define the clinical and histopathological characteristics of premalignancy. In the 1930 proceedings of the Royal Society of Medicine,[125] Jackson led a round table exchange entitled "Discussion on Precancerous Conditions of the Larynx." There was little agreement among the panel members except for the fact that there was a premalignant stage in the biological progression of laryngeal cancer. Shortly thereafter (1932), Broders[126] published his landmark article, "Carcinoma In Situ Contrasted With Benign Penetrating Epithelium." This work effectively established the framework for currently accepted histopathological criteria used to define premalignancy.

In his 1946 publication, "Keratosis of the Larynx," Clerf[127] examined the controversies about terminology (keratosis, hyperkeratosis, leukoplakia, pachydermia) and the biological progression of this disease. He reported four cases of histopathologically aberrant intraepithelial vocal-fold lesions that underwent malignant degeneration within 15 months in one patient and in over 3 years in the other three patients. Although Graham[128] had previously discussed a case report (1942) of a precancerous lesion undergoing malignant degeneration, Clerf's work unequivocally documented the malignant potential of dysplastic vocal-fold mucosa.

Jackson's wisdom stimulated several generations of laryngologists and pathologists to search for reliable diagnostic, clinical, and histopathological criteria for classifying glottal premalignancy and, more recently, for methods to remove that tissue while preserving vocal quality.

The Origin of Vocal Fold Decortication, "Stripping"

Lore,[129,130] in 1934, presented his laboratory experiments on vocal cord stripping in cats as well as in four human cases. Using the analogy that a laryngofissure and cordectomy resulted in a fairly normal appearing neocord, he reasoned that one could easily decorticate the glottal epithelium without significant untoward vocal sequelae. He concluded that establishment of a straight vocal fold edge was the primary goal in the management of noncancerous mucosal disorders. The philosophy of surgical laryngoscopy at the time did not focus on how critically important the relationship of the vocal fold cover to the vocal ligament was for voice quality. He stated clearly that "If necessary one may go as deeply as the thyroarytenoid muscle ..."[129]

Despite this, Lore must be given credit for realizing that there was a natural plane of dissection for vocal fold cover resection. In his initial study, two of four vocal fold strippings were for polypoid corditis/degeneration (Reinke's edema); Putney and Clerf[131] reported on eight of eight patients who underwent treatment for the same indication. The success they reported in the treatment of this disease was, in all likelihood, secondary to the natural distension of Reinke's space (superficial lamina propria [SLP]).

The Body-Cover Theory of Voice Production

While a complete developmental history of voice production theory is beyond the scope of this work, the important contributions to body-cover mucosal wave theory that have influenced phonomicrosurgical concepts are reviewed.

The body-cover mucosal wave theory of voice production was introduced by Bishop[132] in 1836 in his publication, "Experimental Researches into the Physiology of the Human Voice." He stated, "The true vibrating surface of the glottis is the mucous membrane. The vocal cords confer on it the tension, resistance, position, and probably other conditions necessary for vibration." This outstanding and insightful contribution was made without the use of the mirror laryngoscope or the stroboscope; he was, therefore, unable to see the moving glottis.

In 1866, in his comprehensive textbook on voice,[133] Fournie also concluded that the vocal fold mucosa was the major component of the glottal vibration.[134,135]

> The voice is a sound produced by a particular reed having walls modifiable under the influence of muscular action; the vibrating part being furnished by the mucous fold which limits the borders of the glottis. The vibrations are occasioned by the passage of air through the glottis.... For the membranes to vibrate, one tenses them on a frame like the skin of a drum, and they will emit their vibrations transmitting them through the air. They produce a more high pitch shrill sound according to how small and how taut they are.[133]

Hirano[136–138] further developed the body-cover theory of voice production by assimilating information from stroboscopy, gross anatomical evaluations, and his elegant scanning electron-microscopic evaluation of the vocal fold's layered anatomy. These studies of the microanatomy of the vocal fold reveal that there is a cover (epithelium, superficial lamina propria), a transition zone (vocal ligament: medial lamina propria and deep lamina propria), and a body (muscle). The superficial lamina propria is composed of an amorphous substance with few fibroblasts and allows for maximal epithelial pliability for transmission of a vibrational wave.[138] It abates anteriorly as the vocal ligament and mucosa fuse with the anterior commissure tendon, and it disappears posteriorly as the vocal ligament and mucosa join the vocal process of the arytenoid. The medial lamina propria is composed primarily of elastic fibers and the deep lamina propria is composed primarily of collagen fibers. Fibroblasts are more prevalent in the medial and deep lamina propria; as a result, there is concern that there may be excessive scarring of the vocal fold mucosa to these layers when they are surgically disturbed.

Aerodynamic principles of the mucosal wave theory were discussed by Garcia (Fig. 4) in 1855. From his experiments in laryngoscopy, he described the rhythmic release of air by the vocal folds into the supraglottal vocal tract. "The voice is formed by the periodical compressions and dilations which the air experiences when, on reaching the glottis, the latter, by alternate and regular movements, stops or permits its exit."[10]

Current mucosal wave theory suggests that the vocal fold mucosa is stimulated and maintained in a vibrational wave by the pressure differential between the driving force of the subglottal air column and the pressure of the air above the vocal folds. The opening force of the subglottal pressure upon the vocal folds is opposed by the elastic recoil of the vocal folds and Bernoulli's effect. The flexibility and mobility of the musculomembranous vocal-fold epithelium is dependent on submucosal tissue attachment (status of the superficial lamina propria), rheology (tension) of the mucosa, and redundancy of the mucosa.[139] Redundancy of the epithelium is increased and the Bernoulli effect is significant with a shorter vocal fold during chest register. This is in contrast to the minimal Bernoulli effect that occurs during falsetto register when tension and length of the fold are maximized, and redundancy of the mucosa is minimized.[139] Stroboscopic visualization demonstrates increased dynamics of mucosal wave activity with lower pitches. Decreased mucosal wave activity is observed with higher pitches and with scarring of the vocal fold epithelium to the ligament.

Laryngeal Stroboscopy

Visualization of the vibrating vocal fold, which is facilitated by the laryngeal stroboscope, was reported by Oertel[140] in 1895. In essence, a motorized perforated pinwheel disc (Fig. 32) was placed between the artificial light source and the examiner's head mirror. Varying the speed of revolution of the disc allowed for rhythmic interruption of the light that was transmitted from the head mirror to the laryngeal mirror. This provided the effect of slow-motion visualization of the vocal fold.

The device initially did not gain popularity or acceptance for several reasons[141]: *1.* it was necessary

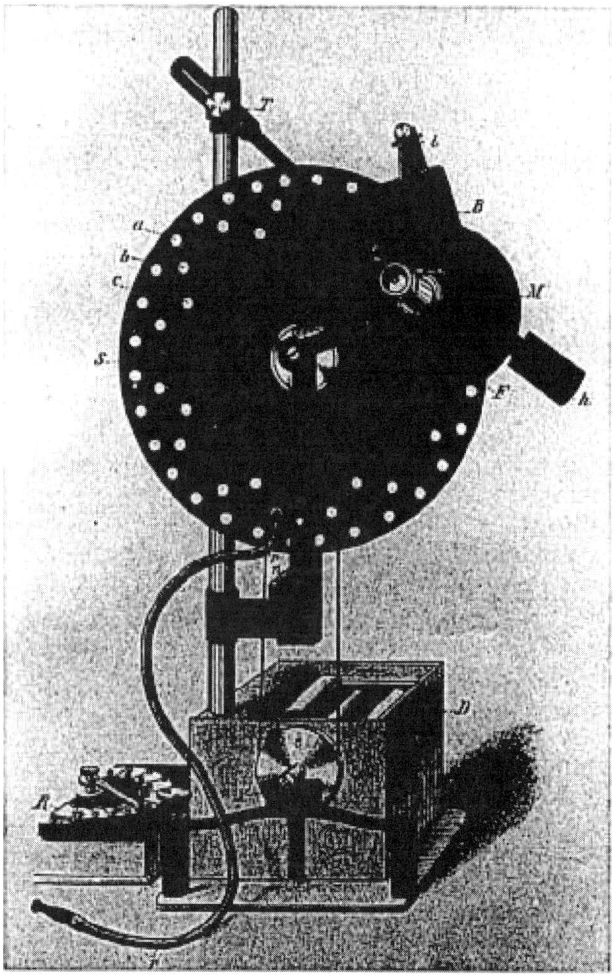

Fig. 32. Max Joseph Oertel's (1835-1897) laryngostroboscope (1895). (From *Archiv fur Laryngologie und Rhinologie.*)

to train the patient to duplicate and maintain a specific pitch that was coordinate with the speed of the rotating disk; *2.* the disk needed to be changed for each frequency; and *3.* finally, the device generated considerable objectionable background noise. Also, whereas in Europe speech and voice science were frequently within otolaryngology departments, in North America, these disciplines were independent and had only limited collaboration with each other.[142] As a result, few laryngostroboscopic investigations[141–148] were done in America throughout much of the 20th century. The recent increase in the number of American multidisciplinary voice and laryngological studies suggests that this trend is changing.

Submucosal Vocal Fold Infusions

Hajek[149] (1891) and later Reinke[150] (1897) published experiments on the submucosal compartments of the larynx. An objective of those experiments was to improve the understanding of the mechanism of laryngeal obstruction from infectious diseases, a common problem of the time. By means of dye infusions, they defined the subepithelial loose connective-tissue compartment of the musculomembranous vocal fold. That particular submucosal space still bears Reinke's name. Hirano[136–138] refers to the loose connective tissue of Reinke's space as the superficial lamina propria.

In the late 1950s, Pressman, *et al.*[151,152] also performed laryngeal dye infusions, which further defined anatomical connective-tissue compartments of the larynx. These studies were designed to delineate intralaryngeal lymphatic flow as a basis for understanding local and regional spread of laryngeal cancer. Like Hajek and Reinke, Pressman, *et al.* observed a submucosal musculomembranous true vocal fold compartment. No mention is made by these authors of this compartment's physiological significance to mucosal-wave theory of voice production. It seems that they were unaware that the compartment they had described supported the loosely attached glottal epithelium that is critical to voice production. This vocal fold epithelium is the vibratory mucosa that Bishop had described in the early 19th century.

INTRODUCTION TO THE INVESTIGATIONS

Four studies were designed to establish surgical methodology that would improve the management of premalignant and microinvasive vocal-fold epithelium. The purpose of the initial study was to determine which patients required biopsy and what surgical approach would most likely result in an accurate diagnosis. Toward this end, an in vivo visual and multiple-section histopathological analysis was performed on vocal fold lesions that had been resected. The second study was done to determine where the vibratory portion of the vocal fold mucosa is located in order to assist in the design and execution of a procedure to resect diseased epithelium. It was deemed important to maximally preserve the vocal fold's layered structure with the hope of optimizing vocal quality. In this study, dye infusions were performed into the superficial lamina propria of vocal folds in cadaver larynges, a technique similar to that described by Hajek,[149] Reinke,[150] and Pressman, *et al.*[151,152] Based on the findings of these two studies, a third study was conducted in which a submucosal infusion with microflap excisional biopsy technique was designed and clinically executed to determine the advantages and disadvantages of the procedure. Finally, a fourth study was conducted to obtain objective acoustic, aerodynamic, visual, and perceptual data from a pilot group that had undergone submucosal infusion and microflap excisional biopsy within the past 24 months.

STUDY 1: Clinical Mapping and Multiple-Section Histopathological Analysis of White and Red Vocal Fold Lesions

MATERIALS AND METHODS

From 1988 to 1993, 52 patients with significant smoking histories underwent suspension microlaryngos-

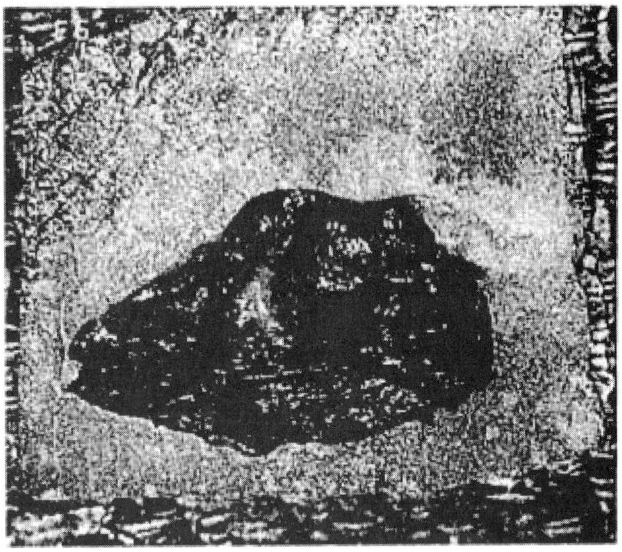

Fig. 33. Vocal fold cover specimen oriented on cucumber mount before paraffin embedding.

copy and en bloc resection of suspected dysplastic or malignant vocal fold epithelium. All patients had agreed to transoral excisional biopsy when it was technically possible. The appropriateness of the lesion for transoral excision was determined by the intraoperative appearance, size, and location of the lesion, as well as by its laryngoscopic exposure.[153]

After intubation with a laser-protected endotracheal tube, the laryngoscope that afforded the greatest glottal exposure was used. In this series, either a Dedo (Pilling Co.) or a triangular (R. Wolf Co.) laryngoscope was used in all cases. All patients were placed in elevated-vector suspension in the Boyce-Jackson position, and the laryngoscope was supported by the Boston University gallows (Pilling Co.). All lesions were evaluated visually under 10×, 25×, and 40× as indicated on the surgical microscope. The true magnification is somewhat less with the use of a 400-mm lens. All lesions were also evaluated by palpation. Excisional biopsy was performed either by cold dissection or carbon dioxide laser resection. The specimens were oriented and flattened on a carrier for fixation, as described by Holinger and Miller[154] (Fig. 33). A map of the location (superior and/or medial vocalizing surface) (Fig. 34), the surface dimensions, and the depth of invasion (lamina propria or muscle) was drawn.

All specimens underwent multiple sectioning and were evaluated independently by a head and neck pathologist. The specimens were subsequently reviewed jointly by the author and the pathologist. Each specimen was analyzed and geographically mapped by the pathologist into a 25-region grid. Each subregion was evaluated for surface appearance and for underlying atypia or invasive cancer. In all, 1300 subregion evaluations were done. For purposes of the first analysis that compared surface to underlying cellular morphology, only the central 9 regions in the 52 specimens (468 subregions) were used becasue the periphery frequently contained a normal margin. Determination of lesion margins was made with clinical and histopathological information.

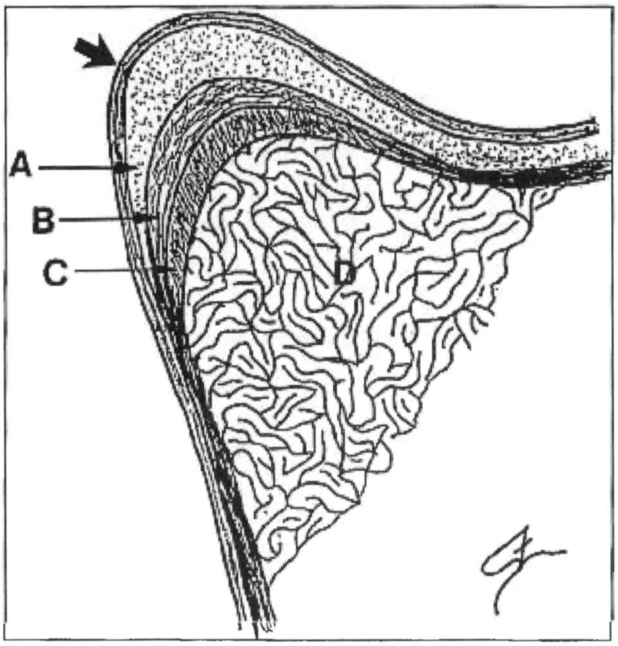

Fig. 34. Schematic coronal section through the vocal fold demonstrating mapping criteria. The arrow correlates with the separation of the superior and medial vocal fold surfaces. A=superficial lamina propria; B=medial lamina propria; C=deep lamina propria; D=vocalis muscle.

Surface characteristics were classified as ulceration, thin parakeratosis, thick parakeratosis, thin orthokeratosis, thick orthokeratosis, and normal. The cellular morphology of the epithelium was classified as follows: *1.* normal, *2.* hyperplastic, *3.* mild atypia, *4.* moderate atypia, *5.* severe atypia, *6.* carcinoma in situ, *7.* microinvasion in the superficial lamina propria, *8.* invasion in the medial lamina propria (vocal ligament), and *9.* invasion into the vocalis muscle. The definitions of these classifications are outlined in Appendix 1.

For the purposes of the second analysis that examined the intralesional variability of each specimen, all 25 subregions of the 52 lesions (1300 subregions) were examined. The cellular morphology was numbered from 1 (normal) to 9 (cancer with muscle invasion). Given a similar surface, the range of cellular morphology within each lesion was documented. The variation in number of cellular morphological categories was then counted for each lesion.

RESULTS

All 52 lesions were confined to the musculomembranous vocal fold. Twenty-seven (52%) of 52 lesions had surface changes on only the superior surface of the fold (Figs. 34, 46); 25 (48%) of 52 lesions had involvement of the superior surface, with extension caudally onto the medial surface (Figs. 34, 48). (Figs. 47, 49, and 50 will be discussed later.)

The most severe histologic finding in the 52 specimens was keratosis with: normal cellular morphology in 5 specimens, hyperplasia in 9 specimens, atypia in 27 specimens, and carcinoma in 11 specimens. The worst grades of atypia in the 27 dysplas-

TABLE I.
Histology of Vocal Fold Lesions.

Cellular Morphology	Number of Specimens
Normal	5
Hyperplasia	9
Mild atypia	10
Moderate atypia	3
Severe atypia	4
Carcinoma in situ	10
Carcinoma	11
Total	52

tic lesions were as follows: mild in 10, moderate in 3, severe in 4, and carcinoma in situ in 10 (Table I). As is standard practice in pathology, the patient's official diagnosis was classified by the worst pathological finding noted and did not necessarily represent the predominant histology. Usually specimens contained areas of less severe atypia.

Surface appearance during microlaryngoscopy revealed that although ulceration was an uncommon finding in this series, it was a reliable indicator of underlying cancer in 6 of 6 subregions (Table II). Otherwise, the surface appearance of the lesion was not a reliable prognosticator of cancer or of the severity of the underlying atypia. This was true whether making the observation between patients or in different areas of the same lesion. Excluding ulceration, all surface types could overlie virtually any underlying cellular histology (Table II) (Figs. 35–40).

The final parameter to be evaluated was the intralesional variability of atypia with a similar surface appearance. In 35 (67%) of 52 lesions, there was at least a three category variation in cellular morphology. Greater variation was noted as the degree of atypia and depth of cancer increased. This is understandable since the number of potential morphological categories increases as the disease worsens.

DISCUSSION

The data from the first investigation suggested that smoking-induced premalignant and microinvasive vocal fold epithelium typically involved the superior/ventricular vocal fold surface. It also frequently involved the medial/vocalizing surface. The surface appearance of these lesions was not a reliable prognosticator of the severity of the underlying atypia. This was true whether considering different areas of the same lesion that had a similar surface appearance or whether considering different patients who had similar appearing lesions. The data indicated that excisional biopsy and three-dimensional histopathological analysis is necessary to obtain an accurate diagnosis.

Patient Presentation With Premalignant Glottal Epithelium

"If we admit, as I think we should, that certain curable laryngeal conditions are in some cases the sequential predecessors of frequently incurable cancer, it is clearly our duty not only to eradicate those incurable precancerous conditions but to contribute to their early recognition ..."

—C. Jackson (1922)[124]

The vocal fold epithelium is unique in the aerodigestive tract in that its degenerative phase quickly results in symptoms (*i.e.*, hoarseness) that can lead to early recognition of metaplastic surface changes. The acoustic voice changes[123,124,127] are often accompanied by vocal fatigue and muscle-strain patterns. Office laryngoscopy typically identifies glottal surface keratosis and/or erythroplasia. Occasionally, early vocal-fold lesions are discovered during a comprehensive head and neck examination for other reasons, such as when a nonlaryngeal primary cancer is being managed.[155]

The Clinical Appearance and Location of Early Vocal Fold Dysplasia and Neoplasia

Vocal fold keratosis and erythroplasia appear

TABLE II.
Surface and Cellular Histology.

Surface Histology	Normal	Ulceration	Thin Ortho-keratosis	Thick Ortho-keratosis	Thin Para-keratosis	Thick Para-keratosis	Total
Normal	6	0	36	4	26	8	80 (17%)
Hyperplasia	20	0	52	26	20	1	119 (25%)
Mild atypia	15	0	13	12	24	4	68 (15%)
Moderate atypia	2	0	6	8	31	7	54 (12%)
Severe atypia	0	0	6	5	16	0	27 (6%)
Carcinoma in situ	3	0	20	14	18	6	61 (13%)
CA: Microinvasion	0	0	3	2	13	4	22 (5%)
CA: Ligament invasion	9	3	0	0	0	9	12 (4%)
CA: Muscle invasion	3	3	0	2	6	2	16 (3%)
Totals	58 (12%)	6 (1%)	136 (29%)	73 (16%)	154 (33%)	41 (9%)	468 (100%)

Note: There were a total of 468 regions analyzed in 52 specimens; 9 regions/specimen. CA = cancer.

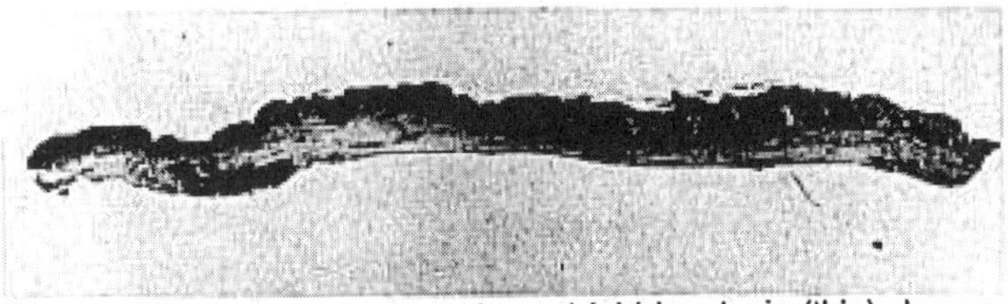

Fig. 35. Whole-mount section of vocal fold keratosis (thin) demonstrating varying atypia (H&E, original magnification × 12).

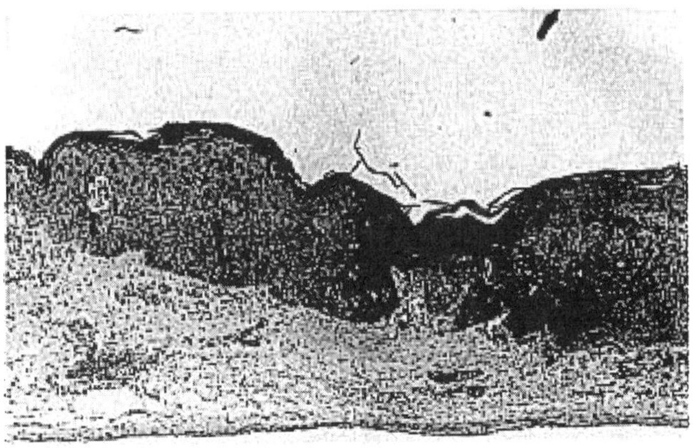

Fig. 36. The same specimen as in Figure 36 demonstrating diffuse variations in atypia (from hyperplasia to severe atypia) despite a uniform keratotic surface (H&E, original magnification × 90).

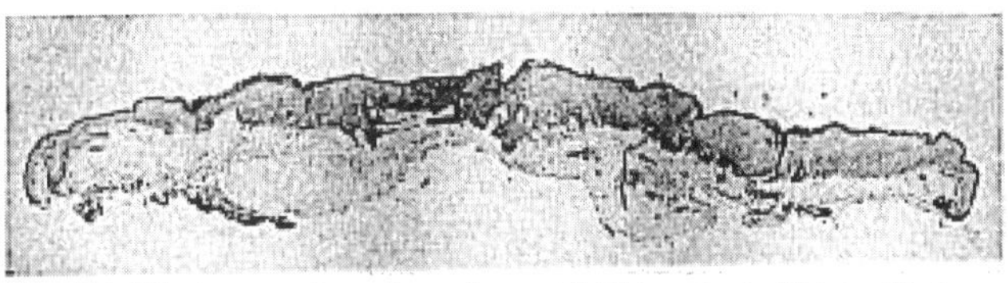

Fig. 37. Whole-mount section of vocal fold keratosis (thin) with hyperplasia and without atypia (H&E, original magnification × 20).

as white and red areas of mucosa. They may occur separately or together, on one or both vocal folds, and may be contiguous or separated geographically (Figs. 46, 48). This is consistent with the concept of Slaughter, *et al.*[156] of mucosal "field cancerization." While keratosis often is accompanied by varied cellular atypia, erythroplasia is likely to represent severe atypia or CIS.[157] Supravital staining with toluidine blue[158] can help define the perimeter of erythroplasia for excisional biopsy, but it is not useful for disclosing cellular atypia that develops underneath keratosis.

There are good data that locate these lesions on the musculomembranous fold;[159,160] there is, however, only anecdotal information that atypia first develops on its superior surface (Fig. 46).[62,123,127] The present study revealed that virtually all specimens demonstrating keratosis with atypia or cancer had involvement of some portion of the superior vocal fold surface. There were some cases (25 of 52) that involved both the medial/vocalizing and the superior/ventricular surface (Fig. 48); there were no cases involving the medial surface alone. This favorable geographic location frequently made it pos-

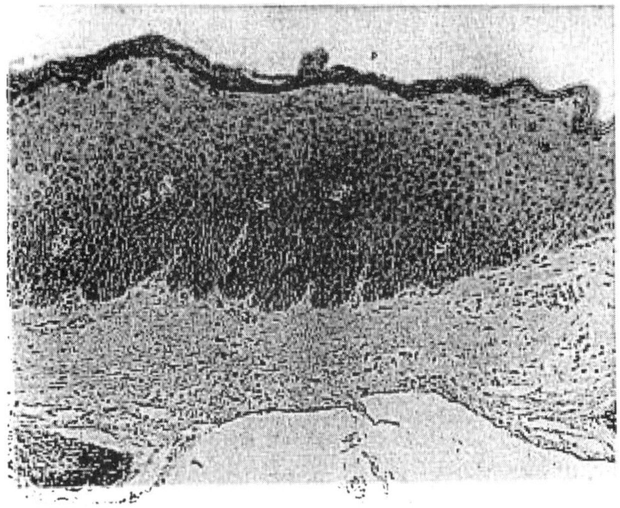

Fig. 38. The same specimen as in Figure 38 with thin keratosis and no atypia (H&E, original magnification × 140).

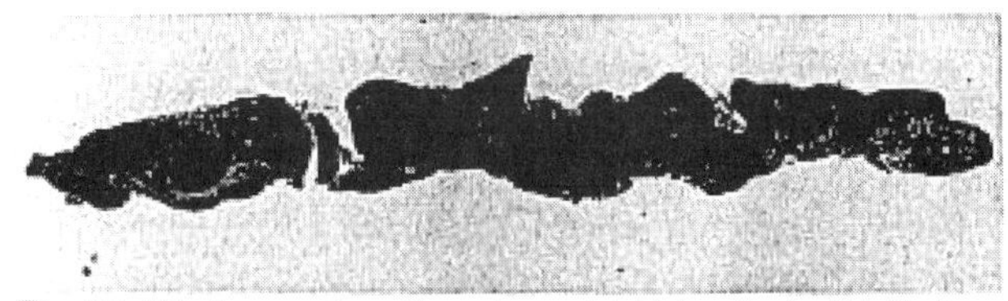

Fig. 39. Whole-mount section of vocal fold keratosis (thick) demonstrating varying atypia (H&E, original magnification × 16).

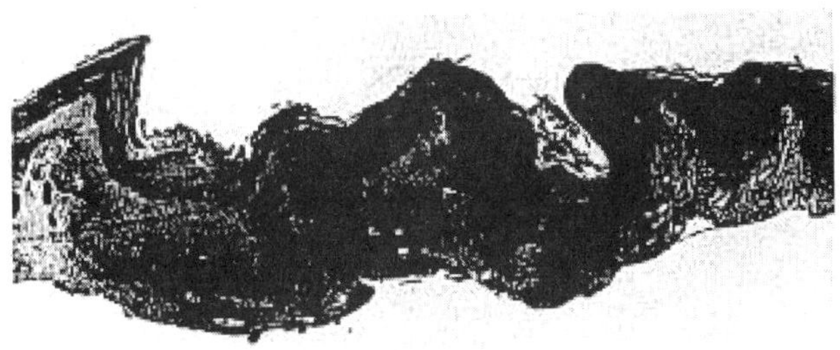

Fig. 40. The same specimen as in Figure 40 demonstrating diffuse variations in atypia despite a uniform thick keratotic surface (H&E, original magnification × 47).

sible to perform excisional biopsy with preservation of the entire vocal-fold layered structure (including the membrane on the medial/vocalizating surface). Hirano[137] has explained that the medial/vocalizing epithelial surface moves principally during vocal fold vibration and is critical to voice production.

The early occurrence of keratosis with atypia on the superior vocal fold surface is not surprising if one considers the pattern of contact of the caustic cigarette smoke with the glottal membrane. Channeling of the smoke past the glottal ledge results in increased exposure of the superior surface of the vocal fold to the carcinogens in the cigarette-smoke condensate.[161,162] Frequently, there will be a line of demarcation between the keratotic epithelium and normal appearing mucosa on the superior/ventricular vocal fold surface. This can be seen well during microlaryngoscopy (Figs. 46, 48). The laryngoscope will usually distend the laryngeal introitus and lateralize the vestibular folds that, in vivo, had protected the lateral superior surface of the vocal fold from smoke exposure.

By analyzing necropsy larynges of smokers and nonsmokers, Ryan, *et al.*[161] and Auerbach, *et al.*[163] were able to demonstrate increased epithelial changes in the true vocal fold as compared to the epithelium in the subglottis.[161] These studies did not compare changes in the mucosa of the medial versus superior surfaces; however, the concept is similar. Likewise, aerodynamic principles of turbulent carcinogenic cigarette-smoke condensate explain why primary tracheal carcinoma is only 1% of tracheobronchial cancers,[164,165] why bronchogenic carcinoma frequently occurs at bronchial bifurcations,[166] and why primary subglottic laryngeal carcinoma is unusual. The location of vocal fold injury is also consistent with descriptions by Ryland,[167] who reported acute caustic glottal mucositis of the musculomembranous vocal folds from inhalation of mustard gas during World War I.

Glottal Keratosis and Erythroplasia: The Incidence of Malignant Degeneration

The concept of glottal premalignancy assumes a phase of mucosal degeneration that has not progressed to invasive cancer. To determine whether microlaryngoscopic resection of these lesions provides benefit to the patient, it is necessary to determine the following: *1.* the frequency of atypia associated with vocal fold keratosis, 2. the frequency of malignant degeneration of the dysplastic epithelium, and *3.* whether the lesions recur or progress to cancer following resection.

Review of the literature reveals that the most reliable parameter for predicting biological aggressiveness for future cancer development is whether epithelial atypia accompanies the surface change.[168-178] A compiling of the data from seven series[168,170,172,174,176-178] revealed that 48 (16.3%) of 295 of the patients who were noted to have atypia with keratotic vocal-fold lesions subsequently developed invasive carcinoma. This is in contrast to a 3% (7 of 221) incidence of malignant degeneration when no atypia was present[168,170,172,176,177]; Bouquot and Gnepp[179] summarized these data. Further, the more recent studies in this report[172,174,177,178] demonstrated a 23% (31/136) incidence of malignant degeneration of dysplastic lesions.[172,174,177,178] The data reported by Hojslet, *et al.*[178] were remarkable in that there was a 40% incidence of malignant degeneration for moderate atypia, a rate that is identical to that of severe dysplasia and carcinoma in situ. In that study, even mild atypia resulted in a 4% incidence of malignant degeneration.

It is extremely difficult to precisely analyze the data from these studies[168-178] for several reasons: *1.* grading the severity of the atypia is not standardized and is quite subjective,[104,157,174,180-183] *2.* as our data suggest, the diagnosis could be erroneous if a limited directed biopsy is performed,[170,180,181,184-186] *3.* in many of these studies, the diagnostic biopsy also treated the lesion,[187,188] *4.* there is varying follow-up time in the various studies, and *5.* there is contradictory evidence about whether smoking cessation affects the rate and incidence of malignant degeneration,[174,186,189] and many studies did not control for this parameter.[170,176-178,180,181,184,185]

In the current study, there was stratification of various grades of atypia into a relatively standard pathological classification scheme. Because of strong historical foundations, it is doubtful that major alterations in this elaborate classification will occur in the near future. However, the author agrees with Bouquot and Gnepp[179] that the simple classification scheme suggested at the Centennial Conference of Laryngeal Cancer (1974) should be employed for clinical management. This scheme would include keratosis and/or erythroplasia—without atypia, with atypia, or with cancer. Lesions showing some cellular atypia should be considered premalignant and managed accordingly.

Glottal Keratosis and Erythroplasia: Patient Selection for Biopsy

If dysplasia is the most reliable parameter by which to prognosticate potential malignant degeneration, the incidence of glottal keratosis with atypia or erythroplasia is crucial. Batsakis[157] stated, "After surveying the reports in the literature, it is obvious that one man's premalignant keratosis is another's benign hyperkeratinization." Reports of atypia with keratotic vocal fold lesions range from 2.8% to 100%.[170-173,176,186,190] Bouquot, *et al.*[190] reported that the diagnosis of carcinoma with glottal keratosis ranged from 3.5% to 66.7%. They attributed some of the discrepancy to the site at which the diagnosis was made, *i.e.*, whether the studied population was hospital-based or not. This seems reasonable; it infers that those who are more experienced with the problem will both see more significant pathology and be more selective with laryngoscopic biopsies under general anesthesia. These types of discrepant data are a reflection of patient and lesion selection[191] rather than of the biology of the disease.

In this study of 52 vocal folds with glottic keratosis and/or erythroplasia, 52% of patients had atypia, while 21% had frank carcinoma. This combined incidence (73%) of vocal fold lesions demonstrating some degree of dysplasia and/or cancer suggests that the location of the lesion is a useful guide to the surgeon for biopsy selection. Superior musculomembranous vocal-fold lesions in smokers[192]

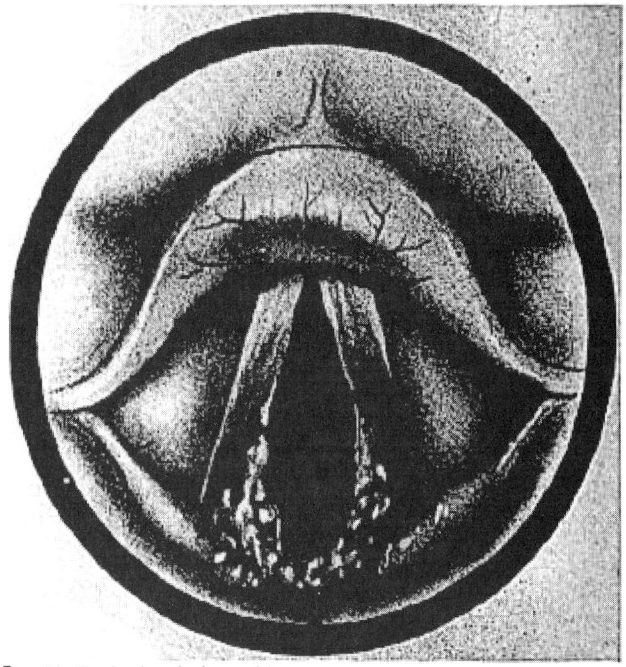

Fig. 41. Pachydermia laryngitis.

should undergo excisional biopsy and multiple-section specimen analysis; those containing some dysplastic cellularity should be considered premalignant and undergo vigilant follow-up. Lesions that appear only on the medial membranous vocal-fold surface, especially in nonsmokers, are likely to be secondary to traumatic hyperfunctional phonation. Similarly, posterior and interarytenoid keratosis, as in classical pachydermia laryngitis (Fig. 41), is more likely to be secondary to vocal hyperfunction and reflux, especially in nonsmokers. For smokers who have medial or posterior glottal lesions, microlaryngoscopic biopsy can be appropriately selected. This selection depends on the glottal epithelial response to the controlling of risk factors (smoking, reflux, and vocal hyperfunction).

The Rationale for Excisional Biopsy

Once the vocal fold lesion is observed, subsequent microlaryngoscopic biopsy may or may not provide an accurate diagnosis, which is fundamental to successful treatment of early vocal-fold lesions. Many have reported that a keratotic vocal fold surface can be accompanied by either normal or a variety of abnormal cellular morphologies.[168,169,173,174,180,182,184,192–194] Furthermore, Norris and Peale,[168] Lederman,[195] and others[180,181,186] have stated that there was unpredictable intralesional variability. Inadequate tissue biopsies, as a result of this variability, would predispose to inappropriate management decisions.[159] Lederman stated, "There is no doubt that many of the problems associated with the diagnosis and treatment of keratosis of the larynx stem from the difficulties of obtaining and interpreting laryngeal biopsy specimens. The larynx does not lend itself as easily for the obtaining of biopsy specimens as do other mucous membranes or the skin. Hence, many of the specimens are inadequate for accurate diagnosis or frankly misleading because they may not be representative of the whole lesion."[195]

The first study in the present report firmly established that a keratotic vocal fold surface does not prognosticate the magnitude of the atypia in the underlying epithelium in different specimens (Figs. 35 through 40) or within the same specimen (Figs. 35, 36, 39, 40). This suggests that multiple-section analysis is necessary to define what tissues need to be removed in order to establish an unequivocal diagnosis.[174,177,180,181,186]

Neither office nor intraoperative microscopic observation of the vocal fold surface was reliable for accurately determining the underlying severity of either epithelial atypia or cancer. The surgeon typically views a white or red lesion consisteing of orthokeratosis, parakeratosis, or ulceration on the superior surface of the vocal fold. The three-dimensional multiple-section analysis demonstrated that the white or red surface did not accurately portend the magnitude of the atypia or microinvasive carcinoma (Table II). Trying to determine the severity of cellular atypia was like trying to determine the depth of a lake by looking at its surface; for both, the surface belies an invisible third dimension. Clinical ulceration proved to be a reliable indicator of underlying carcinoma. All patients presenting with ulceration were clinically thought to have a T1 cancer and this was proven histologically. However, the limits of the cancer were not defined by the limits of the ulcer.

Prior studies have suggested that there is significant intralesional variability of epithelial atypia within the same specimen despite a similar surface appearance.[168,169,173,174,180,182,184,192–194] This supposition was confirmed by the present study's first investigation. Therefore, complete removal of the lesion with multiple-section analysis is necessary for an accurate diagnosis. Also, complete removal obviates the need for a second treatment (XRT or further surgery) that would most likely result in a worse voice,[196] potentially waste a valuable cancer-treatment option (XRT),[182] and not be cost-effective.[160,182,196]

Phonomicrosurgical en bloc transoral excisional biopsy along with controlled microdissection of the lesion and multiple histopathological analyses[171,174,177,180–182,186,197] is a rational management approach for suspected premalignant lesions. This allows for an accurate diagnosis and cost-effective treatment. Definitive cancer treatment options, including further transoral cover resections, remain viable.

The Problems With Directed Biopsy Treatment Approaches

Management approaches to small irregular vocal fold lesions have included the following: *1.* directed biopsies and follow-up, if cancer is not observed in the specimen; *2.* directed biopsies and radiation, if carcinoma in situ or microinvasive cancer is observed; and *3.* directed biopsies and laser vaporization of the residual lesion, if atypia is observed.

Despite microscopic advantage, directed biopsies by visual appearance of the epithelial surface do not ensure accurate diagnostic information about the entire lesion.[171–174,180,181,185,186,197] Exuberant keratosis of the vocal fold may direct a biopsy, but it does not necessarily reflect the severity of intraepithelial atypia. The data from three-dimensional multiple-section analysis of completely resected specimens suggest that surface-directed biopsies are often random sampling. Subsequent management of such lesions with potentially incomplete information about the lesion can misdirect the clinician toward undertreatment or overtreatment.[187] Sir Morell Mackenzie's tragic case with Prince Frederick vividly demonstrated the problematic nature of the laryngeal biopsy for obtaining adequate tissue and assessing its pathology.

It is not uncommon for an individual to have a limited representative biopsy guided by surface appearance. Typically, the specimen is not oriented and may be exiguous with crush artifact from a cup forceps. If hyperplasia, mild atypia, or moderate atypia is noted, the patient is followed. If severe atypia, CIS, or carcinoma is diagnosed, the patient may then undergo a second endoscopic procedure with general anesthesia. However, once the cover has been disrupted, a vocal ligament-sparing, clear, excisional biopsy of the lesion is difficult or impossible. Also, as Hyams[198] has explained, the second specimen is more likely to reflect a misleading dysplastic appearance because of the local changes created by the biopsy-induced ulcer.[168,188,198]

The logic of performing directed biopsies with subsequent laser vaporization of the residual suspicious epithelium is questionable because of the problem of random sampling. The surgical oncological principle of resection with a margin is abandoned for the convenience of the carbon dioxide laser. At the inception of lasers into surgical oncology, Strong[77,199,200] and the Boston University group[201] emphasized that the laser was an efficient cutting instrument and warned that standard surgical principles should not be altered for accommodation with the laser. Another problem with laser vaporization is that it takes great surgical skill to vaporize the mucosal cover without transmitting thermal energy to the superficial and medial laminae propria. This is especially true if the diseased epithelium has extended to the medial vocalizing surface and thereby requires progressive tangential ablation caudally along the curved vocal fold (Figs. 42, 51). In theory, thermal trauma to the laminae propria results in excessive scarring of the regenerated epithelium to the ligament and leads to a poor mucosal wave and poor vocal quality. A final drawback to the laser is simply the availability and expense of a late generation machine.

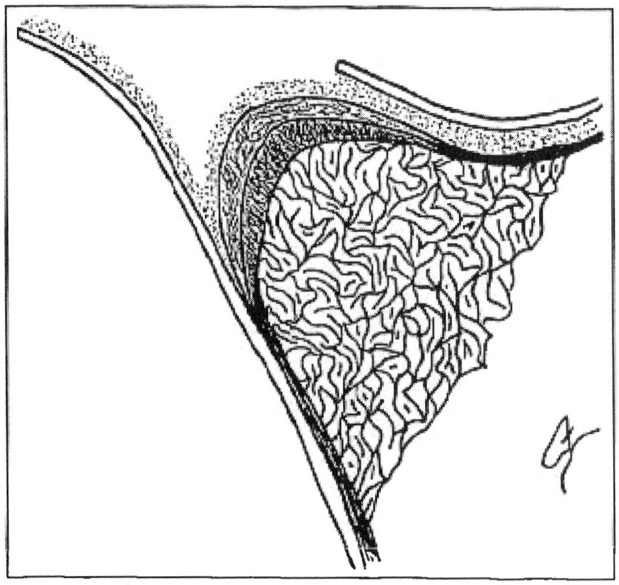

Fig. 42. Caudal tangential dissection of the cover in the plane of the superficial lamina propria along the curved vocal fold.

Another approach, if severe atypia or carcinoma in situ is found in a directed biopsy specimen, is to treat the lesions with radiation therapy. Even if the diagnosis is accurate, irradiating limited dysplastic glottal epithelium would be analogous to firing a cannon at a house to eradicate a mouse living in the kitchen. Along with permanent vocal fold changes that may make office follow-up difficult, there is damage to uninvolved tissue. In addition, a potentially important cancer treatment is permanently excluded. This treatment concept arose in an era when surgical treatment options usually involved some form of transcervical cordectomy or laryngectomy.

Administering full-course radiotherapy to varying grades of atypia to reverse that process or to prevent new lesions is unproven[104,195] and may precipitate malignant degeneration.[168,174,188,202] Miller[202,203] reported an important series which showed that of 100 patients treated for CIS with endoscopic excision, 13% developed invasive carcinoma. Remarkably, of 60 patients treated with XRT for CIS, 30% developed invasive cancer. This is identical to Hellquist, *et al.*[174] and DeSanto,[182] who each reported at 28% incidence of progression to invasive carcinoma for radiation-treated CIS. In contrast, Small, *et al.*[204] recently reported a 95% local control

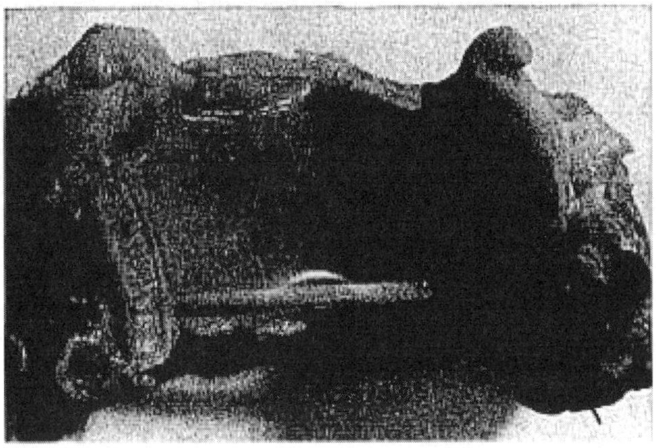

Fig. 43. Medial vocal fold after submucosal infusion of india ink into the superficial lamina propria. Note the convex caudal diffusion of the dye (arrows); the supraglottic larynx has been removed.

rate for CIS (20 of 21 patients) with radiotherapy. In that series no mention was made about the type of biopsy performed, which could have included complete excision. Additionally, three other patients were lost to follow-up.

The rationale and logic that radiotherapy should be administered for an undiagnosed invasive cancer that may be somewhere in the region is curious: it assumes an error in the CIS biopsy diagnosis. Unfortunately, these patients are subjected to a cancer treatment that may be unnecessary since it is not known whether any of them actually have cancer. Further, this treatment may complicate or hamper management of metachronous, aerodigestive-tract cancers.[174,182,195]

STUDY 2: Submucosal Dye Infusions of Reinke's Space (Superficial Lamina Propria)

MATERIALS AND METHODS

In the second study, 7 larynges were harvested from fresh cadavers or from hypopharynx-cancer laryngectomy specimens with no involvement of the medial paraglottic space. Thirteen vocal folds were infused with india ink using a 27-gauge needle. The needle was placed submucosally just anterior to the vocal process on the superior surface of the vocal fold. The dye was infused until resistance and back pressure resulted in retrograde dye-flow from the puncture site. The location of the india ink was noted grossly and mapped. Multiple coronal sections were performed and histologically evaluated with hematoxylin and eosin staining.

RESULTS

There was no significant variability between specimens; the results were consistent with those findings of Reinke a century ago. The hydrostatic dissection of the glottal epithelium resulted in a fusiform swelling, which was limited anteriorly by the anterior commissure tendon and posteriorly by the vocal process (Fig. 43). In the medial glottal region,

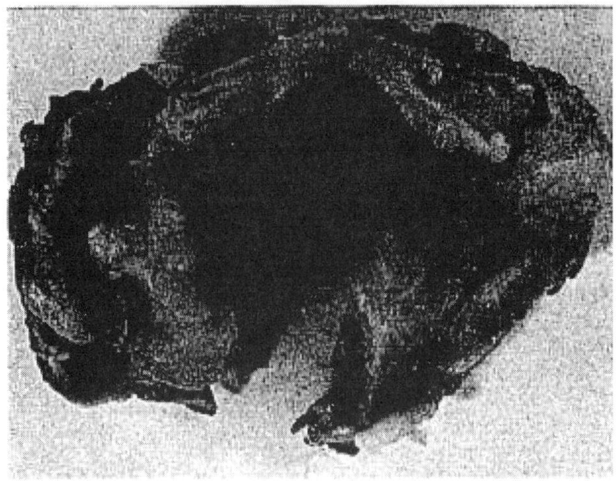

Fig. 44. Superior vocal fold after submucosal infusion of india ink into the superficial lamina propria; the supraglottic larynx has been removed.

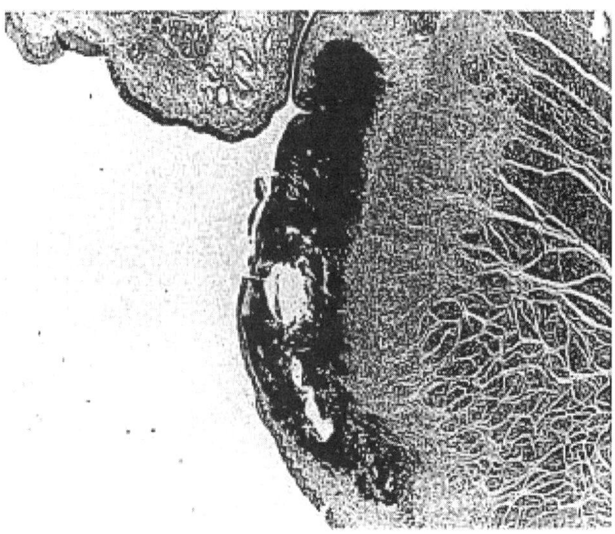

Fig. 45. Cross-sectional view of the vocal fold demonstrating the compartmental hydrodissection of the vocal fold cover from the vocal ligament by distension of the superficial lamina propria (H&E, original magnification × 25).

a caudally directed convex diffusion of the dye was noted; it was seemingly self-limited by attachment of the conus elasticus to the glottal epithelium. The greatest caudal extension was noted in the mid musculomembranous fold. No consistent compartmental limitation of the dye on the ventricular (superior) surface of the vocal fold (Figs. 44, 45) was observed. The magnitude of the extension of the dye toward the ventricle was directly related to the duration of the infusion and the magnitude of the hydrostatic pressure exerted.

The dye infusion separated the epithelial basement membrane from the vocal ligament, and coronal histological vocal-fold section demonstrated a significant increase in the depth of the superior lamina propria (Fig. 45). The linea arcuata inferior

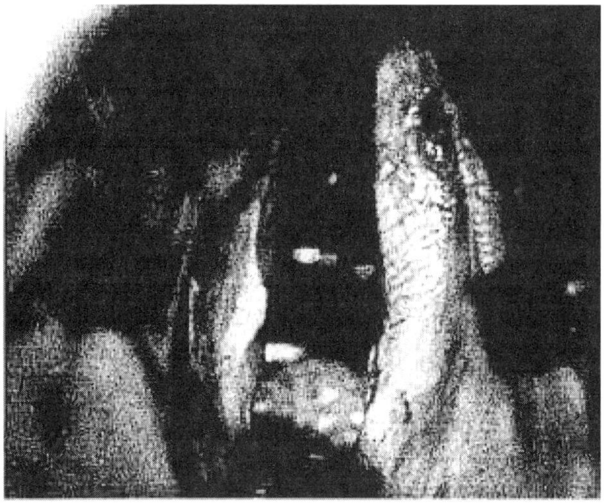

Fig. 46. Keratotic vocal fold lesion on the right superior/ventricular surface (preinfusion).

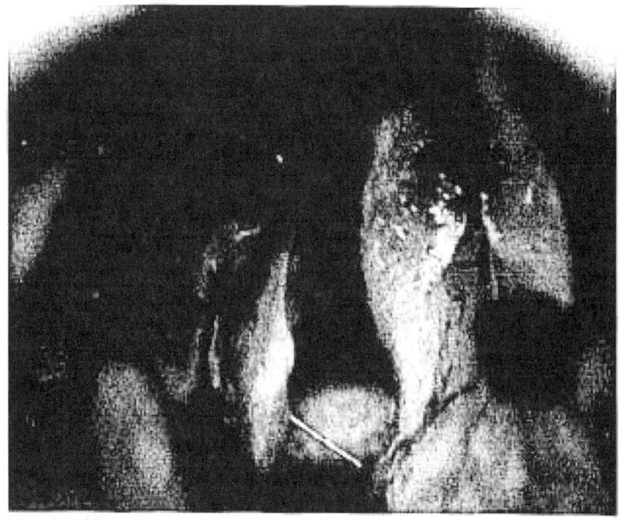

Fig. 47. Keratotic vocal fold lesion on the right superior/ventricular surface (postinfusion). The infusion has exposed more normal ventricular surface epithelium (arrow) to facilitate peripheral incisions. The infusion solution is limited by the vocal process and Broyle's ligament.

(transition from stratified squamous epithelium to pseudostratified epithelium) corresponded with both the caudal limits of the dye infusion and Reinke's space.

DISCUSSION

Submucosal vocal fold infusions done a century ago by Hajek[149] and Reinke[150] were performed to examine mechanisms of infectious laryngeal airway obstruction, which was a common problem of the day. Pressman repeated the infusion experiments 60 years later in an attempt to better understand lymphatic spread of glottic cancer. This current study employed similar infusion techniques to locate the vocal fold mucosa that was supported by the superficial lamina propria and, thereby, help to identify vibratory mucosa involved in voice production.

The dye diffusion (Figs. 43, 45) in the SLP helped to identify the compartment that supports the vibratory vocal fold epithelium by demarcating where the vocal ligament is attached to the vocal fold epithelium. The dye diffusion demonstrated the correspondence between the caudal superficial lamina propria and the linea arcuata inferior. The existence of a compartmentalized SLP allowed for distension of this space. As a result of the infusion, the larynges looked, grossly and histologically, like Reinke's edema. This inspired the application of the infusion technique in a clinical trial (study 3).

Fifty years ago,[129,131] it was discovered that epithelial lesions that occurred in association with polypoid corditis/degeneration (Reinke's edema) were technically easy to resect and resulted in good postoperative vocal quality. Polypoid corditis/degeneration is accompanied by a significantly increased edema of the superficial lamina propria where there is less fibroblast activity for potential scarring.[137,138,205] The increased depth of this space, which is normally approximately 0.3 mm,[137] allowed for greater preservation and less instrumental trauma of the layered vocal-fold structure (medial and deep lamina propria) during resection of the diseased epithelium.

Based on the present study's first investigation, it was determined that complete excisional biopsy was necessary to adequately diagnose and treat keratotic and erythroplastic vocal fold lesions. Resection of keratotic epithelium, supported by Reinke's edema, typically resulted in the most successful outcome. This success was judged by the ease, adequacy, and precision of the excision, as well as by postsurgical vocal quality. This principle was then used to clinical advantage in a patient trial in which initial infusions were made by modifying J. Tucker's 23-gauge mediastinoscopy aspiration needle (Pilling Co.). Ultimately, a 25-gauge needle with a short bevel was designed to improve the ease and quality of the submucosal infusions of the vocal fold.[206]

STUDY 3: Microflap Resection Via the Submucosal Infusion Technique

MATERIALS AND METHODS

After suspension microlaryngoscopy was performed for 42 vocal fold lesions (as described in study 1), a submucosal infusion needle[206] was attached to a 3-mL Luer-Lok syringe that was filled with sterile saline and 1/50,000 epinephrine. The needle was carefully inserted into the superficial lamina propria, anterior to the vocal process on the superior surface of the fold. Care was taken not to disturb the medial lamina propria (vocal ligament). The solution was infused until the compartment was filled and saline began to back out of the puncture site. The saline distended the vibratory vocal fold epithelium and hydrodissected the mucosa (cover) from the underlying vocal ligament and muscle (body) (Figs. 46 through 49).

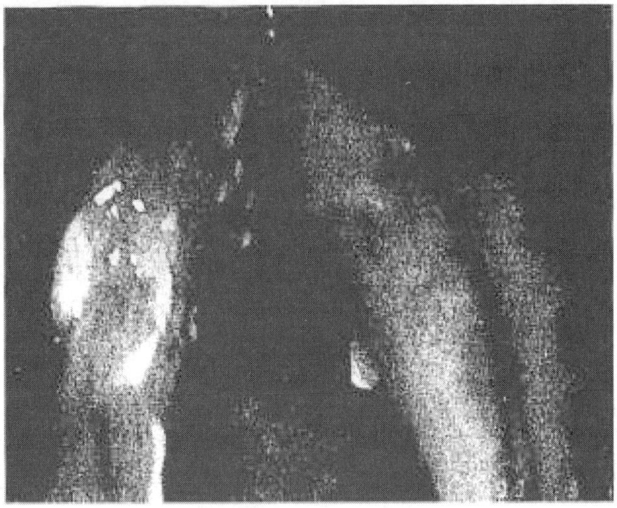

Fig. 48. Keratotic vocal fold lesion on the superior/ventricular and medial/vocalizing surface (preinfusion). Distraction of the left vestibular fold by the triangular laryngoscope reveals a linear perimeter (arrows) of superior surface keratosis.

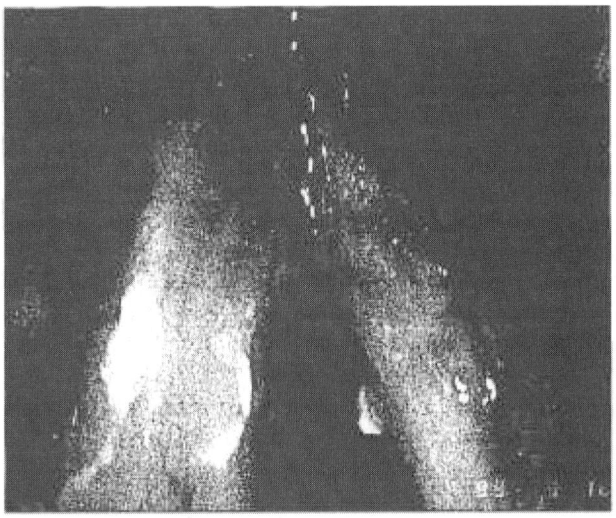

Fig. 49. Keratotic vocal fold lesion on the superior/ventricular and medial/vocalizing surface (postinfusion). The infusion has exposed more normal ventricular surface epithelium (arrows) to facilitate peripheral incisions around the lesion. Note the excellent view of the superior surface of the anterior commissure.

Limiting incisions were made with a sickle blade or a microscissors around the lesion posteriorly, anteriorly, and laterally.[163] This prevented tearing of the microflap into the anterior commissure or into the vocal process. A triangular microflap forceps was used to retract the microflap medially, while a Boucheyer or Ossoff dissector was used to develop a microflap that would encompass the lesion (Fig. 50). The flap was carefully dissected away from the underlying medial lamina propria. To aid hemostasis and visualization, a wet cottonoid with 1/10,000 saline/ epinephrine was placed gently over the fold as needed.

The dissection was carried out inferiorly until the caudal margin of the lesion was reached (Fig. 51). This was checked carefully by redraping the flap (Fig. 52). Once adequately mobilized, the flap was again retracted (Fig. 53) medially and an upturned scissors was used to

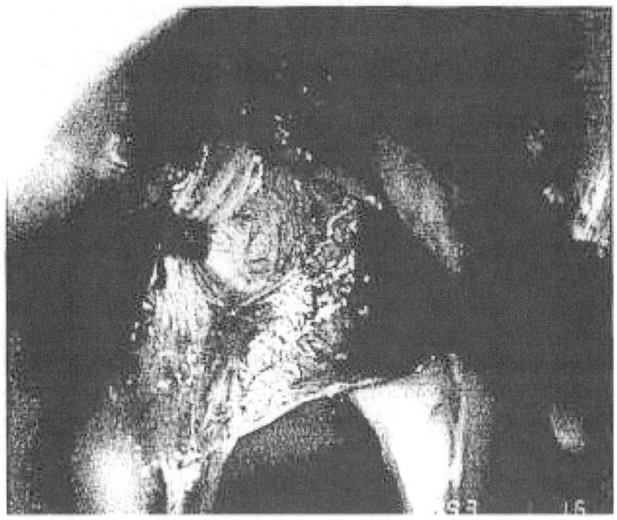

Fig. 50. Blunt microdissection of the vocal fold cover lesion from the medial lamina propria in the superficial lamina propria plane of dissection.

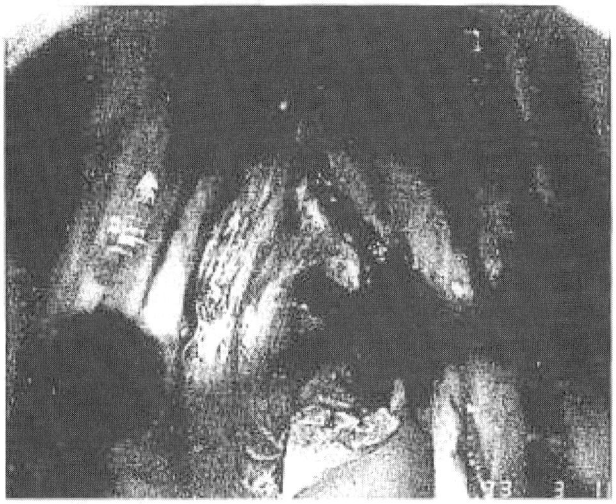

Fig. 51. Caudal dissection of the microflap around the curve of the vocal fold (*cf.* Fig. 42).

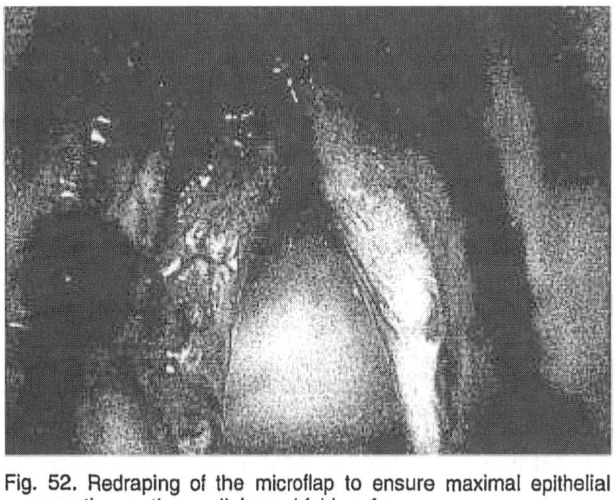

Fig. 52. Redraping of the microflap to ensure maximal epithelial preservation on the medial vocal fold surface.

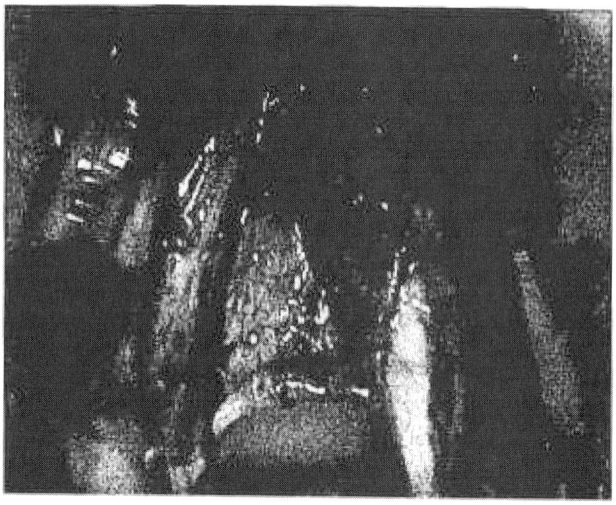

Fig. 53. Completion of the microflap resection.

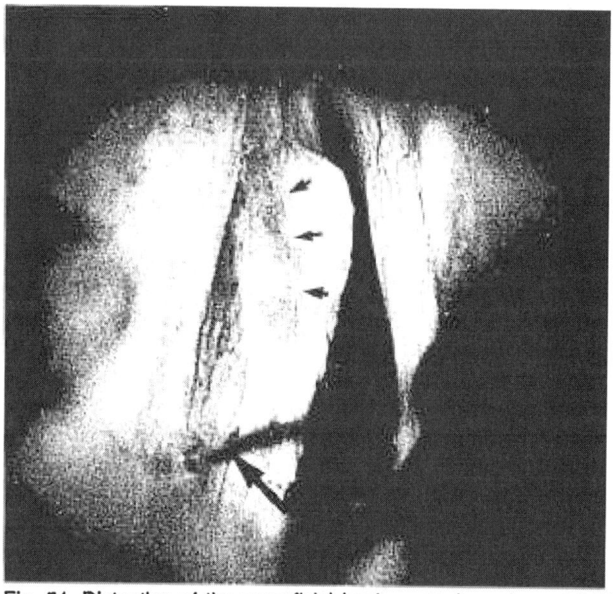

Fig. 54. Distention of the superficial lamina propria and vocal fold cover peripheral to the neoplastic lesion. The small arrows delineate the edge of the edema from the carcinoma which has centrally replaced the superficial lamina propria (the doughnut effect). The large arrow indicates the infusion needle.

complete the excision. Great care was taken to preserve the medial vocalizing membrane as much as was oncologically sound, while leaving the underlying SLP undisturbed. The specimen was then oriented on a carrier as described by Holinger and Miller[164] for multiple-section analysis. Before extubation, the vocal folds were sprayed with 2% lidocaine to reduce the incidence of laryngospasm during emergence from anesthesia.

If the infusion did not dissect the lesion from the vocal ligament, a doughnut effect was observed that demonstrated distension of the SLP peripheral to the central attachment of the neoplastic lesion to the MLP (Fig. 54). From this it was assumed that there was previous surgical scarring or a microinvasive cancer that had transgressed the SLP and invaded the vocal ligament. In this setting, if the patient preferred transoral excision, a

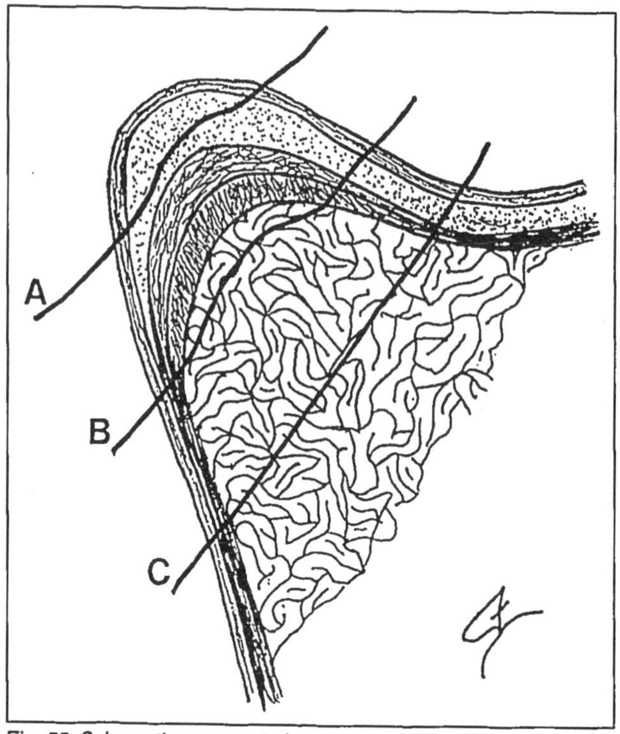

Fig. 55. Schematic representation of three types of vocal fold resections: vocal fold cover (**A**); vocal fold cover and vocal ligament (**B**); and vocal fold cover, ligament, and muscle (**C**).

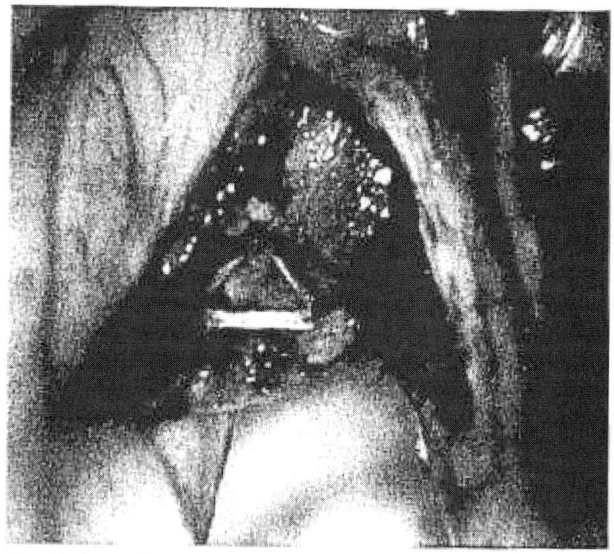

Fig. 56. Resection of an epithelial lesion using the vocal ligament as a connective tissue margin. The vocal ligament and overlying epithelium are contained within the forceps and are being dissected from the vocalis muscle (arrows).

deeper resection was required to obtain adequate margins. This was typically done with the use of a microspot carbon dioxide laser (Fig. 55). There were two types of deep resections performed. If it was thought that the neoplasm had not transgressed the vocal ligament, this structure was utilized as a margin for excision with minimal vocalis-muscle resection (Fig. 56). Margins were adjusted following magnified visualization of the operative site and frozen sections were performed when necessary. If there

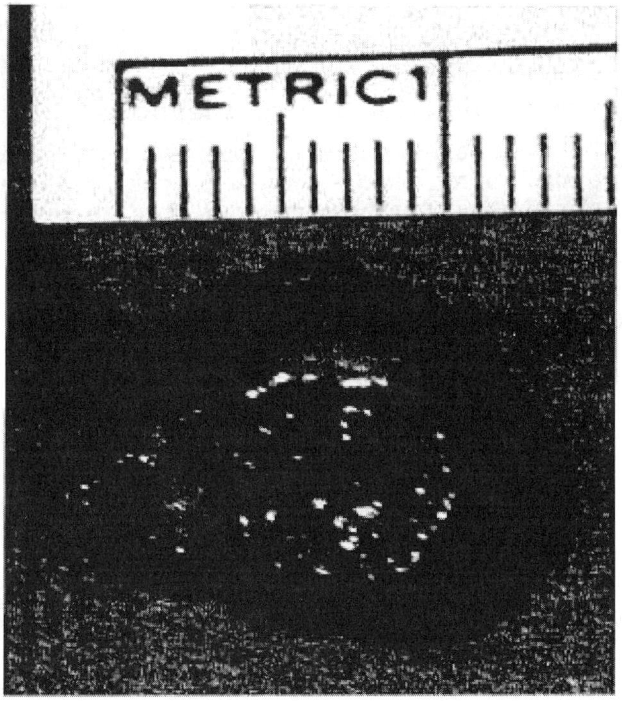

Fig. 57. Excised cordectomy specimen including a significant portion of vocalis muscle.

was muscle invasion, transoral cordectomy was performed (Figs. 55, 57). At the conclusion of the excision, the lesions were mapped according to surface and depth of involvement of the vocal fold. If invasive cancer was suspected and the patient was in favor of radiotherapy, the biopsy was confined to the superior surface of the vocal fold in order not to disturb the medial/vocalizing epithelium.

Postoperatively, patients were strongly admonished about smoking, and those suspected of gastroesophageal reflux were treated aggressively. They were instructed to remain on absolute voice rest for 1 week if it was feasible, and, subsequently, to practice vocal conservation for approximately 3 weeks. Those demonstrating abusive vocal habits or generalized hyperfunction received vocal therapy postoperatively. Objective visual (videolaryngoscopy with stroboscopy), acoustic, and aerodynamic analyses were performed at least 8 weeks later.

RESULTS

Submucosal infusion was performed on 42 vocal folds and clear margins were obtained on all lesions. The margins were evaluated by both whole-mount histological and intraoperative microlaryngeal assessment. Final determination was based on a synthesis of the information from both evaluations. It was not uncommon for a histological specimen to reveal a positive margin because the embedded tissue block was sectioned until the lesion was reached and/or the tissue block was not always exhausted during sectioning.

No patient had residual epithelial disease on microlaryngeal examination and no patient underwent a second operative procedure because of an incomplete resection. Four patients underwent resection of recurrent keratotic lesions at least 6 months following the initial resection. Four patients underwent staged procedures because there was bilateral disease and the resection margin extended to the anterior commissure mucosa. Five patients underwent synchronous bilateral resections, and no postoperative anterior-commissure webs occurred in any patient.

In 6 of the 42 vocal folds, the doughnut effect was observed, indicating that the epithelial lesion was attached to the vocal ligament; an observable superficial lamina propria was not evident in these patients. In 3 lesions, the attachment of the epithelium to the vocal ligament was the result of previous vocal fold surgery; in 2 lesions, there was attachment of a cancer to the vocal ligament; and in 1 patient, the lesion occurred with a sulcus vocalis.

DISCUSSION

Microflap resection, after submucosal infusion, facilitated phonomicrosurgical excision of premalignant epithelium and microinvasive carcinoma. In a subsequent literature review, a passing reference to the use of vocal-fold submucosal infusion was made by Kambic (1978)[171]: "Before excision of the mucous membrane, physiological solution is injected submucosally into the vocal cord so that the mucous membrane is lifted and stripping easily carried out." Therefore, attribution of credit for the technique belongs to Kambic. The membranous vocal fold microflap technique that was described by Yates and Dedo (1984)[207] resulted in good vocal quality after surgical management of polypoid degeneration. The phonomicrosurgical approach, described in study 3, married two concepts, submucosal infusion and microflap resection.

The submucosal infusion technique facilitated phonomicrosurgical resection of diseased vocal fold epithelium by improving visualization of incisions, ease of dissection, and preservation of tissue. The infusion distended the epithelial cover and medialized the lateral border of the lesion away from the vestibular fold. This provided a simpler alternative to vestibulectomy[208] for improved visualization of some lesions. It also provided a less tangential view of the medial/caudal edge of some lesions. The improved visualization of the lesion's perimeter and the hydrostatic tension from the infusion facilitated precise mucosal incisions.

Hirano[137] reported that the average thickness of the vocal fold epithelium and superficial lamina propria was 0.3 mm. The depth of the SLP was markedly increased by the saline and epinephrine submucosal infusion, which performed a hydrodissection of the vocal fold cover from the vocal ligament. This allowed for precise dissection of the microflap with less instrumental trauma of the vocal ligament and epithelium and resulted in maximal preserva-

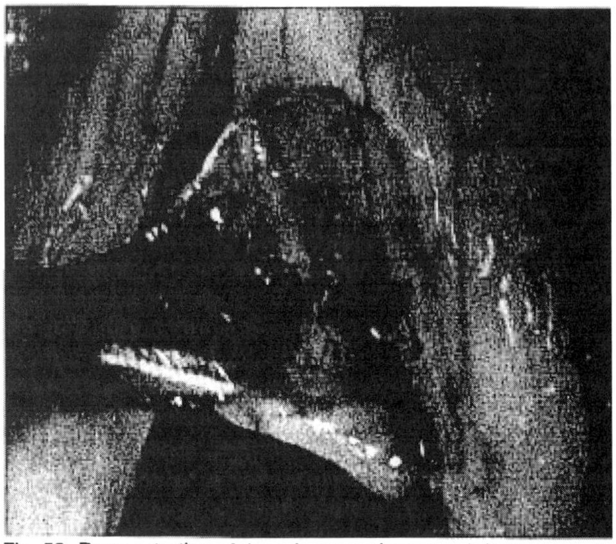

Fig. 58. Demonstration of the microvascular network in the superficial lamina propria during microflap resection. This microvasculature travels tangential to the vocal ligament (medial and deep lamina propria) thereby demonstrating full preservation of the vocal ligament.

tion of the SLP and vocal ligament. Typically, a microvascular network in the SLP can be seen superficial to the medial lamina propria, tangentially crossing the deeper white fibers of the vocal ligament (Fig. 58). Preservation of some of this microvascular network ensures that the vocal ligament has been undisturbed. Hemostasis of this microvascular network is achieved by saline/adrenaline solution both by submucosal infusion and by topical administration. If a microspot carbon dioxide laser is used for the excision, the saline/epinephrine solution acts as a heat sink to prevent thermal trauma to the patient and the specimen.

The ability to predict when microinvasive cancer has invaded the vocal ligament in previously unoperated vocal folds was an unexpected outcome of the infusion technique. Submucosal vocal fold infusion in this setting resulted in a doughnut effect leaving a depression (Fig. 54) where the superficial lamina propria had been replaced by the carcinoma. In one case, the doughnut effect was observed when keratosis occurred in a sulcus vocalis. The submucosal infusion was less effective when the SLP had been obscured by previous surgery. Our experience suggests that if a keratotic lesion occurs on a vocal fold where there is epithelial scarring and loss of the SLP from previous surgery; neither the infusion, palpation, nor stroboscopy will reliably indicate if there is microinvasion into the vocal ligament.

On microlaryngeal examination, no patient had residual intraoperative epithelial disease, and no patient underwent a second operative procedure because of an incomplete resection. The histological slide did occasionally show significant atypia at a margin. This occurred when there were slide preparation problems, such as cutting into the paraffin block to reach the lesion and/or not exhausting the tissue in the block.

Other Techniques for Excisional Biopsy

Vocal fold stripping is a common alternative to controlled microflap resection. Stripping was designed as a one-handed procedure through a monocular glottiscope without magnification or general anesthetic paralysis. Its name accurately depicts the image of imprecise tissue removal. The experienced surgeon can maintain the depth of the excision in Reinke's space (superficial lamina propria); it is difficult to control the excision margins on the ventricular (superior) and vocalizing (medial) surfaces of the vocal fold. Stripping often results in trauma of uninvolved vocalizing membrane and/or of the vocal ligament with subsequent scarring of the regenerated vocal fold cover epithelium to the medial lamina propria. The final outcome is poorer vocal quality that is visualized by a stiff/restricted mucosal wave. Vocal fold stripping may also disrupt the specimen and thus impede histopathological assessment.

Microscopic excisional biopsy may employ the carbon dioxide laser. The primary advantages of the carbon dioxide laser are noncontact precision cutting and hemostasis. Many surgeons find management of the laser's micromanipulator preferable to bimanual cold microsurgical techniques. The carbon dioxide laser has the following disadvantages: *1.* that there is loss of epithelium, albeit small, from both the patient and the specimen, *2.* that tangential caudal dissection around the curved vocal fold is impractical (Figs. 42, 51), and *3.* that there is potential for unintended injury of the laminae propria.

The necessity of impacting and dissecting the tissue in a tangential plane exposes the vocal ligament and specimen to trauma from excessive transmission of thermal energy. Tissue distortion of the specimen can be especially problematic in the deep margin adjacent to the basement membrane. This problem is obviated in cold surgery by curved dissectors. Additional disadvantages of the carbon dioxide laser are the high costs associated with purchasing and maintaining a late-generation machine with a microspot.

Cost-effectiveness of Submucosal Infusion and Microflap Excisional Biopsy

Recent health care cost-containment efforts, including restrictions on insurance reimbursement, capitation, and the introduction of managed competition, have precipitated the need for careful assessment of treatment costs. With the phonomicrosurgical excisional biopsy technique, tertiary care is not required and available medical resources can be utilized more efficiently. In addition, morbidity and the need for rehabilitation are minimized, enabling the individual to return to work as soon as possible. Vaughan, *et al.*[201] have emphasized the cost-effectiveness of microlaryngoscopic treatment of T1 vocal-cord cancer. More recently, Myers, *et al.*[160] presented extrapolated data indicating that the cost of treatment for 100 T1 glottic cancers by microlaryngoscopy, hemilaryngectomy, and radiotherapy was $1.5 million, $3.4 million, and $3.7 million, respectively. In that series, patients in the microlaryngoscopy group underwent an average of two procedures: the first was diagnostic; the second, therapeutic. By performing one endoscopic procedure, Cragle and Brandenburg[209] reported an even greater per patient cost differential between laser resection ($5945) and radiotherapy ($14,151) for treatment of T1 carcinomas. With the submucosal infusion and microflap excisional biopsy technique, patients typically underwent one procedure.

Voice Rest

It is difficult to determine whether absolute postoperative voice rest is advantageous. Koufman and Blalock[210] reported that appropriate vocal therapy was the only variable that resulted in significantly reduced postoperative dysphonia; those patients on absolute voice rest had less postoperative dysphonia than those on vocal conservation, but the difference was not statistically significant. Most patients placed on absolute voice rest are probably only partially compliant, and therefore this approach can only moderate potential abuse. Voice rest is, however, effective in preventing individuals from returning prematurely to vocally demanding workplaces.

STUDY 4: Objective Vocal Assessment of the Submucosal Infusion and Microflap Excisional Biopsy Technique

MATERIALS AND METHODS

In the last phase of the investigation, detailed assessment of postoperative vocal function was made possible by a collaborative effort with a newly established vocal physiology laboratory. Analyses were done on a pilot group of 17 patients who had recently undergone submucosal infusion and microflap resection (*cf.* Appendix 2: two evaluations [PM 7 and PM 8] were done in 1 patient in whom metachronous bilateral resections had been performed; this resulted in a total of 18 evaluations). Along with the pathological diagnosis, the location of the resection was recorded (S, superior/ventricular surface; M, medial/vocalizing surface; L, vocal ligament; V, vocalis muscle).

The evaluations were done in conjunction with a speech scientist who specializes in the use of objective measures to evaluate voice production. The objective measurements of vocal function included acoustic analysis, electroglottography, aerodynamic testing, videolaryngoscopy with stroboscopy, and perceptual assessment. These evaluations were performed at least 2 months after surgery. No patient had undergone vocal therapy.

There were three types of resections: vocal fold cover (type A), vocal fold cover and vocal ligament (type B, PM 12), and vocal fold cover, ligament and vocalis muscle (type C, PM 6). Cold resection was performed if a microflap mucosal resection was necessary; a microspot carbon dioxide laser was used for the deeper cancer resections. In one patient, the lesion was excised as a type B resection just under the vocal ligament (Figs. 55, 56) (Table III, Appendix 2). This patient was included with the epithelial resection group because the volume of vocal cord

TABLE III.
Summary of Acoustic and Aerodynamic Data.

	/a / Phonation				Reading		Maximal Range		Aerodynamic		
Subject	% Jitter	% Shimmer	Spectral Noise	EGG Duty Cycle	F_0	I_0	F_0	I_0	Pressure	Flow	GR
PM1-S	N	N	N	N	N	N	D	N	N	I	N
PM2-S	I	N	I	N/A	N	D	N	D	I	N	N
PM3-S	N	N	N	D	N	N	N	N	I	N	N
PM4-S	N	N	N	D	N	D	D	D	N	D	I
PM5-S	N	N	N	D	N	N	N	N	N	N	N
PM6-SMLV	I	N	I	N/A	N	N	D	D	I	N	I
PM7-SM	N	N	N	N	N	N	D	D	N	I	N
PM8-SM	I	N	N	N	N	N	D	N	N	I	N
PM9-SM	N	N	N	D	N	N	D	N	N	I	N
PM10-S	N	N	N	N	N	N	N	N	I	D	I
PM11-S	N	N	N	N	N	N	N	D	I	N	N
PM12-SML	N	N	N	D	N	I	D	D	I	N	N
PM13-S	N	N	N	D	N	N	N	D	I	N	I
PM14-S	N	N	N	N	N	N	D	D	N	N	N
PM15-SM	N	N	N	N/A	I	N	N	N	I	N	I
PF1-S	I	N	N	N/A	N	N	D	N	I	N	N
PF2-SM	I	N	I	N	D	N	D	D	I	N	N
PF3-SM	I	N	N	N/A	N	N	D	N	I	N	I

EGG = electroglottography; F_0 = frequency; I_0 = intensity; GR = resistance; PM = male evaluation; PF = female evaluation; S = superior surface; SM = superior and medial surfaces; SML = superior and medial surfaces, vocal ligament; SMLV = superior and medial surfaces, vocal ligament, vocalis muscle; N = result within normal limits; I = result had increased above normal levels; D = result had decreased below normal levels; N/A = not obtainable.

muscle resected was not large. For the one patient who had undergone a deep, type C cancer resection (Fig. 57) with a large loss of muscle volume, the measures for many acoustic, aerodynamic, visual, and perceptual criteria (Appendices 2 through 8) were, for understandable reasons, aberrant, and this patient was not considered together with the other patients.

Given the absence of presurgical data, it was decided to compare the results of objective measures with existing normative data. These comparisons were used as a basis for making decisions about the extent to which measures for individual subjects fell within what were defined as normal-range limits. It is readily acknowledged that the quality of some existing normative data is limited by such factors as relatively small sample sizes, methodological variations, etc. However, the same criteria that are routinely used clinically to make judgments about whether the measurements fall within normal limits were employed for this study. Due to the limited numbers in this pilot study, comparison analyses were not done between patients in whom resections were done on one or both vocal folds. More comprehensive studies will be needed to address the issue of bilateral resections.

Acoustic Analysis

Each patient was seated in a sound-treated room (IAC booth) and wore a headband device from which an Electret condenser microphone was suspended at a constant distance of 15 cm from the lips. The output of the microphone was fed to a preamplifier and then recorded on digital audio tape (DAT). A calibration tone of known intensity (dB SPL) was recorded prior to assessing each patient and was used as a reference for acoustic analysis. Recordings were made as each patient performed the following tasks: *1.* read a standard passage; *2.* sustained the vowel "ah" three times, holding pitch and loudness as "steady" (constant) as possible for at least 3 seconds; *3.* produced the "ah" vowel with the highest (including falsetto register) and lowest (excluding pulse register) pitches possible, *i.e.*, maximum pitch range; and *4.* produced the "ah" vowel with the softest (excluding whisper) and loudest voice possible, *i.e.*, maximum intensity range.

The audio recordings of the reading passage (10 kHz sampling rate) and vowels (20 kHz sampling rate) for each patient were digitalized and processed on a 486/33 PC workstation using software that is commercially available (Kay Elemetrics, Inc.), as well as some that was specially developed for this type of analysis. The reading passage was analyzed to yield measures of average fundamental frequency (F_0) and intensity (dB). The steadiest 1-second segment from the midportion of the "best" of the "ah" vowels produced for three seconds (*i.e.*, perceived by the judges to be the steadiest and to have the best quality) was analyzed to yield percent frequency perturbation (jitter), percent intensity perturbation (shimmer), and harmonics-to-noise ratio (dB). Maximum and minimum fundamental frequency (pitch) and intensity (loudness) in dB were also determined for the "ah" vowels produced during the maximum range tasks. The results of the acoustic measures were then compared to normative data.[211]

Electroglottography

Electroglottography (EGG) provides a measure of vocal fold contact during phonation by sensing changes in the electrical impedance of the neck. The EGG was done simultaneously with the audio recordings by having patients wear a neck band that held two opposing EGG surface electrodes against the lamina of the thyroid cartilage. The EGG signal was recorded on the second channel of the DAT recorder.

The EGG signal for the same "ah" vowel that was chosen for perturbation and harmonic-to-noise analysis was digitalized (10 kHz) and assessed using a waveform analysis system (Kay Elemetrics, Inc.). This analysis yielded duty cycle measures that reflect the percentage of time that the vocal folds are apart per vocal fold vibratory cycle. Normal values range from 55% to 65% (Waveform Display System Instruction Manual, Kay Elemetrics, Inc., 1990).

Aerodynamic Testing

Aerodynamic testing was done using an Aerophone system (Kay Elemetrics, Inc.). Patients produced strings of "pah" syllables at a comfortable "normal" level while the following measures were obtained: *1.* oral airflow, using a pneumotachograph mounted in a face mask, and *2.* intraoral air pressure, using a translabially placed catheter connected to a pressure transducer. The flow and pressure signals were digitized and analyzed using the Aerophone system to yield indirect estimates of average glottal airflow rate (l/second), subglottal air pressure (cm H_2O), and glottal resistance (pressure/flow: cm H_2O/L per second). The results of aerodynamic measures were then compared to normative data.[212,213]

Visual: Videolaryngoscopy With Stroboscopy

Standard transoral (rigid) and/or transnasal (flexible) videolaryngoscopy with stroboscopy was performed as each patient sustained "ee" vowels at comfortable "average" pitch and loudness levels. These examinations were recorded on videotape (SVHS format) for subsequent visual evaluation of vocal function including the following: structural integrity, mucosal wave activity, glottal closure, symmetry of vocal fold vibration, and supraglottal characteristics. The visual ratings were recorded on a rating form during a multidisciplinary conference at which both laryngologists and speech pathologists arrived at a consensus opinion.

Perceptual Assessment

Auditory perceptual judging was performed by two American Speech and Hearing Association (ASHA)–certified speech-language pathologists and two otolaryngologists who are experienced in working with voice-disordered patients. From the audio recordings of each patient and of four additional "normal" speakers (two males, NM 1 and 2; two females, NF 1 and 2) (Table IV, Appendix 8), the first three sentences of the reading passage and one of the "ah" vowels (sustained for 3 seconds) were dubbed onto two master tapes in different random orders. These tapes were listened to independently, over headphones, by each of the judges who rated each sentence-vowel combination using the following scales (judges were informed only about the sex of each patient): breathiness—normal, mild, moderate, severe; straining—normal, mild, moderate, severe; hoarseness—normal, mild, moderate, severe; and pitch—too low, normal, too high.

TABLE IV.
Summary of Perceptual Data.

Subject	Breathiness	Straining	Hoarseness	Pitch
NM1	N	N	N	N
NM2	N	N	N	N
PM1-S	N	N	MLD	D
PM2-S	N	N	MLD	N
PM3-S	N	N	N	N
PM4-S	N	N	MLD	N
PM5-S	N	N	MLD	N
PM6-SMLV	MOD	MLD	MOD	N
PM7-SM	N	N	MLD	N
PM8-SM	N	N	MLD	N
PM9-SM	N	N	MLD	N
PM10-S	N	MLD	MLD	N
PM11-S	N	MLD	MLD	D
PM12-SML	N	MLD	MLD	D
PM13-S	N	N	MLD	N
PM14-S	N	N	N	N
PM15-SM	MLD	N	MLD	I
NF1	N	N	N	N
NF2	N	N	N	N
PF1-S	N	N	MLD	N
PF2-SM	N	N	N	N
PF3-SM	MLD	MOD	MOD	N

NM = normal male; NF = normal female; PM = male evaluation; PF = female evaluation; S = superior surface; SM = superior and medial surfaces; SML = superior and medial surfaces, vocal ligament; SMLV = superior and medial surfaces, vocal ligament, vocalis muscle; N = result within normal limits; I = result had increased above normal levels; D = result had decreased below normal levels; MOD = moderate; MLD = mild.

RESULTS

Acoustic, Electroglottographic, and Aerodynamic Measures

Results for the acoustic, electroglottographic, and aerodynamic measures (18 evaluations in 17 patients) are summarized in Table III. In that table, "N" denotes that the measured result was within normal limits, "I" means that it had increased above normal levels, and "D" means that it had decreased below normal levels. The one patient (PM 6) who had undergone a cordectomy, including the excision of a significant amount of vocalis muscle, is not considered in the group analysis. The actual data values for these measures are contained in Appendices 3 through 6.

In the 17 evaluations done on 16 patients who had undergone microflap epithelial resection, none, as shown in Table III, had normal values for all 11 of the measures used. In terms of acoustic assessment, only 3 (18%) of the 17 were normal for all of the acoustic measures that were obtained from sustained vowels, reading, and maximum range tasks. However, a majority of the acoustic measures for "steady" vowel production and reading fell within normal limits. For 12 (71%) of the 17, normal values were obtained for all three vowel-related measures (*i.e.*, jitter, shimmer, and spectral noise). In terms of each parameter, 12 (71%) of the 17 displayed normal jitter (frequency perturbation) while the remaining 5 displayed increased jitter; all of the patients had normal shimmer (amplitude perturbation); and 15 (88%) of the 17 had normal levels of spectral noise, with 2 displaying increased spectral noise (Table III, Appendix 3).

TABLE V.
Acoustic Abnormalities and Resection Surface.

	Acoustic Measure					
	Jitter		Maximal Range: F_0 Pitch/Frequency		Maximal Range: I_0 Loudness/Intensity	
Type of Resection	Abnormal	Normal	Abnormal	Normal	Abnormal	Normal
Superior (10)	2	8	4	6	5	5
Superior and medial (7)	3	4	6	1	4	3
Total No. of resections (17)	5	12	10	7	9	8

F_0 = frequency; I_0 = intensity.

Three of the 5 patients in whom increased jitter was found had undergone superior and medial epithelial resections, while 2 of the 5 had undergone only a superior resection. In this small group of 17 evaluations, increased jitter was more than twice as frequent in the superior and the medial resection group (3 of 7) as in the superior resection group (2 of 10) (Table V). In 4 of the 5 patients in whom increased jitter was found, there was significant supraglottic muscle tension dysphonia (it had been present preoperatively in all 4) (Table III, Appendix 7).

For reading, in 12 (71%) of the 17, the values for both average F_0 (pitch) and average intensity (loudness) were normal. In terms of each parameter: 15 (88%) of the 17 had normal speaking F_0, while 1 had increased F_0 and 1 had decreased F_0; 14 (82%) of the 17 had normal intensity, with 1 displaying increased intensity and 2 displaying decreased intensity (Table III, Appendix 4).

In contrast to the acoustic results for "steady" vowels and reading previously described, a substantial number of the F_0 and intensity measures for the maximum range tasks revealed abnormality (*i.e.*, restricted ranges). Only 4 (24%) of the 17 had values in the normal range for both F_0 (pitch) and intensity (loudness). Seven (41%) of the 17 had a normal maximum pitch range while 10 had decreased ranges for pitch (Table III, Appendix 5). Of those 7, 6 had undergone a superior resection and 1 had undergone a superior/medial resection (Tables III, V). It is noteworthy that 60% (6 of 10) of the superior resection group displayed normal maximal pitch range while only 14% (1 of 7) of the superior/medial resection group did so. Nine (53%) of the evaluations had normal maximum intensity ranges and 8 had decreased ranges (Tables III, V). The type of resection did not appear to be a differentiating factor for maximum intensity ranges in this study (Tables III, V).

It was not possible to obtain a measurable EGG signal for 4 of the 17 evaluations (16 patients). Of the 13 evaluations for which there was usable EGG data, 7 (54%) had normal EGG duty cycle values, while the remaining 6 (46%) displayed decreased (pressed) values (Table III, Appendix 3).

In only 12% of the patient evaluations (2 of 17) were the values for all three of the aerodynamic measures normal. Seven (41%) of the 17 evaluations had normal subglottal pressures. For the majority, 10 (59%), the measured pressures were abnormally high. None of these patients, however, expressed discomfort in conjunction with phonation. Again, the type of resection did not appear to make a difference. Eleven (65%) of the 17 had normal average glottal airflow rates, while 4 displayed increased flow and 2 displayed decreased flow. Glottal resistance (the ratio of pressure to flow) was normal for 12 evaluations (71%) and was increased for 5 (29%) (Table III, Appendix 6).

Visual: Videolaryngoscopy With Stroboscopy

The magnitude (size) of the mucosal wave was normal in 3 of 17 evaluations. All 3 had undergone superior microflap resection (Appendix 7). No patient who underwent a superior/medial resection had a normal mucosal wave. The decrease in mucosal-wave magnitude generally followed the increase in extent of the resection (Appendices 2, 7). The amplitude of vocal fold vibration (excursion) was normal in 12 (71%) of 17 patients (Appendix 7). Eight of the 11 had undergone a superior resection, and 3 had undergone a superior/medial resection. It is noteworthy that 80% of the superior resection group had a normal amplitude of vocal fold vibration, but that only 43% of the superior/medial resection group did so.

Two of 17 evaluations revealed incomplete vocal-fold edge closure in the musculomembranous region, and both of these had undergone a superior/medial resection. Six of 17 demonstrated a vertical phase asymmetry; there were 3 patients from each of the 2 resection groups. Five of 17 developed an irregular vocal fold edge after effective microflap resection. One of the 5 had undergone a superior resection; the other 4 had undergone a superior/medial resection. While only 10% of those in the superior resection group developed an irregular vocal fold edge, 63% of the superior/medial group did so. The irregular edge in patient evaluation PM 7 was secondary to the as yet unresected vocal fold keratosis (Appendices 2 and 7).

Perceptual Measures

It was decided to average the responses of the four judges to yield one rating for each of the four perceptual parameters for each subject (Table IV). Due to the categorical nature of the perceptual responses, there are limitations to this approach. However, given the pilot nature of this work, a simple averaging approach was considered acceptable. Appendix 8 contains the perceptual responses for each judge, average perceptual ratings across judges, and estimates of intrajudge agreement. Intrajudge agreement was simply the percentage (number of times out of 88 total possible judgments [22 subjects × 4 perceptual parameters]) that each judge gave the same rating for both presentations (tape 1 and 2) of each recorded voice. Intrajudgment agreement ranged from 58% to 83%. The vast majority of responses that were not in agreement differed by one category.

Table IV displays a summary of the averaged perceptual responses expressed in terms of the descriptive categories that were originally used by the judges. Average ratings for breathiness, straining, and hoarseness were converted back to descriptive categories as follows: normal (N), 0.0 to 0.9; mild (MLD), 1.0 to 1.9; moderate (MOD), 2.0 to 2.9; and severe (SEV), 3. Average ratings for pitch were converted back to descriptive categories as follows: decreased (D), −1.0 to −0.5; normal (N), −0.4 to 0.4; increased (I), 0.5 to 1.0.

All the averaged ratings for all 4 of the normal subjects fell within the range of values categorized as normal. For the surgical patients, out of the total of 68 averaged perceptual ratings (17 patient evaluations × 4 parameters), 47 (69%) were categorized as normal. For the three vocal quality parameters of breathiness, straining, and hoarseness (17 patients × 3 parameters: 51 averaged ratings), 31 (61%) were categorized as normal, 18 (35%) as mildly abnormal, and 2 (4%) as moderately abnormal. In terms of vocal pitch judgments, 13 (76%) of the averaged ratings were categorized as normal, with 4 (24%) falling outside the normal range (Table IV).

Across all patients, the parameter of hoarseness received the highest (most disordered) averaged ratings. Fourteen (82%) of the 17 patient evaluations revealed some degree of hoarseness, with the majority (13 or 76%) being characterized as mildly hoarse, and the other 1 (6%) categorized as moderately hoarse. Fifteen patient evaluations (88%) demonstrated absence of breathiness, while 2 (12%) were categorized as having mild breathiness. Thirteen patient evaluations (76%) did not reveal strain, while 4 (24%) were categorized as having some degree of straining associated with voice production. Three (18%) were placed into the mild category and 1 was categorized as moderately strained. Of the 4 patients (24%) who displayed averaged ratings for vocal pitch that fell outside of the normal range, 3 were categorized as decreased and 1 was categorized as increased (Table IV).

DISCUSSION

Acoustic, Aerodynamic, and Electroglottography

Overall, a majority of the patients who were evaluated had normal values for acoustic measures related to voice quality (*i.e.*, jitter, shimmer, spectral noise) and/or average speaking pitch and loudness (*i.e.*, average fundamental frequency and SPL for reading). However, during maximum range tasks, most patients were limited (subnormal) in the extent to which they could maximally increase and/or decrease pitch (fundamental frequency) and loudness (SPL). Taken together, these results indicate that most patients had voices that were acoustically within normal limits during average use, and that restrictions or reductions in voice production became apparent only when the vocal mechanism was "stressed" or "pushed" to generate outputs (pitch and loudness) that were at the extremes of the normal ranges. The patients who demonstrated the most frequent average vocal acoustic abnormality, increased jitter, were more likely to be those who had undergone resection of the superior/ventricular and medial/vocalizing glottal surfaces (Table V).

Even though a majority of patients displayed voices that were acoustically within normal limits during average use, aerodynamic and EGG measures indicated a high incidence of abnormalities in underlying physiologic function. Most patients displayed higher than normal subglottal air pressures. This is generally interpreted as being a response to difficulties in producing voice because of vocal fold structural abnormalities and/or heightened levels of vocal fold stiffness, tension, and adduction.[214,215] The possibility that increased vocal fold adduction was associated with increased subglottal pressures was supported by the presence of reduced EGG duty cycles for some patients.

For normal speakers, subglottal air pressure covaries proportionally with vocal SPL, *i.e.*, proportional increases in subglottal pressure accompany increases in SPL.[212,213] Increased pressures, however, did not result in proportionally higher SPLs for the patients in this study. The apparent need for patients to generate higher than normal subglottal pressures to produce normal levels of vocal SPL is indicative of a reduction in the efficiency of the vocal mechanism and undoubtedly underlies the inability of many patients to achieve normal maximum intensity ranges (*i.e.*, maximum air pressure levels are not associated with SPLs of sufficient magnitude to result in a normal range).

The combination of higher than normal subglottal air pressures and reduced EGG duty cycles may also be viewed as indicative of a hyperfunctioning mechanism. Based on these measures, it is not possible to determine whether such hyperfunctional activity was necessary for patients to produce their "best" voices, or if instead, these are persistent hyperfunctional behaviors, which were originally developed by patients in their attempt to compensate for the presence of vocal fold pathology. Probably the only way to determine whether hyperfunction was a necessary component of voice production for these patients would be to observe the effects on vocal function of using voice therapy to reduce hyperfunction. The usefulness of electroglottography was limited by the fact that 5 of 17 patients could not be evaluated because their neck anatomy interfered with obtaining an adequate signal.

Analysis of the patients that demonstrated impaired vocal systems for maximal range tasks revealed that, like jitter (pitch instability) during speech produced at conversational levels, reduced maximal pitch variation was twice as likely with a superior and medial resection as compared to a superior resection alone. However, the nature of the geographic resection had no differential impact on the incidence of impairment in maximal loudness (Table V).

Visual: Videolaryngoscopy With Stroboscopy

Post-treatment: microsurgical. After superior epithelial microflap resection (10 patient evaluations), the stroboscopic evaluations in this series typically revealed minimally affected phase symmetry and minimally decreased amplitude of vocal fold vibration (excursion) (1 of 10). This was so despite the significantly decreased magnitude (size) of the mucosal wave of the superior cordal surface (7 of 10) (Appendix 7). The decreased mucosal wave magnitude is consistent with the data reported by Hirano, *et al.*[205] in 5 patients with a similar depth of resection. These visual findings correlate with the surgically induced, increased stiffness in the vocal mechanism and may also reflect an increase in muscle tension. Increased stiffness and/or tension can lead to the need for increased subglottal driving pressures to produce adequate voice and seems to also underlie impairment of maximal acoustic range tasks in these patients.

The mucosal wave activity of the medial/vocalizing mucosal surface cannot be extrapolated from visualizing the superior/ventricular surface after superior surface microflap resection. Incorrect conclusions about the magnitude of scarring in the medial vocal fold surface occur because the medial membrane and associated SLP have not been violated. Unlike the superior resection group, the patients of Hirano, *et al.*[205] demonstrated a significant decrease in vibrational amplitude. The favorable vibrational amplitude demonstrated by the superior resection group is most likely secondary to preservation of the entire vocal fold layered anatomy on the medial/vocalizing surface. It appears from Hirano's diagram of the resection classification scheme used in their study that no patients had preservation of the medial vocal fold cover.

Microflap resection of both the superior and the medial vocal fold surfaces (seven patient evaluations) frequently resulted in a mild decrease in the amplitude of vocal fold vibration (four of seven) as well as a decrease in the magnitude of the mucosal wave (seven of seven). These visual findings demonstrated more restriction in the vocal systems of these patients as compared to those that had undergone only superior resections. It was also noted that the visual findings of increased stiffness/tension frequently was correlated with maximal acoustic range impairment. These data correlate well to the findings of Hirano, *et al.*[205] on five patients who underwent vocal fold cover resections.

The two patients in the current study in whom deeper cancer resections were performed displayed stiff vocal folds both with regard to the magnitude of the mucosal wave and the amplitude of vocal fold vibration (excursion) (Appendix 7). Generally, there is minimal information reported about vocal function after layered resections; yet, it is becoming increasingly clear that the three-dimensional volume (surface and depth) of resection is probably an important prognosticator of postoperative voice.

There are limitations of stroboscopic postresection evaluations. Stroboscopy is very sensitive in the evaluation of the magnitude of the mucosal wave on the superior/vestibular vocal fold surface as compared with the medial/vocalizing surface. Telescopic and flexible fiberoptic stroboscopy are most effective in evaluating the segment of the mucosal wave motion that moves perpendicular to the plane of visualization. Therefore, with this technology, only tangential visualization of the medial vocal fold surface (which is a primary glottal valving location) is possible. Precise mucosal wave assessment on the medial/vocalizing surface would require that the scope be perpendicular to this region of the glottis, which is impossible.

There are three reasons for the decreased vocal fold mucosal wave magnitude after microflap resections. First, there is simply a loss of volume of mucosa which is typically quite redundant[139,216] (Fig. 59). After resection, there is wound contracture, and regenerating epithelium seals the surface with the least amount of epithelium. Secondly, any technique to resect epithelium will also remove some of the superficial lamina propria, which is crucial to the vibratory characteristics of the mucosal wave. Finally, there will be some degree of scarring of the regenerated epithelium to the underlying tissue depsite optimum phonomicrosurgical technique.

Irregular, postsurgical vocal fold edges, at times resulting in incomplete closure of the musculomembranous vocal fold, were more likely to occur after a superior/medial resection. Phase symmetry seemed to be less strongly correlated to the location of the resection.

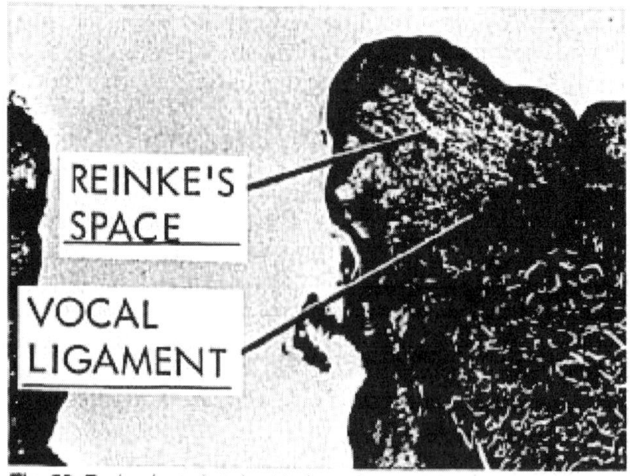

Fig. 59. Redundant glottal epithelium demonstrated on the free edge of the vocal fold. (From Tucker, G.F.: *Human Larynx Coronal Section Atlas*, A.F.I.P. Publishing).

Posttreatment: radiotherapy. Lehman, *et al.*[217] presented compelling evidence about the damaging effect of radiotherapy on the vocal fold. This study of posttreatment vocal function after radiotherapy for early vocal fold cancer revealed that there was a reduced or absent mucosal wave in all vocal folds including all of those uninvolved by neoplasia. They also noted a reduction of the vibrational amplitude in many radiated noncancerous folds. Hirano, *et al.*[205] reported similar reductions in mucosal wave magnitude and vibration in irradiated folds involved by T1 carcinomas. These deleterious effects may well worsen over time with late radiation-induced tissue changes.

Vocal quality is an important parameter for judging the success of treatment of intraepithelial vocal fold atypia just as it is an important factor in the treatment of early vocal-cord cancer. Conceptually, it is troublesome to employ radiation as a treatment option knowing that it will damage tissue uninvolved by the premalignant or neoplastic process.

Pretreatment. Pretreatment stroboscopic data are more frequently discussed than posttreatment results. Stroboscopy has been employed to identify mucosal cancer invasion into the vocal ligament.[205] When neoplastic vocal fold cover epithelium has replaced the superficial lamina propria and has attached to the medial lamina propria, the magnitude and excursion of the mucosal wave may be obscured. However, diagnostic stroboscopy for assessment of cancer invasion is of considerably less value if the patient has had previous surgery. Also, thick keratosis may obscure observation of mucosal wave activity during stroboscopy and therefore impair determination of vocal ligament invasion. This is especially true if the lesion is a large plaque with only small foci of invasion of the vocal ligament.

Stroboscopy is not useful for characterizing the severity of epithelial dysplasia or for identification of carcinoma in situ and microinvasion in Reinke's space. Zhao, *et al.*[218] have reported decreased mucosal wave magnitude and decreased amplitude of vocal fold vibration in hyperplastic and dysplastic vocal fold lesions. They explained that there is an inverse relationship between *a.* the surface involvement and thickness of the keratotic lesion and *b.* the magnitude of the mucosal wave and the amplitude of vocal fold vibration. These abnormal vocal fold vibratory characteristics, which are secondary to increased mass and stiffness, are related to the lesion's volume rather than to its cellular morphology.

Perceptual. Similar to McGuirt, *et al.*,[219] the perceptual ratings used may be interpreted as mild (only a trained listener would detect), moderate (the patient would need to explain his voice to others), and severe (sounds like severe laryngitis).

In terms of the results, there was a wide range of intrajudge agreement. Judge 4 displayed the highest level of point-to-point reliability (83%), and judge 1 displayed the lowest (58%). For the perceptual parameters of breathiness, straining, and hoarseness, the majority of responses varied by only one category for both intrajudge and interjudge comparisons. Interestingly, pitch judgments appeared to be the most unreliable; in many instances, the judges gave all three possible ratings (normal, increased, and decreased) for the same patient.

A majority of the patients' voices were rated as mildly hoarse, but as essentially normal on all other perceptual parameters (breathiness, straining, pitch). In general, these results support the findings that most patients had acoustically normal voices during average speaking tasks. There was not a large difference in the perceptual results between the two types of resection groups (Table IV).

In terms of specific relationships between the results from objective measurement and perceptual evaluation, *1.* all four patients who were categorized as mildly or moderately strained had abnormally high subglottal air pressures, *2.* the two patients who were categorized as moderately hoarse had increased levels of fundamental frequency perturbation (jitter) (one of these was the patient who underwent transmural cordectomy including vocalis muscle), and *3.* only some of the patients who were categorized as mildly hoarse displayed increased levels of perturbation—this is not surprising given the somewhat limited sensitivity of these acoustic measures.[220]

THE HEURISTIC VALUE OF THE HISTORICAL INVESTIGATION

Phonomicrosurgical treatment of premalignant vocal fold epithelium and microinvasive cancer combines principles of surgical oncology with advanced laryngoscopic microsurgical techniques, and it is also guided by mucosal-wave theory of voice production. This treatment approach, which evolved during the past two centuries, is an early example of minimally invasive surgery. Historical analysis helps explain the biases and philosophical differences that have led to the variety of treatment approaches currently in use. It also exposes the importance of determining *1.* what tissue must be excised to obtain an accurate diagnosis and *2.* which laryngoscopic biopsy technique, in conjunction with established anatomical/physiological concepts of voice production, is preferable for attaining optimal vocal function.

Methods of visualizing the vocal folds developed gradually, as did techniques for precise tissue removal. In the 19th century, mirror laryngoscopy was the vanguard of laryngology. In the latter part of that century, laryngeal visualization allowed for routine transoral biopsies. By the end of the 19th and in the early 20th centuries, direct laryngoscopic techniques had replaced indirect biopsy methods. Although Kirstein is credited with discovering direct laryngoscopy in 1895, Green had previously (1852) described both direct visualization of the laryngeal introitus and transoral laryngeal polyp excision. In the early 20th century, Jackson disseminated direct laryngoscopic technique and Killian created suspension laryngoscopy to free surgeons' hands. Although their respective techniques were sound in principle, they were difficult in practice; many surgeons were unable to adopt them. With the subsequent use of general anesthesia and paralysis during laryngoscopy, the importance of their teachings was de-emphasized. Later on, however, with the introduction of larger laryngoscopes (required for stereoscopic magnification) there was a resurgence and marriage of the principles that Killian and Jackson had each espoused.

Rudiments of body-cover mucosal-wave theory of voice production were introduced in the early 19th century but have only recently been incorporated into laryngoscopic glottal surgery (phonomicrosurgery). Currently, methods for excisional biopsy of vocal-fold cover lesions embody the principles of phonomicrosurgery and aim toward maximal preservation of the vocal fold's layered anatomy. Phonomicrosurgical management of premalignant and early malignant vocal fold epithelium is optimized by obtaining the widest glottal surgical operating field possible, especially in the problematic anterior commissure region. To achieve this requires a return to Jackson's and Killian's principles of laryngoscopy that allow for the safe placement of the largest lumened glottiscope possible. This is accomplished by placing the patient in elevated-vector suspension, which requires Boyce-Jackson position, sustained by a modified Killian gallows.

In the 1920s, Jackson also introduced the concept of glottal premalignancy. He suggested that there was a window of opportunity to surgically eradicate precancerous glottal lesions and thus prevent progression to cancer. This theory was temporally coincident with the introduction of the mass production of cigarettes and the gradual decline of infectious membranous laryngeal diseases like tuberculosis. Given these epidemiological factors, many irregular vocal fold lesions found in smokers were presumed to be premalignant or microinvasive cancer, until proven otherwise.

This historical investigation helped formulate the four studies that were conducted for the purpose of developing an effective phonomicrosurgical treatment approach for premalignant and microinvasive glottal epithelium. These studies led to a number of conclusions about current methods for managing this disease process and suggested areas for future research.

CONCLUSIONS

Study 1

1. The initial management goal for vocal fold dysplasia or microinvasive cancer should be to obtain a precise and accurate diagnosis. This cannot be done solely by examining the vocal fold cover surface to determine a site for limited directed biopsy. Excisional biopsy, followed by three-dimensional histopathological analysis, is necessary to provide reliable diagnostic information.

2. Smoking-induced metaplasia and neoplasia typically arise on the superior/ventricular vocal fold surface and often involve the medial/vocalizing surface as well. It is the frequent confinement of these lesions to the superior/ventricular surface that often makes it possible to preserve the vocal fold's layered structure on the medial/vocalizing surface.

Study 2

3. Submucosal vocal fold dye infusions into cadaver larynges help to define where the vocal fold epithlium is supported by the superficial lamina propria and, as a result, help to identify vibratory epithelium.

4. This study also suggests that distension of the superficial lamina propria by submucosal infusion makes it possible to perform microsurgical dissection with minimal instrumental trauma to the vocal fold's layered anatomy.

Study 3

5. Submucosal infusion of saline and epinephrine distends the superficial lamina propria and simulates Reinke's edema. This approach facilitates microflap excisional biopsy and helps preserve the vocal fold's layered anatomy in both surface and depth.

6. Submucosal infusion with microflap excisional biopsy effectively removes dysplastic and microinvasive vocal fold epithelium and provides a tissue specimen suitable for multiple-section histopathological analysis.

7. The submucosal infusion effectively demonstrated when the superficial lamina propria had been replaced by cancer or scar. In patients who had not undergone prior vocal fold surgery, the submucosal infusion enhanced the ability to predict cancer invasion into the vocal ligament and allowed for accurate planning for deep resection margins.

8. Submucosal infusion with microflap excisional biopsy preserves all cancer treatment options. It is also simple, repeatable, and cost-effective.

Study 4

9. Acoustic measures of voice quality (jitter, shimmer, spectral noise) for most patients who had undergone submucosal infusion with microflap excisional biopsy were "normal" during speech tasks produced at conversational levels.

10. The higher than normal subglottal pressures that frequently accompanied the conversational-level speech of these patients suggests that more aerodynamic driving force is necessary to achieve an acoustically normal vocal outcome.

11. These patients do, however, demonstrate limitations in maximal range tasks with regard to both pitch (frequency) and loudness (intensity).

12. Stroboscopy provides only tangential visualization of the vocally critical medial vocal fold surface and cannot, therefore, be used to reliably assess the magnitude of the mucosal wave on that surface.

13. Stiffness of the medial/vocalizing membrane can probably best be assessed by examining the amplitude of vocal fold vibration (excursion).

14. Superior microflap resection typically reveals that vocal fold mucosal-wave excursion and phase symmetry are affected minimally, whereas the magnitude of the mucosal wave on the superior/ventricular surface is decreased significantly.

15. Resection of both superior and medial surfaces results in a decreased amplitude of vocal fold vibration (excursion) in some patients, as well as a decreased magnitude of the mucosal wave on the superior/ventricular surface in most. These visual findings are correlated with the surgically induced increased stiffness of the vocal system.

Future Directions

16. Further investigations are necessary to evaluate the differential impact of varying degrees of three-dimensional vocal fold tissue resections (surface and depth) on vocal outcomes, as well as the differential impact of unilateral versus bilateral resections. Also, the effect of vocal hyperfunction on voice quality and the potential value of therapy for improving postsurgical voice requires further study.

Thus, phonomicrosurgical treatment of premalignant epithelium and microinvasive cancer of the vocal fold, which was examined in this series of studies, integrates principles of surgical oncology with those of voice production. Not only does performing submucosal infusion with microflap excisional biopsy help to establish a definitive diagnosis, but it also treats this spectrum of epithelial diseases without precluding future treatment options. In addition, this approach strives to achieve "normal" voice by preserving the microanatomical layers of the vocal fold.

ACKNOWLEDGMENTS

The author is indebted to his mentors for their thoughtful training and their review of this manuscript: Charles W. Vaughan, MD; M. Stuart Strong, MD; Gerald B. Healy, MD; and Stanley M. Shapshay, MD. This work would not have been possible without the expertise of Gerard Domanowski, MD, and Max Goodman, MD, in pathology and Robert Hillman, PhD, in voice science. Invaluable wisdom and assistance was provided by Matina Horner, PhD, editorial review. The author would also like to thank Geza Jako, MD, and John Tucker, MD, as well as Richard Wolf at the Francis A. Countway Medical Library and Gretchen Worden at the Mutter Museum for their help with the historical investigation. Additional help was provided by Linda Rose, statistical analysis; Andrew Sizeland, MD, computer science; and Andras Mester, MD, language translation. In addition, Richard Cortese and Ralph Kylloe, PhD, provided photographic assistance. The author would also like to thank Dennis DeVona for his clear thinking and Kathleen Reardon for her organizational skills. Finally, the author would like to express his gratitude to Dr. Harry and Natalie Zeitels for their unyielding support.

BIBLIOGRAPHY

1. Wright, J.: Summary. In: *A History of Laryngology and Rhinology*. Lea & Febiger, Philadelphia, p. 333, 1914.
2. Bozzini, P.: *Der Lichtleiter oder Beschreibung einer einfachen Vorichtung, und ihrer Anwendung zur erleucht ung inherer Hohlen, und Zwischenraume des lebenden animaschen Korpers*. Weimar, 1807.
3. Tour, C. d. l. Cited by Fournie,: Physiologie de la voix. *Journal l'Institut*, p. 350, 1825.
4. Senn. Cited by Mackenzie,: The Use of the Laryngoscope in Diseases of the Throat. *Jour. de Progres*, p. 11, 1829.
5. Babington, B.G.: *London Medical Gazette*, 3:555, 1829.
6. Selligue. Cited by Mackenzie,: *The Use of the Laryngoscope in Diseases of the Throat*. p. 17, 1832.
7. Liston, R.: *Practical Surgery*. J. & A. Churchill, London, 1837.
8. Baumes,: Compte Rendu des Travaux de la Societe de Medecine de Lyons. 19:18, 1836–1838.
9. Avery, Cited by Mackenzie,: *The Use of the Laryngoscope in Diseases of the Throat*. p. 25, 1844.
10. Garcia, M.: Observations on the Human Voice. *Proceedings of the Royal Society of London*, 7:397–410, 1855.
11. Wright, J.: The Laryngoscope: Manuel Garcia. In: *A History of Laryngology and Rhinology* (2nd ed.). Lea & Febiger, Philadelphia, p. 207, 1914.
12. Turck, L.: On the Laryngeal Mirror and Its Mode of Employment, With Engravings on Wood. *Zeitschrift der Gesellschaft der Aerzte ze Wein*, 26:401–409, 1858.
13. Czermak, J.: Uber den Kehlkopfspiegel. *Wiener Med. Wocjenschrift*, 8:196–198, 1858.
14. Czermak, J.N.: On the Laryngoscope and Its Employment in Physiology and Medicine. *New Sydenham Society*, 11:1–79, 1861.
15. Turck, L.: *Atlas zur Klinik der Kehlkopfkrankheiten*. Wilhelm Braumuller, Wein, 1860.
16. Stoerk, C.: On the Value of the Laryngo-pharyngeal Mirror. *Zeitschrift der Gesellschaft der Aerzte zu Wein*, 51:797–800, 1858.
17. Mackenzie, M.: *Growths in the Larynx*. J. & A. Churchill, London, 1871.
18. Stoerk, C.: On the Laryngoscope. *Zeitschrift der Gesellschaft der Aerzte ze Wein*, 46:721–727, 1859.
19. Mackenzie, M.: *The Use of the Laryngoscope in Diseases of the Throat with an Appendix on Rhinoscopy*. J. & A. Churchill, London, 1865.
20. Mackenzie, M.: The Laryngoscope and Its Accessory Apparatus; Laryngoscopy; Autolaryngoscopy; Infra-glottic Laryngoscopy; The Laryngoscope Image; Laryngeal Instruments; Dilators of the Larynx. In: *Diseases of the Pharynx, Larynx, and Trachea*. William Wood & Co., New York, pp. 158–195, 1880.
21. Boas, E.: The First Use of the Laryngoscope in the United States. *Journal of the History of Medicine*, 5:452–454, 1950.
22. Elsberg, L.: President's Address: Laryngology in America. *Transactions of the American Laryngological Association*, 1:30–90, 1879.
23. Krackowizer, E.: Church on the Laryngoscope. *New York Academy of Medicine*, 162, 1861.
24. Elsberg, L.: *Laryngoscopal Medication or the Local Treatment of the Diseases of the Throat, Larynx, and Neighboring Organs, Under Sight*. William Wood & Co., New York, 1864.
25. Elsberg, L.: *Laryngoscopal Surgery Illustrated in the Treatment of Morbid Growths Within the Larynx*. Collins, Philadelphia, 1866.
26. Solis-Cohen, J.: Removal of a Fibrous Polyp From the Inferior Surface of the Right Vocal Fold With the Aid of the Laryngoscope. *American Journal of Medical Science*, 404–407, 1867.
27. Elsberg, L.: President's Address: Laryngological Instruction. *Transactions of the American Laryngological Association*, 2:4–8, 1880.
28. Solis-Cohen, J.: *Diseases of the Throat: A Guide to the Diagnosis and Treatment*. William Wood, New York, 1872.
29. Solis-Cohen, J.: President's Address. *Transactions of the American Laryngological Association*, 3:2–4, 1881.
30. Wright, J.: The First Intralaryngeal Operation. In: *A History of Laryngology and Rhinology* (2nd ed.). Lea & Febiger, Philadelphia, p. 214, 1914.
31. Green, H.: Morbid Growths Within the Larynx. In: *On the Surgical Treatment of Polypi of the Larynx, and Oedema of the Glottis*. G.P. Putnam, New York, pp. 56–65, 1852.
32. Kirstein, A.: Autoskopie des Larynx und der Trachea (Laryngoscopia directa, Euthyskopie, Besichtigung ohne Spiegel). *Archiv fur Laryngologie und Rhinologie*, 3:156–164, 1895.
33. Green, H.: On the Subject of the Priority in the Medication of the Larynx and Trachea. *American Medical Monthly*, 1: 241–257, 1854.
34. Green, H.: Report on the Use and Effect of Applications of Nitrate Silver to the Throat, Either in Local or General Disease. *Transactions of the American Medical Association*, 9:493–530, 1856.
35. Brunings, W.: Direct Laryngoscopy: Criteria Determining the Applicability of Autoscopy. In: *Direct Laryngoscopy, Bronchoscopy, and Esophagoscopy*. Bailliere, Tindall, & Cox, London, pp. 93–95, 1912.
36. Clerf, L.H.: Manuel Garcia's Contribution to Laryngology. *Bulletin of the New York Academy of Medicine*, 32:603–611, 1956.

37. Donaldson, F.: The Laryngology of Trousseau and Horace Green. *Transactions of the American Laryngological Association*, 12:10–18, 1890.
38. Lewin, G.: Allgemeine Medicinische Central-Zeitung. 30: 654, 1861.
39. Sands, H.B.: Case of Cancer of the Larynx, Successfully Removed by Laryngotomy; With an Analysis of 50 Cases of Tumors of the Larynx, Treated by Operation. *New York Medical Journal*, 110–126, 1865.
40. Mackenzie, M.: *The Fatal Illness of Frederick the Noble.* Sampson, Low, Marston, Searle and Rivington Ltd., London, 1888.
41. Chalat, N.I.: Sir Morell Mackenzie Revisited. LARYNGOSCOPE. 94:1307–1310, 1984.
42. Delavan, D.B.: A Consideration of the Statistics of the Operations for the Relief of Malignant Disease of the Larynx. *Transactions of the American Laryngological Association*, 22:66–74, 1900.
43. Delavan, D.B.: A History of Thyrotomy and Laryngectomy. Transactions of a Commemorative Meeting in the Honour of Dr. John Edmund Mackenty Held by the Section of Otolaryngology: The New York Academy of Medicine, 1932.
44. Lin, J.I.: Virchow's Pathological Reports on Frederick III's Cancer. *N Engl J Med*, 311:1261–1264, 1984.
45. Solis-Cohen, J. Cited by Wright,: *A History of Laryngology and Rhinology.* p. 330, 1881.
46. Browne, L.: *The Throat and Its Diseases.* Lea and Febiger, Philadelphia, 1878.
47. Semon, F.: In Reference to Transition of Benign Laryngeal Tumors to Malignant Lesions Post Laryngeal Surgery: bezuglich des Ueberganges gutartiger Kehlkopfgeschwulste i bosartige nach intralaryngealen Operatienen. *Internationales Centralblatt fur Laryngologie, Rhinologie, Jahrgang IV*, No. 7:245–246, 1888.
48. Semon, F.: Die Frage de ueberganges gutatiger Kehlkopf-Geschwulster in bosartige, speciell nach intralaryngealen Operation. *Internationales Centralblatt fur Laryngologie, Rhinologie, Jahrgang, IV*, No. 6:271–279, 1889.
49. Butlin, H.T.: *Malignant Disease (Sarcoma and Carcinoma) of the Larynx.* J. & A. Churchill, London, 1883.
50. Fraenkel, B.: The Anatomo Pathologic Diagnosis of Cancer of the Larynx. *Ann Otol Rhinol Laryngol*, 9:276, 1900.
51. Chiari, O.: Contributions to the Diagnosis and Treatment of Laryngeal Cancer. *Ann Otol Rhinol Laryngol*, 7:572–580, 1898.
52. Solis-Cohen, J.: The Surgical Treatment of Laryngeal Cancer. *Transactions of the American Laryngological Association*, 22:75–87, 1900.
53. Mackenzie, J.: A Plea For Early Naked-Eye Diagnosis and Removal of the Entire Organ, With the Neighboring Area of Possible Lymphatic Infection in Cancer of the Larynx. *Transactions of the American Laryngological Association*, 22:56–65, 1900.
54. Mackenzie, J.: Remarks of the Macroscopic Diagnosis and General Indications for Treatment of Cancer of the Larynx. *Ann Otol Rhinol Laryngol*, 15:61–72, 1906.
55. Delevan, D.B.: Recent Advances in the Treatment of Malignant Disease of the Larynx. *Transactions of the American Laryngological Association*, 26:150–170, 1904.
56. Moore, I.: Diagnosis of Intrinsic Cancer of the Larynx. In: *Intrinsic Cancer of the Larynx and the Operation of Laryngofissure.* University of London Press, London, pp. 13–17, 1921.
57. Mackenty, J.: Laryngectomy for Cancer, With Remarks on Seventy Operated Cases. *Transactions of the American Laryngological Association*, 44:205–223, 1922.
58. Jackson, C.: Primary Malignant Disease of the Larynx. LARYNGOSCOPE, 14:590–618, 1904.
59. Jackson, C.: Taking of a Laryngeal Specimen for Diagnosis. In: *Peroral Endoscopy and Laryngeal Surgery.* Laryngoscope Co., St. Louis, pp. 107–110, 1915.
60. Jackson, C. and Jackson, C.L.: A History of the Laryngeal Biopsy. In: *Cancer of the Larynx.* W.B. Saunders, Philadelphia, pp. 231–240, 1939.
61. Jackson, C. and Jackson, C.L.: A History of the Laryngeal Biopsy. In: *Cancer of the Larynx.* W.B. Saunders, Philadelphia, pp. 237, 1939.
62. Fraenkel, B.: First Healing of a Laryngeal Cancer Taken Out Through the Natural Passages. *Archiv fur Klinische Chirurgie*, 12:283–286, 1886.
63. Arslan, A.: Emorragia Laringes. *Archivo Italiano*, 11:390–411, 1901.
64. Ingals, E.F.: Nonrecurrent Carcinoma of the Larynx Removed From the Natural Passages. LARYNGOSCOPE, 17: 370–372, 1907.
65. Sendziac, J.: Treatment of Cancer of the Larynx. *New York Medical Journal*, 86:1042, 1907.
66. Finder: Comments from; The diagnosis and treatment of carcinoma of the larynx. *J Laryngol Otol*, 25:602, 1910.
67. Thompson, S.C.: Intrinsic Cancer of the Larynx-Complete Excision Apparently Effected by the Endo-laryngeal Operation. *Transactions of the American Laryngological Association*, 36:34–44, 1914.
68. Freudenthal, W.: Bernhard Fraenkel—What He Has Done for Rhino-Laryngology. *Ann Otol Rhinol Laryngol*, 15:606–630, 1906.
69. Lynch, R.C.: Suspension Laryngoscopy and Its Accomplishments. *Ann Otol Rhinol Laryngol*, 24:429–446, 1915.
70. Lynch, R.C.: A Resume of My Years Work With Suspension Laryngoscopy. *Transactions of the American Laryngological Association*, 38:158–175, 1916.
71. Lynch, R.C.: Intrinsic Carcinoma of the Larynx, With a Second Report of the Cases Operated on by Suspension and Dissection. *Transactions of the American Laryngological Association*, 40:119–126, 1920.
72. New, G.B. and Dorton, H.E.: Suspension Laryngoscopy in the Treatment of Malignant Disease of the Hypopharynx and Larynx. *Mayo Clin Proc*, 16:411–416, 1941.
73. LeJeune, F.E.: Intralaryngeal Operation for Cancer of the Vocal Cord. *Ann Otol Rhinol Laryngol*, 55:531–536, 1946.
74. Lillie, J.C. and DeSanto, L.W.: Transoral Surgery of Early Cordal Carcinoma. *Transactions of the American Academy of Ophthalmology & Otolaryngology*, 77:92–96, 1973.
75. Jako, G.J.: Laser Surgery of the Vocal Cords. LARYNGOSCOPE, 82:2204–2216, 1972.
76. Strong, M.S. and Jako, G.J.: Laser Surgery of the Larynx: Early Clinical Experience With Continuous CO_2 Laser. *Ann Otol Rhinol Laryngol*, 81:791–798, 1972.
77. Strong, M.S.: Laser Excision of Carcinoma of the Larynx. LARYNGOSCOPE, 85:1286–1289, 1975.
78. Vaughan, C.W.: Transoral Laryngeal Surgery Using the CO_2 Laser. Laboratory Experiments and Clinical Experience. LARYNGOSCOPE, 88:1399–1420, 1978.
79. Blakeslee, D., Vaughan, C.W., Shapshay, S.M., *et al.*: Excisional Biopsy in the Selective Management of T1 Glottic Cancer: A Three-Year Follow-up Study. LARYNGOSCOPE, 94:488–494, 1984.
80. Ossoff, R.H., Sisson, G.A. and Shapshay, S.M.: Endoscopic Management of Selected Early Vocal Cord Carcinoma. *Ann Otol Rhinol Laryngol*, 94:560–564, 1985.
81. Koufman, J.A.: The Endoscopic Management of Early Squamous Carcinoma of the Vocal Cord With the Carbon Dioxide Surgical Laser: Clinical Experience and a Proposed Subclassification. *Otolaryngol Head Neck Surg*, 95:531–537, 1986.
82. Shapshay, S.M., Hybels, R.L. and Bohegian, R.K.: Laser Excision of Early Vocal Cord Carcinoma: Indications, Limitations, and Precautions. *Ann Otol Rhinol Laryngol*, 99: 46–50, 1990.
83. Kirstein, A.: *Autoscopy of the Larynx and Trachea (Direct Examination Without Mirror).* F.A. Davis Co., Philadelphia, 1897.
84. Vaughan, C.W.: Vocal Fold Exposure in Phonosurgery. *J Voice*, 7:189–194, 1993.
85. Jackson, C.: Position of the Patient for Peroral Endoscopy. In: *Peroral Endoscopy and Laryngeal Surgery.* Laryngoscope Co., St. Louis, pp. 77–88, 1915.
86. Boyce, J.W.: Duties of the Second Assistant in Endoscopy Per OS. In: *Tracheobronchoscopy, Esophagoscopy and Gas-*

troscopy. C. Jackson (Ed.). The Laryngoscope Co., St. Louis, pp. 145–147, 1907.
87. Hill, W.: Chevalier Jackson on Per-oral Endoscopy and Laryngeal Surgery. *J Laryngol Rhinol Otol*, 31:164–175, 1916. Book review.
88. Jackson, C. and Jackson, C.L.: Endoscopic Removal of Cancer of the Epiglottis. In: *Cancer of the Larynx*. W.B. Saunders, Philadelphia, p. 52, 1939.
89. Killian, G.: Die Schwebelaryngoscopie. *Archiv fur Laryngologie und Rhinologie*, 26:277–317, 1912.
90. Killian, G.: Suspension Laryngoscopy and Its Practical Use. *J Laryngol Otol*, 24:337–360, 1914.
91. Killian, G.: Suspension Laryngoscopy. In: *Peroral Endoscopy and Laryngeal Surgery*. C. Jackson (Ed.). Laryngoscope Co., St. Louis, pp. 133–154, 1915.
92. Killian, G.: *Die Schwebelaryngoscopie und ihre praktische*. Verwertung, Urban & Schwarzenberg, Wein, 1920.
93. Brunings, W.: Direct Laryngoscopy: Autoscopy by Counterpressure. In: *Direct Laryngoscopy, Bronchoscopy, and Esophagoscopy*. Bailliere, Tindall, & Cox, London, pp. 110–115, 1912.
94. Jackson, C., Jackson, C.L.: *Cancer of the Larynx*. W.B. Saunders, Philadelphia, 1939.
95. Jackson, C. and Jackson, C.L.: *The Larynx and Its Diseases*. W.B. Saunders, Philadelphia, 1937.
96. LeJeune, F.E.: Suspension Laryngoscopy. In: *Diseases of the Nose, Throat and Ear*. C. Jackson and C.L. Jackson (Eds.) W.B. Saunders, Philadelphia, pp. 178–180, 1945.
97. Scalco, A.N., Shipman, W.F. and Tabb, H.G.: Microscopic Suspension Laryngoscopy. *Ann Otol Rhinol Laryngol*, 69: 1134–1138, 1960.
98. Roberts, S.E. and Forman, F.S.: Direct Laryngoscopy—A Simplified Technique With Screw Driven Fulcrum Lift. LARYNGOSCOPE, 57:245–256, 1948.
99. Roberts, S.E.: A Self Retaining Dual Distal Lighted Laryngoscope With Screw Driven Fulcrum Lift. LARYNGOSCOPE, 62:215–221, 1952.
100. King, N.E.: Direct Laryngoscopy Aided by a New Laryngoscope "Stabilizer." *Arch Otolaryngol*, 53:89–92, 1951.
101. Sommers, K.E.: Direct Laryngoscopy and Description of a Self-Retaining Attachment for the Laryngoscope. *Arch Otolaryngol*, 55:484–488, 1952.
102. Lewy, R.B.: Suspension Fixation Gear Power Laryngoscopy (With Motion Pictures). LARYNGOSCOPE, 64:693–695, 1954.
103. Netter, F. and H.: Osteoporosis. In: *The Ciba Collection of Medical Illustrations: Musculoskeletal System*. Ciba-Geigy Co., Summit, pp. 216–227, 1987.
104. Priest, R.E.: Controversial Aspects of the Treatment of Laryngeal Keratosis. LARYNGOSCOPE, 68:766–779, 1958.
105. Thomas, G.K.: Suspension Apparatus for Laryngeal Microsurgery. *Arch Otolaryngol*, 94:258–259, 1971.
106. Grundfast, K.M., Vaughan, C.W., Strong, M.S., *et al.*: Suspension Microlaryngoscopy in the Boyce Position With a New Suspension Gallows. *Ann Otol Rhinol Laryngol*, 87: 560–566, 1978.
107. Jackson, C.: Instruments. In: *Tracheo-Bronchoscopy, Esophagoscopy and Gastroscopy*. The Laryngoscope Co., St. Louis, pp. 15–34, 1907.
108. Killian, G.: Demonstration of an Endoscopic Spatula. *Journal of Laryngology and Rhinology*, 25:549–550, 1910.
109. Israel, S.: The Directoscope of Haslinger (Vienna) in the Diagnosis and Surgery of the Larynx. LARYNGOSCOPE, 33: 945–948, 1923.
110. Jackson, C., Tucker, G. and Clerf, L.H.: Laryngostasis and the Laryngostat. *Arch Otolaryngol*, 1:167–169, 1925.
111. Albrecht, R.: Uber den Wert koloskopischer Untersuchungsmethoden bei Leukoplakien und Carcinomen des Mundes und Kehlkopes. *Arch fur Ohren Nasen und Kehlkopfheilkunde*, 165:459–463, 1954.
112. Jako, G.J.: Laryngoscope for Microscopic Observation, Surgery, and Photography. *Arch Otolaryngol*, 91:196–199, 1970.
113. Jako, G.J.: Laryngeal Endoscopy and Microlaryngoscopy. In: *Otolaryngology*. M. Paparella and D. Shumrick (Eds.). W.B. Saunders, Philadelphia, pp. 2410–2430, 1980.
114. Kleinsasser, O.: Die Laryngomicroscope (Lupenlaryngoskopie) und ihre Bedeutung fur die Erkennung der Vorerkrankungen und Fruhformen des Stimmlipencarcinomas. *Arch fur Ohren Nasen und Kehlkopfheilkunde*, 724–727, 1962.
115. Kleinsasser, O.: Weitere technische Entwicklung und erste Ergebnisse der endolaryngealen Mikrochirurgie. *Z Laryng Rhinol*, 711–727, 1965.
116. Kleinsasser, O.: Development of Microlaryngoscopy and Endolaryngeal Microsurgery. In: *Microlaryngoscopy and Endolaryngeal Microsurgery*. University Park Press, Baltimore, p. 3, 1978.
117. DeSanto, L.W. and Carney, F.W.: Microlaryngoscopic Surgery. *Arch Otolaryngol*, 91:324–326, 1970.
118. Strong, M.S.: Microscopic Laryngoscopy. A Review and Appraisal. LARYNGOSCOPE, 80:1540–1552, 1970.
119. Shapshay, S.M. and Healy, G.B.: New Microlaryngeal Instruments for Phonatory Surgery and Pediatric Applications. *Ann Otol Rhinol Laryngol* 98:821–823, 1990.
120. Castro, J.: Tobacco Road's Dirty Ashtrays. *Time*, 17:52, 1989.
121. MacMahon, B., *et al.*: National Cancer Institute. Health Implications of Smokeless Tobacco Use. *Public Health Rep*, 101:349–354, 1986.
122. Jackson, C.: Malignant Neoplasms of the Larynx. In: *Peroral Endoscopy and Laryngeal Surgery*. Laryngoscope Co., St. Louis, pp. 637, 1915.
123. Pierce, N.H.: Leukoplakia Laryngis. *Ann Otol Rhinol Laryngol*, 29:33–56, 1920.
124. Jackson, C.: Cancer of the Larynx: Is It Preceded by a Recognizable Precancerous Condition. *Transactions of the American Laryngological Association*, 44:182–201, 1922.
125. Jackson, C., Thompson, S., Colledge, L., *et al.*: Discussion on Precancerous Conditions of the Larynx. *Proc R Soc Med*, 24:301–308, 1930.
126. Broders, A.C.: Carcinoma In Situ Contrasted With Benign Penetrating Epithelium. *JAMA*, 99:1670–1674, 1932.
127. Clerf, L.H.: Keratosis of the Larynx. *JAMA*, 132:823–826, 1946.
128. Graham, H.B.: Keratosis of the Larynx. *Arch Otolaryngol*, 36:735–739, 1942.
129. Loré, J.M.: Stripping of the Vocal Cords. LARYNGOSCOPE, 44: 803–816, 1934.
130. Lore, L.M.: Stripping of the Vocal Cords. *Arch Otolaryngol*, 42:378–383, 1945.
131. Putney, F.J. and O'Keefe, J.J.: The Clinical Significance of Keratosis of the Larynx as a Premalignant Lesion. *Arch Otolaryngol*, 62:348–357, 1953.
132. Bishop, J.: Experimental Researches Into the Physiology of the Human Voice. *The London & Edinburgh Philosophical Magazine & Journal of Science*, 1836.
133. Fournie, E.: *Physiologie de la voix et de la parole*. Adrien Delahaye, Paris, 1866.
134. Durant, G.: In: *Hygiene of the Voice: Its Physiology and Anatomy*. G. Shirmer, New York, pp. 22, 1870.
135. Fournie, E.: Proceedings of the International Congress of Laryngology. *Arch Laryngol*, 99:378, 1880.
136. Hirano, M.: Phonosurgery: Basic and Clinical Investigations. *Otologia (Fukuoka)*, 21:239–442, 1975.
137. Hirano, M.: Structure of the Vocal Fold in Normal and Diseased States: Anatomical and Physical Studies. In: *Proceedings of the Conference on the Assessment of Vocal Pathology*. The American Speech-Language-Hearing Association. pp. 11–27, 1981.
138. Hirano, M.: Phonosurgical Anatomy of the Larynx. In: *Phonosurgery*. (Chap. 3). C. Ford and D. Bless (Eds.). Raven, New York, pp. 25–41, 1991.
139. Isshiki, N.: Vibration of the Vocal Folds. In: *Phonosurgery: Theory and Practice*. Springer-Verlag, Tokyo, pp. 7–11, 1989.
140. Oertel, M.: Das laryngo-stroboskop und die Laryngo-Stoboskpische Untersuchung. *Archiv fur Laryngologie und Rhinologie*, 3:1–16, 1895.
141. Von Leden, H.: The Electronic Synchron-Stroboscope: Its Value for the Practicing Laryngologist. *Ann Otol Rhinol*

Laryngol, 70:881–893, 1961.
142. Alberti, P.W.: The Diagnostic Role of Laryngeal Stroboscopy. *Otolaryngol Clin North Am*, 11:3457–354, 1978.
143. Powell, L.S.: The Laryngostroboscope. *Arch Otolaryngol*, 19: 708–710, 1934.
144. Kallen, L.A.: Laryngostroboscopy in the Practice of Otolaryngology. *Arch Otolaryngol*, 16:791–807, 1932.
145. Timcke, R., Von Leden, H. and Moore, P.: Laryngeal Vibrations: Measurement of the Glottic Wave: Part 1. Normal Vibratory Cycle. *Arch Otolaryngol*, 68:1–19, 1958.
146. Timcke, R., Von Leden, H. and Moore, P.: Laryngeal Vibrations: Measurements of the Glottic Wave: Part II. Physiologic Variations. *Arch Otolaryngol*, 69:438–444, 1959.
147. Von Leden, H., Moore, P. and Timcke, R.: Laryngeal Vibrations: Measurements of the Glottic Wave: Part III. The Pathological Larynx. *Arch Otolaryngol*, 71:16–35, 1960.
148. Morrison, M.D.: A Clinical Voice Laboratory, Videotape and Stroboscopic Instrumentation. *Otolaryngol Head Neck Surg*, 92:487–488, 1984.
149. Hajek, M.: Anatomische Untersuchungen uber das Larynxodem. *Archiv fur Kllinsche Chirurgie*, 42:46–93, 1891.
150. Reinke, F.: Uber die Funktionelle Struktur der Menschlichen Stimmlippe mit Besonderer Berucksichtigung des Elastischen Gewebes. (About the Functional Structure of the Human Vocal Cord With Special Reference to the Elastic Tissue). *Anatomische Hefte*, 9:103–117, 1897.
151. Pressman, J., Dowdy, A., Libby, R., *et al.*: Further Studies Upon the Submucosal Lymphatics of the Larynx by Injection of Dyes and Isotopes. *Ann Otol Rhinol Laryngol*, 65: 963–980, 1956.
152. Pressman, J.J., Bertz, M.B. and Monell, C.: Anatomic Studies Related to the Dissemination of Cancer of the Larynx. *Transactions of the American Academy of Ophthalmology & Otolaryngology*, 64:628–638, 1960.
153. Zeitels, S.M.: Microflap Excisional Biopsy for Atypia and Microinvasive Glottic Cancer. In: *Operative Techniques in Otolaryngology—Head & Neck Surgery (Phonosurgery Edition)*, 218–222, 1993.
154. Holinger, L.D. and Miller, A.W. III: A Specimen Mount for Small Laryngeal Biopsies. LARYNGOSCOPE, 92:524–526, 1982.
155. Lundgren, J. and Olofsson, J.: Malignant Tumours in Patients With Non-Invasive Squamous Cell Lesions of the Vocal Cords. *Clin Otolaryngol* 12:39–43, 1987.
156. Slaughter, D.P., Southwick, H.W. and Smejkal, W.: "Field Cancerization" in Oral Stratified Squamous Epithelium: Clinical Implications of Multicentric Origin. *Cancer*, 6: 963–968, 1953.
157. Batsakis, J.G.: "Leukoplakia," "Keratosis" and Intraepithelial Squamous Cell Carcinoma of the Head and Neck. In: *Tumors of the Head and Neck. Clinical and Pathological Considerations.* (Chap. 4). Williams & Wilkins, Baltimore, pp. 121–129, 1982.
158. Strong, M.S., Vaughan, C.W. and Incze, J.I.: Toluidine Blue in Diagnosis of Cancer of the Larynx. *Arch Otolaryngol* 91: 515–519, 1970.
159. Altmann, F., Ginsbery, I. and Stout, A.P.: Intraepithelial Carcinoma (Cancer In Situ) of the Larynx. *Arch Otolaryngol*, 56:121–133, 1952.
160. Myers, E.N., Wagner, R.L. and Johnson, J.T.: Microlaryngoscopic Surgery for T1 Glottic Lesions: A Cost-effective Option. Presented at the American Laryngological Association, 1993.
161. Ryan, R.F., McDonald, J.R. and Devine, K.D.: The Pathological Effects of Smoking on the Larynx. *Arch Pathol*, 60: 472–480, 1955.
162. Proetz, A.W.: Some Preliminary Experiments in the Study of Cigarette Smoke and Its Effect Upon the Respiratory Tract. *Ann Otol Rhinol Laryngol*, 48:176–194, 1939.
163. Auerbach, O., Hammond, E.C. and Garfinkel, L.: Histological Changes in the Larynx in Relation to Smoking Habits. *Cancer*, 25:92–104, 1970.
164. Ranke, E., Presley, S. and Holinger, P.H.: Tracheogenic Carcinoma. *JAMA* 182:519, 1962.
165. Kytta, J., Pulkkinen, K. and Koskiinen, O: Endoscopic Aspects of Bronchogenic Carcinoma. *Ann Chir Gynaecol Fenn*, 51:361, 1962.
166. Marsh, B., Frost, J.K., Erozan, Y.S., *et al.*: Flexible Fiberoptic Bronchoscopy: Its Place in the Search for Lung Cancer. *Ann Otol Rhinol Laryngol*, 82:757–764, 1973.
167. Ryland, A.: The Laryngeal Changes Induced by Mustard Gas. *J Laryngol Rhinol Otol*, 34:153–156, 1919.
168. Norris, C.M. and Peale, A.R.: Keratosis of the Larynx. *J Laryngol Otol*, 77:635–647, 1963.
169. Cracovaner, A.J.: Hyperkeratosis of the Larynx. *Arch Otolaryngol*, 63:287–291, 1959.
170. McGravran, M.H., Bauer, W.C. and Ogura, J.H.: Isolated Laryngeal Keratosis. Its Relation to Carcinoma of the Larynx Based Upon a Clinicopathologic Study of 87 Consecutive Cases With Long-term Follow-up. LARYNGOSCOPE 70: 932–951, 1960.
171. Kambic, V.: Difficulties in Management of Vocal Cord Precancerous Lesions. *J Laryngol Otol*, 92:305–315, 1978.
172. Henry, R.C.: The Transformation of Laryngeal Leukoplakia to Cancer. *J Laryngol Otol*, 93:447–459, 1979.
173. Crissman, J.D.: Laryngeal Keratosis and Subsequent Carcinoma. *Head Neck Surg*, 1:386–391, 1979.
174. Hellquist, H., Lundgren, J. and Olofsson, J.: Hyperplasia, Keratosis, Dysplasia and Carcinoma In Situ of the Vocal Cords—A Follow-up Study. *Clin Otolaryngol*, 7:11–27, 1982.
175. Goodman, M.L.: Keratosis (Leukoplakia) of the Larynx. *Otolaryngol Clin North Am*, 17:179–183, 1984.
176. Gabriel, C.E. and Jones, D.G.: Hyperkeratosis of the Larynx. *J Laryngol Otol*, 87:129–134, 1973.
177. Velasco, J.R., Nieto, C.S. and Bustos, C.P.: Premalignant Lesions of the Larynx; Pathological Prognostic Factors. *J Otolaryngol*, 16:367–370, 1987.
178. Hojslet, P.E., Nielson, V.M. and Palvio, D.: Premalignant Lesions of the Larynx. *Acta Otolaryngol (Stockh)*, 107:150–155, 1989.
179. Bouquot, J.E. and Gnepp, D.R.: Laryngeal Precancer: A Review of the Literature, Commentary, and Comparison With Oral Leukoplakia. *Head Neck Surg*, 13:488–497, 1991.
180. Bauer, W.C.: Concomitant In Situ and Invasive Carcinoma of the Larynx. In: *Workshops From the Centennial Conference on Laryngeal Cancer.* P.W. Alberti and D.B. Bryce (Eds.). Appleton-Century-Crofts, New York, pp. 122–134, 1976.
181. Friedman, I.: Precancerous Lesions of the Larynx. In: *Workshops From the Centennial Conference on Laryngeal Cancer.* P.W. Alberti and D.B. Bryce (Eds.). Appleton-Century-Crofts, New York, pp. 122–126, 1976.
182. DeSanto, L.W.: Selection of Treatment for In Situ and Early Invasive Carcinoma of the Glottis. In: *Workshops From the Centennial Conference on Laryngeal Cancer.* P.W. Alberti and D.B. Bryce (Eds.). Appleton-Century-Crofts, New York, pp. 146–150, 1976.
183. Miller, A.H. and Batsakis, J.C.: Premalignant Laryngeal Lesions, Carcinoma In Situ, Superficial Carcinoma—Definition and Management. In: *Workshops From the Centennial Conference on Laryngeal Cancer.* P.W. Alberti and D.B. Bryce (Eds.). Appleton-Century-Crofts, New York, p. 109, 1976.
184. Putney, F.J. and O'Keefe, J.J.: The Clinical Significance of Keratosis of the Larynx as a Premalignant Lesion. 62: 348–357, 1953.
185. Som, M.L.: Surgery in Premalignant Lesions. In: *Workshops From the Centennial Conference on Laryngeal Cancer.* P.W. Alberti and D.B. Bryce (Eds.). Appleton-Century-Crofts, New York, p. 145, 1976.
186. Gillis, T.M., Incze, J., Strong, M.S., *et al.*: Natural History of Keratosis, Atypia, Carcinoma In Situ, and Microinvasive Cancer of the Larynx. *Am J Surg*, 146:512–520, 1983.
187. Stutsman, A.C. and McGavran, M.H.: Ultraconservative Management of Superficially Invasive Epidermoid Carcinoma of the Vocal Cord. *Ann Otol Rhinol Laryngol*, 80:

507–512, 1971.
188. Norris, C.M. and Peale, A.R.: "Untreated" Carcinoma of the Larynx. *Ann Otol Rhinol Laryngol,* 77:468–475, 1968.
189. Moore, C.: Cigarette Smoking and Cancer of the Mouth, Pharynx and Larynx. *JAMA,* 218:553–558, 1971.
190. Bouquot, J.E., Weiland, L.H. and Kurland, L.T.: Laryngeal Keratosis—It's Relation to Carcinoma in the Rochester, Minnesota Population, 1935–1984. *Cancer Detect Prev,* 15: 83–91, 1991.
191. Weymuller, E.A.: A Surgical Protocol Designed to Improve Outcome Data in Head and Neck Cancer Trials. Presented at the American Laryngological Association, 1993.
192. Muller, K.M. and Krohn, B.R.: Smoking Habits and Their Relationship to Precancerous Lesions of the Larynx. *J Cancer Res Clin Oncol,* 96:211–217, 1980.
193. Wallner, L.J.: Smoker's Larynx. LARYNGOSCOPE, 64:259–270, 1954.
194. Kambic, V. and Gale, N.: Significance of Keratosis and Dyskeratosis for Classifying Hyperplastic Aberrations of Laryngeal Mucosa. *Am J Otolaryngol,* 7:323–333, 1986.
195. Lederman, M.: Keratosis of the Larynx. *J Laryngol Otol,* 77: 651–659, 1963.
196. Greven, K.M., Randall, M.E., McGuirt, W.F., *et al.*: Assessment of Prognostic Factors for Voice Quality in Patients Treated Definitively for Early Glottic Carcinoma. Presented at the Third International Conference on Head and Neck Cancer, 1992.
197. Padovan, I.F.: Premalignant Laryngeal Lesions—A Laryngologist's Viewpoint. In: *Workshops From the Centennial Conference on Laryngeal Cancer.* P.W. Alberti and D.B. Bryce, (Eds.). Appleton-Century-Crofts, New York, pp., 1976.
198. Hyams, V.H.: Premalignant Laryngeal Lesions, Carcinoma In Situ, Superficial Carcinoma—Definition and Management [Discussion]. In: *Workshops From the Centennial Conference on Laryngeal Cancer.* P.W. Alberti and D.B. Bryce (Eds.). Appleton-Century-Crofts, New York, pp. 134–135, 1976.
199. Strong, M.S.: Laser Management of Premalignant Lesions of the Larynx. In: *Workshops From the Centennial Conference on Laryngeal Cancer.* P.W. Alberti and D.B. Bryce (Eds.). Appleton-Century-Crofts, New York, pp. 154–157, 1976.
200. Strong, M.S.: Carcinoma In Situ of the Larynx [Discussion]. In: *Workshops From the Centennial Conference on Laryngeal Cancer.* P.W. Alberti and D.B. Bryce (Eds.). Appleton-Century-Crofts, New York, p. 165, 1976.
201. Vaughan, C.W., Strong, M.S. and Shapshay, S.M.: Treatment of T1 and In Situ Carcinoma: The Transoral Approach. *Otolaryngol Clin North Am,* 13:509–513, 1980.
202. Miller, A.H. and Fisher, H.R.: Clues to the Life History of Carcinoma In Situ of the Larynx. LARYNGOSCOPE, 81: 1475–1480, 1971.
203. Miller, A.H.: Carcinoma In Situ of the Larynx—Clinical Appearance and Treatment. In: *Workshops From the Centennial Conference on Laryngeal Cancer.* P.W. Alberti and D.B. Bryce (Eds.). Appleton-Century-Crofts, New York, 161–163, 1976.
204. Small, W., Jr., Mittal, B., Brand, W., *et al.*: Role of Radiation Therapy in the Management of Carcinoma In Situ of the Larynx. LARYNGOSCOPE, 103:663–667, 1993.
205. Hirano, M., Hirade, Y. and Kawasaki, H.: Vocal Function Following Carbon Dioxide Laser Surgery for Glottic Carcinoma. *Ann Otol Rhinol Laryngol,* 94:232–235, 1985.
206. Zeitels, S.M. and Vaughan, C.W.: A Submucosal Vocal Fold Infusion Needle. *Otolaryngol, Head Neck Surg,* 105:478–479, 1991.
207. Yates, A. and Dedo, H.H.: Carbon Dioxide Laser Enucleation of Polypoid Vocal Cords. LARYNGOSCOPE, 94:731–736, 1984.
208. Kashima, H.K., Lee, D.J. and Zinreich, S.J.: Vestibulectomy in Early Vocal Fold Carcinoma. *Transactions of the American Broncho-Esophagological Association,* 71:28–32, 1991.
209. Cragle, S.P. and Brandenburg, J.H.: Laser Cordectomy or Radiotherapy: Cure Rates, Communication, and Cost. *Otolaryngol Head Neck Surg,* 108:648–653, 1993.
210. Koufman, J.A. and Blalock, P.D.: Is Voice Rest Never Indicated. *J Voice,* 3:87–91, 1989.
211. Baken, R.: Intensity, Vocal Fundamental Frequency, Laryngeal Function. In: *Clinical Measurement of Speech and Voice.* Little Brown & Co., Boston, pp. 95–196, 1987.
212. Holmberg, E.B., Hillman, R.E., Perkell, J.S., *et al.*: Relationships Between Intraspeaker Variation in Aerodynamic Measures of Voice Production and Variation in SPL Across Repeated Recordings. *J Speech Hear Res* (In press.)
213. Holmberg, E.B., Hillman, R.E. and Perkell, J.S.: Glottal Airflow and Transglottal Air Pressure Measurements for Male and Female Speakers in Soft, Normal, and Loud Voice. *J Acoust Soc Am,* 84:511–529, 1988.
214. Hillman, R., Holmberg, E.B., Perkell, J.S., *et al.*: Objective Assessment of Vocal Hyperfunction: An Experimental Framework and Initial Results. *J Speech Hear Res,* 32: 373–392, 1989.
215. Hillman, R., Holmberg, E.B., Perkell, J.S., *et al.*: Phonatory Function Associated With Hyperfunctionality Related Vocal Fold Lesions. *J Voice,* 4:52–63, 1990.
216. Tucker, G.F.: In: *Human Larynx Coronal Section Atlas.* pp. 7–20, 1971.
217. Lehman, J.J., Bless, D.M. and Brandenburg, J.H.: An Objective Assessment of Voice Production After Radiation Therapy for Stage I Squamous Cell Carcinoma of the Glottis. *Otolaryngol Head Neck Surg,* 98:121–129, 1988.
218. Zhao, R., Hirano, M., Tanaka, S., *et al.*: Vocal Fold Hyperplasia. *Arch Otolaryngol Head Neck Surg,* 117:1015–1018, 1991.
219. McGuirt, W.F., Blalock, D., Koufman, J.A., *et al.*: Voice Analysis of Patients With Endoscopically Treated Early Laryngeal Carcinoma. *Ann Otol Rhinol Laryngol,* 101:142–146, 1992.
220. Ludlow, C.L., Bassich, C.J., Connor, N.P., *et al.*: The Validity of Using Phonatory Jitter and Shimmer to Detect Laryngeal Pathology. In: *Laryngeal Function in Phonation and Respiration.* T. Baer and C. Sasaki (Eds.). Little, Brown & Co., Boston, pp. 492–508, 1987.

Appendix 1.
Histopathological Assessment Scheme.

Grade	Layers	Mitosis	Keratin	Basement Membrane	Architecture
Normal	6–9	Confined to lower two cell layers	None	Not breached	Progressive maturation from elongated basal cells to flattened surface cells
Hyperplastic	> 9	Confined to lower two cell layers	None other than top layer	Not breached	Progressive maturation from elongated basal cells to flattened surface cells
Mild atypia	6 or more	In lower layers only	Rare single cell keratin in upper 3 layers	Not breached	Maturation disturbed by occasional abnormal nuclear to cytoplasm ratio and bizarre cells
Moderate atypia	6 or more	In lower 3 or 4 layers	Occasional single cells, down to one half thickness	Not breached	Maturation disturbed by occasional to frequent abnormal nuclear to cytoplasm ratio and bizarre cells
Severe atypia	6 or more	In all but top 2 layers, atypical	Occasional to frequent cells and clusters, down to 2 cell layers from bottom	Not breached	Marked maturation disturbed by frequent abnormal nuclear to cytoplasm ratio and bizarre cells
Squamous cell carcinoma in situ	6 or more	Up to and including top layer, atypical	Occasional to frequent cells and clusters, down to and including basement cell layers	Not breached	Full thickness disturbance of maturation including cells with abnormal nuclear to cytoplasm ratio and bizarre cells
Microinvasive carcinoma	6 or more	Up to and including top layer, atypical	Occasional to frequent cells and clusters, down to and including lowest epithelial cells	Breached, cells and clusters below membrane but not into ligament	May or may not have carcinoma in situ above the cells that break through the basement membrane; cells may or may not be atypical
Invasive squamous cell carcinoma into ligament	6 or more	Up to and including top layer, atypical	Occasional to frequent cells and clusters, down to and including lowest epithelial cells in ligament	Breached, cells and clusters into ligament	May or may not have carcinoma in situ above the cells that invade ligament; cells may or may not be atypical
Invasive carcinoma into muscle	6 or more	Up to and including top layer, atypical	Occasional to frequent cells and clusters, down to and including lowest epithelial cells in muscle	Breached, cells and clusters into muscle	May or may not have carcinoma in situ above the cells that invade muscle; cells may or may not be atypical

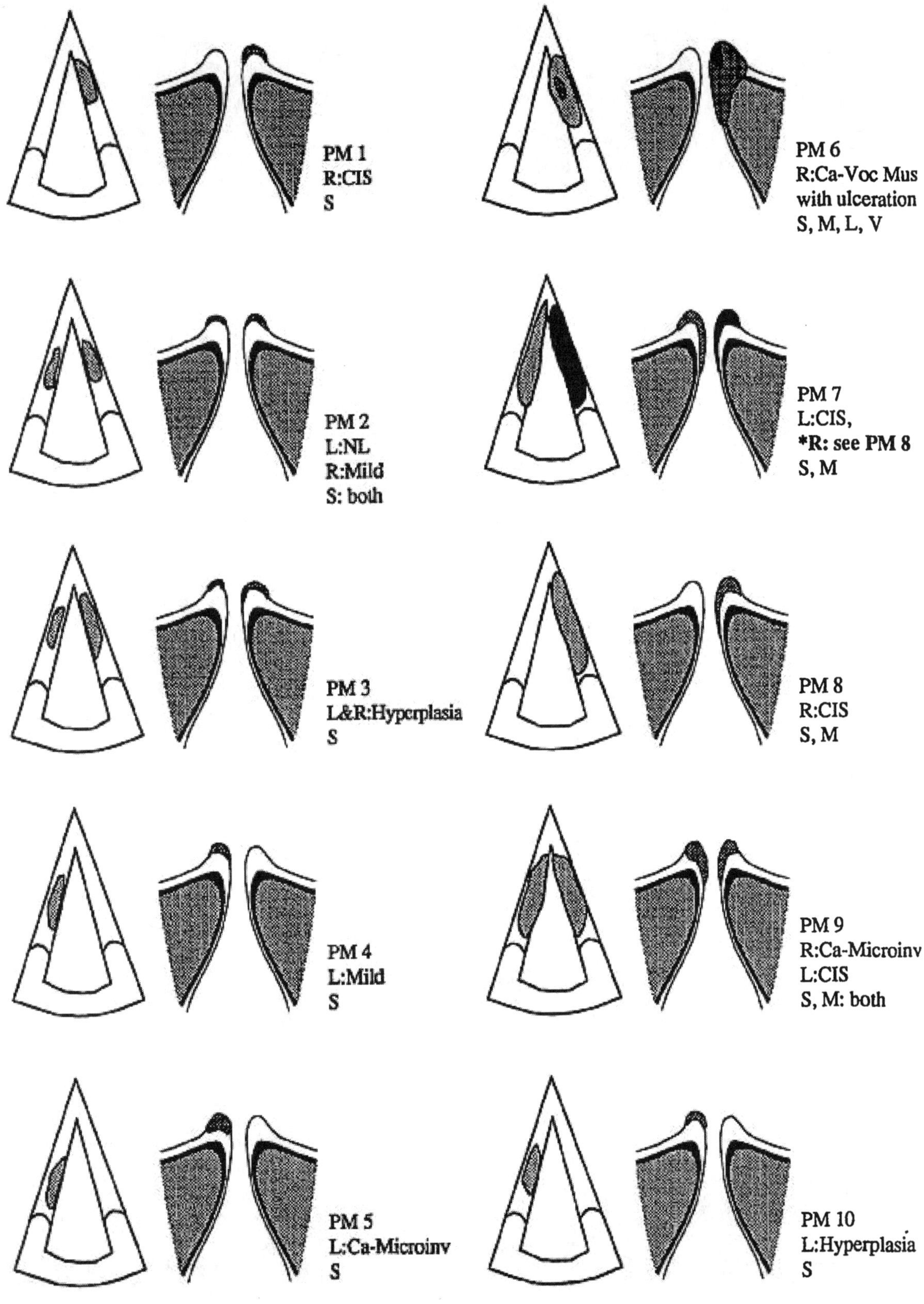
PM 1
R:CIS
S
PM 6
R:Ca-Voc Mus
with ulceration
S, M, L, V
PM 2
L:NL
R:Mild
S: both
PM 7
L:CIS,
*R: see PM 8
S, M
PM 3
L&R:Hyperplasia
S
PM 8
R:CIS
S, M
PM 4
L:Mild
S
PM 9
R:Ca-Microinv
L:CIS
S, M: both
PM 5
L:Ca-Microinv
S
PM 10
L:Hyperplasia
S

Appendix 2.

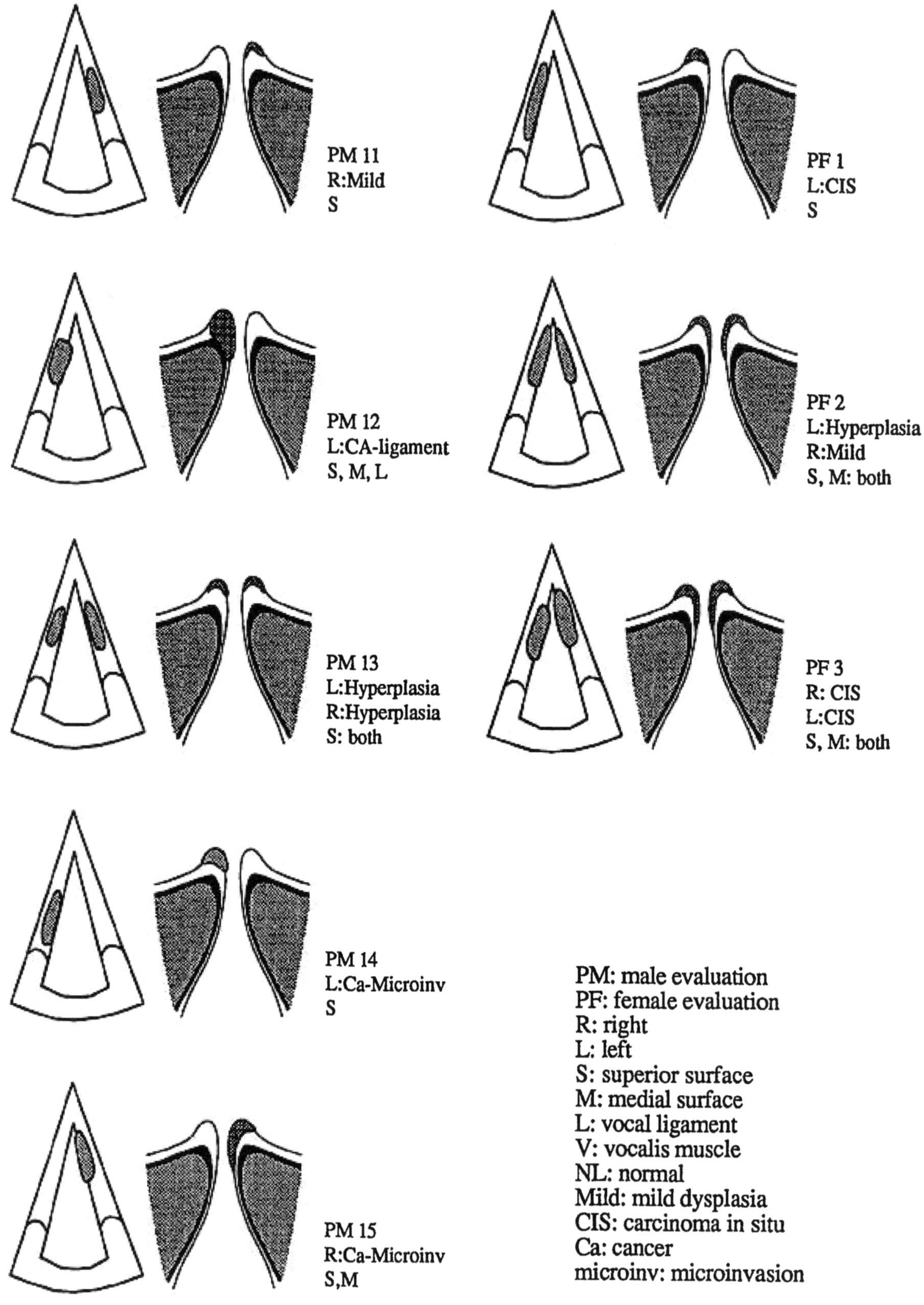
PM 11
R:Mild
S
PF 1
L:CIS
S
PM 12
L:CA-ligament
S, M, L
PF 2
L:Hyperplasia
R:Mild
S, M: both
PM 13
L:Hyperplasia
R:Hyperplasia
S: both
PF 3
R: CIS
L:CIS
S, M: both
PM 14
L:Ca-Microinv
S
PM 15
R:Ca-Microinv
S,M
PM: male evaluation
PF: female evaluation
R: right
L: left
S: superior surface
M: medial surface
L: vocal ligament
V: vocalis muscle
NL: normal
Mild: mild dysplasia
CIS: carcinoma in situ
Ca: cancer
microinv: microinvasion

Appendix 2.

Appendix 3.
Acoustic Data for Sustained Vowels.

Subject	Comfortable Phonation of /a/ F_0 (Hz)	% Jitter	% Shimmer	Spectral Noise s/n (dB)	EGG % Duty Cycle
PM1	111	0.8	0.7	13.2	60
PM2	108	1.4	0.5	4.1	Unanalyzed
PM3	116	0.3	0.2	21.9	47
PM4	104	0.4	0.4	17.7	48
PM5	125	0.5	0.4	18.7	54
PM6	120	3.0	0.6	9.0	Unanalyzed
PM7	93	0.9	0.6	10.5	62
PM8	99	1.7	0.7	13.4	62
PM9	123	0.7	0.3	16.6	53
PM10	109	0.6	0.3	18.2	55
PM11	133	0.6	0.4	21.4	57
PM12	148	0.7	0.2	21.7	47
PM13	109	0.4	0.6	16.7	54
PM14	94	0.6	0.5	15.5	64
PM15	167	0.5	0.2	19.9	Unanalyzed
PF1	205	1.1	0.8	12.4	Unanalyzed
PF2	175	1.3	0.7	9.9	63
PF3	244	1.2	0.3	16.8	Unanalyzed

Normal Values: F_0 (Hz): males, 95–135 Hz
females, 195–235 Hz

% jitter: ≤ 1%

% shimmer: ≤ 1%

Spectral noise (dB): ≥ 10.0 dB

EGG duty cycle (%): 55%–65%

F_0 = frequency; s/n = signal to noise; EGG = electroglottography; PM = male evaluation; PF = female evaluation.

Appendix 4.
Acoustic Data for Reading.

Subject	F_0 (Hz)	Intensity (dB)
PM1	107	73
PM2	108	63
PM3	100	71
PM4	104	64
PM5	122	69
PM6	119	65
PM7	98	69
PM8	98	68
PM9	123	73
PM10	107	73
PM11	99	73
PM12	135	80
PM13	118	72
PM14	122	71
PM15	150	75
PF1	194	68
PF2	163	72
PF3	234	69

Normal Values: F_0 (Hz): males, 95–135 Hz
females, 195–235 Hz

Intensity (dB): 65–75 dB

F_0 = frequency; PM = male evaluation; PF = female evaluation.

Appendix 5.
Acoustic Data for Maximum Range Tasks.

Subject	Maximum F_0 Range (Hz)	Maximum Intensity Range (dB SPL)
PM1	84–297	71–108
PM2	70–353	60–96
PM3	85–525	63–111
PM4	102–298	74–110
PM5	71–350	63–105
PM6	73–208	61–98
PM7	68–276	73–102
PM8	99–289	71–118
PM9	108–340	71–116
PM10	70–461	70–112
PM11	65–446	73–103
PM12	90–316	78–103
PM13	82–513	75–108
PM14	95–312	73–103
PM15	82–584	72–112
PF1	130–359	69–107
PF2	114–413	78–109
PF3	150–417	60–99

Normal Values:

Maximum F_0 range (Hz): > 2 octaves (doubling of $F_0 \times 2$)

Maximum intensity range (dB): > 40 dB

F_0 = frequency; PM = male evaluation; PF = female evaluation.

Appendix 6.
Aerodynamic Data for Comfortable Phonation.

Subject	SPL (dB)	Aerodynamic Data: Subglottal Pressure (cm H_2O)	Glottal Resistance (L/sec_2)	Airflow (L/sec)
PM1	79	7.2	19.05	0.38
PM2	80	10.2	85	0.12
PM3	83	9.9	55	0.18
PM4	80	8.9	177.4	0.05
PM5	82	7.7	28.0	0.27
PM6	60	15.5	97	0.16
PM7	79	8.7	18.13	0.48
PM8	74	8.4	20.79	0.40
PM9	76	7.7	21.4	0.36
PM10	82	13.7	152.22	0.09
PM11	81	13.6	80	0.17
PM12	87	11.0	52.4	0.21
PM13	85	13.3	85.35	0.155
PM14	81	8.4	38.14	0.22
PM15	79	9.7	86.57	0.11
PF1	72	8.1	81	0.10
PF2	72	9.0	64	0.14
PF3	79	16.8	129.23	0.13

Normal Values:

Subglottal pressure: males, 3.8–9.6 cm H_2O
females, 3.2–8.7 cm H_2O

Airflow: males, 0.10–0.35 L/sec
females, 0.09–0.34 L/sec

Glottal resistance: males, 12.3–77.2 L/sec^2
females, 14.2–62.5 L/sec^2

PM = male evaluation; PF = female evaluation.

Appendix 7.
Stroboscopy Ratings.

Subject	Vocal Fold Edge	Glottal Closure	Arytenoid Movement	Amplitude of Vocal Fold Vibration	Mucosal Wave	Phase Symmetry	Ventricular Fold Movement	Other Observations
PM1-S	SM/ST	Comp	Norm	Norm	SLT DCR	Ireg	Mod Comp	Thk Muc
PM2-S	SM/ST	Comp	Norm	Norm	SLT DCR	Reg	FL Comp	MOD A-P Thk Muc
PM3-S	SLT Ireg	Comp	Norm	Norm	SLT DCR	Reg	Norm	Thk Muc
PM4-S	SM/ST	PC (C)	Norm	Norm	Norm	Reg	Norm	MLD A-P Thk Muc
PM5-S	SM/ST	Comp	Norm	R Norm L SLT DCR	Mod DCR	Ireg	SLT Comp	Thk Muc
PM6-SMLV	SLT Ireg	AN CHK	Norm	R SEV DCR L > Norm	R SEV DCR L > Norm	Reg	MOD Comp	MOD A-P Muc Strd Stc As
PM7-SM	SLT Ireg	Comp	Norm	R SLT DCR L Norm	SLT DCR	Reg	MOD Comp	MOD A-P
PM8-SM	SM/ST	PC (C)	Norm	R SLT DCR L Norm	R SLT DCR L Norm	Reg	MOD Comp	MOD A-P Thk Muc
PM9-SM	R SLT Ireg L SM/ST	AN CHK	Norm	Norm	R SLT DCR L MOD DCR	Reg	Norm	Thk Muc
PM10-S	SM/ST	Comp	Norm	Norm	R Norm L SLT DCR	Reg	MOD Comp	MLD A-P Stc As
PM11-S	SM/ST	Comp	Norm	Norm	R SLT DCR L Norm	Reg	Norm	
PM12-SML	SLT Ireg	Comp	Norm	R SLT DCR L SEV DCR	R > Norm L SEV DCR	Ireg	SLT Comp	Thk Muc Stc As
PM13-S	SM/ST	PC (MP)	Norm	Norm	Norm	Ireg	SLT Comp	MLD A-P
PM14-S	SM/ST	Comp	Norm	Norm	R Norm L MOD DCR	Reg	Norm	
PM15-SM	SM/ST	Comp	Norm	Norm	R SLT DCR L Norm	Ireg	Norm	MLD A-P Thk Muc
PF1-S	R SM/ST L SL Ireg	PC (C)	Norm	Norm	Norm	Reg	SLT Comp	SEV A-P Muc Strd
PF2-SM	SM/ST	Comp	Norm	Norm	SLT DCR	Ireg	Norm	Muc Strd
PF3-SM	SLT Ireg	Ireg	Norm	MOD DCR	MOD DCR	Reg	MOD Comp	SEV A-P

Subject
PM = male evaluation
PF = female evaluation
S = superior surface
SM = superior and medial surfaces
SML = superior and medial surfaces, vocal ligament
SMLV = superior and medial surfaces, vocal ligaments, vocalis muscle

Vocal Fold Edge
SM/ST = smooth/straight
SLT Ireg = slight irregularity
SIG Ireg = significant irregularity

Glottal Closure
Comp = complete
HR GLS = hourglass
AN CHK = anterior chink
Ireg = irregular
Bow = bowing
Incomp = incomplete
PC (C) = posterior chink, cartilaginous
PC (MP) = posterior chink, membranous portion

Arytenoid Movement
Norm = normal
SLT RES = slightly restricted
MOD RES = moderately restricted
ABST = absent

Amplitude of Vocal Fold Vibration
> Norm = greater than normal
Norm = normal
SLT DCR = slightly decreased
MOD DCR = moderately decreased
SEV DCR = severely decreased
No Mov = no movement

Mucosal Wave
> Norm = greater than normal
Normal = normal
SLT DCR = slightly decreased
MOD DCR = moderately decreased
SEV DCR = severely decreased
No Mov = no movement

Phase Symmetry
Reg = regular
Ireg = irregular

Ventricular Fold Movement
Norm = normal
SLT Comp = slight compression
MOD Comp = moderate compression
FL Comp = full compression

Other Observations
MLD A-P = mild anterior posterior compression
MOD A-P = moderate anterior posterior compression
SEV A-P = severe anterior posterior compression
VT LEV AS = vertical level asymmetry
Stc As = structural asymmetry
Muc Strd = mucous stranding
Thk Muc = thick mucous

Appendix 8.
Perceptual Data.

		Judge 1		Judge 2		Judge 3		Judge 4		Average Rating
	Subject	T1	T2	T1	T2	T1	T2	T1	T2	
NM1	Breathiness	0	0	0	0	0	0	0	0	0
	Straining	+1	+1	0	0	+1	+1	0	0	+0.5
	Hoarseness	+1	+2	+1	0	0	0	+1	0	+0.6
	Pitch	0	0	0	0	+1	+1	0	0	+0.3
NM2	Breathiness	0	0	0	0	0	0	0	0	0
	Straining	0	0	0	0	0	0	0	0	0
	Hoarseness	+1	+1	0	+1	0	0	0	0	+0.4
	Pitch	−1	0	0	0	0	0	0	0	−0.1
PM1	Breathiness	+1	0	+2	+1	0	+1	0	0	+0.6
	Straining	+1	0	+1	+1	+1	+1	0	0	+0.6
	Hoarseness	+2	+2	+2	+2	+1	+1	+1	+1	+1.5
	Pitch	−1	−1	−1	−1	−1	0	0	−1	−0.8
PM2	Breathiness	0	0	+2	0	0	0	0	0	+0.2
	Straining	0	+1	+2	+1	0	+1	0	0	+0.6
	Hoarseness	+1	+2	+2	+2	+1	+1	0	+1	+1.2
	Pitch	0	−1	−1	−1	+1	+1	0	0	−0.1
PM3	Breathiness	0	0	0	0	0	+1	0	0	+0.1
	Straining	0	0	0	0	0	+1	0	0	+0.1
	Hoarseness	+1	+1	+1	+1	0	0	+1	+1	+0.8
	Pitch	0	−1	0	0	0	0	0	0	−0.1
PM4	Breathiness	+1	0	+1	+1	+1	0	+1	0	+0.6
	Straining	0	0	+1	+1	+1	+1	0	0	+0.5
	Hoarseness	+2	+1	+2	+2	+1	0	+1	+1	+1.2
	Pitch	−1	0	−1	0	+1	0	0	0	−0.1
PM5	Breathiness	+1	+1	0	0	+1	+1	0	0	+0.5
	Straining	0	0	0	0	0	+1	0	0	+0.1
	Hoarseness	+1	+2	+1	+1	0	0	0	0	+0.6
	Pitch	0	0	0	0	0	+1	0	0	+0.1
PM6	Breathiness	+3	+2	+2	+2	+2	+2	+2	+2	+2.1
	Straining	0	+1	+2	+2	+2	+2	+1	0	+1.2
	Hoarseness	+2	+2	+3	+3	+2	+2	+1	+1	+2.0
	Pitch	−1	−1	−1	−1	+1	+1	+1	0	−0.1
PM7	Breathiness	0	+1	+1	0	+1	+1	0	0	+0.5
	Straining	+1	+1	0	+1	+1	+1	0	0	+0.6
	Hoarseness	+1	+2	+2	+2	+1	0	0	+1	+1.1
	Pitch	−1	−1	−1	−1	+1	+1	0	0	−0.2
PM8	Breathiness	0	0	0	0	+1	+1	0	0	+0.2
	Straining	0	0	+1	+1	+1	+1	0	0	+0.5
	Hoarseness	+2	+2	+1	+1	+1	+1	+1	+1	+1.2
	Pitch	−1	0	−1	0	+1	+1	0	0	0
PM9	Breathiness	0	+1	0	0	0	+2	+1	0	+0.5
	Straining	+1	0	+1	0	+1	+2	0	0	+0.6
	Hoarseness	+2	+2	+2	+1	+1	+2	0	+2	+1.5
	Pitch	+1	−1	−1	0	+1	+1	0	0	+0.1

Appendix 8 (continued).
Perceptual Data.

Subject		Judge 1 T1	Judge 1 T2	Judge 2 T1	Judge 2 T2	Judge 3 T1	Judge 3 T2	Judge 4 T1	Judge 4 T2	Average Rating
PM10	Breathiness	+1	0	0	0	0	0	0	0	+0.1
	Straining	+3	+2	+2	+1	+2	+2	+2	+1	+1.9
	Hoarseness	+3	+2	+2	+2	+1	+1	+1	+1	+1.6
	Pitch	+1	+1	−1	0	+1	0	0	0	+0.2
PM11	Breathiness	+1	+1	0	0	0	0	+1	0	+0.4
	Straining	+1	0	+1	+1	+2	+1	+1	+1	+1.0
	Hoarseness	+2	+2	+2	+2	+1	+1	+2	+1	+1.6
	Pitch	−1	−1	−1	−1	0	0	−1	−1	−0.8
PM12	Breathiness	0	+1	+1	0	+1	+1	+1	+1	+0.8
	Straining	+1	0	+2	+1	+1	+1	+1	+1	+1.0
	Hoarseness	+2	+1	+3	+2	+1	+1	0	0	+1.2
	Pitch	−1	−1	−1	−1	0	−1	0	0	−0.6
PM13	Breathiness	0	0	+1	0	+1	+1	0	0	+0.4
	Straining	0	0	+1	0	+1	+1	0	0	+0.4
	Hoarseness	+2	+1	+1	+1	+1	+1	+1	+1	+1.1
	Pitch	0	0	0	0	+1	0	0	0	+0.1
PM14	Breathiness	0	0	0	0	0	0	0	0	0
	Straining	0	0	0	0	+1	+1	0	0	+0.2
	Hoarseness	+2	+2	0	+1	0	0	+1	+1	+0.9
	Pitch	0	−1	0	0	+1	+1	0	0	+0.1
PM15	Breathiness	+1	+1	+2	0	+2	+1	+1	+1	+1.1
	Straining	+1	0	+1	+1	+2	+1	+1	0	+0.9
	Hoarseness	+2	+2	+2	+1	+1	+1	+1	+1	+1.4
	Pitch	+1	−1	+1	+1	+1	0	0	0	+0.4
NF1	Breathiness	0	0	0	0	0	0	0	0	0
	Straining	0	0	0	0	0	0	0	0	0
	Hoarseness	0	+1	0	0	0	0	0	0	+0.1
	Pitch	0	0	0	0	0	0	0	0	0
NF2	Breathiness	0	0	0	0	0	0	0	0	0
	Straining	+1	0	0	0	0	0	0	0	+0.1
	Hoarseness	+2	+1	+1	0	0	0	0	0	+0.5
	Pitch	0	0	−1	0	0	0	0	0	−0.1
PF1	Breathiness	+1	+1	0	0	+1	+1	0	+1	+0.6
	Straining	+1	+1	+1	+1	+1	+1	0	0	+0.8
	Hoarseness	+1	+1	+2	+2	+1	+1	+1	+1	+1.2
	Pitch	0	+1	−1	0	0	0	0	0	0
PF2	Breathiness	0	0	0	0	0	0	0	0	0
	Straining	0	0	+1	0	0	+1	0	0	+0.2
	Hoarseness	+1	+1	+1	+1	0	0	+1	+1	+0.8
	Pitch	0	0	−1	0	−1	0	0	0	−0.2
PF3	Breathiness	+2	+2	+3	+2	+2	+2	+1	+1	+1.9
	Straining	+3	+2	+2	+2	+2	+2	+2	+2	+2.1
	Hoarseness	+3	+2	+3	+3	+3	+2	+2	+2	+2.5
	Pitch	+1	+1	−1	+1	0	+1	−1	0	+0.2
Intrajudge agreement		51/88 (58%)		59/88 (67%)		63/88 (72%)		73/88 (83%)		

NM = normal male; NF = normal female; PM = male evaluation; PF = female evaluation.

11

Vocal Fold Paralysis

Introduction

If there is any hallmark of the modern conception of vocal fold paralysis (VFP), it is the advent and acceptance of an explicitly neurologic understanding of the disorder. What seems self-evident now was not so for nearly a century, during which VFP was seen from a fairly narrow surgical perspective. It was a static condition that compromised the valving functions of the larynx, and the solution was structural rearrangement, either by injection or framework surgery, to restore glottic competence. Furthermore, it was understood to be a relatively homogenous, all-or-none condition, where one case was much like another; after all, the vocal fold could only be either neurologically intact or entirely defunct. Obvious clinical differences were explained initially through Semon's "law," which stated that abductor fibers of the laryngeal nerves were more vulnerable (and thus first affected) than adductor fibers. When that failed to stand up to clinical and anatomic observation, it replaced by the Wagner-Grossman hypothesis—note the retreat from "law," a welcome sign of humility and a hint at the healthy doubt to come—which held vocal fold position to be the product of the integrity of the superior laryngeal nerve.

Close experimental and clinical examination of the latter explanation found it wanting, and in doing so brought down the whole construct. As recounted by Dr. Woodson, experimental evidence contrary to expectations created a need for an alternative explanation for the clinical heterogeneity that was plainly evident in VFP. At the same time, she, Hirano, and others noted by various means the propensity for the denervated vocal fold to reinnervate. The paper accompanying her comments is the clinical half of her Triologic thesis, which carefully and unanswerably deconstructed the old paradigm. With the elucidation of natural reinnervation came an appreciation that vocal fold paralysis was a continuum of neurologic dysfunction, that reinnervation could occasionally be counterproductive, and that it might even be turned to therapeutic use. The 1994 review was a snapshot of the changing field by representatives of the Speech, Voice and Swallowing Committee of the American Academy of Otolaryngology, and captures the fact that the old, fairly well-defined algorithm had evolved into a series of therapeutic options by that date. Dr. Crumley, instrumental over his career not only in therapeutic reinnervation, but also in promoting dialogue and the exchange of ideas in neurolaryngology, further updates that review with a perceptive assessment of the implications of the new knowledge. The analysis of bilateral paralysis, often ignored in the proliferation of therapeutic options for unilateral VFP, by the Holingers continues to stand more than three decades later as the most complete clinical examination of the topic.

In retrospect, it is amazing that an entity that has been long recognized as the result of neurologic compromise should have been thought to be exempt from features common to other neuropathies. That this exceptionalist view has faded into our past is a testament to determined inquiry, interest across specialty boundaries and an understanding of otolaryngology as a broad medical field, all reflected in the papers and commentaries that follow.

Classic Articles

●Reprint of article included in this chapter.
♦Commentary on this article.

●Holinger LD, Holinger PC, Holinger PH. Etiology of bilateral abductor vocal cord paralysis. A review of 389 cases. *Ann Otol Rhinol Laryngol.* 1976;85(4 pt 1): 428–436.

Cavo JW Jr. True vocal cord paralysis following intubation. *Laryngoscope.* 1985;95(11):1352–1359.

Dennis DP, Kashima H. Carbon dioxide laser posterior cordectomy for treatment of bilateral vocal cord paralysis. *Ann Otol Rhinol Laryngol.* 1989;96(12 pt 1):930–934.

●♦Woodson GE. Configuration of the glottis in laryngeal paralysis. I: clinical study. *Laryngoscope.* 1993; 103(11 pt 1):1227–1234.

●♦Benninger MS, Crumley RL, Ford CN, et al. Evaluation and treatment of the unilateral paralyzed vocal fold. *Otolaryngol Head Neck Surg.* 1994;111(4):497–508.

Netterville JL, Koriwchak MJ, Winkle M, Courey MS, Ossoff RH. Vocal fold paralysis following the anterior approach to the cervical spine. *Ann Otol Rhinol Laryngol.* 1996;105(2):85–91.

ETIOLOGY OF BILATERAL ABDUCTOR VOCAL CORD PARALYSIS

A REVIEW OF 389 CASES

LAUREN D. HOLINGER, MD

PAUL C. HOLINGER, MD PAUL H. HOLINGER, MD

CHICAGO, ILLINOIS

SUMMARY – The etiology of 389 cases of partial or complete bilateral abductor vocal cord paralysis has been determined and classified. One hundred and forty-nine were infants and children 12 years of age and under; 240 were adults, age 13 and older. In the infants and children the paralyses were congenital in 82 cases, of which 43 were associated with other congenital anomalies, and 39 were without associated anomalies. Fifty-nine cases were considered acquired, most being secondary to underlying congenital anomalies, particularly the associated findings of meningomyelocele, Arnold-Chiari malformation, and hydrocephalus. Eight cases of paralysis in this age group were of undetermined etiology. Of the 240 adult cases of bilateral vocal cord paralysis, 138 followed thyroidectomy. Fifty-two cases were associated with various neurologic disorders, including poliomyelitis, Parkinson's disease, cerebrovascular accident, Guillain-Barré syndrome, multiple sclerosis, neoplasm, and other miscellaneous neurologic conditions. Sixteen cases were due to malignant neoplasms of the neck and mediastinum. The remaining 34 cases constitute a miscellaneous group which includes foreign bodies, bilateral neck dissection, infection, congenital lesions, trauma, and idiopathic paralyses. The characteristic symptoms of bilateral abductor vocal cord paralysis include normal or near normal phonation with inspiratory stridor which may progress to complete respiratory obstruction. These symptoms are due to the stationary but flaccid midline position of the vocal cords which places them in a phonating position, where they both obstruct the airway and produce a fairly clear voice or cry. This paradoxical combination of symptoms was frequently found to be responsible for a failure or delay in diagnosis.

Bilateral abductor vocal cord paralysis is a distressing condition, often life-threatening, and not infrequently a direct cause of asphyxial death. Yet many times it is unrecognized clinically because the voice or cry of the patient with bilateral paralysis is quite normal and invariably better than that of the patient with unilateral paralysis. This paradox is due to the fact that in bilateral paralysis both cords remain weakly adducted, in which position they vibrate during expiration or phonation, passively but equally. In unilateral paralysis, on the other hand, differences in tension between the normal and the paralyzed cord result in a hoarse, aspirate voice. Patients with bilateral vocal cord paralysis have a limited airway and a persistent, soft, inspiratory stridor which may be barely audible or may increase to a loud, agonal, even terminal crow. Any additional edema of the cords results in extreme dyspnea, for which intubation or tracheotomy may become necessary. Failure to recognize the condition most often occurs in the thyroidectomized adult. Similarly, in the stridorous infant with a major central nervous system (CNS) defect, bilateral paralysis may remain undiagnosed because of a failure to examine the larynx routinely and without anesthesia.

From the Department of Otolaryngology, Abraham Lincoln School of Medicine of the University of Illinois; the Department of Psychiatry, Psychosomatic and Psychiatric Institute, Michael Reese Hospital and Medical Center; the Department of Bronchology, The Children's Memorial Hospital; and the Department of Otolaryngology and Bronchoesophagology, Rush/Presbyterian-St. Luke's Medical Center, Chicago, Illinois.

Presented at the meeting of The American Laryngological Association, Palm Beach, Florida, April 24-25, 1976.

TABLE I

ETIOLOGY OF BILATERAL ABDUCTOR VOCAL CORD PARALYSIS IN INFANTS AND CHILDREN

Congenital				
Without associated anomalies		39		
With associated anomalies				
Neurologic	21			
Laryngeal	10			
Cardiac	8			
Other	4			
		43		
	Total Congenital		82	(55%)
Acquired				
Secondary to congenital anomalies				
Meningomyelocele, A-CM, hydrocephalus	24			
Hydrocephalus unrelated to A-CM	6			
Postoperative for congenital lesion	11			
		41		
Secondary to acquired conditions				
Infectious	7			
Neoplasm	7			
Birth trauma	2			
Guillain-Barré syndrome	2			
		18		
	Total Acquired		59	(40%)
Undetermined		8	8	(5%)
	Total		149	(100%)

METHODS AND MATERIALS

This study reviews the etiology of 389 cases of partial or complete bilateral abductor vocal cord paralysis in infants and children 12 years of age and under, and adults age 13 or older. Diagnosis in all cases was confirmed by mirror or endoscopic examination. In infants, the diagnosis can be established only by direct laryngoscopic examination without anesthesia.[1] The spatulous tip of a standard Jackson pediatric laryngoscope is placed in the vallecula to lift the base of the tongue and epiglottis to evaluate vocal cord mobility. Care must be taken to avoid contact with the vocal cords or arytenoids, which would alter cord mobility. Passive mobility should be evaluated by palpation to rule out midline vocal cord fixation.[2] In adults the examination is made with the laryngeal mirror, not only during the phonation of "e-e-e-e," but especially during inspiration as well.

RESULTS

The data derived from this study are most informative when infants and children are evaluated separately from adults. Bilateral paralysis in infants is largely congenital in origin, or secondary to congenital anomalies of the CNS. In adults the great majority of cases are acquired. Unfortunately, the leading cause is surgical injury to the recurrent laryngeal nerves at thyroidectomy. Neurologic lesions are the second most common cause of bilateral paralysis in adults. A classification based on the two age groups is presented in Tables I and II.

Of the 389 cases, 149 (38%) were present in infants and children under 13 years of age; 240 (62%) were found in adults. There were 146 males and 243 females. Sex distribution was similar among the infants and children (80 males, 69 females), but among the adults there were 66 males and 174 females. This was due to a higher incidence of thyroid disease in females; of 138 cases of bilateral paralysis due to thyroidectomy, only 11 occurred in

TABLE II

ETIOLOGY OF BILATERAL ABDUCTOR VOCAL CORD PARALYSIS IN ADULTS

Thyroidectomy		138	(58%)
Neurologic			
Poliomyelitis	14		
Parkinson's disease	4		
Cerebrovascular accident	4		
Guillain-Barré syndrome	3		
Multiple sclerosis	3		
CNS neoplasm	3		
CNS infection	2		
Charcot-Marie-Tooth	2		
Other	17		
		52	(22%)
Malignancy of the neck		16	(6%)
Miscellaneous			
Foreign bodies	2		
Bilateral neck dissection	3		
Infection	3		
Congenital	3		
Trauma	2		
Substernal thyroid	2		
Idiopathic	8		
Other	3		
Undetermined	8		
		34	(14%)
Total		240	(100%)

males. Tracheotomy was required at some time during the patient's course in 199 cases (51%); 71 cases were in infants and children and 128 in adults; 48% of the infants and children required tracheotomy, as did 53% of adults.

DISCUSSION

Stridor is the most prominent symptom of bilateral abductor vocal cord paralysis. It varies from a soft, high-pitched, inspiratory sound to an extremely loud, distressing crow. Adult patients' families volunteer that often it is easily heard throughout the room or ward and even by neighbors if the windows are open in the summertime. Snoring is especially pronounced when the patient is relaxed during sleep. The voice and speech are somewhat abnormal; a peculiar monotone with long, hurried sentences is interrupted by a stridorous, inspiratory pause as the patient attempts to fill his lungs for continuation of his comment. Laughter is consciously suppressed to avoid the air loss which must be followed by distressing inspiration. Cough is desperately suppressed for the same reason. In infants, while the cry may be clear, stridor is high-pitched and not necessarily accompanied by acute respiratory distress, although marked indrawing of the suprasternal notch and epigastrium is usually apparent. With prolonged obstruction, however, fatigue becomes the major factor precipitating either intubation or tracheotomy.

The degree of aspiration, especially of liquids, helps localize the site of the lesion superior or inferior to the origin of the superior laryngeal nerve. While this should be a fairly accurate diagnostic criterion, patients with aspiration due to superior laryngeal nerve involvement soon learn to control coughing and choking, and the clinical significance of this diagnostic point is lost.

The most serious symptom, of course, is respiratory obstruction, which is evidenced by stridor, dyspnea, retraction, and nasal flaring. Since the airway through the larynx is limited, the least effort, activity, inflammation or edema may result in increasing dyspnea, and even psychiatric symptoms in adults. As obstruction increases, restlessness, the use of the accessory respiratory musculature, and eventually cyanosis become apparent. If unrelieved, total asphyxia follows. Many patients tolerate their condition for considerable lengths of time, remaining marginally compensated until a minimal change in their status renders the airway inadequate. Patients with postthyroidectomy bilateral paralysis usually adapt to a minimal airway over a period of years; yet eventually, even 10 to 20 years later, may require surgical intervention such as a tracheotomy or arytenoidectomy. This may be associated with myxedematous infiltration of the cords due to hypothyroidism or laryngeal spasm associated with the hypocalcemic tetany of hypoparathyroidism. Infants and children may remain stridorous but undiagnosed until an upper respiratory infection leads to obstruction, or a prolonged episode of croup, for which the child is ultimately referred for endoscopic evaluation. The importance of direct endoscopic examination of children with stridor or persistent episodes of croup cannot be overemphasized. In a recent review of subglottic stenosis in infants and children,[3] 34% of 115 cases of congenital subglottic stenosis presented with recurrent or persistent croup.

Infants and Children

Congenital Paralysis. Vocal cord paralysis represents approximately 10% of all congenital anomalies of the larynx.[4] It is the second most common laryngeal anomaly; only laryngomalacia is seen more often. In this series, 82 of the 149 infants and children had congenital bilateral paralysis.

In 39 of the 82 congenital cases the paralysis was without associated anomalies, most of which tended to resolve spontaneously over a period of weeks or months; a closer study of this group is now under way to more accurately determine the outcome. In some of these infants, the arytenoids were observed to move in the absence of any mobility of the vocal cords, which were immobile in the median position. Palpation demonstrated the arytenoids could be moved with forceps.

Forty-three infants and children had other congenital anomalies associated with congenital bilateral paralysis. Twenty-one had associated neurologic lesions. The association between the paralysis and the neurologic disorders had greater etiologic significance in some cases than in others. Congenital bilateral paralysis was seen in six infants with cerebral agenesis, four infants with congenital cranial nerve palsies including X, and one infant with congenital nuclear hypoplasias including X. In these 11 cases the congenital bilateral vocal cord paralysis was apparently secondary to the neurologic lesions. In the remaining ten cases the relationship between the vocal cord paralysis and the neurologic disorder was less well defined. Three of these ten had benign congenital hypotonia, one had Werdnig-Hoffmann disease, another had leukodystrophy (Alexander's disease), and there was one child with scapuloperoneal muscular dystrophy. The exact nature of the neurologic lesion remained obscure in three cases. Congenital bilateral paralysis was found in one patient with Charcot-Marie-Tooth disease; the occurrence of congenital bilateral vocal cord paralysis in families has been documented and is discussed elsewhere.[5-8]

Ten infants and children had other laryngeal anomalies associated with their congenital bilateral vocal cord paralysis; subglottic stenosis was present in six; laryngomalacia in three and laryngocele in one. One of the infants with laryngomalacia had other congenital anomalies, including hypospadias and bilateral dysplasia of the hips; a chromosomal abnormality was documented with karyotype interpretation 46, XY, one of D chromosomes having a short arm.

A wide variety of cardiac anomalies occurred in eight infants and children with congenital bilateral paralysis; these included ventricular septal defect, three; coarctation of the aorta, two; transposition of the great vessels, two; and atrial septal defect, one. Two of these patients also had Down's syndrome.

A miscellaneous group of congenital anomalies comprised the other four cases associated with congenital bilateral paralysis. These included spontaneous pneumothorax, muscular hypertonia and tracheomalacia with a narrow right main bronchus.

Acquired Paralysis. In this series, 59 of the 149 infants and children had acquired bilateral paralysis. In 41, the acquired paralysis occurred secondary to underlying congenital anomalies or was secondary to the surgical treatment of such anomalies. Of these 41, 24 involved infants born with meningomyelocele.

The association of meningomyelocele with paralysis of the vocal cords was noted in 1932,[9] 1939,[10] 1941[11] and again 15 years later.[12,13] Investigators later identified the relationship in more extensive case reports,[14-17] and others have recently probed the pathogenesis of bilateral vocal cord paralysis when related to meningomyelocele.[18-22] Associated meningomyelocele, Arnold-Chiari malformation, and hydrocephalus, as well as the neurosurgical efforts to repair these abnormalities, may result in increased intracranial pressure with subsequent airway obstruction due to bilateral vocal cord paralysis. Arnold-Chiari malformation (Chiari II), documented in 9 of the 24 cases with meningomyelocele, is probably present to some degree in all of these cases.[23] It is a developmental disorder characterized particularly by varying degrees of herniation of the cerebellum and kinking of the medulla oblongata, the causes of which are debated, but for which there may be a genetic background.[24]

In this series, neurosurgical repair of the meningomyelocele was usually accomplished shortly after birth; increased intracranial pressure and hydrocephalus occurred at varying lengths of time thereafter. Shunting procedures were instituted to control the hydrocephalus. The increased intracranial pressure which preceded signs and symptoms of airway obstruction was most frequently associated with malfunctioning or infected shunts. Less frequently, the bilateral paralysis occurred following repair of the meningomyelocele but before a diagnosis of hydrocephalus was made. Some children were later readmitted when the stridor of bilateral paralysis developed as the first sign of increased intracranial pressure due to a malfunctioning or infected shunt. The clinical course and pathophysiology seen in these are reviewed in greater detail elsewhere.[22]

Six cases of infants with bilateral paralyses were seen with hydrocephalus secondary to tumor, meningitis, and other underlying conditions, but without meningomyelocele.

Signs and symptoms of increased intracranial pressure, particularly increased head size, bulging fontanelle, and vomiting, usually preceded evidence of airway obstruction. Stridor and respiratory distress were prominent among the signs and symptoms of the ensuing bilateral paralysis. While associated with increased intracranial pressure, the precise etiology of the bilateral vocal cord paralysis in these cases is uncertain and discussed in detail elsewhere.[21,22] Among the possible hypotheses are brain stem dysgenesis, mechanical compression of the vagus nerve by the herniated posterior fossa contents, stretching of the vagus nerve rootlets during herniation with resulting neuronal degeneration, and circulatory impairment of the brain stem.

Although the etiology of the bilateral vocal cord paralysis in these cases is uncertain, the resulting airway obstruction can be life-threatening, and an airway must be promptly secured by intubation. Subsequent direct laryngoscopy discloses the median or paramedian position of the cords; tracheotomy is frequently necessitated when extubation attempts are unsuccessful. At The Children's Memorial Hospital in Chicago, where nearly all of the infants and children were seen, the neurosurgical service has been acutely aware of the relationship between bilateral vocal cord paralysis and increased intracranial pressure for many years. When stridor develops in a child known to have a potential for increased intracranial pressure, *e.g.*, those with hydrocephalus and meningomyelocele, they are assumed to have bilateral paralysis on the basis of increasing pressure. An endotracheal tube is placed, the cause of the increased pressure treated (it is most often related to an infected or malfunctioning shunt) and the child extubated.

Eleven instances of acquired bilateral paralysis followed surgical repair of congenital lesions which were not related to the CNS. Six became apparent after repair of tracheoesophageal fistula, three following surgery for congenital heart disease. One was diagnosed following the excision of a congenital bronchial cyst and one following craniotomy for craniostenosis.

Eighteen of the 59 children with acquired bilateral paralysis had no associated congenital anomaly. Seven were due to infectious disease: meningitis, encephalitis and poliomyelitis. Neoplasms of the CNS caused the paralysis in six; a seventh patient had Hodgkin's disease of the mediastinum and suffered bilateral paralysis following radiation therapy. Birth trauma was implicated in two cases and Guillain-Barré syndrome in two.

Undetermined Paralysis. The etiology of bilateral abductor vocal cord paralysis was undetermined in 8 of the 149 infants and children.

ADULTS

Two hundred and forty of the patients with bilateral abductor vocal cord paralysis were adults 13 years of age and older. Unlike the infants and children, the overwhelming majority of adults had acquired paralyses. Only three were considered to have congenital paralyses, these on the basis of a history of stridor since infancy. None had ever been examined directly or indirectly until seen at ages 33, 59, and 70, when their obstruction became severe enough to necessitate investigation.

Postthyroidectomy. One hundred and thirty-eight of the acquired adult cases followed thyroidectomy. Many of these had no symptoms of upper airway obstruction until after their second or even third thyroidectomy, although they generally gave a history of voice change following the original operation. In addition to respiratory obstruction, many had signs and findings of hypothyroidism and hypoparathyroidism. The number of cases observed increased during the period of time a total thyroidectomy was recommended for certain cardiac conditions. Psychiatric symptoms associated with hypothyroidism and hypoparathyroidism were freqeunt in this group of 138, and included depression, psychomotor retardation, irritability, and other personality changes.

Hoarseness following thyroidectomy is most often the result of paralysis of one vocal cord, due to trauma to a recurrent laryngeal nerve. The voice is weak and breathy; aspiration is frequent. However, when both nerves are involved, the voice, which may be temporarily affected, soon returns to almost normal, punctuated only by varying degrees of stridor. On examination with a laryngeal mirror during the phonation of "e-e-e-e," the larynx appears quite normal. However, the patient is usually so dyspneic that attempts to watch for the separation of the cords during inspiration are often abandoned.

In a review of 63 cases of bilateral vocal cord paralysis following thyroidectomy reported in 1955,[25] 40% were found to be hypothyroid while 21% were hypoparathyroid. The symptoms are generally manifested by the progressive limitation of the individual's activity, resulting from pulmonary and circulatory involvement as well as the increasing airway obstruction. Bouts of acute respiratory obstruction may be noted after an episode of emotional stress or in association with respiratory tract infections to which these patients are particularly susceptible. When the obstruction becomes sufficiently severe, intubation or tracheotomy must be undertaken to relieve the hypoxia and to protect the circulation: anoxia with its depressant effect on the myocardium can create a circulatory crisis to the extent of precipitating congestive heart failure.

The signs and symptoms of hypothyroidism are readily recognized. The complacent attitude, slowness of response, dull facies, dry skin, marked pallor, coarse hair, and poor tolerance to cold are characteristic. These findings are emphasized to stress their significance in patients who have postthyroidectomy respiratory obstruction from bilateral vocal cord paralysis. The myxedema of hypothyroidism includes the vocal cords and the supporting tissues of the larynx, and thus increases the degree of obstruction. The correction of the laryngeal myxedema with proper thyroid replacement therapy is necessary before surgical intervention is considered, and may obviate the need for surgery.

The symptoms due to hypoparathyroidism may be masked by those of hypothyroidism, and the diagnosis overlooked for this reason. When symptoms of fatigue, muscular weakness, tetany and paresthesias are present in the thyroidectomized patient, hypoparathyroidism should be suspected. Depending upon the degree of hypocalcemia, there may be cramps of the extremities, carpopedal as well as laryngeal spasm; even generalized convulsions may occur. Not uncommonly, these symptoms may be misdiagnosed as psychogenic. Cardiac conduction disturbances relating to calcium metabolism may also be present.

Paralysis Associated with Other Neurological Disorders. The commonest neurologic disorder associated with bilateral paralysis in adults was found to be poliomyelitis. The frequency with which bilateral laryngeal paralysis was caused by bulbar polio has been well documented by Galloway and Seifert.[26] Their description of the life-threatening and fatal complications of not only respiratory obstruction but aspiration of pharyngeal secretions is classic. Similar concepts of management were employed by Ibsen during the great Copenhagen polio epidemic of 1952, through the use of cuffed endotracheal tube and positive pressure ventilation.[27] Our experience in the acute phase[28] is not as extensive as that of Galloway and Ibsen. The 14 cases recorded in this series were encountered during a later stage when the respiratory obstruction of bilatral paralysis was complicated by the atelectasis associated with diaphragmatic and intercostal paralysis. Pharyngeal and laryngeal sensory involvement was thought to complicate the motor paralysis contributing to patients' aspiration of food and fluids, thus increasing the respiratory embarrassment. The resulting respiratory difficulties became extreme and tracheotomy was urgently needed. Yet many physicians who treated poliomyelitis were apparently unaware of the fact that the patient with bilateral vocal cord paralysis is able to phonate without difficulty, although the airway may have been so obstructed that he lapsed into unconsciousness.

In addition to the 14 cases of polio, several other acquired neurologic disorders have been found complicated by bilateral vocal cord paralysis, most with dyspnea so severe that they required tracheotomy. These cases include Parkinson's disease (four), cerebrovascular accident (four), Guillain-Barré syndrome (three), multiple sclerosis (three), CNS tumors (three), encephalitis and meningitis (two), and others (bulbar and pseudobulbar palsies, 17). Also, two patients with Charcot-Marie-Tooth disease, a mother and her son, were both found to have an associated bilateral vocal cord paralysis.

Paralysis Associated with Malignancy of the Neck. Sixteen cases of malignant neoplasms of the thyroid, cervical esophagus, subglottic larynx, neck and upper mediastinum were found to be responsible for bilateral abductor paralysis by pressure or invasion of the vagus or its recurrent branches. Usually one side was affected first; later the dyspnea of bilateral involvement became unmistakable. Mirror laryngoscopy or x-ray studies of the larynx and trachea are necessary to distinguish this symptom from tracheal compression or invasion by the neoplasm.

Miscellaneous Etiology. The 34 remaining patients with bilateral paralysis were found to have a variety of disorders. Foreign bodies in the esophagus were responsible for two cases of bilateral paralysis of the larynx. One was a 2-year-old child who was admitted to the hospital with severe dysphagia and dyspnea. Roentgen studies revealed a large, nonopaque button in the cervical esophagus which the mother was able to identify as having been swallowed nine months previously. Following tracheotomy the button was removed from a bed of scar, granulation tissue, and pus. Laryngoscopy demonstrated the bilateral midline position of the vocal cords. Extensive ulceration of the esophageal walls with periesophageal inflammation, induration, and abscess accounted for the paralysis.[13] The paralysis was permanent and eventually required arytenoidectomy. The second case was an adult who had an extensive cervical mediastinitis following esophageal perforation by a chicken bone.

In three cases in the miscellaneous group the paralysis followed bilateral neck dissection. Three others developed their paralysis following respiratory tract infections. In another three cases discussed previously, the etiology was considered congenital. Two patients had bilateral paralysis due to cervical trauma, and in two others, substernal thyroids involved both recurrent nerves. There was one case each of arthritis, leukemia, and a lesion of the cervical esophagus.

Eight cases in this group of miscellaneous paralyses were seen once in consultation for verification of the diagnosis only, and the etiology was not determined.

Eight adult patients were studied extensively but the etiology of their bilateral vocal cord paralyses was not discovered; these are considered idiopathic. Diagnostic evaluation began with a thorough history, which in many instances led directly to the etiology. Patients were questioned specifically about trauma, previous surgery, the degree and onset of hoarseness, dysphagia, aspiration, stridor and pain. A history of infection or recent upper respiratory infection was sought. Others had had thyroidectomies decades previously with symptoms beginning only weeks or months prior to evaluation; many of these were found to be hypothyroid or hypoparathyroid.

Remaining patients had medical and neurologic evaluations and laboratory studies which usually consisted of CBC, urinalysis, fasting and two-hour postprandial blood glucose, serologic tests for syphilis (VDRL, FTA-abs), erythrocyte sedimentation rate, PBI, T3 and T4. When the etiology remained obscure, thorough head and neck physical examination was extended to include endoscopic evaluation of larynx, trachea, and cervical esophagus. When indicated, these were preceded by special roentgenographic examinations, such as tomography and contrast studies (barium esophagram). Further specialized tests were employed to define associated neurologic lesions.

CONCLUSIONS

The etiology of 389 cases of partial or complete bilateral abductor vocal cord paralysis has been analyzed. There were 149 cases of infants and children 12 years of age and under: in 82, the lesions were congenital in origin, in 59, the etiology was acquired, and in 8, the etiology was undetermined. Two hundred and forty of the patients were adults 13 years of age and older; in all but three the condition was acquired. One hundred and thirty-eight followed thyroidectomy, 52 were neurologic, 16 were due to malignancies of the neck, and 34 were miscellaneous, eight of which were considered idiopathic.

The diagnosis of bilateral vocal cord paralysis is obscured by the paradoxical association of a relatively clear voice or cry with varying degrees of respiratory obstruction. The diagnosis may be overlooked in stridorous infants and children with meningomyelocele, Arnold-Chiari malformation and hydrocephalus, because the larynx is not examined without anesthesia; in such infants the onset of stridor is most often due to bilateral cord paralysis precipitated by increasing intracranial pressure. In adults, mirror examination of the larynx must be made during both phonation and inspiration. While some thyroidectomized adults adapt to the compromised airway of bilateral paralysis, the additional insult of hypothyroid myxedema or hypoparathyroid tetany may upset their compensated state. Conservative management involves correction of the underlying metabolic abnormality before any surgical intervention is undertaken.

REFERENCES

1. Holinger PH: Clinical aspects of congenital anomalies of the larynx, trachea, bronchi and oesophagus. J Laryngol Otol 75:1-44, 1961

2. Cox DJ, Simmons FB: Midline vocal cord fixation in the newborn. Arch Otolaryngol 100:219, 1974

3. Holinger PH, Kutnick SL, Schild JA, *et al*: Subglottic stenosis in infants and children. Ann Otol Rhinol Laryngol, to be published.

4. Holinger PH, Brown WT: Congenital webs, cysts, laryngoceles and other congenital anomalies of the larynx. Ann Otol Rhinol Laryngol 76:744-752, 1967

5. Platt D: Congenital laryngeal – abductor paralysis due to nucleus ambiguus dysgenesis in three brothers. N Engl J Med 271: 593-597, 1964

6. Watters GV, Fitch N: Familial laryngeal abductor paralysis and psychomotor retardation. Clin Genet 4:429-433, 1973

7. Gacek RR: Hereditary abductor vocal cord paralysis. Ann Otol Rhinol Laryngol 85: 90-93, 1976

8. Holinger PC, Holinger LD, Vuckovich MD, *et al*: Familial bilateral abductor vocal cord paralysis in Charcot-Marie-Tooth disease, to be published.

9. New GB, Childrey JH: Paralysis of the vocal cords. Arch Otolaryngol 16:143-159, 1932

10. Heatly CA: The larynx in infancy: A study of chronic stridor. Arch Otolaryngol 29: 90-103, 1939

11. Work WP: Paralysis and paresis of the vocal cords: A statistical review. Arch Otolaryngol 34:267-280, 1941

12. Bigler JA, Holinger PH, Johnston KC, *et al*: Tracheotomy in infancy. Pediatrics 13: 476-486, 1954

13. Holinger PH, Johnston KC: Bilateral recurrent laryngeal nerve paralysis; medical and surgical aspects. Eye Digest 38-45, June 1956

14. Cavanagh F: Vocal cord palsies in children. J Laryngol Otol 69:399-418, 1955

15. Rullan A: Associated laryngeal paralysis. Arch Otolaryngol 64:207-212, 1956

16. Smith MEN: The association of laryngeal stridor with meningomyelocele. J Laryngol Otol 73:188-190, 1959

17. Graham MD: Bilateral vocal cord paralysis associated with meningomyelocele and the Arnold-Chiari malformation. Laryngoscope 73:85-92, 1963

18. Snow JB, Rogers KA Jr: Bilateral abductor paralysis of the vocal cords secondary to the Arnold-Chiari malformation and its management. Laryngoscope 75:316-321, 1965

19. Kirsch WM, Duncan BR, Black FO, *et al*: Laryngeal palsy in association with meningomyelocele, hydrocephalus, and the Arnold-Chiari malformation. J Neurosurg 218: 207-214, 1968

20. Sieben RL, Hamida MB, Shulman K: Multiple cranial nerve deficits associated with the Arnold-Chiari malformation. Neurology 21:673-680, 1971

21. Bluestone LD, Delerme HN, Samuelson GM: Airway obstruction due to vocal cord paralysis in infants with meningomyelocele and hydrocephalus. Ann Otol Rhinol Laryngol 81:778-783, 1972

22. Reichert TJ, Schild JA, Holinger PH: Respiratory obstruction in infants with meningomyelocele and hydrocephalus. Presented at the Third Annual Meeting of Society for Ear Nose and Throat Advances in Children, Mexico City, Mexico, November 8, 1975

23. Emery JL, MacKenzie N: Medullo-cervical dislocation deformity (Chiari II deformity) related to neurospinal dysraphism (meningomyelocele). Brain 96:155-162, 1973

24. Gardner E, O'Rahilly R, Prolo D: The Dandy-Walker and Arnold-Chiari malformations. Arch Neurol 32:393-407, 1975

25. Ranke EJ, Holinger PH: Paralysis of the vocal cords following thyroidectomy. JAMA 158:543-547, 1955

26. Galloway TC, Seifert MH: Bulbar poliomyelitis. Ann Otol Rhinol Laryngol 56:250-263, 1947

27. Ibsen B: Anesthetists' viewpoint on treatment of respiratory complications in poliomyelitis during the epidemic in Copenhagen in 1952. Proc R Soc Med 47:72-74, 1954

28. Holinger PH, Johnston KC: Tracheotomy in acute tracheobronchitis and poliomyelitis. Prog Ophthalmol Otolaryngol 1:590-597, 1952

REPRINTS—Lauren D. Holinger, MD, 700 N. Michigan Avenue, Chicago, IL 60611.

Commentary

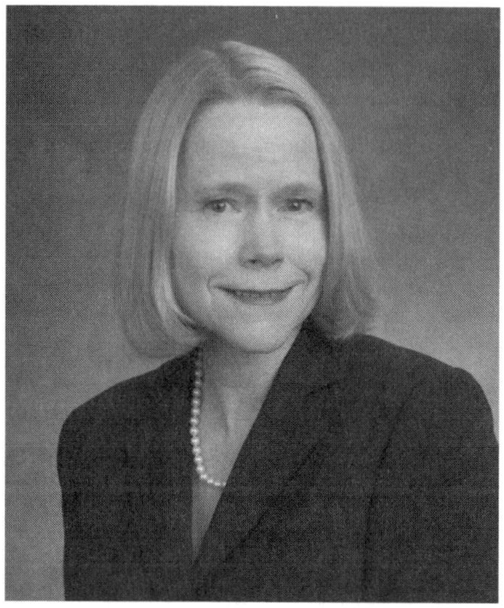

Gayle E. Woodson, MD

Yogi Berra once said, "If you don't know where you are going, you will wind up somewhere else." The research that led me to publish this paper is a clear example of that axiom. When I was a resident, I was taught that the cricothyroid muscle (CT) was the key determinant of laryngeal function after recurrent laryngeal nerve (RLN) injury. The RLN supplies all intrinsic muscles of the larynx except the CT, which is innervated the superior laryngeal nerve (SLN). From lectures, journal articles, textbooks, and test questions I learned that isolated contraction of the CT muscle pulls the vocal fold medially. And this was the widely accepted explanation for why the vocal fold is usually found near the midline after RLN injury. Conversely, when the entire vagus nerve, including SLN fibers, is transected, the vocal fold lies in a more lateral position, similar to that of a cadaveric larynx. This "cadaveric" position was attributed to the lack of CT action.

When only one RLN is injured, a relatively adducted vocal fold position is beneficial, because the opposite, mobile vocal fold can do a better job of closing during speech and swallowing. But when both vocal folds are near the midline, there is significant restriction of airflow during breathing. And so nearly 30 years ago, I reasoned that if I could control activity of the CT, I could greatly influence the symptoms of laryngeal paralysis. For a unilateral injury, I expected that increasing the strength of CT contraction should improve the voice. For bilateral paralysis, suppression of the CT should let the vocal fold move laterally, improving the airway. And if I could achieve fine control of CT activity, I might even be able to restore dynamic motion.

So I began my research career seeking to learn what makes the CT tick. Early on, I was fortunate enough to meet up with Giuseppe and Franca Sant'Ambrogio, world class respiratory physiologists who were also curious about laryngeal respiratory function. I attended a conference where Giuseppe was speaking on respiratory sensation and its influence on laryngeal motion. After the conference, I went up to ask him some questions and before I knew it, he wanted to know when I wanted to begin our collaboration.

I have to say that some of the happiest hours in my life were spent in the Sant'Ambrogio laboratory. Of course, like all research, many hours were slow and dull, and data collection was sometimes tedious. But I learned so much in terms of techniques and theory that the "aha" moments made everything else worthwhile. We studied laryngeal function in an animal model, creating temporary, reversible nerve lesions by cooling RLN and/or nerves to the CT's. We monitored laryngeal muscle EMG and transglottic airflow, and videotaped and analyzed laryngeal motion.

But then we found what we did not expect: that that the CT muscle did not influence vocal fold position or airway resistance across the larynx one whit. This was not what I had expected or hoped to find, and certainly changed my plans for developing a better treatment for my patients. And so I thought, maybe we could not demonstrate an effect of the CT because we were looking in an anesthetized animal with an acute injury. What if, over time, the CT gained strength, and became able to move the vocal fold?

At that time, I relocated from Texas to California, and had to continue this investigation on my own, although well-trained by now. I measured the same parameters of laryngeal function in animals months after a surgical transection of the RLN, comparing results of transecting the RLN alone to the results after cutting both the RLN and the nerve to the CT. I did not just transect the RLN. I removed a long segment by cutting it near its entry into the larynx, pulling the nerve upward, and cutting the near the clavicle, letting the cut end retract back into the mediastinum. I was somewhat dismayed to discover that I could not document an adductor role of the CT in this chronic model either. I was mystified to find that the vocal fold moved from cadaveric to paramedian after 3 to 6 months in both groups of animal, with and without CT paralysis. But I also discovered something that I completely did not expect. In exploring the neck to place a tracheal cannula, I found that the RLN had regenerated across a large gap. Regeneration of a nerve across such a large gap seemed unthinkable. When I stimulated this regenerated nerve, the vocal fold twitched, and when I cut it, the vocal fold became fixed in a more lateral position. In all subsequent experiments, I sought and found this regenerated nerve, and noted the same effects from stimulation and transection. Thus, it seemed that regeneration of RLN nerve fibers were responsible for the medial migration of the vocal fold over time after nerve transection. I reported these results in my Triological Society thesis: "Configuration of the Glottis in Laryngeal Paralysis." The animal experiments were published in the Laryngoscope as "Configuration of the Glottis in Laryngeal Paralysis II: Animal Experiments." This was the companion paper to "Part I: Clinical Study," the paper published in this book.

An ironic encounter occurred just before I moved to California and began the experiments I just described. While I was visiting the University of Wisconsin at Madison, I gave a guest lecture, describing my proposed research. It so happened that Minoru Hirano was also visiting at the same time, and he attended my lecture. Unbeknownst to me, he had already published a landmark article on laryngeal muscle EMG in patients with laryngeal paralysis. Only after I completed my animal studies did I discover his article. It had been originally published in Japanese, but I found it in the Proceedings of a Laryngeal Physiology Conference that had convened in Yale, not a publication that I could have tracked down in Index Medicus. In a series of more than 100 patients, Hirano had found normal TA muscle activity in many patients, demonstrating that a clinically paralyzed larynx is not necessarily denervated. He had also noted that the position of the paralyzed vocal fold was not influenced by the status of the CT muscle, but correlated with the amount of activity detected in the TA muscle. After my talk, I paused to answer questions. Amazingly, Professor Hirano smiled and remained silent although he already had good data indicating that the CT was not the determinant of vocal fold position in laryngeal position. I believe it was his gracious nature that accounts for his silence, and probably his presumption that I would probably find out the truth for myself eventually.

All the while that I was conducting these experiments in animals, I was also treating patients with laryngeal paralysis, and collecting video recordings of their larynges. In many patients, the precise location of the nerve injury could not be determined. Many lesions were idiopathic, or resulted from surgery when the nerve had not been identified. I identified for further analysis a group of patients in whom I conclusively locate the site of lesion, to either the RLN, or the upper vagus. These were patients who had a known surgical disruption of a nerve, or in whom laryngeal EMG demonstrated the site of lesion. Instead of using the usual classification of median, paramedian, and intermediate, I devised more quantitative measures of vocal fold position. As has been classically recorded, I found that the vocal fold was very abducted in patients with a vagus nerve lesion. But in patients with RLN lesions, there was considerable variation in position, ranging from what would be termed cadaveric to paramedian. I concluded, based on these observations, as well as the animal studies, and the previous report by Professor Hirano, which reported that the position of the vocal fold after RLN injury depended on the amount of residual or regenerated innervation of adductor muscles.

My study of these laryngeal images revealed something else. The paralyzed vocal fold was not only immobile, but was also shorter than the normal vocal fold. And the more abducted vocal fold also appeared shorter. Reviewing the literature, I found that this length differential in laryngeal paralysis had been previously noted by Brewer and colleagues. Our subsequent research in excised cadaver larynges indicates that the vocal fold is probably not shorter in laryngeal paralysis, but only seems so, because the vocal process moves upward as it moves outward. This rotates the vocal fold up out of the glottic plane that it *appears* to be shorter.

So my journey to try and control the CT muscle took me somewhere else. My finding that the CT does not adduct the vocal fold has been confirmed by other studies. And there is other evidence to support my finding that the RLN tends to regenerate. But normal function is not recovered because the nerve fibers do not grow back to the correct muscles. The ideal therapy for laryngeal paralylsis has yet to be discovered. My current objective is to find a way to improve the specificity of nerve regeneration. But who knows where that research will lead?

Configuration of the Glottis in Laryngeal Paralysis. I: Clinical Study

Gayle E. Woodson, MD

It is widely accepted in the American literature that the cricothyroid muscle is responsible for the paramedian position of the vocal fold in recurrent laryngeal nerve paralysis. However, support in the literature for this theory is not conclusive, and the cadaveric vocal fold position expected after lesions of the vagus nerve has also been reported in patients with an intact superior laryngeal nerve. This study compares the configuration of the glottis in patients with unilateral paralysis due to known lesions of either the recurrent laryngeal or vagus nerve. Normal subjects were studied as controls. Results indicate that the alteration of glottic configuration in laryngeal paralysis cannot be adequately characterized by standard terms of vocal fold position. The paralyzed vocal fold is shortened, with anterior rotation of the arytenoid. Patients with vagus nerve lesions had a statistically insignificant tendency for a more lateral vocal fold position, but a discrete difference in position between the two groups was not identified. This study also confirms prior observations that paralyzed vocal folds are frequently not denervated. These findings have significant implications for management of laryngeal paralysis.

INTRODUCTION

It has long been recognized that the symptoms of laryngeal paralysis vary considerably. Unilateral paralysis is usually manifested clinically by varying degrees of glottic incompetence, such as vocal breathiness or aspiration, but as many as 30% of patients may be asymptomatic.[1] Symptom severity is in great measure determined by the position assumed by the paralyzed vocal fold, and this varies, not only across subjects over time, but frequently within subjects over time.[2–4] Throughout the years, there has been much discussion in the literature of the factors controlling vocal fold position in laryngeal paralysis. In 1892, Semon amassed a bibliography of 232 papers on the subject![5]

The debate regarding forces responsible for variations in vocal fold position has primarily centered around two conflicting hypotheses. The Semon-Rosenbach hypothesis is that nerve fibers to abductor muscles are more sensitive to injury than those to adductor muscles, so that in a slowly progressive nerve lesion, the vocal fold will assume first a median, and later a lateral position.[4,6] However, clinical cases of vocal fold paralysis are rarely consistent with Semon's Law, and, in fact, vocal fold position is often observed to move from lateral to median with time.[2,3,7,8] The Wagner-Grossman hypothesis holds that in paralysis of the recurrent laryngeal nerve, the vocal fold is maintained near the midline by action of cricothyroid muscle. This theory was based on the observations that bilateral recurrent laryngeal nerve paralysis causes airway obstruction which is relieved by paralysis or removal of the cricothyroid muscle.[9–13] In 1970, Dedo's study of laryngeal paralysis in humans and dogs established general acceptance of the Wagner-Grossman hypothesis.[14] Some methods of treatment for recurrent laryngeal nerve paralysis are based on the assumption that deactivation of the cricothyroid muscle will result in lateralization of the affected vocal fold.[15,16]

The literature casts considerable doubt on the Wagner-Grossman hypothesis. Although initial reports indicated that inactivation of the cricothyroid muscle produced relief of airway obstruction in both clinical and experimental bilateral recurrent laryngeal nerve paralysis, subsequent clinical applications failed to confirm this.[15] There are also many clinical reports of cases of laryngeal paralysis which do not conform to the Wagner-Grossman hypothesis.[17–21] Several reports of electromyography in patients with recurrent laryngeal nerve paralysis have indicated no discernible correlation between the status of cricothyroid innervation and the position of the paralyzed vocal fold.[22–25] In addition, new information on the physiology of the cricothyroid muscle makes it appear unlikely to affect vocal fold position.[26,27]

To determine whether the cricothyroid muscle

Presented, in part, as a Candidate's Thesis to the American Laryngological, Rhinological and Otological Society, Inc., September 1992.

From the Division of Otolaryngology—Head and Neck Surgery, University of California, San Diego. Dr. Woodson is now at the Department of Otolaryngology, University of Tennessee, Memphis.

Research was funded by a VA Merit Review Grant and a Clinical Investigator Development Award (CIDA) from the National Institute of Deafness and Communicative Disorders.

Send Reprint Requests to Gayle E. Woodson, MD, University of Tennessee, Memphis, College of Medicine, Department of Otolaryngology, 956 Court Ave., Room B224, Memphis, TN 38163.

TABLE I.
Clinical Data.

Patient Number	Age	Sex	RvsL	Etiology	Duration	Glottic Angle	Vocal Fold Ratio	Lesion
1	76	M	L	S/P XRT for Lung cancer	1 year	42	.71	RLN
2	39	M	R	Spider bite	7 months	40	.71	RLN
3	35	M	R	Intubation	2 months	42	.68	RLN
4	29	M	L	Intubation	2 months	38	.77	RLN
5	60	M	L	S/P Aortic aneurism resection	2 weeks	46	.70	RLN
6	76	M	R	Tracheal cancer	2 months	49	.56	RLN
7	57	M	L	Lung cancer	2 months	55	.83	RLN
8	62	F	R	Tumor resection/vagus sacrificed	2 months	40	.66	Vagus
9	43	F	L	Tumor resection/vagus injured	2 months	40	.75	Vagus
10	36	M	R	Tumor resection/vagus sacrificed	2 months	49	.47	Vagus
11	48	M	R	Tumor resection/vagus sacrificed	31 years	47	.75	Vagus
12	37	F	R	Tumor resection/vagus sacrificed	1 year	55	.5	Vagus
13	72	M	R	Tumor resection/vagus injured	1 year	80	.5	Vagus
14	53	M	L	Tumor resection/vagus sacrificed	2 months	53	.67	Vagus

S/P = status post; XRT = radiation treatment; RLN = recurrent laryngeal nerve.

has a significant influence on the position of the paralyzed vocal fold, images obtained from videolaryngoscopy were objectively measured to determine glottic configuration in normal subjects as well as patients with known lesions of either the vagus or recurrent laryngeal nerve.

METHODS

Subjects were selected from patients referred to the author for treatment of glottic insufficiency. All patients who presented over a 2-year period, in whom the site of lesion could be determined by either electromyography (EMG), or anatomical demonstration of a lesion, were included in the study. In 6 patients, the upper cervical vagus nerve had been sacrificed during resection of a tumor, and another patient had laryngeal and pharyngeal paralysis after excision of a tumor at the base of the skull, without recognition of direct trauma to the vagus nerve. Electromyography in that patient confirmed incomplete denervation in both the cricothyroid and thyroarytenoid muscles. Six patients had recurrent laryngeal nerve injury. In 4, sparing of the cricothyroid muscle was confirmed by electromyography, and in the other 2, the site of lesion was clearly apparent. In all patients, fixation of the cricoarytenoid joint was ruled out as a cause for the fixation, either by palpation during direct laryngoscopy or open laryngeal surgery, or by observation of return of motion with resolution of the paralysis. Clinical data are summarized in Table I. Normal subjects were randomly selected patients seen during the same time period for problems other than glottic insufficiency.

All subjects were studied with videolaryngoscopy. The larynx was visualized with a rigid Nagashima 70-degree telescope or an Olympus ENF-P3 flexible endoscope coupled to a color video camera (Panasonic WV-CD11A), with illumination provided by a 400-W halogen light source. The image was recorded on a VHS tape recorder. Subjects were observed during quiet breathing, and were then asked to take a deep breath and phonate "ee." This was repeated at least three times in each subject.

The glottic configuration was analyzed during three different prephonatory inspirations in each subject of the video image. Actual measurements were used, as subjective judgments of median and paramedian posterior have been shown to be unreliable.[28] Inspiration was selected because it is known to activate the cricothyroid muscle.[29] Three frames were selected for analysis in each subject, representing the point of maximal abduction in three separate inhalations. Measurements were expressed in degrees of rotation, or a ratios between lengths. The anterior glottic angle was measured to determine the combined abduction of the two vocal folds. As a means of assessing the relative contribution of each vocal fold to the glottal angle, the degree of arytenoid rotation was determined on each side by measuring the angle between the anterior (membranous) and posterior portions of the vocal fold on each side (Fig. 1). Because the vocal fold has been reported to be shorter in cases of unilateral cricothyroid paralysis,[28] the length of the paralyzed and normal sides were compared by determining the ratio of the length of the membranous portion of the paralyzed vocal fold to that of the normal vocal fold.

For each parameter, the mean values in the two groups, vagal and recurrent laryngeal nerve injury, were compared using the unpaired Student's t test. Significance was set at $P<.05$.

RESULTS

The mean measurements of angles are summarized in Figure 2. In the control subjects, the mean anterior glottic angle was 61.5 degrees, with a standard error of 2.2 degrees. Value ranged from 51 to 71 degrees across subjects, but variability within subjects was quite low. Mean vocal fold angle was 110.2 degrees, with a standard error of 1.9 degrees; values ranged from 105 to 115 degrees. In repeated measures in five control subjects, anterior glottic angle was very reproducible. The mean angle was within 1 degree in four subjects, and within 3 degrees in the fifth. The

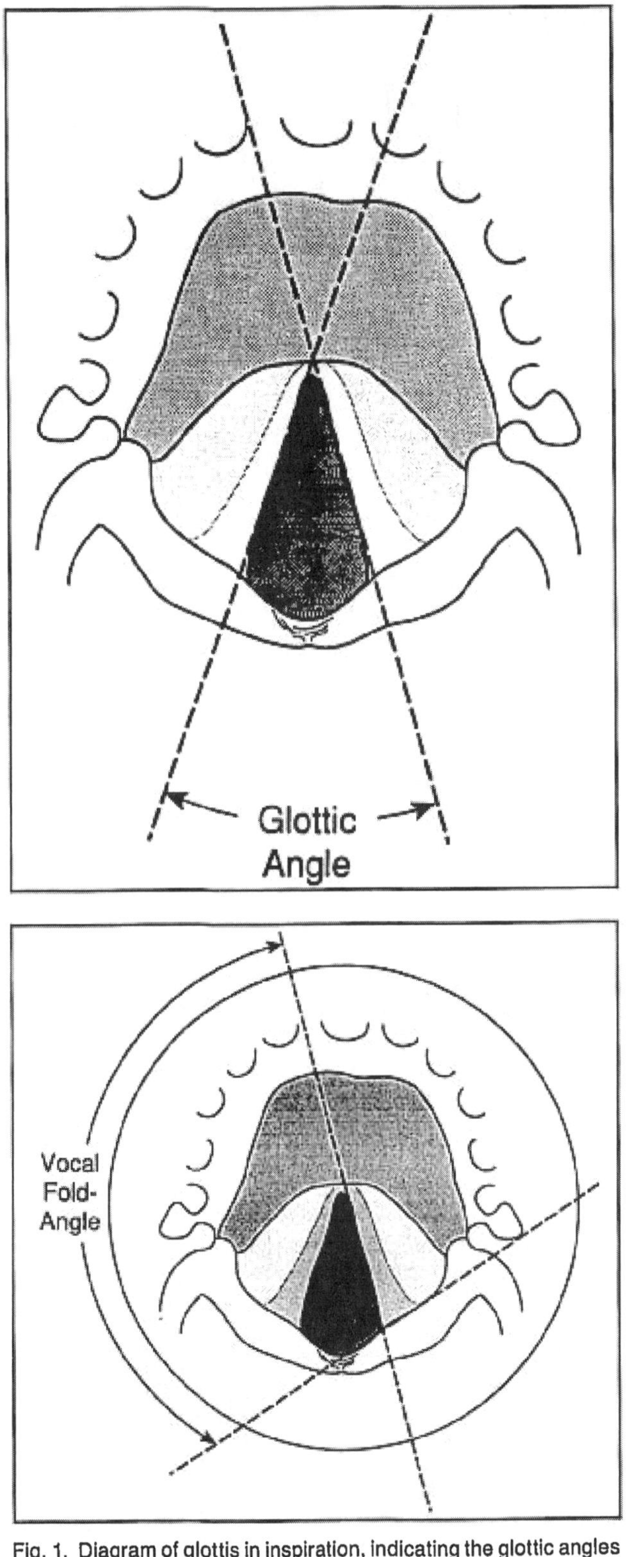

Fig. 1. Diagram of glottis in inspiration, indicating the glottic angles measured in this study. **Top.** Anterior glottic angle is between the membranous portions of the vocal folds. This is determined, even in cases of vocal fold bulging or bowing, by connecting the anterior commissure with both vocal processes. **Bottom.** Vocal fold angle (VFA) is formed by the anterior (membranous) and posterior portions of the vocal fold. The apex is the vocal process which moves laterally during abduction, decreasing the angle. The angle increases with adduction.

vocal-fold–arytenoid angle was somewhat less reliable, varying up to 10 degrees in one subject.

The anterior glottic angle in both patient groups differed significantly from that in control subjects. The mean anterior glottic angle was 52 degrees in the vagal paralysis group, and 41 degrees in patients with recurrent laryngeal nerve lesions; however the difference was not statistically different. The mean value in the vagal group was skewed by one patient with an anterior glottic angle of 80 degrees. The other six patients in that group had glottic angles ranging from 40 to 55 degrees. Angles in the recurrent laryngeal nerve injury group ranged from 30 to 46 degrees.

The vocal fold angle in the mobile vocal fold of patients was not significantly different from that of normal controls. But in every patient, the vocal fold angle was greater on the paralyzed side than on the normal side, and this difference was statistically significant. The mean vocal fold angle was slightly larger in the vagal than in the recurrent laryngeal nerve injury group, 122 versus 118 degrees; however, the difference was not statistically significant. The vocal fold angle was more difficult to measure on the paralyzed side, as the apex of the angle (the vocal process) was frequently obscured by an overhanging arytenoid. In these cases, the angle was extrapolated by extending lines formed by the visible portions of the vocal fold.

In every patient, the arytenoid cartilage on the paralyzed side was tipped anteriorly. Sometimes the membranous vocal fold was partially obscured by the overhanging arytenoid. In such cases, length was interpolated by extending lines from the visible portions of the vocal folds. The ratio of the apparent length of the paralyzed membranous vocal fold to that of the normal side was less than one in every patient. The ratio was smaller in the vagus group, but there was no significant difference between patient groups (Fig. 3). In control subjects, vocal fold length was equal on the two sides.

All patients demonstrated compensatory hyperfunction of the mobile larynx during phonation. Not only did the normal vocal fold consistently cross the midline, but it also shortened so that the vocal processes approached and usually achieved approximation. This process of shortening resulted in considerable anteroposterior compression of the glottis, often with bowing of the normal vocal fold (Fig. 4). In some patients, the paralyzed vocal fold was driven laterally by the hyperadducting force of the normal vocal fold during phonation.

Four patients with recurrent laryngeal nerve injury and one patient with a vagus nerve injury had electromyography. Denervation of involved muscles was evidenced by fibrillation potentials, reduced interference patterns, polyphasic action potentials, and/or bizarre high-frequency discharges. Some degree of voluntary motor-unit activity was present in

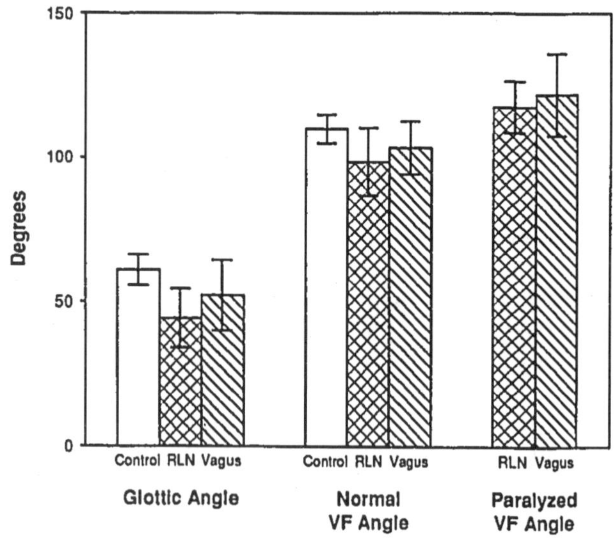

Fig. 2. Laryngeal angles in control subjects and patients with injuries of the recurrent laryngeal nerve (RLN) or vagus nerve (VFA = vocal fold angle.)

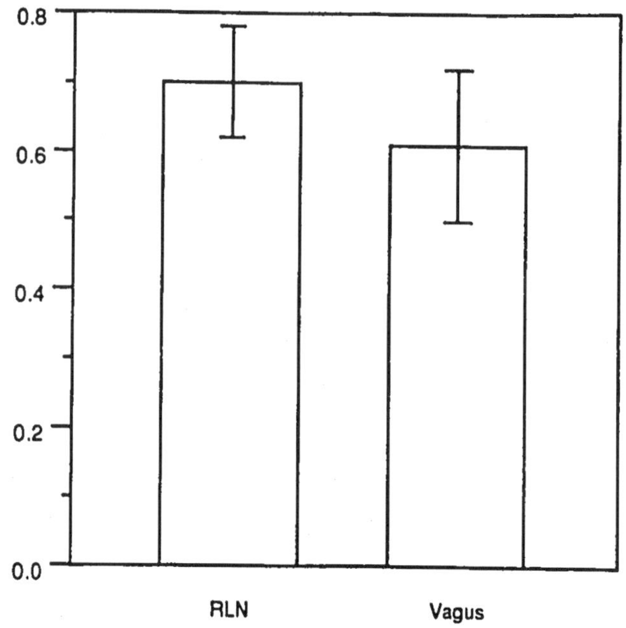

Fig. 3. Vocal fold ratio. Length of the membranous portion of the paralyzed vocal fold expressed as a fraction of that of the normal side (P = .12, unpaired Student's t test).

all patients, despite the clinical findings of immobility.

DISCUSSION

The data do not support the notion that there are distinct "positions" of the paralyzed vocal fold in recurrent laryngeal and vagus nerve injury, and indicate that the cricothyroid muscle is not the determining factor for vocal fold position in laryngeal paralysis. The somewhat larger average glottic angle in patients with vagus nerve paralysis is consistent with the widely accepted clinical impression that vocal fold position tends to be more lateral in these patients. However, the range of values for the anterior glottic angle was broad in each group and there was considerable overlap.

Several prior reports have also failed to demonstrate a dependence of vocal fold position on the cricothyroid muscle. In EMG studies of 114 cases of unilateral laryngeal paralysis by Hirano, *et al.*, only 2 of the 10 patients with evidence of cricothyroid muscle denervation manifested an intermediate vocal fold position.[22] Thus, the majority of patients with cricothyroid involvement actually had a median or paramedian vocal fold. These authors noted a statistically insignificant trend for the paralyzed vocal fold to lie more medially when fewer motor units were affected. A relationship of the degree of voluntary thyroarytenoid motor-unit activity to vocal fold position was more convincingly demonstrated by others.[23,30]

Reviewing the mechanics of the laryngeal skeleton, it seems extremely unlikely that loss of contraction of one cricothyroid muscle would significantly affect position of the ipsilateral vocal fold, and not the other.[23] The cricoid, with which both arytenoids articulate, is a rigid ring, and both vocal folds insert into the same point on the anterior thyroid cartilage. The cricothyroid joints essentially allow rotation in one plane. Thus, even with significant distortion of the thyorid lamina, contraction of one cricothyroid joint should equally affect both vocal folds. And even if physiologic contraction of both cricothyroid muscles could exert a medializing force on a paralyzed vocal fold, loss of one cricothyroid muscle would not completely abolish that force.

The length of the paralyzed vocal fold was shortened in both groups. If the cricothyroid muscle were exerting a significant pull on the paralyzed fold, one might expect a longer vocal fold in patients with an intact cricothyroid muscle, *i.e.*, the recurrent laryngeal nerve injury group. An alternative result of cricothyroid contraction could be an anterior displacement of the paralyzed vocal fold, due to loss of the opposing contraction by the posterior cricoarytenoid muscle. In fact, anterior displacement of the arytenoid was observed in all patients. The mean length ratio was somewhat smaller in the vagus injury group, but this difference was not statistically significant, and as in glottic angle values, the ratios in the two groups were overlapping, not distinct.

The shortening of the paralyzed vocal fold demonstrated in the present study was also recently noted by Brewer, *et al.*[28] They also found, in works by other authors, illustrations which confirmed this observation.[94–95]

In the present study, the shortening of the vocal fold in both groups was associated with anterior displacement of the arytenoid. Phonation was impaired not only by the presence of a glottal gap, but also by

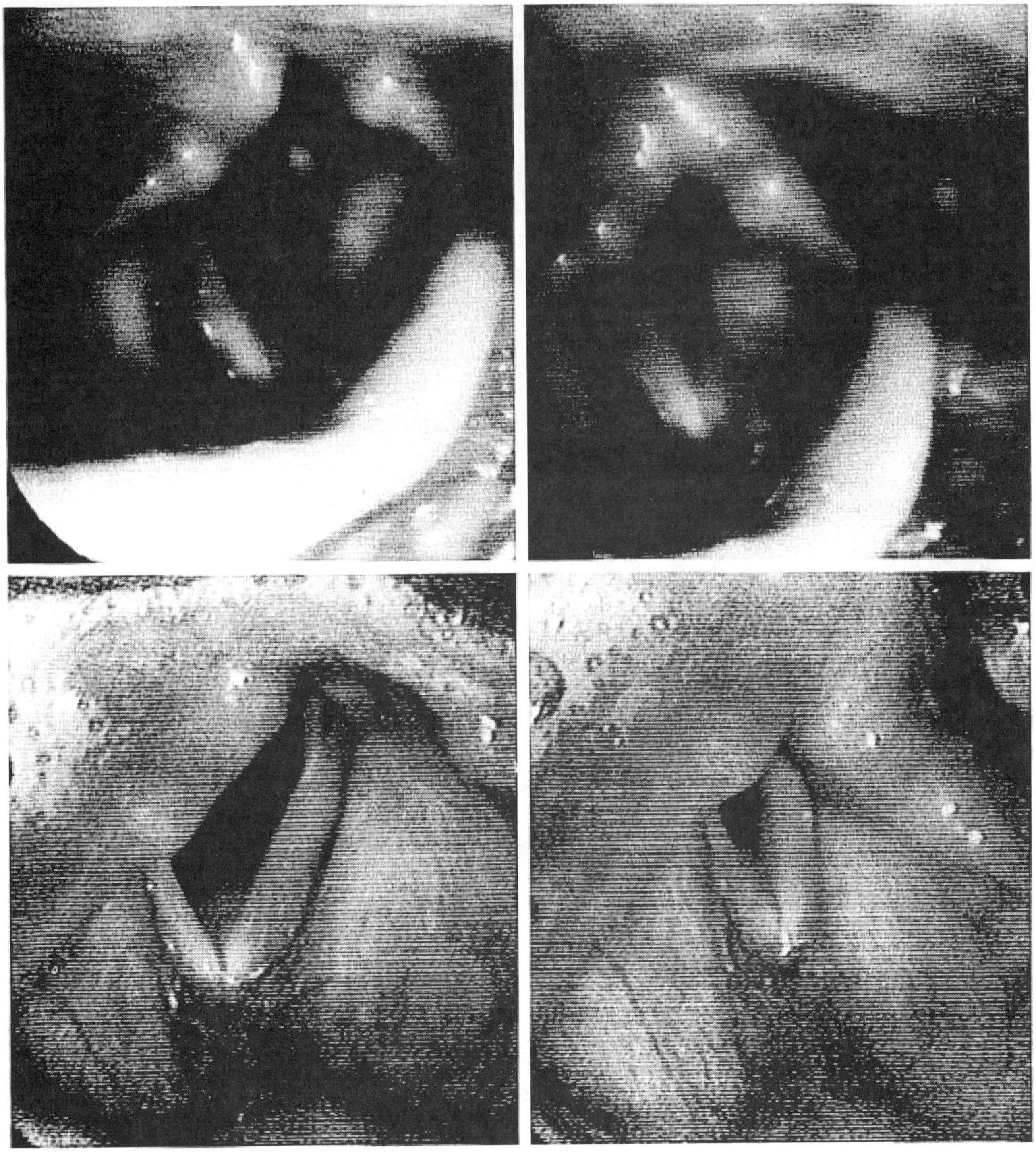

Fig. 4. Videoendoscopic picture of the larynx in patients with chronic paralysis of the recurrent laryngeal nerve **(top)** or vagus nerve **(bottom)**.

the need for the patient to compress the glottis in the plane, to accomplish approximation of the vocal processes. Every patient used this mechanism to accomplish approximation of the vocal processes, so that the length of the membranous vocal folds was equal on the two sides. This maneuver requires increased effort, and frequently results in bowing of the normal vocal fold, thus increasing glottal incompetence. Shortening, and the accompanying compensatory hyperfunction, may limit the success of surgical procedures designed to medialize the paralyzed vocal fold. Neither Teflon® injection nor thyroplasty correct the deficiency in length, and so patients must still use compensatory hyperfunction to achieve glottal closure.

It is difficult to draw conclusions regarding the role of arytenoid rotation in determining vocal fold position and anterior glottic angle. It is of note that the vocal fold angle in the normal vocal fold was quite similar in the two groups, so that differences in abduction of the normal vocal fold does not seem to be responsible for the somewhat larger glottic angle in the vagal-paralysis group. There was a small and statistically insignificant difference in the vocal-fold–arytenoid angle between the two groups of paralyzed vocal folds, but the angle was actually larger in the vagal group. This had not been expected, as active abduction is associated with lateral vocal process rotation and, hence, a narrower vocal fold-to-arytenoid angle. The lack of the expected relationship between rotation and abduction in the paralyzed group is probably related to the fact that the paralyzed vocal fold is lateralized by passive forces, rather than active abduction. It should also be noted that the measured vocal fold angle only represents apparent rotation in a two-dimensional image, and does not account for motion outside of that plane.

What could account for variations in the position of the paralyzed vocal fold? Many factors may be involved. A vagal lesion disrupts much more than the motor nerve supply to the larynx. Pharyngeal muscles are also denervated. Sensory information is disrupted, not only from receptors in the larynx and pharynx, but also from the trachea and lungs. Patients with vagal lesions due to neck surgery may have had disruption of other cranial nerves and are also very likely to have sustained disruption of the nerve supply to the cervical strap muscles. Any of these additional lesions could have an impact on configuration of the glottis.

Another consideration is that 6 of the 7 patients with vagal paralysis in this series had total disruption of the nerve. In contrast, none of the patients with recurrent laryngeal nerve injuries had complete denervation on electromyography, or documentation of complete transection of the nerve. In fact, 2 of the 6 patients with recurrent laryngeal nerve lesions ultimately recovered function. Therefore, differences in vocal fold position may be due to differences in the degree of nerve injury.

A third possibility is that differences in vocal fold position may be affected by the degree of reinnervation. The literature indicates a remarkable propensity for regeneration of the recurrent laryngeal nerve.[33–36] It may be that the likelihood of regeneration, as well as the appropriateness of reinnervation of specific motor units, is influenced by the distance of the lesion from the larynx. That is to say, a patient with a recurrent laryngeal nerve lesion near the larynx may be much more likely to recover by regeneration than one with a lesion of the more remote vagus nerve.

The presence of motor-unit potentials in the absence of mobility, noted in this study, has been previously reported by others.[8,25,37,40] This phenomenon could be accounted for by persisting or regenerated innervation, with either insufficient contractile force to produce movement, or simultaneous synkinetic contractions which result in no net displacement.

The question of whether or not clinically paralyzed laryngeal muscles are in fact denervated has considerable clinical significance in cases where one is considering reinnervation. Crumley has pointed out that an innervated muscle will not accept additional innervation.[41–45] The presence of persisting or regenerated innervation in a paralyzed larynx could well account for the varied clinical success reported with the nerve-muscle pedicle technique of reinnervation. Animal experiments document effectiveness of the technique.[46,47] But any technique of reinnervation would not be expected to be successful in patients whose laryngeal muscles are not, in fact, denervated. Tucker, aware of the fact that the nerve muscle pedicle is unlikely to work if the larynx is not denervated, has recommended palpation of the cricoarytenoid joint to rule out fixation. It would seem prudent to include laryngeal electromyography in the preoperative evaluation of these patients.

There are of course many other factors which can influence the position of the vocal fold in laryngeal paralysis. As the interarytenoid muscle is bilaterally innervated, it has been attributed with exerting a medial pull on the vocal fold in unilateral paralysis, accounting for the paramedian or intermediate position.[4,48,49] This cannot, of course, account for the paramedian position in bilateral paralysis.

Extralaryngeal branching of the recurrent nerve has been reported to be a common occurrence, and one could implicate injury to an isolated abductor branch as a cause of a median or paramedian vocal fold position.[50–58] Other authors have noted the potential role of muscle atrophy in determining vocal fold position.[59–62] The association of muscle atrophy with a lateral vocal fold position has been well demonstrated in autopsy studies.[21,61,63] Other authors have suggested an opposite effect of denervation: that denervation adductor muscles would develop fibrosis and contracture, and pull the vocal fold medially.[50,64] None of these other factors can be ignored, as each could have a significant influence on glottal configuration.

SUMMARY

In view of the numerous factors which can influence the configuration of the glottis in laryngeal paralysis, the statement made by Cody (1946)[65] seems as true today as it was then (*i.e.*, it is impossible to diagnose the site of the nerve lesion on the basis of vocal fold position). Although many questions remain to be answered, there are some conclusions regarding glottic configuration which seem justified on the basis of our present knowledge:

1. Videolaryngoscopy permits quantitative as

sessment of glottic configuration in two dimensions.

2. Vocal fold position in laryngeal paralysis is not determined by the status of innervation of the cricothyroid muscle.

3. Laryngeal paralysis not only affects the rotational position of the vocal fold in the axial plane, but also results in shortening of the membranous vocal fold. Further research is needed to determine three-dimensional changes in glottic configuration.

4. Compensatory hyperfunction in laryngeal paralysis involves not only hyperadduction of the normal vocal fold, but also anterior-posterior compression of the glottis.

5. Type I thyroplasty and Teflon® injection to medialize the paralyzed vocal fold address only the rotation of the vocal fold in the axial plane and do not correct the deficient length.

6. Some degree of voluntary motor-unit activity is common in the paralyzed larynx. This may represent residual or regenerated innervation. Laryngeal EMG should always be performed when laryngeal reinnervation is being considered.

7. Residual or regenerated innervation may be responsible for the variations in vocal fold position and symptoms in patients with laryngeal paralysis.

8. Future development of improved therapy for patients with laryngeal paralysis should take into account the need to correct complex distortion and should address the problems caused by synkinetic reinnervation.

BIBLIOGRAPHY

1. Work, W.P.: Paralysis and Paresis of the Vocal Cords: A statistical review. *Arch Otolaryngol*, 43:267–280, 1941.
2. Arnold, G.E.: Vocal Rehabilitation of Paralytic Dysphonia: III. Present Concepts of Laryngeal Paralysis. *Arch Otol*, 65:317–336, 1932.
3. New, G.B. and Childrey, J.H.: Paralysis of the Vocal Cords: A Study of 217 Medical Cases. *Arch Otol*, 16:143–159, 1932.
4. Rosenbach, O.: Zur Lehre von Dopelseitigen Totalen Lachmung des Nerv. Laryngeus Inferior (Recurrens). *Breslauer Arztliche Zeitschrift*, 2:14–16, 27–30, 1880.
5. Semon, F.: The Study of Laryngeal Paralysis Since the Introduction of the Laryngoscope. *Brain*, 15:471–521, 1892.
6. Semon, F.: Clinical Remarks. On the Proclivity of the Abductor Fibers of the Recurrent Laryngeal Nerve to become Affected Sooner Than the Adductor Fibers or Even Exclusively; in Cases of Undoubted Central or Peripheral Injury or Disease of the Roots or Trunks of the Pneumogastric, Spinal Accessory or Recurrent Nerves. *Arch Laryngol*, 2:197–222, 1881.
7. Smith, A.B., Lambert, V.F. and Wallace, H.L.: Paralysis of the Recurrent Laryngeal Nerves: A Survey of Two Hundred and Thirty-Five Cases. *Edinburgh Med Surg J*, 40:344–354, 1933.
8. Faaborg-Andersen, K.: The Position of Paretic Vocal Folds. *Acta Otolaryngol*, 57:50–54, 1964.
9. Legallois, 1812. Cited by Burger, H.: Zur Stimbandstellung nach recurrens Durchschneidung und zur Frage der Posticuslahmung. *Arch Laryng Rhin*, 9–10:203, 1899–1900.
10. Burger, H.: Zur Stimbandstellung nach recurrens Durchschneidung und zur Frage der Posticuslahmung, *Arch Laryng Rhin* 9–10:203, 1899–1900.
11. Wagner, R.: Die medianstellung der stimmbander bei der rekurrenslahmung. *Arch Pah Anat Physiol* 120:437–549, 1890.
12. Grosman, M.: Experimentelle bietrage zur lehre von der "psticuslahmung." *Arch laryng u Rhin*, 6:282, 1897.
13. Grosman, M.: Contribution to the Mutual Functional Relationships of the Muscles of the Larynx. *Arch Laryngol Rhinol*, 18:463–471, 1906.
14. Dedo, H.H.: The Paralyzed Larynx: An Electromyographic Study in Dogs and Humans. LARYNGOSCOPE, 80:1455–1517, 1970.
15. Tschiassny, K.: Studies Concerning the Action of the Musculus Cricothyreoideus. LARYNGOSCOPE, 54:589–604, 1944.
16. Cohen, S. and Thompson, J.W.: Use of Botulinum Toxin to Lateralize True Vocal Cords: A Biochemical Method to Relieve Bilateral Abductor Vocal Cord Paralysis. *Ann Otol Rhinol Laryngol*, 96:534–541, 1987.
17. Hofer, G.: Unterscuchunngen bei Lahmunger der motorschen kehlkopfnerven. *Acta Otolaryngol*, 43:100–107, 1953.
18. Jaschek, J.: Uber wesheselseitige Funktionsbeziehungen der Kehlkopfumuskulatur. *Arch Ohr Kehlopfhilk*, 163:372, 1953.
19. Lewy, R.B. and Mathews, R.: Immediate Temporary Restoration of the Glottic Valve Function. LARYNGOSCOPE, 75:1348–1351, 1965.
20. Kirchner, J.A.: Intrathoracic Injury to the Motor Nerve Supply of the Larynx. *Acta Otolaryngol*, 67:163–169, 1977.
21. Quiney, R.E. and Michaels, L.: Histopathology of Vocal Cord Palsy from Recurrent Laryngeal Nerve Damage. *J Otolaryngol*, 19:237–241, 1990.
22. Hirano, M., Nozoe, I., Shin, T., *et al.*: Electromyography for Laryngeal Paralysis. In: *Neurolaryngology: Recent Advances*, Hirano, M., Kirchner, J., Bless, D. eds. College-Hill Press, Boston, pp. 232–248, 1987.
23. Hirose, H., Kobayashi, T., Okamura, M., *et al.*: Recurrent Laryngeal Nerve Palsy. *J Otolaryngol Japan*, 70:1–17, 1967.
24. Sawashima, M., Sato, M., Funasaka, S., *et al.*: Electromyography of the Larynx and Its Clinical Applications. *J Otolaryngol Japan*, 61:1357–1364, 1958.
25. Berry, H. and Blair, R.L.: Isolated Vagus Nerve Palsy and Vagal Mononeuritis. *Arch Otolaryngol*, 106:333–338, 1980.
26. Woodson, G.E., Sant'Ambrogio, F., Mathew, O., *et al.*: Effects of Cricothyroid Muscle Contraction on Laryngeal Resistance and Glottic Area. *Ann Otol Rhinol Laryngol*, 98:119–124, 1989.
27. Tully, A., Brancatisano, A., Loring, S.H., *et al.*: Influence of Posterior Cricoarytenoid Muscle Activity on Pressure-Flow Relationship of the Larynx. *J Appl Physiol*, 70:2252–2258, 1991.
28. Brewer, D.W., Woo, P., Casper, J.K., *et al.*: Unilateral Recurrent Laryngeal Nerve Paralysis: A Re-Examination. *J Voice*, 5:178–185, 1991.
29. Woodson, G.E.: Respiratory Activity of the Cricothyroid Muscle in Conscious Humans. LARYNGOSCOPE, 100:49–53, 1990.
30. Ueda, N.: A Clinical Study of the Recurrent Laryngeal Nerve Paralysis Following Surgical Operations. Part II. *Hiroshima J Med Sci*, 16:431–459, 1968.
31. Moore, G.P.: Observations on Laryngeal Disease, Laryngeal Behavior, and Voice. *Ann Otol Rhinol Laryngol*, 85:553–564, 1976.
32. Ward, P.H. and Berci, G.: Observations on So-Called Idiopathic Vocal Cord Paralysis. *Ann Otol Rhinol Laryngol*, 91:558–563, 1982.
33. Crumley, R.L.: Selective Reinnervation of Vocal Cord Adductors in Unilateral Vocal Cord Paralysis. *Ann Otol Rhinol Laryngol*, 93:351–356, 1984.
34. Netterville, J.L., Stone, R.E., Rainey, C., *et al.*: Recurrent Laryngeal Nerve Avulsion for Treatment of Spastic Dysphonia. *Ann Otol Rhinol Laryngol*, 100:10–14, 1991.
35. Wilson, F.B., Oldring, D.J. and Mueller, K.: Recurrent Larynge-

al Nerve Dissection: A Case Report Involving Return of Spastic Dysphonia After Initial Surgery. *J Speech Hear Disord*, 45:112–118, 1980.
36. Schiratzki, H. and Fritzell, B.: Treatment of Spasmodic Dysphonia by Means of Resection of the Recurrent Laryngeal Nerve. *Acta Otolaryngol Suppl (Stockh)*, 449:115–117, 1988.
37. Tomita, H.: An Electromyographic Study of Recurrent Laryngeal Nerve Paralysis. *Nippon Jiblinkoka Gakkai Kaiho*, 70:963–985, 1967.
38. Hiroto, I., Hirano, M. and Tomita, H.: EMG Investigation of Human Vocal Paralysis. *Ann Otol Rhinol Laryngol*, 77:296–304, 1968.
39. Kawano, Y.: Study on Laryngeal Paralysis. *Jpn J Otol*, 67:159–176, 1964.
40. Rodriquez, A.A., Myers, B.R. and Ford, C.N.: Laryngeal Electromyography in the Diagnosis of Laryngeal Nerve Injuries. *Arch Phys Med Rehabil*, 71:587–590, 1990.
41. Crumley, R.: Experiments in Laryngeal Reinnervation. LARYNGOSCOPE, 92(Suppl 30): 1–27, 1982.
42. Elsberg, C.A.: Experiments on Motor Nerve Regeneration and Direct Neurotization of Paralyzed Muscles by Their Own and Foreign Nerves. *Science*, 45:318, 1917.
43. Guth, L.: Neuromuscular Function after Regeneration of Interrupted Nerve Fibers Into Partially Denervated Muscle. *Exp Neurol*, 6:129–141, 1962.
44. Edds, M.V.: Collateral Nerve Regeneration. *Quart Rev Biol*, 28:260–276, 1953.
45. Gwynn, D.G. and Aitken, J.T.: The Formation of New Motor Endplates in Mammalian Skeletal Muscle. *J Anat*, 100:111–126, 1966.
46. Hengerer, A.S. and Tucker, H.M.: Restoration of Function in the Paralyzed Canine Vocal Cord. *Arch Otolaryngol*, 97:247–250, 1973.
47. Neal, D., Cummings, C. and Sutton, D.: Delayed Reinnervation of the Unilateral Vocal Cord Paralysis in Dogs. *Otolaryngol Head Neck Surg*, 89:608–612, 1981.
48. Evoy, M.H.: Paralysis of the Vocal Cords After Thyroidectomy. *Am J Surg*, 102:73–78, 1961.
49. Pressman, J.J. and Keleman, G.: The Larynx. *Physiol Rev*, 35:506–554, 1955.
50. King, B.T. and Gregg, R.L.: An Anatomical Reason for the Various Behaviors of Paralyzed Vocal Cords. *Ann Otol Rhinol Laryngol*, 57:925–944, 1948.
51. Horsley, J.S.: Suture of the Recurrent Laryngeal Nerve. *Southern Surgical and Gynecological Association*, 22:161–167, 1909.
52. Clerf, L.H. and Baltzell, W.H.: Reevaluation of Semon's Hypothesis. LARYNGOSCOPE, 63:693–699, 1953.
53. Bowden, R.E.M. and Scheuer, J.L.: Weights of Abductor Muscles of the Human Larynx. *J Laryngol*, 74:971–980, 1960.
54. Morrison, L.F.: Recurrent Laryngeal Nerve Paralysis: A Revised Concept Based on the Dissections of One Hundred Cadavers. *Ann Otol Rhinol Laryngol*, 61:567–592, 1952.
55. Rustad, W.H.: Revised Anatomy of Recurrent Laryngeal Nerves: Surgical Importance Based on the Dissection of 100 Cadavers. *J Clin Endocrinol Metabol*, 14:87–96, 1954.
56. Arnold, G.E.: Vocal Rehabilitation of Paralytic Dysphonia: IV. Paralytic Dysphonia Due to Unilateral Recurrent Nerve Paralysis. *Arch Otol*, 68:284–300, 1958.
57. Evoy, M.H.: Observations With Certain Experiments on the Paralyzed Vocal Cords in Dogs. LARYNGOSCOPE, 70:1268–1272, 1960.
58. Gregg, R.L.: Experimental Laryngeal Paralysis. *Ann Otol Rhinol Laryngol*, 66:656–678, 1957.
59. Lemere, F.: Innervation of the Larynx IV: Analysis of Semon's Law. *Ann Otol Rhinol Laryngol*, 43:525–540, 1934.
60. Ward, P.H., Berci, G. and Calcaterra, T.C.: Superior Laryngeal Nerve Paralysis: An Often Overlooked Entity. *Trans Am Acad Ophthalmol Otol*, 80:78–89, 1977.
61. Kirchner, J.A.: Atrophy of Laryngeal Muscles in Vagal Paralysis. LARYNGOSCOPE, 76:1753–1765, 1966.
62. Quinney, R.E.: Laryngeal Electromyography: Useful Technique for the Investigation of Vocal Cord Palsy. *Clin Otol*, 14:305–316, 1989.
63. Bridger, G.P.: Unilateral Laryngeal Palsy: A Histopathological Study. *J Laryngol Otol*, 91:303–307, 1977.
64. Meurman, O.H.: Theories of Vocal Cord Paralysis. *Acta Otolaryngol*, 38:460–472, 1950.
65. Cody, C.C., Jr.: Associated Paralysis of the Larynx. *Ann Otol Rhinol Laryngol*, 55:549–561, 1946.

Commentary

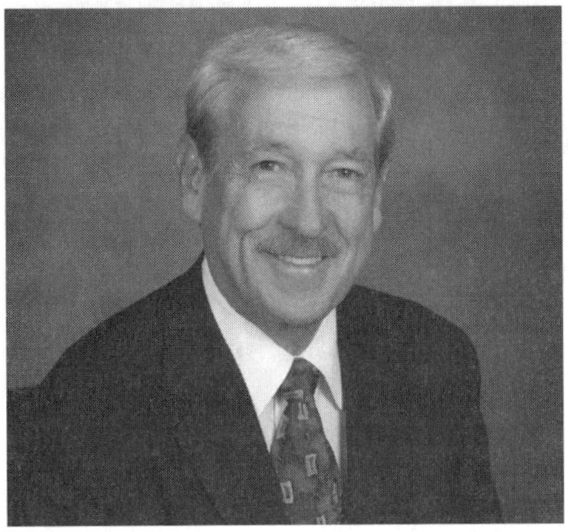

Roger L. Crumley, MD, MBA

The following manuscript (Benninger MS, Crumley RL, Ford C.N., Gould WJ, Hanson DG, Ossoff RH, Sataloff RT. *Otolaryngol Head Neck Surg.* 1994;111(4):497–508) was a good synopsis of the state-of-the-art of the evaluation and treatment of the unilateral paralyzed vocal fold when published in October 1994. Actually, much of this particular publication was received and collated by Dr. Benninger 8 to 12 months prior to publication, so it was in essence "state-of-the-art" in late 1993. Since that time, in my opinion there have been five major changes in the field of neurolaryngology that have resulted in newer viewpoints and understanding of this topic as follows:

- Nomenclature ("paralysis" vs "immobility" vs "motion impairment")
- Laryngeal synkinesis
- Decrease in numbers of medialization laryngoplasty procedures being performed
- Increase in numbers of reinnervation and injection procedures performed
- Other advances in reinnervation relating to bilateral abductor vocal cord paralysis (Holinger, Holinger, Holinger, 1976)

In discussing these areas I was also asked to "offer insight into the more personal and human aspects of scientific investigation innovation . . . " As for the personal "human" side of the story, my own interest in this area was derived by listening to basic and clinical research papers related not to the larynx, but to the facial nerve, in the mid-1970s. I particularly remember several creative reinnervation techniques at the 1976 International Facial Nerve Symposium in Zurich, Switzerland. I don't really remember whether I heard a paper at that symposium or came up with the concept myself, but I do remember soon thereafter in late 1976 and early 1977 performing several procedures where I split the hypoglossal nerve (to spare a portion of the tongue's innervation) in performing hypoglossal-facial anastomosis. It was this splitting concept relating to hypoglossal-facial anastomosis that made me think about application of the principle of nerve splitting to laryngeal reinnervation techniques in managment of "unilateral vocal cord paralysis" (the term used in that era of the late 1970s and early 1980s.). My main focus was to perform animal research using a similar 50% splitting of the phrenic nerve with attachment of a free nerve graft and routing of those phrenic inspiratory nerve fibers to the posterior cricoarytenoid (PCA) muscle. It was hoped that this technique might find value in treating in patients with bilateral vocal cord paralysis and airway impairment. This preliminary series of animal experiments was conducted in the research laboratories of San Francisco General Hospital in the late 1970s. It provided promise for this type of reinnervation procedure for bilateral vocal cord paralysis (motion impairment).[1] I decided to make the continuation of this project the central focus of my Triological thesis, but at the time was still mainly focused on the phrenic nerve to PCA procedure for *bilateral* vocal cord paralysis. It was during the phrenic grafting to PCA experiment that the ansa hypoglossi (now cervicalis) to recurrent laryngeal nerve (RLN) anastomosis was conceived as a treatment for unilateral RLN paralysis.

I remember clearly discussing this during the 1979 Triological Society meeting with Dr. John Kirchner of Yale University, one of the most prolific researchers in laryngeal nerve and muscle innervation (April 1979). He felt that there was potential for this research to be clinically useful some day and encouraged me to proceed. I then decided on how many animals I needed to use and how the experiment would be done. The other important otolaryngologist who allowed this to go forward was Dr. Brian F. McCabe, Professor and Head of the Department of Otolaryngology at the University of Iowa. (I had encountered difficulty in finding pilot research grant money, space, and animals for the project and Dr. McCabe, when learning about the project and my problems in moving it forward, quite simply and clearly told me "just come do it at Iowa.") I will be forever indebted to these two pioneers in our field for their advice, mentoring, role modeling, and support.

This animal research had some unexpected consequences, which could probably be termed serendipitous. Although the original series of dogs described in the Triologic thesis did, in fact, show that there was promise for the phrenic nerve transfer/jump graft technique in reinnervating a single paralyzed PCA muscle, an unexpected side effect was the ability to reinnervate the rest of the muscles of the larynx using ansa hypoglossi (now more correctly called the ansa cervicalis) nerve branches. When subsequently, a patient of mine in San Francisco in the late 1970s asked me what might be able to be done for his vocal cord paralysis, I explained to him how Teflon injection would be the treatment of choice. He refused to have "a foreign substance" injected into his larynx and asked about research into alternative methods. I explained to him that Dr. Harvey Tucker had been using reinnervation techniques for some time and that I was also doing related animal research. I informed him that I could do that sort of reinnervation for him, and also that our canine experiments indicated promise for ansa cervicalis transfer. He requested that I perform the ansa procedure, and indeed it was successful in restoring his voice. This patient had presented with a schwannoma of the vagus nerve, and underwent an extensive cervical vagectomy for schwannoma. EMG had shown that his ipsilateral *cricothyroid muscle* was denervated as well. Being a singer, he told me that his upper register was still absent, even though his speaking voice had been restored from the ansa cervicalis operation. Accordingly, I subsequently reinnervated his paralyzed cricothyroid muscle with a muscle neurotization implant using the opposite ansa cervicalis nerve. He came back to the office and confirmed that his upper register had returned some 6 months after that procedure.

Hence, these early results reinforced my suspicion that these laryngeal reinnervation procedures could be used for *unilateral* paralysis (using the ansa cervicalis-recurrent laryngeal nerve anastomosis), as well as for *bilateral* motion impairment and airway obstruction, using the phrenic nerve-nerve graft-PCA technique.

Now for the five areas of change, refinement, and innovation since 1993 to 1994:

1. Nomenclature

The first aspect of change is in *nomenclature* of "vocal cord paralysis." Since the early 1990s laryngologists and neurolaryngologists (to some degree at the urging of the Neurolaryngology Study Group) have aimed for a more accurate description of the pathophysiology in larynges with immobile vocal folds. Accordingly, from the "vocal cord paralysis" of the 1960s to the 1993 to 1994 version "unilateral paralyzed vocal fold," we have evolved to a more accurate description of what the laryngologist sees. Currently the most common term used in the literature is that of *vocal fold immobility*. It has long been my view that this is not actually an accurate term, simply because a patient might have "vocal fold immobility" and yet show passive *mobility* of the arytenoid on passive mobility testing. ("Immobility" implies that the structure is both passively and actively immobile.) This creates a potential verbal conundrum insofar as a patient may have "vocal fold immobility," and yet still have a normal "passive mobility test" (eg, the cricoarytenoid joint is mobile and yet the vocal fold itself does not actively move secondary to muscular contraction). As a result, it is my own personal opinion that the best description of this clinical finding (the motionless state of one vocal fold) would be *vocal fold motion impairment*, as this means that the vocal fold does not move normally, and yet the results of the passive mobility test can not be in conflict with the term "immobility." In addition, the term *vocal fold motion impairment* makes no statement regarding the presence or absence of apparent (or EMG-confirmed) synkinesis. That is to say, the laryngologist describes a vocal fold that does not have normal abductive and adductive mobility (motion impairment), and yet it remains to be determined whether there is passive mobility as noted above, and as to whether laryngeal synkinesis is present or not.

2. Laryngeal Synkinesis

The second aspect of advancement since 1993 to 1994 is an expanded understanding of laryngeal synkinesis. I think it is correct to say that laryngologists now accept the concept of laryngeal synkinesis, a situation in which a vocal fold does not move normally and yet some form of laryngeal reinnervation has occurred. The laryngologist may observe slight movements either synchronous with the normal VF in abduction or adduction, or asynchronous (causing slight vocal fold abduction during the other side's adductive maneuvers and vice versa). Several scientific papers have introduced and confirmed the concept of laryngeal synkinesis, which results from spontaneous reinnervation of the vocal fold following recurrent laryngeal nerve injuries.[2–5] What is not known at this time is whether the synkinetic reinnervation source is the proximal ipsilateral recurrent laryngeal nerve (which has been injured), or some other neuromuscular source in the neck such as axon sprouting from the cricothyroid muscle and/or its external branch of the superior laryngeal nerve innervation, or as I suspect, some local sprouting from adjacent muscles into the paralyzed laryngeal muscles.

In any event, the synkinesis can be confirmed electrophysiologically by performing laryngeal electromyography. A recent excellent symposium cosponsored by the Neurolaryngology Study Group and the University of Wisconsin drew attention to the increasing role played by electromyography in ascertaining the amount of reinnervation and/or synkinesis that coexists in a patient with vocal fold motion impairment. In the October 1994 Benninger paper, EMG was included and covered. Some would continue to question whether the actual use of EMG has achieved universal acceptance and/or utilization in all patients with vocal fold motion impairment (or immobility syndrome, etc).

3. Decrease in Numbers of Medialization Laryngoplasty Procedures

In planning discussion topics for the Neurolaryngology Study Group, Dr. Lucian Sulica and I decided to cycle through several topic areas over a period of 2 years at our twice-annual meetings. In spring of 2007 at the San Diego meeting of the Neurolaryngology Study Group (in conjunction with the American Laryngological Association), Dr. Sulica and I cochaired a panel consisting of Dr. Harry Hoffman, Dr. Greg Postma, Dr. Paul Flint, and Dr. Clarence Sasaki. I asked them to discuss innovations, enhancements, and current techniques that they used in performing medialization laryngoplasty. In preparing for the 1-hour panel discussion, two of the four notified me that they had virtually stopped using the Isshiki type I medialization laryngoplasty technique. This surprised me and the attendees at the panel, but it was clear that an increase in *injection laryngoplasty* was the main cause and the reason for the decreased numbers of medialization procedures being performed.

To some degree, this has evolved due to the development of simpler and easier outpatient injection procedures. With the evolution of many, many new injectable materials over the last 10 years, longer acting injectibles have become available. Particularly, the introduction of Cymetra® and more recently Radiesse® have made the injection techniques much more user friendly for both laryngologists and for our patients.[6,7] In Europe, there are substances such as Bioplastique®, which are frequently used as vocal fold injectibles, and some practitioners are still fond of such substances as Zyplast® porcine collagen for VF injection.[8,9] Laryngologists have learned further utilization of outpatient injection techniques done in clinics and/or voice laboratories in which patients may have their vocal folds injected with one of these substances and achieve a long lasting (6 to 12 months or longer) treatment of their vocal fold motion impairment, without setting foot in an operating room or requiring general anesthesia.

4. Increase in Numbers of Injection and Reinnervation Procedures

This fourth "change in landscape" has to do with the increase in numbers of reinnervation procedures being performed for unilateral vocal fold motion impairment as well as injection, mentioned above. It would be appropriate to acknowledge the participation of Drs. George Goding, Ramon Esclamado, Randall Paniello, Rob Lorenz, Al Hillel, Nicole Maronian, and several others who have advanced and spread the usage of this technique in the United States.[10–13] In addition, notably Drs. Jean-Paul Marie of Rouen, France, and Prof. Hongliang Zheng in Shanghai, China, have reported large numbers of ansa-RLN reinnervation cases confirming the success rates reported with this technique in the U.S. (Dr. Zheng has performed over 300 ansa cervicalis-recurrent laryngeal nerve anastomoses as of fall 2007, personal communication).[14,15]

Since the 1994 Benninger article was published, my own feelings regarding the central therapeutic role of laryngeal reinnervation for unilateral vocal fold motion impairment have strengthened. Some of this may be because I have found results from medialization thyroplasty to be more variable and less permanent, and sometimes not permanent, accordingly not as dependable as reinnervation. In many patients, injection laryngoplasty is initially very attractive for many patients, and accordingly I often use Cymetra or Radiesse for short-term paralyses within a month or two of the RLN injury, reserving the reinnervation for the subsequently more permanent result. I generally do not perform ansa-RLN reinnervation until at least 9 months have elapsed following RLN injury, unless the RLN injury is well-documented, and the chances for recovery nil. The voices in my own reinnervation series (over 95 cases) suggest to me that it is, indeed, the treatment of choice for anyone who is younger than 40 years of age, or has a quasiprofessional need for their voice (physicians, singers, actors, TV personalities, trial lawyers, public speakers, etc). I have told many colleagues that, if I personally were to sustain the misfortune of having a recurrent laryngeal nerve injury, I would very definitely prefer a reinnervation technique and would find someone to do it for me because I have observed so many normal and near-normal voices from using the technique.

In summary then, numbers 3 and 4 represent the increase in reinnervation and in injection laryngoplasty procedures as being responsible for the decrease in medialization procedures being done. This is not to take anything away from those who are fond of arytenoid adduction. Drs. Steven Zeitels, Gayle Woodson, and James Netterville[16–18] have all popularized arytenoid adduction techniques and demonstrated clearly that there are significant roles for this procedure. I simply have found that, in our own cases, most commonly we see that after using the ansa cervicalis to recurrent laryngeal nerve *main trunk* anastomosis, there is reinnervation of the PCA, the LCA, and the interarytenoid (IA) muscle, which results in appropriate arytenoid adduction and normalization of the arytenoid position atop the cricoarytenoid joint. Accordingly, I do not feel that arytenoid adduction is necessary in most cases of recurrent laryngeal nerve injury with vocal fold motion impairment, since the ansa-RLN procedure produces satisfactory arytenoid adduction with resultant return of normal vertical height to the vocal fold and vocal process.

The last advance, which relates more to the second paper (Holinger, Holinger, Holinger, 1976), is the continued progress regarding selective PCA reinnervation.

5. Selective PCA Reinnervation in Treatment of Bilateral VF Motion Impairment

I find it noteworthy that as we push further into the 21st century, Prof. Jean-Paul Marie in France and Prof. Hongliang Zheng in Shanghai both have demonstrated and published successful human cases using different forms of the phrenic nerve operation for PCA reinnervation.[19,20] Dr. Zheng's technique is modeled somewhat after the Triologic thesis of Dr. Dale Rice, which was published in 1982, in which the phrenic nerve is transsected and sutured to the recurrent laryngeal nerve low in the neck (the downside of this technique and what makes it of less utility in some cases is that it requires RLN continuity from the anastomosis near the thoracic inlet all the way to the PCA muscle).[21] However, it is useful whenever the recurrent laryngeal nerve/lesion occurs in the chest (subclavian artery on the right, aortic arch on the left), as it allows the phrenic nerve axons to traverse the otherwise healthy distal cervical portion of the RLN and into the intrinsic laryngeal muscles. This (Rice, Zheng) technique requires that the adductor division be transected and implanted into the PCA, thus ensuring that all phrenic axons traveling superiorly in the RLN ultimately arrive in the PCA muscle (via PCA abductor nerve branch, and RLN's adductor division) where they enter and innervate PCA abductor muscle.

Many of Dr. Marie's contributions are derived from his impressive Ph.D. thesis in which he further researched the possible utilization of the phrenic nerve procedure for bilateral VF motion impairment. Dr. Marie was bothered by the requirement that the phrenic nerve be transected or partially injured, and hence he desired to reinnervate the PCA with inspiratory axons, but without any diaphragmatic denervation.[22] Accordingly, he was able to demonstrate in rabbits and dogs (and subsequently in humans) that there *was respiratory activity found in certain medial nerve branches related to the brachial plexus.* He showed that these minute branches could be severed and attached to a nerve graft with no resulting denervation of the arm, shoulder, or diaphragmatic muscle ("no donor deficit"). These nerve branches when severed and routed to the ipsilateral PCA muscle were able to incite inspiratory abductor activity (PCA contraction in inspiration.) Dr. Marie further improved the result by illustrating how a nerve graft ("jump graft") could route this inspiratory activity across the midline to the *contralateral* PCA muscle and accordingly in some instances he was able to achieve bilateral PCA inspiratory contraction and VF abduction with a single nerve graft.

In this country, the phrenic-PCA procedure has not to my knowledge been exploited since my initial clinical report. I have not performed many phrenic nerve procedures for bilateral paralysis because I have been awaiting further successes by such investigators as Marie and Zheng. Others in Great Britain, Italy, and the United States have further strengthened this research interest. I think that in the next decade we will see that there are, in fact, ideal cases for this kind of reinnervation to induce inspiratory PCA contraction, and vocal fold abduction in patients with bilateral vocal fold motion impairment. Further advancement in this surgical/scientific area should result from continued advances in molecular biology as well as development of other neurotrophic substances that may promote enhancement of reinnervation results. These new scientific inroads may allow neurolaryngologists to better control vocal fold movements resulting from reinnervation operations. There is promise, in fact, of implantable nerve and/or muscle stimulators for evoking inspiratory abduction, and/or adduction with phonation, swallowing, and coughing. There is, in fact, the possibility that some day a recurrent laryngeal nerve may be controlled by a microchip array, which can be used to stimulate certain axons for adduction during phonation-coughing, while stimulating other axons conversely during inspiratory efforts for abduction mediated by the PCA muscle. I anxiously await further developments in this exciting field of neurolaryngology, and feel deeply honored for the opportunity to contribute to this volume.

References

1. Crumley RL, Horn KL, Clendenning D. Laryngeal reinnervation using the aplit phrenic nerve graft procedure. *Otolaryngol Head Neck Surg.* 1980;88:159–164.
2. Crumley RL. Laryngeal synkinesis: its significance to the laryngologist. *Ann Otol Rhinol Laryngol.* 1989;89(2): 87–92.
3. Maronian NC, Robinson L, Waugh P, Hillel AD. A new electromyographic definition of laryngeal synkinesis. *Ann Otol Rhinol Laryngol.* 2004;113(11):877–886.
4. Blitzer A, Jahn AF, Keidar A. Semon's law revisited: an electromyographic analysis of laryngeal synkinesis. *Ann Otol Rhinol Laryngol.* 1996;105:764–769.
5. Woodson GE. Configuration of the glottis in laryngeal paralysis II: animal experiments. *Laryngoscope.* 1993; 103:1235–1241.
6. Trask DK, MD; Shellenberger DL, Hoffman HT. Transnasal, endoscopic vocal fold augmentation: how I do it. *Laryngoscope.* 2005;115(12):2262–2265.
7. King JM, Simpson CB. Modern injection augmentation for glottic insufficiency. *Curr Opin Otolaryngol Head Neck Surg.* 2007;15(3):153–158.
8. O. Duruisseau Wagner I, Fugain C, Chabolle F. Endoscopic rehabilitation of vocal cord paralysis with a silicone elastomer suspension implant. *Otolaryngol Head Neck Surg.* 2004;131(3):241–247.
9. Luu Q, Tsai V, Mangunta V, Berke G, Chhetri D. Safety of percutaneous injection of bovine dermal crosslinked collagen for glottic insufficiency. *Otolaryngol Head Neck Surg.* 2007;136(3):445–449.
10. Goding GS. Nerve-muscle pedicle reinnervation of the paralyzed vocal cord. *Otolaryngol Clin North Am.* 1991; 24:1239–1252.
11. Lee W, Milstein C, Esclamado R, et al. Results of ansa to recurrent laryngeal nerve reinnervation. *Otolaryngol Head Neck Surg.* 2007;136:450–454.
12. Paniello DC. Laryngeal reinnervation with the hypoglossal nerve: XII. Clinical evaluation and early patient experience. *Laryngoscope.* 2000;110:739–747.
13. Maronian N, Waugh P, Robinson L, Hillel A. Electromyographic findings in recurrent laryngeal nerve reinnervation. *Ann Otol Rhinol Laryngol.* 2003;112(4):314–323.
14. Marie JP. Selective reinnervation of the abductor and adductor muscles of the canine larynx after recurrent nerve paralysis. *Ann Otol Rhinol Laryngol.* 1989;98:530–536.
15. Su W, Hsu Y, Chen H, Sheng H. Laryngeal reinnervation by ansa cervicalis nerve implantation for unilateral vocal cord paralysis in humans. *J Am Coll Surgeons.* 2007;204(1):64–72.
16. Zeitels S. New procedures for paralytic dysphonia: adduction arytenopexy, Gore-TEX* medialization laryngoplasty, and cricothyroid subluxation. *Otolaryngol Clin North Am.* 2000;33(4):841–853.
17. Woodson GE, Murry T. Glottic configuration after arytenoid adduction. *Laryngoscope.* 1994;104:965–969.
18. Netterville JL, Stone RE , Luken ES, et al. Silastic medialization and arytenoid adduction: the Vanderbilt experience. A review of 116 phonosurgical procedures. *Ann Otol Rhinol Laryngol.* 1993;102:413–424.
19. Zheng H, Zhou S, Chen S, et al. Reinnervation of the posterior cricoarytenoid muscle by the phrenic nerve for bilateral vocal cord paralysis in humans. *Zhonghua Er Bi Yan Hou Ke Za Zhi.* 2002;37:210–214.
20. Zheng H (personal communication, R Crumley. Oct 2007).
21. Rice DL. Laryngeal reinnervation. *Laryngoscope.* 1982; 92:1049–1059.
22. S Derrey E, Verin A, Laquerrière A, et al. Restoration of diaphragmatic function after diaphragm reinnervation by inferior laryngeal nerve; experimental study in rabbits. *Respir Res.* 2006;7(1):17.

CLINICAL TUTORIAL

H. BRYAN NEEL III, MD, PhD, and STEPHEN G. HARNER, MD
Clinical Tutorials Associate Editors

Evaluation and treatment of the unilateral paralyzed vocal fold

MICHAEL S. BENNINGER, MD, ROGER L. CRUMLEY, MD, CHARLES N. FORD, MD, WILBUR J. GOULD, MD, DAVID G. HANSON, MD, ROBERT H. OSSOFF, DMD, MD, and ROBERT T. SATALOFF, MD, DMA, Detroit, Michigan, Orange, California, Madison, Wisconsin, New York, New York, Chicago, Illinois, Nashville, Tennessee, and Philadelphia, Pennsylvania

The evaluation and treatment of patients with unilateral vocal fold paralysis have evolved as improvements in objective measurements of phonatory function and new modalities for treatment have developed. A thorough history, physical examination, subjective voice evaluation, objective voice analysis, and electromyography are used to make a diagnosis, determine the cause, and plan treatment. The goal of treatment of the patient with a unilateral vocal fold paralysis is to restore normal phonatory function without aspiration. Multiple modalities have developed to allow for restoration of nearly normal phonatory function, and these include voice therapy alone or in combination with injection medialization, laryngoplastic phonosurgery, or laryngeal reinnervation. Otolaryngologists should be familiar with the incidence, cause, evaluation, and state-of-the-art treatment of unilateral vocal fold paralysis to optimize patient care and avoid suboptimal results often seen with antiquated or inappropriate treatment. (OTOLARYNGOL HEAD NECK SURG 1994;111: 497-508.)

Hippocrates first noted that denervation of the larynx could lead to life-threatening aspiration, and Galen, in the second century, described the anatomic course of the vagus nerve and recurrent laryngeal nerve (RLN). By dividing the RLN in pigs, he concluded that the voice originated in the larynx in contrast to the previously held belief that voice originated in the heart.[1] Despite these early descriptions, the ability to satisfactorily treat the paralyzed vocal fold was limited until the recent increase in interest in the evaluation and treatment of patients with unilateral voice fold paralysis. The new attention to this problem was prompted by the improved ability to objectively measure phonatory function and the popularization of new nonsurgical and surgical treatment options. Although in the past an immobile vocal fold has been described as paralyzed, these are not necessarily synonymous terms. A paralyzed fold implies disruption of the neuromuscular innervation, whereas an immobile vocal fold can be the result of multiple causes including fixation. Members of the Committee on Speech, Voice, and Swallowing Disorders of the American Academy of Otolaryngology–Head and Neck Surgery have noted the growing interest in this subject along with the dynamic changes in the approaches to treatment of unilateral paralysis. The purpose of this article is to describe the etiology and physiology of unilateral laryngeal paralysis, to explore current methods of assessment and objective evaluation, and to describe the roles of the most commonly used surgical and nonsurgical treatments.

From the Committee on Speech, Voice, and Swallowing Disorders American Academy of Otolaryngology–Head and Neck Surgery.

Received for publication Nov. 29, 1993; revision received March 4, 1994; accepted March 11, 1994.

Reprint requests: Michael S. Benninger, MD, Department of Otolaryngology–Head and Neck Surgery, Henry Ford Hospital, 2799 West Grand Blvd., Detroit, MI 48202.

0194-5998/94/$3.00 + 0 **23/1/55734**

ETIOLOGY

The incidence of vocal fold paralysis/immobility has not been established. However, it is safe to say that it is relatively uncommon. It is more common with advancing age because of the increased inci-

Table 1. Unilateral vocal fold immobility: Cause (Henry Ford Hospital 1985-1991)

Cause	No. of patients (%)
Thyroidectomy	16 (10.1)
Trauma/iatrogenic (nonthyroidectomy)	36 (22.7)
Neurologic	14 (8.8)
Malignancy (nonlaryngeal)	39 (24.5)
Miscellaneous (including idiopathic)	54 (33.9)
TOTAL	159 (100)

dence of neurologic and neoplastic disorders, which may affect laryngeal function.

The causes of unilateral immobile vocal folds are varied (Table 1).[2] Traditionally, iatrogenic and thyroid surgery were the most common causes, with resultant injury to the RLN. With refinements in surgical techniques, these causes have decreased in frequency, whereas nonlaryngeal (principally pulmonary) malignancies or their treatment have increased and are now the most common known cause.[2,3] An immobile vocal fold should prompt the otolaryngologist to exclude a nonlaryngeal malignancy. Unilateral laryngeal paralysis in children is rare and is most commonly a result of trauma, surgery, or prolonged intubation. Idiopathic or virus-induced pareses are probably much more common than reported because many of these patients may have temporary dysphonia or aphonia that resolves before they seek medical attention. Although resolution of the immobility might be expected with an idiopathic paralysis, this dictum has not been verified in large reported series.[2] This is likely because of selection bias in that patients with spontaneous resolution are not evaluated. Those with more prolonged dysfunction who are less likely to recover are examined and thus appear in large series.

Vocal fold paralysis can be the result of a central, intracranial disorder or a peripheral process that involves the vagus nerve either above the superior laryngeal nerve (SLN) or more distally without SLN involvement. Central disorders such as a cerebral vascular accident or intracranial brain stem or high skull-base tumors would not be expected to result in a unilateral vocal fold paralysis in isolation. Rather, other neurologic symptoms or cranial nerve involvement is expected. Peripheral lesions, however, often can lead to an isolated unilateral paralysis.

The evaluation of the patient with unilateral vocal fold immobility begins with a thorough local, regional, and systemic history followed by a complete head and neck and laryngeal evaluation. Because undiagnosed nonlaryngeal malignancies are common causes of unilateral immobility, it is incumbent upon the laryngologist to rule out nonlaryngeal causes by evaluating the brain stem, neck, chest, and mediastinum. Appropriate studies might include chest x ray, computed tomography (CT) scan of the skull base, neck, and chest or magnetic resonance imaging (MRI) scanning. The exact evaluation has been a subject of debate and likely will depend on numerous factors including the skill and experience of the otolaryngologist, the presenting history, and the results of the physical examination. A patient who has an immobile fold immediately after neck or thyroid surgery or after neck trauma does not need an extensive workup. Idiopathic paralysis, however, should have an appropriate evaluation to rule out a mass lesion. At Henry Ford Hospital, a review of 159 patients revealed 39 with nonlaryngeal malignancies. All of these patients had lesions large enough to be identified on chest x ray, and in none of the idiopathic paralyses has a subsequent pulmonary or mediastinal lesion been identified. Small skull-base tumors or masses in large necks difficult to palpate may be missed, however. Therefore an appropriate evaluation might include a history and physical examination, CT or MRI of the skull base to the thoracic inlet, and a chest x ray with other studies being dictated by the clinical impressions. Systemic evaluations and blood tests may be achieved if clinically indicated to rule out diabetes, Lyme disease, or other conditions found to be associated with paralyses.

PATHOLOGY

Complete paralysis of one side of the larynx is seen in clinical practice most often after complete resection of the vagal recurrent laryngeal fibers. More commonly, partial injuries to the nerve fibers with paresis are seen after some compensation and reinnervation have taken place. Therefore it is expected that the resting position of the vocal fold and the relative movement and postures of the surrounding structures are variable among patients with unilateral vocal fold paresis.[4]

Unilateral paresis can occur from central lesions and in association with peripheral lesions.[5] Important interconnections occur with the nucleus of the tractus solitarious, the primary sensory nucleus for afferents from the vagal nerve. The basal ganglia and the cerebellum provide important facilitating and inhibitory inputs that expedite the complex coordination of the laryngeal muscles during speech and other voluntary activities. The para-aquaductal grey matter appears to be an important area of interconnecting facilitory and inhibitory inputs to the nucleus ambiguus.[4]

NATURAL COURSE

The natural course of vocal fold pareses depends on the site of the lesion, the severity of the lesion, and the effects of reinnervation and compensation. Complete section of motor nerve fibers in the RLN, SLN, or both results in immediate flaccid paralysis. The muscle fibers that are denervated will subsequently atrophy and will demonstrate random firing denervation or fibrillation potentials on electromyography (EMG). During a period of 6 months to a year, and usually by about 9 months, evidence appears of reinnervation from the cut or injured nerve if it is within several centimeters of the denervated laryngeal muscle.[6] The reinnervated muscle fibers become hypertrophied with reinnervation in the canine, and in both canines and human beings EMG demonstrates polyphasic potentials in the reinnervated muscles.[6,7] Depending on the degree to which appropriate nerve fibers find their way back to the originally innervated muscle group, normal motor unit action patterns may return. This is more likely to occur when there has not been actual interruption of continuity of the nerves. However, motor fibers that originally innervated adductor or abductor fibers do not necessarily reinnervate the appropriate muscles. Therefore it would be unusual that full, appropriate abduction and adduction of the paretic fold returns unless the pathways of the injured nerve fibers were not interrupted.

OBJECTIVE EVALUATIONS

Kinematics

Evaluations or relative movements and the structures of the larynx in respiration, cough, gag, and phonatory tasks will determine whether the vocal fold length and bulk are symmetrical and whether the epithelial cover waves occur in phase and synchrony. Accurate study of relative movements, or kinematic analysis, requires that movement of the structures can be viewed in relation to all of the structures of the hypopharynx. Even the most experienced and skilled examiner can rarely do this adequately with a mirror examination. A 90-degree or 70-degree telescope examination with video documentation is often the examination of choice. Flexible fiberoptic examination has the advantage of allowing viewing during running speech and respiration without limitations imposed by the rigid telescope. A view of the relative movements and positions of the structures in both respiration and phonation permits an understanding of how they are affected by muscle contraction. Often there is some movement of a paretic cord, even after complete recurrent nerve section, because movements of muscles that are still innervated (i.e., interarytenoid fibers and supraglottic muscle fibers) will affect the otherwise paretic vocal fold. Elastic and aerodynamic forces may result in motion on even the completely paralyzed vocal fold.[8]

A brief review of the effects of paresis on specific muscles of the larynx points out the degree to which the specific movements of the vocal fold may vary depending on which motor fibers are injured.[4] In most peripheral laryngeal nerve injuries, a complete segment of the involved nerve has not been resected. Rather, the nerve has been stretched or its vascular supply has been compromised, and some motor fibers may remain intact. Furthermore, effects of variable reinnervation occur after 3 months. Consequently, it is not surprising that the literature reflects some confusion about the specific effects of vocal fold paresis.

Movements of the vocal folds are much more complex than just adduction and abduction. The complex cricoarytenoid joint allows sliding and tilting movements, and there are opposing muscles attached to all three surfaces of the arytenoid cartilages. Therefore the position and movements of the arytenoids depend on the relative balance of the muscles that control their positions. Injury to the motor innervation of the lateral cricoarytenoid results in failure of the vocal process to rotate medially. The arytenoid and its sesamoid cartilages are not fully supported by the paretic lateral cricoarytenoid and will tend to fall medially into the supraglottitis. Injury to the posterior cricoarytenoid motor fibers results in loss of lateral sliding of the arytenoid on the cricoarytenoid joint with loss of abduction of the vocal process. Injury to the thyroarytenoid motor fibers results in atrophy of the body of the fold and differences in mass and internal tension of the body of the fold. It also is associated with the loss of ability to pull the vocal process forward toward the anterior commissure. The effect of this loss of tone in the body is most readily appreciated with stroboscopy. The flaccid paretic fold opens laterally earlier in the glottal cycle and to a greater degree, but it does not have the normal undulating vibration that the normal fold exhibits. When the vocal process of the normal fold is pulled forward, shortening the membranous portion of the vocal fold, the vocal process on the paretic side is not pulled forward, and a difference in length of the membranous portions of the folds can be appreciated. Such asymmetries are often associated with diplophonia. Diplophonia limits the effective voice range of patients who have RLN paresis and who may have fairly normal voice quality in a limited portion of their fundamental frequency range. An RLN injury generally results in a vocal fold positioned in a paramedian position, although some variability can occur, which may be influenced by the mass and size of the larynx, the time from the injury, and the degree of reinnervation.

Isolated unilateral SLN injury results in asymmetrical contraction of the cricothyroid muscles. This effect may be relatively subtle but can be reliably reproduced experimentally.[9] Asymmetrical contraction of the cricothyroid muscles on one side of the larynx results in relative twisting of the cricoid in relation to the thyroid cartilage as an attempt is made to phonate and to raise pitch.[10] The thyroid cartilage also may be slightly tilted toward the side of the intact muscles with the onset of unopposed contraction. The magnitude of these effects will increase with forceful phonation and with higher pitch. The cricothyroid joint allows forward excursion and rotation of the inferior cornu of the thyroid cartilage but limits posterior excursion of the thyroid cornu. Therefore asymmetrical unopposed contraction of the longitudinal and oblique fibers of the cricothyroid muscles results in a relative twisting of the cricoid cartilage in relation to the thyroid. The posterior glottic midline corresponding to the midline of the signet of the cricoid appears to squeeze toward the side of less cricothyroid contraction, or conversely (with spastic paresis or other asymmetrically increased tone), the posterior glottic aperture will appear to shift away from the side of asymmetrically increased cricothyroid tone. SLN paresis results in differing longitudinal tension in the two vocal folds, which may then vibrate out of phase with each other.

If there is a high vagal lesion, the combined effects of RLN and SLN paresis are seen. The vocal folds do not approximate on the same level, and therefore glottic closure is not achieved in phonation. The shift of the posterior glottis to the side of the SLN injury may still be seen. Although a lateralized or cadaveric position of the vocal fold is often described, the position of the vocal fold is variable and frequently is noted to be in the paramedian position. Vocal fold position alone may not allow the otolaryngologist to determine the site of the lesion. Simple medialization of the paretic fold from a high vagal lesion does not accomplish effective glottic closure unless the asymmetrical rostral caudal relationship of the folds is adjusted to symmetrical levels. External laryngeal procedures are more effective in improving voice quality in vagal paralyses than are injection techniques. In addition to the asymmetry of vocal fold position in vagal paralysis, the soft palate may pull toward the intact side, and asymmetrical contraction of the pharyngeal constrictors may occur with the midline pulled toward the side of intact innervation. Voice quality is affected by the soft-palate paresis if closure of the nasopharyngeal port is lacking during running speech.

Upper motor lesions can cause unilateral paresis, but this is usually a spastic paresis. The spasticity slows the movements so that the paretic vocal fold lags in its movements (which may also be reduced). The involved muscles generally have increased tone. The typical findings in a unilateral upper motor neuron paresis after a brain stem stroke may be slowed and reduced range of abduction and adduction of the affected fold in relation to the normal side. There may be a notable shift of the posterior glottic aperture to the normal side with the onset of phonation. This is the opposite of flaccid vagal nerve paresis. In long-standing upper motor neuron vocal fold paresis, the entire larynx may be distinctly rotated toward the side of paresis, in part because of spastic paresis of the pharyngeal constrictor muscles. Prominent spasticity of the cricopharyngeal fibers may occur, which interferes with swallowing in these patients. Therefore the long-term effects of upper motor neuron paresis are opposite those of lower motor neuron injury.

EMG STUDIES

Some laryngologists believe that EMG studies are quite helpful both diagnostically and prognostically in relation to unilateral laryngeal paralysis. The accuracy of EMG data is dependent on placement and type of the recording electrode. Needle electrodes record electrical activity from an area of muscle fibers and may record activity from more than one discrete functional unit. This is a particular problem in the larynx where the muscle bundles are small and overlap and closely adjacent muscle bundles may have different functions. EMG studies, after complete section of motor fibers, show a predictable pattern.[7] Initially, no spontaneous motor unit activity is expected. Within 3 weeks, it is common to see fibrillation potentials of spontaneous random activity. Within 6 months, there may be polyphasic action potentials identified, which signal reinnervation, or there may be return of some normal unit response for the particular muscle indicating reinnervation of appropriate fibers to specific motor groups.[6]

The primary problem with the use of EMG for diagnostic purposes is the problem of sampling. When motor unit activity is not normal it may be difficult to know that the electrode is in the right location. Test/retest reproducibility is difficult because it is impossible to ascertain whether the electrode has been placed in exactly the same spot, making it difficult to compare recordings from one examination with those of another. However, when classic types of motor unit abnormality are identified, the information is diagnostically useful. The primary question in the use of EMG is whether the information gained will actually directly influence the treatment that would be recommended to the patient. Hirano et al.[11] have provided data on EMG findings at various durations after onset of vocal fold paresis. Their data demonstrate a mix of findings at any stage after injury so that roughly a third of subjects may demonstrate any one of the possible findings. That kind of experience makes it difficult to render a strong case for making a firm diagnosis only on the basis of EMG findings.[11] In general, however, identifying evidence of reinnervation is usually associated with a better prognosis, whereas evidence of denervation helps in earlier treatment planning. Furthermore, EMG has been very helpful in distinguishing a high vagal vs. a distal lesion. Further experience will likely improve the ability to use EMG in the assessment and treatment planning of a patient with vocal fold immobility.

Flow and Pressure Evaluations

Airflow and pressure measures are probably the best objective indicators of the effect of vocal fold paresis on vocal food approximation. Flow measures are usually accomplished with a face mask and measure a pressure drop across a known resistance. Subglottal pressure is usually estimated from intraoral pressures during labial interruption of ongoing phonation. For well-defined lesions, pressure and flow data differ for well-documented complete lesions resulting in recurrent vs. vagal paresis.[12]

Figure 1 shows data for estimated subglottal pressure and airflow for several patients with fully compensated complete resection of RLN, SLN, and high vagal nerve compared with normal data and compared with patients with idiopathic paresis that appeared to involve both RLN and SLN and innervation. Compensated recurrent paralysis patients had a slightly higher flow rate compared with normal individuals, whereas high vagal section resulted in a greatly elevated flow rate. Idiopathic paresis and isolated superior pareses were more likely to be associated with phonation produced with high subglottal pressures.

A good functional measure of airflow can be made

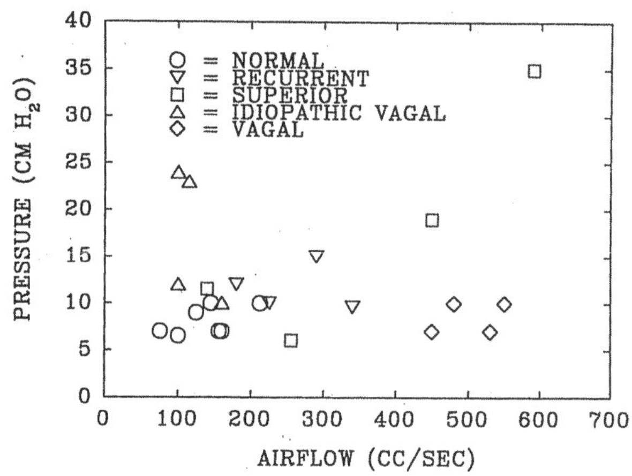

Fig. 1. Pressure and airflow analyses for laryngeal nerve paresis.

by measuring phonation time with a stopwatch. Effects on flow of unilateral vocal fold paresis may be important not only for phonation but also for respiration. Although for sedentary activities inhalation may not be significantly affected by vocal fold paresis, a unilateral deficit can have significant airway effects for rapid inhalations. For example, a unilateral vocal paresis can destroy the career of a concert wind performer. This effect has sometimes not been sufficiently appreciated.

STROBOSCOPY

Stroboscopy is now feasible with a reasonably priced video-recording apparatus. Video documentation is desirable because even with the slowed strobe image it may be difficult to analyze subtle differences in the vibratory patterns of the two folds in real time. Stroboscopy is very effective in demonstrating variations in vibration and excursion of the epithelial wave between the two vocal folds. Stroboscopy is also very valuable in the fixed mode because it can be cued to stop action in the glottal cycle, eliminating the blurring of vibration. This allows better viewing of subtle movements of the vocal processes and body of the vocal folds.

ACOUSTIC MEASURES

Acoustic recording is the simplest means of documenting voice quality. Analysis of the acoustic signal allows for quantification of voice characteristics but is difficult to relate to specific physiologic abnormalities. With unilateral vocal paresis, experience suggests that measures of jitter and shimmer, signal-to-noise measures, and measures of breathiness do correlate with the perceptions of degree of voice abnormality. For a defined study, voice quality can be perceptually rated and quantified with a panel of listeners. However, quantified perceptual ratings are not practical for routine patient care.

TREATMENT OF VOCAL FOLD PARALYSIS

The primary goals of treatment of a patient with unilateral vocal fold paralysis are to eliminate aspiration and improve voice. When aspiration is absent, the physician should recommend intervention based principally on the patient's need and desire for improved voice quality.

Role of Voice Therapy

Objective voice analysis and assessment by a speech-language pathologist specializing in voice are helpful in virtually all patients with dysphonia.[13] In people with unilateral vocal fold paralysis, initial assessment not only quantitates and documents vocal dysfunction but also explores a wide range of potentially useful compensatory strategies. In addition, the speech-language pathologist identifies spontaneous compensatory behaviors that may be counterproductive. For example, although speech pathology textbooks generally classify and treat vocal fold paralysis as a "hypofunctional" disorder,[14,15] undesirable compensatory hyperfunctional behavior is common in these patients. This is responsible for most of the voice strain, neck discomfort, and fatigue that may accompany unilateral vocal fold paralysis. Such gestures can often be eliminated even during the first assessment and trial therapy session, increasing vocal ease and endurance. Moreover, if the assessment reveals improved voice with a different pitch, training in safe pitch modification in combination with other techniques may also provide rapid improvement. Indeed, under good guidance, therapy sometimes produces astonishingly rapid improvements in voice quality despite persistence of the neurologic deficit. In any case, initial assessment is worthwhile to document vocal condition before surgery is considered and to get an estimate of how much the patient's voice can be improved without surgery.

Most often, initial assessment results in modest but noticeable improvement in voice quality and subjectively important improvement in ease and endurance. Generally, several therapy sessions are needed to optimize vocal function. The speech-language pathologist provides patients with educational information about the workings of phonation, about their specific abnormality, and about vocal hygiene. The importance of and rationale for therapy are also explained. Therapy is directed toward avoidance of hyperfunctional compensation and progressive development of optimal breathing, abdominal support, and intrinsic laryngeal muscle strength and agility. Training includes head and neck muscle relaxation exercises, aerobic conditioning, abdominal and thoracic muscle strength and control exercises, attention to respiration, and various voice exercises for muscle development. In general, appropriate exercises are isotonic and analogous to exercises that build limb strength through multiple repetitions with light weights. Forced adduction exercises, often recommended in speech pathology texts,[14,15] such as pushing or pulling on chairs, must be avoided or monitored closely and used with extreme caution. Although such exercises are still in fairly common use, other techniques may be more effective and have less potential for harm.[13] When available, traditional voice therapy combined with a few expert singing lessons may expedite improvement.[13] This is akin to including jogging or running in a rehabilitation program aimed at improving limb strength for walking.

Like surgery, therapy is least successful in combined paralysis. In the majority of patients with unilateral vocal fold paralysis, therapy results in improvement. In many cases, the improvement is sufficient for the patients' needs. When the patients have complied with voice therapy, improvements have reached a plateau, and they feel that their voice quality is not satisfactory, surgery may be indicated.

If preoperative voice therapy has been optimal and if surgery has been successful, the postoperative voice therapy course should be short. Nevertheless, the patient is working with a "new voice." At least a few sessions with a speech-language pathologist generally will help the patient apply effective principles learned in preoperative therapy. It is particularly important for the voice therapist to monitor the patient, avoiding development of abusive habits and stressing the importance of vocal hygiene measures. At the conclusion of therapy, objective voice measures should be repeated.

If the patient is interested in optimizing voice quality, it is reasonable to continue therapy as long as it continues to produce voice improvement. This judgment is usually made jointly by the patient, speech-language pathologist, and laryngologist. In most patients who have had good preoperative voice therapy, this point is reached within 1 to 3 months after surgery.

Voice therapy is invaluable in the management of unilateral vocal fold paralysis. In all cases, the speech-language pathologist can provide detailed preoperative and postoperative assessment. Such assessment is often of diagnostic value. It is also of great help to the surgeon in evaluating objectively the efficacy of treatments. In addition, voice therapy sometimes avoids the need for surgery, saving the patient from exposure to unnecessary surgical risks. Even when surgery is eventually required, preoperative voice therapy helps the patient while surgical decisions are pending, provides training for optimal postoperative phonation, and prepares the patient psychologically for surgery with the knowledge that everything possible has been done to avoid unnecessary operative intervention. This results in superior patient cooperation, motivation, and understanding through educated participation in the voice restoration process. The importance of this factor should not be overlooked in terms of both the art of medicine and medical legal prudence.

SURGICAL THERAPY

After failure of recovery, accommodation, or appropriate voice therapy, surgical intervention may be considered. Many factors may play a role in the determination of the need for intervention, the timing of treatment, and the method of surgical management. The most important consideration is the patients' voice needs and their desire for improvement to accomplish their avocational, occupational, or social functions. Furthermore, other symptoms such as chronic aspiration may prompt more immediate intervention.

The timing of surgery is also dependent somewhat on the patient's voice needs but also requires an evaluation of the cause, likelihood of improvement or resolution, and the success of nonsurgical treatment. After resection of the vagus nerve along with other cranial nerves at the time of skull-base surgery, acute medialization may be advocated particularly if the patient has other chronic or acute illnesses that may predispose to complications associated with a vocal fold paralysis, such as aspiration pneumonia. A patient with a known resection of the vagus or recurrent laryngeal nerves in the neck or chest may still accommodate sufficiently, particularly with voice therapy, and therefore it may be reasonable to allow a few months before advising surgery. With an idiopathic paralysis, many advocate waiting a year before a permanent procedure such as Teflon, although a temporary procedure such as an injection of Gelfoam sterile sponge (Upjohn Co., Kalamazoo, Mich.) or an innervation procedure may be appropriate sooner. EMG has helped evaluate vocal fold denervation and reinnervation and is an aid to determine the likelihood of resolution and can assist in determining whether early surgical intervention is indicated. Finally, the voice demands of some patients may require early intervention even if eventual compensation or recovery is possible or likely. In such a situation a reversible procedure such as Gelfoam or silicone elastomer medialization (M-s) is preferred.

Once surgery is considered, a number of factors may influence the recommendations for the type of procedure. Of critical importance is the training and experience of the surgeon. Many find that they have good results with a particular procedure whereas the results of a different procedure are suboptimal. The surgeon should become well acquainted with the advantages and limitations of any one procedure, and it is best to have experience in more than one surgical approach. Patient factors may also help dictate the recommendations. An elderly patient who has an immobile vocal fold caused by a terminal pulmonary neoplasm or a person with significant other medical problems may benefit from the relative simplicity and quickness of a Teflon injection. A patient with cricoarytenoid joint fixation may not have satisfactory results with a reinnervation procedure. Many now consider M-s as the preferred procedure for obtaining maximal voice results. This is particularly true when combined with other procedures such as reinnervation, refinement injections, or arytenoid adduction (AA) when needed.

Laryngoplastic Phonosurgery Nomenclature

With changes in surgical treatment of vocal disorders, nomenclature that adequately describes such surgeries is lacking. In an effort to standardize nomenclature that is descriptive and capable of being used to compare treatment results, the Committee on Speech, Voice, and Swallowing Disorders of the American Academy of Otolaryngology–Head and Neck Surgery has developed a nomenclature for vocal surgery (Table 2).

Injection Laryngoplasty

Injection in the vocal fold can be used as the primary medialization therapy to correct glottic insufficiency. With a variety of substances now available for injection, it is also possible to use injection as an adjunctive measure to enhance medialization results.

Injection of Teflon (polytef) has been the mainstay of surgical treatment for patients with glottic insufficiency for the past three decades.[16,17] When

Table 2. Nomenclature for laryngoplastic phonosurgery

A. Laryngeal framework surgery (LFS) with
  - Arytenoid adduction (AA)
  - Medialization (M)
  - Lateralization (L)
  - Anterior commissure
    - Retrusion (relaxation) (ACR)
    - Protrusion (tensing) (ACP)
  - Cricothyroid approximation (CTA)

Medialization laryngoplasty can be qualified by method of medialization
  - Medialization laryngoplasty with
    - s = Silicone elastomer
    - c = Cartilage
    - e = Expander
    - o = Other

B. Injection laryngoplasty (IL)
  - D = Direct
  - I = Indirect
  - Injection laryngoplasty with
    - t = Teflon
    - g = Gelfoam sterile sponge
    - col = Collagen
    - f = Fat
    - o = Other

Abbreviations may be used
  - Laryngeal framework surgery with medialization–silicone elastomer (LFS–M-s)
  - Laryngeal framework surgery with arytenoid adduction (LFS-AA)
  - Injection laryngoplasty-direct-Teflon (IL-D-t)

injection is properly performed, particularly in the hands of experienced surgeons, results have been good and complications limited. One of the advantages of Teflon injection for medialization in the paralyzed vocal fold is the ease of introduction. Traditional transoral injection under local anesthesia usually takes less than 10 minutes including anesthetic time.[18] A video-monitored transcutaneous approach has also been described.[19] Failures have often been the result of poor technique but also can develop because of a biologic response to the injected alloplastic material resulting in granuloma formation. Although granuloma removal can be achieved, it is difficult, and subsequent voice results are usually suboptimal. Furthermore, Teflon is not indicated when vocal fold movement may return. Recent interest in medialization laryngoplasty, AA, and reinnervation procedures has prompted a more critical look at medialization injections. For many, Teflon injections remain an important method for correcting glottic insufficiency related to vocal fold paralysis and is a method of choice for many patients with paralysis caused by noncurable pulmonary malignancies or for patients whose medical status makes them poor surgical risks. More temporary substances, such as Gelfoam, can help predict surgical results, facilitate biofeedback training, and provide symptomatic relief while the patient awaits results of surgical reinnervation.

The technique of Teflon injection is important to optimize results and to minimize the risks of complications such as granuloma formation. The bolus should be injected at about the level of the anterior portion of the vocal process of the arytenoid or just anterior to it. The injections should be well into the bulk of the fold, and it is best injected laterally toward the thyroid cartilage in an effort to allow for lateral distribution and medialization of the entire fold as a unit. Injections superficial or medial in the fold, particularly if overinjected, may allow for anterior bulging and a large posterior glottic chink. The procedure is best performed with the patient under a local anesthetic so that voice quality can be assessed and the bolus of injection can be monitored and adjusted accordingly. Overinjection should be avoided to minimize the risk of granuloma formation.

Recently, autogenous fat has been used in treating vocal fold paralysis and to correct previously created surgical defects.[20,21] Fat has the advantage of being readily available, producing minimal to no foreign body reaction, and being easily injected.[20] Unlike Teflon, it may be used even if vocal fold mobility may return. Absorption likely occurs, and long-term studies are lacking. Bioimplants such as collagen can be used to replace connective tissue in a lateralized or atropic vocal fold, to modify contours, and to soften scar tissue. Although collagen is not yet approved for laryngeal use, it has been used safely in large series of patients,[22,23] and it differs from other injectables by integrating into host tissues. Although not preferred in large glottic defects, collagen has been used independently with success in the treatment of patients with minor glottic insufficiencies.[22] Collagen can also soften scar tissue and can be used as an adjunct to other procedures such as M-s or reinnervation. It is important to understand the behavior of injectable substances used in medialization. Proper technique is essential to achieving good results and avoiding complications.

MEDIALIZATION-SILICONE

M-s has become an important method of alleviating glottic insufficiency caused by vocal fold paralysis,[24] and for many has become the method of choice.[25] M-s can also be used with other techniques such as reinnervation with ansa-RLN anastomosis or nerve muscle pedicle transfer. Vocal fold vibration is maintained after M-s.

From April 1987 to August 1992, 139 procedures for glottal incompetence were performed at Vanderbilt University. These procedures included (1) primary M-s (performed with patients under general anesthesia at the time of neural sacrifice); (2) secondary M-s (performed with patients under local anesthesia); (3) bilateral M-s; and (4) AA. Recently ansa-RLN anastomosis has been combined with M-s when indicated. The surgical techniques used for both M-s and AA are modifications of Isshiki's original descriptions.[24,26,27] Although the surgical techniques have been previously outlined, significant changes have evolved during the past 3 years.[28]

M-s, whether unilateral or bilateral, ansa-RLN anastomosis, and AA, are all performed with local anesthesia supplemented by intravenous sedation. A transnasal flexible video laryngoscopy is used on all local procedures to aid in proper implant placement. This continues to give significant feedback to prevent overmedialization of the anterior commissure and the false cord.

The larynx is exposed through a small incision overlying the midportion of the thyroid cartilage, and the perichondrium is elevated from the involved side. The window template, which is 6 × 13 mm, is positioned over the cartilage to mark the window location (Fig. 2). The window is placed parallel to the lower border of the thyroid cartilage. The window is placed as close to the lower border of the laryngeal cartilage as possible, and a strong inferior cartilage strut is left to resist fracture while the implant is placed. In the more obtuse angled cartilage, as seen more often in men the window is moved more posteriorly (about 7 mm) to prevent overmedialization of the anterior commissure. When calcified, the cartilage is removed from the outlined window under magnification with an otologic drill. The inner perichondrium is left intact. In the younger patient with little or no calcification of the cartilage, the freer elevator can be used instead to carefully remove this cartilage island.

It has been proposed that injury to the inner perichondrium would increase the likelihood of graft extrusion.[28] The first 40 procedures were performed with a microscope, and the cartilage was carefully removed and the inner perichondrium left intact. The inner perichondrium was then widely elevated as is most commonly described, and medialization was attempted. Because adequate medialization could often not be accomplished, the perichondrium is now microscopically incised with a

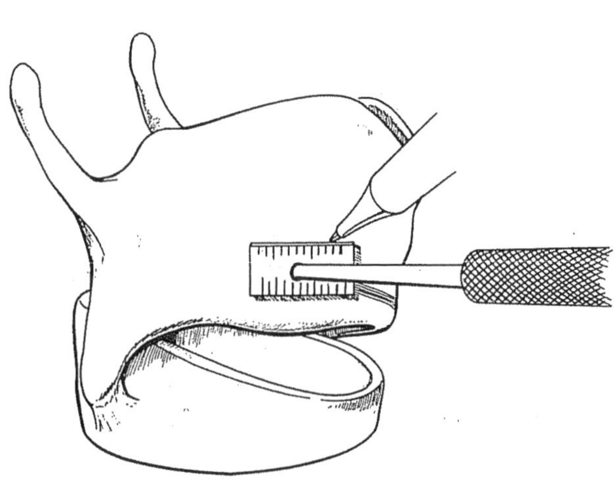

Fig. 2. Window is positioned parallel to the lower border of the thyroid cartilage. A window template is helpful in laying out this window. It is placed 5 to 8 mm back from the anterior commissure and 4 mm up from the inferior border.

small knife at the superior, posterior, and inferior margins of the window. The thyroarytenoid fascia and its underlying vessels are maintained intact. A long laryngeal elevator is then used to elevate the thyroarytenoid muscle fascia away from the inner perichondrium (Fig. 3). The main reason for delayed graft extrusion into the larynx is likely injury to the laryngeal ventricle with implant contamination. This results from rough techniques to create the window. Although most authors advocate avoidance of injury to the inner perichondrium, no extrusions of implants with this technique have occurred thus far.

After the thyroarytenoid muscle elevation has been completed, a depth gauge is used. While the larynx is viewed on the monitor, all aspects of the window are depressed. This information will show the surgeon the relationship of the window to the true and false vocal cords. Usually, medialization at the superior aspect of the window results in movement of the false vocal cord and ventricular mucosa. For this reason, the implant is carved so that the maximum point of medialization is at the lower edge of the window. The larger sloped end of the depth gauge is then used to medialize the cord while the patient is phonating (Fig. 4). These measurements are read off the gauge along the inner aspect of the thyroid cartilage. Care must be taken to prevent overmedialization of the anterior commissure, which results in a strained voice. After the implant dimensions have been acquired, the final implant is carved. It may be divided into two sections to allow for a less traumatic insertion.

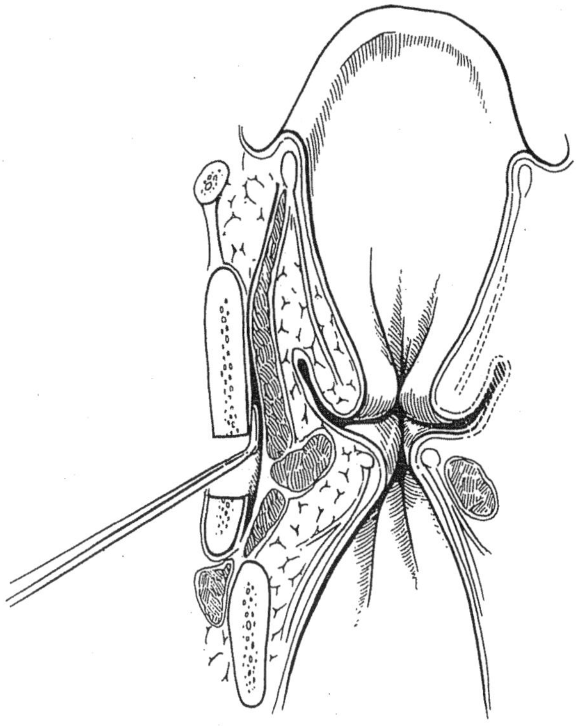

Fig. 3. After perichondrium has been carefully incised along the superior, posterior, and inferior margins of the window, the long laryngeal elevator is used to separate the thyroarytenoid fascia away from the inner perichondrium.

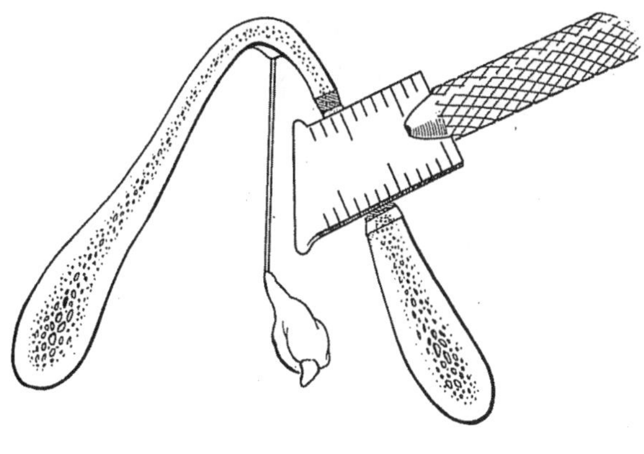

Fig. 4. Depth gauge is very helpful in simulating the medialization needed at both the anterior and posterior aspects of the vocal cord. It is thin enough to move up and down in the window to help prevent over medialization of the false vocal fold. The millimeter markings on the gauge dictate the size of the implant.

Because the female vocal cord is shorter, the distance from the anterior aspect of the window to the maximum point of medialization is less than in a man. In women the implant is approximately 2 mm wide in the front and 5 to 6 mm wide in the posterior aspect. The distance from the anterior edge of the implant to the maximum point of medialization is approximately 10 mm. In men the window is placed further back, about 6 to 7 mm from the anterior commissure. The average implant size is 2 mm in the front and 6 mm in the posterior aspect. The length to the point of maximal medialization is 13 mm. If no return of vocal fold function is possible, a 5- to 6-mm tail on the implant extends medial to the thyroid cartilage and posteriorly to the window. This extension of the implant is tapered to prevent contact with the muscular process of the arytenoid.

If the quality of the voice is not as good as expected, the implant can be removed with two small skin hooks and adjusted appropriately. The time from intralaryngeal elevation to final placement of the implant needs to be as short as possible to allow for voice judgment without the interference of edema. The final shape of the implant provides the maximum plane of medialization at the lower border of the window to prevent medialization of the false vocal cord or the ventricular mucosa (Fig. 5). Such an approach is one method of vocal fold medialization, although variations from this approach may result in equivalent results.

If it is obvious at this point that the posterior glottis cannot be closed, an AA is performed. AA is the only reliable technique that can close large posterior glottic defects. If indicated on the basis of history and intraoperative EMG, reinnervation with a branch of the ansa-hypoglossi-cervicalis system anastomosed to the cut end of the RLN is performed. The major benefit of reinnervation is maintenance of muscle bulk and static tone.

Of the 139 procedures, 16 were revisions with either a larger implant or AA. Forty patients underwent primary M-s at the end of the surgical procedure in which the laryngeal innervation was sacrificed.[29] Primary AA was performed as well in three of the patients. Of this group, five patients have undergone surgical revision, three with larger implants, one with a larger implant and AA, and one with AA only. One of the first three patients with revisions has subsequently undergone a second revision with AA. This group has had no graft extrusions. The voice results in this group have been very good.

Eighty-one patients underwent secondary M-s under local anesthesia. Six of these patients underwent AA as well. Of this group, eight patients have undergone revision surgery, four with larger unilateral implants, two with larger implants plus AA, and two with AA alone. No stridor developed in any of the

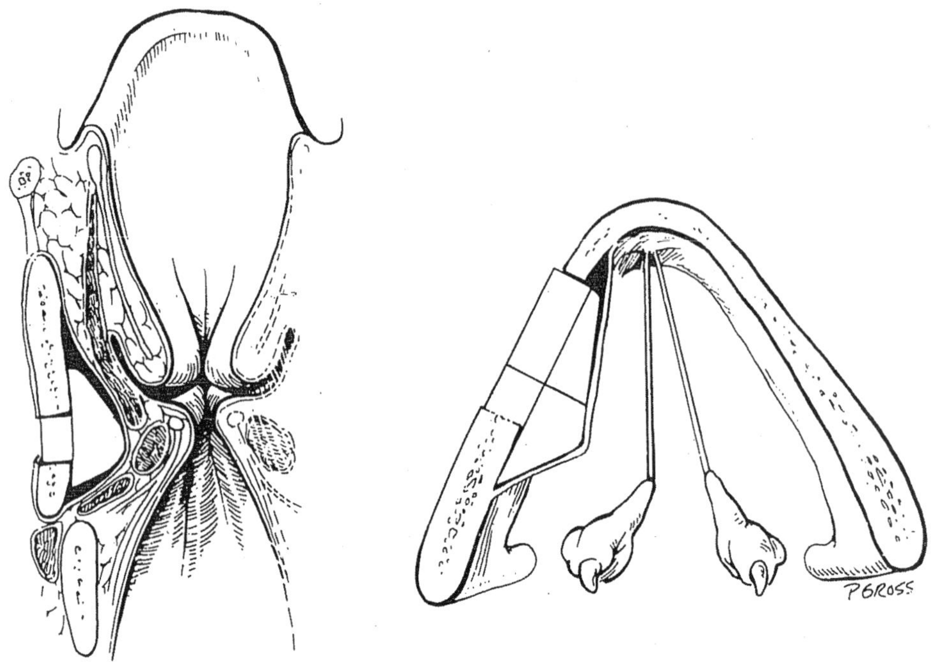

Fig. 5. **A,** Final position of the implant demonstrates the major plane of medialization at the lower margin of the window to prevent medialization of supraglottitis. **B,** Posterior extension of the implant, which can be adjusted, will medialize the vocal process of the arytenoid in most cases.

patients, either immediately or in the postoperative period. The voice quality in this group was judged as "near normal" at 6 months in a majority of the cases. The correlation between five judges was very close in most patients, suggesting validity of the voice scoring system used.

The main advantages of M-s over Teflon are adjustability and reversibility. The adjustability is its single greatest advantage. The reversibility not only allows for future adjustments for anatomical or functional changes that may result in a weaker voice but also allows for its use in several settings that are unsuitable for Teflon, such as vocal cord paresis or correction within the first year after nerve injury.

LARYNGEAL REINNERVATION

Laryngeal reinnervation has been performed by nerve-muscle pedicle or ansa-hypoglossi-RLN anastomosis.[30,31] The principle of reinnervation of paralyzed laryngeal muscle allows for a more physiologic approach to the treatment of the paralyzed vocal fold.

On complete paralysis of the RLN, four ipsilateral endolaryngeal muscles are paralyzed. All of these muscles undergo loss of mass, volume, and muscular tension in the first 14 days after RLN paralysis. The relationships between the paralyzed vocal fold, arytenoid, thyroid cartilage, and opposite fold have been described above. Reinnervation of these four muscles with physiologic normal neurons appears surgically impossible at this time. However, it has been found that reinnervation of the entire distal stump of the RLN and these four intrinsic muscles by ansa cervicalis neurons tends to stabilize the arytenoid cartilage in position, rotating it backward and upward into a more symmetrical location relative to the opposite arytenoid, and more importantly, presents a more normal mass, tension, and symmetry relative to the opposite side.[31] It can be used simultaneously with other methods for treating unilateral vocal fold paralysis such as M-s or injection medialization. This series of 36 ansa cervicalis–recurrent nerve anastomoses performed by Crumley,[31] indicates that this type of reinnervation may provide a better voice than phonosurgery or injection medialization, and he feels that this should be a first consideration in younger individuals or those who have professional uses of their voices. Although reinnervation has shown much promise, it has not been routinely performed in the general otolaryngology community.

SUMMARY

The evaluation and treatment of a patient with a unilateral immobile vocal fold relies on understanding of the pathophysiology, vocal fold positioning, and potential treatment options. A thorough history along with subjective and objective voice assessments should be used, and the patient's desire and need for improved phonatory function are major components in planning treatment. Speech-language pathology assessment and instruction are valuable independently or in association with surgical treatments. Many surgical options are available alone or in combination. The treating physician should become familiar with more than one technique and use techniques most appropriate to each individual patient. When beginning to use new techniques, surgeons should become well trained with appropriate courses and cadaver dissections. They should be critical of their own results, use objective and psychoacoustic analysis to quantify voice function, and stay abreast of new assessments and treatments as they evolve.

REFERENCES

1. Willat DJ, Stell PM. Vocal cord paralysis. In: Paparella MM, Shumrick DA, Gluckman JL, et al., eds. Otolarynology. Philadelphia: WB Saunders Co., 1991:2289-304.
2. Gillen J, Benninger MS. The changing etiology of vocal fold immobility. Laryngoscope, submitted.
3. Terris DJ, Arnstein DP, Nguyen HH. Contemporary evaluation of unilateral vocal cord paralysis. Otolaryngol Head Neck Surg 1992;107:84-9.
4. Hanson DG. Neurological disorders of laryngeal function. Otolaryngol Clin North Am 1991;24:1035-51.
5. Ward PH, Hanson DG, Berci G. Observations on central neurologic etiology for laryngeal dysfunction. Ann Otol Rhinol Laryngol 1981;90:430-41.
6. Shindo M, Herzon G, Sahgal V, Hanson D, Cain D. Effects on reinnervation on laryngeal muscles, a canine model. Laryngoscope 1992;102:663-9.
7. Schaefer SD. Laryngeal electromyography. Otolaryngol Clin North Am 1991;24:1053-7.
8. Fink BR, Demarest RJ. Laryngeal biomechanics. Boston: Harvard University Press, 1978.
9. Berke G, Moore D, Hantke D, Hanson D, Gerratt BR. Laryngeal modeling: theoretical, in-vitro, in-vivo. Laryngoscope 1988;98:871-88.
10. Moore DM, Berke GS, Hanson DG, Ward PH. Videostroboscopy of the canine larynx: the effects of asymmetrical laryngeal tension. Laryngoscope 1987;97:543-53.
11. Hirano M, Nozoe I, Shin T, Maeyama T. Electromyographic findings in laryngeal nerve paralysis. A study of 130 cases. Pract Otol Kyoto 1974;67:231-40.
12. Hanson DG. Phonosurgery: a perspective. In: Cummings C, Fredrickson JM, Harker LA, et al., eds. Otolaryngology—update II. St. Louis: C.V. Mosby, 1990:107-24.
13. Sataloff RT. Professional voice: the science and art of clinical care. New York: Raven Press, 1991.
14. Aronson AE. Clinical voice disorders. 3rd ed. New York: Thieme, Inc., 1990:339-45.
15. Greene MCL, Mathieson L. The voice and its disorders. 5th ed. London: Whurr Publishers, 1989:305-6.
16. Arnold GE. Vocal rehabilitation of paralytic dysphonia. IX. Technique of intracordal injection. Arch Otolaryngol 1962; 76:358-68.
17. Dedo HH, Urrea RD, Lausca L. Intracordal injection of Teflon in the treatment of 135 patients with dysphonia. Ann Otol Rhinol Laryngol 1973;82:661-7.
18. Dedo HH. Injection and removal of Teflon for unilateral vocal cord paralysis. Ann Otol Rhinol Laryngol 1992;101: 81-5.
19. Strasnick B, Gerke GS, Ward PH. Transcutaneous Teflon[R] injection for unilateral vocal cord paralysis: an update. Laryngoscope 1991;101:785-7.
20. Brandenburg MD, Kirkham W, Koschkee D. Vocal cord augmentation with autogenous fat. Laryngoscope 1992;102: 495-500.
21. Mikaelian D, Lowry LD, Sataloff RT. Lipoinjection for unilateral vocal cord paralysis. Laryngoscope 1991;101:465-8.
22. Bless DM, Ford CN, Loftus JM. Role of injectable collagen in the treatment of glottic insufficiency: a study of 119 patients. Ann Otol Rhinol Laryngol 1992;101:237-46.
23. Remacle M, Marbaix E, Hamoir M, Bertrand B, van den Eeckhaut J. Correction of glottic insufficiency by collagen injection. Ann Otol Rhinol Laryngol 1990;99:438-44.
24. Isshiki N, Morita H, Okamura H, Hiramoto M. Thyroplasty as a new phonosurgical technique. Acta Otolaryngol 1974; 78:451-7.
25. Koufman JA. Laryngoplasty for vocal cord medialization: an alternative to Teflon. Laryngoscope 1987;96:726-31.
26. Isshiki N. Recent advances in phonosurgery. Folia Phoniatrica 1980;32:119-54.
27. Isshiki N, Masahiro T, Sawada M. Arytenoid adduction for unilateral vocal cord paralysis: a comparison. Laryngoscope 1988;98:1200-4.
28. Netterville JL, Aly A, Ossoff RH. Evaluation and treatment of complications of thyroid and parathyroid surgery. Otolaryngol Clin North Am 1990;23:529-52.
29. Netterville JL, Jackson CG, Civantos FJ. Thyroplasty in the functional rehabilitation of neurotologic skull base surgery patients. Am J Otol, 1993;14:460-4.
30. Tucker HM. Reinnervation of the unilaterally paralyzed larynx. Ann Otol Rhinol Laryngol 1977;86:789-94.
31. Crumley RL. Update: ansa cervicalis to recurrent laryngeal nerve anastomosis for unilateral laryngeal paralysis. Laryngoscope 1991;101:384-7.

12

Vocal Fold Augmentation

Introduction

In contrast to microlaryngoscopic surgery, both injection augmentation and medialization laryngoplasty have a long history in laryngology. The story of injection augmentation opens in 1911 with Wilhelm Brünings' report of paraffin injection for the relief of symptoms of glottic insufficiency.[1] The aftermath of that report established a familiar pattern. Paraffin provoked a florid inflammatory response in vivo, which could result in catastrophic voice results. Its enthusiasts, led by Brünings (who, after all, had a dueling scar from his university days), vehemently challenged the critics, and claimed that poor outcomes were the result of shoddy technique rather than inherent tissue properties. A cadre of diehards remained committed to paraffin long after it had fallen out of widespread use; one can find papers advocating its injection well into the 1950s.[2] By that time, Godfrey Arnold was experimenting with paraffin's eventual successor, Teflon paste. It had, he claimed, "the quality of being harmless to the patient."[3]

Injection augmentation has never been limited by technical factors; the central problem has been the tissue-filler interaction. The vibratory tissues of the vocal fold are exquisitely sensitive to the tissue changes of inflammation, and the relatively small bulk of the intrinsic muscles of the vocal fold offers little cushioning in which to bury a foreign body so as to prevent any tissue response from spreading medially. This is especially true of the atrophic tissue of a denervated vocal fold. In this respect, Brünings and his allies, as well as the eventual defenders of Teflon, were correct: it does indeed require a fine touch to place an aliquot of an alloplastic material so that it causes no problem.

Collagen and autologous fat are two biological injectables to answers the poor experience with alloplastic material. Dr. Ford's commentary on his landmark work with collagen highlights the preoccupation with tissue response that led to his interest in and clinical success with collagen. There are striking similarities with the considerations that led Dr. Shaw and colleagues to investigate autologous fat. Similar too are the limitations—principally some unpredictability in duration of effect—that have generated continued interest in alloplastic filler. Otolaryngologists would do well to review the specialty's past experience, summarized in the commentaries presented below, as the material of the moment, calcium hydroxylapatite paste, passes into general use.

In addition to the gross glottic insufficiency of paresis and paralysis, local volume loss in small areas of the vocal fold resulting from microsurgery and/or scar has generated interest in injection augmentation as a means of replacing missing or dysfunctional lamina propria. The paper of Chan and Titze illustrates that no currently available material duplicates the critical rheologic properties of that tissue. This sets the stage for the next great challenge for injection augmentation.

References

1. Brunings W. Über eine neue Behandlungsmethode der Rekurrenslähmung. *Verhandl Ver Dtsch Laryngol.* 1911; 17:93.
2. Imre V. Die Rekurrensparesen und ihre Behandlung. *Monatsschr Ohrenheilkd Laryngorhinol.* 1950;84:214–219.
3. Luchsinger R, Arnold GE. *Voice—Speech—Language.* London: Constable; 1963.

Classic Articles

•Reprint of article included in this chapter.
♦Commentary on this article.

Mikaelian DO, Lowry LD, Sataloff RT. Lipoinjection for unilateral vocal cord paralysis. *Laryngoscope.* 1991; 101(5):465–468.

•♦Ford CN, Bless DM, Loftus JM. Role of injectable collagen in the treatment of glottic insufficiency: a study of 119 patients. *Ann Otol Rhinol Laryngol.* 1992;101(3): 237–247.

Brandenburg JH, Kirkham W, Koschkee D. Vocal cord augmentation with autogenous fat. *Laryngoscope.* 1992; 102(5):495–500.

Mikus JL, Koufman JA, Kilpatrick SE. Fate of liposuctioned and purified autologous fat injections in the canine vocal fold. *Laryngoscope.* 1995;105(1):17–22.

Ford CN, Staskowski PA, Bless DM. Autologous collagen vocal fold injection: a preliminary clinical study. *Laryngoscope.* 1995;105(9 pt 1):944–948.

Zaretsky LS, Shindo ML, Rice DH. Autologous fat injection for unilateral vocal fold paralysis. *Ann Otol Rhinol Laryngol.* 1996;105(8):602–606.

•♦Shaw GY, Szewczyk MA, Searle J, Woodroof J. Autologous fat injection into the vocal folds: technical considerations and long-term follow-up. *Laryngoscope.* 1997;107(2):177–186.

Rihkanen H. Vocal fold augmentation by injection of autologous fascia. *Laryngoscope.* 1998;108(1 pt 1):51–54.

•Chan RW, Titze IR. Viscosities of implantable biomaterials in vocal fold augmentation surgery. *Laryngoscope.* 1998;108(5):725–731.

Commentary

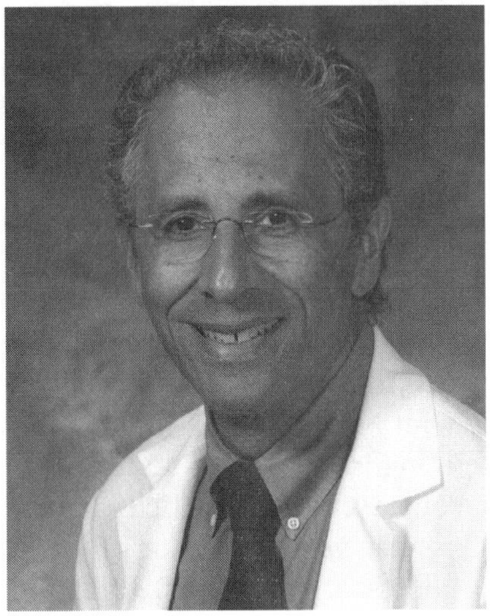

Charles N. Ford, MD

To me, the most meaningful aspect of this report of our 10-year experience with vocal fold collagen injections does not relate to the specific techniques, methodology, or results. With experience, we have since modified techniques, used different materials, and improved our outcome measures. The most meaningful aspect of this report was the introduction of a different paradigm for assessing efficacy of an injectable material in the larynx. Historically, Godfrey Arnold proposed polytetrafluoroethylene (Teflon) paste as an ideal implant because it met 3 essential criteria. It had to be injectable through a Brünings syringe, sufficiently inert to be tolerated by the patient, and persistent over time. Unlike Teflon, injectable collagen (initially we were using the bovine-derived Zyderm preparation) was a biological implant. Unlike alloplastics, success of bioimplants relies on their basic similarity to the implanted tissues, susceptibility to invasion by host cells, and ultimately resorption with replacement by similar host tissues. Although collagen proved easier to inject (it passed easily through a 27-gauge needle affording focal placement) and it was better tolerated (no foreign-body reaction), there remained a concern about persistence. However, the concern became focused on persistence of the correction and vocal fold function, rather than on persistence and stability of the injectate. The emphasis on biological characteristics and activity of the implant has led to development of innovative approaches and materials of variable resorption rates, viscoelastic properties, and long-term impact on the vocal fold composition.

Other meaningful aspects of this paper included the use of objective voice assessments as advocated by my coauthor Diane Bless. Subjective patient self-assessments were complemented with detailed acoustic analyses, aerodynamic measures, blinded perceptual judgments, and assessments of vocal fold motion using the earliest commercially available videostroboscopic equipment by Bruel and Kjaer. I expect that the standard of reporting results using objective voice measures will continue to evolve, incorporating new technologies such as high-speed digital imaging and validated outcome measures. Significantly, our results attested to the overall safety of collagen injections, with no serious side effects or feared allergic reactions. We confirmed that scarred vocal folds and bilateral problems were more difficult to treat but all groups showed objective improvement. Unlike alloplastic materials, collagen could be injected superficially—even into mobile vocal folds—to address focal defects, scars, and atrophy without concern for foreign body granuloma with secondary scar formation. We also designed and introduced a novel injection device that remains a useful multipurpose laryngology instrument.

The inspiration for my initial exploration of collagen was seeing many patients with dysfunctional larynges who had undergone Teflon injections with either immediate or delayed complications due to poor placement, granuloma, and migration. During the early 1980s, my office was next door to Fred Mohs (of Mohs' surgery fame) who often referred patients to me with depressed facial scars after secondary intention healing. I found that repeated injections of bovine Zyderm not only served as filler, but it often softened the scar to allow further augmentation over time. This seemed a favorable property for atrophic or scarred vocal folds and the idea of injecting collagen into a structure that contained collagen (deep lamina propria) was intuitive. Although it was not easy to inject precisely into a vocal ligament plane, the substance proved forgiving in dogs and in preliminary clinical trials, and some scarred vocal folds showed improved pliability. Over the years, I learned that such precision is usually not necessary as I noted that others achieved success with less precise injections of collagen that seemed to spread into multiple tissue planes.

We encountered many problems in our early clinical trials. Some of these continue to have a negative impact on progress. The easiest to overcome was development of an appropriate injection device. With the help of University of Wisconsin engineers and the designers at the Palo Alto-based Collagen Corporation, we designed a prototype laryngeal injector that allowed precise delivery through a disposable 27-gauge needle (currently a Medtronic product). A more difficult step was getting funding and approval from the FDA to use Zyderm, a product approved only for cosmetic applications. With corporate help, an Investigational Device Exemption was approved and the FDA also awarded us a grant through their Orphaned Product Division. This allowed us to conduct preliminary safety and efficacy trials that led to several publications although our efforts proved insufficient to secure NIH funding to support further laboratory or clinical studies. It is interesting to note that current product development is largely driven by the interests of corporations seeking lucrative cosmetic surgery applications. Products such as Zyderm, Cymetra, Cosmoplast, Fascian, Autologen, Restylane, Perlane, Captique, Hylaform, Artefill, and Radiesse were not designed to address vocal fold problems.

After the 1992 publication, I decided to hold off on further collagen-related clinical studies as there was considerable ongoing exploration of injection laryngoplasty with collagen and other bioimplants at other centers. Although other studies supported the use of bioimplants for laryngoplasty, support for collagen use was constrained by skeptics who were either committed to Teflon or anxious to demonstrate the next best alternative. Some continued to deny that Teflon posed a problem and others feared that collagen injection would cause severe allergic reactions, perhaps leading to collagen autoimmune disease. Proponents of Teflon asserted that reports of bad results with Teflon were due to poor technique and stated that concerns over implant migration were overstated. When carefully executed studies demonstrated migration of injected Teflon particles to virtually all organ systems in animal models, they maintained that the small amounts injected for vocal fold augmentation would not act similarly—a position they upheld even when their own research showed Teflon particles having migrated to contralateral cervical nodes in dogs that had only small aliquots injected into their vocal folds. Some Teflon advocates continue to claim that Teflon granuloma formation is rare, when in fact it can be histologically identified anywhere Teflon is injected; although, when deep in laryngeal musculature the fibrous tissue-encased granuloma is asymptomatic. Finally, there continues to be competitive interest in developing the optimal laryngoplasty injectate. Although this is helpful in stimulating creative work and new investigations, it would be useful to have more critical dialogue and focused cooperative studies.

Injection laryngoplasty remains a work in progress. There are at least three pathways being pursued: (1) filler substances provoking minimal reaction while providing bulk to the paraglottic region, (2) substances with viscoelastic properties matching vocal fold lamina propria, and (3) tissue engineering through introduction of growth factors and cultured or stem cells programmed to function like vocal fold tissues. The goal of establishing an ideal filler substance as articulated by Arnold evolved from Teflon and silicone, to bioplastique, polydimethylsiloxane, and, more recently, hydroxylapatite suspension (Radiesse). It is unclear how this will endure with long term follow up but it might represent the current state-of-the-art of that pathway.

I believe our early work with collagen represented a fundamentally different pathway, giving rise to broad interest in bioimplants. Naturally, the scientific process will evolve through phases, retaining proven benefits of some biological implants in laryngoplasty and rejecting materials of limited efficacy. To date, cellular fat, collagen, fascia, and acellular dermal matrix preparations have proven useful bioimplants intended not only to fill space but also to partially match vocal fold viscoelasticity. Interest in the biological properties of implants led to attempts at replicating acellular matrix components of the superficial layer of lamina propria, specifically hyaluronic acid (HA) gels and chemically modified HA derivatives. This is a logical progression as we attempt to produce a more naturally functioning vocal fold, especially in addressing difficult problems like tissue loss and scarring. I expect that continued investigations of biologically active injectable materials will further explore cultured cells, growth factors, stem cell preparations, and evolving tissue engineering concepts.

ROLE OF INJECTABLE COLLAGEN IN THE TREATMENT OF GLOTTIC INSUFFICIENCY: A STUDY OF 119 PATIENTS

CHARLES N. FORD, MD

DIANE M. BLESS, PHD JEAN M. LOFTUS, MD

MADISON, WISCONSIN

Injectable bovine collagen has been used for treatment of glottic insufficiency at the University of Wisconsin Clinical Science Center since 1983. This report reviews our experience in treating 119 patients with a variety of vocal fold disorders manifested by glottic insufficiency. Many of the patients were referred because of prior treatment failures or problems that were impossible to treat with other modalities. Results were assessed by comprehensive voice evaluations using subjective patient self-assessments, perceptual judgments made by a panel of experts who had no prior knowledge of the study, objective assessments, and videostroboscopy. Objective assessment included vocal function measures and acoustic analysis. Results indicate that collagen not only is comparable to other injection filler substances but also has unique advantages as a bioimplant. Collagen injection seems uniquely suited for treatment of several problems, including vocal fold atrophy, focal defects, minimal glottic insufficiency, and scarred vocal folds that are not managed optimally with Teflon injection. Overall there were no serious complications and treatment was effective for a broad spectrum of problems. In most instances the correction persisted, and in those instances in which injected collagen seemed improperly distributed, the vocal fold was recontoured or the implant removed without appreciable damage to the surrounding tissues. Injectable collagen has been extensively studied and deserves to be included in the armamentarium of the laryngeal surgeon.

KEY WORDS — collagen, larynx, vocal fold, voice.

INTRODUCTION

The search for an ideal substance for vocal fold augmentation led Arnold[1] to use Teflon (Polytef Paste), which has become the workhorse method for treating glottic insufficiency. Although Teflon injection has offered tremendous improvement, this alloplastic preparation induces a definite foreign body reaction and focal fibrosis.[2-5] Concerns about complications such as granuloma formation,[6,7] airway obstruction,[8,9] potentially irreversible damage to vocal fold vibratory structure by foreign body reaction and fibrosis,[10] and the possibility of implant extrusion or migration[11,12] have motivated clinicians to look for alternative forms of treatment. Such alternatives have been advocated to enhance voice results and provide greater flexibility without permanently altering vocal fold tissues.[13-15]

Collagen injection differs from other vocal fold medialization approaches in that it is a biological implant, providing more than medial displacement of the vocal fold. The collagen implant consists of bovine collagen modified by solubilization and cross-linking to reduce cellular and humoral host immune response, but it is histologically similar to the deep lamina propria tissues in the vocal fold. Host tolerance of injected collagen is characterized by gradual assimilation starting with ingrowth of vessels and progressive invasion of fibroblasts into the implanted collagen. The events following collagen injection that affect vocal fold function specifically include the gradual variable resorption of injected collagen, the replacement of some resorbed implant by deposition of new host collagen from metabolically active invading host fibroblasts, and the softening of existing scar tissue, probably due to fibroblastic production of collagenase.

The physiologic limitations of alloplastic augmentation and the theoretic advantages of bioimplantable materials have led to experimentation with collagen injection of the vocal fold. Injected soluble bovine collagen has been used successfully to augment dermal defects and to soften depressed scars. We reasoned that this collagen implant might be well tolerated in the collagen-containing layers of the vocal fold and might be useful in treating scarred larynges.

PREVIOUS WORK

These observations prompted us to compare collagen injection to Teflon injection in dog larynges[16] and to look at the long-term histologic fate of different forms of collagen injected into the canine vocal fold.[17] We found that collagen could be injected precisely through a 26-gauge needle into the deep lamina propria of the vocal fold — a site normally composed of dense collagen. The implant was remarkably well tolerated, with no evidence of foreign body or inflammatory reaction; over time there was some peripheral neovascularization and ingrowth of fibroblasts with deposition of scattered

From the Division of Otolaryngology, Department of Surgery (all authors), and the Department of Communicative Disorders (Bless), University of Wisconsin, Madison, Wisconsin. This work was supported in part by grants from the Food and Drug Administration, Orphaned Product Development Division (grant FD-R-000404-02), the Veterans Administration Rehabilitation Research and Development Service, and a General Research Support Grant to the University of Wisconsin Medical School from the National Institutes of Health Division of Research Facilities and Resources (project 133-H529).

Presented at the meeting of the American Laryngological Association, Waikoloa, Hawaii, May 4-5, 1991.

REPRINTS — Charles N. Ford, MD, University of Wisconsin CSC, H4/320, 600 Highland Ave, Madison, WI 53792.

oci of new host collagen within the implant matrix, eplacing some of the assimilated implant. Persis- ence of the implant was noted at intervals up to 1 ear. Similar results were obtained subsequently by)kamoto.[18]

We also looked at the effect of superficially in- ected collagen on vocal fold vibration in the excised arynx and noted that simulated deficiencies could e corrected, with correction resulting in normal assive activation of vibratory activity in response o a steady controlled subglottic air pressure.[19] Re- ent in vivo canine studies have demonstrated im- provement in many vocal function parameters fol- owing injection for simulated vocal fold paralysis.[20]

In 1985 the authors[21] presented the first clinical rials of Zyderm Collagen Implant (Collagen Corp, Palo Alto, Calif) to correct glottic insufficiency in 27 patients. Objective voice analysis demonstrated efficacy, and none of these patients suffered com- plications. Questions were raised regarding long- term persistence of the implant and the possibility of hypersensitivity reactions.[22] A subsequent report with 2-year follow-up data indicated that in most patients, correction evident at 1 to 3 months per- sisted and results stabilized.[23] In this group of 44 pa- tients, there was 1 with a delayed hypersensitivity reaction manifested by development of slight red- ness at the vocal fold and skin test site at 5 weeks. Since 1986 all patients have been injected with cross-linked collagen preparations (generic glutar- aldehyde cross-linked [GAX] collagen, also mar- keted as Zyplast and Phonagel), which are less an- tigenic, diffuse easily, and undergo less initial shrinkage after injection.

Failure to gain Food and Drug Administration (FDA) approval limited clinical trials in this coun- try, but others[24-29] have reported successful results with soluble collagen injections for glottic insuffi- ciency. Most of these investigators made the injec- tions in the superficial mucosal layers of the vocal fold, since it was demonstrated that collagen in- jected deep in vocalis muscle was rapidly resorbed.[17] The issue of resorption was addressed in two post- mortem studies. Remacle and Marbaix[30] reported on the persistence of injected collagen in postmor- tem human larynges up to 5 months postinjection, and Ford et al[31] noted persistence in one patient af- ter 1 year.

It was apparent from these initial studies that col- lagen injection was a successful treatment for a variety of pathologic disorders manifested by glottic insufficiency. The limitations of Teflon injection did not seem to apply to collagen, especially in the treatment of the scarred vocal fold, focal defects, atrophy, and limited glottic insufficiency problems. Efficacy was demonstrated in independent studies of patients with age-related changes in the vocal folds (presbylaryngis)[32] and in those with scarred larynges.[33]

PURPOSE OF STUDY

In an attempt to further explore the potentials of a biologic implant, we initiated a study (suppported by the Orphaned Products Division of the FDA) to treat glottic insufficiency in patients who were not optimal candidates for Teflon injection, and we reviewed the entire group of collagen-injected pa- tients treated at the University of Wisconsin Clin- ical Science Center. Demonstration of efficacy in that select group of patients seemed a sufficiently important endeavor that no attempt was made to compare efficacy of collagen with other modes of treatment.

MATERIALS AND METHODS

Collagen injection of the vocal fold has been per- formed at the University of Wisconsin for manage- ment of glottic insufficiency since 1983. Goals in- cluded improving glottic closure, vocal quality, ease of phonation, and associated laryngeal func- tions in patients with a variety of vocal fold disor- ders. The experimental protocol was initiated in 166 patients, of whom 26 were lost to follow-up, 5 were treated too recently to include, and 2 had non- voice problems. Fourteen patients were not treated: 4 had positive skin tests, 4 declined in favor of alter- native forms of treatment, 3 had marginal airways, and 3 improved with voice therapy.

PATIENTS

The 119 patients reported in this study represent those individuals who were treated and who com- plied with our protocol for follow-up voice assess- ment data collection. The pretreatment age range was 17 to 87 years, with a mean of 56 years, and the male to female ratio was approximately 3:2. Nearly half of the patients treated had scarred larynges, often secondary to laryngeal cancer surgery — a fact reflected in the male preponderance, for laryn- geal cancer remains a predominantly male disease. Patients had experienced voice problems for an av- erage of 6.1 (0.08 to 33.9) years before treatment and 30% had undergone voice therapy prior to col- lagen injection. Some patients underwent more than one injection over a period of months or years. The average length of follow-up was 16.4 (1 to 67) months.

Potential patients were evaluated by a speech pa- thologist and the senior author (C.N.F.) to deter- mine their suitability for treatment. In each case both the protocol and available alternatives to management were described. Those who seriously considered collagen injection were skin-tested with Zyderm, which is generically similar to GAX col- lagen but exhibits greater antigenicity. If the skin test remained negative for 6 weeks, injection was offered. Two patients were injected before 6 weeks because of severe aspiration problems.

Each patient was assigned to one of three vocal fold disorder groups on the basis of those histopathologic findings that seem to affect function and outcome.

Scarred Vocal Fold. The scarred vocal fold group were patients who had evidence of vocal fold scarring manifested by stiffness or decreased mucosal wave on videostroboscopy. Such patients typically had the most impaired vocal fold vibration, often secondary to surgery such as cordectomy, vocal fold stripping, Teflon injection/or removal, and hemilaryngectomy. Other patients had undergone radiotherapy or prolonged endotracheal intubation.

Bilateral Disorder. The bilateral vocal fold disorder group comprised patients who had had some form of bilateral disorder without scar formation. These patients exhibited a variety of diagnoses, including neurologic disorders such as presbylaryngis, Parkinson's disease, and abductor spasmodic dysphonia with bowed vocal folds. Some of these patients showed atrophic changes associated with presbylaryngis as well as bilateral paresis. Bilateral paresis was also attributable to head injuries, respiratory infections, and idiopathic neuropathies.

Unilateral Disorder. The unilateral vocal fold disorder group was made up of patients who had essentially unilateral disorders without evidence of scar formation or contralateral vocal fold disorders. Some had iatrogenic injuries involving the recurrent and/or superior laryngeal nerves. Other patients were paretic or paralyzed as a result of cerebral vascular accident or prolonged intubation, and some cases were idiopathic.

Patients with mixed disorders were assigned to that group typically associated with their greatest impairment of vocal fold function according to the following hierarchy: scarred vocal fold > bilateral disorder > unilateral disorder. The FDA Orphaned Product study was limited to the most severely impaired larynges; these patients had mainly scarred vocal folds or bilateral disorders.

COLLAGEN

The material injected during the initial phase of this study consisted of Zyderm Collagen Implant, a soluble bovine collagen. Since 1986 we have used GAX collagen, an injectable glutaraldehyde cross-linked (0.0075%) fibrillar collagen (Zyplast, Phonagel). It is essentially type I collagen with a residue of 1% to 5% type III collagen, prepared by selective hydrolysis of the nonhelical amino-terminal and carboxy-terminal segments (telopeptides) of the collagen molecule. Antigenicity is reduced by telopeptide cleavage and further reduced during the cross-linking process. GAX collagen remains the preferred material for vocal fold injection because it persists with minimal shrinkage and has reduced antigenicity compared to other forms of injectable collagen.[34]

PROCEDURE

Most of the injections were made by using indirect laryngoscopy and topical anesthesia, but several patients, particularly in the scarred vocal fold group, required direct microlaryngoscopy for proper placement. The material was injected via a device designed by the senior author[35] through the superior surface of the vocal fold into the intermediate and deep lamina propria.[21,23] The 26-gauge needle allowed for precise visual and tactile placement at the plane of the vocal ligament; slight resistance is encountered as the needle is advanced from the superior surface further into the vocal fold tissue.[36] In heavily scarred larynges, an effort was made to get as much collagen injected into the scar as possible with the initial penetration; often this practice resulted in collagen's being dispersed in deeper or more superficial levels than would have been ideal. Subsequent injections were generally easier and more precisely placed. All injections were made on a distinctly more superficial plane than is typical with Teflon, silicone, Gelfoam, or fat. The superficial placement facilitates filling in focal defects without distorting the entire vocal fold, prevents rapid resorption, and allows the implant to be injected at a site in which collagen is normally found.

In some of the more complex cases, collagen injection was used to enhance or correct changes induced by other forms of therapy. For example, patients with fibrotic convex vocal folds secondary to Teflon granulomas were managed by endoscopic removal of Teflon; in those instances in which the medial edge remained irregular, the vocal fold was remodeled with precise injections of collagen. Four patients had sulcus vocalis deformities treated by cordotomy, lysis of the adhesions, and later collagen injection to contour and soften the vocal fold tissues. Several patients were referred because failed attempts at glottic reconstruction following various conservation laryngectomy procedures left them with stiff, scarred larynges incapable of useful phonation. One patient had bilateral vocal fold paralysis and a marginal airway unsafe for any vocal fold augmentation; after successful neuromuscular pedicle transfer to the posterior cricoarytenoid muscle, a small amount of collagen was injected unilaterally in the membranous vocal fold with perceptible improvement in voice and no change in exercise tolerance. Some patients with scarred larynges had large glottic gaps that were initially addressed with thyroplasty surgery, and the scarred vocal fold was treated with collagen injection to soften and restore the contour of the vocal fold.

Postoperatively, patients were observed for airway problems and kept on relative voice rest overnight — talking only when necessary and avoiding extremes in pitch and loudness. Patients returned for full assessment at 1-, 3-, and 6-month and 1-year intervals. Subsequent data were collected on a yearly basis.

ASSESSMENT METHODS

Four general categories of voice assessment were used to measure treatment success: 1) subjective patient self-assessment of voice quality and effort of phonation, 2) perceptual judgments of voice recordings by an impartial panel of experts, 3) laboratory data based on acoustic signal analysis and aerodynamic measures during voice production, and 4) studies of the appearance of vocal fold vibration by videostroboscopy.

Subjective patient self-assessment ratings were included as part of this comprehensive voice evaluation. After treatment, patients were grouped on the basis of their own ratings of their vocal quality and the effort required to produce phonation: 1) voice not improved, 2) voice improved and sustained improvement, 3) transient improvement, and 4) voice worse. Some patients in group 2 (bilateral disorders) noted a very slight decrement in vocal function over time but were convinced that the voice was substantially improved over the pretreatment status. For patients who had multiple injections, the subjective category was based on comparing the most recent evaluation to that immediately before the last injection.

Audiotape recordings were made in a sound-controlled booth with a Nagra tape recorder, as previously described.[21] The test sample recorded included sustained vowels /a/ and /i/ produced at normal pitch and loudness and the sentence "The blue spot is on the key" produced at conversational level. These samples were used for both the acoustic and perceptual analyses.

Perceptual judgments were made from the audio recordings of sustained vowels and the standard sentence. Pretreatment and the most recent posttreatment recordings were randomized and paired on a master tape. Three experienced speech pathologists were asked to make paired comparison judgments to determine which sample, if either, sounded better; they also indicated when there was no appreciable difference. To determine reliability of judgments, 10% of the samples were repeated and 10% of the samples were foils consisting of two identical samples. Foils were used to determine validity of the perceptual ratings. The judges were 100% correct in judging these voices to be the same.

Acoustic analysis of voice production permits quantitative analysis of the multidimensional physical characteristics of the voice signal and inference about the underlying physiologic mechanism. Samples were digitized on an IBM-PC computer with a locally developed software program (C-Speech). Jitter, shimmer, and signal to noise ratio (SNR) were derived by using the least mean square fit of a waveform model to the speech waveform.

TABLE 1. SUBJECTIVE PATIENT SELF-ASSESSMENT REGARDING VOICE QUALITY AND EFFORT

Disorder	*N*	*Sustained Improvement*	*Transient Improvement*	*No Improvement*	*Worse*
Scarred vocal fold	55	39	4	12	0
Bilateral disorder	25	23	1	1	0
Unilateral disorder	39	39	0	0	0

Data are numbers of patients.

Vocal function measures were recorded by means of a face mask attached to the Nagashima PS-77 Phonatory Function Analyzer to obtain maximal intensity (decibels) and mean airflow (milliters per second). Transglottic airflow was assessed during production of /a/ and /i/ during a variety of phonatory tasks. High airflows were considered an indicator of poor laryngeal closure, as might occur in glottic insufficiency. Low airflows generally signified a competent glottis, but were noted to occur also with hyperfunction of laryngeal structures (a common compensatory activity), obstruction, low patient effort, or poor respiratory support.

Vocal fold vibration was observed with a Bruel & Kjaer laryngeal videostroboscope coupled to a rigid 90°-angled Wolfe endoscope and videorecorder. Recordings were used to assess ongoing treatment and to study individual cases over time. Recordings were rated in 15 consecutive cases by trained observers who made qualitative judgments of vocal fold vibration and supraventricular hyperfunction. Parameters observed were symmetry, periodicity, glottic closure, vibration amplitude, mucosal wave, and supraventricular hyperfunction; preoperative and postoperative samples were compared for each patient.

In cases for which preinjection data were available from more than one date, the date closest to injection was selected. Postinjection data were selected from the latest date the patient had been evaluated. When collagen injection was done after thyroplasty, Teflon removal, or reinnervation surgery, baseline measures were taken after the previous operation and before collagen injection.

STATISTICAL ANALYSIS

Efficacy of collagen injections was addressed by asking two questions: 1) Was there a significant change in any of the variables postinjection? and 2) Was there any difference between disorder groups in response to the collagen treatment? To analyze for pretreatment and posttreatment changes in the parameters (acoustic, aerodynamic, perceptual), we used paired t tests to determine whether or not

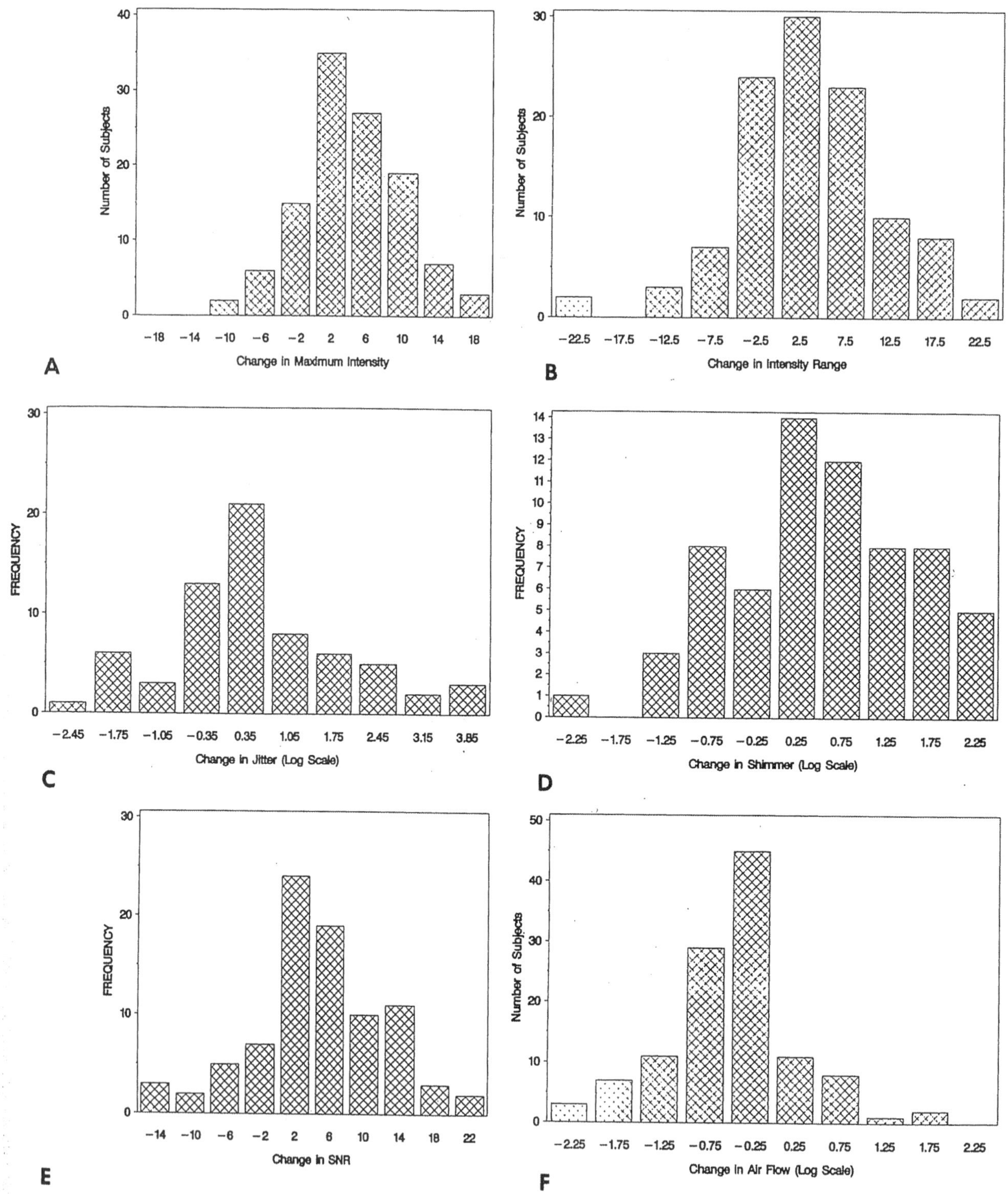

Fig 1. Bar graphs of changes from before to after collagen injection for six measures of vocal function. A) Maximum intensity. B) Intensity range. C) Jitter. D) Shimmer. E) Signal to noise ratio (SNR). F) Airflow.

the mean change was equal to zero. Differences between diagnosis groups were studied by using an analysis of variance. A χ^2 test was used for overall testing of perceptual change within and between groups. For measures with skewed distributions (airflow, jitter, shimmer), the log of the measure was used. These transformed measures had distributions close to normal, thus making the transformation changes nearly equivalent to analyzing percentage changes rather than absolute changes. Pearson's product-moment correlations were used to assess intrajudge and interjudge reliability. Wilcoxon's test was used to test for differences between stroboscopic recordings for select patients. The test

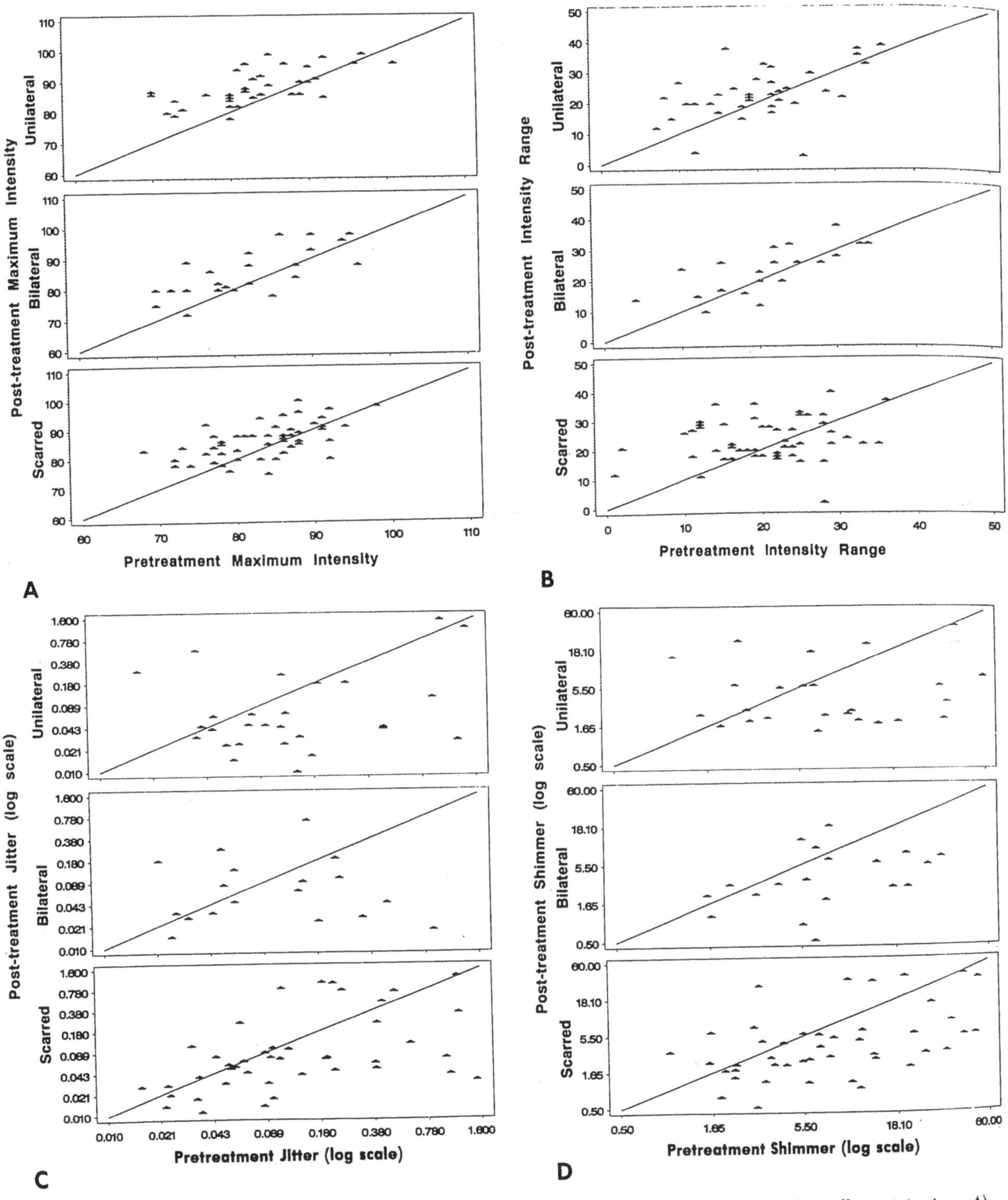

Fig 2. Scatterplots of three treatment groups' performance on measures of vocal function before and after collagen injections. A) Maximum intensity. B) Intensity range. C) Jitter. D) Shimmer. (Continued on next page.)

assumes that the distribution of the data is symmetric about the median.

RESULTS

There were no serious complications or side effects for any of the 119 patients. Two reactions to Zyderm injection in the vocal fold could be considered delayed hypersensitivity reactions. In 1 patient redness was noted at the injection site and developed at the skin test site 5 weeks after the initial skin test and 1 week after vocal fold injection. The second patient developed redness of the injected vocal fold at 1 year postinjection. Neither of these patients experienced any airway compromise and both noted improved voice that persisted. Interestingly, they were both alcoholics, heavy smok-

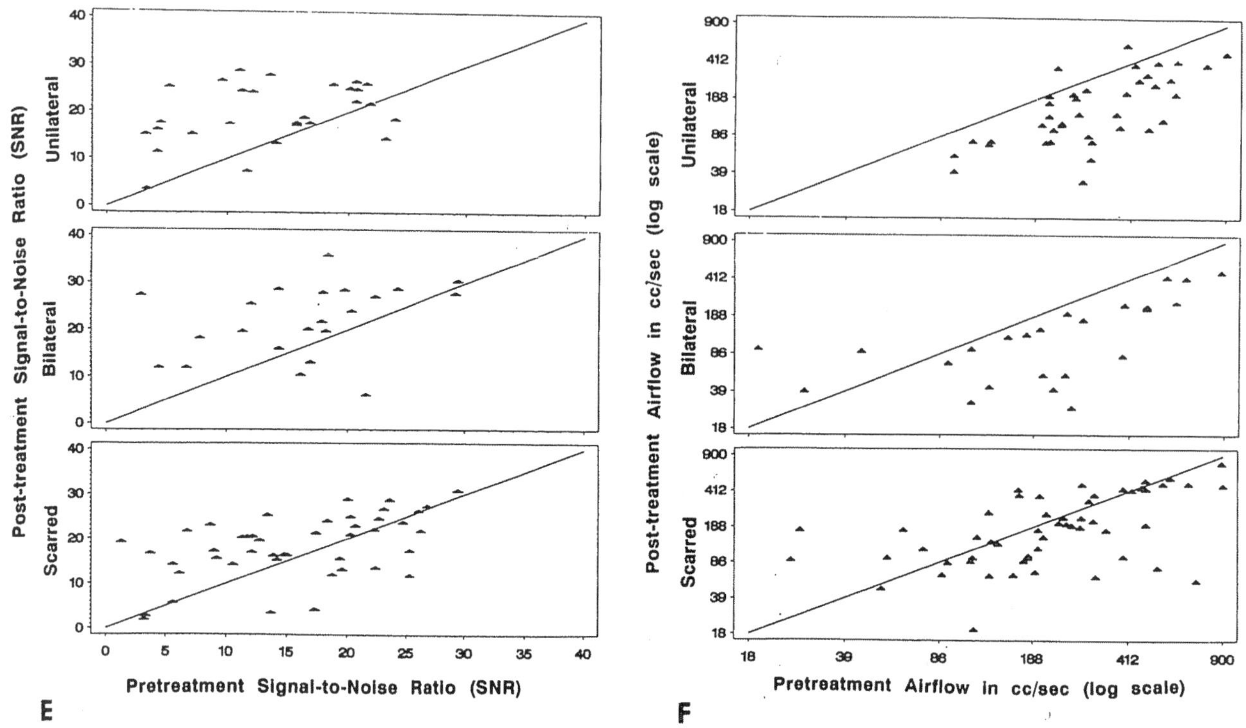

Fig 2, continued. E) Signal to noise ratio. F) Airflow.

ers, and posthemilaryngectomy men who had been injected with Zyderm in 1984. There have been no apparent hypersensitivity reactions to GAX collagen injections.

In the subjective patient assessment (Table 1), those in the unilateral paralysis group all rated their voices improved, and improvement over preinjection status was noted throughout the follow-up period. Those with scarred larynges had the worst ratings, with 12 patients noting no appreciable improvement. No patient felt the voice was worse following collagen injection. In 3 patients with scarred larynges, the surgeon noted qualitative changes such as diplophonia and inappropriately elevated pitch that appeared to be related to focal loculations of implanted collagen at superficial sites. In each of those patients a small incision was made over the implant bleb and the material easily aspirated; this procedure resulted in improved contour and subjective vocal quality. Improvement was noted by perceptual judgments, and the significance varied by diagnostic group. In comparing pretreatment to posttreatment assessments the overall improvement was significant at $p = .00023$ (unilateral $p = .021$, bilateral $p = .71$, and scarred $p = = .0009$).

Acoustic measures evaluated from pretreatment to posttreatment included maximum intensity, intensity range, jitter, shimmer, airflow, and SNR (Figs 1 and 2). In general, maximum intensity, intensity range, shimmer, and SNR increased and jitter and airflow decreased. Results were predicted (Table 2) as a function of the anatomic changes achieved through the collagen injections.

Successful injection for glottic insufficiency should result in improved glottic closure such that there is less wasted airflow during phonation. Although some patients have a tendency to compensate for glottic insufficiency by supraglottic valving, which also decreases flow, reduced airflow following injection was generally considered to indicate success. Low preoperative flows (<80 mL/s) increased (Fig 2F), and high flows (>200 mL/s) decreased, regardless of the disorder classification.

Significant differences were determined for all groups for six objective parameters (Table 3). One of the greatest changes for the unilateral group was airflow. Both the bilateral and scarred groups also showed significant airflow changes, but the significance in the scarred group was marginal. Maximum

TABLE 2. SELECTED VOCAL PARAMETERS AND HOW THEY SHOULD CHANGE AS FUNCTION OF TREATMENT GOALS

Treatment Goal	*Intensity*	*Airflow*	*Frequency*	*Jitter*	*Shimmer*	*SNR*
Improved closure	+	−	−	−	−	+
Decreased stiffness	+	−	−	+	0	+
Improved vocal fold contour	+	−	0	−	0	+
Reduced hyper-function	0	+	0	+	0	0

SNR — signal to noise ratio, plus — should increase, minus — should decrease, zero — no predictable change.

TABLE 3. SIGNIFICANT DIFFERENCES FOR THREE DISORDER GROUPS ON SIX OBJECTIVE VOCAL PARAMETERS

Vocal Parameters	Disorder Groups: Scarred	Bilateral	Unilateral
Airflow	+	++	++
Maximum intensity	++	++	++
Signal to noise ratio	++	++	++
Intensity range	++	−	+
Jitter	++	−	++
Shimmer	++	++	++

Two pluses — significantly different, one plus — significantly different but marginally so, minus — not significantly different.

TABLE 4. LARYNGEAL VIDEOSTROBOSCOPIC ASSESSMENT OF 15 CASES BY WILCOXON'S TEST OF MEDIAN EQUAL TO 0.000000 VERSUS MEDIAN NOT EQUAL TO 0.000000

Parameters	No. of Cases	Estimated: p	Median
Supraglottic hyperfunction	15	.001	1.000
Periodicity	14*	.281	0.000
Glottic gap	15	.001	1.000
Amplitude vibration	14*	.022	0.500
Mucosal wave	14*	.022	0.500
Symmetry	15	.234	0.500
Overall function based on above	15	.001	3.000

*One subject could not be rated on vibratory activity because of malfunction of strobe light, so that subject was rated only on supraglottic activity, glottic gap, and symmetry.

intensity and SNR increased significantly for all three groups. For the scarred group, intensity range, jitter, and shimmer also increased significantly. Both jitter and shimmer were significantly increased for the unilateral disorder group.

Videostroboscopy was particularly helpful in assessing individual patients and in guiding initial placement and modification. It was difficult to objectively assess results of collagen injections by using videostroboscopy, because the medialized vocal fold was usually obvious in the postoperative sample. Recognition of the postinjection samples did not interfere with ratings of supraglottic hyperfunction, waveform periodicity, glottic gap, amplitude of vibration, mucosal wave, and vocal fold symmetry. These measures were rated on preoperative and postoperative videotapes and the results subjected to statistical analysis with Wilcoxon's test (Table 4). These data suggest a significant improvement in all videostroboscopic parameters.

DISCUSSION

SUBJECTIVE MEASURES

In this study, voice improvement was determined by both subjective and objective measures. Patient self-assessments were, overall, higher than the perceptual judgments of the panel of experts; the professional did not note improvement unless the voice was less hoarse, whereas the patient self-assessment included not only quality, but also effort and loudness.

In many patients the primary concern was the extreme effort and dyspnea of phonation; another frequent concern was inadequate vocal volume. After successful treatment, patients perceived a louder voice as improved because they could carry on a more normal life talking over noise in restaurants, cars, etc. Improved closure would often result in increased intensity levels even when quality was not changed. Although such changes may not have been apparent to the listener, for the speaker they were very important.

The patient self-assessments related well to the measures of airflow, SNR, and intensity. One might be tempted to explain the difference between the patient self-assessment and professional perceptual ratings on the probability that the patient expects changes to result from therapy, and therefore rates his or her voice as improved. The correlation of self-assessment ratings with objective measures and analysis of ratings in different disorder groups suggest more fundamental differences. The scarred group had the worst voice both preoperatively and postoperatively, but the panel of speech pathologists noted more individuals with improved voice in this group than in the other two. Some of these patients started out aphonic or nearly aphonic with very high harmonics. Thus, any treatment resulting in some voice or reduction in the higher harmonics would be rated by the speech pathologist as improved. The bilateral group generally began with some voice, though often characterized by weakness, breathiness, and poor control. This group also had the most individuals with other neurologic and respiratory problems that were often not treated and that continued to contribute to the overall quality of voice. Following treatment, the voice was louder and therefore rated as better by the patient, but not necessarily by the speech pathologist, who was more attuned to the absence of changes in quality.

OBJECTIVE MEASURES

It is interesting that airflow significantly decreased for all three groups. Even more interesting is the observation that individuals with low preoperative flows increased flow following treatment. In other words, the treatment tended to normalize values. It was anticipated that increased glottic closure would result in increased intensity and an improved SNR, as proved true for all three disorder groups. It was also assumed that increased closure would result in better vocal control, less aerodynamic turbulence, and decreased perturbation values. Contrary to expectations, jitter and shimmer increased significantly, not only in the unilateral group but in the scarred group as well. The bilateral groups showed a similar response, but only shimmer was significantly changed.

Although laryngeal videostroboscopy is extremely useful in assessing disease and in observing the effect of treatment, it is difficult to objectively quantify these results to assess efficacy. It is possible to observe the effect of injection on vocal fold vibration and to determine the degree of correction of glottic closure; one can also grossly quantify the amplitude of vibration, mucosal wave, and periodicity. Unfortunately, it is difficult to mask the treated larynx because of the obvious displacement and whitish color often found in the injected fold. It is therefore not possible to objectively compare random preoperative and postoperative samples to eliminate judgment bias.

PHYSIOLOGIC ASPECTS OF COLLAGEN INJECTIONS

In addressing any particular type of disorder of the vocal fold, one must consider the components contributing to the dysphonia, including respiratory support and the vibratory structure. Often subtle changes in vocal fold composition affect vibratory properties, so that it is undesirable to lump all patients with paralysis or glottic insufficiency into the same group. For example, simply adding mass to a deficient vocal fold does not assure adequate vibration; in some instances it may increase stiffness and thereby impede vibration. The physical properties of GAX allowing superficial precise placement in focal defects and the biologic properties rendering it effective in the scarred larynx make collagen useful in addressing complex vocal fold problems associated with discrete tissue loss or scarring.

Resorption is reduced when collagen is injected into more superficial vocal fold levels (superficial lamina propria) and, in many patients, a superficially injected implant could be seen easily through the transparent mucosa years after injection. The recent use of GAX collagen has drastically reduced the amount of resorption,[25,26] but it may still occur in some patients. Usually it is very gradual and only minimal. In most of these patients, such resorption is not accompanied by a decrement in voice function. It is likely that some degree of resorption occurs in all patients, but this is quantitatively offset by deposition of host collagen. Functionally such change may be insignificant as long as the functional correction remains. Those patients who actually lose correction but maintain voice improvement deserve comment.

We hypothesize that the patient receives immediate relief after injection, and if the implant is properly placed in the lamina propria, gradual resorption and replacement allow the vocal mechanism to compensate incrementally for small changes. In other words, some neuromuscular retraining is occurring over time as the patient adjusts to these small changes, allowing the patient to hit the vocal target even with an inadequate vocal fold structure. This biologic successive approximation training is an example of alteration of the nervous system through biofeedback. Such nervous system plasticity may be an important mechanism in the success of collagen injection in some patients (H. Okamura, personal communication, 1989).

Reviewing selected patients' videostroboscopic studies reveals four patterns of change: 1) correction persists with negligible perceptible change, 2) correction decreases over the first few weeks and then stabilizes within 1 to 3 months, 3) correction persists months to years and then suddenly, usually after an upper respiratory tract infection, resorption occurs, and 4) rapid resorption occurs in a few patients within weeks. This last group consists mainly of patients with other medical problems such as Parkinson's disease. It is not totally clear why these patients are so resistant to correction. Problems with neuromotor control might explain their inability to adapt, but it is not at all clear why they should be susceptible to implant resorption.

In those patients for whom the implant persists but the contour or distribution is not ideal, it is possible to redistribute superficially placed collagen for several months after injection. In patients with less than ideal contour, voice, and stroboscopic findings following injection, visible collagen was nudged from an anterior to a more posterior location with the edge of the injection device; such procedures were done within 2 weeks of injection, by using topical anesthesia and indirect laryngoscopy in the outpatient clinic. In three patients we easily removed small focal blebs of injected collagen, within 1 year of injection, by placing a small incision over the collagen and aspirating with a small suction tip. No apparent scar tissue or inflammatory tissue developed, and in each case the voice improved with loss of diplophonia and decreased roughness.

No patients treated with GAX collagen injection experienced airway compromise, focal redness, swelling, or other signs of allergic reactions. Delayed onset of erythema at the injection site in two patients — one of whom also developed redness at the skin test site — occurred early in our series when Zyderm (not GAX collagen) was used. Overall, GAX preparations are less antigenic and persist longer.[37] Zyderm, Phonagel, and Zyplast are qualitatively different from other available forms of collagen (Koken Atelocollagen, Gelfoam, Collastat, and Avitene), and their biologic characteristics seem most favorable for vocal fold injection.[34] Other studies may not be comparable if different materials are used for injection.

ROLES OF COLLAGEN

Factors that determine the efficacy of collagen injection include the degree of glottic insufficiency and the specific vocal fold disorder. In some instances conditions may be best treated by combining collagen injection with other modalities such as thyroplasty. Our experience suggests that collagen injection may be used to treat many different conditions, but it is particularly useful in four situations.

Atrophied Vocal Fold. Examples include patients with high vagal lesions showing loss of recurrent and superior laryngeal nerves, presbylaryngis with loss of vocal fold connective tissue bulk and a characteristic arrowhead-shaped residual glottic gap during phonation, congenital hypoplasia in which there is failure of development of the layers of vocal fold such as in sulcus vocalis, and isolated superior laryngeal nerve paralysis. In all of these examples there is loss of fullness of the vocal fold, often associated with a medial furrow. Since collagen can be injected effectively in a superficial plane, it is possible to fill out such folds and recontour the vocal fold to match the contralateral side.

Scarred Vocal Fold. Scarring of the membranous vocal fold is a difficult problem, because the functional integrity of the tissue is destroyed, and even with perfect displacement, restoration of vibratory activity will not occur unless the tissues undergo some biologic transformation. No procedure or material besides collagen has been shown to address this problem. Collagen injection has been demonstrated to soften scar tissue in the dermis[38] and also in vocal folds.[33] Such changes have allowed for additional augmentation and restoration of the body-cover relationship required for vocal fold vibration. This effect of collagen is based theoretically on the biologic activity of the implant affecting the scar tissue–amino acid equilibrium to allow remodeling over time. Unfortunately, it is difficult to inject anything into scar tissue, and optimal results may take many injections over several years. For now, there are no suitable alternatives.

Minimal Glottic Insufficiency. In patients with relatively minimal glottic insufficiency who are bothered by weak, breathy voice production, collagen injection has proven a relatively safe and successful method of treatment. Many patients with presbylaryngis, with bilateral paresis from neurologic disease or trauma, and with bowing due to cricothyroid muscle weakness fit in this group. We found that small amounts (0.05 to 0.20 cm^3) of GAX collagen injected in the plane of the vocal ligament and the intermediate layer of the lamina propria were successful at producing improved voices.[32] These cases may represent instances in which some gradual resorption occurs as the patient develops improved phonation strategies.

Focal Vocal Fold Defects and Adynamic Segments. Focal loss of tissue or scarring confined to a limited area of the membranous vocal fold requires precise placement of a filler substance. Often the scarring may be so subtle as to escape detection on routine examination but will appear as an adynamic segment, with absence of a mucosal wave, on laryngeal videostroboscopy. Collagen can be injected with extreme precision at the site of the defect in mucosal and immediate submucosal tissues. This is a unique advantage over Teflon, which must be injected deep into the thyroarytenoid muscle.

Each of the four conditions can coexist with additional vocal fold disease that might be more suitably handled with a different form of treatment such as thyroplasty, reinnervation, or arytenoid adduction. In some of these instances, collagen injection might be considered as an adjunctive measure.

In addition to patient selection, the most important factor in determining the success of collagen injection is proper technique. All those who have reported successful management of glottic insufficiency by collagen injection have described placement of the implant at a superficial level in the vocal fold. This is quite different from the placement of Teflon. Deep injection of collagen results in poor correction of the defect and rapid resorption of the implant. If the material fails to be distributed as intended, it is possible to modify the contour by rubbing the edge of the vocal fold with the injector device. Scarred vocal folds may require injection at different levels to facilitate maximal distribution of the implant.

SUMMARY AND CONCLUSIONS

This study and other clinical data indicate that collagen injection is relatively safe and useful in treating atrophic, scarred, or focally damaged vocal folds, and that it is helpful in relieving symptoms in patients with a small degree of glottic insufficiency. Some conditions treatable with collagen cannot be handled effectively with other treatment modalities, and other conditions might benefit from collagen injection as an alternative or adjunctive measure. While there is no reason to claim that collagen injection is the single best treatment for glottic insufficiency, these data support inclusion of GAX collagen injection in the armamentarium of the phonosurgeon engaged in treating glottic insufficiency problems. Collagen differs from other injectables in that it is a bioimplant with the capacity to be assimilated into the host tissues and soften scar tissue. A collagen implant can be redistributed or removed after injection without harmful effects. No patients have exhibited allergic reactions to the newer GAX collagens (Zyplast or Phonagel).

Acceptance, however, has been hampered by concerns over safety and efficacy that do not seem justified on the basis of worldwide experience and the data presented in this study. Ironically, Gelfoam has never been approved by the FDA for laryngeal injection, and yet it is commonly injected into vocal folds by laryngologists to determine if a patient is a suitable candidate for Teflon injection.

A GAX collagen generically identical to Zyplast is commercially available, but use in the larynx has not been approved.

The immediate challenge is to make collagen injection available to patients in need. Collagen injection has been studied more extensively than many other currently used substances. Our results on 119 patients showing it to be relatively safe, well tolerated, and effective are consistent with those of other researchers. Collagen can be used to treat a variety of conditions for which there are no good alternatives, and it can be considered a useful adjunctive measure in treating complex vocal fold problems.

ACKNOWLEDGMENTS — The authors thank Thomas D. Cook for his assistance in statistical analysis, Joseph F. Bollettierri for data processing, Celeste Kirk for editorial advice, Loree A. Ketner for typing the manuscript, and Danna Koschkee, Edie Swift, and Dawn Biever-Lowery for assisting in data collection.

REFERENCES

1. Arnold GE. Vocal rehabilitation of paralytic dysphonia. Arch Otolaryngol 1962;76:358-68.

2. Toomey JM, Brown BS. The histological response to intracordal injection of Teflon paste. Laryngoscope 1967;77:110-20.

3. Stone JW, Arnold GE. Human larynx injected with Teflon paste. Histologic study of innervation and tissue reaction. Arch Otolaryngol 1967;86:550-61.

4. Stone JW, Arnold GE, Stephens CB. Intracordal Polytef (Teflon) injection. Histologic study of three further cases. Arch Otolaryngol 1970;91:568-74.

5. Dedo HH, Carlsöö B. Histologic evaluation of Teflon granulomas of human vocal cords. A light and electron microscopic study. Acta Otolaryngol (Stockh) 1982;93:475-84.

6. Tucker HM. Complications after surgical management of the paralyzed larynx. Laryngoscope 1983;93:295-8.

7. Wenig BM, Heffner DK, Johnson FB. Teflonomas of the larynx and neck. Hum Pathol 1990;21:617-23.

8. Solomons NB, Livesey JR. Acute upper airway obstruction following Teflon injection of a vocal cord: the value of nebulized adrenaline and a helium/oxygen mixture in its management. J Laryngol Otol 1990;104:654-5.

9. Lewy RB. Teflon injection of the vocal cord: complications, errors, and precautions. Ann Otol Rhinol Laryngol 1983; 92:473-4.

10. Watterson T, McFarlane S, Menicucci A. Vibratory characteristics of Teflon-injected and noninjected paralyzed vocal folds. J Speech Hear Disord 1990;55:61-6.

11. Malizia AA, Reiman HM, Myers RP, et al. Migration and granulomatous reaction after periurethral injection of Polytef (Teflon). JAMA 1984;251:3277-81.

12. Ellis JC, McCaffrey TV, DeSanto LW, Reiman HV. Migration of Teflon after vocal cord injection. Otolaryngol Head Neck Surg 1987;96:63-6.

13. Isshiki N, Morita H, Okamura H, Hiramoto M. Thyroplasty as a new phonosurgical technique. Acta Otolaryngol (Stockh) 1974;78:451-7.

14. Kaufman JA. Laryngoplasty for vocal cord medialization: an alternative to Teflon®. Laryngoscope 1986;96:726-31.

15. Crumley RL, Izdebski K, McMicken B. Nerve transfer versus Teflon® injection for vocal cord paralysis: a comparison. Laryngoscope 1988;98:1200-4.

16. Ford CN, Martin DW, Warner TF. Injectable collagen in laryngeal rehabilitation. Laryngoscope 1984;94:513-8.

17. Ford CN. Histologic studies on the fate of soluble collagen injected into canine vocal folds. Laryngoscope 1986;96:1248-57.

18. Okamoto K. A fundamental study of injectable collagen in vocal rehabilitation. J Otolaryngol Jpn (Tokyo) 1987;90:394-403.

19. Ford CN, Bless DM, Campbell D. Studies of injectable soluble collagen for vocal fold augmentation. Rev Laryngol Otol Rhinol (Bord) 1987;108:33-6.

20. Trapp TK, Berke GS, Bell TS, Hanson DG, Ward PH. Effect of vocal fold augmentation on laryngeal vibration in simulated recurrent laryngeal nerve paralysis: a study of Teflon and Phonogel. Ann Otol Rhinol Laryngol 1989;98:220-7.

21. Ford CN, Bless DM. A preliminary study of injectable collagen in human vocal fold augmentation. Otolaryngol Head Neck Surg 1986;94:104-12.

22. Spiegel JR, Sataloff RT, Gould WJ. The treatment of vocal fold paralysis with injectable collagen: clinical concerns. J Voice 1987;1:119-21.

23. Ford CN, Bless DM. Clinical experience with injectable collagen for vocal fold augmentation. Laryngoscope 1986;96:863-9.

24. Remacle M, Clerin M, Dubois P, Ryckaert M, Bertrand B, Hamoir M. Exploration of glottic function before and after injection of collagen for rehabilitation of the vocal cord. Acta Otorhinolaryngol Belg 1986;40:405-20.

25. Remacle M, Marbaix E, Hamoir M, Declaye X, van den Eeckhaut J. Initial long-term results of collagen injection for vocal and laryngeal rehabilitation. Arch Otorhinolaryngol 1989;246: 403-6.

26. Remacle M, Marbaix E, Hamoir M, Bertrand B, van den Eeckhaut J. Correction of glottic insufficiency by collagen injection. Ann Otol Rhinol Laryngol 1990;99:438-44.

27. Okamoto K, Kawamura Y, Yumoto E, Okamura H. The application of injectable collagen in vocal rehabilitation. Proc Int Assoc Logopedics Phoniatrics 1986;1:484-5.

28. Joussen K. Soluble collagen as a bioimplant to remove glottic insufficiency. Proc Int Assoc Logopedics Phoniatrics 1986; 1:476-8.

29. Yumoto E, Okamoto K, Kawamura Y, Okamura H. Injection of atelocollagen to augment the paralyzed vocal cord. J Jpn Bronchoesophagol Soc 1988;39:271-4.

30. Remacle M, Marbaix E. Collagen implants in the human larynx, pathological examination of two cases. Arch Otorhinolaryngol 1988;245:203-9.

31. Ford CN, Gilchrist KW, Bartell TE. Persistence of injectable collagen in the human larynx: a histopathologic study. Laryngoscope 1987;97:724-7. [Erratum, Laryngoscope 1987;97: 1042.]

32. Ford CN, Bless DM, Pratt S, Peppard R, Collins MJ, Collins MT. Bovine collagen injections in the senile larynx [Abstract]. ASHA 1988;30:96.

33. Ford CN, Bless DM. Collagen injection in the scarred vocal fold. J Voice 1987;1:116-8.

34. DeLustro F, Contell RA, Nguyen MA, McPherson JM. A comparative study of the biologic and immunologic response to medical devices derived from dermal collagen. J Biomed Mater Res 1986;20:109-20.

35. Ford CN. A multipurpose laryngeal injector device. Otolaryngol Head Neck Surg 1990;103:135-7.

36. Ford CN. Laryngeal injection techniques. In: Ford CN, Bless DM, eds. Phonosurgery: assessment and surgical management of voice disorders. New York, NY: Raven Press, 1991:123-41.

37. Kligman AM, Armstrong RC. Histologic response to intradermal Zyderm and Zyplast (glutaraldehyde cross-linked) collagen in humans. J Dermatol Surg Oncol 1986;12:351-7.

38. Stegman SJ, Tromovich TA. Implantation of collagen for depressed scars. J Dermatol Surg Oncol 1980;6:450-3.

Commentary

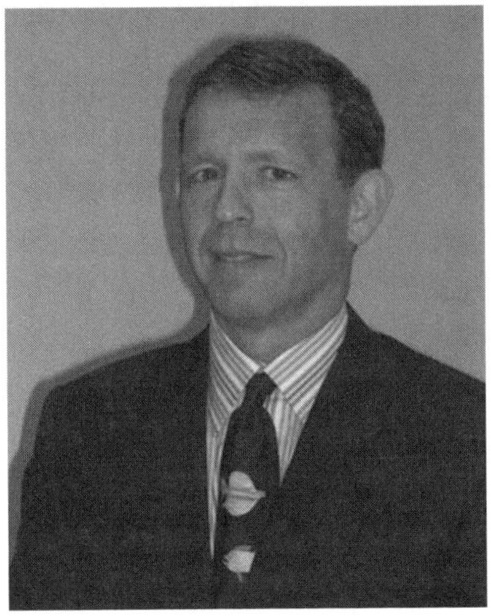

Gary Y. Shaw, MD

From the 1960s through the 1980s, the injection of Teflon dominated as the injection laryngoplasty material of choice. As a junior resident in the mid-1980s, I was fortunate to be taught the technique by a senior ENT who had published extensively on the technique of Teflon injections into the vocal folds. Dr. Robert Lewy (of Lewy suspension fame), was impressed with the ease of injection with immediate improvement and great patient satisfaction. Unfortunately, as sometimes occurs in medicine, the deleterious long-term side effects (ie, Teflon metastasis, giant cell granulomas, difficulty in removing after overinjection) were not widely reported until the late 1980s. With the introduction of medialization Type I thyroplasty in 1974 by Isshiki, the approach to vocal fold medialization was unequivocally altered and the need for injection laryngoplasty diminished. Nevertheless, it was evident to most in the field that there were still indications for injection laryngoplasty. Among these included small glottic defects, scarring, and mobile but atrophied vocal folds. Furthermore, the improved understanding of the microanatomy of the vocal fold and its contribution to the mucosal wave combined with the widespread availability of the videostoboscope led to intensified search of biocompatible materials that would not only medialize but also help restore the mucosal wave. The search of an ideal injection material is still ongoing but by the early 1990s three studies were published utilizing autologous fat as a promising material. Our group noted that these reports were generally small series, nonblinded, and relied predominantly on subjective assessments of immobile vocal folds. Furthermore, follow-up seemed very short (5 months) for a material that was well known in the plastic surgery literature to lose volume over time. Additionally there was considerable research (particularly in the French plastic surgery literature) on techniques to preserve transplanted fat which we felt would be of benefit to report in our specialty. Finally, as it turned out, our first patient (LB) injected with our technique and serially followed for a year succumbed to a massive myocardial infarction. His wife, who happened to be a prominent neurologist in town, was aware of our research and graciously allowed early autopsy and histologic evaluation of the injected vocal fold. This allowed a rare opportunity to evaluate the viability of injected fat into the vocal folds after nearly 2 years. For all these reasons, we felt it worthwhile to report our study.

Since our publication other reports have commented on the unpredictability of autologous fat volume loss. The search for an ideal injection material has continued. Calcium hydroxyapatite (Radiance®), micronized acellular compound (Cymetra®), autologous fascia, among others have been introduced, each with its advantages and drawbacks. In my practice, I continue to use autologous fat in patients with a glottic gap less than 5 mm on maximal adduction especially if the volume loss has a component of scarring or to augment an atrophied vocal fold medialized by type 1 thyroplasty.

I would be remiss not to include my coauthors Mark Szewczyk, a third-year resident at the time whose enthusiasm and frequent questions only helped in my clarity of purpose; Janet Woodruff, a pathologist who dealt expertly in the special circumstance of our cadaver specimen; and finally, my speech pathologist and friend, Jeff Searle, now a well-published PhD in his own right, whom I have been fortunate to continue to collaborate with on number of voice related research since that time.

Autologous Fat Injection into the Vocal Folds: Technical Considerations and Long-Term Follow-up

Gary Y. Shaw, MD; Mark A. Szewczyk, MD; Jeff Searle, CCC-SLP; Janet Woodroof, MD

Numerous materials have been used over the years for vocal fold augmentation. Early use of bioreactive compounds, such as paraffin, gave way to relatively inert substances, such as Teflon. More recently biocompatible materials, such as collagen and autologous fat, have gained wider acceptance. Autologous fat, in particular, is an easily obtainable source for potential rehabilitation of scarred, paralytic, and atrophic vocal folds. However, long-term systematic follow-up has been lacking. Since 1991 we at the University of Kansas Center for Voice and Swallowing Disorders have employed autologous fat for vocal fold augmentation, primarily for either paralysis or repair of a volume-deficient vocal fold segment. Twenty-two patients have completed ≥1 year of follow-up studies, including graded videolaryngostroboscopy, electroglottography, computerized acoustic analysis, and blinded perceptual analysis by two speech-language pathologists. Statistically significant improvement was demonstrated in many parameters tested, frequently improving with time. Although the volume-deficient group had more "normal" values, the paralysis group had greater improvement in many variables using fat injection. We conclude that while autologous fat injections of the vocal fold may have long-term benefits, certain technical considerations and criteria of selection of patients are critical for success.

Key Words: Vocal fold augmentation—Volume-deficient vocal fold—Paralysis—Autologous fat—Follow-up—Scarred vocal folds.

***Laryngoscope*, 107:177–186, 1997**

Presented at the Meeting of the Middle Section of the American Laryngological, Rhinological and Otological Society, Inc., Dearborn, MI, January 20, 1996.

From the Departments of Otolaryngology (G.Y.S., M.A.S.), Speech and Hearing (J.S.), and Pathology (J.W.), University of Kansas Medical Center, Kansas City, Kansas, U.S.A.

Send Reprint Requests to Gary Y. Shaw, MD, Department of Otolaryngology—Head and Neck Surgery, University of Kansas Medical Center, 3901 Rainbow Blvd., Kansas City, KS 66160, U.S.A.

INTRODUCTION

The use of autologous fat to correct various defects was first described by Neuber (1) in 1893. He reported failure when large tissue blocks were employed but success with smaller samples. Lexer (2) was the first to report success in correcting head and neck defects. Peer (3,4) carefully studied the transplantation of free fat and dermal fat grafts. He concluded that small-volume free fat grafts can survive by osmotically obtaining a nutrient supply until a vascular supply is established. A variable percentage of cells, though, underwent phagocytosis and eventual fibrosis. Autologous fat injections into various body defects since that time have met with variable degrees of success. The use of fat to augment a vocal fold was first alluded to by Dedo and Rowe (5), who described augmentation of a scarred vocal fold by an open laryngo-fissure approach.

Mikaelian et al. (6) reported on three other patients with vocal fold paralysis treated by fat injection. All had immediate subjective improvement, although follow-up was short term. Brandenburg et al. (7) employed autologous fat in 12 patients, 11 with some form of laryngeal nerve paralysis and one with a "scalloped" vocal fold defect. All procedures were reported to be objectively (aerodynamic) and subjectively (voice rating) successful with prolonged follow-up (≥5 months). To date, these are the only published clinical studies, and little can be said about the success of this therapy for glottal insufficiency in nonparalyzed vocal folds. We employed autologous fat to correct glottic insufficiency of various etiologies, including paralysis, volume deficiency, and scarring of the vocal folds. We then objectively and subjectively compared results of therapy between the paralyzed and nonparalyzed groups at regular intervals over a 12-month period.

TABLE I.
Subject Profiles for Patients Treated with Autologous Fat Injection to the Vocal Folds.

Patient's no.	Subject's initials	Age	Sex	Etiology	Postop visit (days) No. 1	No. 2	No. 3
Paralysis group							
1	LB	58	M	s/p vagal neuroma excision	14	130	320
2	BT	53	F	Idiopathic	18	152	317
3	AS	28	F	Idiopathic	21	126	332
4	KM	44	F	s/p multiple CVA	3	17	350
5	LM	35	F	s/p base of skull/carotid tumor excision	12	132	302
6	JH	71	M	Idiopathic	10	120	307
7	CE	73	M	Idiopathic	19	136	310
8	LS	81	F	s/p thyroid mass excision	23	124	281
9	CD	41	F	s/p thyroid mass excision	11	137	296
10	DR	53	F	s/p lobectomy	14	117	308
11	RS	64	M	Idiopathic	9	132	312
Volume-deficient group							
1	DH	51	M	s/p excision of SQCC of TVC	22	115	295
2	MC	67	F	s/p vocal cord stripping	13	121	306
3	EB	62	M	s/p Teflon granuloma excision	14	125	326
4	CW	50	M	s/p vocal cord stripping	21	131	336
5	KA	23	F	s/p vocal nodule removal	12	139	340
6	DA	67	M	s/p Teflon granuloma excision	17	119	289
7	IV	57	F	s/p vocal cord stripping	13	123	303
8	LS	56	F	s/p polyp excision	14	166	321
9	RR	39	M	s/p vocal cord mass excision	11	140	300
10	LS	54	F	s/p Teflon granuloma excision	10	120	296
11	RT	42	F	s/p vocal cord mass excision	23	113	341

s/p, status post; CVA, cerebral vascular accident; SQCC, squamous cell cancer; TVC, true vocal chord.

MATERIALS AND METHODS

Selection of Patients

From August 1991 to November 1994, 22 patients (nine men and 13 women) were treated with autologous fat injection into their vocal folds. These patients were divided into two groups. Eleven patients received the injections for augmentation of a volume-deficient fold segment (volume-deficient group) that resulted from postsurgical trauma. The second group was treated for vocal fold paralysis (paralysis group); six resulted from postsurgical trauma to the Recurrent Laryngeal Nerve, one stemmed from a brain stem infarct, and five were idiopathic. Of 47 patients who underwent medialization procedures for unilateral vocal fold paralysis, 11 qualified for autologous fat injection. These were patients with paralyzed folds in the paramedian position, where the maximum glottic gap was felt to be ≤5 mm, as determined by videolaryngostroboscopy. Subject profiles for each group are listed on Table 1.

Data Collection

Measurements were obtained from each patient on four occasions: preoperatively, post 1 (4 weeks postop), post 2 (6 months), post 3 (1 year). At each visit several measurements were recorded, described herein.

Acoustic Analysis. Subjects were seated upright in a quiet room for audiotape recording. Recordings were made using a Telex headset microphone (model PH-91; Telex, Evanston, IL, U.S.A.) and a Marantz recorder (model PMD 201; Marantz, Chatsworth, CA, U.S.A.). A constant mouth-to-microphone distance of 1.5 inches was maintained. Subjects were asked to sustain the vowel /i/ for 5 s at three pitch levels: habitual, highest, and lowest. Two productions at each pitch level were recorded.

The tape-recorded signal was routed from the Marantz, recorded to an analog signal-processing board (model SA-415; SA Instrumentation, Encinitas, CA, U.S.A.), then to a Data Translation I/O board (model 2821; Marlboro, MA), and, ultimately, to a Zenith 386/25 personal computer (St. Joseph, MI). CSpeech software (version 3.1, Milenkovic, Madison, WI) was used to analyze the acquired waveform. The middle 500 msec of each vowel production was used for acoustic analysis. The following measures were obtained: fundamental frequency (F_0), jitter (frequency perturbation), shimmer (amplitude perturbation), and signal-to-noise ratio (SNR). Jitter, shimmer, and SNR reported values are from the habitual pitch productions. Mean values of each measure were calculated from the two productions. F_0 range was calculated by subtracting a subject's mean low F_0 from their mean high F_0.

Electroglottography. The electrodes of a two-channel electroglottograph (model MC2-1; Glottal Enterprises, Syracuse, NY) were placed on either side of the thyroid alae and were held with an elastic collar. Subjects were instructed to sustain the vowel /i/ at a comfortable pitch and loudness level. The glottographic waveform was monitored on-line through a digital storage oscilloscope (model 2211; Tektronix, Beaverton, OR, U.S.A.). The glottographic signal was routed to a signal-processing board (SA-415; SA Instrumentation), where it was low-pass-filtered at 1,500 Hz and routed to a Data Translation I/O board (model 2821), which fed the signal into a Zenith 386/25 personal computer. CSpeech software was used to mark/measure glottal wave form. The signal was differentiated by the software and then used to identify the point of initial glottal opening, the point of peak opening, and the point of closure, as reported by Murty et al. (8) and Hanson et al. (9). From these points, two measures of interest were recorded: the opening quotient (time open/time of entire cycle) and the speed quotient (opening time/closing time).

Videolaryngostroboscopy. Initial evaluation consisted of videolaryngostroboscopic testing using a modified Bless-Hirano grading system (10). Videolaryngostroboscopy was performed with a Kay 70° rigid telescope (model Sn0296; Kay Instruments, Lincoln Park, NJ, U.S.A.) attached to a CCD camera (model 1k-C30A; Toshiba, Osaka, Japan) and stroboscopic light source (model 4914; Bruel and Kjaer, Marlboro, MA, U.S.A). Recordings were performed on a super VHS video recorder (model BV-1000; Mitsubishi, Cypress, CA, U.S.A). The video signal was then routed to a high-resolution monitor (model PVM-1343MD; Sony, Tokyo, Japan). After positioning of the telescope, the patient was asked to produced a sustained /i/ at normal pitch. Stroboscopy was performed and recorded. Two of the authors (G.Y.S. and J.A.S) independently rated glottal closure and mucosal wave.

Perceptual Ratings. An independent speech-language pathologist who was blinded to the patient's diagnosis made perceptual ratings of voice quality using a standard GRBAS scale. These ratings were done based on the audiotaped recordings of patients' production of a sustained /i/. The parameters of grade (overall dysphonia severity), roughness, breathiness, asthenia ("weakness"), and strain were rated on a 5-point scale, with 1 = none and 5 = severe.

Patients' Ratings. Patients were asked to complete a short questionnaire rating three aspects of voice using a 5-point scale with 1 = none/normal and 5 = severe. These aspects were effort in voice production, sound of their voice to them, functional interference (interference their voice creates for them in their daily activities).

Surgical Technique

Harvest and preparation of fat graft were identical for both paralyzed and scarred vocal folds. The patient is intubated with a 5.0-diameter endotrachael tube and placed under general anesthesia. The left greater trochanter is palpated, and a 3-cm vertically oriented incision is made after administration of local anesthetic (1% lidocaine with 1:100,000 epinephrine). A 3- to 4-cm^3 piece of fat is harvested using an atraumatic technique. The fat is then cut into smaller pieces of 2–3 mm (3), removing any fibrous tissue. A purification technique previously described by Niechajev and Sevcuk (11) is then employed. The fat is placed in a large capped syringe with 30 ml of injectable saline, which is gently agitated for 3 min in order to separate the fat from blood, free fatty acids, and cellular debris. The supernatant is removed, and this cleansing process is repeated four to six times until the fat appears homogeneous without traces of blood and the saline suspension is clear.

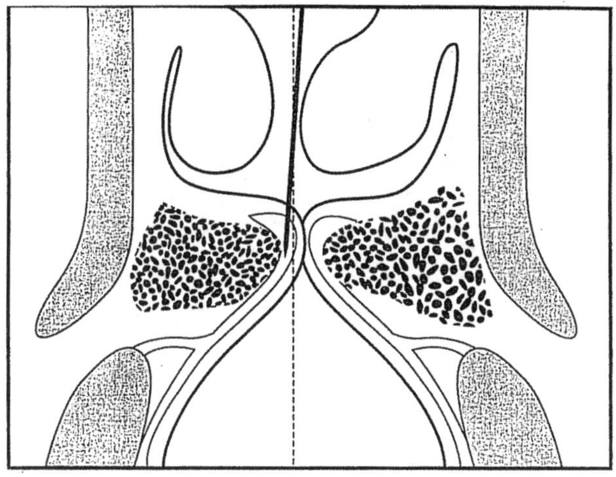

Fig. 1. Schematic depicts vocal fold site of autologous fat injection for patients in the volume-deficient group.

The small fat grafts are placed in a human insulin suspension (Humulin) of 100 U/ml for ≥5 min. The purified fat is then drained over a gauze sponge. The fat graft is loaded into a Brüning-type micro-injection ratchet gun cartridge. An 18-gauge bayonet injection needle is attached, and the injection gun handle is squeezed until fat emanates from the needle point. The patient then undergoes laryngoscopy employing an adult Dedo laryngoscope with Lewy suspension. Using a 4-mm-diameter 36-cm length Hopkins rod telescope for magnification, the injection needle is placed in the laryngoscope. At this juncture the injection technique for scarred vocal folds differs from that for paralyzed vocal folds. For scarred vocal folds the involved area of vibrating surface, which was carefully determined preoperatively by videolaryngostroboscopy, is pierced on the superior surface of the fold. The needle is advanced only to the submucosal space (Fig. 1). Fat is then injected.

Typically, only one or two ratchet clicks are necessary. For the paralyzed vocal fold the preoperative videolaryngoscopy is again consulted. At maximal adduction the area of greatest glottal gap is appreciated. Typically this is the central third of the vocal fold. The injection needle is then placed in the superior surface of the vocal fold and directed into the thyroarytenoid muscle (Fig. 2). Fat is injected into this area, often at two or three sites, until the deficient area is overcorrected by approximately one third. A 4% cocaine pledget is placed on the vocal fold injection site to control hemostasis and reduce the chance of postoperative laryngospasm. The trochanteric donor site is irrigated, and any persistent bleeding is controlled with cautery. The wound is closed in three layers: a deep layer of 3-0 Vicryl (Ethicon, Somerville, NJ) to close dead space, a buried subcutaneous

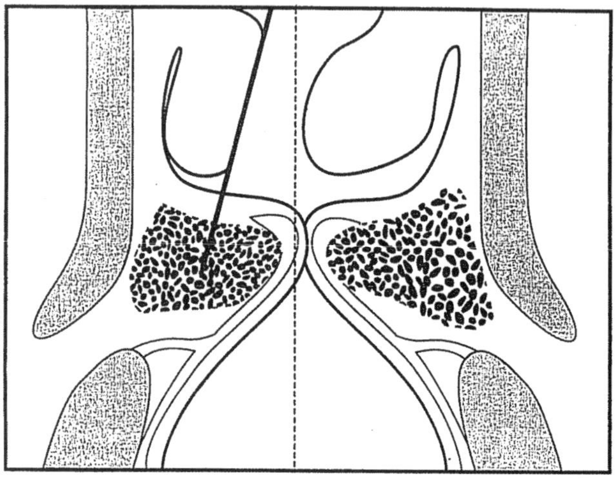

Fig. 2. Schematic depicts vocal fold site of autologous fat injection for patients with vocal cord paralysis.

layer of 4-0 Vicryl horizontal mattress, and a running subcuticular layer of 5-0 nylon. A pressure dressing is applied. Patients are encouraged to wear Lycra compression shorts or a girdle for 3 days postsurgery. A broad-spectrum antibiotic and mucolytic are prescribed, as well as intense humidification. Relative voice rest (e.g., no whispering, screaming, or excessive talking) is encouraged for 2 weeks.

Statistical Testing

A 2 × 4 repeated-measures analysis of variance was used to examine the group mean values for each variable. Differences within the groups over time (between preop and postop visits) as well as differences between groups (volume deficient vs. paralytic) were studied. Post hoc testing was then conducted using the Scheffe test. Statistical significance was defined as $p < 0.05$.

RESULTS

Acoustic Analysis

Group mean values for acoustic measurements are graphed for the paralysis group (Fig. 3) and for the volume-deficient group (Fig. 4).

Modal F_0. In neither group did this measure achieve statistical significance over time, nor was there a significant difference between the two groups.

F_0 Range. The paralysis groups change was statistically significant at visits post 2 and post 3. The change in the volume-deficient group was significant at post 3. There was no significant difference between groups.

Jitter. The paralysis group change was statistically significant at post 2 and post 3 visits. The vol-

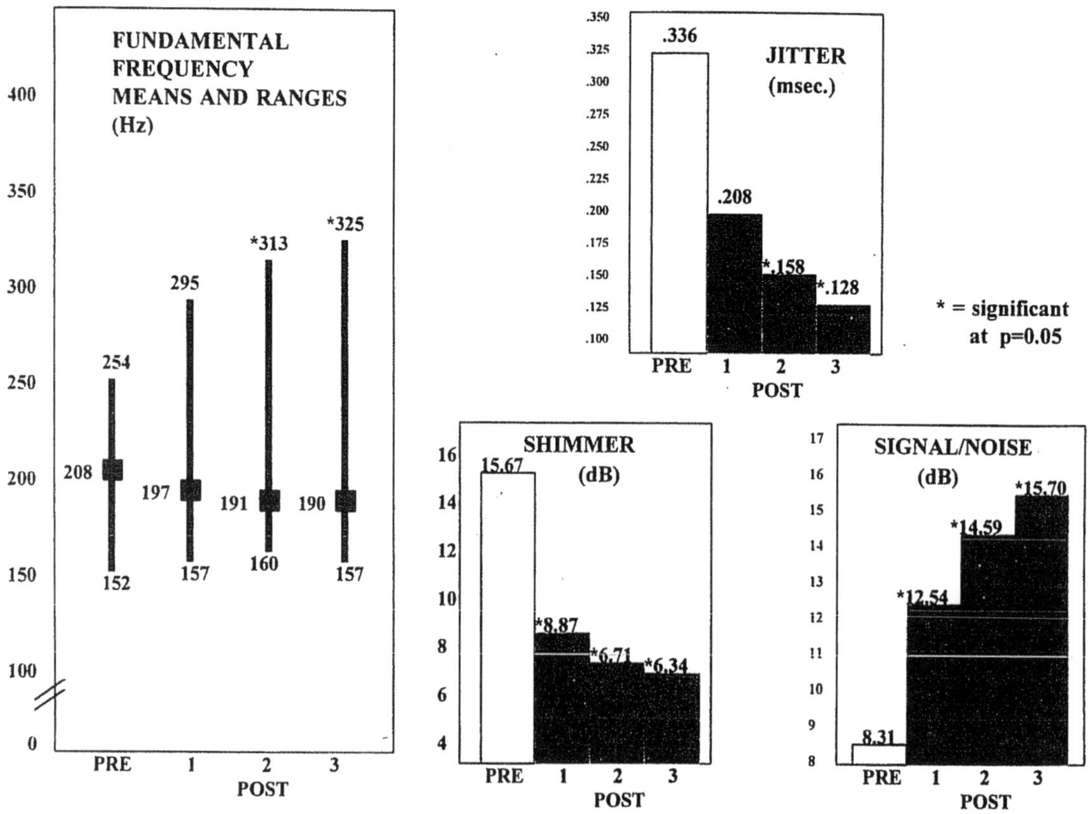

Fig. 3. Group means in paralysis group are shown for acoustical data. Asterisks designate means with statistically significant improvement.

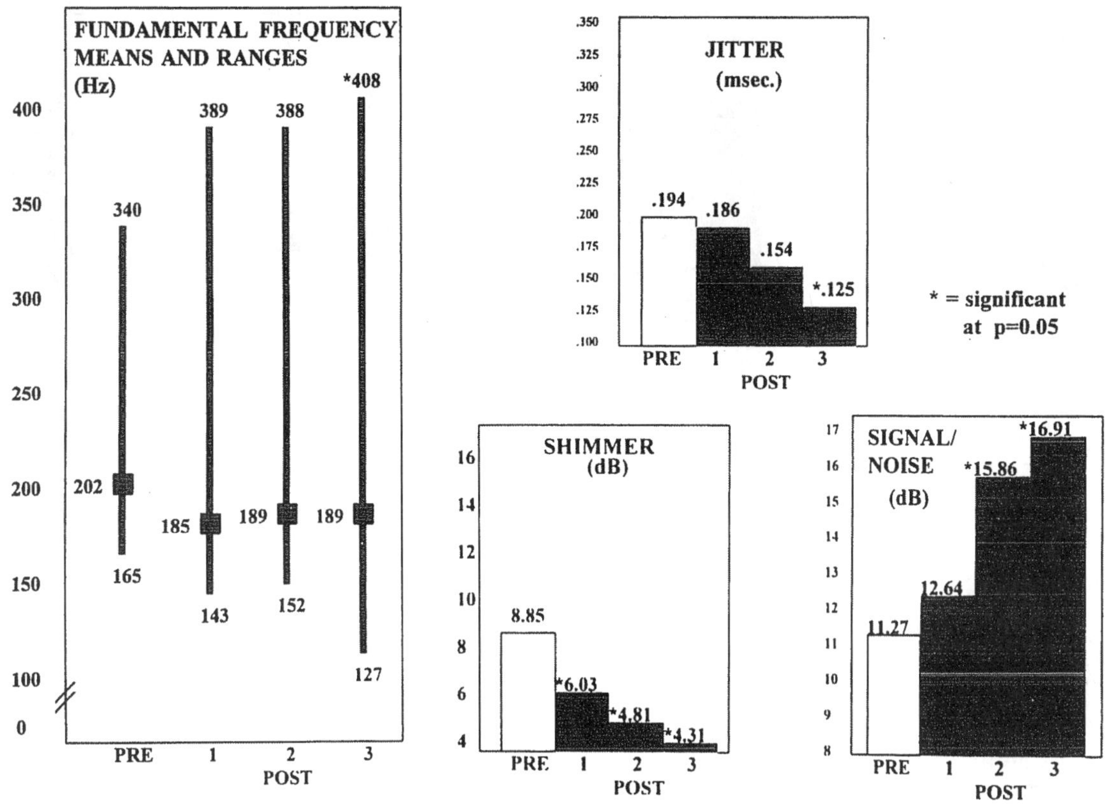

Fig. 4. Group means in volume-deficient group are shown for acoustical data. Asterisks designate means with statistically significant improvement.

ume-deficient group change was significant at the post 3 visit. Moreover, the paralysis group improved significantly more than the volume-deficient group at each postop visit. Neither group had means that reached expected normal values (≤0.075).

Shimmer. The volume-deficient group corrected to expected normal values (≤6) on post 2 and post 3 visits. Both groups had statistically significant decreases on all postop visits. There was no significant difference between groups.

SNR. The paralysis group's change was statistically significant on all postop visits. The volume-deficient group reached significance on post 2 and post 3 visits. Neither group achieved expected normal values (≥20). The paralysis group evidenced a significantly greater improvement at each postop visit compared with the volume-deficient group (p = 0.017).

Electroglottography

Group means for electroglottographic measurements are graphed for the paralysis group (Fig. 5) and the volume-deficient group (Fig. 6).

Open Quotient. Neither group achieved expected normal values (0.60–0.35). Both groups showed significant reductions at all postop visits. There was no significant difference between groups.

Speed Quotient. There was no significant decrease in speed quotient in either group compared with preop values, nor was there a significant difference between groups.

Videolaryngostroboscopy

There were no surgical complications, including granuloma formation. The true vocal folds remained somewhat full but did not appear edematous or inflamed. Group means for videolaryngostroboscopy measurements are graphed for the paralysis (Fig. 7) and the volume-deficient (Fig. 8) groups.

Glottal Closure. Both groups showed statistically significant improvement in their mean ratings at all postop visits. There was no significant difference between groups.

Mucosal Wave. Neither group had significant improvement at any postop visit, nor was there a significant difference between groups.

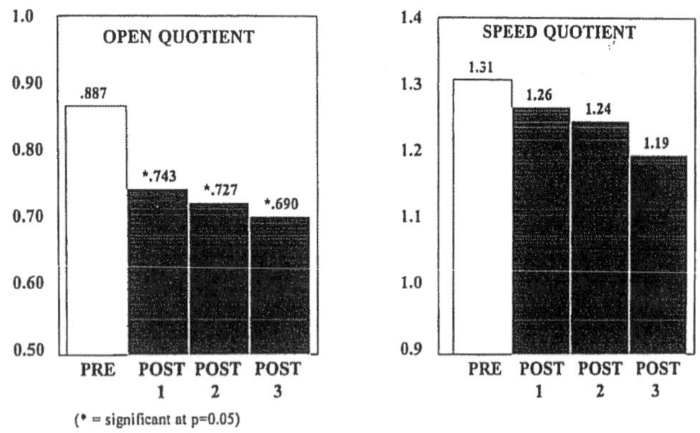

Fig. 5. Group means in paralysis group for electroglottographic data. Asterisks designate means with statistically significant improvement.

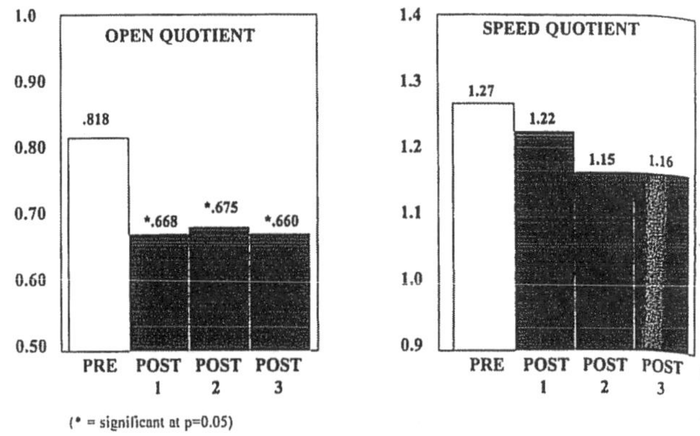

Fig. 6. Group means in volume-deficient group for electroglottographic data are shown. Asterisks designate means with statistically significant improvement.

Perceptual Ratings

Group means for the perceptual ratings and patients' ratings are graphed for the paralysis (Fig. 9) and the volume-deficient (Fig. 10) groups.

Grade. Both groups showed statistically significant improvements at all visits. There was no significant difference between groups.

Roughness. The paralysis group showed significant improvement at all postop visits. The volume-deficient group had significant improvement at post 2 and post 3 visits. The paralysis group showed significantly more improvement than the volume-deficient group. No other comparisons were significant.

Breathiness. Both groups showed statistically significant improvement on all postop visits. There was no significant difference between groups.

Asthenia. The volume-deficient group's improvement was not statistically significant. The paralysis group showed significant improvement at all postop visits. Moreover, the paralysis group had a statistically significantly greater improvement than the volume-deficient group at all postop visits.

Strain. Both groups had significant improvement on all postop visits. There was no significant difference between groups.

Patients' Ratings

Effort. Both groups had significant improvement at all postop visits. There was no significant difference between groups.

Sound. The paralysis group had significant improvement on all postop visits. The volume-deficient group had significant improvement on post 2 and post 3 visits. There was no significant difference in improvement between groups.

Functional Interference. Both groups achieved statistically significant improvement compared with preop conditions at post 2 and post 3 visits. There was no significantly different effect between groups.

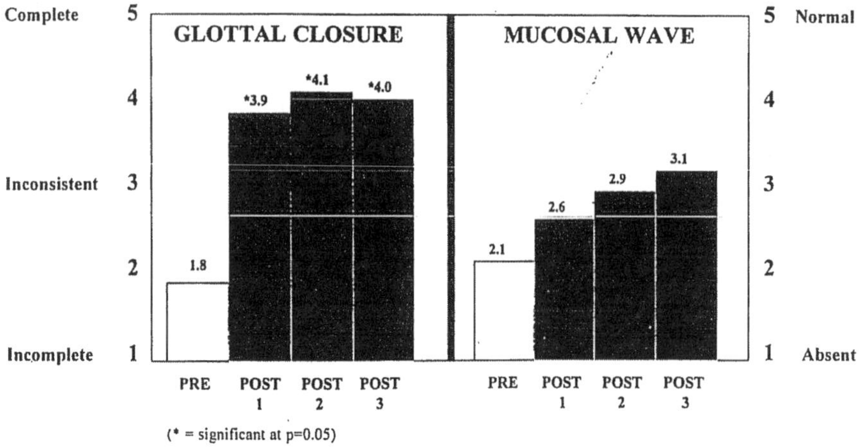

Fig. 7. Group means in paralysis group for videostroboscopic data are given. Asterisks designate means with statistically significant improvement.

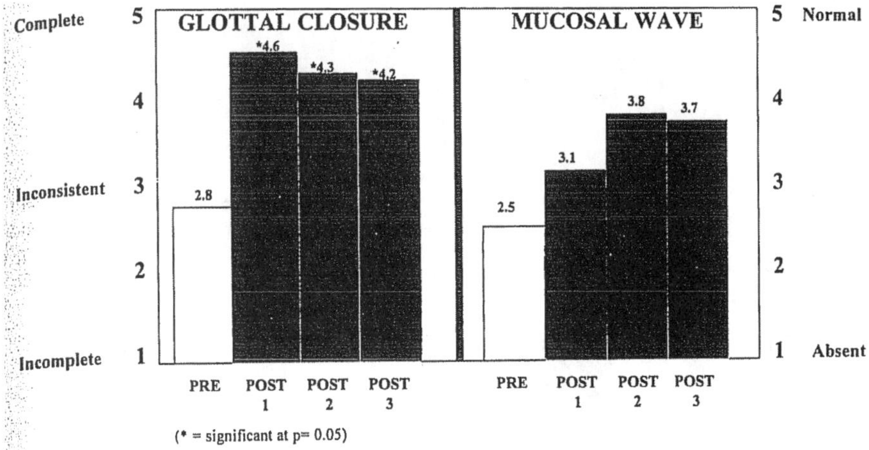

Fig. 8. Group means in volume-deficient group for electroglottographic data are given. Asterisks designate means with statistically significant improvement.

DISCUSSION

Neuber (1) first described using autologous fat to correct various types of defects in 1893. He reported failure when large tissue blocks were employed but success with smaller samples. Lexer (2) was first to report success in correcting head and neck defects. Peer (3,4) carefully studied the transplantation of fat and dermal fat grafts. Peer concluded that small-volume free fat grafts can survive by osmotically obtaining a nutrient supply until a vascular supply is established and called the phenomena the "cell survival theory." A variable percentage of cells, though, underwent phagocytosis and eventual fibrosis (3,4). Autologous fat injections into various body defects since that time have met with variable degrees of success.

Autologous fat has been employed experimentally in canine larynges. Jiang et al. and Wexler et al. (12,13) surgically implanted fat autografts submucosally via a midline laryngo-fissure approach to the cords in five dogs 6–8 weeks after mucosal excision. After excision of the larynges, they noted improvement in laryngeal pressures, glottal efficiency, and acoustic stability. Published reports on the use of autologous fat to augment vocal folds in humans have been limited. Dedo and Rowe, in 1983, briefly alluded to employing free fat grafts to augment a scarred vocal fold. (5) In 1991, Mikaelian et al. (6) reported its use in three patients with vocal fold paralysis. All three experienced good results subjectively (although one patient required a second injection because too little fat was injected on the first treatment). Videolaryngostroboscopic examination and acoustic analysis in these patients were encouraging.

Brandenburg et al. (7) treated 12 patients, 11 for vocal fold paralysis and the other for a scarred fold. Most of these patients were evaluated with videolaryngostroboscopy (VLS) before and after treatment and were scored using a GRBAS scale. Some were also evaluated with additional aerody-

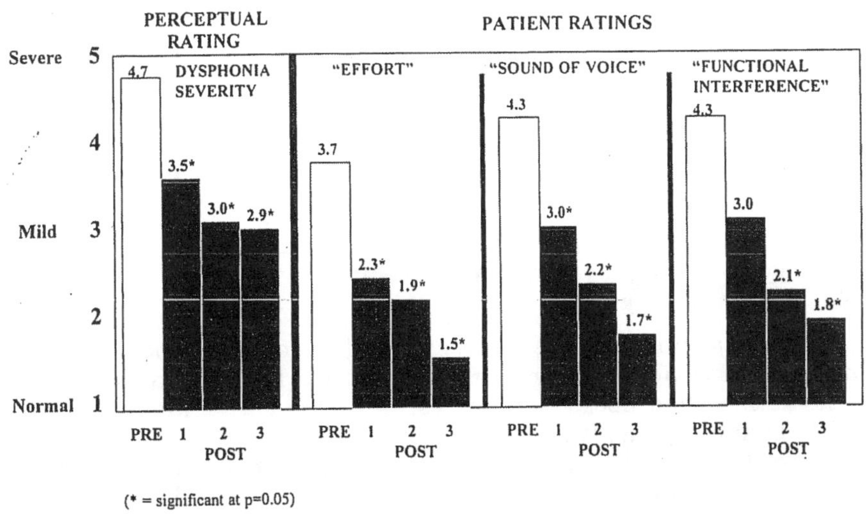

Fig. 9. Group means in paralysis group are given for perceptual ratings and patients' subjective ratings. Asterisks designate means with statistically significant improvement.

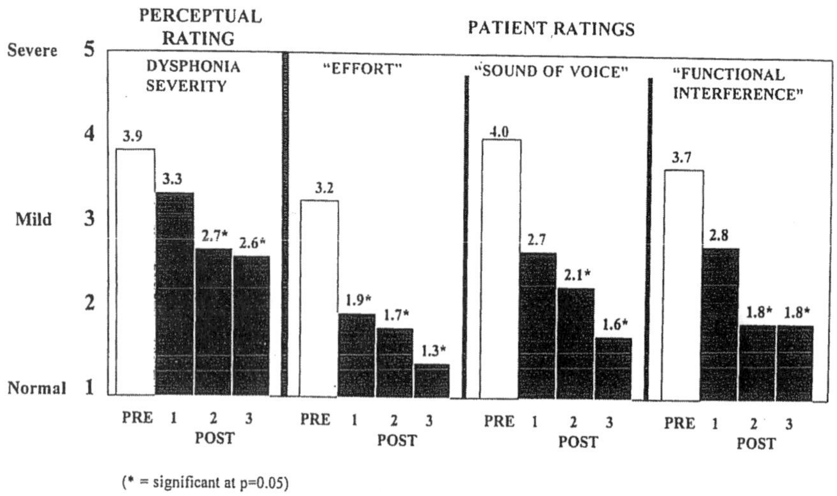

Fig. 10. Group means in volume-deficient group are shown for perceptual ratings and patients' subjective ratings. Asterisks designate means with statistically significant improvement.

namic and acoustic tests. VLS ratings of glottal closure and perceptual ratings found improvement in 80% of patients treated. Aerodynamic and acoustic measures improved, although these improvements did not reach statistical significance.

Studies have previously shown that autologous fat transplants survive after injection into the vocal folds. Most were in canine studies. In 1991, Hill et al. (14) injected five dog vocal folds and then studied them histologically at 48 h and 3 weeks. They found that the fat demonstrated revascularization, normal morphology, and volume maintenance. Similarly, Zaretsky et al. (15) in 1995 studied eight dogs after autologous fat injection into their vocal folds. They reported maintenance of bulk for ≤3 months and viable fat cells at 6 months. Mikus et al. (16) studied 13 dogs histologically from 3 to 12 weeks after autologous fat injection into their vocal folds. Viable fat cells were confirmed to be present.

A histologic study in humans after autologous fat injection into vocal folds was reported by Bauer et al. (17). Their patient, who had suffered a brain stem infarction, underwent total laryngectomy for chronic aspiration 5 months after autologous fat injection. Histologic examination revealed normal-appearing fat boluses with evidence of revascularization. In our series, patient 1 (L.B.) had undergone autologous fat injection for a paralyzed vocal fold after excision of a vagal neuroma. Eighteen months later he died of a myocardial infarction. Postmortum histologic sectioning of the larynx also confirmed viable fat deposits (Fig. 11).

Several techniques have been employed to maximize fat survival. We prefer surgically excised fat grafts rather than liposuction harvest. Kononas et al. (18) studied 30 rabbits, in whom they transferred fat from the groin to the ears. On one side the fat was harvested surgically and on the other through liposuction. After 9 months, they reported that surgically excised grafts maintained more volume ($p < 0.05$) than liposuctioned grafts. In 1990, Hudson et al. (19) attempted to determine the best site for fat graft harvest based on the assumption that larger cell size and increased lipogenic enzyme adipose tissue lipoprotein lipase (ATLPL) activity would increase viability. They found that the trochanteric region had a greater average lipocyte diameter and increased ATLPL activity. Thus, we chose this as our site of graft harvest. The purification technique used is that described by Niechajev and Sevcuk (11). Their study demonstrated that gentle washing, as opposed to centrifugation, results in more viable fat cells. After purification, we equilibrate our grafts in insulin to block lipolytic enzymes, as described by Illouz (20). Throughout the procedure, the fat graft is handled delicately to prevent excessive trauma to the lipocytes.

Results showed statistically significant improvement in 14 of 17 measured parameters for the paralysis group and 13 of 17 for the volume-deficient group. In addition, these improvements lasted at least a year and often were actually better at 1 year than immediately postop. This may have stemmed from our initial overinjection of the involved fold by one third, which led to subsequent loss of fat volume and allowed for a more effective glottal closure. In nearly all measurements, the absolute values of the volume-deficient group remained better than the paralysis group postop. However, the paralysis group had statistically significantly greater improvement than the volume-deficient group in three measurements: jitter (acoustic), signal-to-noise ratio (acoustic), and asthenia (perceptual rating). It is significant to note that despite improvement in many phonatory parameters, injection of autologous fat into scarred areas of the vocal fold did not significantly improve mucosal

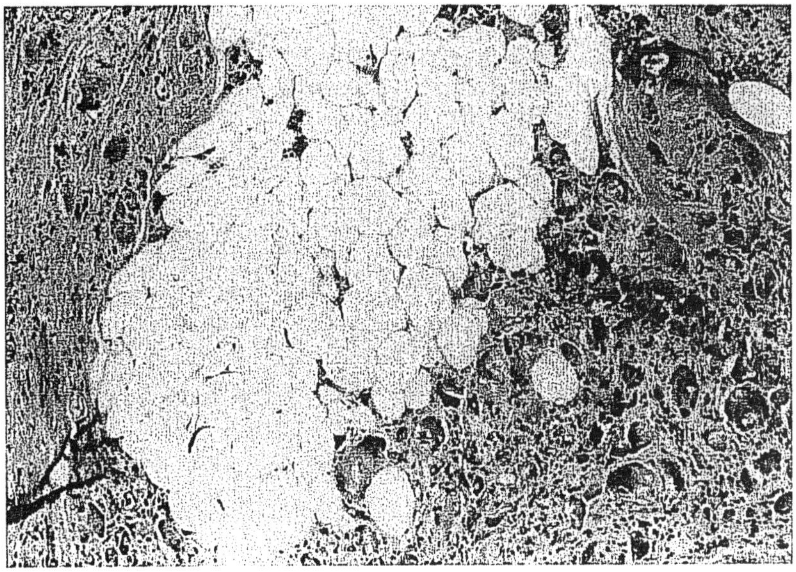

Fig. 11. Photomicrograph shows viable fat in sectioned larynx 18 months after autologous fat injection (H & E, original magnification ×400).

wave. However, this finding may be related to technical considerations of fat injection. Wexler et al. (12) employed a laryngo-fissure approach to create a submucosal pocket in scarred canine vocal folds. They found mucosal wave restoration close to normal in the operated folds. Sataloff et al. (21) have recently described similar findings in humans.

CONCLUSION

In select patients requiring augmentation of the vocal fold, injection of autologous fat offers advantages over existing techniques. It is readily available. There appears to be minimal risk of foreign body reaction, hypersensitivity, granuloma formation, or graft rejection. The procedure requires no external incisions on the neck. Most important, results appear to be long-lasting, which has been confirmed objectively and subjectively. Longer follow-up is planned for these patients to ascertain if their improvement is maintained; however, the histological evidence that fat remains viable 18 months after injection is encouraging.

This study did not attempt to compare phonatory parameters of other medialization techniques (i.e., type I thyroplasty, arytenoid adduction, etc.) with those of fat injection. Our goal was simply to determine if autologous fat injection offers long-term improvement in patients with impaired glottal closure from vocal fold paralysis due to a small (≤5 mm) glottal defect or from a scarred or bowed vocal fold. To this end, our results seem to indicate that a long-term phonatory advantage can be expected employing this technique. Larger glottal gaps and severely atrophic vocal folds may need other procedures, which may very well complement fat injection. The treatment of scarred vocal folds, in particular, remains a clinical problem. While injection of autologous fat clearly offers some improvement, problems remain (i.e., poor restoration of the mucosal wave). The search for an ideal material and technique to restore scarred vocal folds remains an active area of research.

ACKNOWLEDGMENT

The authors acknowledge Dr. Irene Bettinger for assistance in obtaining the cadaveric larynx and Terri Bustetter for preparation of this article.

BIBLIOGRAPHY

1. Neuber GA. Fettransplantation. *Verh Dtsch Ges Chir* 1893;22:66.
2. Lexer E. Free fat grafting. *Dtsch Med Wochenschr* 1910;36:640.
3. Peer LA. The neglected "free fat graft": its behavior and clinical use. *Am J Surg* 1956;92:40.
4. Peer LA. Loss of weight and volume in human fat grafts. *Plast Reconstr Surg* 1950;5:217.
5. Dedo HH, Rowe LD. Laryngeal reconstruction in acute and chronic injuries. *Otol Clin North Am* 1983;16:373–89.
6. Mikaelian DO, Lowrey LD, Sataloff RT. Lipoinjection for unilateral vocal cord paralysis. *Laryngoscope* 1991;101:465–8.
7. Brandenburg JH, Kirkham W, Koschkee D. Vocal cord augmentation with autogenous fat. *Laryngoscope* 1992;102:495–500.
8. Murty GE, Carding PN, Kelly PJ, Lancaster P. The effect of frequency on combined glottography. *Clin Otolaryngol* 1991;16:298–301.
9. Hanson DG, Gerratt BR, Ward PH. Glottographic measurement of vocal dysfunction: a preliminary report. *Ann Otol Rhinol Laryngol* 1983;92:413–20.
10. Hirano M, Bless D. *Videostroboscopic examination of the larynx*. San Diego: Singular Publishing Co., 1993.
11. Niechajev I, Sevcuk O. Long-term results of fat transplantation: clinical and histologic studies. *Plast Reconstr Surg* 1994;96(3):496–506.
12. Wexler DB, Jiang JJ, Gray SD, Titze IR. Phonosurgical studies: fat-graft reconstruction of injured canine vocal cords. *Ann Otol Rhinol Laryngol* 1989;98:668–73.

13. Jiang, JJ, Titze IR, Wexler DB, Gray SD. Fundamental frequency and amplitude perturbation in reconstructed canine vocal folds. *Ann Otol Rhinol Laryngol* 1994;103:145–8.
14. Hill DP, Meyers AD, Harris J. Autologous fat injection for vocal cord medialization in the canine larynx. *Laryngoscope* 1991;101:344–8.
15. Zaretsky LS, DeTar M, Shindo ML, Rice DH. Autologous fat injection for vocal cord paralysis: long-term histologic evaluation. *Ann Otol Rhinol Laryngol* 1995;104:1–4.
16. Mikus JL, Koufman JA, Kilpatrick SE. Fate of liposuctioned and purified autologous fat injections in the canine vocal fold. *Laryngoscope* 1995;105:17–22.
17. Bauer CA, Valentino J, Hoffman HT. Long-term results of vocal cord augmentation with autogenous fat. *Ann Otol Rhinol Laryngol* 1995;104:871–4.
18. Kononas TC, Bucky LP, Hurley C, May JW. The fate of suctioned and surgically removed fat after reimplantation for soft-tissue augmentation: a volumetric and histologic study in the rabbit. *Plast Reconstr Surg* 1993;91(5):763–8.
19. Hudson DA, Lambert EV, Bloch CE. Site selection for fat autotransplantation: some observations. *Aesth Plast Surg* 1990;14:195–7.
20. Illouz YG. Present results of fat injection. *Aesth Plast Surg* 1988;12:175–81.
21. Sataloff RT, Spiegel JR. Autologous fat implantation for vocal fold scar. Presented at the Voice Foundation's 24th Annual Symposium on Care of the Professional Voice, Philadelphia, PA, June 11, 1995.

Viscosities of Implantable Biomaterials in Vocal Fold Augmentation Surgery

Roger W. Chan, BSc; Ingo R. Titze, PhD

Vocal fold vibration depends critically on the viscoelasticity of vocal fold tissues. For instance, phonation threshold pressure, a measure of the "ease" of phonation, has been shown to be directly related to the viscosity of the vibrating mucosa. Various implantable biomaterials have been used in vocal fold augmentation surgery, with implantation sites sometimes close to or inside the mucosa. Yet their viscosities or other mechanical properties are seldom known. This study attempts to provide data on viscosities of commonly used phonosurgical biomaterials. Using a parallel-plate rotational rheometer, oscillatory shear experiments were performed on implantable polytetrafluoroethylene (Teflon or Polytef; Mentor Inc., Hingham, MA), collagen (Zyderm; Collagen Corp., Palo Alto, CA), glutaraldehyde cross-linked (GAX) collagen (Phonagel or Zyplast; Collagen Corp.), absorbable gelatin (Gelfoam; Upjohn Co., Kalamazoo, MI), and human abdominal subcutaneous fat. Samples of human vocal fold mucosal tissues were also tested. Under sinusoidal oscillatory shear at 10 Hz and at 37°C, the dynamic viscosity was 116 Pascal-seconds (Pa-s) for polytetrafluoroethylene, 21 Pa-s for gelatin, 8-13 Pa-s for the two types of collagen, 3 Pa-s for fat, and 1 to 3 Pa-s for vocal fold mucosa. Results extrapolated to 100 Hz also show similar differences among the biomaterials, but all values are an order of magnitude lower because of the typical inverse frequency relation (shear thinning effect) for polymeric and biologic materials. The data suggest that the use of fat for vocal fold augmentation may be more conducive to the "ease" of phonation because of its relatively low viscosity, which is closest to physiologic levels. This implication is probably the most relevant in predicting initial outcome of the postoperative voice before there is any significant assimilation (e.g., resorption and fibrosis) of the implanted biomaterial.

***Laryngoscope*, 108:725–731, 1998**

Presented in part at the First International Conference on Voice Physiology and Biomechanics, Evanston, Illinois, May 31, 1997.

From the Department of Speech Pathology and Audiology, National Center for Voice and Speech, The University of Iowa, Iowa City, Iowa.

Supported by a grant (No. P60 DC00976) from the National Institute on Deafness and Other Communication Disorders, National Institutes of Health.

Editor's Note: This Manuscript was accepted for publication July 31, 1997.

Send Reprint Requests to Roger W. Chan, Department of Speech Pathology and Audiology, 330 WJSHC, The University of Iowa, Iowa City, IA 52242, U.S.A.

INTRODUCTION

Injection laryngoplasty is a common practice in phonosurgery. The usual objective is to medialize a paralyzed vocal fold, to soften a scar, or to augment an atrophic vocal fold. In the management of scarring or atrophy the injection or implantation is close to or directly into the vibrating vocal fold mucosa, to repair focal defects, to smooth the vocal fold margin, and to soften the stiffened scar tissue.[1,2] A number of synthetic implantable materials have been used historically in vocal fold augmentation surgery, including paraffin, polytetrafluoroethylene (Teflon [Polytef; Mentor Inc., Hingham, MA]), and silicone (in Japan). Today, the use of biologic materials is becoming more popular, primarily because of the promising results, but also because of persisting problems associated with synthetic materials like Teflon.[3,4]

Implantable collagen and fat have been the most widely used biologic materials, while gelatin is a common biomaterial used for temporary vocal fold medialization. Bovine dermal collagen suspension (Zyderm Collagen Implant; Collagen Corp., Palo Alto, CA) was first used by Ford et al.[5] in phonosurgery and was shown to be a viable alternative to Teflon.[2,6] Glutaraldehyde crosslinked (GAX) collagen (Phonagel or Zyplast; Collagen Corp.) was better tolerated immunologically and was more stable against gradual postsurgical resorption.[6,7] More recently, autologous collagen has been harvested from patients' own abdominal skin, which has virtually eliminated any immunologic risk.[8] Autologous fat from abdominal liposuction or excision has also been used clinically for augmenting paralyzed vocal folds, with encouraging results.[9–11] Favorable results have also been reported in fat-graft reconstruction of injured canine vocal fold mucosa[12,13] and scarred human vocal fold mucosa.[11,14] Gelatin (Gelfoam; Upjohn Co., Kalamazoo, MI) paste was first used by Schramm et al.[15] as a biomaterial for the temporary restoration of glottal competence (e.g., before radiation therapy).[16]

Many factors must be considered when choosing an appropriate biomaterial for implantation into the vocal folds. Some of the more important considerations include potential malposition and overinjection, and resorption and stability of the implant. The overriding consideration, however, is the ability of the repaired vocal fold to return to normal or near-normal vibration, which depends critically on the viscoelasticity of vocal fold tissues. Viscous and elastic properties are both affected by the introduction of the foreign biomaterial, especially in the management of vocal fold scarring. It has been shown that the *phonation threshold pressure* for vocal fold oscillation is directly related to the viscosity of the vocal fold mucosa.[17] This pressure has been defined as the minimum subglottal pressure required to produce vocal fold oscillation.[17,18] It is an objective indicator of the "ease" of phonation and can be useful as a diagnostic parameter of vocal function. Titze[17] showed analytically that phonation threshold pressure increases with viscosity of the vibrating vocal fold mucosa. The validity of this relationship has been verified by different kinds of experiments, using excised larynges,[19] a physical model,[20] and human subjects.[21,22]

Few data on viscosity or other mechanical properties of the commonly used biomaterials are available in the voice and laryngology literature. This study attempts to remedy this situation by presenting measurements of the *dynamic viscosity* of implantable polytetrafluoroethylene, collagen, gelatin, fat, and human vocal fold mucosa. Dynamic viscosity characterizes the internal friction of a material during oscillatory deformation around an equilibrium position and can be defined in the context of sinusoidal oscillatory shear.[23] When a sinusoidal oscillatory shear stress is applied to a sample of viscoelastic material, a steady-state condition can be reached (for linear small-amplitude oscillations) where the sinusoidal shear stress will have a constant relation to the sinusoidal shear strain (deformation) at a given frequency of oscillation. The strain amplitude will be proportional to the stress amplitude, and a constant phase lag will exist. Dynamic viscosity can be derived from this phase lag and the ratio of stress to strain amplitude. Mathematically, dynamic viscosity is defined as the real part of the complex dynamic viscosity and can be described as follows by the analytic relationship between shear stress, strain, and strain rate for a Kelvin-Voigt viscoelastic model[23,24]:

$$\tau = \mu\,\gamma + \eta\,\dot{\gamma} \tag{1}$$

where τ is shear stress (in Pa), γ is shear strain (in radians), $\dot{\gamma}$ is strain rate (in s^{-1}), μ is elastic shear modulus (in Pa), and η is dynamic viscosity (in Pascal-seconds [Pa-s]). In the engineering literature, elastic shear modulus is often represented by G', since it is the real part of the complex dynamic shear modulus G^*. Likewise, dynamic viscosity is often represented by η', since it is the real part of the complex dynamic viscosity η^*.

MATERIALS AND METHODS

Samples

Teflon samples were obtained in form of an injectable paste suspended in glycerin (740 mg/mL). Three samples (each of approximately 0.5 mL) were taken and tested in a mechanical testing machine (rheometer). Implantable collagen samples included both 0.0075% GAX bovine dermal collagen suspension and the lized, purified, and reconstituted preparations of type I collagen suspended in a phosphate-buffered saline solution (35 mg/mL) and were contained in syringes ready for injection.[5–7] For each type of collagen, three samples (each 0.5 mL) from three different syringes were tested. Autologous collagen was not included in the present study but may be tested in future studies. Three injectable gelatin samples were prepared by mixing 0.375 g of Gelfoam absorbable gelatin powder with 1.5 mL (0.9%) saline solution, resulting in a gelatin suspension of 250 mg/mL, a concentration also used in phonosurgery.[15,16]

Fat samples were harvested from a 70-year-old female cadaver from autopsy approximately 24 hours postmortem. A block of approximately 4 cm^3 of subcutaneous fat tissue was excised from the periumbilical area of the cadaver's anterior abdomen. Computed tomography (CT) observations have shown two layers of abdominal subcutaneous fat, superficial and deep,[25] but it was not known from which layer the sample was harvested. Possible differences between the two may be studied in future experiments. The block of fat was minced into smaller pieces (approximately 0.1 to 0.3 cm^3), and any fascia and fibrous tissue was removed. It was then rinsed thoroughly with saline solution to remove any remaining debris. Three 0.5-mL samples were taken from the pieces and tested. This procedure of fat-graft preparation was similar to one described for phonosurgery.[11] It was recognized that different surgeons prepare their fat samples somewhat differently and that might have an effect on mechanical properties, in addition to biologic effects.[14] Possible differences may be studied in the future.

Samples of vocal fold mucosa were also tested. They were obtained from two excised larynges (62-year-old male and 72-year-old male cadavers) approximately 24 hours postmortem from autopsy. Mechanical properties of the mucosa might have been affected by postmortem changes, but fresher human tissues were not available at the time of testing. The mucosa consisted of the superficial layer of lamina propria and the epithelium, which remained attached to the superficial layer during testing and hence served as a natural boundary of attachment to the rheometer. Two samples of mucosa were obtained from each larynx, one from the left and the other from the right vocal fold. The volume of each sample was approximately 0.1 mL.

Rheometer and Oscillatory Shear Experiments

Rheologic or viscometric measurements were made with a Bohlin controlled stress (CS-50) rheometer, controlled by a computer with commercial CS oscillation data acquisition and analysis software. A plate-on-plate (parallel-plate) testing geometry was used, with a stationary lower plate and a rotating upper plate (diameter, 20 mm). The parallel-plate geometry was used so that the sample volume required to fill the gap could be adjusted by the gap size. To match a sample volume of 0.1 mL (typical of mucosal tissue samples), the gap size was 0.3 mm. Complete sample filling of the gap was ensured by first mounting samples with slightly larger volume than that of the gap (0.1 mL). Excessive material was then wiped off the rim of the gap while care was taken to prevent removing any material between the plates.

The sample was subject to a precisely controlled sinusoidal torque from the upper plate, driven by a motor (torque range 0.001 to 10 mNm, resolution < 0.0002 mNm). The resulting angular displacement and angular velocity of the upper plate were monitored by a sensitive transducer (linear angular deflection range, resolution approximately 2×10^{-5} rad) as a function of time. Sinusoidally varying shear stress, shear strain and strain rate were calculated from the preset torque and the measured angular velocity by the computer. From the shear stress and strain rate functions, the CS oscillation software calculated dynamic viscosity using the linear viscoelasticity theory mentioned above. Measurements of dynamic viscosity were made at a frequency range of 0.01 to 15 Hz, covering 32 frequencies over three decades. Testing at higher frequencies was not performed because linearity of the underlying viscoelasticity theory could not be ensured when the rotor (upper plate) and sample inertial effects become significant at high frequency. Linearity was also maintained by using small-amplitude oscillation with the shear strain amplitude set at 0.01 rad throughout the experiments. This target shear strain was located by strain (or stress) sweep tests performed before frequency sweep experiments, where steady dynamic viscosity was obtained at low strain up to at least 0.01 rad.

Calibration of the rheometer was performed by the manufacturer and was double checked by measuring the steady-shear viscosities of standard polydimethylsiloxane solutions (Dow Corning [Midland, MI] 360 Medical Fluids) with known viscosities of 0.1, 0.35, 1, and 12.5 Pa-s at 20°C. The measured viscosities showed a less than 6% deviation from the stated viscosities at all strain rates in all cases. Throughout the experiments, the sample under test was maintained at a temperature of 37°C ± 0.1°C by a Bohlin temperature control unit, which circulated water into the mounting of the lower plate. The vocal fold mucosa samples were kept viable during testing by bathing in physiologic saline solution.

RESULTS

Figure 1 shows the dynamic viscosity of three samples of injectable gelatin (Gelfoam) as a function of oscillation frequency, on a log-log scale. Because the three gelatin samples came from a single source of preparation, discrepancies in results between them reflect an estimation of the experimental error or repeatability of the oscillatory shear experimental procedure. Possible sources of errors include differences in the process of sample mounting (e.g., during the removal of excessive sample material) and the rheometer (e.g., errors in torque output and measurement of angular displacement). According to the largest differences between the results in Figure 1 (between samples 1 and 3), experimental error or repeatability of the experimental procedure is estimated to be within 10% of the measured dynamic viscosity values across all frequencies.

Figure 2 shows the dynamic viscosity of human vocal fold mucosa plotted against frequency on a log-log scale. Results of two samples from each larynx are shown, one from the left and one from the right vocal fold. It can be seen that discrepancies in results between the left and the right halves for both larynges are at approximately the same magnitude as those in Figure 1 (i.e., the discrepancies can mostly be accounted for by the experimental error). Thus the larynges were basically symmetric in terms of dynamic viscosity. Discrepancies in results between the two larynges, on the other hand, are much larger than the magnitude of the experimental error, shown in Figure 1. Age is probably one of many factors that could contribute to this intersubject difference.

Figure 3 plots the average values of dynamic viscosity of all five implantable biomaterials and vocal fold mucosal tissues, again as a function of frequency on a log-log scale. As is the case in most biomacromolecules and polymeric materials,[23] the dynamic viscosities of implantable biomaterials and vocal fold mucosal tissues are a monotonically decreasing function of frequency (known as a shear thinning effect). Moreover, the decrease in frequency is approximately linear on the log-log scale, which indicates that the relationship between dynamic viscosity and frequency can be modeled by a power law:

$$\eta = k f^n \quad (2)$$

or

$$\log \eta = \log k + n \log f \quad (3)$$

where f is frequency and k and n are constants. Data for each material shown in Figure 3 were fitted to equation (3) by simple linear least-squares regression. Table I summarizes the results of curve-fitting by giving the values of k, n, and the square of the correlation coefficient r for different materials. Data are very well matched by the regression equation, yielding correlation coefficients above

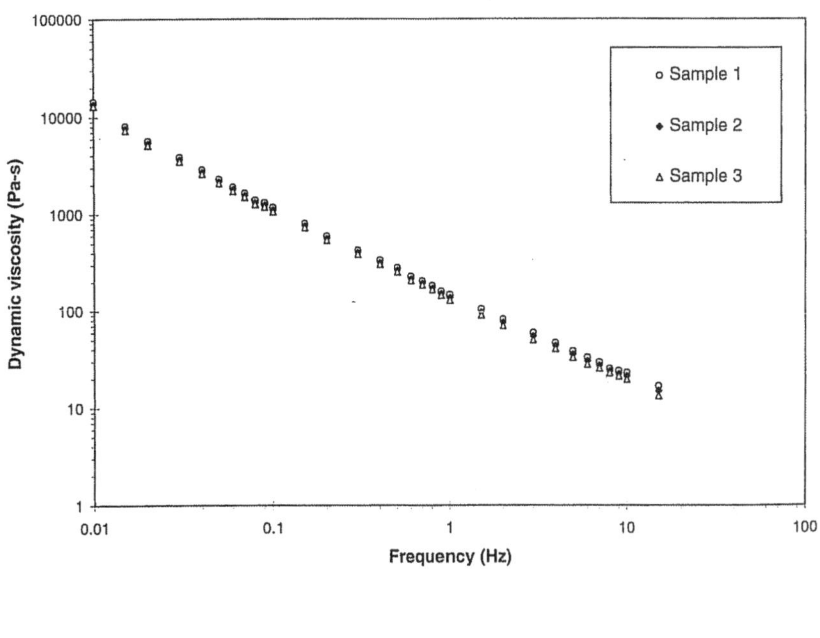

Fig. 1. Dynamic viscosity of injectable gelatin (Gelfoam) as a function of frequency.

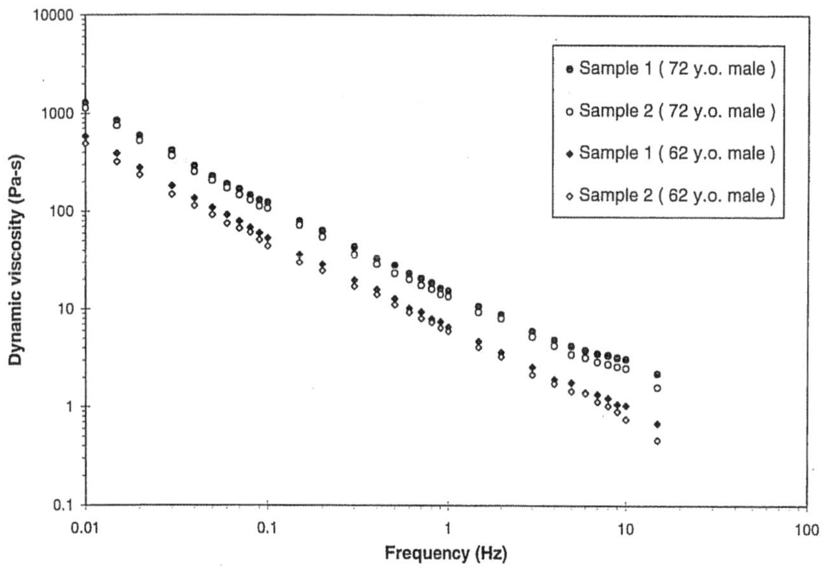

Fig. 2. Dynamic viscosity of human vocal fold mucosa (superficial layer of lamina propria) as a function of frequency.

0.99. Dynamic viscosity decreased with frequency at approximately the same rate for different materials, with very similar slopes *(n),* as shown clearly in Figure 3.

The main difference between the materials can be described by the vertical separation of the curves in Figure 3 or the difference in the values of k in Table I. Polytetrafluoroethylene is the most viscous, followed by gelatin, GAX collagen, noncrosslinked collagen, fat, and vocal fold mucosa. Figure 3 also shows the results of data extrapolation to 100 Hz, a typical male vocal fold vibration frequency, based on the regression equation [equation (3)]. Table II summarizes the measured dynamic viscosity values at 10 Hz and the extrapolated values at 100 Hz. Results show that the order and magnitude of differences among the materials in dynamic viscosity extrapolated to 100 Hz are approximately the same as for the measured frequencies, because of the similarity in the slopes of the curves. However, it should be noted that a deviation from this similarity in slope is possible at frequencies higher than 15 Hz, especially for vocal fold mucosal tissues that show some degree of "nonlinearity" (on the log-log scale) when higher frequencies are approached. Unfortunately, the highest frequency of oscillation allowed in the rheometer is limited by inertia of the rotating plate and sample inertia, as mentioned above. In future studies, measurements made at higher frequencies are needed to validate the extrapolation.

DISCUSSION

The viscosity of a material is a measure of its resistance to shear flow and is always associated with dissipation of internal energy, typically as heat. A material with a low viscosity flows easily, with little internal energy being dissipated in the shearing process. A highly viscous material flows more slowly and dissipates more energy in the process.

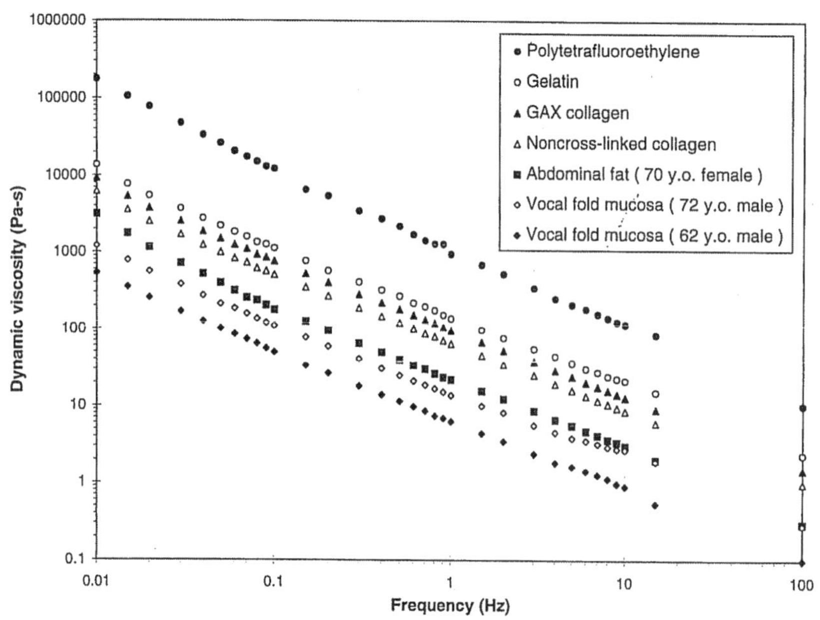

Fig. 3. Dynamic viscosity of implantable biomaterials and human vocal fold mucosa as a function of frequency. Data points are averages of two samples (for vocal fold mucosal tissues) and three samples (for the rest). The values at 100 Hz are extrapolated by linear least-squares regression (equation 3).

TABLE I.
Results of Linear Least-Squares Regression Curve-Fitting (Equation 3).

Material Sample	k	n	r^2
Polytetrafluoroethylene (Teflon)	1151.9	−1.0267	0.997
Gelatin (Gelfoam)	149.39	−0.9030	0.997
GAX collagen (Phonagel or Zyplast)	99.851	−0.9145	0.998
Noncrosslinked collagen (Zyderm)	66.395	−0.9154	0.998
Human abdominal subcutaneous fat (70-year-old woman)	23.576	−0.9508	0.994
Vocal fold mucosa (72-year-old man)	15.758	−0.8741	0.995
Vocal fold mucosa (62-year-old man)	6.5601	−0.9109	0.998

The resistance to flow for a viscoelastic material is quantified by dynamic viscosity. At the microscopic level, this resistance depends on the ease of relative shear or slippage between molecules of the material, which is determined by different kinds of intramolecular and intermolecular interactions. Some of the most significant molecular interactions include physical entanglement, electrostatic forces (e.g., hydrogen bond), hydrophilic and hydrophobic interactions, and chemical interactions (e.g., covalent crosslink formation).[26] The stronger the molecular interactions, the more resistant the molecules are to slippage, and the higher the viscosity. These interactions are especially important in polymeric materials (the biomaterials tested in this study), where long chains of molecules occupy a large space relative to their atomic dimensions. More densely packed, longer and more highly charged polymeric chains are more likely to have physical entanglements, chemical crosslinks, and more significant electrostatic interactions. Hence *concentration, molecular weight,* and *molecular structure* of the macromolecules are all important in dictating material viscosity.[26]

Our results show that the synthetic polymer Teflon is much more viscous than the other (biologic) materials (Fig. 3; Table II), probably because of the extensive molecular interactions resulting from a close packing of polymeric chains. Being a denatured or partially hydrolyzed collagen, gelatin has a higher dynamic viscosity than collagen. It may be explained by the fact that gelatin exists as a heterogeneous aggregate of partially hydrolyzed fragments of collagen fibrils and tropocollagen molecules. These fragments of gelatin molecules are basically randomly coiled together with intramolecular and intermolecular interactions, like physical entanglements, hydrogen bonds, and covalent crosslinks.[27] In addition, the gelatin samples used were prepared with a higher concentration (250 mg/mL) than that of collagen (37 mg/mL). These two factors probably contributed to the higher viscosity of gelatin. Owing to their relatively high viscosities, Teflon and gelatin can be used for medialization of paralyzed vocal folds, but probably not for implantation into any vibrating portion of the vocal fold. This is especially true for Teflon, since it cannot be assimilated easily by body tissue reactions.

The chemically crosslinked GAX collagen showed a higher dynamic viscosity than noncrosslinked collagen, as expected from the formation of many covalent crosslinks in tropocollagen molecules after glutaraldehyde treatment. Therefore molecular interactions between and within the collagen fibrils are probably stronger for GAX collagen, hence its higher viscosity.

Fat is stored in droplets in cellular adipocytes of subcutaneous adipose tissue. The typical lipid molecules are the highly nonpolar and hydrophobic triacylglycerols. Our results show that fat has a lower dynamic viscosity than collagen, probably because of its very different molecular

TABLE II.
Dynamic Viscosity of Implantable Biomaterials and Human Vocal Fold Mucosal Tissues Measured at 10 Hz and Extrapolated to 100 Hz.

	Dynamic Viscosity (Pa-s)	
Material Sample	Measured at 10 Hz	Extrapolated to 100 Hz
Polytetrafluoroethylene (Teflon)	116.144	10.186
Gelatin (Gelfoam)	21.297	2.335
GAX collagen (Phonagel or Zyplast)	12.844	1.480
Noncrosslinked collagen (Zyderm)	8.563	0.980
Human abdominal subcutaneous fat (70-year-old woman)	3.026	0.296
Vocal fold mucosa (72-year-old man)	2.702	0.281
Vocal fold mucosa (62-year-old man)	0.897	0.099

Extrapolation was based on simple linear least-squares regression (see Equation 3).

structure. Unlike collagen molecules, fat molecules do not have significant electrostatic forces between them, particularly for fatty acids with relatively saturated hydrocarbon chains. Collagen, including "noncrosslinked" collagen, also has numerous covalent crosslinks among individual molecules, while the relatively inert fat molecules do not have reactive functional groups to form crosslinks. Therefore it is likely that fat has relatively weak molecular interactions and a lower viscosity.

Since the vocal fold mucosal tissues tested in this study were obtained 24 hours postmortem, there may well be considerable postmortem changes (possibly stiffening) in their mechanical properties after 24 hours. Nevertheless, the dynamic viscosity of vocal fold mucosa measured at 10 Hz was around 1 Pa-s, with a considerable difference between the two subjects. The vocal fold mucosa of the 72-year-old male cadaver was approximately three times more viscous than that of the 62-year-old male cadaver. This finding alone is interesting and consistent with the observations of significant intersubject differences in molecular constituents of the lamina propria.[28,29] The dynamic viscosity of canine vocal fold mucosa reported by Kakita et al.[30] at 0.1 Hz and 19°C was approximately 400 Pa-s, compared with 50 Pa-s and 100 Pa-s for our two subjects. Their much higher viscosity was probably due to the fact that the deep layer of lamina propria (instead of the superficial layer) was tested at a lower temperature. Besides, the use of human versus canine tissues is certainly a major difference between the two studies.

Vocal fold molecular composition has been investigated to some depth previously.[28,29,31–33] Cellular structures found in the lamina propria include mainly fibroblasts and macrophages, while the extracellular matrix of lamina propria consists of fibrous proteins (collagen and elastin), glycosaminoglycans (e.g., hyaluronate, chondroitin sulfate, keratan sulfate, heparan sulfate), proteoglycans (glycosaminoglycans covalently attached to a protein core [e.g., versican, decorin, fibromodulin]), and structural glycoproteins (e.g., fibronectin).[28,29,31–33] As cellular structures are sparse in the superficial layer of lamina propria, the extracellular matrix probably plays an important role in metabolism, as well as mucosal vibration.[33] Among the many constituents found in the extracellular matrix, hyaluronate (conjugate base of hyaluronic acid at pH 7.0 to 7.4) and proteoglycans are important mechanically because of their huge size and potential for molecular interactions. However, their concentrations and molecular weights in the superficial layer are not known at present, making the correlation between molecular structure and mechanical properties difficult.

Balazs and Gibbs[34] measured the complex dynamic shear modulus of hyaluronate solution (5.59 mg/mL) from the human umbilical cord. From their results, dynamic viscosity of hyaluronate is estimated to be 0.3 to 0.5 Pa-s at 10 Hz. The viscosity of a hyaluronate solution depends strongly on its molecular weight and concentration,[35] as expected from the differences in molecular interactions attributable to different polymeric chain lengths and closeness of packing. Dynamic viscosity of link-stable proteoglycan aggregate solution (40 mg/mL) is estimated to be 0.2 to 0.4 Pa-s at 10 Hz, from the dynamic shear modulus data reported by Zhu and Mow[36] and Zhu et al.[37] Considerable difference was found between proteoglycan aggregates and monomers and between aggregates with and without stabilizing link-proteins. This again shows that differences in molecular interactions correspond to differences in mechanical properties.

Our data on dynamic viscosity of vocal fold mucosal tissues are quite different from those of the molecular constituents, namely collagen, hyaluronate, and proteoglycans. Collagen suspension has the highest dynamic viscosity, followed by vocal fold mucosa, then hyaluronate and proteoglycan solutions (Table II). It is likely to be a result of the complex molecular interactions among collagen, hyaluronate, and proteoglycans that have yet to be fully understood. As in many other extracellular matrices, collagen and elastin probably form a fibrous scaffolding mesh in the superficial layer of lamina propria, showing various molecular interactions (e.g., electrostatic) with hyaluronate and proteoglycans.[38] Hyaluronate with its large size, extended shape, and high charge density and proteoglycans with their branching and charge might physically entangle with the mesh and become "space fillers." These molecular interactions contribute to the shear elasticity and viscosity and may explain why viscosity of vocal fold mucosa is higher than that of hyaluronate and proteoglycans. On the other hand, interactions among collagen molecules (e.g., covalent crosslinks) might be somewhat weakened by the infiltration of hyaluronate and proteoglycan molecules (e.g., with a decrease in number of entanglement interaction sites in the collagen-proteoglycan matrix[37]), rendering the fibrous mesh more susceptible to shear than the crosslinked molecules in pure collagen suspension, thus producing a lower viscosity.

CONCLUSION

The dynamic viscosity of five commonly used implantable biomaterials for vocal fold augmentation surgery was measured by sinusoidal oscillatory shear experiments using a parallel-plate rotational rheometer. The biomaterials included polytetrafluoroethylene paste in glycerin (Teflon), noncrosslinked type I bovine dermal collagen suspension (Zyderm collagen implant), glutaraldehyde crosslinked (GAX) collagen (Phonagel or Zyplast), absorbable gelatin suspension (Gelfoam), and human abdominal subcutaneous fat. Results show that polytetrafluoroethylene is the most viscous, followed by gelatin, GAX collagen, noncrosslinked collagen, and fat. The dynamic viscosity of fat is closest to that of the vocal fold mucosa (epithelium and superficial layer of lamina propria), while the viscosities of two key constituents of the superficial layer of lamina propria, hyaluronic acid and proteoglycans, are lower than that of the vocal fold mucosa according to the literature.

Our results suggest that the use of fat or other materials with relatively low viscosity may be more conducive to the "ease" of phonation, especially in phonosurgery involving implantation into the vocal fold mucosa (e.g., repair of vocal fold scarring or atrophy). Use of materials with relatively high viscosity would make vocal fold vibration more difficult, especially if the materials are not easily assimilated (e.g., absorbed or resorbed) by body tissue reactions. The mechanical properties of materials are important and should be considered together with medical and other concerns (in particular, short- and long-term biologic tissue response) in the choice of materials for vocal fold augmentation surgery.

ACKNOWLEDGMENT

The authors thank Dr. Brad H. Story of the Wilbur James Gould Voice Research Center, Denver Center for the Performing Arts, for his contributions in viscometric measurements.

BIBLIOGRAPHY

1. Benninger MS, Alessi D, Archer S, et al. Vocal fold scarring: current concepts and management. *Otolaryngol Heck Neck Surg* 1996;115:474–82.
2. Ford CN, Bless DM. Collagen injection in the scarred vocal fold. *J Voice* 1987;1:116–8.
3. Horn KL, Dedo HH. Surgical correction of the convex vocal cord after Teflon injection. *Laryngoscope* 1980;90:281–6.
4. Rubin HJ. Misadventures with injectable Polytef (Teflon). *Arch Otolaryngol* 1975;101:114–6.
5. Ford CN, Martin DW, Warner TF. Injectable collagen in laryngeal rehabilitation. *Laryngoscope* 1984;94:513–8.
6. Ford CN, Bless DM, Loftus JM. Role of injectable collagen in the treatment of glottic insufficiency: a study of 119 patients. *Ann Otol Rhinol Laryngol* 1992;101:237–47.
7. Remacle M, Dujardin JM, Lawson G. Treatment of vocal fold immobility by glutaraldehyde–cross-linked collagen injection: long-term results. *Ann Otol Rhinol Laryngol* 1995; 104:437–41.
8. Ford CN, Staskowski PA, Bless DM. Autologous collagen vocal fold injection: a preliminary clinical study. *Laryngoscope* 1995;105:944–8.
9. Mikaelian DO, Lowry LD, Sataloff RT. Lipoinjection for unilateral vocal cord paralysis. *Laryngoscope* 1991;101:465–8.
10. Brandenburg JH, Kirkham W, Koschkee D. Vocal cord augmentation with autogenous fat. *Laryngoscope* 1992;102: 495–500.
11. Shaw GY, Szewczyk MA, Searle J, Woodroof J. Autologous fat injection into the vocal folds: technical considerations and long-term follow-up. *Laryngoscope* 1997;107:177– 86.
12. Wexler DB, Jiang J, Gray SD, Titze IR. Phonosurgical studies: fat-graft reconstruction of injured canine vocal cords. *Ann Otol Rhinol Laryngol* 1989;98:668–73.
13. Jiang JJ, Titze IR, Wexler DB, Gray SD. Fundamental frequency and amplitude perturbation in reconstructed canine vocal folds. *Ann Otol Rhinol Laryngol* 1994;103: 145–8.
14. Sataloff RT, Spiegel JR, Hawkshaw MJ, Rosen DC, Heuer RJ. Autologous fat implantation for vocal fold scar: a preliminary report. *J Voice* 1997;11:238–46.
15. Schramm VL, May M, Lavorato AS. Gelfoam paste injection for vocal fold paralysis: temporary rehabilitation of glottic incompetence. *Laryngoscope* 1978;88:1268–73.
16. Hoffman HT, Sullivan MJ, Winter P. Gelfoam injection for vocal cord paralysis prior to radiation therapy. *Ear Nose Throat J* 1991;70:385–6.
17. Titze IR. The physics of small-amplitude oscillation of the vocal folds. *J Acoust Soc Am* 1988;83:1536–52.
18. Titze IR. Phonation threshold pressure: a missing link in glottal aerodynamics. *J Acoust Soc Am* 1992;91:2926–35.
19. Finkelhor BK, Titze IR, Durham PL. The effect of viscosity changes in the vocal folds on the range of oscillation. *J Voice* 1987;1:320–5.
20. Titze IR, Schmidt SS, Titze MR. Phonation threshold pressure in a physical model of the vocal fold mucosa. *J Acoust Soc Am* 1995;97:3080–4.
21. Verdolini K, Titze IR, Fennell A. Dependence of phonatory effort on hydration level. *J Speech Hear Res* 1994;37:1001–7.
22. Verdolini-Marston K, Titze IR, Druker DG. Changes in phonation threshold pressure with induced conditions of hydration. *J Voice* 1990;4:142–51.
23. Ferry JD. *Viscoelastic Properties of Polymers.* New York: Wiley; 1970:1–33.
24. Whorlow RW. *Rheological Techniques.* Chichester, West Sussex: Ellis Horwood; 1980:243–307.
25. Johnson D, Cormack GC, Abrahams PH, Dixon AK. Computed tomographic observations on subcutaneous fat: implications for liposuction. *Plast Reconstr Surg* 1996;97: 387–96.
26. Barnes HA, Hutton JF, Walters K. *An Introduction to Rheology.* Amsterdam: Elsevier; 1989:97–114.
27. Ward AG, Courts A. *The Science and Technology of Gelatin.* London: Academic Press; 1977:137–77.
28. Hammond TH, Zhou R, Hammond E, Pawlak A, Gray S. The intermediate layer: a morphologic study of the elastin and hyaluronic acid constituents of normal human vocal folds. *J Voice* 1997;11:59–66.
29. Matsuo K, Watanabe S, Hirano M, Kamimura M, Tanaka Y, Takazono I. Acid mucopolysaccharide and glycoprotein in the vocal fold: alterations with aging. *Practica Otol Kyoto* 1984;77:817–22.
30. Kakita Y, Hirano M, Ohmaru K. Physical properties of the vocal fold tissue: measurements on excised larynges. In: Stevens KN, Hirano M, eds. *Vocal Fold Physiology.* Tokyo: University of Tokyo Press; 1981:377–97.
31. Gray SD, Hirano M, Sato K. Molecular and cellular structure of vocal fold tissue. In: Titze IR, ed. *Vocal Fold Physiology: Frontiers in Basic Science.* San Diego: Singular Publishing Group; 1993:1–35.
32. Hirano M. Structure of the vocal fold in normal and disease states anatomical and physical studies. In: Ludlow CL, Hard MO, eds. *Proceedings of the Conference on the Assessment of Vocal Pathology.* Rockville: American Speech-Language-Hearing Association; 1981:11–30.
33. Pawlak AS, Hammond TH, Hammond EH, Gray SD. Immunocytochemical study of proteoglycans in vocal folds. *Ann Otol Rhinol Laryngol* 1996;105:6–11.
34. Balazs EA, Gibbs DA. The rheological properties and biological function of hyaluronic acid. In: Balazs EA, ed. *Chemistry and Molecular Biology of the Intercellular Matrix.* vol 3. New York: Academic Press; 1970:1241–53.
35. Bothner H, Wik O. Rheology of hyaluronate. *Acta Otolaryngol (Stockh)* 1987;442:25–30.
36. Zhu WB, Mow VC. Viscometric properties of proteoglycan solutions at physiological concentrations. In: Mow VC, Ratcliffe A, Woo S, eds. *Biomechanics of Diarthrodial Joints.* New York: Springer-Verlag; 1990:313–44.
37. Zhu W, Iatridis JC, Hlibczuk V, Ratcliffe A, Mow VC. Determination of collagen-proteoglycan interactions in vitro. *J Biomechanics* 1996;29:773–83.
38. Lehninger AL, Nelson DL, Cox MM. *Principles of Biochemistry.* New York: Worth Publishers; 1993:298–321.

13

Laryngeal Framework Surgery

Introduction

Framework surgery will probably stand definitively as the most sophisticated and versatile means of treatment of glottic insufficiency until dynamic means of rehabilitation are perfected. A truly successful outcome, with full restoration of voice volume and projection, is a particular satisfaction for the laryngeal surgeon because of the precision and responsiveness of the technique.

The reinvention of laryngeal framework surgery in the late 1960s and early 1970s is largely due to the efforts of Dr. Nobuhiko Isshiki. "Reinvention" because the concept—thyroplasty specifically—had been introduced by Ernst Payr in 1915. Technical modifications to the original surgery were made by several surgeons, Muerman of Helsinki and Opheim of Oslo prominent among them, in the ensuing decades. Despite encouraging results, the technique did not achieve popularity, in part because the cartilage that provided the primary medialization bulk in this operation presented some of the same unpredictability in long-term survival and implant stability that it does elsewhere in the head and neck, in part because the procedure requires some technical finesse, and perhaps in greatest part because the widespread adoption of Teflon for injection augmentation essentially transferred considerable momentum from medialization laryngoplasty to injection augmentation.

"Reinvention" also because Isshiki's innovation was not simply a matter of introducing silastic as an adjunct material to cartilage. He reimagined medialization, instead of as simple problem-oriented technique, as part of a rational approach to adjusting vocal fold positions and properties by altering their supporting framework. Even though his type I operation—medialization—sees the most use, it should not be overlooked that Isshiki's approach was systematic and visionary. His 1989 monograph *Phonosurgery*, now sadly out of print, remains revelatory and not one bit dated; in it he anticipates virtually every refinement of technique that has been introduced since and a few that have yet to be tackled.

In the commentary accompanying his truly classic descriptions of thyroplasty and arytenoid adduction, Isshiki reveals the origin of his insights and provides a window into his approach and thinking, as well as into some unrealized potentials for his techniques. The theme that emerges is that successful laryngeal manipulation depends on a deep understanding of its physiology. That is an observation reinforced for the surgeon by every medialization laryngoplasty performed, especially when it is necessary to adjust a suboptimal result intraoperatively. The report of the Vanderbilt experience remains the largest series published and reinforces the observations of Dr. Isshiki. It is remarkable for its results as well as its technical and conceptual insights. Together with Isshiki's papers, these offer a remarkably complete picture of the re-establishment of framework surgery as a mainstay in the laryngological armamentarium.

Classic Articles

● Reprint of article included in this chapter.
♦ Commentary on this article.

●♦Isshiki N, Morita H, Okamura H, Hiramoto M. Thyroplasty as a new phonosurgical technique. *Acta Otolaryngol.* 1974;78(5–6):451–457.

Isshiki N, Okamura H, Ishikawa T. Thyroplasty type I (lateral compression) for dysphonia due to vocal cord paralysis or atrophy. *Acta Otolaryngol.* 1975;80(5–6): 465–473.

●Isshiki N, Tanabe M, Sawada M. Arytenoid adduction for unilateral vocal cord paralysis. *Arch Otolaryngol.* 1978;104:555–558.

Koufman JA. Laryngoplasty for vocal cord medialization: an alternative to Teflon. *Laryngoscope.* 1986;96:726–731.

Koufman JA, Isaacson G. Laryngoplastic phonosurgery. *Otolaryngol Clin North Am.* 1991;24(5):1151–1177.

●Netterville JL, Stone RE, Luken ES, Civantos FJ, Ossoff RH. Silastic medialization and arytenoid adduction: the Vanderbilt experience. A review of 116 phonosurgical procedures. *Ann Otol Rhinol Laryngol.* 1993;102(6): 413–424.

Cummings CW, Purcell LL, Flint PW. Hydroxylapatite laryngeal implants for medialization: preliminary report. *Ann Otol Rhinol Laryngol.* 1993;102(11):843–851.

Commentary

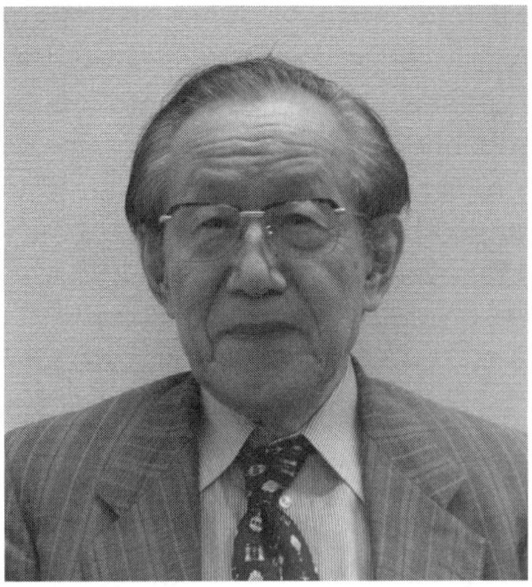

Nobuhiko Isshiki, MD

The thyroplasty paper reproduced here that actually constitutes the theoretical initiation of laryngeal framework surgery is based on experiments using excised human and canine larynges. The basic concept for laryngeal framework surgery originated in my mind while performing a variety of experiments to simulate normal and abnormal voice using human or canine larynges. The initial purpose of these experiments was to reveal the mechanism underlying hoarse voice production. While doing research on the aerodynamics of voice in 1962 to 1964 with Dr. Hans von Leden at the Laryngeal Research Laboratory at UCLA, I became more and more convinced that the major causative factor for hoarseness must be imperfect closure of the glottis during phonation, creating aerodynamic noise. On the other hand, imperfect closure does not always cause hoarseness, as for example in falsetto. A question arose: what is the threshold value of glottal closure deficits to produce a hoarse voice? On returning to Japan, I started experiments on artificial voice production using the model originally designed by van den Berg: the vocal folds in an excised larynx were adducted and stretched by applying varying weights simulating muscle contraction of the adductor and cricothyroid muscles. Humidified airflow was presented from below to bring the vocal folds into vibration. The experiment revealed that the glottal chink, when greater than a certain critical value (threshold value), produced a hoarse voice regardless of other conditions, such as tension of the vocal folds or airflow rate. This was simply a matter of course; nothing about it was either exciting or surprising.

About that time, a patient, a karate (Loochoo art of self-defense) expert visited our clinic at Kyoto University, complaining of a deformity of the larynx allegedly due to karate hand blows. His voice was quite normal. The prominent deviated Adam's apple was simply reduced to the patient's satisfaction, without affecting the voice at all. This experience led me to the idea that deliberately created deformity of the laryngeal framework could improve the voice in some cases. This concept turned over a new leaf in phonosurgery. A variety of deliberate deformations of the laryngeal framework were evaluated for the potential to address a variety of inadequate glottal closures and vocal fold tensions, such as those that may occur in laryngeal paralysis and so on.

The deformations of the laryngeal framework, or thyroplasties, were classified into four types on the basis of their functional effects on position and tension of the vocal folds. These are (1) medialization, (2) lateralization, (3) relaxation, and (4) tensing of the vocal fold. The classification has remained unchanged so far. What I did not anticipate was that excessively tight closure of the glottis produced a rough and hoarse voice as well, but there was no way to express the degree of tightness of the closure under the experimental conditions; this was left to the future studies (type 2 thyroplasty). The effect of the dry vocal fold mucosa also surpassed my assumptions, indicating how important the rheological features (stiffness, mobility) of the vocal fold mucosa are for the Bernoulli effect to be effective. Most of the data obtained in the model experiment still remain as particles in chaos in my mind, each probably increasingly charged with new information. I preferred not to publish the data in a way rationally arranged by statistical measure. I was afraid that a rational rearrangement might lose chaotic energy to spark a new concept when I might come across a new problem.

Thyroplasty Type 1 (Lateral Compression) for Dysphonia due to Vocal Fold Paralysis or Atrophy

Around this time, I happened to be in charge of a patient with severe dysphonia resulting from laryngeal trauma. What impressed me most was how difficult it was to treat scar of the vocal fold. One of the lessons I learned then was that a wide surgical intervention into the vocal fold proper should be avoided whenever possible. On the other hand, I had great hopes that this new type of laryngeal framework surgery might be capable of somehow replacing a direct intervention into the vocal fold, thereby avoiding the development of incurable scar. However, there were a number of obstacles to clear before it became a clinical reality. The first was a strict concept of reductionism: the basic concept of surgery then consisted of removal or repair of the lesion responsible for the disease. Surgical intervention in the laryngeal framework, which is not contributing to or causing dysphonia, seemed inconceivable in the light of this prevailing concept of surgery at that time. We had long been constrained by this idea of direct treatment of the lesion. The second problem was whether the lesion causing the hoarseness is clearly evident or not. Type 1 thyroplasty was fairly easily accepted because its effects can easily be identified after operation; the laterally displaced vocal fold was effectively brought to the median position, restoring the voice by this surgery.

What about spasmodic dysphonia (SD)? It is difficult to differentiate between adequate complete closure of the glottis and an excessively tight closure. In the experiment using the excised larynx, it was incidentally found that too tight a closure of the glottis also produced rough sounds. This has led to an idea of utilizing type 2 thyroplasty as a treatment for SD. Another example of a difficult to appreciate finding that can lead to a wrong concept and frequent misdiagnosis, such as functional dysphonia, is related to the scar. We have to have an insight to see the reality beyond the initial appearance. By way of example, an excessive fat injection into an atrophic vocal fold results in severely breathy voice because, although the appearance may be corrected, reducing the glottal chink on phonation, the consequent maximal expansion of the mucosa results in immobility or extremely high stiffness of the vocal fold. Occasionally, we see such patients. The surgeon must have appreciated the anatomical appearance only, and failed to see beyond it—the advantage of thyroplasty over fat injection.

At the time the above clinical paper was published, most neck surgeries were performed under general anesthesia, and phonosurgery or laryngeal framework surgery under local anesthesia was entirely unpopular and took time to be accepted. My previous experiences with Woodman's operation, for instance, had already shown me that there was no problem in doing such surgery under local anesthesia. Surgery under local anesthesia made it possible to adjust the surgical procedures to obtain the best voice. This adjustability is the greatest advantage of the laryngeal framework surgery, different from the vocal fold injection or from any procedure under general anesthesia.

Arytenoid Adduction for Unilateral Vocal Fold Paralysis

The first step in the model experiment for arytenoids adduction was to set the vocal fold to the phonatory position by pulling the muscular process anterolaterally along the vector of lateral cricoarytenoid muscle. After repetitions of the procedures for each experiment, it didn't take much time for me to understand the use of this procedure as an effective treatment for vocal fold paralysis with a large glottal chink. One of the advantages of this operation that is often overlooked is that no big foreign body is used for medialization of the vocal fold, and therefore no persistent pressure is applied to the surrounding tissues. Therefore, there is no chance for atrophy or necrosis (pressure sore) of the tissue, which would lead to migration of the foreign body and return of symptoms. Arytenoid adduction is certainly difficult technically, compared with type 1 thyroplasty, but worth the effort, for the medialization effect is greater without using a big prosthesis. Often, a combination of arytenoid adduction with type 1 thyroplasty will yield the best voice result. The keys to the success in laryngeal framework surgery are: (1) technical precision, including use of the exact instruments necessary to realize the intended mechanical change of the laryngeal framework, and (2) right navigation (the next step to be taken) toward the goal, based on the right understanding of the problem when initially faced with unsatisfactory voice result during surgery. Although type 2 thyroplasty for SD has not gained popularity yet, and is therefore very infrequently cited, this would become a surgery of choice for SD if it were performed in a correct as well as precise manner, using a proper titanium bridge. So far we have performed type 2 thyroplasty on 140 SD patients with great success without recurrence. Surgical tips for the surgery will be reported soon.

THYROPLASTY AS A NEW PHONOSURGICAL TECHNIQUE

N. Isshiki, H. Morita, H. Okamura and M. Hiramoto

From the Department of Otolaryngology, School of Medicine, Kyoto University, Kyoto, Japan

(Received February 13, 1974)

Abstract. In an attempt to examine the surgical possibility of changing the vocal cord position and tension by reforming the thyroid cartilage, an experimental study was made using 10 adult dogs. Hoarseness produced by section of the recurrent laryngeal nerve was generally much improved by vertical incision on the thyroid ala and slipping in of the lateral cartilage segment. Four types of thyroplasty were proposed from the functional viewpoint. Their effects on the vocal cord are (1) lateral compression, (2) lateral expansion, (3) relaxation (shortening) and (4) stretching (lengthening) respectively. Possible indications for each type of thyroplasty were described with reference to specific laryngeal diseases. The advantages of thyroplasty were emphasized namely, that the intervention inside the thyroid cartilage is minimal and therefore fine and reliable adjustment is possible during surgery. Thyroplasty thus offers a new possibility in phonosurgery.

The aim of treatment for laryngeal diseases is most frequently to attain a normal voice, although this becomes secondary in such cases as laryngeal carcinoma or bilateral recurrent nerve paralysis. Phonosurgery, defined as surgery for better voice, is at present almost limited to removal of a benign tumor on the vocal cord or reduction of the glottal chink by teflon injection or cartilage implantation for unilateral recurrent nerve paralysis. Despite the recent development of laryngo-microsurgical technique, direct intervention on the vocal cord itself, z-plasty for sulcus vocalis for instance, has not yet been performed.

There may be several factors which prevent direct surgical intervention on the vocal cord. Surgical techniques which can be used through a suspension laryngoscope are naturally limited and fine suturing as is necessary for z-plasty is virtually impossible. Laryngofissure, which would then be required for such a technique, poses another unsolved problem—postoperative development of granuloma at the anterior commissure. The greatest obstacle we encounter, however, is the inevitable postoperative scarring of the mucosa, which reduces the compliance of the vocal cord mucosa, thus greatly hindering vibration of the vocal cord.

As a result, phonosurgery at present is quite incompetent for laryngeal diseases such as mutational voice disorders, hyperfunctional dysphonia, vocal cord hypertrophy due to anabolic hormones, sulcus vocalis, vocal cord atrophy, and traumatic laryngeal deformities. We laryngologists should thus break away from conventional vocal cord polypotomy. As a stage prior to direct surgical intervention on the vocal cord, we attempted to change the position and physical property of the vocal cord by actively reforming the cartilaginous frame-work on which vocal cords are suspended.

A search of the literature fails to reveal any similar systematic investigation on how the reformation of the thyroid cartilage affects the vocal cord and the voice. This preliminary report deals with the experimental results of thyroplasty in dogs. Several clinical cases will be reported in detail later.

EXPERIMENTAL PROCEDURE

Ten adult dogs were used for the experiment. The dogs were anesthesized by intraperitoneal injection of Pentobarbital Natrium (Mintal) 125 mg, and fixed supine for laryngeal surgery. Un-

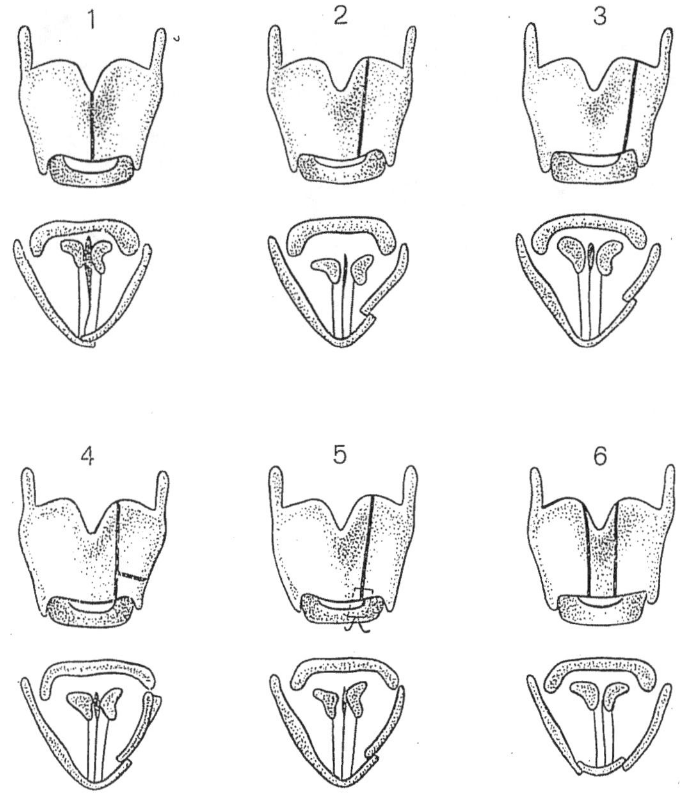

Fig. 1. Schematic demonstration of varied thyroplasties performed on dogs.

der local anesthesia with 1% Xylocaine, the larynx and left recurrent laryngeal nerve were exposed. For better visualization of the vocal cord, supraglottic laryngectomy was performed. Voicing was evoked by pain stimuli. For each experimental condition mentioned below, laryngeal pictures—black and white, color photographs, and 16 mm cinefilm—were taken during respiration and phonation. The voice was recorded by tape-recorder for later acoustic analysis. Before sectioning of the recurrent laryngeal nerve, the vocal cord movement and voice were confirmed to be normal. Any dog whose respiratory movement of the vocal cord was asymmetrical was excluded from the analysis of the experimental results.

After section of the left recurrent laryngeal nerve, thyroplasty was performed: vertical incision of the left lamina was made at 1. the median line, 2. anterior one third, 3. middle, and the lateral part of the cartilage lamina was slipped underneath the medial part and fixed by 4–0 Nylon suture. The two laminae were overlapped 2–4 mm width depending on the case. In addition to the recurrent laryngeal nerve, the external branch of the left superior laryngeal nerve was also cut in two dogs. Two parallel vertical incisions on the thyroid cartilage and depression of the median cartilage were done in one dog. Incisions and fixation of the thyroid cartilage used in the present experiment are schematically shown in Fig. 1.

EXPERIMENTAL RESULTS

1. *Median incision on thyroid cartilage and repositioning of left lamina (1 in Fig. 1, Dog no. 1)*

The hoarse voice caused by section of the left recurrent laryngeal nerve was somewhat improved by the above procedure but still re-

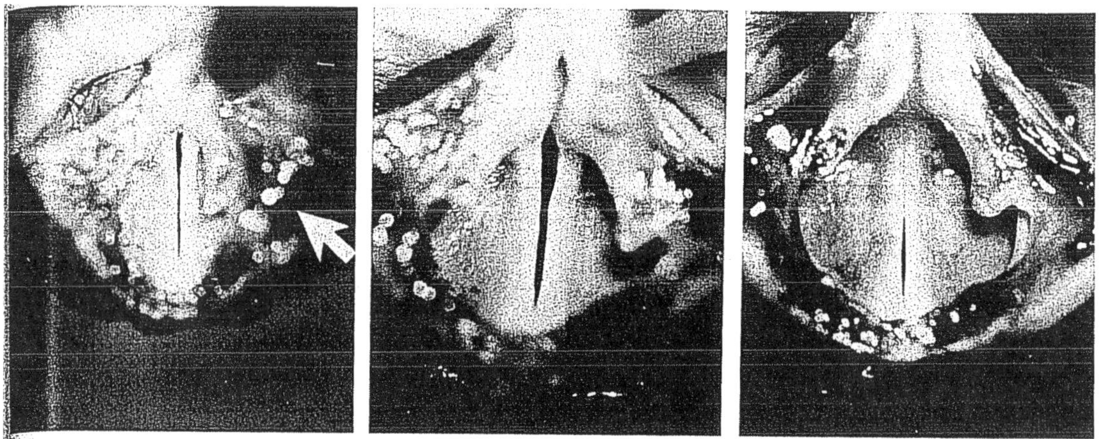

Fig. 2. *Left*: control, during phonation; *middle:* after section of the left recurrent laryngeal nerve, during phonation; *right*: after thyroplasty during phonation. The arrow indicates the site of repositioning.

remained rough. The procedure resulted in the shift of the paralysed vocal cord slightly toward the midline, with the decrease of glottal slit during phonation. Nevertheless a noticeable chink remained at the posterior glottis (cartilaginous portion). The voice was lowered in pitch by slipping in the left lamina.

2. *Vertical incision of left lamina at anterior middle third and shift of lateral (posterior) lamina underneath the median (anterior) lamina (2 in Fig. 1, Dogs 2, 4, 7, 8, 9, 10)*

Hoarseness due to recurrent nerve section was remarkably improved, particularly in dogs 4 and 9, whose voices became quite normal (Fig. 2). In general, there remained a narrow slit at the cartilaginous portion. The vocal pitch did not change markedly. In dog no. 8, the inner perichondrium was separated over a wide area from the thyroid lamina along the vertical incision line so that the lateral part could be slipped far anteriorly underneath the median part. This wide perichondrium separation and overlapping of the laminae resulted in prominent bulging of the vocal cord, and the voice remained hoarse and low-pitched. The excessive increase in thickness seemed to have arrested the vibration of the vocal cord.

3. *Vertical incision at antero-posterior mid-line and shift of lateral part (3 in Fig. 1, Dog no. 3)*

The hoarseness was not much improved by this procedure. A slit remained not only at the cartilaginous portion but also at the anterior glottis.

4. *Vertical incision at anterior middle third supplemented by horizontal incision and shift of upper lateral part (4 in Fig. 1, Dog no. 2)*

A slit always remained at the cartilaginous portion even following the procedures 1–3 in Fig. 1. It was assumed that the inferior horn or cricothyroid joint was in the way of the lateral lamina shifting medially. For this reason, an additional incision was placed horizontally above (cranially) the cricothyroid joint to shift the posterior part of the lamina more medially.

This tilted T-shaped incision (|—) unexpectedly ineffectuated the function of the cricothyroid muscle, because the muscle attachment on the thyroid cartilage was indirectly disconnected with the anterior commissure. Consequently the vocal cord was shortened and slightly abducted. The slit did not become narrower, and the resultant voice improvement was not remarkable.

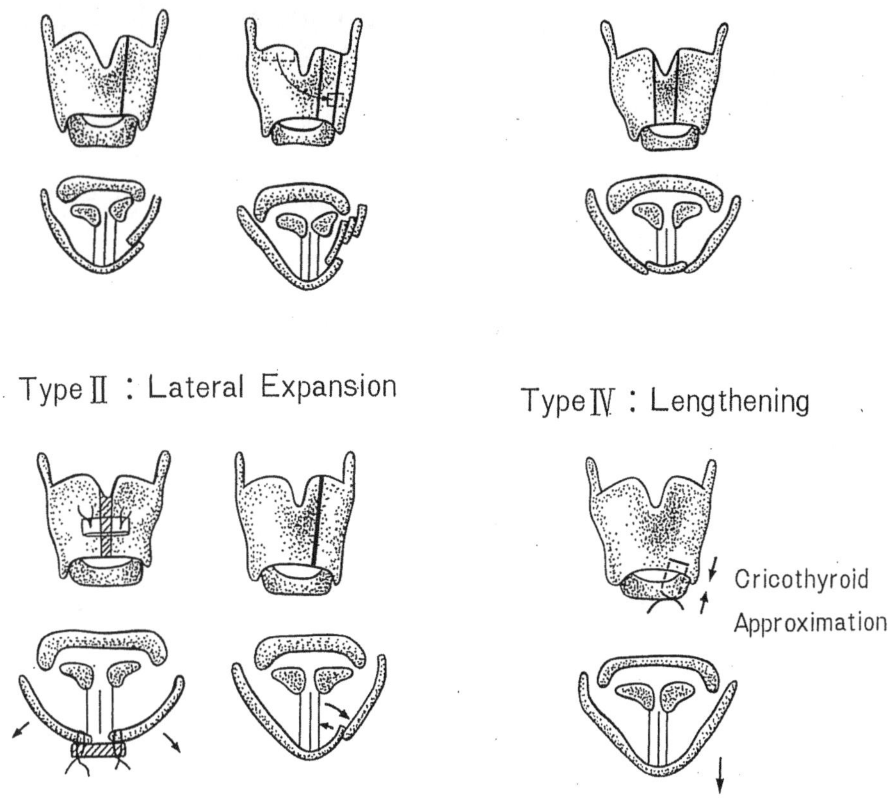

Fig. 3. Four types of thyroplasty.

5. *Vertical incision at anterior middle third and anterior approximation of cricothyroid distance (5 in Fig. 1, dogs 6 and 9)*

The recurrent laryngeal nerve and the external branch of the superior laryngeal nerve on the left were cut first. The consequent glottal chick during phonation was not sufficiently eliminated by mere vertical incision at the anterior middle third of the thyroid lamina. The difference in level between the bilateral cords remained, with the left cord positioning higher than the right. The left cord was so lax that it vibrated only at the initial stage of phonation but soon remained open without vibration. The voice, which started with a rough quality, soon became breathy with a widening glottal chink during phonation.

Then, the cricoid cartilage was approximated to the thyroid by 4–0 Nylon suture just as in the case of a contraction of the cricothyroid muscle. The result was excellent: the voice was improved almost to the normal with only a slight posterior glottal slit (dog no. 6) or without any slit (dog no. 9).

6. *Parallel vertical incision on thyroid cartilage on each side of midline and about 1 cm from it (6 in Fig. 1, dog no. 5)*

In this case, the recurrent laryngeal nerve was not sectioned. After the parallel incisions, the median segment was depressed to slip in. The voice was much lowered in pitch but not hoarse. Pulling up and fixing the median segment back in the original position resulted in a rise of pitch up to the previous level.

DISCUSSION

The results of the present experiment indicated that re-formation of the thyroid cartilage can quite effectively modify the position and tension of the vocal cord. Clinical indications for the techniques may therefore include insufficient glottal closure or excessive tension of the vocal cord. Treatment of dysphonia due to unilateral vocal cord paralysis, which seems most relevant to the present thyroplasty is reviewed below to evaluate the technique.

1. *Surgical treatment of dysphonia due to unilateral vocal cord paralysis*

In 1911, Brünings first developed a method of narrowing the glottis by paraffin injection in case of a unilateral recurrent nerve paralysis. Despite his success, this method had long been abandoned, probably because of the side effects such as paraffinoma. Recently, Arnold (1962 and 1964) and many others revived this approach with new synthetic materials such as teflon, tantalum powder, and silicone.

In 1915 Payr utilized a tilted U-shaped incision on the thyroid ala to make a pedicled cartilage flap, which was then depressed inward to shift the vocal cord medially. Probably because of the pedicle, the shift effect was limited and the technique did not gain popularity.

It was Meurman (1952) who first utilized cartilage implant for this purpose. The implant taken from the costal rib was inserted between the thyroid cartilage and the inner perichondrium. Opheim (1955) used an incised segment of the thyroid cartilage instead, which was inserted inside the inner perichondrium at the level of the vocal cord. Direct intervention on the soft tissue just lateral to the vocal cord gave rise to postoperative edema, eventually requiring tracheotomy. Sawashima et al. (1968) inserted an incised segment of the thyroid cartilage between the thyroid ala and inner perichondrium, with excellent results in voice. Kamer & Som (1972) inserted a piece of the thyroid cartilage from the lower rim of the thyroid cartilage in case of traumatic vocal cord paralysis.

An experimental attempt was made by Bernstein & Holt (1967) to reposition the vocal cord by inserting the bipedicled vital sternohyoid muscle between the thyroid cartilage and inner perichondrium. Transposition or rotation of the arytenoid cartilage (Morrison's reverse King operation, 1948, and Montgomery's Arthrodesis, 1966) for this purpose does not seem very popular because of its technical difficulty. Mündnich (1970) pulled and fixed the arytenoid toward the lower horn of the thyroid cartilage without fenestration of the thyroid cartilage for tensing and median shifting of the vocal cord.

At present, injection of various synthetic materials appears most popular as the treatment of hoarseness in unilateral recurrent nerve paralysis. Percutaneous injection methods were recently reported by Hurst (1972) and Sato et al. (1971).

As Bernstein & Holt (1967) described, there seem to be many problems left unsolved in the above treatments: the possibilities are neoplastic response or eventual rejection by the tissue of the synthetic materials, migration or absorption of the implanted tissue, local stiffening of the vocal cord due to injection and so on.

On account of the advantage that our procedure is rather simple and easy to perform and does not intervene inside the thyroid cartilage, the thyroplasty seems to have a place in treating dysphonia of vocal cord paralysis in man.

2. *From the functional view-point, thyroplasty (Isshiki) can be classified into the following 4 types (Fig. 3)*

Type I: Lateral Compression

This type would be of widest application. Depending on the antero-posterior location and the degree of the glottal chink, incision and overlapping can be adjusted: rather anterior incision may be used for anterior chink, and a wedge may be inserted between the overlapping cartilage laminae to reinforce the median shift of the vocal cord. An added horizontal incision or rectangular incision may also be a further possibility to be considered.

Type II: Lateral Expansion

There would be few indications for this type of procedure. It also seems rather difficult to widen the angle of the thyroid cartilage. Indications for this type in hyperfunctional dysphonia such as dysphonia plica ventricularis would be a future problem to be examined.

Type III: Relaxation (Shortening) of Vocal Cord

Too high pitch as in mutational voice disorder or sulcus vocalis may be a good indication for this type of thyroplasty. Niimi et al. (1973) already reported that a square incision around the anterior commissure and depression of the segment was effective for treating dysphonia in sulcus vocalis.

Type IV: Stretching (Lengthening) of Vocal Cord

We attempted to lengthen the thyroid cartilage horizontally by squeezing a cartilage segment into the vertical incision crevice, but failed. For this purpose, approximation of the anterior cricothyroid distance by mattress sutures was much easier and more effective. Possible late loosening of the knot is a problem worthy of due consideration.

Mixed types of the above are naturally possible. Actually, we clinically adopted a mixed type I and III for mutational voice disorder and I and IV for combined paralysis of the recurrent laryngeal nerve and the external branch of the superior laryngeal nerve. The details of the clinical cases will be reported later but the advantage is that we can select the type and adjust the extent of reformation during operation by the produced voice quality.

3. *Limitation of present experiment*

The cartilaginous portion of the vocal cord is relatively much longer in the dog than in man. It is therefore assumed that the deficient glottal closure at the cartilaginous portion remaining after thyroplasty may be less important in the human case. Present experiments are all acute. In clinical cases of vocal cord paralysis, further consideration may be required on the problem of accompanying vocal cord atrophy or compensatory movement of the intact vocal cord. However, the present experiment provided a fair prospect of clinical application of thyroplasty.

Together with metrological study on the human cadaver larynx now under way, clinical application has already been started. Thyroplasty as we proposed offers a new possibility in phonosurgery.

ZUSAMMENFASSUNG

Die Frage, ob sowohl die Stellung als auch die Spannung der Stimmbänder durch die Umgestaltung des Schildknorpels verändert werden können, wurde anhand von experimentellen Tierversuchen mit 10 erwachsenen Hunden untersucht. Durch die vertikale Abschneidung des Schildknorpelflügels und die mediale Verlagerung seines lateralen Stückchens wurde die mittels Durchtrennung des N. recurrens hervorgerufene Heiserkeit im allgemeien ausgezeichnet verbessert.

Vom funktionellen Standpunkt aus wurden 4 Typen von der Thyreoplastik vorgeschlagen, die jeweils folgende Wirkung auf die Stimmbänder haben: 1. Laterale Kompression, 2. Laterale Expansion, 3. Erschlaffung (Verkürzung), 4. Spannung (Verlängerung). Ihre Operationsindikation wurde für jede Kehlkopfkrankheit erstellt. Als Vorteile der Thyreoplastik beurteilen wir, dass der operative Eingriff in das Innere des Schildknorpels minimal ist, und dass daher die feine und sichere Regulierung intraoperativ ohne weiters durchgeführt werden kann.

Die Thyreoplastik setzt dehalb ihre grosse Hoffnung auf die Phonochirurgie.

REFERENCES

Arnold, G. E. 1962. Vocal rehabilitation of paralytic dysphonia. *Arch Otolaryngol 76*, 358.

— 1964. Further experiences with intrachordal teflon injection. *Laryngoscope 74*, 802.

Bernstein, L. & Holt, G. P. 1967. Correction of vocal cord abduction in unilateral recurrent laryngeal nerve paralysis by transposition of the sternohyoid muscle. *Laryngoscope 77*, 876.

Brünings, W. 1911. Über eine neue Behandlungsmethode der Rekurrenslähmung. *Verh Verl Deutsch Laryngol 18*, 93.

Hurst, W. B. 1972. Percutaneous injection of a vocal cord with teflon. *J Laryngol Otol 86*, 633.

Kamer, F. M. & Som, M. L. 1972. Correction of the traumatically abducted vocal cord. *Arch Otolaryngol 95*, 6.

Lewy, R. B. 1963. Glottic reformation with voice rehabilitation in vocal cord paralysis. *Laryngoscope 73*, 547.

Meurman, Y. 1952. Operative mediofixation of the vocal cord in complete unilateral paralysis. *Arch Otolaryngol 55*, 544.
Montgomery, W. W. 1966. Cricoarytenoid Arthrodesis. *Ann Otol Rhinol Laryngol 75*, 380.
Morrison, L. F. 1948. The "Reverse King operation". *Ann Otol Rhinol Laryngol 57*, 945.
Mueller, P. B. 1973. Paralytic dysphonia. *Folia Phoniatr* (Basel) *25*, 104.
Mündnich, K. 1970. Eine einfache und verläßliche Methode zur Spannung und Verlagerung des Stimmbandes medianwärts bei Dys-und Aphonie mit phonatorische Dyspnoe. *Arch Klin Exp Ohren Nasen Kehlkopfheilkd 196*, 324.
Niimi, S., Takemoto, K. & Shidara, T. 1973. A surgical method for sulcus vocalis. *Jap Otol* (Tokyo) *76*, Suppl. *43*.
Opheim, O. 1955. Unilateral paralysis of the vocal cord. Operative treatment. *Acta Otolaryngol* (Stockh) *45*, 226.
Payr, 1915. Plastik am Schildknorpel zur Behebung der Folgen einseitiger Stimmbandlähmung. *Dtsch Med Wochenschr 43*, 1265.
Rubin, H. J. 1965. Intracordal injection of silicone in selected dysphonia. *Arch Otolaryngol 81*, 604.
Sato, T., Yamamoto, K., Utsumi, S. & Takayama, M. 1971. The present status of cancer of the thyroid gland and its treatment. *Pract Otolog* Kyoto *65*, 514.
Sawashima, M., Totsuka, G., Kobayashi, T. & Hirose, H. 1968. Surgery for hoarseness due to unilateral vocal cord paralysis. *Arch Otolaryngol 87*, 289.

N. Isshiki, M.D.
Dept. of Otolaryngology
School of Medicine
Kyoto University
Sakyo-ku
Kyoto, 606
Japan

Arytenoid Adduction for Unilateral Vocal Cord Paralysis

Nobuhiko Isshiki, MD; Masahiro Tanabe, MD; Masaki Sawada, MD

• The arytenoid adduction technique was devised and performed under local anesthesia on five patients with unilateral vocal cord paralysis. It is especially indicated for the case of a wide, glottal chink and a difference in the level of the two cords. The muscle process is pulled by two 3-0 nylon sutures in simulation of the functions of the lateral cricoarytenoid muscle and the lateral thyroarytenoid muscle. Improvement of voice after surgery was dramatic in all of the patients who were operated on.

The surgical procedure is rather simple, easy, and allows adjustment of the degree of arytenoid adduction during surgery to produce the best voice obtainable.

(*Arch Otolaryngol* 104:555-558, 1978)

Accepted for publication Jan 12, 1978.

From the Voice Science Laboratory, Departments of Plastic Surgery (Drs Isshiki and Sawada) and Otorhinolaryngology (Dr Tanabe), Kyoto University School of Medicine, Japan.

Read before the general meeting of the Japan Society of Otorhinolaryngology, as a special report, Fukuoka, Japan, May 21, 1977, and before the Julliard Meeting, New York, June 17, 1977.

Reprint requests to Department of Plastic Surgery, Kyoto University School of Medicine, Kyoto 606, Japan (Dr Isshiki).

In previous studies,[1,2] it has been reported that thyroplasty type I, that is, lateral compression of the vocal cord, is useful for medial shifting of the paralyzed vocal cord.

Through experience with thyroplasty type I in 24 patients, however, we gradually become aware of a certain limitation of that type of surgery especially when the glottal chink is very wide, and there is a difference in the levels of the two vocal cords. In two cases of a wide, glottal chink due to unilateral vocal cord paralysis, a sizable glottal chink remained posteriorly after thyroplasty type I. Moreover, the difference in the levels of the vocal cords[3] was not effectively corrected by thyroplasty type I or combined I and IV. As is well known, the cricoid cartilage overlaps the thyroid cartilage posteriorly, thus blocking inward displacement of a cartilage piece of the thyroid ala. The posterior part of a glottal chink cannot effectively be reduced by thyroplasty type I. Another drawback of thyroplasty type I is that it cannot contribute toward correcting a difference in the levels of the two cords.

Many previous investigators[4,5] demonstrated that the vocal process moves downward on adduction and upward on abduction mainly because of the cylindrical shape of the cricoarytenoid joint.

These two facts led us to the realization that arytenoid adduction in the physiologic condition will effectively adduct the vocal cord and lower the level of the paralyzed vocal cord (Fig 1).

INDICATION FOR ARYTENOID ADDUCTION

Arytenoid adduction is indicated when dysphonia due to unilateral vocal cord paralysis is particularly associated with a large, glottal chink and with a level difference between the two cords during phonation.

SURGICAL PROCEDURES

Surgery is performed under local anesthesia with 1% lidocaine (Xylocaine) hydrochloride. The patient is in the supine position with the head extended and

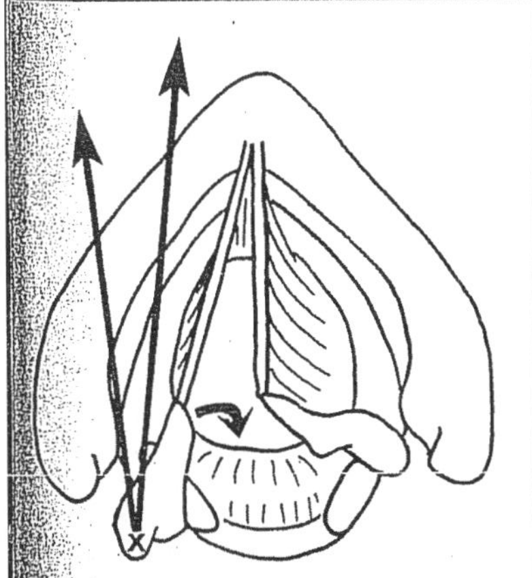

Fig 1.—Principle of arytenoid adduction for unilateral vocal cord paralysis. Pull of muscle process in directions shown by arrows results in adduction and caudal displacement of vocal cord.

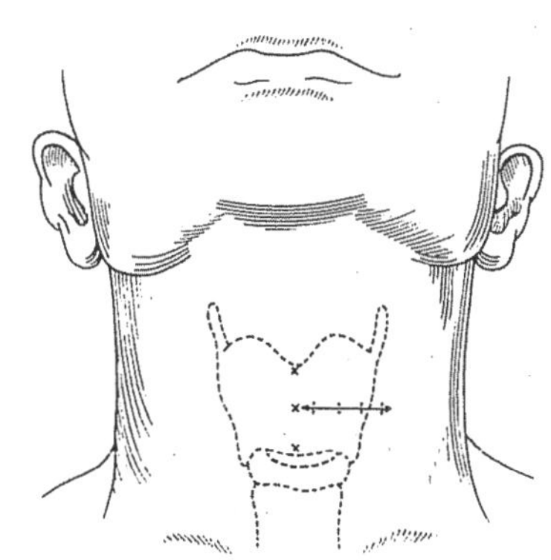

Fig 2.—Incision for arytenoid adduction.

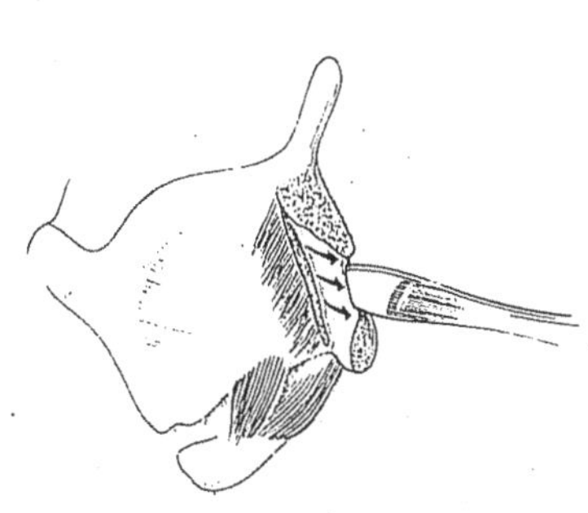

Fig 3.—Thyropharyngeal muscle is sectioned and elevated to expose posterior margin of thyroid cartilage.

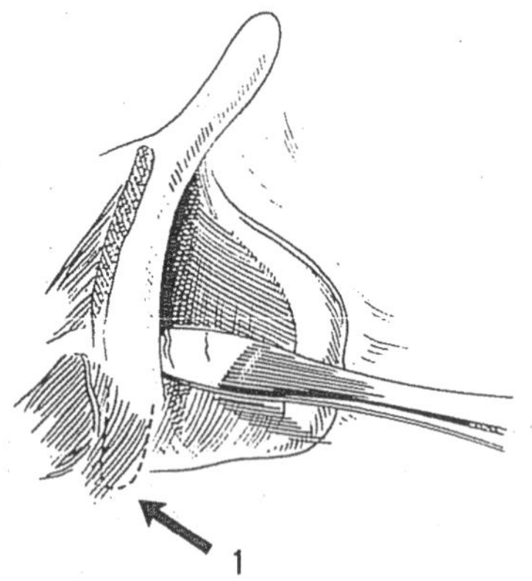

Fig 4.—Inner surface of thyroid cartilage is subperichondrially elevated. Dislocation of cricothyroid joint (1).

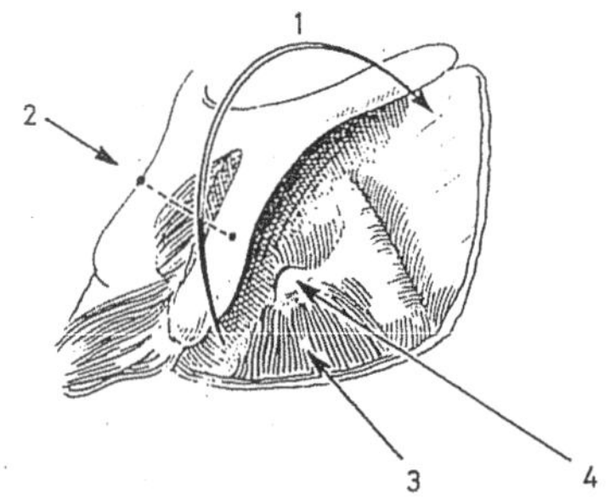

Fig 5.—Turnover of mucosa that covers pyriform recess (1). Care should be taken not to enter airway. Muscle process (4) is on same level as vocal cord (2). Posterior cricoarytenoid muscle (3).

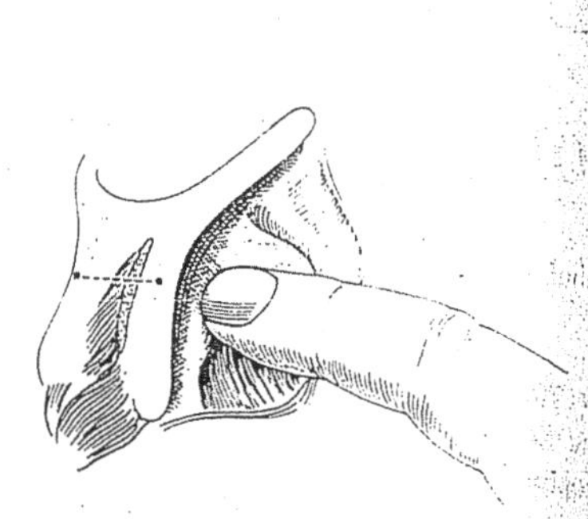

Fig 6.—Muscle process is palpated by finger.

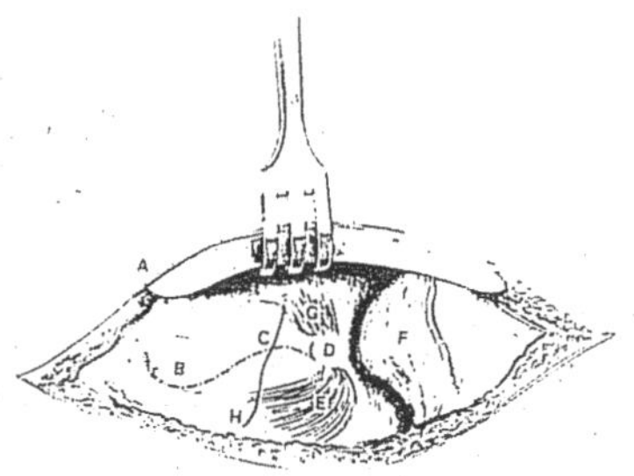

Fig 7.—A indicates thyroid cartilage; B, surface of cricothyroid joint on cricoid cartilage; C, concavity on ridge between lateral and posterior surface of cricoid cartilage; D, muscle process; E, posterior cricoarytenoid muscle; F, mucosa of pyriform recess now elevated; G, lateral cricoarytenoid muscle; H, branch of recurrent laryngeal nerve innervating adductor muscles.

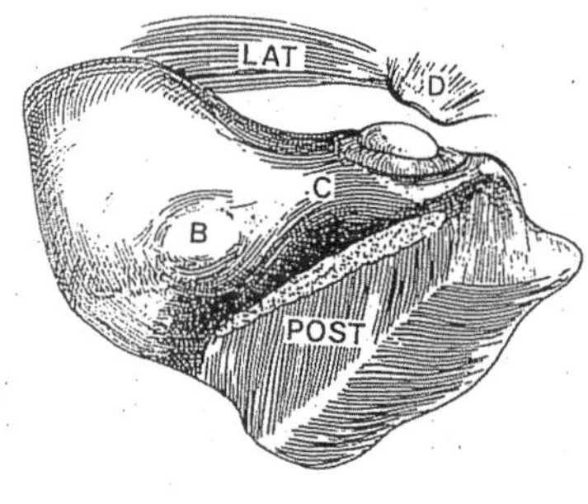

Fig 8.—Cricoid cartilage seen from posterior upward direction. Cricoarytenoid joint D can be reached from B via C. LAT indicates lateral cricoarytenoid muscle; POST, posterior cricoarytenoid muscle.

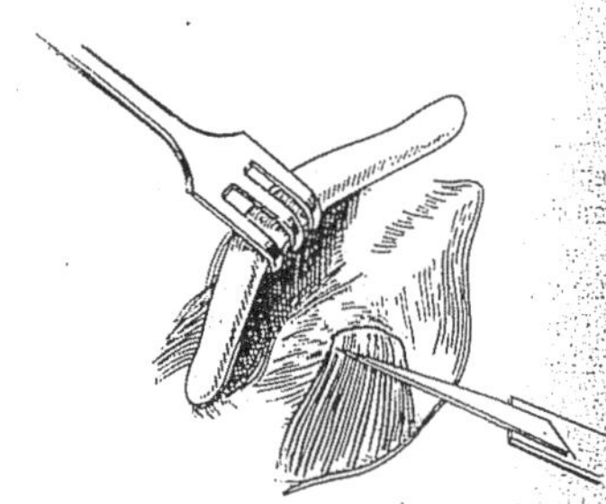

Fig 9.—Small incision is made on posterior cricoarytenoid muscle to open cricoarytenoid joint; it can be opened bluntly too.

twisted a little toward the intact side. The incision is made horizontally on the anterior portion of the neck at the level of the midpoint between the thyroid notch and the lower margin of the thyroid cartilage, extending over the posterior margin of the thyroid cartilage on the paralyzed side (Fig 2). The thyroid cartilage is exposed down to the posterior margin. The thyropharyngeal muscle is elevated and sectioned as illustrated in Fig 3. Elevation is continued to the inner surface of the thyroid cartilage, and the cricothyroid joint is dislocated (Fig 4). This procedure provides a wide view of the surgical field. The mucosa that covers the pyriform recess, which lies more caudally than the muscle process, is elevated upward, with special care being taken not to enter the laryngeal inner cavity. To maintain the surgical field aseptic, invasion into the pyriform recess should strictly be avoided (Fig 5).

The next step is to approach the muscle process. Three criteria are taken into consideration in the procedure to reach the muscle process as follows:

1. The muscle process is almost on the same level as that of the vocal cords. The anterior commissure is about the midway between the thyroid notch and the lower margin of the thyroid cartilage, or slightly (within 1 mm) higher than that point. The projection of the vocal cord runs from this point parallel to the horizontal line that can be drawn along the lower margin of the thyroid cartilage, neglecting the convex part of the inferior thyroid tubercle.

2. The muscle process can be identified as a minute prominence by finger palpation, when the thyroid ala is sufficiently rotated toward the intact side (Fig 6).

3. The simplest way to approach the muscle process is to search for the process by direct vision, starting from the cricothyroid joint and going obliquely upward on

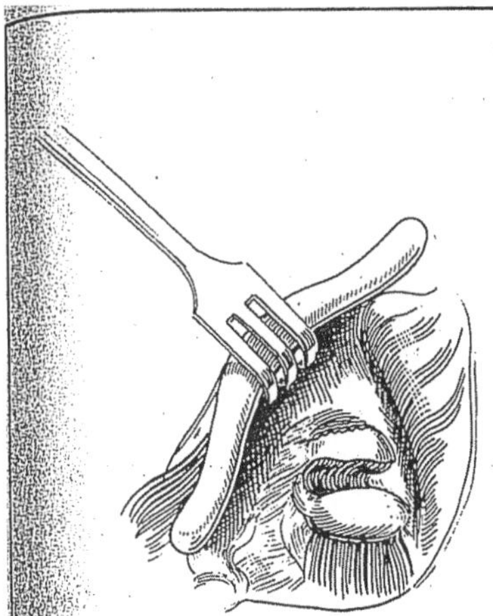

Fig 10.—Joint is open, with convex white joint surface appearing.

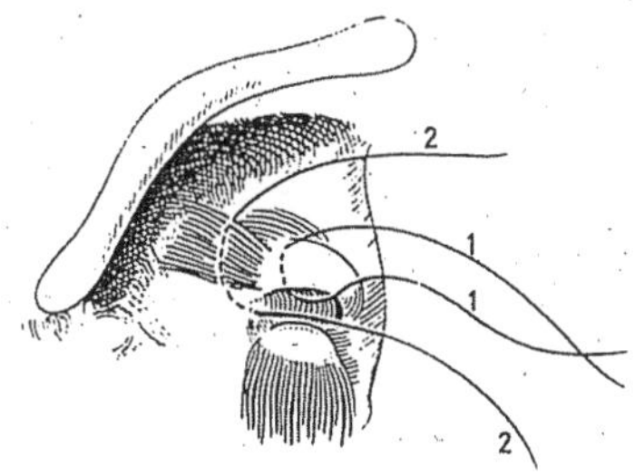

Fig 11.—Two nylon (3-0) sutures are used to grasp muscle process. One suture (2) mainly grasps soft tissue (lateral cricoarytenoid muscle).

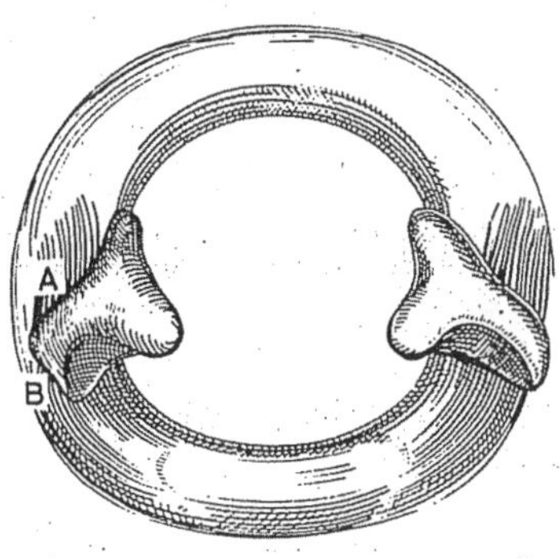

Fig 12.—Position of inserting sutures partly determines degree of adduction. Suture at point B will result in enhanced adduction of vocal cord.

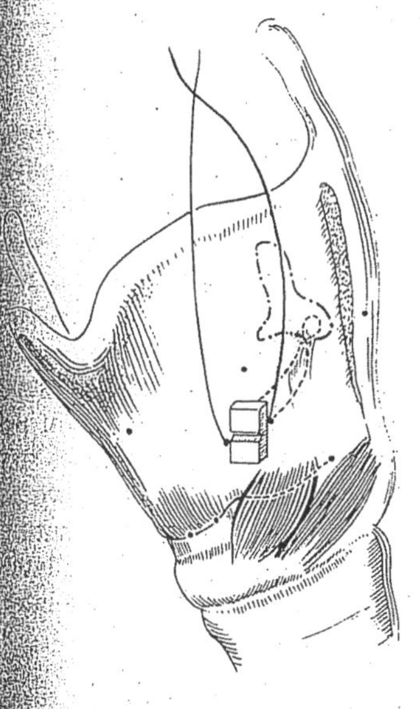

Fig 13.—Sutures inserted around muscle process are tied there to prevent slipping and pulled in anteromedial direction as illustrated. Suture should not be tied too tightly. Usually, bolster is not needed, although it is shown here.

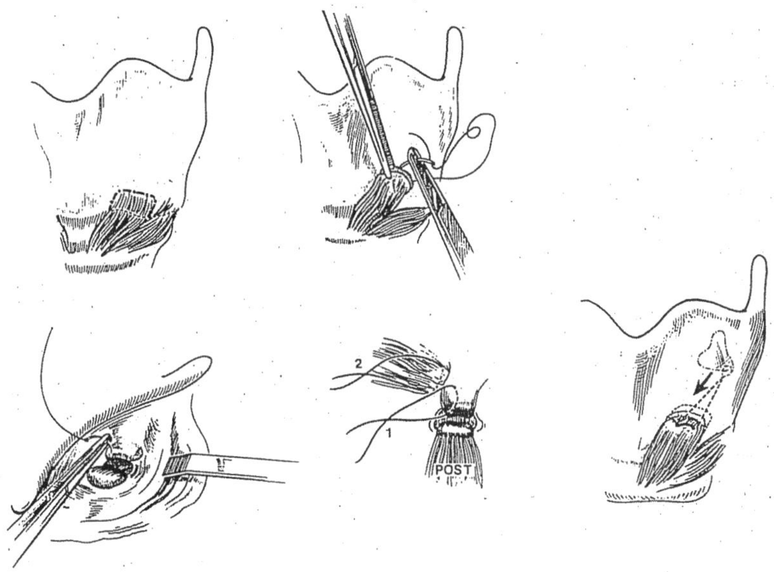

Fig 14.—Transposition of cricothyroid muscle (pars recta) to muscle process. POST indicates posterior cricoarytenoid muscle.

cricoid cartilage as shown in Fig 7 and

The cricoarytenoid joint is opened after small incision has been made on the posterior cricoarytenoid muscle (Fig 9). Then, the white and smooth surface of the cricoarytenoid joint appears as final identification of the joint (Fig 10). Two 3-0 nylon sutures are tied across the muscle process.

Since the arytenoid cartilage is rather fragile in aged patients, the sutures should hold not only the muscle process but also a sufficient amount of the soft tissues around the muscle process. The usual places of sutures insertion are shown in Fig 11 and 12.

When enhanced adduction of the vocal cord is needed, it is better to insert one suture rather posteriorly as indicated by B in Fig 12. Two sutures are tied to prevent

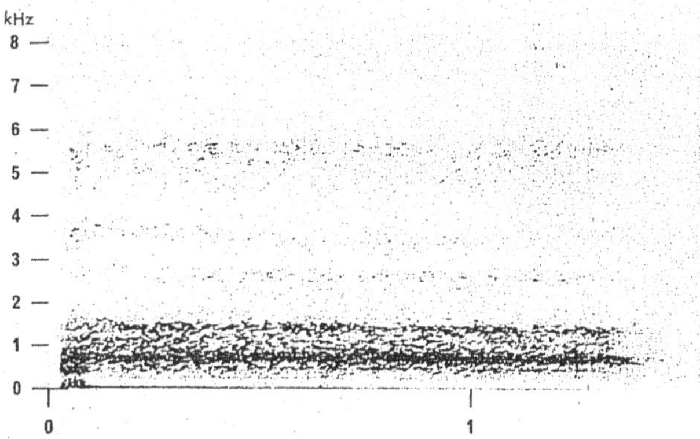

Fig 15.—Sound spectrogram (narrow-band filter) for voice *a* before surgery.

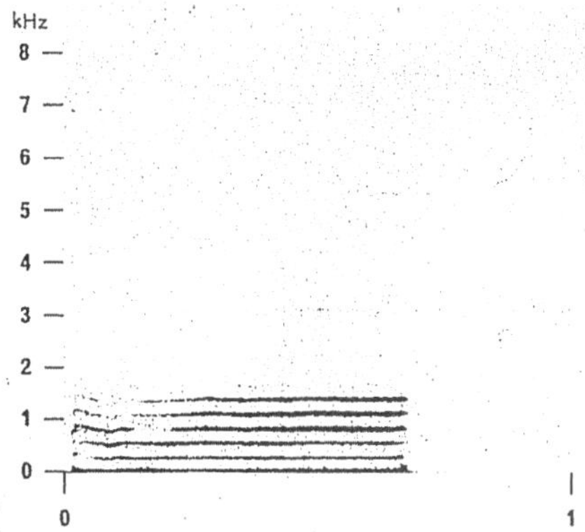

Fig 16.—Sound spectrogram for voice *a* after surgery.

slipping of the sutures around the muscle process. The sutures are then pulled out with the use of a large, sharp gently curved needle through the thyroid ala. In male patients with advanced calcification of the thyroid cartilage, holes should be made on the thyroid ala by a drill or engine burr before the above procedure. Then the patient is asked to phonate to adjust the degree of pull-force of the sutures. Too much adduction usually results in a strenuous, pressed, and rough voice that somehow resembles hyperfunctional or spastic dysphonia. Excessive force is unnecessary when tying the sutures on the thyroid ala. Since the tension of the suture is rather moderate, a bolster is not required except in the case of a fragile or thin thyroid cartilage (Fig 13). Actually, a bolster was used only in one out of the five cases. A drain is inserted for two or three days after the operation to reduce swelling of the arytenoid region.

RESULTS

Arytenoid adduction was performed on five patients with vocal cord paralysis. Two of them had undergone thyroplasty type I first, whose voices had improved remarkably but were still hoarse due to a posterior glottal chink that remained during phonation. The other three patients had had an extremely breathy and asthenic voice due to a wide, glottal chink, and they underwent arytenoid adduction as the first surgery. In one patient, surgical treatment of transposition of the cricothyroid muscle (pars recta) to the muscle process was also included as illustrated in Fig 14, but no vocal cord movement was obtained after surgery. Improvement of the voice after arytenoid adduction was dramatic to the extent that the voice can be considered normal in all of the five cases. The rather few cases of this surgery do not allow a conclusive statement, but it appears that arytenoid adduction is superior to thyroplasty type I, so far as vocal improvement in cases of a wide, glottal chink is concerned. Edema in the arytenoid region or pyriform recess was noted for about a week in all of the cases. The paralyzed vocal cord, now fixed at the midline, gave us the impression of being rather tense after surgery. There was almost no pain, spontaneous or on swallowing in these patients. Figures 15 and 16 exemplify the sound spectrogram of the voices before and after surgery.

COMMENT

Two surgical procedures have been previously reported, which aimed at shifting the arytenoid cartilage in unilateral vocal cord paralysis. In 1948, Morrison[6] described a surgical technique called "the reverse King operation," which displaces the arytenoid cartilage toward the midline under general anesthesia. The technique of fixation of the arytenoid cartilage at this position does not seem simple. In 1966, Montgomery[7] reported "cricoarytenoid arthrodesis," which is performed via a laryngofissure approach. Because of the stainless steel pin, which has to be used to fix the arytenoid and cricoid cartilages at the new position, this surgery does not seem to have gained popularity.

Although the chordal injection technique is useful for unilateral vocal cord paralysis with a narrow, glottal chink, it does not guarantee good results in cases of a wide, glottal chink and cannot correct a difference of the levels of the two cords if one exists.

The arytenoid adduction technique that we performed is rather simple, safe, and also capable of adjusting the degree of adduction to obtain the best voice under local anesthesia. As to the long-term effect of surgery, the rather short follow-up period, six to eight months, does not allow any definite conclusion at present. However, since the force to pull the muscle process of the arytenoid cartilage is rather slight (less than 50 g), the recoil of the arytenoid cartilage to the original position of paralysis is quite unlikely to occur. We think that the once-opened cricoarytenoid joint would show ankylosis several months after surgery. For this reason, the cricoarytenoid joint must be opened or had better be opened and scratched superficially. The optimal direction of pulling the muscle process remains to be studied further. At present, we pull the muscle process by two sutures, simulating the function of the lateral cricoarytenoid muscle and the lateral thyroarytenoid muscle.

References

1. Isshiki N, Morita H, Okamura H, et al: Thyroplasty as a new phonosurgical technique. *Acta Otolaryngol* 78:451-457, 1974.

2. Isshiki N, Okamura H, Ishikawa T: Thyroplasty type I (lateral compression for dysphonia due to vocal cord paralysis or atrophy). *Acta Otolaryngol* 80:465-473, 1975.

3. Isshiki N, Ishikawa T: Diagnostic value of tomography in unilateral vocal cords paralysis. *Laryngoscope* 86:1573-1578, 1976.

4. Sonesson B: Die funktionelle Anatomie des Cricoarytenoidgelenkes. *Z Anatomie Entwicklungsgeschichts* 121:292-303, 1959.

5. Von Leden H, Moore P: The mechanics of the cricoarytenoid joint. *Arch Otolaryngol* 73:541-550, 1961.

6. Morrison LF: The "reverse King operation." *Ann Otol Rhinol Laryngol* 57:945-956, 1948.

7. Montgomery WW: Cricoarytenoid arthrodesis. *Ann Otol Rhinol Laryngol* 75:380-391, 1966.

SILASTIC MEDIALIZATION AND ARYTENOID ADDUCTION: THE VANDERBILT EXPERIENCE

A REVIEW OF 116 PHONOSURGICAL PROCEDURES

JAMES L. NETTERVILLE, MD

R. E. STONE, PHD
ELIZABETH S. LUKEN, MS

FRANCISCO J. CIVANTOS, MD
ROBERT H. OSSOFF, DMD, MD

NASHVILLE, TENNESSEE

From April 1987 to April 1992, 116 phonosurgical procedures were performed to treat glottal incompetence. The initial numbers of these surgical procedures included the following: 29 primary Silastic medializations, 3 primary Silastic medializations with arytenoid adduction, 53 secondary Silastic medializations, 4 secondary Silastic medializations with arytenoid adduction, and 11 bilateral Silastic medializations. These procedures are useful in treating unilateral true vocal cord paralysis, scarring, bowing, or paresis, as well as bilateral true vocal cord bowing. Of the initial 100 patients, 16 later underwent a revision with either a larger implant's being placed or an arytenoid adduction. Primary Silastic medialization is the placement of an implant under general anesthesia in the same surgical setting in which laryngeal innervation is sacrificed. Secondary Silastic medialization is the placement of an implant under local anesthesia for a preexistent vocal cord malfunction. In either case, overall voice results for unilateral paralysis are very good. Primary Silastic medialization significantly decreases the postoperative rehabilitation period in skull base patients because of the immediate postoperative glottal competence and decreased use of perioperative tracheotomy. Bilateral implants yielded good results in 6 patients with presbylaryngis, but 6 other patients with bowing from other causes experienced only moderate improvement in speech quality. There were no implant extrusions; however, 1 implant was removed secondary to a persistent laryngocutaneous fistula in a patient who had previously undergone laryngeal irradiation. This was the only complication in this series.

KEY WORDS — arytenoid adduction, glottis, medialization, phonosurgery, Silastic, thyroplasty, vocal cord.

INTRODUCTION

Silastic medialization (SM; thyroplasty type I) and arytenoid adduction (AA) have provided significant improvement to the care of patients with glottal insufficiency due to paralysis, paresis, scarring, or bowing of the true vocal cords (TVCs). Two review articles on this subject by Koufman[1] and Koufman and Isaacson[2] provide an excellent historical background. Although several series had been previously reported, medialization did not receive significant attention as a treatment for vocal cord paralysis until Isshiki et al[3,4] advanced the technique using Silastic as the implant. Isshiki deserves credit as the author of the surgical procedure most used today. Koufman[5] helped to popularize the procedure within the United States, as well as adding further refinements to the surgical techniques. Series by Maves et al[6] and Tucker[7] supported the high-quality results provided by the procedure, yet pointed out its limitations and potential complications. The purpose of this paper is to review the results of our series derived over the last 5 years and discuss further refinements in surgical technique and instrumentation. By drawing on otologic surgical techniques, we developed a less traumatic and more accurate procedure for implant placement. The patients will be divided into different procedure categories for more accurate comparison and assessment.

PATIENT EVALUATION AND SURGICAL TECHNIQUE

From April 1987 to April 1992, 116 procedures for glottal incompetence were performed at our institution. These procedures included primary SM (performed under general anesthesia at the time of neural sacrifice), secondary SM (performed under local anesthesia), bilateral SM, and AA. Recently, ansa–recurrent laryngeal nerve (RLN) transfer has been combined with SM when indicated. The surgical techniques we use for both SM and AA are modifications of the original descriptions of Isshiki et al.[3,4,8] Although we have outlined our surgical techniques before, we would like to amplify these to demonstrate the significant changes that have evolved over the last 3 years.[9]

Patients presenting with preoperative voice deficiency received an extensive evaluation, which included a complete head, neck, and chest examination. Patients who present with idiopathic paralysis undergo a magnetic resonance imaging scan to evaluate the entire course of the ipsilateral vagus nerve. If an abnormality is suspected at the level of the skull base,

From the Department of Otolaryngology, Vanderbilt Medical Center, Nashville, Tennessee.

Presented at the meeting of the American Laryngological Association, Palm Desert, California, April 11-12, 1992.

REPRINTS — James L. Netterville, MD, Dept of Otolaryngology, Vanderbilt University Medical Center, S-2100 Medical Center North, Nashville, TN 37232-2559.

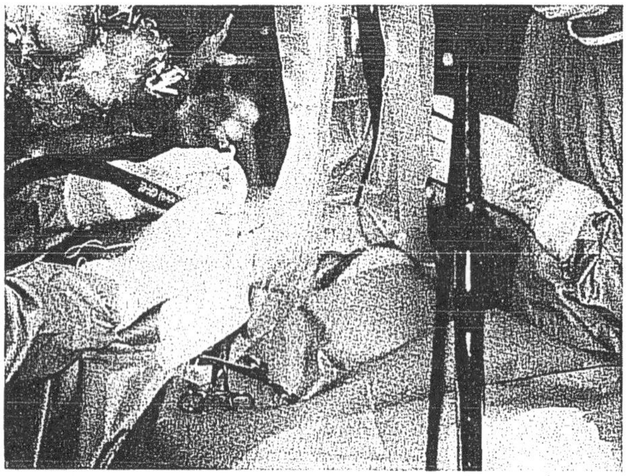

Fig 1. Flexible nasopharyngoscope is attached to intravenous pole for support and sterilely draped so surgeon can manipulate it during procedure to maintain best view of true vocal cords.

a computed tomography scan is used for higher resolution of the bone–soft tissue interface. Laryngeal function tests, videostroboscopic evaluation, and voice analysis are also performed. The composition of this evaluation has matured as our series has progressed. Many of the early patients did not undergo laryngeal function tests or voice analysis. Although the human ear remains the most accurate judge of improvement in voice quality, it is quite difficult to objectively quantify this improvement for presentation. Therefore, over the last 2 years we have tried to identify which objective tests in the laryngeal function and voice analysis battery best correlate with improvement in voice quality.

The preoperative videostroboscopy demonstrates the position of the paralyzed TVC. If during phonation the mobile vocal process comes into contact with the paralyzed vocal process, then usually SM alone results in marked improvement. If there is a wide posterior glottic gap with the vocal processes widely spaced, then the patient is prepared for SM with the possible addition of AA.

Silastic medialization (either unilateral or bilateral), ansa-RLN transfer, and AA are all performed with local anesthesia, supplemented by intravenous sedation. Patients are monitored by the anesthesiology service throughout the procedure. It is not necessary for the success of the procedure to use transnasal flexible videolaryngoscopy. The size of the laryngeal implant, or the degree of adduction, is mainly dependent on the quality change in the voice obtained during the procedure. We, however, continue to use intraoperative laryngeal video monitoring on all local procedures (Fig 1). It provides excellent feedback to demonstrate the position of the TVC in relation to the window created in the thyroid cartilage, and helps to prevent overmedialization of the false vocal cord (FVC) or the ventricle. It is particularly helpful during AA to prevent overadduction of the vocal process. The same feedback can be obtained by intermittent observation of the larynx with the nasopharyngoscope by either the surgeon or an assistant. If video monitoring is used, the patient should receive atropine and topical nasal anesthesia preoperatively to decrease excess pharyngeal secretions that would block the view of the nasopharyngoscope.

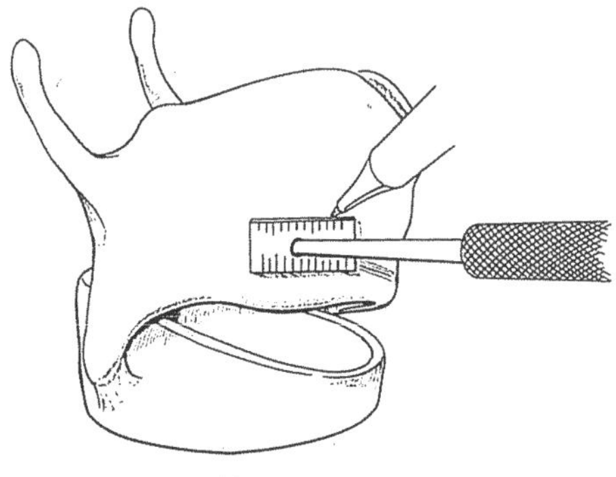

Fig 2. Window is positioned parallel to lower border of thyroid cartilage. Window template is helpful in laying out this window; it is placed 5 to 8 mm back from prow of larynx and 3 mm up from inferior border.

The larynx is exposed through a small incision overlying the midportion of the thyroid cartilage, and the perichondrium is elevated from the involved side. The window template, which is 6 x 13 mm, is positioned over the cartilage to mark the window location (Fig 2). The window is placed parallel to the lower border of the thyroid cartilage. The plane forming the lower border of the thyroid cartilage is formed between the anterior lower edge and the portion behind the muscular process. The inferior extension of the muscular process at the anterior third of the lower border of the thyroid cartilage is quite variable.

If the plane between the anterior point of the thyroid cartilage and the maximum inferior extension of the muscular process is used as the parallel line for the lower border, the window may be tilted too far inferiorly at its posterior point. The window should be placed as close to the lower border of the laryngeal cartilage as possible, while leaving a strong inferior cartilage strut to resist fracture while placing the implant. The distance from the anterior commissure back to the anterior edge of the window is determined by the shape of the cartilage. In the more obtuse-angled cartilage, as seen more often in women, the window is placed closer to the prow of the larynx (Fig 3A). When the laryngeal angle is more acute, as seen most often in men, the window is moved more posterior to prevent overmedialization of the anterior third of the cord. When calcified, the cartilage is removed from the outlined window under magnification, by means of an otologic drill with a 2- to 3-mm cutting bur (Fig 4A). The internal perichondrium is left intact at this point. In the younger patient, with little or no calcification of the cartilage, a sharp elevator can be used to remove this cartilage island.

By removing all of the cartilage from the window,

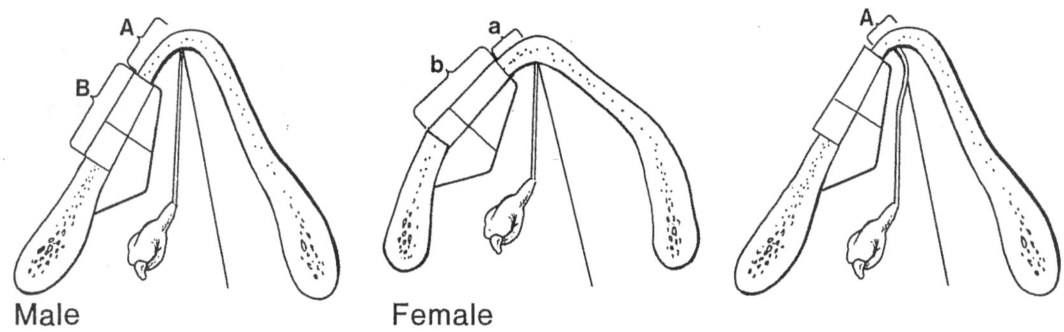

Fig 3. A) Although either laryngeal shape can be seen in either sex, women usually have more obtuse anterior angle, and men more acute anterior angle, of thyroid cartilage. Average window setback from anterior commissure is 7 mm in men (A) and 5 mm in women (a). This will prevent overmedialization of anterior commissure. Length of window (B,b) is same, 13 mm, in both men and women. B) Overmedialization of anterior commissure results in strained voice, even if posterior commissure is wide open. This can occur when window is placed too close to anterior commissure (A), or when too-large implant is placed.

greater accuracy in medialization can be achieved. The cartilage island, if left in place during medialization, can shift when the inverted Silastic T is positioned. If the island shifts superiorly, as we have seen in 1 patient referred to us for revision, then the FVC is medialized, resulting in poor vocal quality. If the island is pushed straight in, often the medialization is still too high, and ventricular mucosal prolapse occurs. If the cartilage island shifts inferiorly when the implant is placed, then good voice quality can occur; however, care must be taken to prevent overmedialization of the anterior TVC, which results in a strained vocal quality. Histologic evidence of this is seen in a recent case report by Isaacson et al.[10] One month after SM was performed, with an inverted Silastic T used to medialize the cartilage island, the patient died. Whole organ sectioning of the larynx demonstrated the overcompensation of the anterior half of the vocal cord by the cartilage island.[10] Because of this we prefer to remove the entire cartilage island. This allows the shaped implant to control more accurately the degree of medialization.

The short laryngeal elevator is used to begin elevation of the perichondrium from the inner surface of the thyroid cartilage. The inner edge of the cartilage window is smoothed with a small bur or an otologic curette. In several previous discussions of this procedure, the integrity of the inner perichondrium has been stressed, implying that injury to it would increase the likelihood of graft extrusion.[1,4,7] However, the operative techniques recommended in those same reports for creating the cartilage island included the use of the oscillating saw or a sharp surgical knife. We were fearful that these methods would not only injure the inner perichondrium, but would also cut through the thyroarytenoid fascia and the underlying distal branches of the superior laryngeal vessels.

There is a likelihood of opening into the laryngeal ventricle with these techniques, as well. To firmly establish this principle, we performed the first 40 procedures with an operating microscope, carefully removing the cartilage and leaving the inner perichondrium intact. The inner perichondrium was then widely elevated, and medialization was attempted. Rarely could adequate medialization be accomplished. Because of this finding, we microscopically incise the perichondrium with a small knife at the superior, posterior, and inferior margins of the window, making it a flap. The thyroarytenoid fascia and its underlying vessels are maintained intact. The long laryngeal elevator is then used to separate the thyroarytenoid muscle fascia from the inner perichondrium (Fig 4B). The distal superior laryngeal vessel branches can be seen lying under this fascia. At this point very accurate medialization can be accomplished. We feel the main reason for delayed graft extrusion into the larynx is injury to the laryngeal ventricle with implant contamination. For this reason we feel it is risky to use a paramedian incision adjacent to the anterior commissure for implant placement rather than using a window. The ventricle, which is adjacent to the inner perichondrium at the anterior commissure, can easily be injured with any paramedian cartilage incision. Several papers that have outlined this approach in the past have reported implant extrusions secondary to implant contamination.[1,11]

Even with the perichondrium sectioned, a capsule is formed around the implant, further preventing its extrusion (Fig 5). Using this technique we have had no extrusion of implants thus far. After the thyroarytenoid muscle elevation has been completed, the depth gauge (Fig 6) is employed. While viewing the larynx on the monitor, one can use the small end of the gauge to discretely medialize the tissue in the anterior, middle, and posterior aspects of the window. This is performed at the superior and inferior edges of the window in each of these positions, the resultant information showing the relationship of the window to the TVCs and FVCs. Usually, medialization at the superior aspect of the window results in movement of

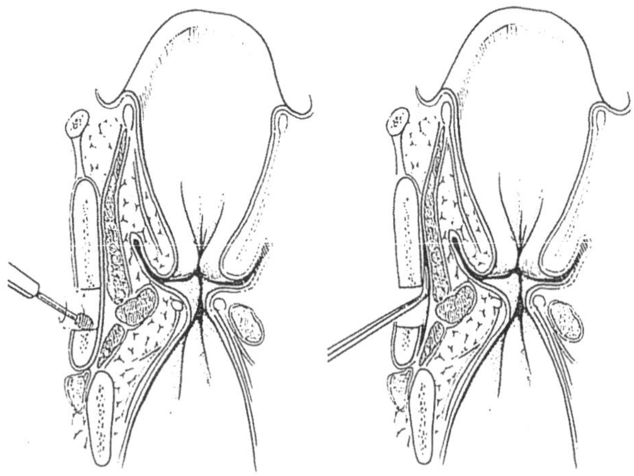

A B

Fig 4. A) Under magnification, 2- to 3-mm cutting bur is used to remove cartilage from window. This can be done without injury to inner perichondrium. B) After perichondrium has been carefully incised along superior, posterior, and inferior margins of window, long laryngeal elevator is used to separate thyroarytenoid fascia away from inner perichondrium.

the FVC and ventricular mucosa. For this reason, the implant is carved so that the plane of maximum medialization is at the lower edge of the window. The larger, sloped end of the depth gauge is then used to medialize the cord while the patient is phonating. The gauge can be moved or angled in any position to define the depths of the anterior and posterior aspects of the implant needed to acquire the best voice. These measurements are read off the gauge from the inner aspect of the thyroid cartilage. If the inner edge cannot be seen well, then the distance to the outer edge is recorded. The smaller end of the gauge can then be used to measure the anterior and posterior widths of the cartilage, which are subtracted from the measurements just acquired. Care must be taken to prevent overmedialization of the anterior third of the TVC, which results in a strained, spastic voice (Fig 3B).

After the implant dimensions have been acquired, the final implant is carved. We hope that a precarved implant will soon be released that requires only minor modifications for each patient's needs. Until then we continue to carve implants from Silastic block (Fig 7). Several implants are partially carved ahead of time to prevent lengthy carving during surgery.

Because of the shorter female vocal cord, the distance from the anterior aspect of the window to the maximum point of medialization is less in women. This, combined with the more obtuse shape of the female thyroid cartilage, results in an implant that is more equilateral in its two laryngeal surfaces. From the anterior edge of the implant to the maximum point of medialization is approximately 10 mm in women and 13 to 14 mm in men. If no return of vocal cord function is possible, then a 5- to 6-mm tail extends

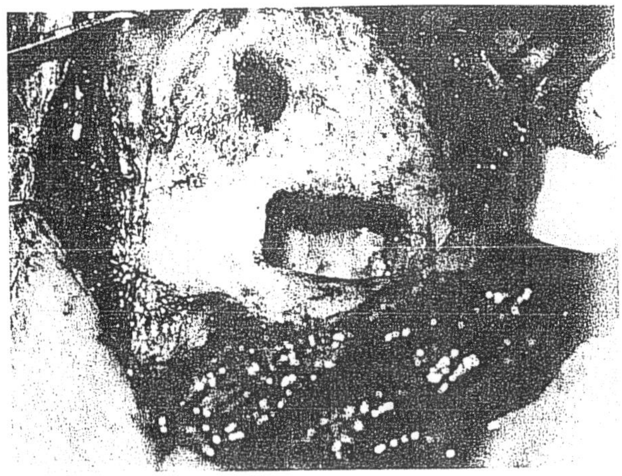

Fig 5. This view through thyroid cartilage window during revision operation in which larger implant was placed demonstrates fibrous capsule that develops around implant after placement.

medially to the thyroid cartilage and posteriorly to the window. This extension of the implant is tapered to prevent contact with the muscular process of the arytenoid. Contact on the anterior surface of that process would prevent adduction of the process, working contrary to its proposed mechanism. If there is still a possibility of functional return of the vocal cord or the implant is being placed deep to a mobile cord because of paresis, scarring, or bowing, then the posterior extension may be decreased to ensure no interference with arytenoid movement.

To standardize our records we use the formula a x b x c...d to document the size in millimeters of the implants placed; "a" stands for anterior medialization, "b" for posterior maximal medialization, "c" for the overall length, and "d" for the length from the front of the implant back to the point of maximal medialization. A typical implant placed in a male larynx would be 2 x 6 x 18...13 mm. The implant is often divided into two pieces to allow a more gentle insertion (Fig 8A).

After the lower edge is placed into the window, the implant is rotated into position (Fig 8B). The posterior portion is placed first and moved back partially posterior to the window, after which the anterior half then locks the posterior segment in place. If the quality of the voice is not as good as expected, then the implant can be removed with two small skin hooks and adjusted appropriately. The time from intralaryngeal elevation to final placement of the implant needs to be as short as possible to allow for voice evaluation without the interference of edema. The final shape of the implant usually provides the maximum plane of medialization at the lower border of the window to prevent medialization of the FVC or the ventricular mucosa (Fig 9).

If it is obvious at this point that the posterior glottis cannot be closed, then an AA is performed. We perform this in a very similar manner to the original

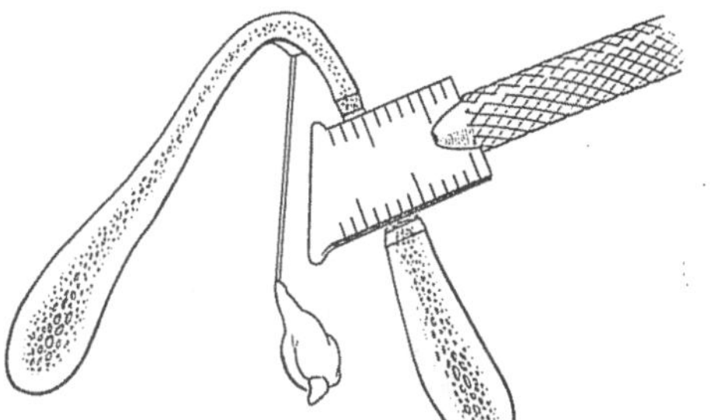

Fig 6. Depth gauge is very helpful in simulating medialization needed at both anterior and posterior aspects of vocal cord. It is thin enough to move up and down within window to identify level that will move true cord into position without medialization of false cord. Millimeter markings on gauge dictate anterior and posterior dimensions of implant.

description of Isshiki et al.[8] The posterior border of the thyroid cartilage can be approached by either dissecting lateral to the strap muscles and cutting through the inferior constrictor to expose the cartilage, or continuing the elevation of the outer perichondrium until the entire ala of the thyroid cartilage can be seen.

After the lateral edge of the thyroid cartilage is isolated, either the cricothyroid joint is opened for better access, or a portion of the posterior rim of the thyroid cartilage is removed to expose the muscular process of the arytenoid. The pyriform mucosa is carefully elevated until the posterior aspect of the arytenoid can be palpated. The posterior cricoarytenoid muscle can be removed from the muscular process of the arytenoid as needed for mobility of the cartilage. We rarely open the cricoarytenoid joint capsule as described by Isshiki et al.[8] This can lead to prolapse of the arytenoid cartilage into the laryngeal lumen with overadduction of the posterior commissure. A 3-0 Prolene suture is passed twice through the muscular process and the surrounding tissue and brought forward to reproduce the pull of the thyroarytenoid muscle on the muscular process. Arytenoid adduction is most often performed in conjunction with, or delayed after, SM; thus, the suture is passed through the paraglottic space and the Silastic implant. Only a gentle pull is necessary to adduct the vocal process. We move the arytenoid back and forth until the correct position is identified. The suture is tied over either the anterior portion of the implant or the lower border of the thyroid cartilage, about 5 to 8 mm back from the prow of the larynx.

If indicated after completion of SM, reinnervation as described by Crumley[12] is performed to suture a branch of the ansa-hypoglossal-cervicalis system to the cut end of the RLN. This, along with SM and AA, can easily be performed under local monitored anesthesia with intravenous sedation. The goal of this procedure is not the return of normal function, which is highly unlikely, but to maintain muscle bulk and provide static muscle tone within the laryngeal muscles. Many injuries to the RLN or the vagus nerve that produce TVC paralysis are the result of stretch or crush injuries with a high likelihood of delayed reinnervation. Often this regrowth does not result in physiologic motion of the cord, but activity on electromyography (EMG) confirms the reinnervation. This regrowth will maintain the muscle bulk and provide tone, making nerve transfer unnecessary. If division of the RLN or vagus nerve is known to have occurred within 2 years of the potential date of repair, then reinnervation is indicated if no spontaneous regrowth has occurred.

This determination is confirmed with either preoperative or intraoperative EMG. If normal EMG activity is absent and no reinnervation potentials are seen, then nerve transfer is performed along with SM. If neural injury has occurred more than 2 years from the surgery date, reinnervation is unlikely to add any benefit secondary to chronic denervation muscle atrophy. The decision-making process becomes more confusing if one schedules the patient for SM within the first year, as we often do. Spontaneous nerve regeneration through an intact but injured nerve may not have had time to manifest itself on EMG. Tucker[7] uses a nerve-muscle pedicle placed through the cartilage window to reinnervate the thyroarytenoid only. This has the potential advantage of leaving the RLN intact for the possibility of regrowth, while providing an alternate neural supply to the thyroarytenoid muscle. These concepts on nerve transfer are only a rough guide. Hopefully, as we obtain longer follow-up on our patients with intraoperative EMG, we can suggest more concrete guidelines.

RESULTS

From April 1987 until April 1992, 116 procedures were performed on 100 patients. There were 123 Silastic implants placed, and 14 AAs performed. Several of these were performed at the same surgical setting and were considered as one procedure. The procedures used are outlined in Table 1.

Primary Silastic Medialization. Thirty-two patients underwent primary SM at the end of the surgical procedure in which the laryngeal innervation was sacrificed. There were 18 men and 14 women ranging in age from 22 to 75 years. Primary AA was performed as well in 3 of the patients. The cause of vagal sacrifice was either a skull base or high vagal nerve tumor in 26 patients, while 5 patients underwent cervical excision of both the carotid artery and vagus nerve secondary to involvement by squamous cell carcinoma (SCC). One further patient, with unilateral paralysis, presented with an extensive anterior cervical osteophyte impinging on the RLN at the cricothyroid junction. Primary SM was performed after the osteophytes were removed. Of this group, 5 patients have undergone surgical revision, 3 with larger implants placed, 1 with both a larger implant

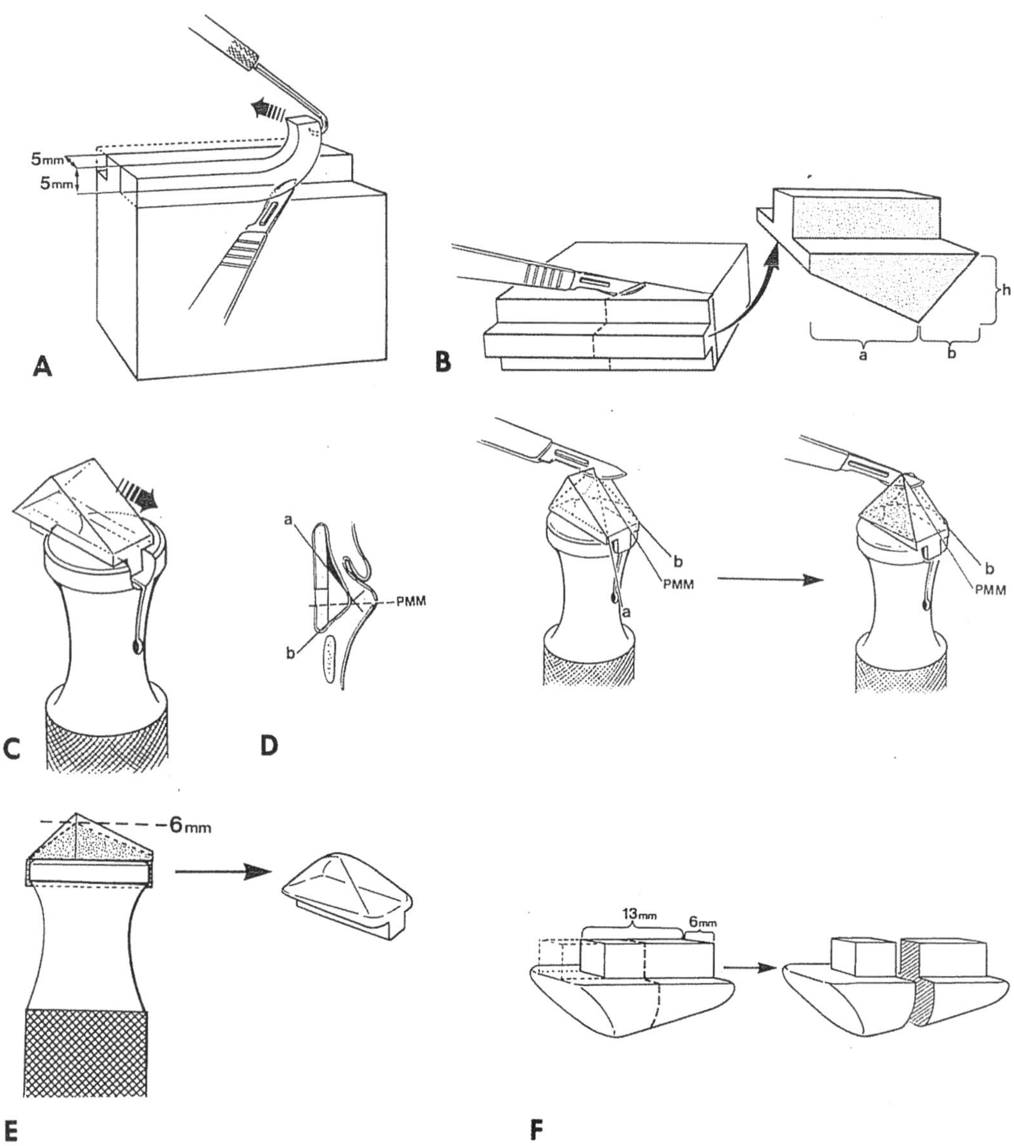

Fig 7. A) Medium-softness Silastic block is prepared by removing two lateral strips, leaving central 5 x 5-mm ridge. B) Rough implant is outlined and cut from block. Distance from front of implant back to point of maximum medialization (a) is determined during voice testing with depth gauge. Residual distance to posterior aspect of implant (b) is 5 mm. Height of rough implant (h) is usually outlined 1 to 2 mm greater than final implant height. C) Rough implant slides into implant holder for final shaping. D) Plane of maximum medialization (PMM) is outlined on implant at level determined by depth gauge during voice testing. This plane is usually at lower level of cartilage window. Excess Silastic is removed from implant by carving from PMM along cuts a and b. E) Final height or medialization point (6 mm in this example) is outlined, and excess Silastic is further removed. All sharp edges are rounded to decrease trauma to paraglottic space during placement of implant. F) After removal from holder, lateral strut is outlined to fit window and excess is removed. Final implant is divided into two pieces to further decrease trauma of insertion.

and AA, and 1 with AA only. One of the first 3 patients with revisions has subsequently undergone a second revision with AA. There have been no graft extrusions in this group.

In the 6 patients who received primary SM secondary to neck surgery, 4 underwent a tracheotomy at the same time to prevent airway compromise after composite resection for SCC. The fifth patient, who underwent radical neck dissection only, and the sixth patient, who underwent resection of the cervical osteophytes, did well with no tracheotomy. Even with early glottal competence provided by the primary SM, 4 of the 5 patients presenting with SCC have performed poorly with swallowing rehabilitation. This is probably due to the surgical alteration of the laryngopharyngeal tissue, as well as the significant sustained edema that accompanies the combination of these ablative procedures and radiotherapy.

Of the 26 patients who received a primary SM secondary to skull base surgery, the first 5 also underwent a tracheotomy. This was standard procedure prior to primary SM to protect the airway from aspiration and provide pulmonary toilet. After we gained confidence in primary SM, the following 21

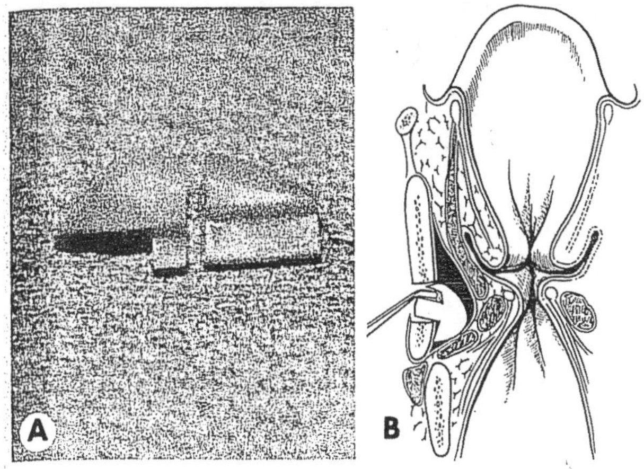

Fig 8. Carved Silastic implant. A) Ready to insert into larynx. It has been divided in half for ease of insertion. B) Lower edge of implant is rolled into window, and upper edge is slowly compressed until it snaps under thyroid cartilage. Posterior half is placed first and moved back into position; anterior piece locks it in place.

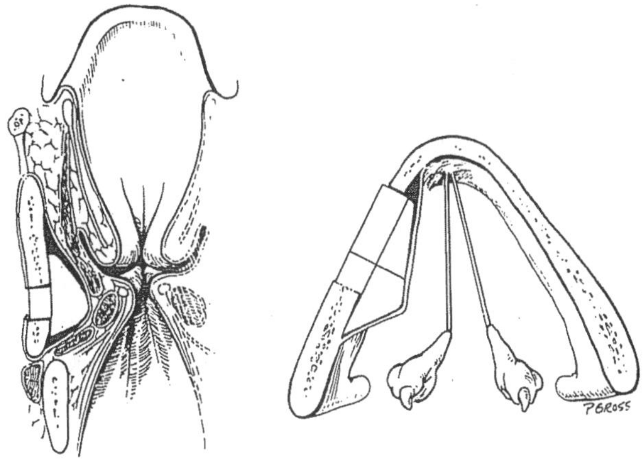

A B

Fig 9. A) Final position of implant demonstrates maximum plane of medialization at lower margin of window to prevent medialization of false cord and ventricle. B) Posterior extension of implant, which can be adjusted, will medialize vocal process of arytenoid in most cases.

patients underwent medialization only at the time of skull base surgery.

Two of these 21 patients subsequently underwent a tracheotomy. The first, a 75-year-old man, lost cranial nerves IX, X, XI, and XII secondary to a complete temporal bone resection for SCC. Cranial nerves IX and X were positive for carcinoma at the brain stem. The patient never regained his preoperative level of mental status. Postoperatively he was lethargic but arousable and underwent a tracheotomy 2 weeks later after severe aspiration pneumonia further compromised his health. He died of his disease 8 months later.

The second, a 56-year-old woman who underwent primary SM along with excision of an extensive vagal paraganglioma, developed increasing stridor postoperatively. On laryngoscopic examination we could see that the implanted cord was nicely positioned in the midline; however, the contralateral TVC was paralyzed as well, necessitating a tracheotomy to relieve airway obstruction. Her clinical course was further complicated by subacute bacterial endocarditis. Two months later, after normal function of the contralateral TVC returned, she was decannulated and oral nutrition was resumed.

The other 19 patients have progressed through their postoperative period without the need for tracheotomy. Initial oral intake and adequate oral intake occurred earlier in these patients who did not undergo a tracheotomy, as compared to patients who underwent tracheotomy alone or tracheotomy along with primary SM. We recently reviewed this group of patients to assess the improvements in postoperative rehabilitation by the use of primary SM.[13] To prevent redundancy, the reader is referred to that work for an in-depth discussion of the results. The voice results in this group are difficult to report objectively. When trained speech evaluators were asked to judge the quality of the voice of these primary SM patients, the quality and projection of the voice was frequently underappreciated because of the hypernasality and articulation deficits resulting from high resection of cranial nerves IX, X, and XII. For this group a simple rating scale included four divisions. Patients with follow-up tapes were evaluated. Fourteen of the 21 patients who returned to Nashville for follow-up were judged to have normal or near-normal voice. Five patients developed either moderate breathiness with good projection or significant raspiness. Two patients had a significant air leak and could not communicate in a loud environment. No patients developed a whisper voice. The voice quality continues to improve for up to 1 year after the procedure. There were no delayed complications in this group.

Secondary Silastic Medialization. Fifty-seven patients underwent secondary SM under local anesthesia. Four of these patients underwent AA as well. This group consisted of 36 men and 20 women who ranged in age from 24 to 85 years. Of this group 8 patients have undergone revision surgery, 4 with larger unilateral implants, 2 with larger implants plus AA, and 2 with AA alone. The causes of the unilateral paralysis or paresis are outlined in Table 2. No stridor developed in any of the patients, either acutely or in the postoperative period. All except 2 presented with unilateral paralysis. One of these 2 was a 31-year-old man who presented with a 2-year history of poor communication with a breathy voice. He was struggling to keep his job as foreman of the night shift at a local factory. The voice alteration occurred after a severe bout of laryngitis. Examination demonstrated bilateral motion with significant notching of the anterior half of the right TVC. After unilateral SM his voice returned to near normal, with excellent projection. The second patient presented with significant

TABLE 1. PHONOSURGICAL PROCEDURES USED FOR GLOTTAL INCOMPETENCE

Procedure	*No.*
Primary unilateral implant	29
Primary unilateral implant with arytenoid adduction	3
Secondary unilateral implant	62
Secondary unilateral implant with arytenoid adduction	7
Arytenoid adduction	4
Bilateral implants	11
Total	116

unilateral paresis; a unilateral implant failed to improve his condition. The arytenoid on the weaker side, although mobile, failed to come to midline. During attempted revision it was obvious that if a large enough implant were placed to medialize the arytenoid, its function would be impaired. This may have been indicated for voice improvement, but not fully understanding the cause of his paresis, we were hesitant to harm unilateral function for fear that the opposite TVC might be affected in a similar manner in the future. The only complication in the series occurred in a man who presented with a lateralized fixed hemilarynx. Fifteen years prior he had undergone radiotherapy to his right TVC for SCC. This resulted in a breathy voice with mild aspiration. During the surgical procedure, after the cartilage window had been removed, the paraglottic space was found to be fibrotic with scar tissue. The ventricle was inadvertently entered during the elevation of this fixed tissue. The operation was completed with perioperative antibiotic coverage. The patient was initially pleased with the voice improvement, but a draining sinus to the skin developed several weeks later. After a lengthy trial of antibiotics failed to bring improvement, the patient refused to allow removal of the implant. Although his voice was very raspy, he was pleased with the improvement in swallowing resulting from the implant. Finally, 6 months postoperatively the implant was removed. He went on to develop chondritis of the thyroid cartilage, which resolved after debridement.

To gain a more objective approach to the analysis of the postoperative voice quality, several different parameters were considered. Although maximum phonation time and mean airflow have a great deal of variation, these may be the best tests to demonstrate improved glottal competence. Our early data were sketchy in this area, and we continued to try to apply these tests in a meaningful way to determine the degree of voice improvement. A subjective review of the available voice tapes using a simple evaluation of postoperative voice yielded 23 patients with normal or near-normal voice, 11 patients with slight breathiness or significant raspiness, 2 patients with weak voice, and no patients with a whisper voice.

In an attempt to better quantify these findings, one of the senior authors (R.E.S.) set up a computer model in which matched pairs of preoperative and postoperative voice samples were recorded on a computer disk. The preoperative and postoperative voice samples of each patient were randomly presented so that the listener was blinded as to whether samples were preoperative or postoperative. The samples were then played in pairs to each of 5 voice listeners. The listeners assigned a value (1 to 50) to the "desirability" of voice quality. Eighteen patients with good-quality preoperative and postoperative tapes were selected from this group. Sixteen of these patients were judged to have a better postoperative voice, while 2 were judged to have a better preoperative voice. The summary of the scores of the 5 judges are shown in Fig 10. A score of 40 or above was judged to show a near-normal or normal voice. This graph demonstrates a significant sustained improvement in a majority of the patients. The correlation between the scores of the 5 judges was very close on most patients, lending a greater validity to the accuracy of the voice score.

TABLE 2. CAUSE OF VOCAL CORD PARALYSIS OR PARESIS IN PATIENTS UNDERGOING SECONDARY SILASTIC MEDIALIZATION WITH OR WITHOUT ARYTENOID ADDUCTION

Cause	*No.*
Unilateral paresis	
Laryngitis	1
Idiopathic	1
Unilateral paralysis	
Skull base surgery	10
Chest surgery	10
Chest neoplasm	8
Trauma	4
Recurrent laryngeal nerve avulsion for spastic dysphonia	4
Thyroid surgery	4
Other neck surgery	3
Neck cancer	2
Laryngeal surgery	2
Idiopathic	6
Unknown	2

Bilateral Silastic Medialization. Eleven patients underwent bilateral SM for glottal incompetence. This incompetence was most often manifested in the patient by a weak, breathy voice along with mild aspiration. The disorders that resulted in this condition are listed in Table 3. There have been no complications in this group. One of the earlier patients developed mild stridor on the first postoperative morning due to bilateral vocal cord edema with slight unilateral intracordal bleeding. After treatment with intravenous steroids and observation, he was asymptomatic within 48 hours. Only 1 of the 11 patients has undergone a revision, with a larger implant placed on 1 side only.

The 6 patients who underwent surgery for presbylaryngis were all improved, with increased volume and projection, as well as improvement in deglutition

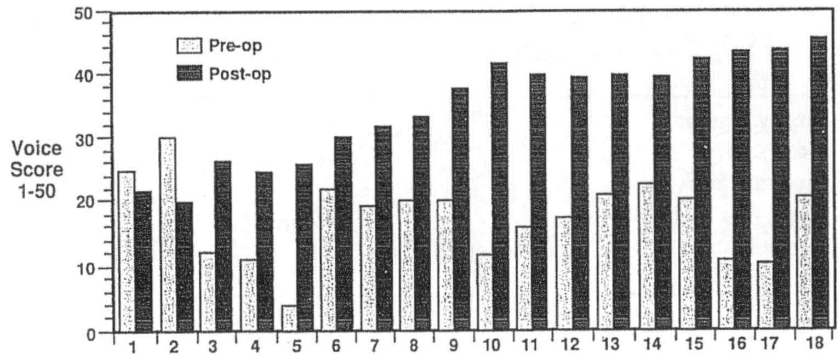

Fig 10. Summary voice scores for preoperative and postoperative voice in 18 patients who underwent unilateral secondary Silastic medialization demonstrate voice improvement in 16 of 18 patients. Voices were rated from 1 to 50 on basis of quality of communication and voice desirability. Scores above 40 were given for normal or near-normal voice.

with decreased aspiration. There were 5 men and 1 woman in this group, with an average of 71 years. The remaining 5 patients, 3 women and 2 men with a mean age of 35 years, were the least improved group in this series.

The configuration in all of these larynges demonstrated bowing of the vocal cords, greater in the posterior third than the anterior aspect of the glottal opening. Moderate improvement with decrease in breathiness was seen in 2 patients, who presented, respectively, with a history of strangulation and severe upper respiratory tract infection.

Minimal differences were seen in the postoperative voice in the remaining 3. The first, who had suffered a cerebrovascular accident secondary to fat embolism, presented with a weak whisper voice and poor articulation. Her examination showed a 2- to 3-mm open posterior glottic chink. Bilateral implants 2 x 5 x 13...10 failed to close the gap, and minimal change in voice was noted. She has, however, continued to gain further volume over the first postoperative year.

The second patient, a 40-year-old man, presented with the same laryngeal configuration, along with slight breathiness in the voice that prevented him from singing. A test with bilateral Gelfoam injections resulted in an excellent, strong voice. Conservative implants were placed bilaterally, but little improvement was seen. He was sent to another center for collagen injections, which also failed to improve the voice.

The final patient presented with a 2- to 3-mm gap between the cords and a spastic, strained quality to the voice. He had received a diagnosis of spastic dysphonia; however, on examination his vocal cords did not touch. We felt that the spastic quality might be a compensation for his glottal incompetence, and he underwent bilateral implants of 2 x 5 x 13...13. He continued to have mild spasticity, but his voice quality improved. In retrospect, larger implants might have been more helpful in these 5 patients. We were very conservative at first, for fear the implant would impair the normal arytenoid movement.

Voice analysis was performed by the panel of listeners judging the random blinded voice pairs, as described, for 8 patients in this category. This is outlined in Fig 11. One of the patients, who had suffered strangulation, was felt to have a worse voice postoperatively. Although the patient felt her communication and especially swallowing function were greatly improved, the quality of her voice was quite variable over time.

DISCUSSION

Many have been the detractors of SM, citing the ease of injection and long-term record of Teflon and implying that SM offers no advantage over the use of Teflon. As we have begun to take a closer look at Teflon, the problems are more evident. Because most otolaryngologists lack adequate experience with this procedure, they doubt that good results can predictably be obtained with Teflon injection. It is difficult to predict the migration of the Teflon during the injection within the TVC. We are beginning to see, with increasing frequency, granuloma formation within the injected TVC, which is devastating to voice quality and eventually causes airway compromise.

We feel that SM has several significant advantages over Teflon. First, good-quality voice results are highly reproducible. Compared to Teflon, the quality of improvement is more predictable, depending on the preoperative condition. Second, it is much easier to train other physicians in its use. It is impossible to teach someone the correct feel for the injection of Teflon into the TVC. This must be learned by experience, which is gained at the expense of patients until the technique has been perfected.

Most often, attending physicians in training programs will personally perform their own Teflon injections, because it is one of the few procedures that if performed wrong is uncorrectable. On the other hand, the techniques and judgments in SM can be readily conveyed to a pupil. All the residents leaving our program are fully trained and comfortable with this procedure.

The real difference in the two procedures is mainly due to the third and fourth advantages of SM, adjustability and reversibility. The adjustability is its single greatest advantage over Teflon. With a depth

TABLE 3. CAUSE OF GLOTTAL INCOMPETENCE IN PATIENTS RECEIVING BILATERAL IMPLANTS

Cause	*No.*
Presbylaryngis	6
Head injury	1
Strangulation	1
Laryngitis	1
Idiopathic	2
Total	11

gauge, the medialization can be simulated prior to implant placement, allowing for the rapid testing of multiple positions of cord displacements to acquire the best voice. If further adjustments are needed after the implant placement, it can be removed, adjusted, and replaced as necessary. The reversibility not only allows for future adjustments for anatomic or functional changes that may result in a weaker voice over time, but also allows for its use in several settings that are unsuitable for Teflon. First, it is inappropriate to inject Teflon in patients who have an intact vagal-RLN system who present within the first year of the paralysis, if there is any chance that vocal cord function may return. If vocal cord movement returns, the Teflon would prevent normal function of the injected cord. An exception to this would be in the terminally ill patient who might benefit from the brevity of the procedure for Teflon medialization. Because of the reversibility of SM, it can be placed relatively safely within this first year, as the severity of the symptoms dictate, in the knowledge that removal of the implant is possible if function returns. Second, it can be placed deep to a mobile TVC, augmenting the adducted TVC position without significant effect on its motion or vibratory function.

Besides voice improvement, the second major benefit of cord medialization is improvement in deglutition with a decrease in aspiration. Even if the voice was not brought back to its normal premorbid state, aspiration was universally improved. In 3 patients who had previously suffered a cerebrovascular accident from either a traumatic head injury or a postoperative complication from a neurosurgical procedure, the voice results were disappointing. Although the projection and the volume that developed were reasonable, the oropharyngeal incoordination led to such poor articulation that it shadowed the voice improvement. Aspiration, however, was significantly improved in all 3.

A consistent pattern of voice improvement has been seen in most patients. The initial voice improvement acquired on the operating table rapidly changes in the recovery room as perioperative edema develops. Although the voice is usually much stronger, it is raspy for several days to weeks after surgery. Often, however, the voice quality is quite good within the first week after surgery. Surprisingly, a second raspy phase occurs at 4 to 6 weeks after surgery. This usually subsides, however, within 2 more weeks.

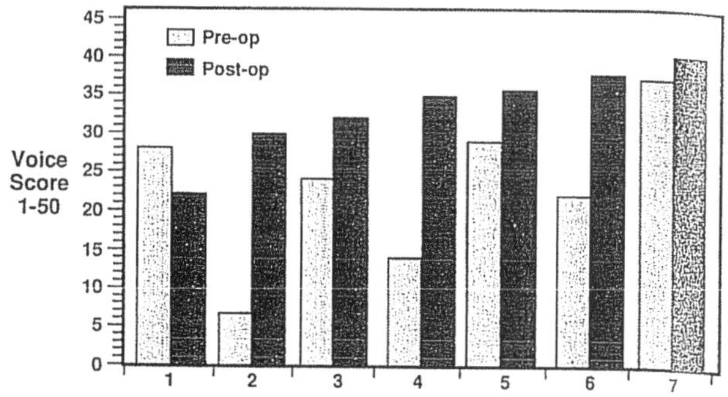

Fig 11. Results of "desirability rating" are outlined for preoperative and postoperative voice scores in 7 patients who underwent bilateral Silastic medialization.

Voice quality continues to improve in some patients for up to 1 year after surgery. Because of this postoperative cycle, voice samples recorded before 3 months after the date of surgery may not be representative of the long-term voice quality. It is important to inform patients and their family of this postoperative voice cycle, to prevent disappointment with their voice results over the first several postoperative months.

There are only 2 relative contraindications to SM. First, patients who have previously undergone a vertical hemilaryngectomy often develop a weak, breathy voice. Teflon injection has been recommended to augment the scarred surgical side to improve glottal closure. We were consulted to perform a revision in 1 such patient who had developed no voice improvement from SM after a vertical hemilaryngectomy. Without the buttress of the thyroid cartilage there is probably not enough lateral support for the Silastic implant to hold the scarred band of the larynx in a medialized position. Thus, placement of an implant would only lateralize the cervical soft tissue, rather than effecting medialization of the scarred side of the larynx. Second, previous laryngeal irradiation is a relative contraindication. If the larynx is still soft and supple, with minimal scarring, then careful surgery may be indicated. If the ventricle is violated during the procedure, placement of the implant should be delayed until mucosal healing has occurred.

The ansa-RLN transfer and SM have been compared as mutually exclusive procedures for repair of unilateral paralysis.[14] We, however, perceive the ansa-RLN transfer and SM not as alternate procedures exclusive of each other, but as surgical companions, both functioning by different mechanisms to conjointly return laryngeal function to its normal state. Even with excellent initial success with SM, if the laryngeal muscles are denervated, the atrophy of the muscles may lead to delayed glottal incompetence within 1 to 2 years in the postoperative period. In any patient undergoing SM within the first year of paralysis, whose vagus nerve or RLN is known to be sectioned, an ansa-RLN is now performed if spontaneous reinnervation cannot be demonstrated by EMG. After skull base surgery in which the vagus and hypoglossal nerves are sacrificed, the posterior branch of the ansa arising from the cervical plexus can be used for neural anastomosis with the RLN. Since we have less than 1 year's follow-up on the group of patients who have undergone nerve transfer, it will be several years before we can make significant statements based on the results of the procedure.

Primary SM under general anesthesia is a natural outgrowth of Silastic medialization performed under local anesthesia. The main reason for initiation of its use in this fashion was to eliminate the need for tracheotomy and to decrease the postoperative rehabilitation phase of patients undergoing loss of multiple cranial nerves at the time of skull base surgery. It is obvious that immediate glottal competence in the early postoperative period will allow for better pulmonary protection, with earlier swallowing rehabilitation. This immediate glottal competence also decreases the need for tracheotomy in most skull base procedures in which the pharynx has been denervated and not surgically altered. Tracheotomy, which is often performed in this situation for airway protection, causes significant problems in deglutition secondary to laryngotracheal fixation to the skin and reflex TVC hypomotility secondary to the decrease in laryngeal airflow. Thus, the combination of immediate glottal closure from the primary implant and the prevention of the complications caused by tracheotomy significantly improves the postoperative rehabilitation effort.

A conservative approach was taken initially with primary SM. The first implants were made small for fear of causing airway obstruction. The laryngeal edema that develops from intubation over a 12-hour period added further concern to the potential for airway compromise. However, in time, with no postoperative obstruction due to the implants, they have been enlarged to the same size as secondary implants placed for the same laryngeal configuration. One patient, who was very short and heavy, developed peripheral edema over her 11-hour procedure. She was left intubated for 4 days until the edema subsided and then was extubated; no airway complications were noted postextubation. Prior to primary SM, a preoperative computed tomography scan can aid in identifying thyroid cartilage anatomy and help to predict implant size. In patients with a more obtuse larynx, most often women, the implant is approximately 2 x 5 x 15...10 mm. In the more acute-angled larynx, most often seen in men, the window is placed further back, as previously described. The average size of the the implant is 2 x 6 x 18...13 mm. The initial postoperative voice, although strong, is usually hoarse for several weeks. We continue to see voice improvement for up to 1 year after all of these procedures. Of the 6 revisions performed in this group, 4 were to enlarge some of the earlier small implants. The usefulness of AA in conjunction with these patients will be discussed later.

The degree of improvement of voice quality has not been as consistent in patients presenting with presbylaryngis or bilateral bowing of different causes. Even though the results were not as good as we had hoped, the presbylaryngis patients were quite satisfied with the voice improvement. The major preoperative complaint in this patient group was the inability to communicate well over the telephone or in any public setting with background noise. All patients reported a significant improvement in their communication skills. The second most frequent complaint, mild aspiration, was significantly improved also. This was judged from the patients' history only, with no preoperative or postoperative swallowing tests. Earlier in the series, undersize implants were placed for fear of interfering with arytenoid movement. These early patients have not developed as much volume as the later patients. One of the earlier patients underwent a revision replacing one of his original implants, which was 2 x 4.5 x 13...13 mm, with a new implant that was 2 x 7 x 15...13 mm. This resulted in moderate voice improvement. He may undergo replacement of the opposite, smaller implant in the future. The posterior slope of the implant is designed so that there is no interference with the rocking motion of the arytenoid in and out of the larynx. A man with a large larynx underwent bilateral implants that were 2 x 6.5 x 15...13 mm, with no alteration of arytenoid function. When the larynx is viewed postoperatively in the fully abducted position, one can appreciate the mild decrease in glottal opening secondary to the implant. This decrease, however, is not symptomatic in the geriatric population in which presbylaryngis develops.

A review of the other 5 patients presenting with bilateral bowing not secondary to presbylaryngis is less encouraging. Although initial improvements were minimal in the patients who presented with strangulation and paresis secondary to a severe upper respiratory tract infection, both have shown further improvement over the course of 2 years. It is difficult to know whether this improvement should be credited to the implants or to a slow resolution of the underlying problem. A posterior glottal opening of 3 mm was initially seen in a 30-year-old patient who had undergone a stroke secondary to fat embolism. This posterior glottic gap is probably secondary to incomplete adduction of the vocal processes of the arytenoid. These are difficult to medialize without interference with the arytenoid function. Medializing the paraglottic tissue failed to improve this patient or the two middle-aged patients who presented with idiopathic TVC bowing. Oropharyngeal discoordination and articulation problems, often seen after head injury or stroke, further obscure any improvement in voice that is acquired from the implant. Although we were initially discouraged with the results in this group, the numbers are far too small to draw any conclusions.

The choice to use AA is not as clear-cut as that of SM. In theory, AA would add tension and help bring the vocal cord into a more physiologically correct phonating position. However, the complex interaction of the intralaryngeal muscles, which results in adduction of the arytenoids, is impossible to simulate with a single suture pulling forward on the muscular process. Our experience with 14 patients undergoing AA alone or in conjunction with SM is again too limited to draw more than early inferences. The recommended indications for AA are 1) a very wide glottal chink in which the vocal processes do not come into contact during phonation and 2) a difference in the level of the TVCs during phonation. Certainly, AA is useful in closing a wide glottic gap, but it is not always necessary. We use AA only after the intraoperative evaluation demonstrates incomplete closure of the larynx with SM. In several patients in whom the adjunctive use of AA was anticipated, the Silastic implant alone, with its posterior extension, was able to medialize the posterior commissure very well. If the posterior commissure is still open after SM has been performed, we progress to AA.

In Isshiki's original description, the joint capsule of the cricoarytenoid joint was opened prior to the AA. We routinely performed this in our earlier cases. Although the initial voice result was good, the postoperative video demonstrated overmedialization of the vocal process, which may represent subluxation of the arytenoid into the larynx. In spite of continued good vocal projection, all these patients have developed raspiness of the voice. The joint capsule was opened in only 1 of the more recent 10 patients. Joint fixation in this patient necessitated drilling open the joint with a microcutting bur in order to accomplish adduction. This patient's voice never returned to normal, but significant improvements occurred in the form of increased volume and decreased aspiration. None of the remaining 9 patients have developed raspiness at this time. In this group the average follow-up is 16 months. Arytenoid adduction is an excellent addition to SM for selected patients. Long-term follow-up with voice analysis will be necessary to indicate its real usefulness.

SUMMARY

After this complete review of our first 100 patients undergoing SM and/or AA, we are very encouraged with the improvements in communication derived from these two procedures. The addition of ansa-RLN transfer, when indicated, may prevent muscle atrophy and further sustain the initial voice improvement. These procedures, however, are still in their infancy in regard to development. There is still much to be learned from long-term follow-up of these patients in a multicenter cooperative effort to compare results, performed as the surgical techniques continue to improve.

ACKNOWLEDGMENT — The authors thank Britt Hissong and Xomed Treace for their help in the design and development of the surgical instruments described in this article.

REFERENCES

1. Koufman JA. Laryngoplastic phonosurgery. In: Johnson JT, ed. Instructional courses. American Academy of Otolaryngology–Head and Neck Surgery. St Louis, Mo: CV Mosby, 1988:339-50.

2. Koufman JA, Isaacson G. Laryngoplastic phonosurgery. Otolaryngol Clin North Am 1991;24:1151-77.

3. Isshiki N, Morita H, Okamura H, Hiramoto M. Thyroplasty as a new phonosurgical technique. Acta Otolaryngol (Stockh) 1974;78:451-3.

4. Isshiki N. Recent advances in phonosurgery. Folia Phoniatr (Basel) 1980;32:119-34.

5. Koufman JA. Laryngoplasty for vocal cord medialization: an alternative to Teflon. Laryngoscope 1986;96:726-30.

6. Maves MD, McCabe BF, Gray S. Phonosurgery: indications and pitfalls. Ann Otol Rhinol Laryngol 1989;98:577-80.

7. Tucker HM. Combined laryngeal framework medialization and reinnervation for unilateral vocal cord paralysis. Ann Otol Rhinol Laryngol 1990;99:778-81.

8. Isshiki N, Tanabe M, Sawada M. Arytenoid adduction for unilateral vocal cord paralysis. Arch Otolaryngol 1978;104:555-8.

9. Netterville JL, Aly A, Ossoff RH. Evaluation and treatment of complications of thyroid and parathyroid surgery. Otolaryngol Clin North Am 1990;23:529-52.

10. Isaacson G, Kim JH, Kirchner JC, Kirchner JA. Histology of Isshiki thyroplasty type I. Ann Otol Rhinol Laryngol 1990; 99:42-5.

11. Meurman Y. Operative mediofixation of the vocal cord in complete unilateral paralysis. Arch Otolaryngol 1952;55:544-53.

12. Crumley RL. Update. Ansa-cervicalis to recurrent laryngeal nerve anastomosis for unilateral laryngeal paralysis. Laryngoscope 1991;101:384-8.

13. Netterville JL, Jackson GC, Civantos F. Thyroplasty in the functional rehabilitation of neurotologic skull base surgery patients. Am J Otolaryngol (in press).

14. Crumley RL, Izdebski K, McMicken B. Nerve transfer versus Teflon injection for vocal cord paralysis: a comparison. Laryngoscope 1988;98:1200-4.

14

Laryngeal Dystonia

Introduction

Within the time encompassed by the articles in this collection, spasmodic dysphonia metamorphosed from a psychiatric condition resulting from anxiety, stress, and neurosis to a neurologic disorder with medical treatment. That it could have existed as a psychiatric disease for a century since its original, recognizable descriptions by Traube and Schnitzler—generating 100 years of patients who not only obtained no relief, but were told with authority and confidence that they had a mental problem—should be humbling and thought provoking to today's physician.

The suggestions that spasmodic dysphonia was organic began with neurologists' observations that the characteristic voice sometimes occurred in conjunction with other involuntary motion of better established neurologic origin. Therapeutic frustration—well expressed in his heartfelt commentary—drove Dr. Dedo to attempt his ultimately successful nerve block. Its results led him to perform recurrent laryngeal nerve section for treatment. The resulting paper, reproduced herein, amounted not only to a significant therapeutic advance for the disorder, but also provided a vindication for thousands of patients heretofore considered to be "emotionally fragile" or worse.

Spasmodic dysphonia is now well established as a focal dystonia. Unfortunately, the good results that Dedo reported in his 1976 paper proved difficult to attain over the long term, probably because of the vocal fold's robust tendency to reinnervate. In his recollection, Dr. Blitzer describes the circumstances and the path that led him to the notion to use botulinum toxin for treatment, which has now become the most extensively studied and widely recommended treatment for spasmodic dysphonia.

The accompanying papers are, like that of Dedo, carefully observed descriptions of a fascinating disorder with highly variable symptoms. They also present closely reasoned rationales for treatment that acknowledge the central nervous system origin of the dystonia. As Blitzer points out, herein lies the weakness of both surgical and chemical denervation: by targeting the end organ, existing approaches to treatment do not affect the abnormality directly, and are likely to prove inadequate for full, permanent symptom relief.

The next shift in this disorder may be from laryngologic treatment to neurologic treatment. The discovery of molecular and genetic determinants of generalized dystonia, the advent of implantable basal ganglia stimulators, the evolution of better pharmaceutical agents may yet transform the disease again, to the benefit of the patient. Time will tell what contribution otolaryngologists and voice scientists have to make to such advances.

Classic Articles

● Reprint of article included in this chapter.
♦ Commentary on this article.

●♦Dedo HH. Recurrent laryngeal nerve section for spastic dysphonia. *Ann Otol Rhinol Laryngol.* 1976;85(4 pt 1):451–459.

Blitzer A, Brin MF, Fahn S, Lovelace RE. Localized injections of botulinum toxin for the treatment of focal laryngeal dystonia (spastic dysphonia). *Laryngoscope.* 1988;98(2):193–197.

Blitzer A, Brin MF, Fahn S, Lovelace RE. Clinical and laboratory characteristics of focal laryngeal dystonia: study of 110 cases. *Laryngoscope.* 1988;98(6 pt 1):636–640.

●♦Blitzer A, Brin MF. Laryngeal dystonia: a series with botulinum toxin therapy. *Ann Otol Rhinol Laryngol.* 1991;100(2):85–89.

Donati F, Meistelman C, Plaud B. Vecuronium neuromuscular blockade at the adductor muscles of the larynx and adductor pollicis. *Anesthesiology.* 1991;74(5):833–837.

Truong DD, Rontal M, Rolnick M, Aronson AE, Mistura K. Double-blind controlled study of botulinum toxin in adductor spasmodic dysphonia. *Larygoscope.* 1991;101(6 pt 1):630–634.

Zwirner P, Murry T, Swenson M, Woodson GE. Effects of botulinum toxin therapy in patients with adductor spasmodic dysphonia: acoustic, aerodynamic, and videoendoscopic findings. *Laryngoscope.* 1992;102(4):400–406.

Ludlow CL, Naunton RF, Sedory SE, Schulz GM, Hallett M. Effects of botulinum toxin injections on speech in adductor spasmodic dysphonia. *Neurology.* 1998;38(8):1220–1225.

Blitzer A, Brin MF, Stewart CF. Botulinum toxin management of spasmodic dysphonia (laryngeal dystonia): a 12-year experience in more than 900 patients. *Laryngoscope.* 1998;108(10):1435–1441.

Commentary

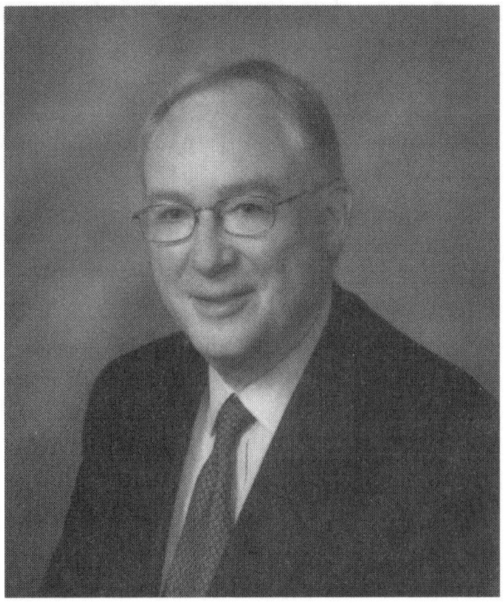

Herbert H. Dedo, MD

In my residency (1959–1963), we were taught "hysterical spastic dysphonia" was a psychiatric disorder to be treated by voice therapy and or tranquilizers. In 1974, Dr. Seymour Brockman called me from Los Angeles to refer Mrs. Mildred Younger, wife of the then Attorney General of California, for severe spastic (now spasmodic is preferred) dysphonia. (She can be named because she later discussed her case on television and in *Time* magazine). I asked why he was referring her to me and not a voice therapist as we had been taught. He said voice therapy never cures this and I then recalled the three patients I had sent for voice therapy had not returned cured. *Observation 1:* Voice therapists and doctors generally do not write papers about disorders they cannot cure. Mrs. Younger had seen 29 of the best ENT doctors and voice therapists in the United Stated in the prior 19 years with no relief (unless she shouted, sang all words in falsetto voice, or whispered). Furthermore, she had severe face grimaces when she tried to talk.

I said, in that case, we need to do better. First, I suggested tying back one vocal fold so they could not hyperadduct but immediately dismissed that idea because the suture would cut rapidly through a mobile vocal fold. Then I suggested paralyzing one vocal fold to mate a breathy weak phonatory voice with the overly tight voice of spasmodic dysphonia. Dr. Brockman was shocked but because I already had injected Teflon in many paralyzed vocal folds, it was not a fearsome disorder to me and I knew it would be easy to reposition the paralyzed vocal fold if her voice became too breathy.

Then, just before her first visit, I had my second inspiration—to test my idea with Xylocaine injection of one recurrent nerve. It took three injections of 3 cc, 1% Xylocaine before I succeeded in paralyzing the right recurrent nerve adjacent to the cricothyroid joint. Her voice then immediately became nonspasmodic, phonatory, slightly soft (low in volume, but it had been soft while spasmodic), and breathy and her face grimaces ceased. She then worked with a waiting voice therapist to try to relearn how to talk easily but the spasticity began to return after 25 minutes and on indirect laryngoscopy, the right vocal fold was just beginning to recover motion. *Observation 2:* It was already clear to me this was not a psychiatric, stress, or hysterical disorder. Neither she nor I knew when the vocal fold was going to be paralyzed or for how long. Thus, the dramatic voice improvement was only during paralysis, not while she expected it to be paralyzed. I repeated the Xylocaine temporary paralysis four more times over a period of several months to make sure it was not a fluke. The results were consistent. So, on September 9, 1975, I tied a silk ligature tightly around the right recurrent laryngeal nerve so I could remove it if she developed hysterical transference ("old ideas die hard"). Postoperatively, her voice was nonspasmodic; it was phonatory, slightly soft and breathy, and her face was relaxed. She and her husband were delighted. The last time I heard her voice 18 years later it was still excellent. Word spread rapidly; I did several more RLN sections and reported it with pre- and post-op voice recordings to demonstrate the dramatic results at the American Laryngological Association Meeting in April 1976. My colleagues were shocked and several assured me this operation was just psychosurgery.

It was fascinating to review the literature. Traube in 1871 in Vienna first described this well enough (tight strangled voice) to be sure he was referring to SD. By 1874, he announced it was hysterical for several reasons:

1. The majority are women. (True, about two-thirds are but how could males have hysteria without a uterus to send vapors to the brain as was then thought to be the cause going back to Roman concepts.)
2. There is no visible pathology in the larynx so the cause must be in the brain. (True, but we now know the pathology is with control of vocal fold muscle tension in the basal ganglia not the forebrain as in hysteria. Some may be of viral etiology because we had a group of patents whose voice symptoms started after Hong Kong Flu in 1966.)
3. These spasmodic dysphonia patients, no matter how severe, can still sing clearly, and even talk in a falsetto or singsong voice and "everyone knows with hoarseness the singing voice goes first." (True, but with visible lesions on the vocal folds, which they already had noted did not exist here.).

For over 100 years, in over 400 books, papers, and articles authors just kept copying the same material with one change; hysterical etiology was changed to stress by some (but not here at the University of California San Francisco) in about the 1920s. *Observation 3:* Doctors hate to admit they do not know the etiology of a disorder. If they no longer blame them on hysteria, humor imbalance or planet misposition as they did in the 1800s they now substitute stress, viruses, or allergy. Lately, for vocal fold disorders they have added GERD (gastroesophageal reflex disorder) even without proof of cause, shursh (patient aware of reflux) and without cure with treatment based on these assumptions.

I have now done over 700 recurrent laryngeal nerve sections with good results.[1] We have had *partial* recurrence of spasticity in about 18% after 6 to 30 months. This has been eliminated by vocal fold thinning or re-resection of the recurrent laryngeal nerve high near the cricothyroid joint. Eight patients were presented at the ALA Meeting in 2003, but this has not been published yet. None of these had recovered any vocal fold motion but presumably nerve fibers grew into the distal recurrent laryngeal nerve stump and "bulked up" the thyroarytenoid muscle slightly. Also, we have observed partial recurrence of spasticity is mainly in patients who had moderately severe and severe spasticity prerecurrent laryngeal nerve section.[2] This probably explains why Mayo Clinic had a higher recurrence rate (about 66% of some spasticity rather than our 18%—because of selection). They only operated on severe spasmodic dysphonia cases (personal communication, Dr. Lawrence De Santo).

The disorder is bilateral. We have sectioned the left recurrent laryngeal nerve since about 1979 because the theoretical possibility of a later spontaneous paralysis of the remaining recurrent nerve is greater on the left as it is longer, so we section it to start with.

In the early 1980s, Dr. Turner, then at Baylor and later at Tulane, suggested injecting botulinum toxin into a vocal cord to paralyze it for spasmodic dysphonia. Dr. Blitzer has since written much on this. This is using our paralysis principle but it is not an effective treatment with 18% or even 66% recurrence but rather 100% recurrence of spasticity. Spasticity recurs after 3 to 6 months in all these patients. Ten to 50% fail even the initial injection and require a repeat injection. So the injection has to be repeated every 3 to 6 months the rest of the patient's life with a "roller-coaster voice" as one patient described it. Dr. Krzysztof Izdebski and I have seen many who have required more than 15 to 20 injections at large expense and trouble. In my opinion, it is simply a prolonged diagnostic test and some patients are beginning to agree and have the RLN Section.

Secondary surgical procedures can be done after recurrent laryngeal nerve section if necessary for "fine tuning" of the voice. If the voice is too breathy after post-op (not pre-op) voice therapy, when it can be very helpful, and 1 year delay for the voice to stabilize, *underinjection* of Teflon has been successful in reducing this breathiness and weakness. However, if enough is injected to bring the paralyzed fold edge to the midline in an attempt to eliminate all breathiness, spasmodic dysphonia will return, not surprisingly. If spasticity recurs (6 to 30 months post-op), the paralyzed vocal fold can be thinned as is done for a Teflon over injected vocal fold[3] or the RLN can be re-resected (presented at the 2003 Western Section, Triological Society Meeting, but not yet published).

References

1. Dedo HH, Behlau MS. Recurrent laryngeal nerve section for spastic dysphonia: 5 to 14 year preliminary results in the first 300 patients. *Ann Otol Rhinol Laryngol.* 1991;100(4):274–279.
2. Dedo HH, Izdebski K. Evaluation and treatment of recurrent spasticity after recurrent laryngeal nerve section. A preliminary report. *Ann Otol Rhinol Laryngol.* 1984;93:343–345.
3. Horn KL, Dedo HH. Surgical correction of the convex vocal cord after Teflon injection. *Laryngoscope.* 1980;90:281–286.

RECURRENT LARYNGEAL NERVE SECTION FOR SPASTIC DYSPHONIA

HERBERT H. DEDO, MD

SAN FRANCISCO, CALIFORNIA

SUMMARY – Spastic dysphonia is a severe vocal disability in which a person speaks with excessively adducted vocal cords. The resulting weak phonation sounds tight, as if he were being strangled, and has also been described as laryngeal stutter. It is often accompanied by face and neck grimaces. In the past it has been regarded as psychoneurotic in origin and treated with speech therapy and psychotherapy with disappointing results. Because of laboratory and clinical observation that recurrent nerve paralysis retracts the involved vocal cord from the midline, it was proposed that deliberate section of the recurrent nerve would improve the vocal quality of patients with spastic dysphonia. In 34 patients the recurrent nerve was sectioned after Xylocaine® temporary paralysis showed significant improvement in vocal quality. Several patients have been advised against this operation because of the type of voice they developed with one vocal cord temporarily paralyzed. With nerve section plus postoperative speech therapy, approximately half of the patients have returned close to a "normal" but soft phonatory voice. The rest had varying degrees of improvement, but all, so far, have been pleased with the improvement in ease and quality of phonation and reduction or elimination of face and neck grimaces. Two men have a breathy component in their phonatory voices, and one woman has variable pitch.

The first description of a spastic form of psychogenic hoarseness was made by Traube[1] in 1871. Four years later the Viennese laryngologist, Schnitzler,[2] provided a detailed description of spastic dysphonia and coined the diagnostic term. Berendes[3] defined spastic dysphonia as a disorder of phonation which is characterized by a strained, creaking, and choked vocal attack, a tense and squeezed voice sound which is accompanied by extreme tension of the entire phonatory system. He noted that the stressed vowels may be broken into two portions and that the disorder disturbs primarily the communicative function of speech with variations in intensity. Often the patient can speak to himself, whisper, laugh, achieve a falsetto singing tone and sometimes phonate isolated vowels or whole sentences with a normal phonatory voice. During indirect laryngoscopy, the structure of the larynx and vocal cords appears normal. While silent respiration is normal, the frustrated vocal effort causes severe obstruction to expiration of air from the lungs causing aching fatigue of the upper anterior chest muscles.

Spastic dysphonia has been repeatedly described as "stuttering with vocal cords."[3] It is often accompanied by associated spastic or grimacing type contractions of the neck and facial muscles, causing complete closing of the eyes at times. In some people there is superimposed stuttering of the lips and tongue and palate as an extreme form of an already serious disability. It ordinarily starts in people over the age of 40 years, but one patient in our series had the onset in her 20s.

Virtually all of the contributors to this subject in the last hundred years have stated that spastic dysphonia is an expression of psychoneurosis. According to the early psychiatric teaching, such conditions were regarded as hysterical.[1] In a most exhaustive review by Ber-

From the Department of Otolaryngology, University of California, San Francisco, San Francisco, California.

Presented in part at the meeting of the American Laryngological Association, Palm Beach, Florida, April 24-25, 1976.

endes in 1939, spastic dysphonia was regarded as a typical neurosis without hysterical traits.[3] Robe *et al*[4] and Aronson *et al*[5,6] were among the exceptional authors who suggested that spastic dysphonia is due to some organic pathology of the nervous system, rather than hysteria or psychogenic disorder or reaction to stress. These investigators also were among the few who admitted the singular ineffectiveness of voice therapy and psychotherapy in spastic dysphonia.

Multiple treatments have been tried without achieving consistent permanent cure of vocal spasticity. Brodnitz comments that psychotherapy has not been too helpful.[7] It may help the patient to gain better insight into his psychological background but he still will exhibit a marked degree of dysphonia; only one of his patients improved "significantly." He adds that it is one of the characteristics of the disorder that many of the patients react violently to the suggestion of psychiatric counseling. One only has to give such advice to lose the patient immediately. Brodnitz further states that voice training alone has proved to be of only very limited value. Cooper reported that of 41 patients, 22 entered speech therapy and only 6 of them completed therapy with results described as excellent – one; good – three; and fair – one.[8] Even this much improvement required a minimum of 1½ years. Boone comments that with speech therapy "progress has been erratic and limited, with no one patient experiencing a permanent restoration of normal voice. The problem of spastic dysphonia still remains both a diagnostic and etiologic unknown, which, of course, makes the development of an effective therapeutic approach impossible."[9]

In the spring of 1975 I was asked to see M.Y. in consultation. I feel that because of the special nature of her problem, including the tenacity with which she continued to seek help after 17 years of disappointment, and her willingness to knowingly undergo experimental procedures, she and her husband deserve credit for participating in the discoveries which were made. She had treatment by more than 29 doctors, including laryngologists, speech therapists, psychiatrists, and hypnotists in the United States. She continued to be disabled by severe dysphonia which was accompanied by marked associated grimaces of the face and neck during her attempts to talk. Speech therapists confirmed that their modality could not offer her the chance to return to normal. Because of the disruption of her life caused by her being a vocal cripple, there was considerable encouragement to develop a new approach to help her. I proposed that we again try temporary topical and local paralysis of the internal branch of the superior laryngeal nerve which had earlier given her only partial, temporary relief and if this failed, to test the effects of paralysis of the recurrent nerve. Diligent review of the literature did not provide any support for such a proposal. In fact, the only report of surgery for this disorder was that of Rethi,[10] in which he reported some success in one patient with dividing the stylopharyngeus muscle, which is considerably different than deliberately paralyzing the recurrent laryngeal nerve (RLN).

RATIONALE

Laryngeal research in dogs and humans with electromyography and still and motion pictures has confirmed that paralysis of one recurrent laryngeal nerve in the normal individual not only paralyzes the vocal cord but sets it in the paramedian position so that the normal (unparalyzed) cord fails to reach it as firmly as usual, causing a breathy but often phonatory soft voice.[11] It has long been recognized that the voice can sound nearly normal, although soft in some persons, if the normal vocal cord can compensate by crossing the midline to reach a paralyzed vocal cord. In patients with Teflon®* injections of paralyzed vocal cords, many had a brief period of spas-

* Polytef paste for injection; Mentor Division, Codman & Shurtleff, Inc., Randolph, MA.

tic or tight phonation for a few moments after the injection before the mobile vocal cord quit compensating across the midline. It seemed possible that if a recurrent laryngeal nerve were paralyzed in a patient with spastic dysphonia, the other vocal cord might prove to be "precompensated" so that its excessively strong adduction would carry it across the midline to the deliberately paralyzed cord, giving a relatively normal phonation. After describing the above hypothesis, it was proposed to M.Y. that one recurrent laryngeal nerve be paralyzed temporarily with lidocaine since paralysis of the superior laryngeal nerve had temporarily improved her voice by only 10% or 15%. She and her husband agreed, and to our amazement and delight, once the recurrent nerve had been thoroughly paralyzed by the injection of 1% lidocaine, she was able to talk with a phonatory voice without vocal spasticity. Furthermore, as soon as she found she had a consistent phonatory sound, she was able to stop the neck and facial grimaces and special respiratory efforts. Although her voice at this point had a raspy or husky sound, Dr. Lucie Lawson, speech therapist, was rapidly able to help her raise the pitch and bring the sound "up in the front of her mouth," largely clearing the huskiness. Unfortunately, as soon as the lidocaine wore off, the spasticity of voice and face and neck returned. When this had been repeated four more times with identical results, she and her husband agreed to surgical section of the recurrent nerve to try to make the vocal improvement permanent, even though there was no guarantee what would happen to her voice or psyche. Although she did not appear hysterical or psychoneurotic when her vocal cord was temporarily paralyzed and she was able to phonate properly, there was some trepidation about whether she would develop hysterical phenomena such as paralysis or numbness of a limb, since the literature had stressed the psychiatric etiology of this disease for over a hundred years. However, when the right recurrent nerve was sectioned on September 9, 1975, she had an uneventful convalescence. Her speech and facial movements were dramatically better on awakening from the anesthetic. With speech therapy she regained an essentially normal voice within weeks, and she was able to stop the associated movements of her face or neck. She has now even resumed her political, radio, and television career after an 18-year hiatus.

TREATMENT TECHNIQUE

Diagnosis. There are several different types of spastic dysphonic speech. The basic type has a constant, very tight, hoarse, soft, barely phonatory sound which may vary slightly with fatigue and stress. Several have resorted to a stage whisper voice, inspiratory speech, or even the small buzzer* used by laryngectomees to talk, and when requested to phonate they can only produce a soft, harsh, tight sound low in the back of the throat. A second type has frequent breaks in the tight sound caused by momentary vocal cord abductions which produce a quavering, spastic dysphonic sound low in the back of the throat. Considerable variation in the spasticity can occur in one patient. Some are able to achieve a clear, normal phonatory voice with occasional single words, phrases or sentences. In one patient, within one sentence the voice went from a whisper through clear phonatory, to spastic phonatory, back through clear phonatory to a whisper. (Her spastic dysphonia had been present less than two years, and in the majority of patients who had had the disorder longer than this, the voice did not have such remarkable variability.) There is often throat clearing or groaning phonations made between words in an attempt to obtain a clear phonatory sound. Many of these patients can laugh and sing a falsetto musical note or phonate some vowels such as "e" and "o" with a clear phonatory sound. There is considerable variation between patients on the amount of associated grimacing

* Western Electric buzzer available through local telephone company.

movements of the face and neck and oral tics which they have, similar to that of a severe oral stutterer. Indirect laryngoscopy ordinarily shows that there are no lesions on the vocal cords. Naturally it is essential to rule out benign or malignant tumors of the vocal cords and unilateral or bilateral voice cord paralysis by indirect laryngoscopy before proceeding.

Two patients were noted to have mobile vocal cords which were bowed during phonation but created a spastic type of phonation. Although the initial reaction was that Teflon® injection was indicated as with previous patients with bowed mobile vocal cords and breathy voices,[12] it was found that paralysis of one recurrent laryngeal nerve with lidocaine dramatically improved the voice by clearing the spasticity. However, this made the voice worse in one patient with bowed mobile cords during phonation and a breathy voice. Therefore, it appears that patients with spastic dysphonia *and* bowed mobile vocal cords during phonation actually have adopted the technique of cricothyroid relaxation in their attempts to achieve a nonspastic voice. They can benefit by recurrent nerve section if indicated by lidocaine test paralysis. Teflon® injection of *one* vocal cord should be reserved for bowed mobile vocal cord with *breathy* phonation.[12]

Preoperative Evaluation. The voice is tape-recorded and evaluated by a speech therapist and the surgeon. Temporary paralysis is then achieved by injecting 1% lidocaine, 3-6 ml adjacent to the cricothyroid joint. Paralysis is then confirmed after two to four minutes by repeat indirect laryngoscopy. The risks of this lidocaine, of course, are explained to the patient. Although they are unlikely, they include the possibility of severing the nerve with the needle, entering the carotid artery or jugular vein or the trachea. The temporary paralysis wears off in 7 to 30 minutes, sometimes before the patient can break through the old speech therapy relaxation training and hear and feel the improvement.

The patient must be prepared to accept this voice as the minimum achievable voice after surgery in case speech therapy does not achieve maximum potential improvement. As soon as the recurrent nerve has been temporarily paralyzed, the voice is tape-recorded again and the speech therapist, the surgeon and the patient decide whether enough improvement has been obtained to justify permanent section of the recurrent laryngeal nerve. Ordinarily these procedures are performed on the right side because the laryngeal nerves and vocal cords are symmetrical and it is technically preferable on the right. Several patients have been refused recurrent nerve section because they or the surgeon were not satisfied they had achieved the typical and proper change in their voice. The voice change during lidocaine paralysis differs somewhat from that obtained after permanent recurrent nerve paralysis. This is because the adjacent external branch of the superior laryngeal nerve and therefore the right cricothyroid muscle is often paralyzed by the lidocaine but not the surgery. (This is shown by posterior rotation of the larynx to the left.) They often have a temporary Horner's syndrome and a "lump" sensation in the throat during lidocaine paralysis which disconcerts them during the usual 10 to 15 minutes they have to determine whether the recurrent laryngeal nerve paralysis should be made permanent. Thus, the temporary lidocaine paralysis only approximates the vocal improvement which can be obtained by recurrent nerve section. However, even though this has usually been exceeded by surgical division of one recurrent nerve, especially when supplemented by speech therapy, it is emphasized that the voice, while likely to be improved, will not necessarily be completely normal after permanent section.

Surgical Technique. Under general anesthesia a collar incision is made one finger-breadth below the cricoid cartilage. Dissection is carried down to the anterior surface of the trachea and around its right side to the tracheoesophageal groove. The recurrent nerve is identified ordinarily at the level of the inferior pole of the right thyroid gland 1 cm lateral to the trachea. It is sometimes necessary for adequate exposure to divide the isthmus and resect the upper portion of the thyroid gland off of the trachea with resultant extra bleeding. Direct laryngoscopy is then performed so that the right vocal cord can be observed while an assistant crushes the presumed recurrent nerve with a hemostat. If the vocal cord contracts abruptly at the instant of crushing, the structure is presumed to be the whole recurrent nerve and is ligated with a 2-0 silk ligature. A 1 cm segment is then removed adjacent to the inferior pole of the thyroid gland about 3 - 4 cm below the cricoid. Care needs to be taken to avoid injury to the trachea, thyroid gland, parathyroid glands, carotid artery, cervical esophagus, cervical sympathetics and, especially to the recurrent nerve on the other side. (It is possible to dissect through the party wall between the trachea and esophagus and reach the left recurrent laryngeal nerve.) It is *not* necessary or desirable to section both recurrent nerves. Care must also be taken to avoid injury to the innominate artery and vein which are nearby in the upper mediastinum in some patients.

The incision is closed with gut subcutaneous sutures and Steri-strips®* to the skin with a drain in place. A pressure dressing is installed. When the endotracheal tube is removed and the patient awakens, it is usually possible to hear marked improvement in the voice, even in the recovery room. One exception was a patient in whom a small amount of arytenoid and vocal cord edema resulted from the intubation or direct laryngoscopy so that an injection of cortisone was necessary, and improvement was delayed for several days.

RESULTS

We have now temporarily paralyzed the right recurrent laryngeal nerve in 41 patients and have surgically sectioned 34 recurrent laryngeal nerves. All of these patients have been pleased with the improvement (loss of spasticity) in their voices and decrease or clearance of associated tics and grimaces. However, several of the patients have spoken with a mild residual hoarseness (huskiness or raspiness or a soft low pitch), and one has had some intermittent mild spastic phonation and pitch variability after surgery. Two have breathy but phonatory voices when tired or they have to push their voices in a noisy environment. Although clarity of tone, good pitch control and elimination of associated face, neck and chest movements (grimaces, tics, oral stuttering, and chest muscle fatigue) have been achieved by some patients spontaneously after surgery, most have benefited by speech therapy varying from a few days to several weeks. So far there has been no reversion to the severe preoperative spastic dysphonia and no hysterical conversions. Three patients had been receiving psychotherapy, including one who had a complete nervous breakdown five months before surgery and two who had attempted suicide. They are reported by their psychiatrists as doing much better because the disability of spastic dysphonia had been causing or increasing their emotional disturbances, rather than the reverse situation which has generally been the one described in the literature.

DISCUSSION

Etiology. If the etiology for a disorder is unknown, it is ordinarily blamed on psychoneurotic reaction to stress, or on viruses, or on allergy. In the past, most authors stated that spastic dysphonia was caused by emotional stress.[13] This just increased the patient's problems and resentments because psychotherapy has been singularly ineffective in treating this disorder. Psychotherapy should be used, if necessary, for other emotional problems which may be present, but not in an attempt to treat the spastic dysphonic since it has not been useful in the past. It just adds to these patients' problems by suggesting they are benefiting from their terrible speech dis-

* 3M, Minnesota Mining and Manufacturing Co., St. Paul, MN.

ability and they can talk normally if they just will try.

The fanciful psychodynamics in the psychiatric reports sent with these patients is incredible. It is interesting that when Aronson[5,6] used the Minnesota Multiphasic Personality Test (MMPT) to evaluate patients with spastic dysphonia, he found a lower incidence of repressed anger and compulsive personality traits than were present in the general medical population at Mayo Clinic. This whole concept that spastic dysphonia was due to hysteria or psychoneurosis apparently was based on the clinical observation that even though these patients could get a clear phonatory sound with singing and laughing, they spoke with spastic dysphonia when required to talk "with emotional content."[1] Furthermore, the spasticity was variable and, in some, increased with stress or fatigue or seemed to start originally after some special stress. Therefore, it was assumed that this was a conscious attempt to penalize family members or coworkers and that all that was necessary was to trick or analyze the patient out of the problem. This was reinforced by occasional observations that spastic dysphonic patients could speak with a clear, phonatory voice while awakening from general anesthesia or if they were plied with enough alcohol to make them drunk. None of these are useful observations since it is not possible to remain in a drunken or drugged state from alcohol or general anesthetic agents and to continue to function with full effectiveness. In fact, in discussions with psychiatrists who were seeing three of these patients, they readily agreed that the spastic dysphonia had increased the emotional problems rather than the emotional problems being the cause of the spastic dysphonia.

Only a few authors have suggested that spastic dysphonia was caused by organic disorder of the neuromuscular system. Moore and his coworkers[4] found that 10 of 14 patients with spastic dysphonia had abnormal electroencephalograms. Aronson *et al*[5,6] then exhaustively reviewed 31 spastic dysphonia patients seen at Mayo Clinic. Of 27 patients given neurologic examinations, 20 had one or more neurologic signs, including tremor, hyperreflexia, reduced alternate motion rate and faciolingual asymmetries. (Only one of our patients has had organic neurologic defects elsewhere, and her spinocerebellar degeneration was far advanced before spastic dysphonia appeared.) These signs occurred with greater frequency than would be expected in normal population. They hypothesized that spastic dysphonia has a neurologic substrate and may be related to the essential tremor syndrome. Of the 29 patients given psychiatric interviews, 18 were judged to have some emotional problems, and 11 did not. Although as a group they gave the impression of being compulsive, of overcontrolling their anger, and of being quite unaggressive verbally, it is suggested that these traits are not exclusively characteristic of spastic dysphonia. It should be remembered that these traits are present in a vast number of people who show no signs of spastic dysphonia.

I would now like to suggest that this disease is caused by a disturbance in the proprioceptive control of the vocal cords. Specifically, it is proposed that neurotropic viral infection damages the a & c fibers either peripherally or in the central nervous system while sparing the larger diameter motor nerve fibers to the intrinsic laryngeal muscles. Neurotropic viral injury of the large motor nerve fibers is invoked for many cases of paralysis of the facial nerve causing Bell's palsy. Viral damage of the large motor nerve fibers unilaterally or bilaterally is given as the present best explanation of spontaneous recurrent laryngeal nerve paralysis. Proprioceptive control of the vocal cord muscles is poorly understood because even with electroneurophysiology techniques now available, it is difficult to study in the normal human and dog. Furthermore, there is no good animal model for spastic dysphonia. It is interesting that over half of these patients had a clinically apparent viral illness of the respiratory or gastrointestinal system at, or shortly before, the onset of spastic dysphonia. In fact, it was easier to elicit this than a history of specific stress at or about the time of onset. One patient had poliomyelitis some time before, and one had a temporary partial paralysis of the right facial nerve which started at the same time as the spastic dysphonia. An advantage of using this hypothesis is that there is no specific treatment for viral infection so the patient's money is not wasted on psychotherapy.

It is striking that these patients do not appear hysterical or emotionally disturbed after the recurrent laryngeal nerve has been cut and they are able to resume reasonably normal phonation. In every patient a control injection to test the Psychoneurotic Etiology Hypothesis was performed by injecting Xylocaine®* subcutaneously and beside the cricoid cartilage or for two to four minutes after placing it on the nerve sheath. There was no change in the voice even though the patient was unable to see precisely where the Xylocaine® was being placed. The spasticity left the voice only when the recurrent laryngeal nerve became fully paralyzed by the lidocaine, as confirmed by indirect laryngoscopy. Furthermore, the spasticity returned as soon as the lidocaine began to wear off, in spite of the fact that these patients did not know exactly how long the lidocaine effect would last. If their spastic dysphonia were on a voluntary or hysterical basis, at least some of them would have cleared with the combination of suggestion, and an injection of a powerful medicine in the neck or the improvement should have lasted after the lidocaine wore off. Only one patient has had an hysterical manifestation elsewhere in the body (a brief glove anesthesia of one hand one month before surgery). None have had postoperative hysterical conversion reactions or increase in emotional problems. In fact, there has been a striking decrease in manifestation of emotional disorders after their voices have returned to normal or to even near-normal status. Intensive speech therapy during temporary lidocaine paralysis of the vocal cord did not achieve permanent resolution of the spastic dysphonia in a single patient. Associated movements of the face, neck and throat, clearing of the throat, whisper voice, bowed mobile vocal cords during phonation, and even use of a W.E. Buzzer to achieve phonation were all caused by conscious attempts to achieve phonatory sound. When consistent, reliable glottic phonation became possible and apparent to these patients after lidocaine injections and later when recurrent laryngeal nerve section had repositioned the cord, these associated problems usually cleared rapidly. If the patient had really been trying to use the disease for psychological or social reasons, these voluntary manifestations would be expected to continue or to increase. Usually after section of the recurrent laryngeal nerve, the pitch is low "in the back of the throat," showing they were trying to relax the vocal cords before the paralysis.

There is no reliable clinical or experimental evidence for classifying spastic dysphonia as a psychoneurotic or hysterical disease. In fact, it just causes time and money to be wasted on psychotherapy, at least for the vocal disorder itself, and it increases the patient's guilt and emotional stress. Proprioceptive disturbance by neurotropic viral infection has as solid a theoretical and clinical basis as psychoneurosis and causes less expense (for ineffective psychotherapy) and less social opprobrium.

Treatment. Psychotherapy, allergy treatment, hypnosis, acupuncture, special diets, vitamins, cortisone and tranquilizers had all been tried repeatedly on these patients and have no place in the treatment of spastic dysphonia. Speech therapy before recurrent laryngeal nerve section had only helped *some* patients *partially* and then it took 1½ years or more at considerable cost and constant deliberate effort which always continued to be necessary.

* Astra Pharmaceutical Products, Inc., Worcester, MA.

The speech therapists who have seen this group of patients have now agreed that speech therapy is not useful or effective if spastic dysphonia has been present three months or more. In fact, we are still looking for an established spastic dysphonic who has been returned to a normal voice by speech therapy. Therefore, patients in whom spastic dysphonia has been present more than three months are advised to have the lidocaine paralysis test of the RLN, and if there is the typical improvement in the voice, a RLN section. The advantage of this approach is that the RLN can be paralyzed temporarily with lidocaine before the surgery so the patient and family can determine whether they wish to make it permanent. This kind of inexpensive diagnostic test is not possible with any of the other modalities, such as speech therapy alone, psychotherapy, hypnosis, acupuncture, special diets, tranquilizers, allergy treatment and cortisone shots. The surgery is a low risk, general anesthetic procedure and is rapidly effective in one or two hours, instead of one or more years. Postoperative speech therapy is provided when the patient is not able to spontaneously return to a relatively normal, clear, soft phonatory voice. The chest muscle fatigue (from pushing against the tightly closed glottis during phonation) is eliminated. Most importantly, these persons are able to stop being vocal cripples and even to forget about their voices and just proceed to talk. It is not necessary for them to make an enormous effort to learn to speak in an unnatural way. In fact, the biggest problem in resuming "normal" phonatory speech so far has been in the patients who have had the most effective preoperative speech therapy or who have developed a lot of associated movements in their desperate attempt to speak. Even the worst of these, however, were dramatically better within minutes after the lidocaine injection and within an hour after surgery (*i.e.*, as soon as they were awake enough to talk in the recovery room).

Theoretically, a vocal cord could also be repositioned slightly away from the midline and preserve the recurrent nerve by placing a silk suture between the arytenoid and the thyroid ala. Since there is a limit to how far the mobile cord can adduct, this would tie it back so the mobile one could just reach it at the end of its excursion, preventing the overtight closure and vocal spasticity. However, it is more difficult to reposition a cord in the ideal paramedian position with a tie-back suture than by sectioning a recurrent nerve. Furthermore, the suture would soon cut through the cartilage because of the strong persistent adduction, which is not present in the patients who require Woodman operations for bilateral recurrent nerve paralysis. Speech therapy has then improved the voice further when necessary. It is designed to get the patient to do three things:

1. Raise the pitch from the back of the throat ideally to a clear phonatory level (which may well not equal the prespastic dysphonic "normal"). This pitch adjustment is sometimes necessary to minimize or eliminate diplophonia, which is present in some of these patients postoperatively because of the slightly different vocal cord tension on the two sides. (The diplophonia can be minimized or eliminated by matching the mobile vocal cord frequency to that of the paralyzed vocal cord.)

2. Resume normal volume and pressure of air flow through the larynx.

3. Eliminate the associated face and neck movements and throat clearing, which all the patients so far have been able to do rapidly once they were able to achieve reliable, easy laryngeal phonation.

If the vocal cord were to atrophy and move too far from the midline, Teflon® injection could be used to reposition it. If the cord did not end up far enough lateral from the midline to prevent the other vocal cord from reaching it too tightly, a direct laryngoscopy and excision of some of the free edge of the vocal cord could be performed. So far neither of these secondary procedures has been necessary.

The main problem now is getting used to the idea of sectioning a recurrent nerve for a disease widely considered to be psychoneurotic. However, severing the facial nerve for blepharospasm must have been just as shocking initially.

Many of these people have had difficulty retaining jobs and friends and some have become recluses. The satisfying part of this surgical procedure, which has been as dramatic as with many patients after repair of severe hearing loss by stapedectomy, is seeing these patients resume normal, happy lives. Just as stapedectomy can provide a dramatic improvement in hearing and be successful without return to "normal" (0 dB), recurrent nerve section can dramatically improve a spastic dysphonic voice even when it does not return completely to "normal." However, deliberate surgical section to achieve permanent unilateral recurrent nerve paralysis is not yet standard treatment for even as disabling a disease as spastic dysphonia; it should not be done without careful preparation and evaluation.

REFERENCES

1. Traube, cited by Arnold GE: Spastic dysphonia: I. Changing interpretations of a persistent affliction. Logos 2:3-14, 1959

2. Schnitzler, cited by Arnold GE: Spastic dysphonia: I. Changing interpretations of a persistent affliction. Logos 2:3-14, 1959

3. Berendes, cited by Arnold GE: Spastic dysphonia: I. Changing interpretations of a persistent affliction. Logos 2.3-14, 1959

4. Robe E, Brumlik J, Moore P: A study of spastic dysphonia. Neurologic and electroencephalographic abnormalities. Laryngoscope 79:219-245, 1960

5. Aronson AW, Brown JR, Litin EM, *et al*: Spastic dysphonia. I. Voice, neurologic, and psychiatric aspects. J Speech Hear Dis 33:203-218, 1968

6. Aronson AW, Brown JR, Litin EM, *et al*: Spastic dysphonia. II. Comparison with essential (voice) tremor and other neurologic and psychogenic dysphonias. J Speech Hear Dis 33:219-231, 1968

7. Brodnitz FS: Spastic dysphonia. Ann Otol Rhinol Laryngol 85:210-214, 1976

8. Cooper M: *Modern Techniques of Vocal Rehabilitation*, ed 2. Springfield, Ill., Charles C. Thomas, 1974

9. Boone DR: *The Voice and Voice Therapy*. Englewood Cliffs, N.J., Prentice-Hall, Inc., 1971

10. Rethi A: Role des stylopharyngealen muskelsystems im Krankheitsbild der Taschenbandstimme und der dysphonia spastica. Folia Phoniatr (Basel) 4:201-216, 1952

11. Dedo HH: The paralyzed larynx: An electromyographic study in dogs and humans. Laryngoscope 80:1455-1517, 1970

12. Dedo HH, Urrea RD, Lawson L: Intracordal injection of Teflon® in the treatment of 135 patients with dysphonia. Ann Otol Rhinol Laryngol 82:661-667, 1973

13. Bloch P: Neuro-psychiatric aspects of spastic dysphonia. Folia Phoniatr (Basel) 17: 301-364, 1965

ACKNOWLEDGMENTS—The author wishes to express appreciation to Francis A Sooy, MD, Joseph H. Ogura, MD, Roger Boles, MD, and the Nationl Institutes of Health for providing the training, support, and milieu which made this work possible.

REPRINTS—Herbert H. Dedo, MD, Department of Otolaryngology, University of California, 400 Parnassus Ave., San Francisco, CA 94143.

Commentary

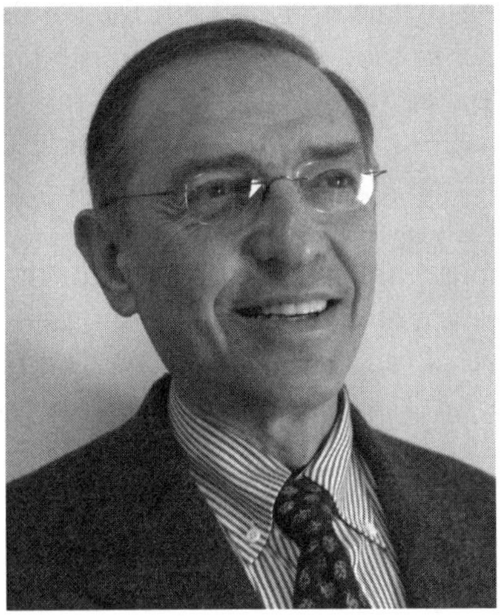

Andrew Blitzer, MD, DDS, FACS

In 1975, I did my first recurrent laryngeal nerve section at the Mt. Sinai Hospital in New York City with my mentor, Dr. Hugh Biller. Spastic dysphonia was a strange disorder that I really didn't understand. Dr. Herb Dedo designed this operation as a way of treating the symptom. He gets tremendous credit for having taken a disorder that was considered psychogenic, and returned these patients to the laryngologist. He noted that injecting an anesthetic agent near the recurrent nerve, temporarily paralyzing the vocal fold, could eliminate the strain-strangled voice in many of the patients.

Later, Dr. Max Som, another of my mentors and giant in the field of laryngology, told me that the operation violated a basic concept in laryngeal and head and neck surgery. The surgeon should always protect and defend the recurrent laryngeal nerve. He then developed an alternative, the recurrent laryngeal nerve "crush" procedure. His thought was that it would temporarily paralyze the nerve, but would regain function after several months, and perhaps eliminate the symptom by altered reinnervation. Max Som, Hugh Biller, and Bill Lawson published a few cases utilizing this technique in 1983. A few years later, they published another paper stating that all of the patients had a return of symptoms, and therefore they did not any longer recommend the operation.

Arnold Aronson at the Mayo Clinic, further characterized SD into adductor (strain-strangled) type and abductor (whispering) type. Cannito et al reported that all of the SD patients were "mixed" with a predomination of one type or the other, and that some patients would switch types or present with both. This further reinforced the concept of a central etiology.

Aronson later reported the Mayo Clinic experience with RLN section and found after 3 years that only 30% of the patients still were symptom free. My series also showed a great number of initial successes, with later failures. The nature of this disorder as well as the failures was still elusive. I began performing laryngeal EMGs on these patients in hopes of finding some of the answers. We found a number of variables that suggested hyperfunction, but nothing that was diagnostic. In the early 1980s, annual meeting of the Voice Foundation had a panel dedicated to the subject "Spastic Dysphonia." Dr. George Gates, the chair of the panel, challenged us to try to decipher the pathophysiology of the disorder. The panel posed more questions than answers. We agreed that this was probably not a psychogenic disorder, and that it should be termed "spasmodic dysphonia" because it wasn't a spastic disease.

The challenge of the panel, and the new questions led me to Dr. Stan Fahn, Director of the Movement Disorders group at the Neurological Institute in New York City. It also led to my collaboration with Dr. Mitchell Brin (a movement disorders neurologist). This became a long friendship and a wonderful and productive academic team. Drs. Fahn and Brin had a number of children and some adults with known generalized dystonia, who also had voices like the "spasmodic dysphonia" patients that I evaluated. We performed EMGs, laryngoscopies, and voice analysis on these patients too, and they seemed very similar to ours. We postulated that my patients had a "focal" dystonia, much like writer's cramp, torticollis, or blepharospasm. At about the same time, Dr. David Marsden's group (movement disorders neurology at Queen's Square Hospital in London) published their analysis of Meige disease patients and suggested that Meige disease was a multifocal cranial dystonia and that a number had laryngeal involvement. They further speculated that isolated focal laryngeal disease could be represented as "spastic dysphonia." The findings of our group and of Marsden's group now put the disorders in the central nervous system (probably at the basal ganglia), and helped to explain the phenomenology and failures of local treatments for focal dystonias. These included nerve sections, myotomies, injection of caustic agents, peripheral nerve stimulators, and others. The link between the temporal lobe, which generated electrical signals for a particular activity, was discoordinated in the brainstem before it got to the muscles needed for a particular function.

Now with this new information, how does one treat these patients? Believing that this was a central nervous system disorder, we began giving many oral agents that were used for dystonia treatment (eg, tranquilizers, baclophen, artane). Some patients had benefit, but the side effects of the agents (sleepiness and forgetfulness in particular) made using these agents for a focal symptom difficult.

In the late 1970s, Dr. Alan Scott, a pediatric ophthalmologist at UCSF, was working on agents that could be used to improve the results in strabismus surgery. He looked at the possibility of using an injectable muscle-weakening agent, and studied cobra venom, alpha bungarotoxin, botulinum toxin, and others and found that small amounts of botulinum toxin could predictably weaken muscle for a long period of time. He did animal studies, and then human clinical trials. Once finding an agent that could predictably weaken the muscles of the eye, Dr. Scott applied this to other disorders of the eye with muscle hyperfunction, namely, blepharospasm and hemifacial spasm. In 1983, the FDA awarded grants to Drs. Stan Fahn (Columbia), Joe Jankovic (Baylor), and Mark Hallet (NIH), all movement disorders neurology experts, to see if injections of botulinum toxin could be applied to other focal and generalized dystonia patients.

In 1983, I injected the first jaw patient (oromandibular dystonia) and in April of 1984 the first spasmodic dysphonia patient. The SD patient had blepharospasm and was treated by Dr. Scott with botulinum toxin successfully. He then developed SD, and wanted the same agent injected into his vocal folds. The consent process involved myself, three neurologists, a research nurse, and lawyers from the hospital and the university. It was video recorded. I had no idea of dose, so we tried to calculate the volume of the orbicularis oculi muscle and the dose for that muscle and compare it to the thyroarytenoid muscle. I injected only one vocal fold with 3 units of toxin. The patient was then taken to the ICU with a tracheostomy set at the bedside. Over the next 2 days, no change was noted. I then added another 3 units and, at about 1 week, he had a relatively normal voice.

Over the next several years we continued to acquire additional patients who also achieved improvement in their ability to speak. I reported this first group of patients to the Triological Society in 1987 and published it in 1988. The response ranged from some who thought it was a curiosity to others who questioned why I was trying to inject patients who had a "surgical" disease. Soon after, Bob Miller's group, Charles Ford's group, and Christy Ludlow's group all reported variation in technique, but similar successful treatments. We extended the treatments to the abductor type, injecting the posterior cricoarytenoid muscle via an external cervical and a transcricothyroid membrane approach. We also identified other varieties of the laryngeal syndrome who only had their spasms when breathing (adductor respiratory dystonia) or those whose singing voice was primarily involved, adductor "singer's" dystonia.

Since the initial reports, over 100 papers have been published on botulinum toxin treatments for SD and it is available in just about every city in the United States, and many other parts of the world. Debates continue on whether to treat one vocal fold, both, other muscles, dosing, and ancillary treatments. Other surgical treatments and implantable stimulators have been reported. None of these treat the cause (brainstem) and therefore fail as the brain reacts to the surgical change. We reported a group of recurrent laryngeal nerve section failures, which were then treated with botulinum toxin. These failures were from in growth of motor fibers from other muscles giving tone, or a central processing reorganization exaggerating the dystonic behavior of the functional laryngeal muscles.

Our philosophy has been to individualize treatment, because we are only treating symptom. We have patients who receive unilateral, bilateral, bilateral staggered, and mini doses. Many are also on small amounts of oral agents that work centrally. A few of our generalized dystonia patients who also have SD have undergone deep brain stimulator surgery. Most have had improvement of their voices as well as of other body parts. Eventually, treatment will be able to chemically or genetically treat the central nervous system.

Our group in conjunction with Ozellius' group helped to find the DYT1 gene at the 9q34 locus. Two new neural proteins were found to be produced by this gene, called torsin A and torsin B. Much work had been done since then, trying to identify the location and function of these neural proteins in the brain. In addition to genetic transmission of the disorder, there may be viral or idiopathic mutations also producing these mutant neural proteins. New and interesting work has already been done to perform allele-specific silencing of these mutant proteins. This is the very beginning of changing brain function with control of neural proteins, thereby normalizing signal to the periphery and abolishing dystonic activity. Once we are able to change the brain function by altering mutant neural proteins, peripheral treatment of the larynx for SD will be unnecessary.

Recommended Readings

Dedo HH. Recurrent laryngeal nerve section for spastic dysphonia. *Ann Otol Rhinol Laryngol.* 1976;85:451–459.

Biller HF, Som ML, Lawson W. Laryngeal nerve crush for spastic dysphonia. *Ann Otol Rhinol Laryngol.* 1983; 92:469.

Aronson AE, DeSanto LW. Adductor spastic dysphonia: three years after recurrent laryngeal nerve section. *Laryngoscope.* 1983;93:1–938.

Scott AB. Clostridial toxins as therapeutic agents. In: Simpson LL, ed., *Botulinum Neurotoxin and Tetanus Toxin.* New York, NY: Academic Press; 1989:399–412.

Blitzer A, Brin MF, Fahn S, et al. Localized injections of botulinum toxin for the treatment of focal laryngeal dystonia (spastic dysphonia). *Laryngoscope.* 1988;96: 193–197.

Ozelius LJ, Hewett JW, Page CE, et al. The early-onset tortion dystonia gene (DYT1) encodes an ATP-binding protein. *Nat Genet.* 1997;17:40–48.

Gonzales-Alegre P, Miller VM, Davidson BL, et al. Toward therapy for DYT1 dystonia: allele-specific silencing of mutant TorsinA. *Ann Neurol.* 2003;53:781–787.

Blitzer A, Lovelace RE, Brin MF, et al. Electromyographic findings in focal laryngeal dystonias (spastic dysphonia). *Ann Otol Rhino Laryngol.* 1985;94:591–594.

Friedman M, Toriumi DM, Grybauskas VT, Applebaum EL. Implantation of a recurrent laryngeal nerve stimulator for the treatment of spastic dysphonia. *Ann Otol Rhinol Laryngol.* 1989;98:130–134.

Isshiki N, Haji T, Yamamoto Y, Mahieu HF. Thyroplasty for adductor spasmodic dysphonia: further experiences. *Laryngoscope.* 2001;111:615–621.

Berke GS, Blackwell KE, Gerratt BR, et al. Selective laryngeal adductor denervation-reinnervation: a new surgical treatment for adductor spasmodic dysphonia. *Ann Otol Rhinol Laryngol.* 1999;108:227–231.

Cannito MO, Johnson P. Spasmodic dysphonia: a continuum disorder. *J Commun Disord.* 1981;14:215–223.

Grillone GA, Blitzer A, Brin MF, Annino DJ, Saint-Hilaire MH. Treatment of adductor laryngeal breathing dystonia with botulinum toxin type A. *Laryngoscope.* 1994;104:30–32.

Marsden CD, Sheehy MP. Dysphonia, Meige disease, and tortion dystonia. *Neurology.* 1982;32:1202–1203.

Chitkara A, Meyer T, Keidar A, Blitzer A. Singer's dystonia: first report of a variant of spasmodic dysphonia. *Ann Otol Rhinol Laryngol.* 2006;115(2):89–92.

LARYNGEAL DYSTONIA: A SERIES WITH BOTULINUM TOXIN THERAPY

ANDREW BLITZER, MD, DDS MITCHELL F. BRIN, MD

NEW YORK, NEW YORK

Laryngeal dystonia is a syndrome characterized by action-induced, involuntary spasms of the laryngeal muscles. Most patients have involvement of the adductor laryngeal muscles producing uncontrolled spasms during phonation, and a "strain-strangle" speech pattern commonly termed "spastic dysphonia." Other patients have involvement of the abductor muscles producing "whispering dysphonia." Rare patients have paradoxical vocal cord motion during respiration with adductor spasms on inspiration. Over the past 5 years we have used botulinum toxin (BOTOX) to treat more than 200 patients with laryngeal dystonia. This group includes patients with adductor involvement (phonatory dystonia, recurrent laryngeal nerve section failure, respiratory dystonia) and those with abductor involvement (whispering dystonia). Patients received benefit within 24 to 72 hours, with sustained improvement for 2 to 9 months with an average of 4 months. Patients improved to an average of 90% of normal function. Clinically significant adverse effects included extended breathy dysphonia and mild choking on fluids. BOTOX has become our treatment of choice for dystonic conditions of the larynx.

KEY WORDS — botulinum toxin, laryngeal dystonia, spastic dysphonia.

Laryngeal dystonia is a neurologic disorder of central motor processing characterized by action-induced spasms of the vocal cords. The spasms are poorly controlled by the patient, and the symptoms are exacerbated by stress. These spasms produce a clinical voice syndrome often termed spasmodic dysphonia (SD) or spastic dysphonia, which is characterized by a choked, constrained voice pattern with breaks in vocalization.[1,2] In addition, the voice pattern may also be tremulous with inhalation phonation, harshness, and audible grunts. In addition to the adductor form of laryngeal dystonia, approximately 10% of patients will present with the abductor form. In this form of phonation, the cords will have a spasmodic motion of the posterior cricoarytenoid (PCA) muscles, producing a breathy voice. The history of observations of SD has previously been reported.[2-8] Our group and others[9-12] have linked SD to dystonia, a central nervous system disorder. Dystonia may manifest itself in other focal and segmental presentations, including blepharospasm (forced, involuntary eye closure), oromandibular dystonia (face, jaw, or tongue involvement), torticollis (twisting of the neck), and writer's cramp (action-induced dystonic contractions of the hand muscles).[13-16] Laryngeal dystonia may present focally or in association with other dystonic movements.

Vocal analysis of the adductor SD patients reveals harshness, usually a tremor, inappropriate pitch or pitch breaks, groaning, breathiness, and glottal fry.[17,18] The voice arrests come from hyperadduction of the true and false vocal cords. Some of the patients with tremor have synchronous involvement of the pharynx, face, masticatory muscles, etc.[19,20] The abductor SD patients were described by Aronson et al[10] in 1968 as a group with a whispering dysphonia or aphonia. This may be the earliest report of the true abductor SD. Many of these patients may be misdiagnosed as having a vocal cord paralysis.

Our electromyography (EMG) data also showed 17% of patients with enlarged potentials, as well as 11% with polyphasic potentials.[9,21] This finding is indicative of some reorganizational activity, perhaps denervation and reinnervation.

In addition we have identified two other variations of presentation. The term compensatory abductor dysphonia refers to those patients with such severe adductor spasms that they voluntarily produce a breathy voice by not contracting their vocal cords in order to prevent the spasms and the broken speech pattern. Patients with compensatory adductor dysphonia are those severe abductors who try to prevent the breathiness by tightly contracting their vocal cords.[1]

Psychotherapy, speech therapy, and biofeedback are generally unsuccessful methods of treating SD. Recurrent laryngeal nerve section has a long-term success rate of about 36%,[22] with continued vocal cord paralysis. We have postulated[20] that this failure rate is related to hyperfunction of the opposing hyperfunctional dystonic muscle, which usually exaggerates the dystonic symptoms. Our series[1] has shown poor results of treatment of adductor dystonia with medication, although there was a 33% response rate in the abductor type. We therefore established a program of treatment of laryngeal dystonia with botulinum toxin (BOTOX) injections.

From the Departments of Otolaryngology (Blitzer) and Neurology (Brin) and the Dystonia Clinical Research Center (both authors), Columbia-Presbyterian Medical Center, New York, New York. Supported in part by a grant from the Dystonia Medical Research Foundation.

Presented at the meeting of the American Laryngological Association, Palm Beach, Florida, April 28-29, 1990.

REPRINTS — Andrew Blitzer, MD, DDS, Dept of Otolaryngology, Columbia-Presbyterian Medical Center, 630 W 168th St, New York, NY 10032.

METHODS

CLINICAL DATA

This study (approved by our Institutional Review Board) consists of a group of 260 primary and 60 secondary laryngeal dystonia patients, of whom 210 patients had the presumptive diagnosis of SD (adductor or abductor laryngeal dystonia) when referred. Patients were evaluated with a detailed history and physical examination including direct fiberoptic laryngoscopy with video recording, a complete neurologic examination, and laryngeal EMG; some had brain stem audiometric evoked response and magnetic resonance imaging scans. In questionable cases, the videotapes were reviewed to confirm the diagnosis. Patient data are stored in a Foxbase data base.

Initially we only invited patients who had previously failed treatment with pharmacotherapeutic agents. BOTOX has been so successful as compared to other modalities, with few clinically significant side effects, that we began to offer BOTOX as primary therapy. We also have offered BOTOX therapy to patients who have failed surgical therapy (recurrent laryngeal nerve section and anterior commissure release procedures), patients with abductor laryngeal dystonia, and patients with dystonic respiratory laryngeal dysrhythmias.

INJECTION TECHNIQUE

Adductor. Each patient had injections that were individualized with doses of 1.25 U to 3.75 U. Injections were given percutaneously with EMG guidance as we have previously reported.[23]

Abductor. The first abductor patient was initially treated with BOTOX via a direct laryngoscopy and injection into the PCA muscle. This was not possible to do with EMG control, and besides the patient discomfort, very little improvement was noted. We next began EMG-guided percutaneous injection. The larynx is manually rotated away from the side of intended injection and the hollow EMG needle with syringe is placed posterior to the posterior edge of the thyroid lamina. The needle is advanced to the cricoid cartilage and then moved out under EMG guidance to the optimum position in the PCA muscle.

RATING

Patient's voices were scored in a nonblinded fashion by means of a subjective rating scale estimating the percent of normal speech, with 0% representing no speech or full disability and 100% representing normal speech. Patients scored themselves before each injection, and a videotaping and voice recording were performed. In addition, the physicians made a similar rating and the most conservative rating was recorded and used as the percent improvement in all cases. Patients kept diaries of vocal function, noting the time of onset of vocal weakness, peak weakness, duration of breathy hypophonia, duration and severity of choking with liquids, and any other notable events. No correlation was made between the observed improvement and vocal cord paralysis, since with our technique, paralysis is very rare. Postinjection EMG studies were performed on the 2-week follow-up visit in a limited number of patients early in our study. The studies were not carried out in all patients since they did not appear to have direct clinical relevance.

DYSTONIA AT COLUMBIA-PRESBYTERIAN MEDICAL CENTER

	Laryngeal Dystonia (N = 320)		*All Dystonia (N = 1,926)*	
	Primary	*Secondary*	*Primary*	*Secondary*
N	260 (81%)	60 (19%)	1,356 (70%)	570 (30%)
F	152 (58%)	36 (60%)	813 (60%)	326 (57%)
M	108 (42%)	24 (40%)	543 (40%)	244 (43%)
F:M	1.4	1.5	1.5	1.3
Jewish	60 (23%)	13 (22%)	325 (24%)	112 (20%)
Non-Jewish	200 (77%)	47 (78%)	1,031 (76%)	458 (80%)
J:NJ	0.30	0.28	0.32	0.25
Positive family history	44 (17%)	5 (8%)	248 (18%)	48 (8%)
Focal	168 (65%)	15 (25%)	770 (57%)	168 (30%)
Segmental cranial	43 (17%)	6 (10%)	191 (14%)	55 (10%)
All segmental /hemidystonia	70 (27%)	18 (30%)	431 (32%)	203 (36%)
Generalized	20 (8%)	23 (38%)	138 (10%)	138 (24%)

RESULTS

CLINICAL CHARACTERISTICS

Laryngeal Dystonia Data. Of the 1,926 cases of dystonia registered at the Dystonia Clinical Research Center, 320 cases (16.6%) had vocal involvement. Of these 320 patients, 260 (81%) had primary dystonia and 60 (19%) had secondary dystonia (see Table). Of the primary group, 152 (58%) were female and 108 (42%) were male. This is very similar to the 60% female/40% male ratio found in the entire group of primary dystonias. The Jewish/non-Jewish ratio for primary laryngeal dystonia was 23%/77%, which is consistent with the 24%/76% found in the entire primary dystonia group.

In the group of 320 patients with laryngeal dystonia, 270 (84.4%) had adductor vocal involvement ("spastic dysphonia"); 47 (14.6%) had abductor vocal involvement ("whispering dysphonia"); and 3 (1%) had adductor breathing dystonia. The average age at onset of SD patients was 38. The three patients with laryngeal adductor breathing dystonia were 27, 55, and 56 years of age at onset. Of interest was the fact that 27 patients of the primary dystonia group (10.4%) had laryngeal involvement first and then went on to have involvement of another neuromuscular system. The importance of family history is illustrated by the fact that 44 of the 260 (17%) patients who had primary laryngeal dystonia had a family history of dystonia.

BOTULINUM TOXIN THERAPY

Adductor Laryngeal Dystonia. Of the 320 cases of laryngeal dystonia recorded in our data base, we have injected 210 patients since April 1984. At the inception of our study, there were no previous guidelines for laryngeal BOTOX injections and therefore our dose schedule was empiric. Recognizing that the vocalis-thyroarytenoid complex consists of small muscles, we planned small doses with the goal of minimizing adverse effects and vocal trauma. Our first approach was to inject 2.5 U into one vocal cord. This injection had little effect. We then gave an additional 7.5 U, which caused a vocal cord paresis and a period of breathy dysphonia but 90% improvement of vocal function. In keeping with our goal of minimizing the total exposure to BOTOX, we decided to explore bilateral, low-dose injections. This decision also paralleled our theory that weakening or paralyzing one vocal cord stresses the remaining vocal cord and exaggerates the dystonic symptoms. We therefore initiated a first-treatment program of injecting both vocalis muscles with 3.75 U. All patients experienced benefit. Initially there was an effect within the first 24 hours, followed by a hypophonia that was maximum at the third post-injection day. This breathy speech typically lasted 4 to 14 days and was mild, but lasted 57 days in one patient. Some patients also experienced a mild choking sensation when drinking fluids, although there were no cases of aspiration. Patients found that drinking slowly compensated adequately for this symptom until it resolved. Patients' speaking improved from 60% to 100% of normal function with a mean of 90%, and the duration of effect was from 3 to 4 months. Patients often requested reinjection before returning to their pretreatment level of functioning. When we performed 2-week follow-up laryngeal EMG, occasional evidence of denervation could be found.

Owing to the prolonged period of breathy hypophonia in some of the patients receiving 3.75 U per vocal cord, we modified our first treatment protocol by reducing the dose to 2.5 U per vocal cord. Although there was a trend for decreased duration of breathiness, choking, and duration of benefit at 2.5 U, the differences were not statistically significant. Two patients, however, failed to have any noticeable effect at the lower dose and had to be reinjected. Because of the lack of significant difference in the duration or degree of benefit of these two doses, our current protocol is to initially inject 2.5 U per cord except when the patient finds it impossible to make a return visit in 2 weeks should the injection have no effect. In these patients a dose of 3.75 U per cord is given. For repeat injections, we initially injected either 3.75 or 2.5 U per cord. We have begun to give some patients 2.5 U unilaterally or 1.25 U bilaterally on follow-up to minimize the length of hypophonia, since there often appears to be some residual weakness at the time of the follow-up injection.

The adverse effects from laryngeal BOTOX injections included a mild breathy dysphonia for a short period of time in 45% of patients and mild choking on fluids for the first several days in 22%. Several patients hyperventilated and became dizzy trying to speak while hypophonic. Several patients coughed up blood-tinged sputum and/or had a sore throat. One patient had itching but no rash.

Nerve Section. Of the adductor vocal group, nine were patients who had failed a recurrent laryngeal nerve section. This group, previously reported,[20] included four men and five women ranging in age from 36 to 62 with a mean of 50. They all failed RLN section from 0 to 4 years postoperatively (mean, 1.8 years). Four of the patients had more than one procedure performed on the nerve or vocal cord to try to turn failure into success. Laryngeal EMG was performed on all patients; most showed signs of chronic denervation with few and very small potentials and occasional fibrillation potentials. We injected most of the patients with 2.5 U unilaterally. This was given in the functional cord in most patients with an improvement of 0% to 100% with a mean of 81% as compared to 10% to 80% with a mean of 59% when the paralyzed cord was injected.

Anterior Commissure Release. In addition to the nerve section failures we have treated three patients who failed an anterior commissure release procedure. In these patients the larynx appeared foreshortened, but the adductor spasms were as intense as in the nonoperated group. These patients were also given 2.5 U per vocal cord, and all experienced benefit. The spasms remitted, but because of the laxity of the vocal cord from the release, most noticed a narrowed pitch range. The duration of the breathy hypophonia also was extended in this group.

Abductor Laryngeal Dystonia. With our growing experience, we cautiously elected to treat abductor laryngeal dystonia with injection of BOTOX into the PCA muscle. We informed the patients that excessive weakening of the PCA muscle might cause airway distress and might necessitate a temporary tracheostomy. Doses of 1.25 to 5 U were given in one to four treatments to weaken one or both PCA muscles in 12 patients. Marked improvement was seen in 8, with a mean improvement to 57% and a return of mean maximal functional performance to 80% of normal. Follow-up treatments required smaller toxin doses. The adverse effects included brief choking on fluids without aspiration and mild stridor on exertion in 2 patients. There were no significant breathing difficulties, even in the cases in which both PCA muscles were injected.

Adductor Laryngeal Breathing Dystonia. In addition to the patients who had phonatory symptoms due to laryngeal dystonia, we identified three patients who had paradoxical motion of the vocal cords during respiration. These patients were not hypoxic, but produced moderate to severe inspiratory stridor. This symptom disappeared as soon as the patients went to sleep, and took a short while after awakening in the morning to reappear. After a thorough otolaryngologic, neurologic, and pulmonary workup, we treated two of these patients with BOTOX with decrease or cessation of the symptoms. A complete description of these patients and their test results will be published separately.

DISCUSSION

The data from our previous publications,[1,9,15,19-21,23] our current series, and reports of other authors support the conclusion that "spastic dysphonia" and "whispering dysphonia" are focal laryngeal forms of dystonia. Our data on age of onset, sex preponderance, Jewish/non-Jewish ratio, family history, and involvement of other body parts are consistent with those of other authors and with those of our total dystonia group.

The average age at onset in our entire group was 38 for both the adductor and abductor forms. The average age of patients who had primary dystonia of the larynx and another body part was 31, since patients with early-onset disease are more likely to have more than one site involved.

Of the 260 patients who had the larynx as their primary site of onset, 27 (10.4%) had spread to another body part. These data suggest that patients should be advised of possible spread and be followed and reexamined on a regular basis for signs of other dystonic involvement. The family history was also significant, with 44 of 260 patients (17%) with primary laryngeal dystonia having a family history of dystonia. Family studies of childhood onset idiopathic dystonia show an autosomal dominant inheritance with reduced penetrance. A gene locus marker located on the 9q chromosome has just recently been established by our group and others, and this finding opens new doorways for the understanding and possible treatment of the disorder.[24] Therefore, it is of paramount importance to obtain a family history and have genetic counseling provided where necessary.

Recurrent laryngeal nerve section originally seemed to be the treatment of choice for SD. However, many late failures were found leaving a poor voice with a continued paralyzed vocal cord. We believe that the return of symptoms in these patients is due to stressing the remaining functioning vocal cord, thereby intensifying the dystonic symptoms.

Ludlow et al[25] and Miller et al[26] have injected higher doses of toxin (up to 60 U over three visits) into one vocalis muscle in patients with SD. Since the goal of this treatment method is unilateral vocal cord paralysis, we see little advantage of this technique over recurrent laryngeal nerve section. We have theorized that surgical therapy may ultimately fail because the contralateral functioning vocal cord hyperadducts. This hyperadduction stresses the remaining functional vocal cord and exaggerates the underlying dystonic state, causing additional dysfunction and a return of the dysphonia.

Our experience with 210 patients has shown that local injections of BOTOX into laryngeal muscles is a relatively safe and effective mode of therapy for laryngeal dystonia. In contrast to surgical therapy, BOTOX injections have the advantage of being given on an ambulatory basis; both vocal cords can be treated; and the toxin is given under EMG control for precise localization of the most active part of the muscle complex. Graded weakening can be achieved by using low dosages and repeating the injections to achieve the optimum weakness desired. If too much weakness is produced, the strength gradually returns with time. The procedure is very acceptable to patients with very satisfactory vocal results. It is too soon to tell whether patients will become refractory to this form of therapy. To date we have not found anyone who has become refractory with laryngeal injections or sustained a disability from laryngeal toxin injections.

CONCLUSION

Laryngeal dystonia is a disorder of central motor processing that can cause adductor spasms ("spastic dysphonia"), abductor spasms ("whispering dysphonia"), and adductor breathing dystonia. Laryngeal BOTOX injections are performed percutaneously, on an ambulatory basis under EMG control. Graded weakening can be achieved by using small dosages and injecting additional toxin as needed. If too much weakness is produced, the strength gradually returns with time. Our data suggest that BOTOX injection is the treatment of choice for dystonic symptoms of the larynx.

REFERENCES

1. Blitzer A, Brin MF, Fahn S, Lovelace RE. Clinical and laboratory characteristics of focal laryngeal dystonia: study of 110 cases. Laryngoscope 1988;98:636-40.

2. Traube L. Spastiche Form der nervosen heiserkeit. Gerammelte Beitr Pathol Physiol 1871;2:677.

3. Fraenkel B. Ueber die beschaeftigungsschwaeche der stimme: mogiphonie. Dtsch Med Wochenschr 1887;13:121-3.

4. Critchley M. Spastic dysphonia ("inspiratory speech"). Brain 1939;62:96-103.

5. Bloch P. Neuro-psychiatric aspects of spastic dysphonia. Folia Phoniatr (Basel) 1965;17:301-64.

6. Marsden CD, Sheehy MP. Spastic dysphonia, Meige disease and tortion dystonia. Neurology 1982;32:1202-3.

7. Golper LAC, Nutt JG, Rau MT, Coleman RO. Focal

cranial dystonia. J Speech Hear Disord 1983;48:128-34.

8. Schaefer SD. Neuropathology of spasmodic dysphonia. Laryngoscope 1983;93:1183-204.

9. Blitzer A, Lovelace RE, Brin MF, Fahn S, Fink ME. Electromyographic findings in focal laryngeal dystonia (spastic dysphonia). Ann Otol Rhinol Laryngol 1985;94:591-4.

10. Aronson AE, Brown JR, Litin EM, Pearson JS. Spastic dysphonia II. Comparison with essential (voice) tremor and other neurologic dysphonias. J Speech Hear Disord 1968;33:219-31.

11. Dedo HH, Izdebski K. Problems with surgical (RLN section) treatment of spastic dysphonia. Laryngoscope 1983;93: 268-71.

12. Feldman M, Nixon JV, Finitzo-Hieber T, Freeman FJ. Abnormal parasympathetic vagal functions in patients with spastic dysphonia. Ann Intern Med 1984;100:491-5.

13. Fahn S, Marsden CD, Calne DB. Classification and investigation of dystonia. In: Marsden CD, Fahn S, eds. Movement disorders 2. London, England: Butterworths, 1987:332-58.

14. Fahn S. The varied clinical expressions of dystonia. Neurol Clin 1984;2:541-54.

15. Brin MF, Fahn S, Moscowitz C, et al. Localized injections of botulinum toxin for the treatment of focal dystonia and hemifacial spasm. Movement Disord 1987;2:237-54.

16. Brin MF, Blitzer A, Fahn S, Ramig LO, Stewart C. Laryngeal motion disorders. In: Blitzer A, Brin MF, Fahn S, Sasaki CT, Harris K, eds. Neurological disorders of the larynx. New York, NY: Thieme Medical Publishing (in press).

17. Aronson AE, Hartman DE. Adductor spastic dysphonia as a sign of essential (voice) tremor. J Speech Hear Disord 1981;45: 52-8.

18. Ludlow CL, Naunton RF, Bassich CJ. Procedures for the selection of spastic dysphonia patients for recurrent laryngeal nerve section. Otolaryngol Head Neck Surg 1984;92:24-31.

19. Brin MF, Blitzer A, Fahn S, Gould W, Lovelace RE. Adductor laryngeal dystonia (spastic dysphonia): treatment with local injections of botulinum toxin (Botox). Movement Disord 1989;4:287-96.

20. Blitzer A, Brin MF, Fahn S. Botulinum toxin therapy for recurrent laryngeal nerve section failure for adductor laryngeal dystonia [Abstract]. Trans Am Laryngol Assoc 1989;110:206.

21. Lovelace RE, Blitzer A, Szmidt-Salkowska E. Percutaneous laryngeal electromyography for evaluation of neurologic disorders, myopathies, and spastic dysphonia. Electroencephalogr Clin Neurophysiol 1985;61:576.

22. Aronson AE, DeSanto LW. Adductor spastic dysphonia: three years after recurrent nerve section. Laryngoscope 1983;93: 1-8.

23. Blitzer A, Brin MF, Fahn S, Lovelace RE. Localized injections of botulinum toxin for the treatment of focal laryngeal dystonia (spastic dysphonia). Laryngoscope 1988;98:193-7.

24. Bressman SB, de Leon D, Brin MF, et al. Idiopathic dystonia among Ashkenazi Jews: evidence for autosomal dominant inheritance. Ann Neurol 1989;26:612-20.

25. Ludlow CL, Naunton RF, Sedory SE, Schultz GM, Hallett M. Effects of botulinum toxin injection on speech in adductor spasmodic dysphonia. Neurology 1988;38:1220-5.

26. Miller RH, Woodson GE, Jankovic J. Botulinum toxin injection of the vocal fold for spasmodic dysphonia. Arch Otolaryngol Head Neck Surg 1987;113:603-5.

≈

15

Laryngeal Transplant

Introduction

As of this writing, laryngeal transplant remains a singular achievement, completed in the face of no small amount of skepticism and resistance. Dr. Strome offers a revealing commentary alongside his description of the case, in which he reflects on challenges and personal doubts encountered in pursuing his goal. It is frankly difficult to decide whether his account of the path to success or his vision of the future is the more inspiring.

Classic Article

- ●Reprint of article included in this chapter.
- ♦Commentary on this article.

●♦Strome M, Stein J, Esclamado R, Hicks D, et al. Laryngeal transplantation and 40-month follow-up. *N Engl J Med.* 2001;344(22):1676–1679.

Commentary

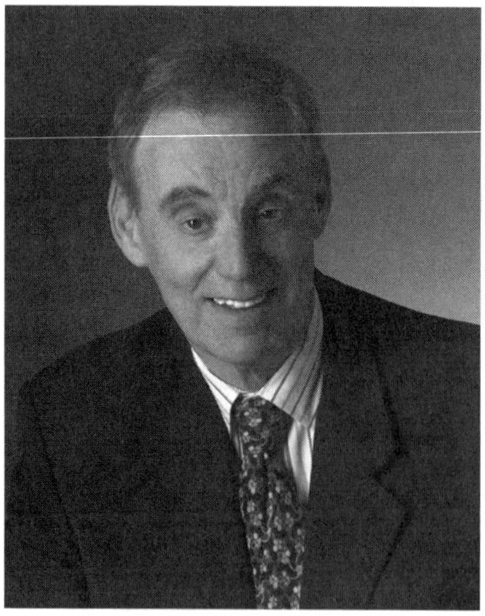

Marshall Strome, MD

The Dream, the Reality, and the Vision

"Dreams never die until we let them."

MS

To date, all measures save one for restoration of the varied laryngeal functions have failed to provide such. The first total human laryngeal transplantation now with more than a decade of viability continues to provide near normal voice, normal swallowing, and clearing of laryngotracheal secretions and restored sense of smell. It represents the only organ transplantation performed for the first time in concert with an immunosuppressive regimen to maintain viability for a decade. The patient's quality of life has dramatically improved and he remains pleased with his decision.

We ride on the shoulders of giants—Ogura, Boles, Work, and Silver, who in the late 1960s dreamed of the potential to replace a larynx with another. Their dreams became mine following two chance occurrences—the first my second total laryngectomy as resident, who, 2 weeks following discharge, committed suicide. Then, as a young resident I became acutely aware of the morbidities and social stigma associated with the procedure. The dream was born. The second chance occurrence was a brief conversation at a meeting with Dr. Ogura. I queried: "Do you think it will ever be possible to transplant a larynx?" Lowering his glasses on his nose, he peered over them. His eyes focusing directly on mine, he said. "If you have the guts, the determination and the intellect it could be you."

A partial transplant in the late 1960s, performed for cancer, was followed by a rapid recurrence with the patient succumbing to the malignancy. The event had significant negative repercussions for both the surgeon and the field. Many prominent surgeons over the next 2 decades publicly stated that laryngeal transplantation should never again be considered for ethical and moral reasons. Others believed normal swallowing without aspiration to be improbable, if not impossible.

In the 1980s the development of cyclosporine transformed the field of transplantation. Starting with dogs, then goats, and ultimately rats, I developed a viable reproducible animal model. This afforded my laboratory the ability to assess rejection, viability parameters, adjunctive irrigants, and a host of immunosuppressive regimens. After a decade of defining the essential parameters to proceed with a human experience, the ideal recipient and donor were identified. I share with you that, on the night the phone call came that a satisfactory match had been identified, my emotions were conflicted. Phone in hand, I had to accept or reject the organ.

Thirty years of dreaming and the guts of which Dr Ogura had spoken, something I was certain I had until the moment was at hand, inexplicably began to fail me. It wasn't as if I hadn't considered the issues on multiple prior occasions—graft failure, recipient death with severe negative repercussions from colleagues, the effects of failure on my family. I simply wanted to hang up the phone, do my research, and leave it to others to do the procedure. In the background, I heard my wife: "Take it, get on the plane, you can make it happen. If it fails which it won't, we can live happily together on an island." The rest is history.

Lost in the success of the larynx transplant is that associated were the first vascularized tracheal, thyroid, and pharynx transplants. Eighty percent of the recipients' current thyroid function is from the transplanted organ. The parathyroids were also transplanted. In the accompanying article, based on the best consultative information available at the time, it is stated that the parathyroids were not viable. Subsequent research in my laboratory has shown that reestablishing parathyroid perfusion within 3 hours leads to viability and near-normal parthormone production in 48 hrs. We now use parthormone levels as a measure of organ viability in our animal model. In the decade following the transplant, much data have emerged from our patient and our laboratory. An in-depth consideration is beyond the scope of this discussion. However, we have shown that a 7-day course of Tacrolimus and alpha beta TCR prevents rejection for 100 days. Furthermore, we have demonstrated that short additional pulses of the same regime at 90 and 180 days can sustain viability for 270 days. To summarize, 15 total days of immunosuppression led to transplanted organ viability at 9 months.

Our current work based on Everolimus, an antiproliferative, vascular-sparing immunosupressant has shown that it is possible to suppress the growth of squamous cell cancer using an immunosuppressant. Our laboratory is now in the process of attempting to identify an adjunctive immunosuppressant that will afford the tumor suppressive effects of Everolimus while supporting laryngeal viability. Some measure of success seems to be evolving with unique dosing of Everolimus and Mycophenolate.

Immature dendritic cells have shown promise as being toleragenic. To work in this realm a change in our animal model was requisite. Over the past year, we have developed a viable mouse model. Technically far more demanding, it requires the anastamosis of submillimeter vessels for success. Currently, rejection parameters have been defined and dosing sequences of varied products are being evaluated.

The future of laryngeal transplantation is bright. Surgeons in Columbia from 2003 to present have performed 18 laryngotracheal transplants. This work represents proof of concept. Head and neck transplantation is with us and is our future. In the early 1990s in Paris during the first presentation of our rat model, I stated that a successful larynx transplant could occur before the turn of the century. Appropriately, there was considerable skepticism.

I now believe that in the next decade it will be possible to transplant a larynx in the face of malignancy, suppress tumor growth, and maintain organ viability. To paraphrase Winston Churchill, It is not the end, it is not the beginning of the end but it is the end of the beginning.

"Vision is conceptualizing the impossible,
leadership is implementing it."

MS

I will always be grateful to the host of young physicians who chose to spend a year with me doing research and my technician without whom none of this would have been possible.

Brief Report

Laryngeal Transplantation and 40-Month Follow-up

Marshall Strome, M.D., Jeannine Stein, M.D., Ramon Esclamado, M.D., Douglas Hicks, Ph.D., Robert R. Lorenz, M.D., William Braun, M.D., Randall Yetman, M.D., Isaac Eliachar, M.D., and James Mayes, M.D.

TOTAL laryngectomy and total occlusion of the larynx with tracheostomy are associated with an impaired sense of taste and smell, an increased incidence of tracheobronchial infections, stomal encrustations, loss of nasal respiration, and loss of a human-sounding voice. A fundamental consideration in treating a patient whose larynx has been irreparably damaged is whether the goals of surgery should include replacement of the larynx to improve the patient's quality of life. An early attempt to treat laryngeal cancer with a partial laryngeal transplant[1] was accompanied by rapid recurrence of the tumor, an outcome that quashed interest in the procedure for nearly two decades. Similarly, tracheal transplantation has had only limited success.[2,3]

In 1987, we initiated a program to explore the potential of laryngeal transplantation. The program addressed four issues critical to successful transplantation: revascularization, reinnervation, rejection, and the ethics of transplanting an organ considered by some to be nonvital. In rats, the rate of success of laryngeal transplantation was nearly 100 percent.[4,5] In these studies in animals, we classified the histologic features of laryngeal rejection[6]; determined the maximal tolerable period of ischemia; evaluated preservative solutions[5]; determined doses of cyclosporine,[7] prednisone, and adjunct in vitro radiation[8]; and studied the use of sirolimus and tacrolimus.[9]

In 1998, we performed a total laryngeal transplantation in a man who had sustained a severe traumatic injury to the larynx and pharynx.[10] We describe the procedure and report the results in detail here.

CASE REPORT

The Patient and the Donor

The patient was a 40-year-old man who had been in a motorcycle accident 20 years earlier. His larynx and pharynx had been crushed, leaving him aphonic. He lost his sense of smell and taste a year after the injury. He used an external device (Cooper-Rand Electrolarynx) to speak. Despite attempts at another institution to reconstruct his larynx, it was totally stenotic and shortened, with immobile arytenoid cartilages and a fragmented cricoid cartilage. A barium swallow revealed narrowing of the pharynx and upper esophagus and a pharyngolaryngeal fistula. The supraglottis was bathed in oropharyngeal secretions.

Other than mild essential hypertension that was treated with valsartan and hydrochlorothiazide, the patient was healthy. Although he had mild dysphagia, his nutritional status was normal. He did not smoke. Serologic tests for cytomegalovirus and Epstein–Barr virus were negative, and his serum creatinine concentration was normal. With the exception of the tracheal stoma and the aforementioned laryngeal, tracheal, and pharyngeal abnormalities, the results of a physical examination were normal.

After surgery was proposed, the patient was interviewed once by a psychiatrist and four times by members of the surgical team and a speech pathologist. All those involved agreed that the patient understood the risks and agreed that his motivation was appropriate. The procedure was approved by the institutional review board of the Cleveland Clinic Foundation, and the patient gave written informed consent.

A donor larynx was found after a six-month search. The donor, a 40-year-old man who had died from a ruptured cerebral aneurysm, had had no coexisting illnesses and had not smoked. Serologic tests for cytomegalovirus and Epstein–Barr virus were negative. HLA matching between the donor and the recipient was complete. The donor had been intubated for less than 48 hours before his death.

The entire pharyngolaryngeal complex, including six tracheal rings and the thyroid and parathyroid glands, was removed; most of the associated vasculature remained intact (Fig. 1). The left internal jugular vein was injured during removal, limiting subsequent anastomosis on the left side to the middle thyroid vein. The larynx was stored in University of Wisconsin solution and ice until implantation 10 hours later. The duration of ischemia was thus well within the acceptable 20-hour window.[5]

Surgical Procedure

Before surgery, the patient received cyclosporine, azathioprine, and methylprednisolone. During surgery, his laryngeal vasculature and innervation were delineated. The strap muscles, hyoid bone, and preepiglottic fat were removed from the donor's larynx, and perfusion was established before the recipient's larynx was removed (Fig. 1). We anastomosed the donor's right superior thyroid artery to that of the patient and the proximal end of the donor's right internal jugular vein to the end of the patient's relatively large common facial vein. The distal end of the donor's jugular vein was oversewn. Blood flow through the transplant — including the transplanted thyroid gland, the six tracheal rings, the larynx, and the pharynx — was seen within 30 minutes after clamp release.

We then performed a narrow-field laryngectomy and removed the portion of the patient's trachea above the upper half of the tracheal stoma. We split the patient's thyroid and repositioned the segments laterally. We left the patient's hyoid bone in place to ensure that the tongue base and laryngeal elevation were relatively normal. The pharynx had two midlevel strictures and one stricture at the esophageal inlet. Believing that a tight suture line would increase the risk of a fistula, we widened the patient's pharynx substantially by including in the transplant 75 percent of the donor's pharynx. We placed three permanent sutures, 1 cm apart, between the patient's hyoid bone and the donor's thyroid cartilage and then elevated and fixed the larynx to the hyoid bone (Fig. 1). The central suture incorporated the epiglottis to prevent prolapse.

Five tracheal rings were needed to reach the patient's tracheal stoma. The back of the tracheal wall was sutured to that of the donor, and the stoma was recreated superiorly. The left superior thyroid arteries were anastomosed in an end-to-end fashion. The left middle thyroid vein of the transplant was anastomosed in an end-to-side fashion to the patient's left internal jugular vein. Both

From the Departments of Otolaryngology (M.S., J.S., R.E., D.H., R.R.L., I.E.), Nephrology and Hypertension (W.B.), and Plastic and Reconstructive Surgery (R.Y.), Cleveland Clinic Foundation, Cleveland; and Lifelink Transplant Institute, Tampa, Fla. (J.M.). Address reprint requests to Dr. Strome at the Department of Otolaryngology, Cleveland Clinic Foundation, 9500 Euclid Ave., Cleveland, OH 44195.

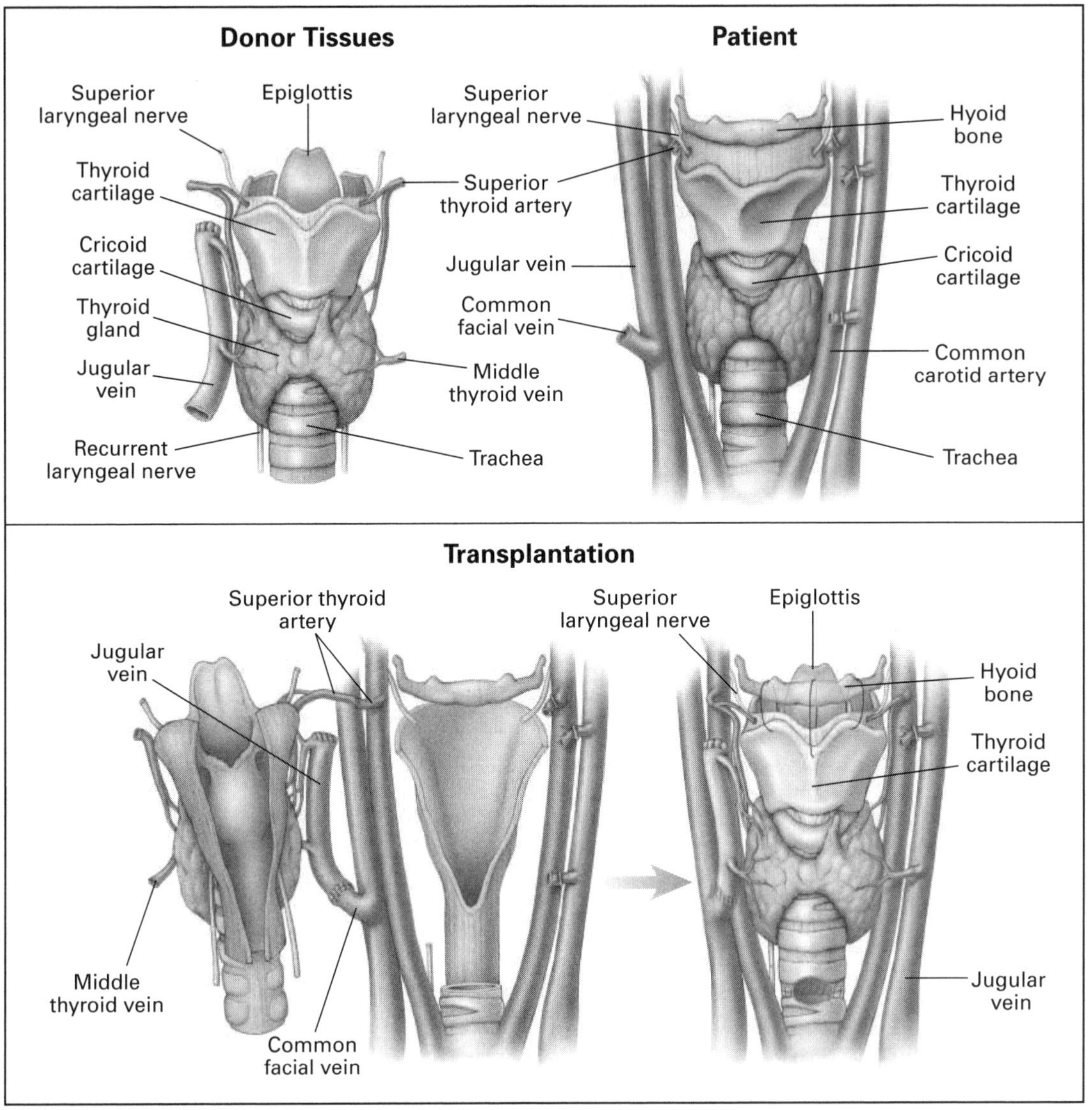

Figure 1. Transplantation of the Pharyngolaryngeal and Tracheal Complex.

The upper left panel shows the tissues obtained from the donor, including a portion of the trachea, the thyroid gland, the pharynx, the larynx, both superior laryngeal nerves, both superior thyroid arteries, both recurrent laryngeal nerves, a segment of the right jugular vein with contributions from the larynx and the pharynx, and the middle thyroid vein. The upper right panel shows the tissues removed from the patient (purple areas). The thyroid gland was split in the midline and retracted laterally. The lower left panel shows the pharynx and upper esophagus of the transplant split posteriorly in the midline, with the right superior thyroid artery anastomosed to that of the patient and the right jugular vein anastomosed to the patient's right common facial vein. The lower right panel shows the donor tissues after transplantation in the patient. The tracheal stoma is permanent and self-sustaining. Three circumferential sutures secure the thyroid cartilage to the hyoid bone, elevating the larynx. The midline suture also includes the epiglottis and pulls it anteriorly. Both superior thyroid arteries and superior laryngeal nerves are juxtaposed. The transplanted left middle thyroid is anastomosed in an end-to-side fashion to the patient's left jugular vein.

superior laryngeal nerves and the right recurrent laryngeal nerve of the transplant were sutured to those of the patient. The patient's left recurrent laryngeal nerve was not identified.

Postoperative Course

The tracheostomy tube and operative drains were removed the day after surgery. We prepared for the possibility of aspiration because all the motor and sensory nerves in the pharynx had been transected. Glycopyrrolate and atropine were administered to reduce salivary secretion. The patient was fed through a gastrostomy tube for 14 weeks, after which time he was able to swallow adequately. During the first week after surgery, he was given muromonab-CD3 (5 mg per day), cyclosporine (500 mg per day), methylprednisolone (50 mg per day, with the dose decreased to 20 mg per day by postoperative day 4), and mycophenolate mofetil (1 g twice daily).

Subsequently, the patient received cyclosporine, mycophenolate mofetil, and prednisone in progressively decreasing doses, with his responses monitored by measurements of plasma drug concentrations and biopsies of the transplanted tracheal mucosa. None of the tracheal biopsy specimens revealed signs of rejection. At one month, the transplanted trachea was normal both on endoscopic examination and on microscopical examination of the biopsy specimens. Cyclosporine was given in doses needed to maintain trough plasma concentrations of 400 ng per milliliter. Six months after surgery, the patient's blood pressure and serum creatinine concentration had increased. Administration of additional antihypertensive drugs and a reduction in the dose of cyclosporine resulted in the resolution of these symptoms within six months.

The patient had one episode of rejection 15 months after transplantation. The quality of his voice declined over a period of several days until he became aphonic, at which time he sought treatment. His larynx was edematous. High doses of prednisone were administered, and his larynx returned to normal within three days. Tacrolimus was then substituted for cyclosporine, and he has had no further rejection episodes. He currently takes 7.5 mg of prednisone per day, 1 g of mycophenolate mofetil daily, and 4 mg of tacrolimus twice daily. His blood pressure and renal function are stable.

RESULTS

Voice Quality

On the third postoperative day, the patient uttered his first laryngeal speech in 20 years (the word "hello"). At one month, both vocal folds were lateral, creating a voice that was breathy with vibration generated by the aryepiglottic folds. At four months the right vocal fold was midline, and at six months the left vocal fold was just adjacent to the midline. We believe that the left recurrent laryngeal nerve of the transplant was reinnervated by the patient's small regional motor nerves. Electromyography confirmed that both vocal folds and the cricothyroid muscles had been reinnervated.

Subjective and objective measures of phonation improved steadily and became stable at normal or near-normal levels 16 months after transplantation. These measures included pitch, jitter (vocal quality), intensity (loudness), maximal phonation time, respiratory volume, and airflow (a measure of the efficiency of phonation). At 16 months, the pitch of the patient's voice changed, increasing its natural quality, as confirmed by a trained listener. At 36 months, the characteristics of his speech were all within the normal range. His voice sounded normal, and it served all his verbal communication needs. He was very pleased with the results and reported that his quality of life had improved "immeasurably." Unemployed before the transplantation, he has since become a motivational speaker.

Respiration and Swallowing

We initially planned to close the tracheal stoma one year after laser cordotomy of the left vocal fold. Closure would leave a serviceable airway without markedly affecting voice quality. The procedure is currently being actively considered. Attempts to provide a self-closing external valve at the site of the tracheal stoma were not successful. At 40 months, the stoma was self-sustaining, and it has not become crusted or granulated during 34 months of follow-up. Stimulation of the right side of the upper trachea through the stoma with a flexible laryngoscope elicited a sensation of touch but no cough, whereas there was no response on the left side.

Three months after transplantation, the supraglottis and vocal folds were sensitive to touch, which initiated a severe cough. Purposeful swallowing returned soon thereafter, and full oral alimentation was possible. A barium swallow revealed no aspiration of solids or liquids. The patient's sense of taste and smell returned.

Infection

The patient had a mild case of oropharyngeal thrush three weeks after transplantation, which subsided with decreasing doses of atropine and oral nystatin. He subsequently had three episodes of tracheobronchitis, at 16 and 18 weeks and at 15 months, that were successfully treated with oral amoxicillin clavulanate. Examinations with a fiberoptic laryngoscope through the stoma during each episode of tracheobronchitis suggested that infection, rather than aspiration, was the cause. During the first episode, the patient inexplicably stopped taking the trimethoprim–sulfamethoxazole given routinely after transplantation and had *Pneumocystis carinii* pneumonia, which cleared rapidly with intravenous antibiotic therapy.

Thyroid Effects

We also transplanted the donor's thyroid and parathyroid glands. The patient's serum calcium, phosphate, and thyroid hormone concentrations remained normal. Four months after transplantation, the four-hour uptake of iodine-123 by the thyroid was 5 percent (normal range, 5 to 15 percent). Imaging revealed that 83 percent of the activity was in the transplanted thyroid lobes and that 17 percent was in the patient's thyroid lobes. It is unlikely that the donor's parathyroid glands were functional after a 10-hour period of ischemia. Therefore, we think that the patient's own parathyroid glands were functioning normally.

DISCUSSION

This patient underwent transplantation of the larynx, trachea, pharynx, and thyroid and parathyroid glands, and the transplant has remained viable for 40 months. He has a human-sounding voice with inflection, range, and qualities unique to him, and he can swallow normally. Transplanting 75 percent of the donor pharynx did not compromise swallowing. Thus, when transplantation is a reconstructive procedure, a constricted pharynx can be widened without impairing swallowing, as long as sensation is restored.

The results in this patient show that laryngeal transplantation is feasible. We propose that potential candidates for transplantation include aphonic patients with laryngeal trauma, patients with large benign chondromas requiring laryngectomy, and patients who have undergone laryngectomy for cancer and who remain disease-free after five years.

Supported by the Cleveland Clinic Foundation.

We are indebted to the many staff members of the Cleveland Clinic Foundation who contributed to this patient's care and to Mr. Tom Lang for critical appraisal and editing services.

REFERENCES

1. Kluyskens P, Ringoir S. Follow-up of a human larynx transplantation. Laryngoscope 1970;80:1244-50.
2. Rose KG, Sesterhenn K, Wustrow F. Tracheal allotransplantation in man. Lancet 1979;1:433.
3. Jacobs JP, Quintessenza JA, Andrews T, et al. Tracheal allograft reconstruction: the total North American and worldwide pediatric experiences. Ann Thorac Surg 1999;68:1043-52.
4. Strome S, Sloman-Moll E, Samonte BR, Wu J, Strome M. A rat model for a vascularized laryngeal allograft. Ann Otol Rhinol Laryngol 1992;101:950-3.
5. Strome M, Wu J, Strome S, Brodsky G. A comparison of preservation techniques in a vascularized rat laryngeal transplant model. Laryngoscope 1994;104:666-8.
6. Strome S, Brodsky G, Darrell J, Wu J, Strome M. Histopathologic correlates of acute laryngeal allograft rejection in a rat model. Ann Otol Rhinol Laryngol 1992;101:156-60.
7. Strome M, Strome S, Darrell J, Wu J, Brodsky G. The effects of cyclosporin A on transplanted rat allografts. Laryngoscope 1993;103:394-8.
8. Barthel SW, Dan O, Myles J, Strome M. Effect of in vitro irradiation of donor larynges on cyclosporine requirements and rejection rates in rat laryngeal transplantation. Ann Otol Rhinol Laryngol 2001;110:20-4.
9. Strome M, Wu J, Jalisi H, Strome S. Laryngeal transplantation: a systematic approach to establish efficacy. In: Fried MP, ed. The larynx: a multidisciplinary approach. 2nd ed. St. Louis: Mosby–Year Book, 1996:625-9.
10. Birchall MA. Human laryngeal allograft: shift of emphasis in transplantation. Lancet 1998;351:539-40.